HEMATOLOGY REFERENCE RANGES – PEDIATRIC

Assay	0-1d	2-4d	5-7d	8-14d	15-30d	1-2mo	3-5mo	6-11mo	1-3y	4-7y	8-13y	Common units	SI UNITS
RBC	4.10-6.10	4.36-5.96	4.20-5.80	4.00-5.60	3.20-5.00	3.40-5.00	3.65-5.05	3.60-5.20	3.40-5.20	4.00-5.20	4.00-5.40	x 10⁶/µL	x 10¹²/l
HGB (Hb)	16.5-21.5 (165-215)	16.4-20.8 (164-208)	15.2-20.4 (152-204)	15.0-19.6 (150-196)	12.2-18.0 (122-180)	10.6-16.4 (106-164)	10.4-16.0 (104-160)	10.4-15.6 (104-156)	9.6-15.6 (96-156)	10.2-15.2 (102-152)	12.0-15.0 (120-150)	g/dL	(g/L)
HCT	48-68	48-68	50-64	46-62	38-53	32-50	35-51	35-51	34-48	36-46	35-49	%	L/L
MCV	95-125	98-118	100-120	95-115	93-113	83-107	83-107	78-102	76-92	78-94	80-94	fL	fL
MCH	30-42	30-42	30-42	30-42	28-40	27-37	25-35	23-31	23-31	23-31	26-32	pg	pg
MCHC	30-34	30-34	30-34	30-34	30-34	31-37	32-36	32-36	32-36	32-36	32-36	%	g/dL
RDW	11.5-14.5	11.5-14.5	11.5-14.5	11.5-14.5	11.5-14.5	11.5-14.5	11.5-14.5	11.5-14.5	11.5-14.5	11.5-14.5	11.5-14.5	%	%
RETICs	1.5-5.8	1.3-4.7	0.2-1.4	0-1.0	0.2-1.0	0.8-2.8	0.5-1.5	0.5-1.5	0.5-1.5	0.5-1.5	0.5-1.5	%	%
NRBCs	2-24	5-9	0-1	0	0	0	0	0	0	0	0	/100 WBC	/100 WBC
WBC	9.0-37.0	8.0-24.0	5.0-21.0	5.0-21.0	5.0-21.0	6.0-18.0	6.0-18.0	6.0-18.0	5.5-17.5	5.0-17.0	4.5-13.5	x 10³/µL	x 10⁹/L
PMNs	37-67	30-60	27-51	22-46	20-40	20-40	18-38	20-40	22-46	30-60	23-53	%	%
BANDs	4-14	3-11	3-9	1-9	0-5	0-5	0-5	0-5	0-5	0-5	0-5	%	%
LYMPHs	18-38	16-46	24-54	30-62	41-61	42-72	45-75	48-78	37-73	29-65	23-53	%	%
MONOs	1-12	3-14	4-17	4-17	2-15	3-14	2-11	2-11	2-11	2-11	2-11	%	%
EOs	1-4	1-5	2-6	1-5	1-5	1-4	1-4	1-4	1-4	1-4	1-4	%	%
BASOs	0-2	0-2	0-2	0-2	0-2	0-2	0-2	0-2	0-2	0-2	0-2	%	%
ANC	3.7-30	2.6-17.0	1.5-12.6	1.2-11.6	1.0-9.5	1.2-8.1	1.1-7.7	1.2-8.1	1.2-8.9	1.5-11.0	1.6-9.5	x 10³/µL	x 10⁹/L
PLTs	150-450											x 10³/µL	x 10⁹/L

From Riley Hospital for Children, Clarian Health Partners, Indianapolis, IN.

HGB – hemoglobin
HCT – hematocrit
MCV – mean cell volume
MCH – mean cell hemoglobin
MCHC – mean cell hemoglobin concentration
RDW – relative distributive width

Polys – polymorphonuclear neutrophils
Lymphs – lymphocytes
Monos – monocytes
Eos – eosinophils
Basos – basophils
ANC – absolute neutrophil count, includes polys and band

NRBC – nucleated red blood cells
Retic – reticulocyte count
PLTs – platelets

BONE MARROW ASPIRATE

WBC differential	Range (%)	Erythrocyte Series	Range (%)
Blasts	0-3		
Promyelocytes	1-5	Pronormoblasts	0-1
N. myelocytes	6-17	Basophilic NB	1-4
N. metamyelocytes	3-20	Polychromatophilic NB	10-20
N. bands	9-32	Orthochromic NB	6-10
N. segmented (polymorphonuclear)	7-30		
Eosinophils	0-3	*Other*	
Basophils	0-1	M:E ratio	1.5-3.3:1
Lymphocytes	5-18	Megakaryoctyes	2-10/lpf
Plasma cells	0-1		
Monocytes	0-1		
Histiocytes (macrophages)	0-1		

N – Neutrophilic
NB – Normoblast
M:E – Myeloid:Erythroid
lpf – low power field

HEMATOLOGY

Clinical Principles and Applications

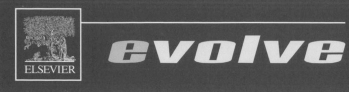

ELSEVIER

evolve

HEMATOLOGY
Clinical Principles and Applications
Third Edition

Bernadette F. Rodak, MS, CLSpH(NCA)
Professor
Clinical Laboratory Science Program
Department of Pathology and Laboratory Medicine
Indiana University School of Medicine
Indianapolis, Indiana

George A. Fritsma, MS, MT(ASCP)
Associate Professor
Pathology and Clinical Laboratory Sciences
University of Alabama at Birmingham
Birmingham, Alabama

Kathryn Doig, PhD, CLS(NCA), CLSp(H)
Director and Professor
Medical Technology Program
Michigan State University
East Lansing, Michigan

SAUNDERS

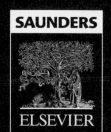

ELSEVIER

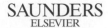

11830 Westline Industrial Drive
St. Louis, Missouri 63146

Notice

Previous editions copyrighted 2002, 1995.

ISBN-13: 978-1-4160-3006-5
ISBN-10: 1-4160-3006-9

Publishing Director: Andrew Allen
Executive Editor: Loren Wilson
Developmental Editor: Ellen Wurm
Publishing Services Manager: Pat Joiner
Project Manager: Jennifer Clark
Senior Designer: Julia Dummitt

Printed in China.

Last digit is the print number: 9   8   7   6   5   4   3   2

Contributors

Larry D. Brace, MS, PhD, MT(ASCP)SH
Emeritus Associate Professor
University of Illinois at Chicago
Clinical Pathology/Laboratory Consultant
Chicago, Illinois
Adjunct Associate Professor of Pathology
University of North Dakota
Grand Forks, North Dakota
Thrombocytopenia and Thrombocytosis; Qualitative Disorders of Platelets and Vasculature

Carol A. Bradford, BS, MT(ASCP)SH
Education Coordinator, Department of Medicine,
Division of Hematology/Oncology, Indiana Cancer Pavilion,
Indiana University Medical Center
Indianapolis, Indiana
Cytochemistry

Sarah Burns, MS, MT(ASCP)
Michigan State University
East Lansing, Michigan
Quality Assurance

Michelle Butina, MS, MT(ASCP), CLS(NCA)
Assistant Professor
Department of Medical Technology
Armstrong Atlantic State University
Savannah, Georgia
Glossary

Deanne H. Chapman, BS, MT(ASCP)SH
Technical Sales Manager
Bayer HealthCare LLC, Diagnostics Division
Tarrytown, New York
Automated Cell Counting Instrumentation and Point of Care Testing

Mary Coleman, MS, CLSpH(NCA)
Assistant Professor
University of North Dakota
Grand Forks, North Dakota
Hemoglobin Metabolism; Iron Metabolism

Leilani Collins, MS, MT(ASCP)SH, CLS(NCA)
Assistant Professor
University of Tennessee Health Science Center
Memphis, Tennessee
Body Fluids in the Hematology Laboratory

Magdalena Czader, MD, PhD
Assistant Professor
Department of Pathology and Laboratory Medicine
Indiana University School of Medicine
Indianapolis, Indiana
Flow Cytometric Analysis in Hematologic Disorders; Mature Lymphoid Neoplasms

Kathryn Doig, PhD, CLS(NCA), CLSp(H)
Director and Professor
Medical Technology Program
Michigan State University
East Lansing, Michigan
Erythrocyte Production and Destruction; Metabolism of the Erythrocyte; Examination of the Peripheral Blood Smear and Correlation with the Complete Blood Count; Disorders of Iron and Heme Metabolism; Anemias Caused by Defects of DNA Metabolism; Introduction to Increased Destruction of Erythrocytes

Peter D. Emanuel, MD
Professor of Medicine, Division of Hematology/Oncology
Senior Scientist, Comprehensive Cancer Center
University of Alabama at Birmingham
Birmingham, Alabama
Introduction to Leukocyte Neoplasms

Sheila A. Finch, CHFP, CHMM, MT(ASCP)
Corporate Director/ISO Administrator
Environment of Care
Detroit Medical Center
Detroit, Michigan
Safety in the Hematology Laboratory

George A. Fritsma, MS, MT(ASCP)
Associate Professor
Pathology and Clinical Laboratory Sciences
University of Alabama at Birmingham
Birmingham, Alabama
An Overview of Clinical Laboratory Hematology; Platelet Production, Structure, and Function; Normal Hemostasis and Coagulation; Hemorrhagic Coagulation Disorders; Thrombosis Risk Testing; Laboratory Evaluation of Hemostasis; Monitoring Anticoagulant Therapy

Margaret Fritsma, MA, MT(ASCP)SBB
Associate Professor
Clinical Laboratory Science Program
School of Health Professions
University of Alabama at Birmingham
Birmingham, Alabama
Normal Hemostasis and Coagulation

John A. Griep, MD
Medical Director
St. Catherine Hospital
East Chicago, Indiana
Clinical Professor
Department of Pathology and Laboratory Medicine
Indiana University School of Medicine
Indianapolis, Indiana
Metabolism of the Erythrocyte; Myeloproliferative Disorders

Teresa G. Hippel, BS, MT(ASCP)SH
Laboratory Resource Manager
Baptist Memorial Hospital Memphis
Memphis, Tennessee
Routine Testing in Hematology

Cynthia S. Johns, MSA, MT(ASCP)SH
Supervisor
Esoterix, Inc.
Lakeland, Florida
Coagulation Instrumentation

Elaine M. Keohane, PhD, CLS(NCA), CLSpH
Professor, Department of Clinical Laboratory Sciences
School of Health Related Professions
University of Medicine and Dentistry of New Jersey
Newark, New Jersey
Bone Marrow Failure

John R. Krause, MD
Chairman and Professor of Pathology
Department of Pathology and Laboratory Medicine
Tulane University Health Science Center
Director of Laboratories
Tulane University Hospital and Clinic
New Orleans, Louisiana
Bone Marrow Overview

Mark E. Lasbury, MS, PhD
Assistant Scientist
Department of Pathology and Laboratory Medicine
Indiana University School of Medicine
Indianapolis, Indiana
Molecular Diagnostics in the Clinical Laboratory

Susan J. Leclair, PhD, CLS(NCA)
Chancellor Professor
Department of Medical Laboratory Science
University of Massachusetts Dartmouth
Dartmouth, Massachusetts
Leukopoiesis; Morphologic and Distributive Leukocyte Disorders; Acute Leukemias

Sharral Longanbach, MT(ASCP)SH
Hematology Technical Support Specialist
Bayer HealthCare LLC, Diagnostics Division
Tarrytown, New York
Automated Cell Counting Instrumentation and Point of Care Testing

Lynn Maedel, MS, CLS(NCA), MT(ASCP)SH
Executive Director
Colorado Association for Continuing Medical Laboratory Education, Inc. (CACMLE)
Denver, Colorado
Examination of the Peripheral Blood Smear and Correlation with the Complete Blood Count

Marisa B. Marques, MD
Associate Professor
Division of Laboratory Medicine
Department of Pathology
University of Alabama at Birmingham
Birmingham, Alabama
Hemorrhagic Coagulation Disorders; Thrombosis Risk Testing

Roslyn McQueen, PhD
Certified Clinical Research Coordinator
Hematology Specialist
Hurley Medical Center
Flint, Michigan
Pediatric and Geriatric Hematology

Rakesh P. Mehta, MD
Assistant Professor of Clinical Medicine
Division of Hematology/Oncology
Department of Medicine
Indiana University School of Medicine
Indianapolis, Indiana
Anemias: Red Blood Cell Morphology and Approach to Diagnosis; Thalassemias

Martha K. Miers, MS, MBA, MT(ASCP)
Vice Chair, Finance and Administration
Assistant Hospital Director, Diagnostic Laboratories
Vanderbilt University Medical Center
Nashville, Tennessee
*Automated Cell Counting Instrumentation and Point of Care
Testing*

**Carole A. Mullins, MPA, CLDir (NCA), BS,
MT(ASCP)**
Adjunct Faculty
Nursing and Human Services
Southwestern Michigan College
Dowagiac, Michigan
Specimen Collection

Keila Poulsen, CLS(NCA)H, MT(ASCP)H,SH
Hematology/Histology Supervisor
Eastern Idaho Regional Medical Center
Idaho Falls, Idaho
Morphology and Function of Cellular Components

Tim R. Randolph, MS, MT(ASCP), CLS(NCA)
Assistant Professor
Department of Clinical Laboratory Science
Doisy College of Health Sciences
Saint Louis University
St. Louis, Missouri
Hemoglobinopathies (Structural Defects in Hemoglobin)

Vishnu V.B. Reddy, MD
Professor of Pathology
Department of Pathology
University of Alabama at Birmingham
Section Head, Hematology ABM Laboratory
University of Alabama at Birmingham Hospitals
Birmingham, Alabama
*Intracorpuscular Defects Leading to Increased Erythrocyte
Destruction; Extracorpuscular Defects Leading to Increased
Erythrocyte Destruction—Nonimmune Causes; Extracorpuscular
Defects Leading to Increased Erythrocyte Destruction—Immune
Causes*

Bernadette F. Rodak, MS, CLSpH(NCA)
Professor
Clinical Laboratory Science Program
Department of Pathology and Laboratory Medicine
Indiana University School of Medicine
Indianapolis, Indiana
Care and Use of the Microscope; Myelodysplastic Syndromes

Larry Smith, PhD
Assistant Attending Scientist, Associate Director
Memorial Sloan-Kettering Cancer Center
New York, New York
Hematopoietic Theory

Gail H. Vance, MD
Professor
Department of Medical and Molecular Genetics
Department of Pathology and Laboratory Medicine
Indiana University School of Medicine
Indianapolis, Indiana
Cytogenetics

Karen Bourlier Waldron, MS, CLS(NCA)
Clinical Performance Specialist
Office of Clinical Quality and Safety
Henry Ford Health System
Detroit, Michigan
*Automated Cell Counting Instrumentation and Point of Care
Testing*

Preface

Advances in the study of medicine have enhanced the ability to recognize diseases at earlier stages, as well as the ability to treat diseases more effectively. Several of these advances have affected the diagnosis and treatment of hematologic disorders, and these advances are covered in this edition.

This book will appeal to students and educators in clinical laboratory science because of its logical organization. Its readability also lends itself to laboratory practitioners and medical residents, who may need to find information quickly.

ORGANIZATION

The book begins with an overview of hematology to provide a preview to the material. Several topics common to all areas of the laboratory, including safety, specimen collection, and quality assurance follow the overview. Then, a review of general cell morphology is given, with chapters covering development, maturation, and function of each cell line. Manual testing in hematology is then discussed, which is followed by a chapter that details the preparation, staining, and systematic evaluation of the peripheral blood film.

In order to set the stage for the study of hematologic disorders, a chapter on bone marrow evaluation is included. This is followed by an overview of body fluid examination in the hematology laboratory and includes excellent photomicrographs of cells and crystals that might be encountered. The next group of chapters provides a general approach to anemias, detailing various types of anemias from both a morphologic view and a pathophysiologic view. Anemias caused by nutritional deficiencies, hemolysis, structural hemoglobin defects, and thalassemias are also covered.

Chapter 28 begins a discussion of leukocyte disorders with nonmalignant changes in white blood cells, including storage disorders. Although morphology is the initial suggestion of malignancy, other studies contribute to the diagnosis. Thus, the next chapters cover those areas of study: cytochemistry, molecular genetics, cytogenetics, and flow cytometry.

The next section addresses hematologic neoplasia with chapters on myeloproliferative disorders, myelodysplastic syndromes, acute leukemias, and mature lymphocytic malignancies.

Brought back from the first edition, a new chapter on pediatric and geriatric hematology highlights the differences in these populations from the general adult reference ranges. The final chapter in the hematology section covers the major lines of automated cell counters. A new section on Point of Care Testing concludes this part.

The last section of the text is devoted to hemostasis and thrombosis and includes several new chapters and new authors.

DISTINCTIVE FEATURES

The logical organization of the text is enhanced by high-quality figures in full color, as well as tables that support the material in the text. Students will benefit by attempting to answer questions following each chapter's case studies and by using the objectives and review questions to guide their test preparation. Material in tables and figures also provide important material and often summarize information from within the text.

NEW TO THIS EDITION

- Objectives and review questions written by noted CLS educator, Dr. Kathryn Doig (Michigan State University).
- Thrombosis and hemostasis section coordinated and edited by George A. Fritsma (University of Alabama at Birmingham), well-known for his expertise. Two new authors have been added to this section.
- Point of Care Testing—now more readily available and more widely used.
- Chapter 38, Pediatric and Geriatric Hematology
- Chapter 46, Monitoring Anticoagulant Therapy
- Substantial revision of chapters on hematopoiesis, thalassemias, hemoglobinopathies, and flow cytometry.

LEARNING AIDS

Each chapter contains:
- **Learning objectives** cover all three levels of the cognitive domain.
- One or two **case studies** at the beginning of each chapter pique the readers' interest.
- A **"Chapter at a Glance"** bulleted summary provides a quick review of essential material.
- **Review questions** that end each chapter are written to match the chapter objectives, and they are given in the format used by certification examinations.

ANCILLARIES

With the third edition, Evolve offers several assets for instructors and students.

For the Instructor

- **Test bank:** An ExamView test bank of 900 multiple-choice questions features rationales, cognitive levels, and page number references to the text. This can be used as in-class review or for test development.
- **Instructor's manual:** The instructor's manual includes one chapter for every chapter in the text and contains key terms, objectives, outlines, and study questions. This can be used in preparation for classes and during lecture.
- **Case studies:** Some 54 case studies feature images and questions. These can be used in class for review of material, for practical exams, or for students' class presentations.

- **PowerPoint presentations:** One PowerPoint presentation per chapter can be used "as is" or as a template to prepare lectures.
- **Image Collection:** All of the images from the book are available as JPEGs and can be downloaded into PowerPoint presentations. These can be used during lecture to illustrate important concepts.
- **Glossary:** The glossary from the book is also available on the Evolve site in PDF format and can be used as a quick reference to look up unfamiliar terms.

For the Student

- **Weblinks:** Links to places of interest on the web specifically for hematology.
- **Content Updates:** The latest information on relevant issues in the field.

Acknowledgments

This manuscript is the result of the contributions of many dedicated professionals. I would like to thank those who contributed new chapters and those who revised and updated chapters from the previous edition. A special note of appreciation goes to those who accepted additional assignments with a very tight timeline.

I am most grateful to George A. Fritsma and Kathryn Doig, who collaborated on this edition—for their expertise, diligence, and energy.

Ellen Wurm, developmental editor, deserves a huge gold star for the management of this edition. Additionally, I would like to thank the staff of Elsevier who encouraged, supported (and sometimes prodded) me through this process, especially Jen Clark, Loren Wilson, and Jennifer Presley.

Finally, I express my appreciation to Linda Kasper and Linda Marler, faculty colleagues, in the Science program at Indiana University, Indianapolis, for their understanding and support.

Bernadette F. Rodak, MS, CLSpH(NCA)

Contents

additional unit from 2nd edition

HEMATOLOGY

Clinical Principles and Applications

An Overview of Clinical Laboratory Hematology

1

George Fritsma

The average human possesses five liters of blood. Blood transports oxygen from lungs to tissues; clears tissues of carbon dioxide; transports glucose, proteins, and fats; and moves wastes to the liver and kidneys. The liquid portion is plasma, which transports coagulation enzymes that protect vessels and maintain the circulation. Plasma carries and nourishes blood cells. There are three families of blood cells: red blood cells (RBCs), or erythrocytes; white blood cells (WBCs), or leukocytes; and platelets, or thrombocytes. Hematology is the study of blood cells. By expertly staining, counting, analyzing, and recording the appearance of all three types of cells, the clinical laboratory scientist is able to predict, detect, and diagnose blood diseases and many systemic diseases that affect blood cells. Physicians rely on hematology laboratory test results to select and monitor therapy for these disorders.

HISTORY

Early scientists such as Athanasius Kircher in 1657 described "worms" in the blood, and Antony van Leeuwenhoek in 1674 gave an account of RBCs,[1] but it was not until the late 1800s that Giulio Bizzozero described platelets as a *"petites plaques."*[2] The development of Wright stain by James Homer Wright in 1902 opened a new world of examination of the blood through the microscope. Although many automated instruments now enumerate and differentiate blood cells, Wright's Romanowsky-type stain (mixture of acidic and basic dyes), and modifications thereof, remain the "heart" of the examination of blood smears under the microscope.

RED BLOOD CELLS

RBCs, or erythrocytes, are anucleate biconcave cells filled with a reddish protein, hemoglobin (HGB), which transports oxygen and carbon dioxide (Chapter 10). In the hematology laboratory, blood cell appearance is analyzed by 1000× light microscopy examination of cells fixed to a glass microscopic slide and stained with a polychromatic dye called *Romanowsky stain, Wright stain,* or *Wright-Giemsa stain* (Chapter 15). RBCs appear pink to red and are 6 to 8 μm in diameter with a zone of pallor covering one third of their center (Fig. 1-1A), reflecting their biconcavity (Chapters 8 and 9). The scientific term for cell appearance is *morphology,* a term that encompasses cell color, size, shape, and inclusions (Chapters 8 and 18).

Since before 1900, physicians and clinical laboratory scientists counted RBCs in measured volumes to detect anemia or polycythemia. *Anemia* means loss of oxygen-carrying capacity and is often reflected in a reduced RBC count (Chapters 14 and 18). *Polycythemia* means an increased RBC count related to increased body RBC mass, a condition that leads to hyperviscosity (Chapter 34). To count RBCs, laboratory scientists carefully pipetted a tiny aliquot of whole blood and mixed it with 0.85% (normal) saline. This saline concentration matches the osmolality of normal blood; consequently, the suspended RBCs closely retained their native morphology, neither swelling nor shrinking. A 1:200 dilution was typical for RBC counts, and a glass pipette designed to provide this dilution, the Thoma pipette, was used routinely until the advent of the Unopette dilution system in 1962.[3] The Thoma pipette is still available from clinical laboratory supply companies, although it is seldom used.

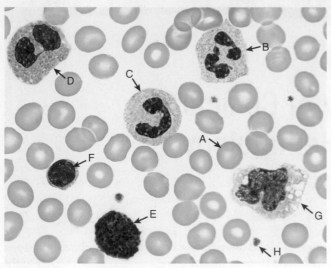

Figure 1-1 Cell types in peripheral blood as they would appear under the microscope with Wright stain. The ratio of leukocytes to erythrocytes and platelets is greater than would be observed under normal conditions. **A,** erythrocyte; **B,** polymorphonuclear neutrophil; **C,** band neutrophil; **D,** eosinophil; **E,** basophil; **F,** lymphocyte; **G,** monocyte; **H,** platelet.

Using the Unopette, the diluted blood is transferred to a counting chamber or hemacytometer (see Figure 14-1). The clinical laboratory scientist observes and counts RBCs in selected areas of the hemacytometer, applies a mathematical formula based on the dilution and the area of the hemacytometer counted, and reports the RBC count in cells per microliter (µL), milliliter (mL) (also cubic millimeter), or liter (L).

Visual RBC counting was developed before 1900 and, although never accurate, was the only way to count RBCs until 1958, when automated particle counters became available in the clinical laboratory. The first electronic counter, patented in 1953 by Joseph and Wallace Coulter of Chicago, Ill., was used so widely that today automated cell counters are often called "Coulter counters," although many high-quality competitors exist (Chapter 39). The Coulter principle of direct current electrical impedance is the principle still used for RBC counting in many automated hematology profiling instruments.

Hemoglobin, Hematocrit, and Red Blood Cell Indices

RBCs also are measured for HGB concentration and hematocrit (HCT) (Chapters 10 and 14). HGB measurement relies on a weak solution of potassium cyanide and potassium ferricyanide, called *Drabkin solution.* An aliquot of whole blood is mixed with a measured volume of Drabkin solution, HGB is converted to stable cyanmethemoglobin (hemiglobincyanide), and the solution is placed in a photometer with incident light at 540 nm. The color intensity is compared with a reagent blank and a known standard and mathematically converted to HGB concentration. Drabkin reagent is used in manual and most automated applications, although some automated

hematology profiling instruments use a formulation of the ionic surfactant (detergent) sodium dodecyl sulfate to reduce environmental cyanide.

HCT is the ratio of RBCs to whole blood and is determined by transferring blood to a graduated plastic tube, centrifuging, and measuring the column of RBCs and RBCs plus plasma. The normal ratio approaches 50%. HCT is also called *packed cell volume,* the packed cells referring to RBCs. Often one can see a light-colored layer between the RBCs and plasma. This is the *buffy coat* and contains WBCs and platelets. The clinical laboratory professional may use the three numerical results, RBC count, HGB, and HCT, to compute the RBC indices mean cell volume (MCV), mean cell HGB (MCH), and mean cell HGB concentration (MCHC). The MCV reflects RBC diameter on a Wright-stained blood film; the MCHC reflects its staining intensity or degree of pallor. The MCH expresses the mass of HGB and is seldom used diagnostically, although it is a stable measure used for quality control. A fourth RBC index, RBC distribution width (RDW), expresses the variation in RBC volume. Extreme RBC volume variability is visible on the Wright-stained blood film as variation in diameter and is called *anisocytosis.*

Few laboratory scientists now use the microscope to count RBCs in peripheral blood; nevertheless scientists routinely use 1000× visual examination (Chapter 4) to review RBC morphology, commenting consistently on RBC diameter, color or hemoglobinization, shape, and the presence of inclusions (Chapter 18). All these parameters—RBC count, HGB, HCT, indices, and RBC morphology—are used to detect, diagnose, assess severity of, and monitor treatment of anemia, polycythemia, and numerous systemic conditions that affect RBCs. Automated hematology profiling instruments are used in nearly all laboratories to generate these data, although examination of the Wright-stained blood film is still essential.

Reticulocytes

In the Wright-stained film, 1% to 2% of RBCs exceed the 6-8 µm average diameter and stain slightly blue-gray. These are polychromatophilic erythrocytes, newly released from the RBC production site, the bone marrow (Chapter 8). Polychromatophilic erythrocytes are closely observed because they indicate bone marrow regeneration during blood loss and certain anemias. Special stains, called *nucleic acid stains* or *vital stains,* are used to differentiate carefully and count these young cells, also called *reticulocytes.* Reticulocyte counting was a tedious visual chore until the development of automated reticulocyte counting by the Toa Corporation (presently Sysmex Corporation, Kobe, Japan) in 1990. Now essentially all automated profiling instruments provide an absolute reticulocyte count and a particularly sensitive measure of bone marrow function, the immature reticulocyte count or immature reticulocyte fraction.

WHITE BLOOD CELLS

WBCs, or leukocytes, are not really blood cells; they are a loosely related category of cell families dedicated to protecting their host from infection and injury (Chapters 12 and 28). WBCs "hitch a ride" in the blood from their source, bone marrow or lymphoid tissue, to their tissue destination. They are so named because they are nearly colorless in an unstained cell suspension. In chronic leukemia, an extreme increase in the WBC count imparts a milky appearance to the blood (Chapters 29, 34, and 37).

WBCs may be counted visually using a microscope, hemacytometer, and a Thoma pipette or Unopette. The technique is the same as RBC counting, but the typical dilution is 1:20, and the diluent includes dilute acetic acid that causes RBCs to lyse or rupture. Without the acetic acid, RBCs would obscure the WBCs, whose count ranges from 5000/μL to 11,000/μL. Visual WBC counting has been largely replaced by automated hematology profiling instruments but is accurate and useful in situations in which no automation is available.

A decreased WBC count is called *leukopenia,* and an increased WBC count is called *leukocytosis,* but the WBC count alone has modest clinical usefulness. The laboratory scientist must differentiate the types of WBCs found in the blood using a Wright-stained blood film and light microscopy (Chapter 15). The types of WBCs are as follows:

- Polymorphonuclear neutrophils (PMNs, or segmented neutrophils, SEGs) (see Fig. 1-1B). PMNs are phagocytic cells whose sole purpose is to engulf and destroy bacteria that are labeled as harmful by the immune system. An increase in PMNs is called *neutrophilia* and often signals bacterial infection. A decrease is called *neutropenia* and often is caused by long-term drug administration or a viral infection.
- Band neutrophils (BANDs) (see Fig. 1-1C). Bands are part of the PMN family; they are less differentiated or less "mature" than PMNs. A BAND increase also signals bacterial infection and is customarily called a *left shift.* The cytoplasm of SEGs and BANDs contains submicroscopic, pink-staining granules filled with bactericidal secretions.
- Eosinophils (EOs) (see Fig. 1-1D). EOs are cells with bright-orange, regular granules filled with antihistamine. An elevated EO count is called *eosinophilia* and signals a response to allergy or parasitic infection.
- Basophils (BASOs) (see Fig. 1-1E). BASOs are cells with dark-purple, irregular cytoplasmic granules that obscure the nucleus. An elevated BASO count is called *basophilia.* Basophilia is rare and often signals a hematologic disease, such as leukemia.
- PMNs, BANDs, EOs, and BASOs are collectively called *granulocytes* because of their prominent cytoplasmic granules, although their functions differ. The distribution of EOs and BASOs in blood is so small compared with PMNs that the terms *eosinopenia* and *basopenia* are theoretical and unused.
- Lymphocytes (LYMPHs) (see Fig. 1-1F). LYMPHs are a complex system of cells that provide for host immunity. LYMPHs recognize foreign antigens and mount antibody (humoral) and cell-mediated antagonistic responses. Most LYMPHs are nearly round, slightly larger than RBCs, with round feature-less nuclei and a thin rim of nongranular cytoplasm. An increase in the LYMPH count is called *lymphocytosis* and often is associated with viral infections. An abnormally low LYMPH count is called *lymphopenia* or *lymphocytopenia* and

is associated with long-term drug therapy or immuno-deficiency.
- Monocytes (MONOs) (see Fig. 1-1G). The MONO is an immature macrophage passing through the blood from its point of origin, usually the bone marrow, to a tissue location. Macrophages are the most abundant cell in the body, more abundant than RBCs or skin cells. They occupy every body cavity; some are motile and some immobilized. Their task is to identify and phagocytose foreign particles and assist the LYMPHs in mounting an immune response through the assembly and presentation of immunogenic epitopes. MONOs have a slightly larger diameter than other WBCs, gray cytoplasm, and a lobulated nucleus. An increased MONO count may signal a hematologic disease, such as leukemia, and is called *monocytosis.* Scientists seldom document a decreased MONO count, so the theoretical term *monocytopenia* is seldom used.

PLATELETS

Platelets, or thrombocytes, are true blood cells that maintain blood vessels by initiating repairs (Chapter 13). Platelets move to the scene of blood vessel damage, adhere to the damaged surface, form aggregates with neighboring platelets to plug the vessel, and secrete substances that trigger thrombosis, or clot formation. Platelets are the cells that control *hemostasis,* a series of cellular and plasma-based mechanisms that seals wounds, repairs vessel walls, and maintains vascular patency. Platelets are only 2-4 μm in diameter, round or oval, anucleate, and slightly granular (see Fig. 1-1H). Their small size makes them appear insignificant, but they are essential to life and are extensively studied for their complex physiology.

The clinical laboratory professional counts platelets using the same technique used in counting WBCs on a hemacytometer, although the typical dilution is 1:100 in an ammonium oxalate diluent, and the counting usually is confined to the center square millimeter. Owing to their minuscule volume, platelets are hard to distinguish in the hemacytometer. In the laboratories that employ visual platelet counting, phase microscopy provides for easier visualization and greater specificity. Automated profiling instruments have largely replaced visual platelet counting.

One important advantage of automated profiling instruments is their ability to generate a mean platelet volume (MPV), which is unavailable through visual methods. The presence of predominantly larger platelets generates an elevated MPV, sometimes signaling a regenerative bone marrow response to platelet consumption (Chapter 43).

Elevated platelet counts, called *thrombocytosis,* signal inflammation or trauma but carry small intrinsic significance. Essential thrombocythemia is a rare condition characterized by extremely high platelet counts and uncontrolled platelet production. Essential thrombocythemia is a life-threatening hematologic disorder (Chapter 34).

A low platelet count, called *thrombocytopenia,* is a common consequence of drug treatment and may be life-threatening. Because the platelet is responsible for normal blood vessel maintenance and repair, thrombocytopenia usually is accompanied by easy bruising and uncontrolled hemorrhage (Chapter 43). Accurate platelet counting is essential to patient safety in many therapeutic regimens.

COMPLETE BLOOD COUNT

The clinical laboratory scientist may collect a blood specimen for the complete blood count (CBC); a phlebotomist, nurse, or patient care technician also may collect the specimen (Chapter 3). In all cases, the scientist is responsible for the integrity of the specimen and ensures it is free of clots, hemolysis, and inappropriate anticoagulant-to-specimen ratios known as "short draws." The clinical laboratory scientist also ensures the specimen is fresh enough for accurate analysis (Chapter 5), then accurately registers the specimen in the worklist, a process known as specimen "accession."

Although all laboratory scientists are equipped to perform visual RBC, WBC, and platelet counts using dilution pipettes, hemacytometers, and microscopes, most laboratories employ profiling instruments to generate the CBC parameters listed in Box 1-1. More sophisticated profiling instruments provide comments on RBC, WBC, and platelet morphology. When one of the results from the profiling instrument is abnormal, the instrument provides an indication, sometimes called a "flag." In this case, the scientist performs a blood film examination (Chapter 15).

The blood film examination is a specialized, demanding, and central CBC activity. Nevertheless, if all profiling instrument results are normal, the blood film examination is omitted from the CBC. The blood film examination is waived in 50% to 80% of cases, depending on the facility's case mix. Acute care facilities report more normal CBCs than specialized or tertiary care facilities.

Blood Film Examination

To accomplish a blood film examination, the clinical laboratory scientist prepares a "wedge-prep" blood smear on a glass microscope slide; allows it to dry; and fixes and stains it using Romanowsky, Wright, or Wright-Giemsa dyes (Chapter 15). The scientist affixes the slide to the microscope stage and examines the RBCs and platelets for abnormalities of shape, diameter, color, or inclusions using the 100× oil immersion lens to generate 1000× magnification (see Chapter 4). The WBC count and platelet count are estimated for comparison with the instrument counts, and all abnormalities are carefully recorded. The scientist systematically reviews, identifies, and tabulates 100 (or more) WBCs to determine their percent distribution. This process is called the *WBC differential* ("diff"). This individualized activity is highly reliant on the scientist's skill, visual acuity, and integrity because it provides extensive diagnostic information. Clinical laboratory scientists pride themselves on their technical skills in performing the blood film examination. The results of the CBC, including all profiling and blood film examination parameters and interpretive comments, are provided on a single page or computer screen for physician review, with abnormal results highlighted.

ENDOTHELIAL CELLS

Because they are structural and do not flow in the bloodstream, endothelial cells, the endodermal cells that form the inner surface of the blood vessel, are seldom studied by clinical laboratory scientists in the hematology laboratory. Nevertheless, endothelial cells are important in maintaining normal blood flow, in snaring platelets during times of injury, and in enabling WBCs to escape from the vessel to the surrounding tissue. Increasingly refined laboratory methods will enable clinicians to examine fully at least the secretions of these important cells.

COAGULATION

Most hematology laboratories include a blood coagulation testing section (Chapters 42 and 45). Coagulation is one component of hemostasis; another is platelets, as reviewed previously. The coagulation system employs a complex sequence of at least 16 plasma proteins, some enzymes and some enzyme cofactors, to produce clot formation in blood vessel injury. Another six to eight enzymes exert control on the coagulation mechanism, and a third system of enzymes and cofactors digests clots to restore vessel patency, a process called *fibrinolysis*. Bleeding and clotting disorders are manifold and complex, and the coagulation section of the hematology laboratory provides a series of plasma-based laboratory assays reflecting complex interactions of hematologic cells with plasma proteins (Chapters 40, 42, and 45).

The clinical laboratory scientist focuses especially on blood specimen integrity for the coagulation laboratory because minor blood specimen defects, including clots, hemolysis, lipemia, plasma bilirubin, and short draws, render the specimen useless (Chapters 3 and 40). High-volume coagulation tests suited to the acute care facility include the platelet count and MPV as described previously, prothrombin time and partial thromboplastin time (or activated partial thromboplastin

---

BOX 1-1   Measurements Generated by Automated Hematology Profiling Instruments

RBC Parameters	WBC Parameters	Platelet parameters
RBC count	WBC count	Platelet count
HGB	PMN count: % and absolute	MPV
HCT	BAND count: % and absolute	
MCV	LYMPH count: % and absolute	
MCH	MONO count: % and absolute	
MCHC	EO and BASO counts: % and	
RDW	absolute	
Retic		

time), thrombin time (or thrombin clotting time), fibrinogen assay, and D-dimer assay. The prothrombin time and partial thromboplastin time are particularly high-volume assays. These tests assess each arm of the coagulation pathway for deficiencies and are used to monitor anticoagulant therapy. Another 30 to 40 low-volume assays are available in specialized or tertiary care facilities. The specialized or tertiary care coagulation laboratory, with its interpretive complexities, is a haven for advanced clinical laboratory scientists with specialized knowledge and communication skills.

ADVANCED HEMATOLOGY PROCEDURES

In addition to the CBC, the hematology laboratory provides bone marrow examinations, flow cytometry, cytogenetic analysis, and molecular diagnosis. These specialties may require advanced preparation or particular dedication by clinical laboratory scientists with a desire to specialize.

Clinical laboratory scientists assist physicians with bone marrow collection and prepare, stain, and microscopically review bone marrow smears (Chapter 16). Bone marrow aspirates and biopsy specimens are collected and stained to analyze cells that are precursors to blood cells. Cells of the erythroid series are precursors to RBCs (Chapter 8); myeloid series cells mature to form BANDs and PMNs, EOs, and BASOs (Chapter 12); and megakaryocytes produce platelets (Chapter 13). Scientists, clinical pathologists, and hematologists review Wright-stained aspirate smears for morphologic abnormalities, high or low bone marrow cell counts, and inappropriate cell line distributions. An increase in the erythroid cell line may indicate bone marrow compensation for abnormally increased RBC consumption during blood loss (Chapter 18). The biopsy specimen, enhanced by the hematoxylin and eosin stain, may reveal abnormalities in bone marrow architecture indicating leukemia, aplastic anemia, or a host of additional hematologic disorders. Examination results of bone marrow aspirates and biopsy specimens are compared with CBC results generated from the peripheral blood to look for anomalies.

In the bone marrow laboratory, special cytochemical stains may be employed to differentiate abnormal myeloid, erythroid, and lymphoid cells (Chapter 30). These stains include myeloperoxidase, Sudan black B, nonspecific and specific esterase, periodic acid–Schiff stain, the tartrate-resistant acid phosphatase stain, and the alkaline phosphatase stain. The cytochemical stains are time-honored and may be gradually replaced by flow cytometry immunophenotyping, cytogenetics, and molecular diagnosis (Chapters 30-33). Since 1980, immunostaining methods have enabled the identification of selected cell lines with certainty. An example of immunostaining is an immune-based dye for antibodies against factor VIII, which are present in megakaryoblastic leukemia.

There are two kinds of flow cytometers—quantitative clinical flow cytometers that have grown from the original Coulter principle and qualitative, laser-based instruments that have grown from research applications (Chapter 33). The former devices are automated clinical profiling instruments that generate the quantitative parameters of the CBC through applications of electrical impedance and laser or light beam interruption (Chapter 39). Qualitative laser-based flow cytometers are mechanically simpler but technically more demanding. They are used to analyze cell populations by measuring the effects of individual cells on light, such as forward angle light scatter and right angle light scatter, and by immunophenotyping for cell membrane epitopes. The qualitative flow cytometry laboratory is indispensable to leukemia and lymphoma diagnosis.

Molecular diagnostic techniques are beginning to enhance and even replace some of the advanced hematologic methods. Polymerase chain reaction, real-time polymerase chain reaction, and isothermal amplification and detection systems enable laboratory scientists to detect mutations such as the Philadelphia chromosome and translocation 15;17 that signal specific forms of leukemia and establish their therapeutic profile and prognosis (Chapters 31 and 32).

ADDITIONAL HEMATOLOGY PROCEDURES

Clinical hematologists in the hematology laboratory provide many specific whole-blood methods to support diagnosis. The *osmotic fragility* test uses various concentrations of saline solutions to detect abnormal spherocytic RBCs in anemia (Chapter 23). Likewise, the glucose-6-phosphate dehydrogenase assay tests for a common RBC enzyme deficiency causing severe acute hemolytic anemia. The sickle cell solubility assay and its follow-up test, HGB electrophoresis, are used to detect and diagnose sickle cell anemia and other common inherited HGB abnormalities and thalassemias (Chapters 26 and 27). One of the oldest hematology tests, the erythrocyte sedimentation rate, detects inflammation and provides a rough estimation of its intensity (Chapter 14).

Finally, the hematology laboratory scientist reviews the cellular counts, distribution, and morphology from body fluids other than blood (Chapter 17). These include cerebrospinal fluid, synovial (joint) fluid, pericardial fluid, pleural fluid, and peritoneal fluid, where RBCs and WBCs may be present in disease and where additional malignant cells require specialized detection skills. Analysis of nonblood body fluids is always performed on an emergency basis because cells in these hostile environments rapidly lose their integrity. The conditions leading to a need for body fluid withdrawal are invariably acute.

HEMATOLOGY QUALITY ASSURANCE AND QUALITY CONTROL

Clinical laboratory scientists in the hematology laboratory employ particularly complex quality control systems (Chapter 5). The measurement of cells and biologic systems defies standardization in the chemical sense and requires elaborate validation, matrix effect examination, linearity, and reference interval determinations. An internal standard methodology known as the "moving average" is peculiar to hematology.

Laboratory scientists compare methods through clinical efficacy calculations that produce clinical sensitivity, specificity, and positive and negative predictive values for each assay performed. Scientists must monitor specimen integrity and test ordering patterns and ensure the integrity of reports, including numerical and narrative statements and reference interval comparisons. Similar to most branches of laboratory science, the hematology laboratory places an enormous responsibility for accuracy, integrity, judgment, and timeliness on the clinical laboratory professional.

REFERENCES

1. Wintrobe MM: Hematology, The Blossoming of a Science. Philadelphia: Lea & Febiger, 1985.
2. Bizzozero J: Ueber einem neuen formbestandtheil des blutes und dessen rolle bei der thrombose und der blutgerinnung. Virchows Arch Pathol Anat Physiol Klin Med 1882;90:261-332.
3. Freundlich MH, Gerarde HW: A new, automatic, disposable system for blood counts and hemoglobin. Blood 1963;21:648-655.

Safety in the Hematology Laboratory

Sheila A. Finch

OUTLINE

Universal [Standard] Precautions
Occupational Hazards
Developing a Safety Management Program

OBJECTIVES

After completion of this chapter, the reader will be able to:

1. Define universal [standard] precautions.
2. List infectious materials included in universal [standard] precautions.
3. Describe the safe practices required in the "Occupational Exposure to Bloodborne Pathogens" standard.
4. Identify occupational hazards that exist in the hematology laboratory.
5. Identify the requirements of the "Occupational Exposure to Hazardous Chemicals in Laboratories" standard.
6. Discuss the development of a safety management program.
7. Describe the principles of a fire prevention program, including details such as the frequency of testing equipment.
8. Name the most important practice to prevent the spread of infection.
9. Given a written laboratory scenario, assess it for safety hazards, and recommend corrective action.
10. Select the proper class of fire extinguisher for a given type of fire.
11. Define Material Safety Data Sheets (MSDSs), list information contained on MSDSs, and determine when MSDSs would be used in laboratory activity.
12. Name the specific practice during which most needle stick injuries occur.

CASE STUDIES

After studying the material in this chapter, the reader should be able to respond to the following case study:

Hematology Services, Inc., had a proactive safety program. Quarterly safety audits were conducted by members of the safety committee. The following statements were recorded in the safety audit report. Which statements are considered good work practices, and which statements represent deficiencies? List the corrective actions that should be taken.

1. A hematology technologist was observed removing gloves and immediately left the laboratory for a meeting. The clinical laboratory professional did not remove the laboratory coat.
2. Food was found in the specimen refrigerator.
3. Syringes were found in the proper sharps container. On further investigation, 50% of the attached needles were recapped.
4. Hematology technologists were seen in the lunchroom wearing laboratory coats.
5. Fire extinguishers were found every 75 ft of the laboratory.
6. Fire extinguishers were inspected quarterly and annually.
7. One fire drill was conducted in the last 8 months.
8. Unlabeled bottles were found at the workstation.
9. A 1:10 solution of bleach was found near the electronic cell counter. On further investigation, the bleach was made 6 months ago.
10. Gloves were worn by the staff receiving specimens.
11. MSDSs were obtained by fax.
12. Chemicals were stored alphabetically.
13. Fifty percent of the staff interviewed had not participated in a fire drill.

The author acknowledges the assistance of Debra Walters, safety officer at Clarian Health Partners, Indianapolis, Ind., for review of this chapter.

Many conditions in the laboratory have the potential for causing injury to staff and damage to the building or to the community. Patients' specimens, needles, chemicals, electrical equipment, reagents, and glassware all can be potential causes of accidents or injury. Managers and employees must be knowledgeable about safe work practices and incorporate these practices into the operation of the hematology laboratory. The key to prevention of accidents and laboratory-acquired infections is a well-defined safety program.

Safety is a broad subject and cannot be covered in one chapter. This chapter simply highlights some of the key safe practices that should be followed in the laboratory. Omission of a safe practice from this chapter does not imply that it is not important or that it should not be considered in the development of a safety curriculum or a safety program.

UNIVERSAL [STANDARD] PRECAUTIONS

One of the greatest risks associated with the hematology laboratory is the exposure to blood and body fluids. In December 1991, the Occupational Safety and Health Administration (OSHA) issued the final rule for the "Occupational Exposure to Bloodborne Pathogens" standard. The standard that specifies universal [standard] precautions to protect laboratory workers and other healthcare professionals became effective on March 6, 1992. *Universal* was the original term; OSHA's current terminology is *universal [standard] precautions*. Throughout this text, the term *standard precautions* is used to encompass universal precautions and body substance isolation.

Standard precautions, which require that all human blood, body fluids, and tissues be treated as if they were infectious, must be adopted by the laboratory. Standard precautions apply to the following potentially infectious materials: blood, semen, vaginal secretions, cerebrospinal fluid, synovial fluid, pleural fluid, any body fluid with visible blood, any unidentified body fluid, unfixed slides, microhematocrit clay, and saliva from dental procedures. Past practice was to label specimens from patients known to have infectious diseases; however, experience has shown that patients without visible symptoms can have infectious diseases. Labeling such specimens also jeopardizes patient confidentiality. Adopting standard precautions lessens the risk of healthcare worker exposures to blood and body fluids, decreasing the risk of injury and illness.

Bloodborne pathogens are pathogenic microorganisms that, when present in human blood, can cause disease. They include, but are not limited to, hepatitis B virus (HBV), hepatitis C virus, and human immunodeficiency virus (HIV). This chapter does not cover the complete details of the standard; it covers only the sections that apply directly to the hematology laboratory. Additional information can be found in the references at the end of this chapter.

Applicable Safety Practices Required by the OSHA Standard

The following standards are applicable in a hematology laboratory and must be enforced:

1. *Handwashing* is one of the most important safety practices. Hands must be washed with soap and water. If water is not readily available, alcohol hand gels (minimum 62% alcohol) may be used. Hands must be thoroughly dried. The proper technique for handwashing is as follows:
   a. Wet hands *and wrists* thoroughly under running water.
   b. Apply germicidal soap and rub hands vigorously for at least 15 seconds, including between the fingers and around and over the fingernails.
   c. Rinse hands thoroughly under running water in a downward flow from wrist to fingertips.
   d. Dry hands with a paper towel. Use the paper towel to turn off the faucet handles.
   Hands must be washed:
   a. Whenever there is visible contamination with blood or body fluids
   b. After completion of work
   c. After gloves are removed and between glove changes
   d. Before leaving the laboratory
   e. Before and after eating and drinking, smoking, applying cosmetics or lip balm, changing contact lens, and using the lavatory
   f. Before and after all other activities that entail hand contact with mucous membranes, eyes, or breaks in skin
2. *Eating, drinking, smoking, and applying cosmetics or lip balm must be prohibited* in the laboratory work area.
3. Hands, pens, and other fomites must be kept away from the worker's mouth and all mucous membranes.
4. *Food and drink, including oral medications and tolerance-testing beverages* must not be kept in the same refrigerator as laboratory specimens or reagents or where potentially infectious materials are stored or tested.
5. *Mouth pipetting* must be prohibited.
6. Needles and other sharp objects contaminated with blood and other potentially infectious materials should not be manipulated in any way. Such manipulation includes resheathing, bending, clipping, or removing the sharp object. Resheathing or recapping is permitted only when there are no other alternatives or when the recapping is required by specific medical procedures. Recapping is permitted by use of a method other than the traditional two-handed procedure. The one-handed method or resheathing device is often used (Chapter 3). Documentation in the exposure control plan should identify the specific procedure by which resheathing is permitted.
7. *Contaminated sharps* (including, but not limited to, needles, blades, pipettes, syringes with needles, and glass slides) must be placed in a puncture-resistant container that is appropriately labeled with the universal biohazard symbol (Fig. 2-1) or a red container that adheres to the standard. The container must be leak-proof (Fig. 2-2).
8. Procedures such as removing caps when checking for clots, filling hemacytometer chambers, making slides, discarding specimens, making dilutions, and pouring specimens or fluids must be performed so that splashing, spraying, or production of droplets of the specimen being manipulated is prevented. These procedures may be performed behind

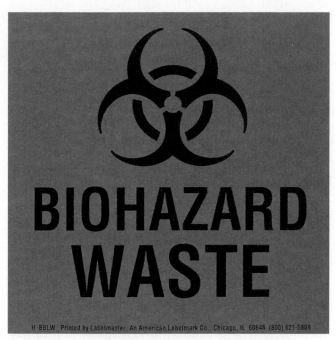

Figure 2-1 Biohazard symbol.

a barrier, such as a plastic shield, or protective eyewear should be worn (Fig. 2-3).

9. *Personal protective clothing* and equipment must be provided to the worker. The most common forms of personal protective equipment (PPE) are as follows:

a. *Outer coverings,* including gowns, laboratory coats, and sleeve protectors, should be worn when there is a chance of splashing or spilling on work clothing. The outer covering must be made of fluid-resistant material, must be long-sleeved, and must remain buttoned at all times. If contamination occurs, the PPE should be removed immediately and treated as infectious material.

Laboratory coats may be worn. If cloth coats are worn, the coats must be laundered inside the laboratory or hospital or by a contracted laundry service. Laboratory coats used in the laboratory while performing laboratory analysis are considered personal protective equipment and are not to be taken home.

All protective clothing should be removed before the worker leaves the laboratory; it should not be worn into public areas. Public areas include, but are not limited to, break rooms, storage areas, bathrooms, cafeterias, offices, and meetings outside the laboratory.

A second laboratory coat can be made available for use in public areas. A common practice is to have a different-colored laboratory coat that can be worn in public areas. This second laboratory coat may be provided at the expense of the employer and would be laundered by the employee.

b. *Gloves* must be worn when the potential for contact with blood or body fluids exists (including removing and handling bagged biohazardous material and when

decontaminating benchtops) and when venipuncture or finger sticks are performed. Gloves provided to the laboratory workers must accommodate latex allergies. Alternative gloves must be readily accessible for any laboratory worker with a latex allergy. Gloves must be changed after each contact with a patient, when there is visible contamination, or if physical damage occurs. Gloves should not be worn when "clean" areas, such as a copy machine or a "clean" telephone, are used. Gloves must not be worn again or washed. After one glove is removed, the second glove can be removed by sliding the index finger of the ungloved hand between the glove and the hand and slipping the second glove off. This technique prevents contamination of the "clean" hand by the "dirty" second glove.[1] Contaminated gloves should be disposed of according to applicable federal or state regulations.

c. *Eyewear,* including face shields, goggles, and masks, should be used when there is potential for aerosol mists, splashes, or sprays to mucous membranes (mouth, eyes, or nose). Removing caps from specimen tubes, working at the cell counter, and centrifuging specimens are examples of tasks that could result in aerosol mist.

10. *Phlebotomy trays* should be appropriately labeled to indicate potentially infectious materials. Specimens should be placed into a secondary container, such as a resealable biohazard-labeled bag.

11. If a *pneumatic tube system* is used to transport specimens, the specimens should be placed into a special leak-proof bag, appropriately labeled with the biohazard symbol. If there is potential for leakage, a secondary container should be used. Requisition forms should be placed outside of the secondary container to prevent contamination if the specimen leaks.

When specimens are received in the laboratory, they should be handled by someone wearing gloves, a laboratory coat, and other protective clothing, in accordance with the type and condition of specimen. Contaminated containers or requisitions must be decontaminated or replaced before being sent to the work area.

12. When *equipment* used to process specimens becomes visibly contaminated or requires maintenance or service, it must be decontaminated, whether service is performed within the laboratory or by a manufacturer repair service. Decontamination of equipment at a minimum would consist of flushing the lines and wiping the exterior and interior of the equipment. If it is difficult to decontaminate the equipment, it must be labeled with the biohazard symbol to indicate potentially infectious material. *Routine cleaning* should be performed on equipment that has the potential for splashes and sprays, such as inside the lid of the microhematocrit centrifuge.

Housekeeping

Blood and other potentially infectious materials can contaminate work surfaces easily. Contamination can be in the

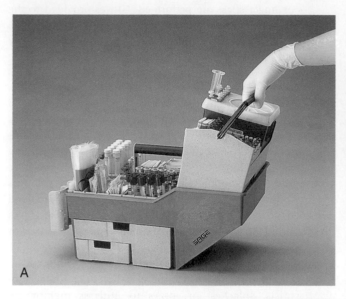

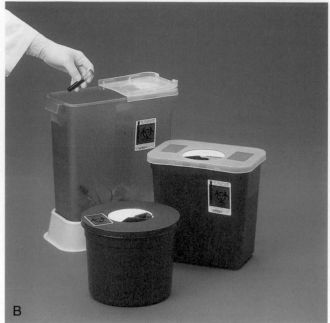

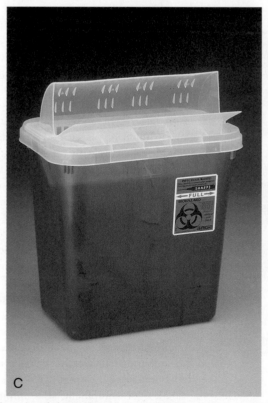

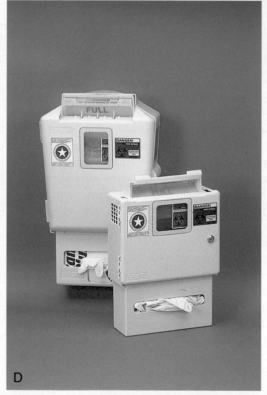

Figure 2-2 Examples of sharps disposal systems. **A,** Compact stat tray. **B,** Multipurpose containers with rotor and hinged lids. **C,** Multipurpose container with horizontal drop lid. **D,** In Room® System Wall Enclosures. (Courtesy of Sage Products, Crystal Lake, IL.)

form of splashes, poor work practices, and droplets of blood on the work surface. To prevent contamination, all work surfaces should be cleaned at the completion of the procedures and whenever the bench area or floor becomes visibly contaminated. An appropriate disinfectant solution is household bleach, used in a 1:10 volume/volume dilution (10%), which can be made by adding 10 mL of bleach to 90 mL of water or

$2\frac{1}{2}$ cups of bleach per 1 gallon of water, to achieve the recommended concentration of chlorine of 5500 ppm. Because this solution is not stable, it must be made fresh *daily*. The container of 1:10 solution of bleach should be labeled properly with the name of the solution, the date/time prepared, date/time of expiration (24 hours), and the initials of the preparer. Bleach is not recommended for aluminum surfaces. Other

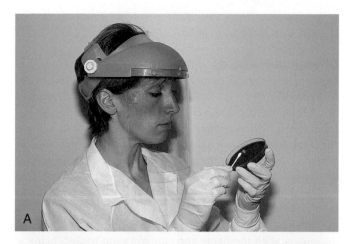

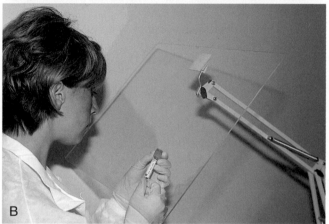

Figure 2-3 Examples of safety shields. **A,** Face shield. **B,** Adjustable swing arm shield. (Courtesy of Steve Kasper.)

solutions used to decontaminate include, but are not limited to, Amphyl, tuberculocidal disinfectants, and 70% ethanol. All paper towels used in the decontamination process should be disposed of as biohazardous. Documentation of the disinfection of work areas and equipment after each shift is required.

Laundry

If nondisposable laboratory coats are used, they must be placed in appropriate containers for transport to the laundry at the facility or contract service and not taken to the employee's home.

Hepatitis B Virus Vaccination

Laboratory workers should receive the HBV vaccination series at no cost before or within 10 days after beginning work in the laboratory. An employee must sign a release form if he or she refuses the series. The employee can request and receive the hepatitis vaccination series, however, at any time. If an exposure incident (needle puncture or exposure to skin, eye, face, or mucous membrane) occurs, postexposure evaluation and follow-up, including prophylaxis and medical consultation, should be made available at no cost to the employee. Employees should be encouraged to report all exposure inci-

dents, and such reporting should be enforced as standard policy.

Training and Documentation

Hematology staff should be properly educated in epidemiology and symptoms of bloodborne diseases, modes of transmission of bloodborne diseases, use of protective equipment, work practices, ways to recognize tasks and other activities that may result in an exposure, and the location of the written exposure plan for the laboratory. Education should be documented and should occur when new methods, equipment, or procedures are introduced; at the time of initial assignment to the laboratory; and at least annually thereafter.

Waste Management

Specimens from the laboratory are identified as regulated waste. State and local regulations for disposal of medical waste must be followed. In 1988 OSHA developed a Medical Waste Tracking Act that required generators (producers) of medical waste to be responsible for the handling and disposal of that waste. Waste from the hematology laboratory should be disposed of according to applicable regulations.

OCCUPATIONAL HAZARDS

Four important occupational hazards in the laboratory are discussed in this chapter: fire hazard, chemical hazards, electrical hazard, and needle puncture. There are other hazards to be considered when a safety management program is developed, and the reader is referred to the Department of Labor section of the Code of Federal Regulations for detailed regulations.[2]

Fire Hazard

Because of the numerous flammable and combustible chemicals used in the laboratory, fire is a potential hazard. Complying with standards established by the National Fire Protection Association, OSHA, the Joint Commission on the Accreditation of Healthcare Organizations, the College of American Pathologists, and other organizations can minimize the dangers. A good fire safety/prevention plan is necessary and should consist of the following:
1. Enforcement of a no-smoking policy.
2. Installation of appropriate fire extinguishers. Several types of extinguishers, most of which are multipurpose, are available for use for specific types of fire.
3. Placement of fire extinguishers every 75 ft (22.9 m). A distinct system for marking the locations of fire extinguishers enables quick access when they are needed. Fire extinguishers should be checked monthly and maintained annually. Not all fire extinguishers are alike. Each fire extinguisher is rated for the type of fire that it can suppress. It is important to use the correct fire extinguisher for the correct class of fire. Laboratory workers should be trained on how to recognize the class of extinguisher and proper use of a fire extinguisher. Table 2-1 summarizes the fire extinguisher classifications. The fire extinguishers used in the laboratory

TABLE 2-1 Fire Extinguisher Classifications

Class Type of Extinguisher	Type of Fire
A	Use class A extinguishers on ordinary combustibles such as wood, cloth, or paper
B	Use class B extinguishers on flammable liquids, gases, or grease
C	Use class C extinguishers on energized (plugged-in) electrical fires. Examples are household appliances, computer equipment, fuse boxes, or circuit breakers
ABC	ABC extinguishers are multipurpose extinguishers that handle class A, B, and C fires

are portable extinguishers and are not designed to fight large fires. In the event of a fire in the laboratory, the local fire department must be contacted immediately.

4. Placement of adequate fire detection systems (alarms, sprinklers), which should be tested every 3 months.
5. Placement of manual fire alarm boxes near the exit doors. Travel distance should not exceed 200 ft (61 m).
6. Written fire prevention and response procedures, commonly referred to as the *fire response plan*. All staff in the laboratory should be knowledgeable about the procedures. Workers should be given assignments for specific responsibilities in case of fire, including responsibilities for patients' care, if applicable. Total count of employees in the laboratory should be known for any given day, and a buddy system should be developed in case evacuation is necessary. Equipment shutdown procedures should be addressed in the plan, as should responsibility for implementation of those procedures.
7. Quarterly fire drills should be conducted so that response to a fire situation is routine and not a panic response. All laboratory staff members should participate in the fire drills. Proper documentation should be maintained to show that all phases of the fire response plan were activated. If patients are in the hematology laboratory, evacuation can be simulated, rather than evacuating actual patients. The entire evacuation route should be walked to verify the exit routes and clearance of the corridors. A summary of the laboratory's fire response plan can be copied on a quick reference card and attached to workers' identification badges to be readily available in a fire situation.
8. Written storage requirements for any flammable or combustible chemicals stored in the laboratory. Chemicals should be arranged according to hazard class and not alphabetically.
9. A well-organized fire safety training program. This program should be completed by all employees. Activities that require walking evacuation routes and locating fire extinguishers and pull boxes in the laboratory area should be scheduled. Types of fires likely to occur and use of the fire

extinguisher should be discussed. Local fire departments work with facilities to conduct fire safety programs.

Chemical Hazards

Some of the chemicals used in the hematology laboratory are considered hazardous and are governed by the standard on "Occupational Exposure to Hazardous Chemicals in Laboratories." This standard requires laboratories to develop a chemical hygiene plan that outlines safe work practices to minimize exposures to hazardous chemicals. The full text of this standard can be found in the July 1, 1998, *Federal Register*.[2]

General principles that should be followed in working with chemicals are as follows:

1. Label all chemicals properly, including secondary containers, with the name and concentration of the chemical preparation or fill date, expiration date (time, if applicable), initials of preparer (if done in-house), and chemical hazards (e.g., poisonous, corrosive, flammable). Do not use a chemical that is not properly labeled as to identity or content.
2. Follow all handling and storage requirements for the chemical.
3. Store alcohol and other flammable chemicals in approved safety cans or storage cabinets at least 5 ft away from a heat source (e.g., Bunsen burners, paraffin baths). Limit the quantity of flammable chemicals stored on the workbench to 2 working days' supply. Do not store chemicals in a hood or in any area where they could react with other chemicals.
4. Use adequate ventilation, such as fume hoods, when working with hazardous chemicals.
5. Use personal protective equipment, such as gloves (e.g., nitrile, polyvinyl chloride, rubber—appropriate for chemical in use), rubber aprons, and face shields. Safety showers and eye wash stations should be available every 100 ft or within 10 seconds of the work area where the hazardous chemicals are used.
6. Use bottle carriers for bottles containing more than 500 mL.
7. Use alcohol-based solvents, rather than xylene or other particularly hazardous substances, to clean microscope objectives.
8. The wearing of contact lenses should not be permitted when an employee is working with xylene, acetone, alcohols, formaldehyde, and other solvents. Many lenses are permeable to chemical fumes. Contact lenses can make it difficult to wash the eyes adequately in the event of a splash.
9. Spill response procedures should be included in the chemical safety procedures, and all employees must receive training in these procedures. Absorbent material should be available for spill response. Multiple spill response kits and absorbent material should be stored in various areas and rooms other than only in the area where they are likely to be needed. This prevents the necessity of walking through the spilled chemical to obtain the kit.
10. Material Safety Data Sheets (MSDSs) are written by the manufacturers of the chemicals to provide information on

the chemicals that cannot be put on a label. When an MSDS is received in the laboratory, it must be retained and reviewed with laboratory personnel. The MSDS provides information on the following:

a. Manufacturer—name, address, emergency phone number, date prepared
b. Hazardous ingredients—common names, worker exposure limits
c. Physical and chemical characteristics—boiling point, vapor pressure, evaporation rate, appearance, and odor under normal conditions
d. Physical hazards—data on fire and explosion hazard and ways to handle the hazards
e. Reactivity—stability of the chemical and with what chemicals it would react
f. Health hazards—signs and symptoms of exposure, such as eye irritation, nausea, dizziness, and headache
g. Precautions for safe handling and use—what to do if the chemical spills, disposal of the chemical, and equipment required for cleanup
h. Control measures—how to reduce the exposure to the chemical and protective clothing or equipment, such as respirator, gloves, and eye protection, that should be used in handling the chemical. See Appendix A for a sample MSDS. Use this sample to review the information that can be found on the MSDS.

An MSDS management system should be considered to track the incoming MSDSs received in the laboratory. When new or revised MSDSs are received, a notice should be posted to alert the hematology staff that new or revised MSDSs have been received. MSDSs may be obtained electronically by means of computer, fax, Internet, CD-ROM, and microfiche machines. If an electronic device is used in the laboratory to receive and store MSDSs, each employee must be trained on the use of the device. The training must include emergency procedures for power outages and malfunctions of the device. The device must be reliable and readily accessible during the hours of operation. In the event of emergency, hard copies of the MSDSs must be accessible to medical staff. MSDSs are required to be kept for 30 years post employment of the last employee who has used the chemicals in the work area, and they should be dated when the chemical is no longer used in the laboratory.

Electrical Hazard

Electrical equipment and outlets are other sources of hazards. Faulty wiring may cause fires or serious injury. Guidelines include the following:

1. Equipment must be grounded or double insulated. (Grounded equipment has a three-prong plug.)
2. Use of "cheater adapters" (adapters that allow three-pronged plugs to fit into a two-pronged outlet) should be prohibited.
3. Use of gang plugs (plugs that allow several cords to be plugged into one outlet) should be prohibited.

4. Use of extension cords should be avoided.
5. Equipment with loose plugs or frayed cords should not be used.
6. Stepping on cords, rolling heavy equipment over them, and other abuse of cords should be prohibited.
7. When cords are unplugged, the plug, not the cord, should be pulled.
8. Equipment that causes shock or a tingling sensation should be turned off, the instrument unplugged and identified as defective, and the problem reported.
9. Before repair or adjustment is attempted on electrical equipment, the following should be done:
   a. Unplug equipment.
   b. Make sure hands are dry.
   c. Remove jewelry.

Needle Puncture

Needle puncture is a serious occupational hazard for laboratory workers. Handling procedures should be written and followed, with special attention to phlebotomy procedures and disposal of contaminated needles. Other items that can cause a puncture similar to a needle puncture include sedimentation rate tubes, applicator sticks, capillary tubes, glass slides, and transfer pipettes.

Disposal procedures should be followed and enforced. The most frequent cause of a needle puncture or a puncture from other sharp objects is improper disposal. Failure to check sharps containers on a regular basis and to replace them when they are no more than three-quarters full encourages overstuffing them, which sometimes leads to injury. Portable bedside containers are available for workers when performing venipunctures or capillary punctures. Wall-mounted needle disposal containers also are available and make disposal convenient. As mentioned previously, all needle punctures should be reported to the health services or proper authorities within the institution.

DEVELOPING A SAFETY MANAGEMENT PROGRAM

Every accredited laboratory is required to have a safety management program. A safety management program is a program identifying the guidelines necessary to provide a safe working environment free from recognizable hazards that can cause harm or injury. Many clinical laboratory scientists assume positions as supervisors or laboratory safety officers. Responsibilities in these positions require knowledge of the safety principles and the development of a laboratory safety program. This section provides an overview of the elements that should be considered in developing a safety program.

Beginning Stages: Research

Awareness of the standards and regulations that govern laboratories is a required step in the development of a safety program. Taking the time to become knowledgeable about the regulations and standards that relate to the procedures performed in the hematology laboratory is an essential first step. Some regulatory agencies that have standards, requirements, and guidelines are listed in Box 2-1. Sorting through the regulatory maze can be frustrating, but the government agencies and voluntary organizations are willing to assist employers in complying with their standards.

Safety Program Elements

A proactive program should include the following ingredients:

Written safety plan—written policies and procedures that explain the steps to be taken for all of the occupational hazards that exist in the laboratory.

Training programs—conducted annually for all employees. New employees should receive safety information on the first day that they are assigned to the hematology laboratory.

Job safety analysis—identifies all of the tasks performed in hematology, the steps involved in performing the procedures, and the risk associated with the procedures.

Safety awareness program—promotes a team concept and encourages employees to take an active part in the safety program.

Risk assessment—proactive risk (identification) assessment of all the potential safety or occupational hazards that exist in the laboratory. The assessment should be conducted at least annually and when a new risk is added to the laboratory. After conducting the risk assessment, policies and procedures should be developed to prevent the hazard from injuring a laboratory worker. Some common risks are exposure to bloodborne pathogens; exposure to chemicals; needle punctures; slips, trips, and falls; and ergonomics issues.

Safety audits and follow-up—a safety checklist should be developed for the hematology laboratory.

Reporting and investigating of all accidents, "near misses," or unsafe conditions—the causes of all incidents should be reviewed and corrective action taken, if necessary.

Emergency drill and evaluation—periodic drills for all potential internal and external disasters. Drills should address the potential accident or disaster before it occurs and test the preparedness of the staff for an emergency situation. Planning for the accident and practicing the response to the accident reduces the panic that results when employees do not know the correct response to a situation.

Emergency management plan—emergencies, sometimes called *disasters* (anything that prevents normal operation of the laboratory), do not occur only in the hospital-based laboratories. Freestanding laboratories, physician office laboratories, and university laboratories can be affected by emergencies that occur in the building or in the community. Emergency planning is crucial to being able to sustain an emergency situation and recover enough to continue the daily operation of the laboratory. Similar to the safety risk assessment, a hazard vulnerability analysis should be conducted. Hazard vulnerability analysis helps to identify all of the potential emergencies that may have an impact on the laboratory. Emergencies such as a utility failure—loss of power, water, or telephones—can have a great impact on the laboratory's ability to perform procedures. Emergencies in the community, such as a terrorist attack, plane crash, flood,

---

BOX 2-1 Government Regulatory Agencies Providing Laboratory Safety Standards

Department of Labor: 29 Code of Federal Regulations Parts 1900-1910

Hazard Communication Standard (right to know)—29 CFR 1910.1200

Occupational Exposure to Bloodborne Pathogens Standard—29 CFR 1910.1030

Occupational Exposure to Hazardous Chemicals in Laboratories Standard—29 CFR 1910.1450

Formaldehyde Standard—29 CFR 1910.1048

Air Contaminants: Permissible Exposure Limits—29 CFR 1910.1000

Occupational Noise Level Standard—29 CFR 1910.95

Hazardous Waste Operations and Emergency Response Standard—29 CFR 1910.120

Personal Protective Equipment—29 CFR 1910.132

Eye and Face Protection—29 CFR 1910.133

Respiratory Protection—29 CFR 1910.134

Department of Interior: Environmental Protection Agency: 40 Code of Federal Regulations Parts 200-399

Resource Conservation and Recovery Act (RCRA)

Medical Waste Tracking Act

Clean Air Act

Clean Water Act

Toxic Substances Control Act (TSCA)

Comprehensive Environmental Response, Compensation, and Liability Act (CERCLA)

Superfund Amendments and Reauthorization Act (SARA)

SARA Title III: Community Right to Know Act

Voluntary Agencies/Accrediting Agencies

Joint Commission on the Accreditation of Healthcare Organizations (JCAHO)

College of American Pathologists (CAP)

State Public Health Departments

Centers for Disease Control and Prevention (CDC)

CFR, Code of Federal Regulations.

---

or civil disturbances, can affect the laboratory workers' ability to get to work and can affect transportation of crucial supplies or equipment. When the potential emergencies are identified, policies and procedures should be developed and practiced so that the laboratory worker knows the backup procedures and can implement them quickly during an emergency/disaster situation. The emergency management plan should cover the four phases of response to an emergency, as follows:

1. Mitigation—measures to prevent the emergency
2. Preparedness—design of procedures, identification of resources that may be used, and training on the procedures

---

BOX 2-2 Emergency Management Activities: Planning for Response to a Fire

Mitigation Activities
Fire alarm pull box
Emergency code to notify workers
Smoke detectors
Fire/smoke doors
Audible and visual alarms
Fire exit lights
Sprinkler system

Preparedness Activities
Training of workers
Fire drills
Fire response procedure
Annual and monthly fire extinguisher checks

Response Activities
Fire response plan
Specific assignments during the actual event

Recovery Activities
Communication of "all clear"
Documentation of response to the fire
Damage assessment
Financial accounting of response activities
Restocking of supplies
Stress debriefing for workers

---

3. Response—actions that will be taken when responding to the emergency
4. Recovery—procedures to assess damage and restock supplies so that the laboratory can return to normal operation

An example of an emergency management plan is shown in Box 2-2. The Clinical and Laboratory Standards Institute document on "Planning for Challenges to Clinical Laboratory Operations During a Disaster" provides detailed actions to prepare for an emergency/disaster. The document also provides some valuable websites for additional resources.[3]

Safety committee/department safety meetings—to communicate safety policies to the employees.

Review of equipment and supplies purchased for the laboratory—for code compliance and safety features.

Annual evaluation of the safety program—review of the regulations for compliance in the laboratory.

CHAPTER at a GLANCE

- The responsibility of a clinical laboratory professional is to perform analytic procedures accurately, precisely, and safely.
- Safe practices must be incorporated into all laboratory procedures and should be followed by every employee.
- The laboratory must adopt universal [standard] precautions, which require that all human blood, body fluids, and tissues be treated as if they were infectious.
- One of the most important safety practices is handwashing.
- Occupational hazards in the laboratory include fire, chemical, and electrical hazards and needle puncture.
- Some common-sense rules of safety are as follows:
  - Be knowledgeable about the procedures being performed. If in doubt, ask for further instructions.

- Wear protective clothing and use protective equipment when required.
- Clean up spills immediately.
- Keep workstations clean and corridors free from obstruction.
- Report injuries and unsafe conditions. Review accidents and incidents to determine their fundamental cause. Take corrective action to prevent further injuries.
- Maintain a proactive safety management program.

Now that you have completed this chapter, go back and read again the case study at the beginning and respond to the questions presented.

REVIEW QUESTIONS

1. Universal [standard] precautions apply to all of the following *except:*
   a. Blood
   b. Cerebrospinal fluid
   c. Semen
   d. Concentrated acids

2. The *most important* practice in preventing the spread of disease is:
   a. Wearing masks during patient contact
   b. Proper handwashing
   c. Wearing disposable laboratory coats
   d. Identifying specimens from known or suspected HIV and HBV patients with a red label

3. The appropriate dilution of bleach to be used in laboratory disinfection is:
   a. 1:2
   b. 1:5
   c. 1:10
   d. 1:100

4. How frequently should fire alarms and sprinkler systems be tested?
   a. Weekly
   b. Monthly
   c. Quarterly
   d. Annually

5. Where should alcohol and other flammable chemicals be stored?
   a. In an approved safety can or storage cabinet away from heat sources
   b. Under a hood and arranged alphabetically for ease of identification in an emergency
   c. In a refrigerator at 2° C to 8° C to reduce volatilization
   d. On a low shelf in an area protected from light

6. The most frequent cause of needle punctures is:
   a. Patient movement during venipuncture
   b. Improper disposal of phlebotomy equipment
   c. Inattention during removal of needle after venipuncture
   d. Failure to attach needle firmly to syringe or tube holder

7. Under which of the following circumstances would an MSDS be helpful?
   a. A phlebotomist has experienced a needle puncture with a clean needle.
   b. A fire extinguisher failed during routine testing.
   c. A pregnant laboratory staff member has asked whether she needs to be concerned about working with a given reagent.
   d. During a safety inspection, an aged microscope power supply is found to have a frayed power cord.

8. It is a busy evening in the City Hospital hematology department. One staff member called in sick, and there was a major auto accident that has one staff member tied up in the blood bank all evening. Mary, the clinical laboratory scientist covering hematology, is in a hurry to get a stat sample on the analyzer but needs to pour off an aliquot for another department. She is wearing gloves and a gown. She carefully covers the stopper of the well-mixed ethylenediamine tetraacetic acid (EDTA) tube with a gauze square and tilts the stopper toward her so it opens away from her. She pours off about 1 mL into a prelabeled tube, replaces the stopper of the EDTA tube, and puts it in the sample rack and sets it on the conveyor. She then runs the poured sample off to the other department. How would you assess Mary's safety practice?
   a. Mary was careful and followed all appropriate procedures.
   b. Mary should have used a shield when opening the tube.
   c. Mary should have poured the sample into a sterile tube.
   d. Mary should have wiped the tube with alcohol after replacing the stopper.

9. A class C fire extinguisher would be appropriate to use on a fire in a chemical cabinet.
   a. True
   b. False

10. According to OSHA standards, all of the following statements about laboratory coats are true *except* that laboratory coats must be:
    a. Water resistant
    b. Made of cloth fabric that can be readily laundered
    c. Long sleeved
    d. Worn fully buttoned

REFERENCES

1. Garza D, Becan-McBride K: Phlebotomy Handbook, 7th ed. Upper Saddle River, NJ: Pearson Prentice Hall, Appleton & Lange, 2005.
2. Department of Labor: 29 Code of Federal Regulations Parts 1900-1910. Federal Register, July 1, 1998. Available at: www.access.gpo.gov/nara/cfr/waisidx____98/29cfrv5____98.html.
3. CLSI: Planning for challenges to clinical laboratory operations during a disaster, a report. X4-R, vol 23, no 29.

ADDITIONAL RESOURCES

Comprehensive Accreditation Manual for Hospitals: Environment of Care Standards, 2005.
National Fire Protection Association: Laboratories Using Chemicals, NFPA 45.
Resource for occupational hazards found in the laboratory and other related regulations. Available at: www.osha.gov/SLTC/etools/hospital/lab/lab.html.
Resource for four phases of emergency planning and up-to-date disaster information. Available at: www.fema.gov.
Resource for regulatory health guidelines. Available at: www.osha.gov/SLTC/healthguidelines.
NIOSH pocket guide for chemical hazards. Available at: www.cdc.gov/niosh/npg.

Specimen Collection

3

Carole A. Mullins

OBJECTIVES

After completion of this chapter, the reader will be able to:

1. Describe the application of standard precautions to the collection of blood samples.
2. List collection equipment used for venipuncture and skin puncture.
3. Correlate tube stopper color with additive, if any, and explain the purpose of the additive and use of that tube in the laboratory.
4. Discuss selection of a vein for venipuncture, and name the vein that is preferred in most instances.
5. List in order the steps recommended by the Clinical and Laboratory Standards Institute (CLSI) for venipuncture in adults, including recommended order of collection for tubes with various additives.
6. Discuss complications encountered in blood collection and proper response of the phlebotomist.
7. Explain appropriate use of skin puncture equipment and procedure to be followed, including sites for infants, children, and adults.
8. Discuss essentials of quality assurance in specimen collection.
9. List reasons for specimen rejection.
10. Given the description of a specimen and its collection, determine acceptability.
11. Recognize deviations from the recommended venipuncture practice in a written scenario, and describe corrective procedures.
12. Name the most important step in the venipuncture procedure.
13. List reasons for inability to obtain a blood specimen.
14. Summarize legal issues that need to be considered in specimen acquisition.

CASE STUDIES

After studying the material in this chapter, the reader should be able to respond to the following case studies:

Case 1

A phlebotomist asks an outpatient, "Are you Susan Jones?" After the patient says "yes," the phlebotomist proceeds by labeling the tubes and drawing the blood. What is wrong with this scenario?

Case 2

A patient must have blood drawn for a complete blood count (CBC), potassium (K^+), prothrombin time (PT), and type and screen (T&S). The phlebotomist draws the following tubes in this order:

1. SST or serum separation tube
2. PT light-blue tube
3. CBC lavender tube
4. K^+ green tube

The physician questions the results of the K^+ and PT. Why?

SAFETY

Standard precautions must be followed in the collection of blood, and all specimens must be treated as potentially infectious for bloodborne pathogens (e.g., hepatitis B virus, hepatitis C virus, and human immunodeficiency virus [HIV]). Regulations from the Occupational Health and Safety Administration (OSHA) that took effect on March 6, 1992, outlined in detail what must be done to protect healthcare workers from exposure to bloodborne pathogens, such as the pathogens that cause hepatitis C, hepatitis B, hepatitis D, syphilis, malaria, and HIV.[1]

Bloodborne pathogens may enter the body via an accidental injury by a sharp object, such as a contaminated needle, a scalpel, broken glass, or anything else that can pierce the skin. Cuts, dermatitis, abrasions, and mucous membranes (of the mouth, eyes, and nose) may provide a portal of entry. Indirect transmission can occur when a person touches a contaminated surface or object and then touches the mouth, eyes, nose, or nonintact skin without washing the hands. Hepatitis B virus can survive on inanimate or dried surfaces at room temperature for at least 1 week.[2]

Handwashing is the most important procedure to prevent the spread of infectious diseases. The phlebotomist should wash his or her hands with a nonabrasive soap and running water between patients and every time gloves are removed. If handwashing facilities are unavailable, an antiseptic hand cleanser or an antiseptic towelette may be used as a temporary measure. *Gloves* are essential protective equipment and must be worn when venipunctures are performed. When gloves are removed, it is important that no substances from the soiled gloves come in contact with the hands. Glove removal is covered in detail in Chapter 2.

Contaminated sharps and infectious wastes should be placed in designated puncture-resistant containers. The red or red-orange *biohazard* sign (see Fig. 2-1) indicates that a container holds potentially infectious materials. Biohazard containers should be easily accessible and not be overfilled.

RESPONSIBILITY OF PHLEBOTOMIST IN INFECTION CONTROL

Because phlebotomists interact with patients and staff throughout the day, they potentially could infect numerous people. Phlebotomists should become familiar with and observe infection control and isolation policies. Violations of policies should be reported. A phlebotomist must maintain good personal health and hygiene, making sure to have clean clothes, clean hair, and clean fingernails. Standard precautions must be followed at all times, with special attention to the use of gloves and handwashing.

PHYSIOLOGIC FACTORS AFFECTING TEST RESULTS

Certain physiologic factors specific to the patient may affect results of laboratory testing. These factors include posture (supine or erect), diurnal rhythms (day or night), exercise, stress, diet (fasting or not), and smoking (Box 3-1).[3-5] It is important that the phlebotomist adhere to requests for specimens to be drawn at a specific time and to record the time of collection.

VENIPUNCTURE

Collection Equipment for Venipuncture

The most common means of collecting blood specimens is with the use of an evacuated tube system (Fig. 3-1). The system includes a tube, which can be either plastic or glass; a needle; and an adapter, which is used to secure the needle and the tube. For safety, plastic tubes are recommended by OSHA whenever possible. Most glass tubes are coated with silicone to help decrease the possibility of hemolysis and to prevent blood from adhering to the sides of the tube. All tubes come in various sizes and may contain a variety of premeasured additives.

Although there are several manufacturers of evacuated tubes, all follow a universal color code in which the stopper

---

BOX 3-1 Physiologic Factors Affecting Test Results

Posture
Changing from a supine (lying) to a sitting or standing position results in a shift of body water from inside the blood vessels to the interstitial spaces. Larger molecules cannot filter into the tissues and concentrate in the blood. There are significant increases in test values for lipids, enzymes, and proteins.

Diurnal Rhythm
Diurnal pertains to daylight, and *diurnal rhythm* refers to daily body fluid fluctuations that occur. Certain hormone levels, such as cortisol and adenocorticotropic hormone, decrease in the afternoon. Other test values, such as iron and eosinophils, increase in the afternoon.

Exercise
Muscle activity elevates creatinine, protein, creatine kinase, aspartate transaminase, and lactate dehydrogenase test values. Research also suggests that exercise activates coagulation and fibrinolysis and increases platelet and white blood cell counts.

Stress
Anxiety can cause a temporary increase in white blood cells and an acid-base imbalance.[6]

Diet
Fasting means no food or beverages except water for 8 to 12 hours before a blood draw. If a patient has eaten recently (<2 hours prior), there will be a temporary increase in glucose and lipid content in the blood. As a result, the serum or plasma may appear cloudy or turbid (lipemic), which interferes with testing, especially with tests such as glucose, sodium, and complete blood counts.

Smoking
Patients who smoke before blood collection may have increased white blood cell counts and cortisol levels. Long-term smoking can lead to decreased pulmonary function and result in increased hemoglobin levels. Skin punctures may be more difficult to obtain as a result of impaired circulation.

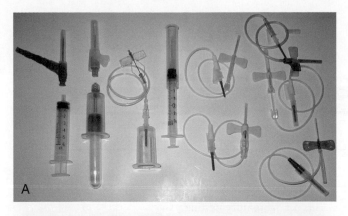

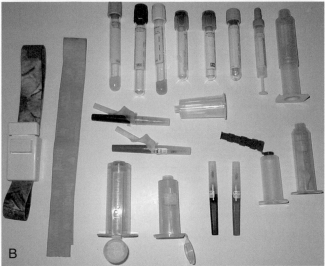

Figure 3-1 A, Butterfly equipment. **B,** A variety of tubes, needles, and tourniquets. (Courtesy of Rich Mullins.)

color indicates the type of additive contained within the tube. Figure 3-2 shows a summary of collection tubes.

Additives in Collection Tubes

Antiglycolytic Agent. An antiglycolytic agent inhibits the use of glucose by blood cells. Such inhibition may be necessary if testing for glucose level is delayed. Examples of antiglycolytic agents are sodium fluoride and lithium iodoacetate. Tubes containing sodium fluoride alone yield serum. Sodium fluoride is combined with potassium oxalate or potassium ethylenediamine tetraacetic acid (K_2EDTA), both anticoagulants, to yield plasma for more rapid testing.

Anticoagulant. An anticoagulant prevents blood from clotting. The mechanism by which clotting is prevented varies with the anticoagulant. EDTA, citrate, and oxalate remove calcium by forming insoluble salts, whereas heparin prevents the conversion of prothrombin to thrombin. If calcium is removed or thrombin is not formed, coagulation does not occur. Examples of anticoagulants are EDTA, sodium citrate, and lithium or sodium heparin. Tubes must be inverted gently several times to ensure proper mixing *immediately* after collection, according to the manufacturer's instructions.

Clot Activator. A clot activator helps initiate or enhance the clotting mechanism. Clot activators include glass or silica particles that provide increased surface area for platelet activation and a clotting factor such as thrombin.

Separator Gel. Separator gel is an inert material that undergoes a temporary change in viscosity during the centrifugation process, enabling it to serve as a separation barrier between the liquid (serum or plasma) and cells. Because this gel may interfere with some testing, serum or plasma from these tubes cannot be used with certain instruments or for blood bank procedures.

Needles

Sterile needles come in a variety of lengths and gauges (bore or opening size). Needles are made to be screwed into the evacuated tube holder or to be attached to the tips of syringes. Evacuated tube needles are double pointed and have a plastic cap covering the long, narrow, pointed end that punctures the patient's skin and a short beveled point at the other end covered by a rubber sleeve that punctures the rubber stopper of the evacuated tube. The rubber sleeve prevents blood from dripping into the holder when tubes are changed. On syringes, "single-sample" needles are used. The end of the needle that is inserted into the vein has a point with a slanted side (bevel), which must be facing up when the needle is inserted. Needle tips should be examined for burrs or bends before a venipuncture is performed. Gauge numbers are related inversely to the bore size: the smaller the gauge number, the larger the bore. Needle gauges for drawing blood range from 20 gauge to 25 gauge. The most common needle size for adult venipuncture is 21 gauge with a length of 1 inch. The advantage of using a 1-inch needle is that it provides better control.

Several new needles and holders have been designed to comply with the revised "Occupational Exposure to Bloodborne Pathogens" (effective April 18, 2001) and its required implementation of safer medical devices. These needles and holders are as follows:

1. The Punctur-Guard (Bio-Plexus, Inc., Vernon, Conn.) needle assembly comprises a blunt cannula, called a *blunting member,* placed within an otherwise standard needle that is blunted before removal from the patient's vein.

2. The Vacutainer Eclipse Blood Collection Needle (Becton Dickinson, Franklin Lakes, N.J.) provides single-handed activation after performing the venipuncture, by pushing the safety shield forward with the thumb until an audible click is heard. The Becton Dickinson Eclipse needle should be used with a single-use tube holder. After activating the safety shield, the entire assembly should be discarded intact into the sharps container.

3. The Vacu-Pro Venipuncture Needle Protection Device (Concord Portex, Keene, N.H.) allows the Vacu-Pro sheath to be snapped over the needle with one hand after completing the venipuncture. The entire device is disposed of into the sharps container.

BD Vacutainer® Venous Blood Collection
Tube Guide

For a full line of BD Vacutainer® Specimen Collection Products, visit www.bd.com/vacutainer.

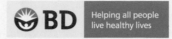

BD Vacutainer® Tubes With Hemogard Closure	BD Vacutainer® Tubes With Conventional Stopper	Additive	Inversions at Blood Collection*	Laboratory Use	Your Lab's Draw Volume/Remarks
Gold	Red/Black	• Clot activator and gel for serum separation	5	BD Vacutainer® SST™ Tube for serum determinations in chemistry. Tube inversions ensure mixing of clot activator with blood. Blood clotting time: 30 minutes.	
Light Green	Green/Gray	• Lithium heparin and gel for plasma separation	8	BD Vacutainer® PST™ Tube for plasma determinations in chemistry. Tube inversions prevent clotting.	
Red		• None (glass) • Clot activator (plastic)	0 5	For serum determinations in chemistry, serology, and immunohematology testing (ABO grouping, Rh typing, antibody screening, red cell phenotyping and DAT testing). Tube inversions ensure mixing of clot activator with blood and clotting within 60 minutes.	
Orange	Gray/Yellow	• Thrombin	8	For stat serum determinations in chemistry. Tube inversions ensure complete clotting, which usually occurs in less than 5 minutes.	
Royal Blue		• Sodium heparin (glass) • Na$_2$EDTA (glass) • No additive (glass serum) • Clot activator (plastic serum) • K$_2$EDTA(plastic)	8 8 0 5 8	For trace-element, toxicology and nutritional-chemistry determinations. Special stopper formulation provides low levels of trace elements (see package insert)	
Green		• Sodium heparin • Lithium heparin	8 8	For plasma determinations in chemistry. Tube inversions prevent clotting.	
Gray		• Potassium oxalate/sodium fluoride • Sodium fluoride/Na$_2$ EDTA • Sodium fluoride (serum tube)	8 8 8	For glucose determinations. Oxalate and EDTA anticoagulant will give plasma samples. Sodium fluoride is the antiglycolytic agent. Tube inversions ensure proper mixing of additive and blood.	
Tan		• Sodium heparin (glass) • K$_2$EDTA (plastic)	8 8	For lead determinations. This tube is certified to contain less than .01 µg/mL(ppm) lead. Tube inversions prevent clotting.	
Yellow		• Sodium polyanethol sulfonate (SPS) • Acid citrate dextrose additives (ACD): **Solution A -** 22.0g/L trisodium citrate, 8.0g/L citric acid, 4.8g/L dextrose **Solution B -** 13.2g/L trisodium citrate, 4.8g/L citric acid, 14.7g/L dextrose	8 8 8	SPS for blood culture specimen collections in microbiology. Tube inversions prevent clotting. ACD for use in blood bank studies, HLA phenotyping, DNA and paternity testing.	
Lavender		• Liquid K$_3$EDTA (glass) • Spray-coated K$_2$EDTA (plastic)	8 8	K$_3$EDTA for whole blood hematology determinations. K$_2$EDTA for whole blood hematology determinations and immunohematology testing (ABO grouping, Rh typing, antibody screening). Tube inversions prevent clotting.	
White		K$_2$EDTA with gel	8	For use in molecular diagnostic test methods (such as but not limited to polymerse chain reaction (PCR) and/or branched DNA (bDNA) amplification techniques).	
Pink		• Spray-coated K$_2$EDTA	8	For whole blood hematology determinations and immunohematology testing (ABO grouping, Rh typing, antibody screening). Designed with special cross-match label for required patient information by the AABB. Tube inversions prevent clotting.	
Light Blue	Clear	• Buffered sodium citrate 0.105M (~3.2%)glass 0.109M (~3.2%)plastic • Citrate, theophyline, adenosine, dipyridamole (CTAD)	3-4 3-4	For coagulation determinations. NOTE: Certain tests may require chilled specimens. Follow your institution's recommended procedures for collection and transport. CTAD for selected platelet function assays and routine coagulation determination. Tube inversions prevent clotting.	
Clear		• None (plastic)	0	For use as a discard tube or secondary specimen collection tube.	

Partial-draw Tubes (2ml and 3ml: 13 x 75 mm)   **Small-volume Pediatric Tubes** (2ml: 10.25 x 47mm, 3ml: 10.25 x 64 mm)

		Additive	Inversions	Laboratory Use	
Red		• None	0	For serum determinations in chemistry and serology. Glass serum tubes are recommended for blood banking. Plastic tubes contain clot activator and are not recommended for blood banking. Tube inversions ensure mixing of clot activator with blood and clotting within 60 minutes.	
Green		• Sodium heparin • Lithium heparin	8 8	For plasma determinations in chemistry. Tube inversions prevent clotting.	
Lavender		• Liquid K$_3$EDTA (glass) • Spray-coated K$_2$EDTA (plastic)	8 8	K$_3$EDTA and K$_2$EDTA for whole blood hematology determinations and immunohematology testing (ABO grouping, Rh typing, antibody screening). Tube inversions prevent clotting.	
Light Blue		• .105M sodium citrate (~3.2%)	3-4	For coagulation determinations. Tube inversions prevent clotting. NOTE: Certain tests may require chilled specimens. Follow your institution's recommended procedures for collection and transport of specimen.	

BD Diagnostic
Preanalytical Systems
1 Becton Drive
Franklin Lakes, NJ 07417 USA

BD Global Technical Services: 1.800.631.0174
BD Customer Service: 1.888.237.2762
www.bd.com/vacutainer

* Invert gently, do not shake

BD, BD Logo and all other trademarks are the property of Becton, Dickinson and Company. ©2005 BD.
Printed in USA   01/05   VS5229-6

Figure 3-2 Vacutainer Tube Guide. (Courtesy and © Becton, Dickinson and Company.)

Needle Holders

Needle holders usually are made to fit a specific manufacturer's needles and tubes and, for best results, should not be interchanged. The holders are disposable and must be discarded after a single use with the needle still attached as per OSHA.[5] Because needle sticks continue to be a safety concern, several new needle holders on the market have sheaths that lock into place after use. Examples include Safety-Lok Needle Holder (Becton Dickinson) and Saf-T Clik holder (Winfield Medical, San Diego, Calif.).

Tourniquet

A tourniquet is used to provide a barrier against venous blood flow to help locate a vein. A tourniquet can be a disposable latex strap, a heavier Velcro strap, or a blood pressure cuff. The tourniquet should be applied 2 to 4 inches above the venipuncture site and left on for no longer than 1 minute before the venipuncture is performed. Latex-free tourniquets are available for individuals with a latex allergy.

Syringes

Syringes consist of a barrel that is graduated in milliliters and a plunger. Syringe needles have a point at one end and an open hub at the other end that attaches to the barrel. Syringes come with different types of needle attachments and in different sizes. It is important to attach the needle securely to the syringe to prevent air from entering the system. Syringes may be useful in drawing blood from pediatric, geriatric, or other patients with tiny, fragile, or "rolling" veins that would not be able to withstand the vacuum pressure from evacuated tubes. With a syringe, the amount of pressure exerted is controlled by the phlebotomist. After the syringe needle is shielded, removed, and discarded in a sharps container, a syringe blood transfer

device (Becton Dickinson or Tyco Healthcare/Kendall Co) is attached to the syringe, and a vacuum tube is inserted into the transfer device. The blood is transferred from the syringe into the tube using the tube's vacuum.

Winged Infusion Sets (Butterflies)

A butterfly is an intravenous device that consists of a short needle and a thin tube with attached plastic wings. The butterfly can be connected to evacuated tube holders, syringes, or blood culture bottles with the use of special adapters. Butterflies are useful in collecting specimens from children or other patients from whom it is difficult to draw blood. Butterflies now come with resheathing devices to minimize the risk of needle stick injury (e.g., Vacutainer brand SAFETY-LOK and Becton Dickinson Vacutainer Push Button Blood Collection Set [Becton Dickinson], and Angel Wing Safety Needle System [Tyco Healthcare/Kendall Co], Surshield Safety Winged Blood Collection Set [Terumo Medical Corp], VACUETTE Safety Blood Collection Set [Greiner Bio-One]).

Solutions for Skin Preparation

The most common skin cleanser is 70% isopropyl alcohol. It can be applied by a commercially prepared alcohol pad or by a cotton ball or piece of gauze soaked in the alcohol. The site should be cleaned in a circular motion, beginning in the center and working outward. It is important to allow the area to air dry before the venipuncture is performed so that the patient does not experience a burning sensation and to prevent contamination of the specimen. When a sterile site is prepared for collection of blood cultures, a two-step procedure is used in which isopropyl alcohol is followed by iodine. Some healthcare facilities use a one-step application of chlorhexidine gluconate/isopropyl alcohol. To avoid contamination when

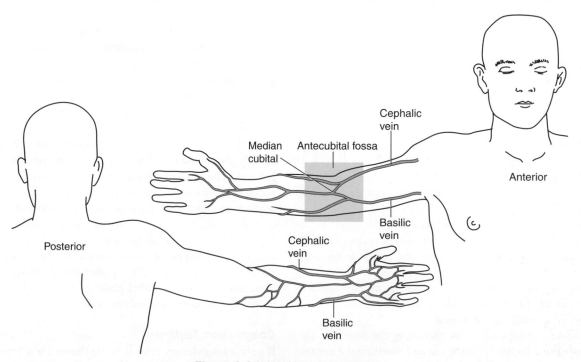

Figure 3-3 Veins of forearm (two views).

legal blood alcohol level is measured, benzalkonium chloride (Zephiran Chloride) or a nonalcohol antiseptic is used.

Selecting a Vein for Routine Venipuncture

The superficial veins of the antecubital fossa are the most common sites for venipuncture. The three primary veins that are used are (1) the cephalic vein, located on the upper forearm and on the thumb side of the hand; (2) the basilic vein, located on the lower forearm and the little finger side of the hand; and (3) the median cubital vein, which connects the basilic and cephalic veins in the antecubital fossa (bend in elbow). The median cubital vein is the vein of choice (Fig. 3-3).

If necessary, the phlebotomist should have the patient make a fist after application of the tourniquet; the vein should become prominent. The patient should not do any vigorous pumping of the fist because it may affect some of the test values. The phlebotomist should palpate (examine by touching) the vein with his or her index finger to determine vein depth, direction, and diameter. If a vein cannot be located in either arm, it may be necessary to examine the veins in the dorsal side of the wrist and hand.

The feet should not be used if the patient is diabetic or prone to developing blood clots. Some facilities require physician permission before drawing blood from feet. The policy in some institutions is to request that a second phlebotomist attempt to locate a vein in the arm before one of these three alternate sites is used.

Routine Venipuncture Procedure

The phlebotomist should practice standard precautions, which include applying gloves and washing hands at the beginning of the procedure and removing gloves and washing hands at the end of the procedure. The following steps are recommended by the Clinical and Laboratory Standards Institute (CLSI):[3]

1. Prepare the accession order.
2. Identify the patient by having the patient verbally state his or her name and confirm with patient's identification number (i.e., medical records number, birth date, or Social Security number).
3. Verify any diet restrictions (i.e., fasting, if appropriate), and check for any sensitivity to latex.
4. Assemble supplies and put on gloves.
5. Reassure the patient.
6. Position the patient.
7. Verify paperwork and tube selection.
8. If necessary, to help locate the vein, ensure that the patient's hand is closed.
9. Select an appropriate venipuncture site.
10. Cleanse the venipuncture site with 70% isopropyl alcohol, working in concentric circles from the inside to outside. *Allow to air dry.*
11. Apply the tourniquet 2 to 4 inches above the selected puncture site for no longer that 1 minute.
12. Inspect the needle and equipment.
13. Perform the venipuncture by anchoring the vein with the thumb 1 to 2 inches *below* the site and inserting the needle, bevel up, with a 15- to 30-degree angle between the needle

and the skin. Collect tubes using the correct order of draw, and invert each tube containing any additive *immediately* after collection. A particular order of draw is recommended when drawing multiple specimens from a single venipuncture. Its purpose is to avoid possible test result error because of cross-contamination from tube additives. The recommended order of draw is as follows:

1. Blood culture or sterile tubes (i.e., yellow stopper)
2. Coagulation tube (i.e., light-blue stopper)
3. Serum tube with or without clot activator or gel (i.e., red, gold, or red-gray marbled stopper)
4. Heparin tubes (i.e., green or light-green stopper)
5. EDTA tubes (i.e., lavender stopper)
6. Oxalate/fluoride tubes (i.e., gray stopper)

14. Release and remove the tourniquet as soon as blood flow is established or no longer than 1 minute.
15. Ensure that the patient's hand is open.
16. Place the gauze lightly over the puncture site without pressing down.
17. After the last tube has been released from the back of the multisample needle, remove the needle and activate safety device as per manufacturer's directions.
18. Apply direct pressure to the puncture site.
19. Bandage the venipuncture site *after* checking to ensure that bleeding has stopped.
20. If a syringe has been used, fill the tubes.
21. Dispose of the puncture equipment and other biohazardous waste.
22. Label the tubes with the correct information. The minimal amount of information that must be on each tube is as follows:
    1. Patient's full name
    2. Patient's unique identification number
    3. Date of collection
    4. Time of collection (military time)
    5. Collector's initials or code number
23. Perform any special handling requirements (i.e., chilling or protection from light).
24. Eliminate any diet restrictions and thank patient.
25. Send the properly labeled specimens to the laboratory.

The most crucial step in the process is patient identification. The patient must verbally state his or her name, or someone must identify the patient for the phlebotomist. A hospitalized patient also must be identified by his or her identification bracelet. The patient's name and identification number or Social Security number must match the information on the test requisition. Any discrepancies must be resolved before the procedure can continue. Failure to confirm proper identification could result in a life-threatening situation for the patient and possible legal ramifications for the phlebotomist. All tubes should be labeled immediately after the blood specimen has been drawn, with the label attached to the tube before the phlebotomist leaves the patient's side.

Coagulation Testing

If only a coagulation tube is to be drawn for a prothrombin time or an activated partial thromboplastin time, the *first* tube drawn may be used for testing. It is no longer necessary to draw a 3-mL discard into a nonadditive tube before collecting for routine coagulation testing. Tubes for coagulation must be filled to the correct level to maintain a 9:1 ratio of blood to anticoagulant to ensure accurate test results. Underfilling tubes results in prolonged test values. When using a butterfly to draw a single blue top tube, a nonadditive or another light-blue tube must be used to clear the dead space in the tubing before collecting the tube to be used for testing. For special coagulation testing, however, the second or third tube drawn should be used.[3]

Venipuncture Procedure in Children and Infants

Pediatric phlebotomy requires experience, special skills, and a tender touch. Excellent interpersonal skills are needed to deal with distraught parents and with crying, screaming, and scared children. Ideally, only experienced phlebotomists should draw blood from children; however, the only way to gain experience is through practice. Through experience, one learns what works in different situations. Frequently, smaller-gauge (23 gauge or 25 gauge) needles are used. Syringes or butterflies may be advantageous with some infants' veins. No matter what equipment is used, the real secret to a successful venipuncture is a good child holder! The child's arm should be immobilized as much as possible to get the needle successfully into the vein and be able to keep it there if the child tries to move. Use of special stickers or character bandages as rewards may serve as incentive for cooperation; however, protocol of the institution with regard to their distribution must be followed.

Complications Encountered in Blood Collection

Ecchymosis (Bruise)

Bruising is the most common complication encountered in obtaining a blood specimen. It is caused by leakage of a small amount of fluid around the tissue. The phlebotomist can prevent bruising by applying direct pressure to the venipuncture site, instead of having the patient bend the arm at the elbow.

Syncope (Fainting)

Fainting is the second most common complication. Before drawing blood, the collector always should ask the patient whether he or she has had any prior episodes of fainting during or after blood collection. The CLSI recommends that ammonia inhalants no longer be used because they may trigger an asthma attack or a sudden, exaggerated response that could lead to patient injury. The phlebotomist should follow the protocol at his or her facility.

If the patient begins to faint, the phlebotomist should remove the needle immediately, lower the patient's head, and apply cold compresses to the back of the patient's neck and loosen any constrictive clothing. The patient should take some deep breaths and be offered some orange juice or cold water to drink. The patient should sit for at least 30 minutes before leaving. The incident always should be documented.

Hematoma

A hematoma results when leakage of a large amount of fluid around the puncture site causes the area to swell. If swelling begins, the needle should be removed immediately and pressure applied to the site for at least 2 minutes. Hematomas may result in bruising of the patient's skin around the puncture site if adequate pressure is not maintained. Blood that leaks out of the vein under the patient's skin may clot and result in nerve compression and permanent damage to the patient's arm. A hematoma most commonly occurs when the needle goes through the vein, when the bevel of the needle is only partially in the vein, and when the phlebotomist fails to apply enough pressure after venipuncture.

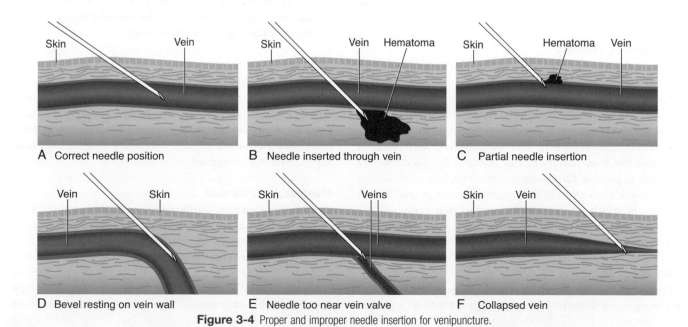

Figure 3-4 Proper and improper needle insertion for venipuncture.

Failure to Draw Blood

One reason for failure to draw blood is that the vein is missed, often because of improper needle positioning. The needle should be inserted completely into the vein with the slanted side (bevel) up, at an angle of 15 to 30 degrees. Figure 3-4 shows reasons for unsatisfactory flow of blood. It is sometimes possible to enter the vein by redirecting the needle, but only an experienced phlebotomist should attempt this because such manipulation can cause discomfort to the patient.

Occasionally, an evacuated tube has insufficient vacuum, and insertion of another tube yields blood. Keeping extra tubes within reach during blood collection can prevent a recollect when the problem is a technical issue associated with the tubes (i.e., inadequate vacuum).

Petechiae

Petechiae are small red spots indicating that small amounts of blood have escaped into the skin epithelium. Petechiae indicate a possible coagulation problem and should alert the phlebotomist to be aware of possible prolonged bleeding.

Edema

Swelling caused by an abnormal accumulation of fluid in the intercellular spaces of the tissues is termed *edema*. The most common cause is infiltration of the tissues by the solution running through an incorrectly positioned intravenous catheter. Edematous sites should be avoided for venipuncture because the veins are hard to find and the specimens may become contaminated with the tissue fluid.

Obesity

In obese patients, veins may be neither readily visible nor easy to palpate. Sometimes the use of a blood pressure cuff can aid in locating a vein. The cuff should not be inflated any higher than the patient's diastolic pressure and should not be left on the arm for longer than 1 minute. It is not advisable to probe blindly in the patient's arm because muscle or nerve damage may result.

Intravenous Therapy

Drawing blood from an arm with an intravenous catheter should be avoided if possible. The arm opposite the intravenous arm should be used. If there is no alternative, blood should be drawn *below* the catheter with the tourniquet placed *below* the catheter site. It is preferable to have the nurse stop the infusion for 2 minutes before the specimen is drawn. The CLSI recommends that 5 mL of blood be drawn for discard before samples to be used for testing are obtained. It is important to note on the requisition that the specimen was obtained from an arm in which an intravenous solution was running.[2] The phlebotomist always should follow the protocol established at his or her facility.

Hemoconcentration

Hemoconcentration is an increased concentration of larger molecules and analytes in the blood as a result of a shift in water balance. Hemoconcentration can be caused by leaving the tourniquet on the patient's arm for too long or by probing or massaging the site. It is recommended that the tourniquet not remain on for more than 1 minute before venipuncture. If it is left on for a longer time because of difficulty in finding a vein, it should be removed for 2 to 3 minutes and reapplied before the venipuncture is performed.[4]

Hemolysis

The rupture of red blood cells (RBCs) with the consequent escape of hemoglobin—a process termed *hemolysis*—can cause the plasma or serum to appear pink or red. Hemolysis can occur if too small a needle was used during a difficult draw; if the phlebotomist pulls back too quickly on the plunger of a syringe, forces blood into a tube from a syringe, or shakes a tube too hard; or if contamination by alcohol or water occurs at the venipuncture site or in the tubes. Hemolysis also can occur physiologically as a result of hemolytic anemias or severe renal problems. Testing hemolyzed specimens can alter test results, such as potassium and enzymes, which can have a negative impact on patient outcome.

Burned, Damaged, Scarred, and Occluded Veins

Burned, damaged, scarred, and occluded veins should be avoided because they do not allow the blood to flow freely and may make it difficult to obtain an acceptable specimen.

Seizures and Tremors

Patients occasionally experience seizures because of a pre-existing condition or as a response to the needle stick. If a seizure occurs, the needle should be removed immediately. The patient's safety should be ensured by preventing injury from nearby objects.

Vomiting and Choking

If the patient begins vomiting, the patient's head must be positioned so that he or she does not aspirate any vomit. During vomiting or choking, the phlebotomist should prevent the patient from hitting his or her head.

Allergies

Some patients may be allergic to skin antiseptic substances other than alcohol. Adhesive bandages and tape also may cause an allergic reaction. Hypoallergenic tape should be used or pressure applied manually until the bleeding has stopped completely. Sensitivity to latex should be determined before any phlebotomy procedure.

Mastectomy Patients

The phlebotomist should follow the protocol established at his or her facility and by the patient's physician when drawing blood from a patient with a mastectomy (removal of one or both breasts). The pressure on the arm that is on the same side as the mastectomy from a tourniquet or blood pressure cuff can lead to pain or lymphostasis from accumulating lymph fluid. The other arm should be used whenever possible. In cases of a double mastectomy, the phlebotomist should perform a skin puncture or draw from the back of the hand without using a tourniquet.

Inability to Obtain a Blood Specimen

Each institution should have a policy covering proper procedure when a blood specimen cannot be collected. If two unsuccessful attempts at collection have been made, the nurse in charge of the patient and the phlebotomy supervisor should be notified. Another individual can make two attempts to obtain a specimen. If a second person is unsuccessful, the physician should be notified.

The patient has the right to refuse to give a blood specimen. If gentle urging does not persuade the patient to allow blood to be drawn, the phlebotomist should alert the nurse, who either talks to the patient or notifies the physician. The phlebotomist must not try to force an uncooperative patient to have blood drawn; it can be unsafe for the phlebotomist and for the patient. In addition, forcing a patient of legal age and sound mind to have blood drawn against his or her wishes can result in charges of assault and battery or unlawful restraint.

If the patient is a child and the parents offer to help hold the child, it is usually all right to proceed. Any refusals or problems should be documented for legal reasons. If the patient is not in his or her room, the absence should be reported to the nursing unit so that the nurses are aware that the specimen was not obtained.

SKIN PUNCTURES

Skin punctures often are performed in newborns; in pediatric patients younger than 2 years old; in adults who are severely burned, and whose veins are being reserved for therapeutic purposes; and in elderly patients with fragile veins. When peripheral circulation is poor, however, accurate results may not be obtained with specimens acquired by skin puncture.

Capillary blood is actually a mixture of venous blood, arterial blood, and tissue fluid. When the puncture site is warmed, the specimen more closely resembles arterial blood. Because capillary specimens may generate slightly different test results, a notation should be made when the specimen is obtained by skin puncture.[7] White blood cell counts in specimens obtained by skin puncture may be 15% to 20% higher than the counts in venous specimens.[8] Clinically significantly higher glucose values are found in specimens obtained by skin puncture compared with those obtained by venipuncture.[7] This is especially important to note when a glucose tolerance test is performed or when glucometer results are compared with findings from venous samples.

Collection Sites

In most patients, skin punctures may be performed on the heel, big toe, or finger. In infants, the finger should not be punctured because the lancets could cause serious injury to the bones in the fingers. The site of choice in infants is the lateral (outside) or medial (inside) surface of the plantar side

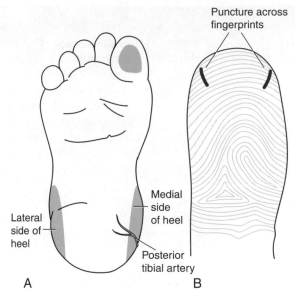

Figure 3-5 Areas for skin puncture specimens: heel **(A)** and finger **(B)**.

(bottom) of the heel, although there have been some problems with using the medial heel surface and puncturing the posterior tibial artery (Fig. 3-5A). The plantar surface of the big toe is recommended for after the child has started walking and the fingers are too small. In older children and adults, the palmar surface of the distal portion of the third (middle) or fourth (ring) finger may be used; the third finger is the recommended site.[7] The puncture on the finger should be made perpendicular to the fingerprint lines when a puncture device with a blade is used (Fig. 3-5B). Warming can increase the blood flow sevenfold. The site can be warmed with a warm washcloth or a commercial heel warmer. The site should be warmed to a temperature no greater than 42° C for no longer than 2 to 5 minutes, unless the collection is for capillary blood gases. The skin puncture site should be cleansed with 70% isopropyl alcohol and allowed to air dry. Povidone-iodine should not be used because of possible blood contamination, which would produce falsely elevated levels of potassium, phosphorus, or uric acid.

Skin Puncture Technique

The finger or heel must be securely immobilized. Punctures should not be made more than 2 mm deep because of the risk of bone injury and possible infection (osteomyelitis). In premature infants, it is advisable to use a puncture device with even less depth. Most devices on the market for performing skin punctures come in varying depths. The use of plastic tubes or Mylar-coated glass tubes is recommended by OSHA to avoid broken glass and exposure to biohazardous materials.

The phlebotomist should not puncture an area that is swollen or bruised or already has been punctured. The first drop of blood should be wiped away to prevent contamination of the specimen with tissue fluid and to facilitate the free flow of blood.[7]

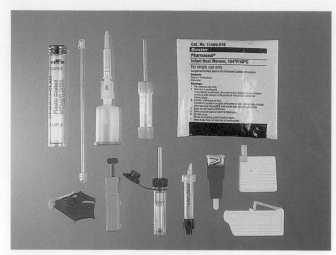

Figure 3-6 Examples of equipment used for skin puncture specimens: (left to right) capillary tubes, Unopette, heel warmer, microcollection devices, and skin puncture devices. (Courtesy of Steve Kasper.)

Devices for Collecting Blood from Skin Puncture

Devices for collecting blood from skin puncture include capillary tubes, microcollection tubes, and unopettes.[7] *Capillary tubes* (Fig. 3-6) of various sizes are available with or without heparin added. *Microcollection tubes* have virtually replaced Caraway/Natelson tubes, which are large-bore glass collecting tubes. Microcollection tubes are available with or without additives, and the cap colors on the tubes correspond with the colors on vacuum tubes. The order of drawing is different for microcollection tubes. The EDTA microcollection tube should be collected first to ensure adequate volume and accurate hematology results, especially for platelets, which tend to aggregate at the site of puncture. Other tubes containing anticoagulants should be collected next, followed by serum tubes. *Unopettes,* which are available in various dilutions and with varied diluents, come with their own calibrated micropipettes and are used in the preparation of specimens for cell counting (Chapter 14).[4] Labeling for capillary specimens should contain the same information as for vacuum tubes.

Skin Puncture Procedure

Standard precautions, which include applying gloves and washing hands at the beginning of the procedure and removing gloves and washing hands at the end of the procedure, should be practiced. The following steps are recommended by the CLSI:[7]

1. Obtain and examine the requisition form.
2. Assemble equipment and supplies.
3. Greet the patient (and parents); identify the patient by having the patient verbally state his or her name and confirm with patient's identification number (i.e., medical records number, birth date, or Social Security number).
4. Verify any diet restrictions (i.e., fasting), and check for any sensitivity to latex.
5. Position the patient and the parents or designated holder as necessary.

6. Put on gloves.
7. Organize equipment and supplies.
8. Select the puncture site.
9. Warm the puncture site. Warming increases the blood flow sevenfold. Use a commercial heel warmer or warm washcloth (40° C to 42° C) for 2 to 5 minutes.
10. Cleanse the puncture site with 70% isopropyl alcohol using concentric circles, working from the inside to outside. *Allow to air dry.*
11. Perform the puncture. Puncture depth should not exceed 2 mm.
12. *Wipe away the first drop of blood.* This removes any residual alcohol and any tissue fluid contamination.
13. Make blood smears if requested.
14. Collect the specimens and mix as needed. If an insufficient sample has been obtained because the blood flow stopped, repeat the puncture at a different site with all new equipment. *Order of collection* is as follows:
    1. Blood gases
    2. Slides, unless made from the EDTA microcollection tube
    3. EDTA microcollection tube
    4. Other microcollection tubes with anticoagulants (i.e., green or gray)
    5. Serum microcollection tubes
15. Elevate the puncture site and apply pressure until bleeding has stopped.
16. Label the specimens with the required information.
17. Perform appropriate specimen handling.
18. Thank the patient and parents.
19. Dispose of all puncture equipment and biohazardous materials.
20. Complete paperwork and indicate "skin puncture collection."
21. Deliver the properly labeled specimens to the laboratory.

PREPARATION OF BLOOD SMEARS

Blood smears can be made directly from capillary blood or from venous blood by wedge or coverslip method. In either method, the phlebotomist must remember to wipe away the first drop of blood and use the second drop to make the smear, if blood from a finger or heel stick is used (Chapter 15).

QUALITY ASSURANCE IN SPECIMEN COLLECTION

To ensure accurate patient test results, it is essential that the blood collection process, which includes specimen handling, be monitored. Patient diagnosis and medical care are based on the outcomes of these tests. The following areas should be monitored in specimen collection.

Technical Competence

The individual performing phlebotomy should be trained properly in all phases of blood collection. Certification is recommended. Continuing education is encouraged to keep current on all the changes in the field. Competency should be assessed and documented on an annual basis for each employee performing phlebotomy.

Collection Procedures

Periodic review of collection procedures is essential to maintaining quality specimens. Proper patient preparation and correct patient identification are crucial. The correct tube or specimen container must be used.

Anticoagulants and Preservatives

The manufacturer's instructions must be followed with regard to mixing of *all* tubes with additives to ensure accurate test results and that no microclots form in the tubes. All tubes should be checked for cracks and expiration dates. The additives should be observed for discoloration or cloudiness, which could indicate contamination. New lot numbers of tubes must be checked to verify draw and fill accuracy. Blood collected in the light-blue tube for coagulation must maintain a 9:1 ratio of blood to anticoagulant to ensure accurate results. Specimens must be stored and handled properly before testing.

Requirements for a Quality Specimen

Requirements for a quality specimen are as follows:
1. Proper patient identification
2. Proper patient preparation
3. Specimens collected in the correct order and labeled correctly
4. Correct anticoagulants and preservatives used
5. Specimens not hemolyzed
6. Fasting specimens collected in a timely manner
7. Timed specimens drawn at the correct time

Blood Collection Attempts

One individual should not attempt to obtain a specimen successfully from the patient more than twice. If two individuals have each tried twice, the physician should be contacted. There should be written procedures for what to do when the patient is unavailable for a blood draw or when the patient refuses.

Collection of Blood Cultures

Each facility should monitor its blood culture contamination rate and keep that rate less than 3% as recommended by the American Association of Microbiology.[9,10] Failure to do so could indicate a problem in the quality of all procedures being performed.

Quality Control and Preventive Maintenance on Specimen Collection Instruments

Thermometers used in refrigerators and freezers where specimens are stored should be calibrated annually, or only thermometers certified by the National Bureau of Standards should be used. If bleeding times are performed, the blood pressure cuff should be checked for leaks and accuracy. Centrifuges should be maintained following the manufacturer's instructions as to cleaning and timing verification.

BOX 3-2   Reasons for Specimen Rejection

- The test order requisition and the tube identification do not match.
- The tube is unlabeled, or the labeling, including patient identification number, is incorrect.
- The specimen is hemolyzed.
- The specimen was collected at the wrong time.
- The specimen was collected in the wrong tube.
- The specimen was clotted, and the test requires whole blood.
- The specimen was contaminated with intravenous fluid.
- The specimen is lipemic.*

*Lipemic specimens cannot be used for certain tests; however, the phlebotomist has no control over this aspect. Collection of a fasting specimen may be requested to try to reduce the potential for lipemia.

Reasons for Specimen Rejection

A laboratory procedure is only as good as the specimen provided. At times a specimen does not yield accurate results and must be rejected. Box 3-2 lists reasons for specimen rejection.

SPECIMEN HANDLING

Proper handling of specimens begins with the initiation of the test request and ends when the specimen is finally tested. Accurate test results depend on what happens to the specimen during that time. This pretesting period is referred to as the *preanalytical phase* of the total testing process.

Routine specimens must be adequately inverted to mix the additive and blood. Shaking can result in hemolysis of the specimen and lead to specimen rejection or inaccurate test results. Specimens should be transported in an upright position to ensure complete clot formation and reduce agitation, which could result in hemolysis.

Exposure to light can cause falsely decreased values in tests such as bilirubin, carotene, RBC folate, and urine porphyrins. For certain tests, the specimens need to be chilled, not frozen, and should be placed in an ice-water bath to slow down cellular metabolism. These tests include blood gases, ammonia, lactic acid, and certain coagulation tests. Other specimens must be kept warm to ensure accurate results. The cold agglutinin test is one such test; if the specimen is refrigerated before the serum is removed, the antibody is reabsorbed onto the RBCs.

Most specimens for routine testing should be delivered to the laboratory within 45 minutes to 1 hour of collection for processing. To ensure accurate results, less time is recommended for tests such as glucose, potassium, cortisol, and some enzymes. The CLSI recommends that the maximum time limit for separating serum and plasma from cells be 2 hours (120 minutes) from the time of collection.

LEGAL ISSUES IN PHLEBOTOMY

There are many daily practices in healthcare that, if performed without reasonable care and skill, could result in a lawsuit.

Phlebotomists have been and will continue to be held legally accountable for their actions in blood collection. Two areas of particular concern to phlebotomists are breach of patient confidentiality and patient misidentification. Unless there is a clinical need to know or a patient has given written permission, no one has a right to patient information. A patient will never be misidentified if correct procedures for specimen collection are followed. Phlebotomists often are called to testify in court in cases involving blood alcohol levels. The phlebotomist is asked about patient identification procedures and skin antisepsis. No antiseptics containing alcohol should be used for skin antisepsis. Soap and water may be used if no other cleaners are available.

To minimize the risk of legal action, the phlebotomist should do the following:
1. Follow up on all incident reports
2. Participate in continuing education
3. Become certified in the profession
4. Know the extent of liability coverage
5. Follow established procedures
6. Always exhibit professional, courteous behavior
7. Always obtain proper consent
8. Respect and honor the patient's bill of rights
9. Maintain proper documentation

CHAPTER at a GLANCE

- Laboratory test results are only as good as the specimen tested.
- Standard precautions must be followed in the collection of blood to prevent exposure to bloodborne pathogens.
- Physiologic factors affecting test results include posture, diurnal rhythm, exercise, stress, diet, and smoking.
- Although there are several manufacturers of evacuated tubes, all follow a universal color code in which the stopper color indicates the type of additive contained in the tube.
- The gauge numbers of needles relate inversely to bore size: the smaller the gauge number, the larger the bore.
- The three primary veins used for phlebotomy are the cephalic, basilic, and median cubital veins.

- CLSI guidelines should be followed for venipuncture and skin puncture.
- Common complications of blood collection include bruising, fainting, and hematoma.
- Each institution should establish a policy covering proper procedure when a blood specimen cannot be obtained.
- Following established procedures and documenting all incidents minimize the risk of liability when performing phlebotomy.

Now that you have completed this chapter, go back and read again the case studies at the beginning and respond to the questions presented.

REVIEW QUESTIONS

1. The vein of choice for performing a venipuncture is the:
   a. Basilic
   b. Cephalic
   c. Median cubital
   d. Femoral

2. The most important step in phlebotomy is:
   a. Cleansing the site
   b. Patient identification
   c. Proper needle length
   d. Using the correct evacuated tube

3. Failure to obtain blood by venipuncture may occur because of all of the following *except*:
   a. Incorrect needle positioning
   b. Tying the tourniquet too tightly
   c. Inadequate vacuum in the tube
   d. Collapsed vein

4. The needle should be inserted into the arm with the bevel facing:
   a. Down
   b. Up
   c. To either side
   d. Makes no difference

5. What is the proper angle of needle insertion for phlebotomy?
   a. 5 degrees
   b. 15 degrees
   c. 35 degrees
   d. 45 degrees

6. What is the recommended order of drawing when the evacuated tube system is used?
   a. Gel separator, nonadditive, coagulation, and blood culture
   b. Additive, nonadditive, gel separator, and blood culture
   c. Nonadditive, blood culture, coagulation, and other additives
   d. Blood culture, coagulation, nonadditive, and gel separator or other additives

7. Acceptable sites for skin puncture on infants are:
   a. Middle of the heel and tip of the big toe
   b. Lateral or medial surface of the bottom of the heel and plantar surface of the big toe
   c. Inside of the heel, close to the arch of the foot, and any of the toes, close to the tip
   d. Middle of the bottom of the heel and middle of the big toe

8. An anticoagulant is an additive placed in evacuated tubes to:
   a. Make the blood clot faster
   b. Dilute the blood before testing
   c. Prevent the blood from clotting
   d. Ensure the sterility of the tube

9. You are evaluating a new phlebotomist on his venipuncture performance. He performed the following steps in the order listed:
   - Asked the outpatient his name and date of birth and compared those with the requisition
   - Applied tourniquet and selected a prominent vein in the center of the antecubital fossa
   - Released the tourniquet, collected needed equipment, and assembled it all
   - Cleansed venipuncture site and allowed it to dry
   - Applied tourniquet, unsheathed needle, stretched the skin below the proposed venipuncture site, and inserted the needle into the selected vein within the cleansed area
   - Pushed tube onto the holder while holding the needle still, withdrew the tube from the holder, removed needle from the arm, and engaged the safety device
   - Immediately applied a gauze pad to the site and released the tourniquet
   - Applied pressure to the site while gently mixing the specimen
   - Verified that the patient was not bleeding and applied a bandage
   - Labeled tube appropriately

   What is your assessment or the phlebotomist's technique?
   a. All steps were performed acceptably in the proper order
   b. The phlebotomist should have labeled the tubes before collecting the specimen.
   c. The phlebotomist should have cleansed the arm while the tourniquet was in place.
   d. The phlebotomist should have removed the tourniquet before removing the needle from the arm.

10. A patient was to have a complete blood count (hematology) and a prothrombin time (coagulation) performed. The phlebotomist collected a lavender top and a green top tube. Are these specimens acceptable?
    a. Yes, EDTA is used for hematology, and heparin is used for coagulation.
    b. No, although EDTA is used for hematology, citrate, not heparin, is used for coagulation.
    c. No, although heparin is used for hematology, citrate, not EDTA, is used for coagulation.
    d. No, hematology requires citrate and coagulation requires a clot, so neither tube is acceptable.

11. Which step in the CLSI procedure for venipuncture is part of standard precautions?
    a. Wearing gloves
    b. Positively identifying the patient
    c. Cleansing the site for the venipuncture
    d. Bandaging the venipuncture site

REFERENCES

1. Rules and regulations: bloodborne pathogens. Fed Reg 1991;56:64175-64182.
2. McCall RE, Tankersley CM: Phlebotomy Essentials, 3rd ed. Philadelphia: Lippincott Williams & Wilkins, 2003.
3. Clinical and Laboratory Standards Institute (formerly NCCLS): Procedures for the Collection of Diagnostic Blood Specimens by Venipuncture, 5th ed (NCCLS Document H3-A5). Wayne, PA: NCCLS, 2003.
4. Garza D, Becan-McBride K: Phlebotomy Handbook, 7th ed. Upper Saddle River, NJ: Pearson Prentice Hall, Appleton & Lange, 2005.
5. Occupational Safety and Health Administration (OSHA), US Department of Labor: OSHA Safety and Health Information Bulletin (SHIB): Re-use of blood tube holders. October 15, 2003.
6. Vora S: Isoenzymes of human phosphofructokinase: biochemical and genetic aspects. In Rattazz MC, Scandalios JG, Whitt GS (eds): Isozymes: Current Topics in Biological and Medical Research, 2nd ed. New York: Alan R Liss, 1983:119-167.
7. Clinical and Laboratory Standards Institute (formerly NCCLS): Procedures and Devices for the Collection of Diagnostic Capillary Blood Specimens, 5th ed (NCCLS Document H4-A5). Wayne, PA: NCCLS, 2004.
8. Geller J (presenter): Effect of sample collection on laboratory test results (ASCP Spring 1992 Teleconference). American Society of Clinical Pathologists, Chicago, 1992.
9. Strand CL, Wajsbort RR, Sturmann K: Effect of iodophor vs. tincture skin preparation on blood culture contamination rate. JAMA 1999;269:1004-1006.
10. Schifman RB, Strand CL, Meier FA, et al: Blood culture contamination: a College of American Pathologists Q-Probes study involving 640 institutions and 497,134 specimens from adult patients. Arch Pathol Lab Med 1998;122:216-221.

4

Care and Use of the Microscope

Bernadette F. Rodak

OBJECTIVES

After completion of this chapter, the reader will be able to:

1. Given either a diagram or an actual brightfield light microscope, identify the component parts.
2. Explain the function of each component of a brightfield light microscope.
3. Define *achromatic, planachromatic, parfocal,* and *parcentric* as applied to lenses and microscopes; explain the advantages and disadvantages of each; and recognize examples of each from written descriptions of microscope use and effects.
4. Explain the purpose of adjusting microscope light using a procedure such as Koehler illumination.
5. List the steps, in proper order, to adjust a brightfield light microscope using Koehler illumination.
6. Given the procedure provided in the text and a brightfield light microscope with appropriate components, properly adjust a brightfield light microscope by use of Koehler illumination.
7. Describe the proper steps to view a stained blood film with a brightfield light microscope, including use of oil immersion lenses, and recognize deviations from these procedures.
8. Given the procedure provided in the text and a brightfield light microscope with appropriate lenses, focus a stained blood film, with dry and oil immersion objectives.
9. Describe proper care and cleaning of microscopes and recognize deviations from these procedures.
10. Given the procedures described in the text and a microscope, properly clean the microscope after routine use.
11. Given the magnification of lenses in a compound microscope, calculate the total magnification.
12. Given a problem with focusing a slide using a brightfield light microscope, suggest possible causes and their correction.
13. For each of the following, describe the components of the microscope that differ from a standard light microscope, what the differences accomplish, and the uses and benefits of each type in the clinical laboratory:
    Phase-contrast microscope
    Polarized light microscope
    Darkfield microscope

CASE STUDY

After studying the material in this chapter, the reader should be able to respond to the following case study:

A Wright-stained peripheral blood smear focuses under 10× and 40× but does not come into focus under the 100× oil objective. What steps should be taken to identify and correct this problem?

Microscopes available today reflect improvement in every aspect since the first microscope of Anton van Leeuwenhoek (1632-1723).[1] Advanced technology as applied to microscopy has resulted in computer-designed lens systems, sturdier stands, perfected condensers, and built-in illumination systems. Continued care and proper cleaning ensure the use of a powerful diagnostic instrument. The references listed at the end of this chapter address the physical laws of light and illumination as applied to microscopy.

PRINCIPLES OF MICROSCOPY

By the use of the compound microscope, an intermediate image of the illuminated specimen is formed by the objective

The author acknowledges the work of M. Ann Wallace, who authored this chapter in the second edition.

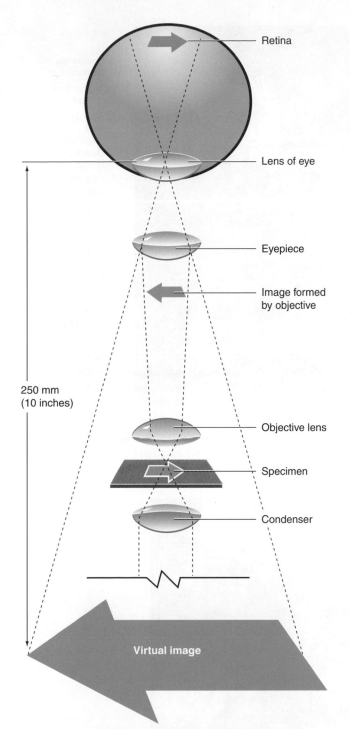

Figure 4-1 Compound microscope. (From Abramowitz M: The Microscope and Beyond, Vol 1. Lake Success, NY: Olympus Corp., 1985:2. Reprinted courtesy of Eastman Kodak Company, Rochester, N.Y.)

lens in the optical tube. This image is magnified and viewed through the eyepieces (Fig. 4-1).

An example of a *simple microscope* is a magnifying lens that enlarges objects that are difficult to view with the unaided eye. Movie theater projection units incorporate this system efficiently.

The *compound microscope* employs two separate lens systems, the product of which produces the final magnification. In standard microscopes, the brightfield illumination system, which passes light directly through the transparent specimen, is used.

COMPONENT PARTS AND FUNCTION OF EACH PART

Component parts and function of each part of the microscope are summarized as follows (Fig. 4-2):

1. The *eyepieces,* or *oculars,* usually are equipped with 10× lenses (degree of magnification is 10×). The lenses magnify the intermediate image formed by the objective lens in the optical tube; they also limit the area of visibility. Microscopes may have either one or two adjustable oculars. Both should be used correctly for optimal focus (see section on operating procedure). Eyepieces should not be interchanged with the eyepieces of other models of microscopes. The eyepieces in a pair are optically matched.

2. The *interpupillary control* is used to adjust the lateral separation of the eyepieces for each individual. When properly adjusted, the user should be able to focus both eyes comfortably on the specimen and visualize *one* clear image.

3. The *optical tube* connects the eyepieces with the objective lens. The intermediate image is formed in this component. The standard length is 160 mm, which, functionally, is the distance from the real image plane (eyepieces) to the objective lenses.

4. The *neck,* or *arm,* provides a structural site of attachment for the revolving nosepiece.

5. The *stand* is the main vertical support of the microscope. The stage assembly, together with the condenser and base, is supported by the stand.

6. The *revolving nosepiece* holds the objectives and allows for easy rotation from one objective lens to another. The working distance between the objectives and the slide varies with the make and model of the microscope.

7. There are usually three or four *objective lenses* (Fig. 4-3), each with a specific power of magnification. Engraved on the barrel of each objective lens is the power of magnification and numerical aperture (NA). The NA is related to the angle of light collected by the objective; in essence, it indicates the light-gathering ability of the objective lens. Functionally, the larger the NA, the greater the *resolution* or the ability to distinguish between fine details of two closely situated objects.

Four standard powers of magnification/NA used in the hematology laboratory are 10×/0.25 (low power), 40×/0.65 or 45×/0.66 (high power, dry), 50×/0.90 (oil immersion), and 100×/1.25 (oil immersion). The smaller the magnification, the larger the viewing field; the larger the magnification, the smaller the viewing field. Total magnification is calculated by multiplying the magnification of the eyepiece by the magnification of the objective lens; for example, 10× (eyepiece) multiplied by 100× (oil immersion) is 1000× total magnification.

Microscopes employed in the clinical laboratory are used with achromatic or planachromatic objective lenses,

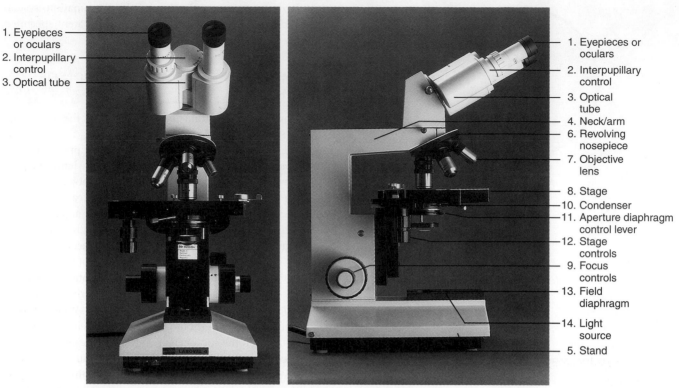

1. Eyepieces or oculars
2. Interpupillary control
3. Optical tube

1. Eyepieces or oculars
2. Interpupillary control
3. Optical tube
4. Neck/arm
6. Revolving nosepiece
7. Objective lens
8. Stage
10. Condenser
11. Aperture diaphragm control lever
12. Stage controls
9. Focus controls
13. Field diaphragm
14. Light source
5. Stand

Figure 4-2 Components of a microscope. (Courtesy of Commercial Imaging & Design, Inc., Royal Oak, Mich.)

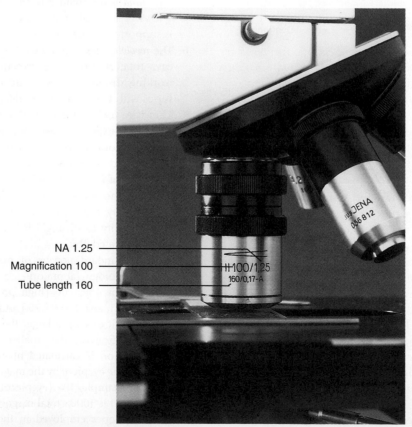

NA 1.25
Magnification 100
Tube length 160

Figure 4-3 Microscope objective lens. (Courtesy of Commercial Imaging & Design, Inc., Royal Oak, Mich.)

whose function is to correct for chromatic and spheric aberrations. *Chromatic aberrations* are caused by the spheric surface of the lens, which acts as a prism. As the various wavelengths pass through the lens, each focuses at a different point, causing concentric rings of color near the periphery of the lens. *Spheric aberrations* result as light waves travel through the varying thicknesses of the lens, blurring the image. The *achromatic objective lens* brings light of two colors into focus, partially correcting for the aberrations. When achromatic objective lenses are used, the center of the field is in focus, whereas the periphery is not. A *planachromatic lens,* which is more expensive, also corrects for curvature of the field, which results in a flat field with uniform focus.[2,3] Planachromatic lenses sometimes are referred to as "flat field" lenses. For critical microscopy, a *planapochromatic lens,* which brings light of three colors into focus and almost completely corrects for chromatic aberration, may be used. This objective lens is fairly expensive and rarely needed for routine laboratory use.

A set of lenses with corresponding focal points all in the same plane is said to be *parfocal.* As the nosepiece is rotated from one magnification to another, the specimen remains in focus, and only minimal fine adjustment is necessary.

8. The *stage* supports the prepared microscope slide to be reviewed. A spring assembly secures the slide to the stage.

9. The *focus controls* (or adjustments) can be incorporated into one knob or can be two separate controls. When a single knob is used, moving it in one direction engages the coarse control, while moving in the opposite direction engages the fine control. One gradation interval of turning is equivalent to 2 μm. Many microscopes are equipped with two separate adjustments: the coarse and the fine. The order of usage is the same: engage the coarse adjustment first and then fine-tune with the fine adjustment.

10. The *condenser,* consisting of several lenses in a unit, may be permanently mounted or vertically adjustable with a rack-and-pinion mechanism. It gathers, organizes, and directs the light through the specimen. Attached to and at the bottom of the condenser is the *aperture diaphragm,* an adjustable iris containing numerous leaves that control the angle and amount of the light sent through the specimen. The angle, also expressed as an NA, regulates the balance between *contrast* (ability to enhance parts within a cell) and *resolution* (ability to differentiate fine details of two closely situated objects). The best resolution is achieved when this iris is used fully open, but there is some sacrifice in image contrast. In practice, this iris is closed only enough to create a slight increase in image contrast. Closing it beyond that point leads to a loss of resolution.

Some microscopes are equipped with a swing-out lens immediately above or below the main condenser lens. This lens is used to permit a wider field of illumination when the NA of the objective lens is less than 0.25 (e.g., the 4×/0.12 objective lens).[4] If the swing-out lens is *above* the main condenser, it should be *out* for use with the 4× objective lens and *in* for lenses of magnification 10× and greater. If it is *below* the condenser, it should be *in* for use with the 4× objective lens and *out* for lenses of magnification 10× and greater.

The stage and condenser (Fig. 4-4) consist of (1) a control lever for a swing-out lens, (2) an aperture diaphragm control lever, (3) a vertical adjustment of the condenser, and (4) a condenser diaphragm.

11. The *control lever* swings the condenser top lens out of position.

12. The *stage controls* located under the stage move it along an *x* or a *y* axis.

13. The *field diaphragm* is located below the condenser within the base. When it is open, it allows a maximal-size circle of light to illuminate the slide. An almost closed diaphragm, when low power is used, assists in centering the condenser apparatus by the use of two centering screws. Some microscopes have permanently centered condensers, whereas in others the screws are used for this function. The glass on top of the field diaphragm protects the diaphragm from dust and mechanical damage.

14. Microscopes depend on electricity as the primary source for illumination power. There are two types of *brightfield illumination:* (1) critical illumination, in which the light source is focused at the specimen, resulting in increased but uneven brightness, and (2) the Koehler (or Köhler) system, in which the light source is focused at the condenser aperture diaphragm. The end result of Koehler illumination is a field of evenly distributed brightness across the specimen. Tungsten-halogen light bulbs are used most frequently as the illumination source. They consist of a tungsten filament enclosed in a small quartz bulb that is filled with a halogen gas. Tungsten possesses a high melting point and gives off bright yellowish light. A blue (daylight) filter should be used to eliminate the yellow color emitted by tungsten.[5] The light control knob turns on the light and should be used to regulate the intensity of the light needed to visualize the specimen. Although the field diaphragm also may be used to reduce light intensity, the aperture diaphragm should never be used for this purpose because closing it reduces resolving power.[6]

OPERATING PROCEDURE WITH KOEHLER ILLUMINATION

This procedure applies to microscopes with a nonfixed condenser.[5] The following steps should be included at the start of each laboratory session using the microscope:

1. Connect the microscope to the power supply.
2. Turn on the light source.
3. Open all diaphragms.
4. Revolve the nosepiece until the 10× objective lens is directly above the stage.
5. Adjust the interpupillary control so that looking through both oculars yields one clear image.
6. Place a stained blood film on the stage and focus on it, using the fixed ocular, while covering the other eye. (Do

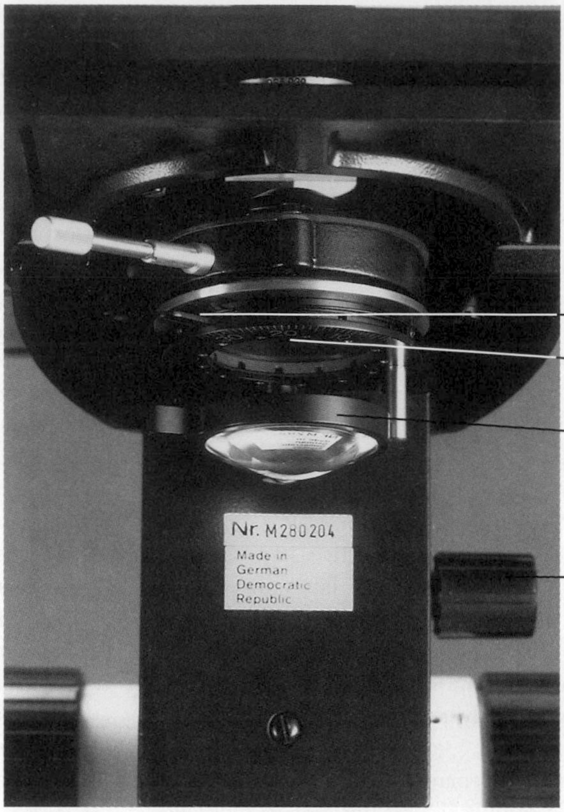

Figure 4-4 Condenser. (Courtesy of Commercial Imaging & Design, Inc., Royal Oak, Mich.)

2. Aperture diaphragm control lever
4. Condenser diaphragm
1. Swing-out lens
3. Vertical adjustment of condenser

not simply close the other eye because this would necessitate adjustment of the pupil when you focus with the other ocular.)

7. Using the adjustable ocular and covering the opposite eye, focus on the specimen. Start with the eyepiece all the way out, and adjust inward. If using two adjustable oculars, focus each individually.
8. Raise the condenser to its upper limit.
9. Focus the field so that the cells become sharp and clear. Concentrate on one cell and place it in the center of the field.
10. Close the field (lower) diaphragm. Look through the eyepieces. A small circle of light should be seen. If the light is not in the center of the field, center it by using the two centering screws located on the condenser. This step is essential because an off-center condenser would result in uneven distribution of light. Adjust the vertical height of the condenser so that you see a sharp image of the field diaphragm, ringed by a magenta halo. If the substage condenser is raised too much, the halo is orange; if it is lowered too far, the halo is blue.
11. Reopen the field diaphragm until the image is nearly at the edge of the field, and fine-tune the centering process.
12. Open the diaphragm slightly until the image just disappears.
13. Remove one ocular and, while looking through the microscope (without the ocular), close the condenser diaphragm completely. Reopen the condenser diaphragm until the leaves just disappear from view. Replace the ocular.
14. Rotate the nosepiece until the 40× objective lens is above the slide. Adjust the focus (which should be minimal) and find the cell that you had centered. If it is slightly off

center, center it again with the stage *x-y* control. Note the greater amount of detail that you can see.
15. Move the 40× objective out of place. Place a drop of immersion oil on top of the slide. Rotate the nosepiece until the 100× objective lens is directly above the slide. Avoid moving a non-oil objective through the drop of oil. Adjust the focus (which should be minimal) and observe the detail of the cell: the nucleus and its chromatin pattern; the cytoplasm and its color and texture. The objective lens should dip into the oil slightly.

Considerations

1. When revolving the nosepiece from one power to another, rotate it in such a direction that the 10× and 40× objective lenses never come into contact with the oil on a slide.
2. *Parcentric* refers to the ability to center a cell in question in the microscopic field, rotating from one magnification power to another while retaining the cell close to the center of the viewing field. Recentering the cell at each step is minimal. Most laboratory microscopes have this feature.
3. In general, when the 10× or 40× objective lenses are used, the light intensity should be low. When the 50× or 100× objective lenses are used, increase the intensity of light by using *only* the light control knob or by varying neutral density filters. Neutral density filters are used to reduce the amplitude of light and are available in a variety of densities.[5,6]
4. Do not change the position of the condenser or the aperture lever to regulate light intensity. The condenser should always be in its upward position. The aperture lever is used only to achieve contrast of the features of the specimen being viewed.

IMMERSION OIL AND TYPES

Immersion oil is required when the 100× objective lens is used to increase the *refractive index*. The refractive index is the speed at which light travels in air divided by the speed at which light travels through a substance. This oil, which has the same properties as glass, allows the objective lens to collect light from a wide NA, providing high resolution of detail.

Three types of immersion oil, differing in viscosity, are employed in the clinical laboratory:

1. *Type A* has very low viscosity and is used in fluorescence and darkfield studies.
2. *Type B* has high viscosity and is used in brightfield and standard clinical microscopy. In hematology, this oil is routinely used.
3. *Type C* has very high viscosity and is used with inclined microscopes with long-focus objective lenses and wide condenser gaps.

Bubbles in the oil tend to act as prisms and subsequently reduce resolution. Bubbles may be created when oil is applied to the slide. They are caused more often by lowering of the objective immediately into the oil. Sweeping the objective from right to left in the oil eliminates bubbles.[2]

CARE OF THE MICROSCOPE

Care of the microscope involves the following details:

1. When not in use, the microscope always should be covered or protected in a cabinet.
2. Before use, inspect the component parts. If dust is found, use an air syringe, a camelhair brush, or a soft nonlint cloth to remove it. Lens paper used directly on a dirty lens without removal of the dust first may scratch the lens.
3. Avoid placing fingers on the lens surface. Fingerprints affect the contrast and resolution of the image.
4. Use solvent sparingly. The use of xylene is discouraged because it contains a carcinogen component (benzene). Xylene is also a poor cleaning agent, leaving an oily film on the lens. Lens cleaner or 70% isopropyl alcohol employed sparingly on a cotton applicator stick can be used to clean the objective lenses. Alcohol should be kept away from the periphery of the lenses because alcohol can dissolve the cement and seep into the back side of the lens.
5. When fresh oil is added to residual oil on the 100× objective lens, there may be loss of contrast. Clean off all residual oil first.
6. Do not use water to clean lenses. Your condensed breath on the lens surface may be useful in cleaning slightly soiled lenses.
7. When transporting the microscope, place one hand under the base as support and one hand firmly around the arm.

BASIC TROUBLESHOOTING

Most common problems are related to inability to focus. After the operator has ensured that he or she is not trying to obtain a "flat field" using an objective lens that is not planachromatic, the following checklist aids in identifying the problem:

- Oculars
  Clean?
  Securely assembled?
- Objective lens
  Screwed in tightly?
  Dry objective free of oil?
- Condenser
  Adjusted to proper height?
  Free of oil?
- Slide
  Correct side up?
- Coverslip
  Correct side of smear?
  Only one coverslip on slide?
  Free of mounting media?
- Light source
  Fingerprints on bulb?
  Bulb need changing?
  Light source aligned correctly?

MICROLOCATOR SLIDE

Some microscope stages include locator values for *x* and *y* on the stage, allowing the operator to take coordinates of a cell so that it can be located easily for review. When locator values are not incorporated into the stage, a microlocator slide or microslide field finder can be used.

The field finder slide is a commercially manufactured standard glass slide with a precise etched coordinate grid running along the *x* and *y* axes. Figure 4-5 shows one example of such a slide.

1. When a microscopist locates a cell of interest on a prepared slide, the cell should be centered under high dry or oil and then under the 10× objective lens. *Note whether the feathered edge of the blood film faces right or left.*
2. Carefully remove the slide from the spring assembly, taking care not to disturb the position of the stage.
3. Place the microlocator slide onto the stage.

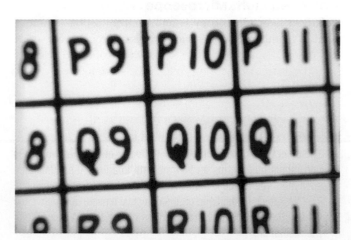

Figure 4-5 Microlocator slide.

4. View the microlocator through the eyepiece, and record the letter-number combination.

5. To relocate the cell, place the microlocator onto the stage and place the recorded letter-number combination in the center of the stage.

6. Remove the locator slide carefully and replace it with the initial blood smear. The cell of interest should be in the field.

OTHER MICROSCOPES USED IN THE CLINICAL LABORATORY

Phase-Contrast Microscope

The ability to view a stained specimen by the use of brightfield microscopy is affected by two features: (1) the ability of the specimen to absorb the light impacting it and (2) the degree to which light waves traveling through the specimen remain in phase (⟨⟨⟨⟩⟩⟩).

Specimens that are transparent or colorless, such as unstained cells, are not clearly visualized with brightfield microscopy. Phase-contrast microscopy, through the installation of an *annular diaphragm* placed in the condenser, together with a *phase-shifting element*, creates excellent contrast of a cell against its surrounding background.

The principle of phase contrast involves the index of refraction and thickness of a specimen, which produce differences in the optical path. Light passing through a transparent specimen travels slightly slower than the light that is unobstructed. The difference is so small that it is not noticeable to the viewer. When a transparent phase plate is placed into the microscope, however, the change in phase can be increased to half a wavelength, making the otherwise transparent objective visible (⟨⟨⟨⟩⟩⟩). This phase difference produces variation in light intensity from bright to dark, creating contrast in the image. Often the objects appear to have "haloes" surrounding them.

In hematology, phase-contrast microscopy is employed in counting platelets, which are difficult to visualize and count using brightfield microscopy. It also can be used to view formed elements in unstained urine sediments.

Polarized Light Microscope

Polarized light microscopy is another contrasting technique used to identify substances such as crystals in urine and other body fluids (Chapter 17). With brightfield microscopy, light vibrates in all directions. If a polarizer (filter) is placed in the light path, the light vibrates in only one direction or plane, creating polarized light. To convert a brightfield microscope to a polarizing one, two filters are needed. One filter (the polarizer) is placed below the condenser and allows only light vibrating in the east-west direction perpendicular to the light path to pass through the specimen. The second filter (the analyzer) is placed between the objective and the eyepiece and allows only light vibrating in a north-south direction to pass to the eyepiece. When these two filters have their transmission axes oriented at right angles, no light can pass through the pair to the eyepiece. When polarized light (vibrating in east-west direction) passes through an optically active substance, however, such as a monosodium urate crystal, the light is refracted into two beams, one vibrating in the original direction (east-west) and one vibrating in a plane 90 degrees to it (i.e., north-south). The refracted light, vibrating in the north-south direction, can pass through the second filter (the analyzer) and is visible at the eyepiece. The magnified crystal appears white against a black background. If a first-order red compensator filter also is placed in the light path below the stage, the background becomes pink-red, and the crystal appears yellow or blue depending on its physical orientation relative to the incident light path (east-west). Some crystals can be specifically identified based on their unique birefringent (doubly refractive) characteristics when using polarizing microscopy (see Figs. 17-25 and 17-26).

Darkfield Microscope

Darkfield microscopy is a contrasting technique that employs a special condenser. The condenser sends light up toward the specimen in a hollow cone. Because of the high angle of this cone, none of the illuminating rays enter the objective lens. Without the specimen in place, the field would appear black because of the absence of light. When the specimen is in place and if fine detail exists in the specimen, light is diffracted in all directions. This diffracted light is picked up by the objective lens and appears as bright detail on a black background. Darkfield microscopy is helpful in microbiology in the identification of spirochetes. When combined with the use of fluorochrome dyes, darkfield fluorescence microscopy can be used to identify lymphocyte subsets.

CHAPTER at a GLANCE

- The compound microscope, through the use of an objective lens in the optical tube, forms an intermediate image of the illuminated specimen. The image is magnified and viewed through the oculars.
- The NA, which is engraved on the objective lenses, designates the light-gathering ability of the lens. The higher the NA, the greater the resolution.

- Achromatic lenses maintain the center of the field in focus, whereas planachromatic lenses also correct for the curvature of a field, providing uniform focus.
- The condenser gathers and directs the light across a specimen.
- Koehler illumination establishes a field of evenly distributed brightness across the specimen.

CHAPTER at a GLANCE—cont'd

- Microscopes should be carefully handled and maintained. Solvents should not be used to clean lenses; lens cleaner or 70% isopropyl alcohol is recommended.
- Phase-contrast microscopy uses the effect of index refraction and thickness of specimen; these two features affect light waves by retarding a fraction of the wavelength, resulting in a difference in phase. This allows transparent or colorless objects to become visible.
- Polarizing microscopes use two polarizing lenses to cancel the light passing through the sample. If the object is able to polarize light, as in some crystals, the light passing through rotates and becomes visible.

- Darkfield microscopes use a high angle from the condenser to the sample, directing the light at an angle away from the objective lens. If the sample has fine detail, it causes the light to bend back toward the objective, allowing it to be viewed against an otherwise dark background.

Now that you have completed this chapter, go back and read again the case study at the beginning and respond to the question presented.

REVIEW QUESTIONS

1. Use of which of the following objective lenses causes the center of the microscope field to be in focus, while the periphery is blurred?
   a. Planachromatic
   b. Achromatic
   c. Planapochromatic
   d. Flat field

2. Which of the following gathers, organizes, and directs light through the specimen?
   a. Ocular
   b. Objective lens
   c. Condenser
   d. Optical tube

3. After focusing a specimen by using the 40× objective, the laboratory professional switches to a 10× objective. The specimen remains in focus at 10×. Microscopes with this characteristic are described as:
   a. Parfocal
   b. Parcentric
   c. Compensated
   d. Parachromatic

4. The objective with the greatest degree of color correction is the:
   a. Achromatic
   b. Planapochromatic
   c. Bichromatic
   d. Planachromatic

5. The total magnification obtained when a 10× ocular and a 10× objective lens is used is:
   a. 1×
   b. 10×
   c. 100×
   d. 1000×

6. After a microscope has been adjusted for Koehler illumination, light intensity should *never* be regulated by using the:
   a. Rheostat
   b. Neutral density filter
   c. Koehler magnifier
   d. Condenser

7. The recommended cleaner for removing oil from objectives is:
   a. 70% alcohol or lens cleaner
   b. Xylene
   c. Water
   d. Benzene

8. Which of the following types of microscopes is valuable in the identification of crystals that are able to rotate light?
   a. Compound brightfield
   b. Darkfield
   c. Polarizing
   d. Phase-contrast

9. A laboratory science student has been reviewing a hematology slide using the 10× objective to find a suitable portion of the slide for examination. He moves the 10× objective out of place, places a drop of oil on the slide, rotates the nosepiece so that the 40× objective passes through the viewing position, and continues to rotate the 100× oil objective into viewing position. This practice should be corrected in which way?
   a. The stage of a parfocal microscope should be lowered before the objectives are rotated.
   b. The 100× oil objective should be in place for viewing before the oil is added.
   c. The drop of oil should be in place and the 100× objective lowered into the oil, rather than having the objective swing into the drop.
   d. The objectives should be rotated in the opposite direction so that the 40× objective does not risk entering the oil.

10. Darkfield microscopes create the dark field by:
    a. Using two filters that cancel each other out, one above and the other below the condenser
    b. Angling the light at the sample so that it misses the objective unless something in the sample bends it backward
    c. Closing the condenser diaphragm entirely, limiting light to just a tiny ray in the center of the otherwise dark field
    d. Using a light source above the sample and collecting light reflected from the sample, rather than transmitted through the sample, so that when there is no sample in place, the field is dark

REFERENCES

1. Asimov I: Understanding Physics: Light, Magnetism, and Electricity. London: George Allen & Unwin, 1966.
2. Oldham AD: Care and use of the microscope. In Wentworth BB (ed): Diagnostic Procedures for Mycotic and Parasitic Infections, 7th ed. Washington, DC: American Public Health Association, 1988:567-597.
3. Benford JR: The Theory of the Microscope, 4th ed. Rochester, NY: Bausch & Lomb, 1965.
4. Leitz E: Leitz Teaching and Routine Microscope-Operating Instructions. Wetzlar, Germany: E. Leitz, undated.
5. Bradbury P: Introduction to Microscopy. Richmond, British Columbia, Canada: Steveston Scientific Publications, 1990.
6. Murphy DB: Fundamentals of Light Microscopy and Electronic Imaging. New York: Wiley-Liss, 2001.

ADDITIONAL RESOURCES

http://www.olympusmicro.com/primer/index.html.
Brunzel NA: Microscopy. In: Fundamentals of Urine and Body Fluid Analysis, 2nd ed. Philadelphia: Saunders, 2004:1-23.

Quality Assurance

5

Sarah Burns

OUTLINE

OBJECTIVES

After completion of this chapter, the reader will be able to:

1. Define terms commonly used in quality control and recognize examples of each when provided with data and descriptions of test performance.
2. Calculate mean, standard deviation, coefficient of variation, and confidence intervals when given necessary data.
3. Describe the use of the statistics involved in describing populations and interpret their results.
4. Describe how reference ranges are derived, and calculate the same when given necessary data.
5. Select calculations to measure the clinical efficacy of a test method, describe their use, and interpret results.
6. Distinguish between types of errors in test systems or methods when given data on test performance.
7. Discuss and identify possible sources of error in testing processes when given a description of a situation or the data from test performance.
8. Differentiate among internal, external, and equivalent quality control.
9. Discuss several methods used to monitor internal quality control.
10. Interpret results of internal quality control monitors and suggest follow-up action.
11. Discuss the importance of external quality control procedures.
12. Discuss the role of continuing education in maintaining a quality laboratory.
13. Briefly discuss the role that quality control plays in a total quality assurance program.

CASE STUDIES

After studying the material in this chapter, the reader should be able to respond to the following case study:

On a multichannel automated analyzer, controls are performed every 8 hours. On a 4:00 P.M. run, all levels of hemoglobin control read 2 g/dL more than the upper limit of the acceptable range. The technologist checks the last 10 patient results and notices that the delta checks on most of the hemoglobin values are 1.8 to 2.2 g/dL more than previously reported.

1. What do you call the type of error detected in this case?
2. Can you continue to run patient specimens as long as you subtract 2 g/dL from the results?
3. What should you investigate when troubleshooting this problem?

In the healthcare arena today, the emphasis is on the implementation of quality assurance procedures to monitor the delivery of healthcare in the presence of rapidly rising healthcare costs. Congress passed the Clinical Laboratory Improvement Amendments (CLIA) in 1988 to ensure the accuracy and reliability of clinical laboratory test results. The Joint Commission on Accreditation of Healthcare Organizations (JCAHO) focuses on the comprehensiveness of quality assurance programs to evaluate the quality of medical care delivered by all providers. This chapter is limited to quality assurance and quality control procedures in the clinical laboratory and in particular the clinical hematology laboratory. Readers who desire more detailed explanations of quality control may find them at the Clinical and Laboratory Standards Institute website at http://www.clsi.org/.

Quality assurance is the coordinated effort to organize all the various activities in the laboratory to provide the best possible service to the patient and to the physician. It is not a single activity; rather, it includes controlling and monitoring the competence of staff, quality of materials, methods, reagents, instruments, reporting of test results, patient and physician satisfaction, and the financial costs attributable to the laboratory. *Quality control* involves procedures for monitoring and evaluating the characteristics of the testing system. Quality control is exercised by analyzing control samples along with the patient samples and applying appropriate statistical methods to the results to establish accuracy and precision, which are benchmarks for determining acceptability of results. It also involves taking any necessary corrective actions to bring the results into conformance. Quality control is an important part of the quality assurance program.

DEFINITIONS

The following key terms are commonly used in the monitoring of quality control in the clinical laboratory.

Control

A *control* is a material that has a predetermined assay value and typically the same matrix as the patient samples. It is tested alongside patient specimens to monitor the performance of the assay.

Primary Standard

A *primary standard* is a reference material that is used to calibrate an instrument or prepare standard curves for manual assays. It is of fixed and known composition and capable of being prepared in essentially pure form. The matrix may or may not be the same as the patient samples. The term also is used for any certified reference material that is generally accepted or officially recognized as the unique standard for the assay, regardless of its level of purity. In hematology, the cyanmethemoglobin standard is one such standard.

Secondary Standard

A *secondary standard* is a reference material in which the analyte concentration has been ascertained by reference to a primary standard and can be used as a primary standard.

Calibrator

In hematology, only the Hb assay is based on a standard. All other hematology parameters count or analyze cells by relying on calibrators. The same is true of clot-based coagulation tests that measure enzyme activity. A calibrator is a preserved human or surrogate cell suspension whose hematology parameters have been determined by multiple reference laboratories and monitored daily by the distributor.

Accuracy

Accuracy describes the closeness of a measurement to the true or actual value.

Precision

Precision describes the closeness of results obtained from repeated analysis of the same sample. The precision of a test, or its *reproducibility,* may be expressed as standard deviation or the coefficient of variation. A method may yield results that are precise but not accurate. Results that are accurate and precise are desirable (Fig. 5-1).

Delta Checks

A *delta check* involves comparing the result from the analysis of a sample with the result from the previous sample for the same analyte for the same patient. The name derives from the use of the Greek *delta* as a symbol for change. Because patient values are expected to be consistent unless there is a treatment affecting the test, a delta check assesses change. A test result that fails a delta check not due to a significant change in the patient's condition may indicate an analytical error or a mislabeled sample. Test results from a sample with a failed delta check should not be reported until an investigation has occurred to determine the cause of the failure. Analytes that have little intraindividual variation should be used to monitor delta checks. In the hematology laboratory, these include mean cell volume, mean platelet volume, and red blood cell (RBC) distribution width (RDW; see Chapter 14). Evaluating the precision or accuracy of a method can be done this way by

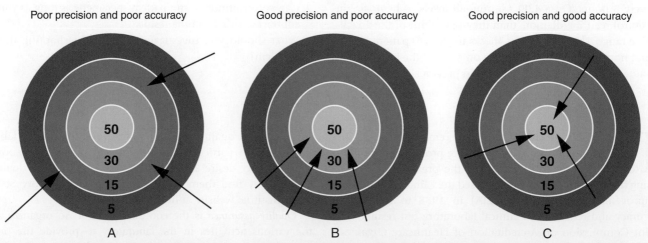

Figure 5-1 Examples of precision and accuracy. In these examples, the target value is 50. Arrows designate individual results. **A,** Poor precision and poor accuracy because the points are neither close to each other nor close to the target value. **B,** Good precision because all values are close to each other, but poor accuracy because they miss the target value. **C,** Good precision and good accuracy because all values are close to each other and hit the target value.

defining delta check limits in the laboratory information system. The laboratory information system flags results when the limit is exceeded.

Reliability

Reliability refers to the extent to which a method is able to maintain accuracy and precision over time. All aspects of a testing system (instrument, method, reagents, and ancillary quality control materials) must be monitored to ensure a high degree of reliability.

Reference Interval

The term *reference interval,* or reference range, describes the range of values for an analyte in healthy individuals. This is sometimes called the "normal range"; however, there is always some vagueness about what "normal" or healthy is, and so the term *reference interval* is more appropriate. A reference population is a group of individuals from whom the data were obtained to establish the reference interval. Each laboratory must define its own reference intervals for the test method or instrument that it uses and for the population that it serves. Reference intervals should be determined for men, women, and children. Within the pediatric group, reference values may change dramatically over short age intervals, and it is appropriate to determine reference intervals for newborns, infants, and subsequent pediatric age groups. This is particularly true for hematology values, as is evident in the reference interval tables on the inside cover of this book. The changes in hematology parameters warrant different reference intervals within the first days and weeks after birth (Chapter 38).

STATISTICAL DESCRIPTION OF POPULATIONS

A single laboratory measurement is inexact. If a single specimen is repeatedly analyzed under identical conditions, a series of nonidentical results is obtained. These nonidentical values arise from the random variation that is present in all measured parameters. When numerous results are obtained from the repeated analysis, their frequency distribution approximates a normal, or *gaussian,* distribution (Fig. 5-2). Distribution of many medical measurements in populations approximates the gaussian curve. The value at the center of a gaussian distribution is the *mean* ($\bar{x}$), or average. The mean is a measure of central tendency and is calculated by dividing the sum of all results by the number of results.

The distribution of data about the mean is expressed as the *standard deviation* (*s* or SD), which is a statistical measurement of the imprecision or variability among analytical results. In general, the standard deviation increases as results become more variable around the mean. The absolute value of the standard deviation can be misleading, however. An *s* of 10 for one population is larger than an *s* of 5 for another population if the mean of the two populations is the same. If the means are different, the conclusion of greater variability of an *s* of 10 may not be correct.

The *coefficient of variation* (CV) can be used to allow comparisons of the precision of assays with different means. It is a unitless number that is calculated as $s/\bar{x}$, although more often the CV is calculated as $100(s/\bar{x})$ and expressed as a percentage. The smaller the CV value, the more precise the analytical method. Table 5-1 presents examples of the calculations for the terms just described.[1]

According to Figure 5-2, 68.26% of the results are located within the interval bounded by the $x \pm 1.0s$ line, 95.46% are within the $\bar{x} \pm 2.0s$ lines, and 99.73% are within the $\bar{x} \pm 3.0s$ lines. These intervals represent specific *confidence intervals.* The $\bar{x} \pm 2.0s$ interval is the 95.5% confidence interval, which means there is a 95.5% probability that any given result would fall within the $\bar{x} \pm 2.0s$ line. If a population has a gaussian distribution, only the mean and standard deviation are necessary to describe the population. Virtually all quality control procedures in the clinical laboratory assume a gaussian distribution. Causes of deviation from normal include outliers, shifts, nonrandom variation, and instability of the analytical method, some of which are described later in this chapter.

REFERENCE INTERVAL DETERMINATION

It may be acceptable to use a previously established reference interval for an analyte if the study population and methodology used in the reference interval determination are the same or comparable to that of the laboratory.[2] In most instances, however, it is necessary for a laboratory to establish the

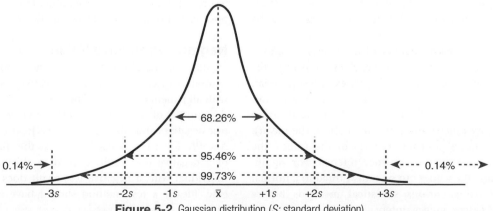

Figure 5-2 Gaussian distribution (*S;* standard deviation).

TABLE 5-1 Example of Selected Calculations Used in Quality Control

Hemoglobin Value (g/dL)	$x - \bar{x}$	$(x - \bar{x})^2$
12.2	0.1	0.01
12.3	0	0.01
12.5	0.2	0.04
12.5	0.2	0.04
11.9	−0.4	0.16
12.5	0.2	0.04
12.8	0.5	0.25
12.3	0	0.01
11.8	−0.5	0.25
12.2	0.1	0.01
12.7	0.4	0.16
12.4	0.1	0.01
11.9	−0.4	0.16
12.2	−0.1	0.01

Confidence Intervals

$1s$ (65% of values) = 12-12.6
$2s$ (95% of values) = 11.7-12.9
$3s$ (99% of values) = 11.4-13.2

Mean $(\bar{x}) = \dfrac{\Sigma x}{n}$, where Σx = sum of values and n = number of values; $\bar{x} = \dfrac{172.2}{14}$

= 12.3.

Standard deviation $(s) = \sqrt{\dfrac{+\, \Sigma(x - \bar{x})^2}{n - 1}}$; $s = \sqrt{\dfrac{1.14}{13}} = 0.3$. (Use n if number of observations is ≥ 30, $n - 1$ if <30.)

Coefficient of variation (CV) $= 100\left(\dfrac{s}{\bar{x}}\right)$; CV $= 100\left(\dfrac{0.3}{12.3}\right) = 2.4\%$.

---

reference interval by performing a reference value study. A *reference sample group* (the individuals from the reference population used to determine the reference interval) must be carefully selected to ensure that they are healthy, as defined by a set of predetermined criteria. Specimens from each subject are collected, managed, and treated as patient specimens. Disagreement exists concerning the number of individuals needed for a reference value study. A minimum of 120 individuals is suggested to be included in the reference sample group[2]; however, statistical calculations may be used to determine the necessary number of individuals. The sexes should be equally represented.

After samples from each member of the reference sample group have been analyzed, the results are assessed using statistical methods. If the values, when plotted, exhibit a gaussian distribution, the mean ± 2 standard deviations may be calculated to determine the reference interval. If the data are slightly skewed (asymmetrically distributed about the mean), by excluding the upper and lower 2.5% of the values, the remaining 95% represent the reference interval. For significantly skewed data, the values can be transformed to a normal distribution by using various statistical methods before selecting the 95% confidence interval. For instance, many biological analytes have a log-normal distribution in which the curve is skewed to the right, for example RBCs and reticulocytes. To establish a Gaussian distribution, the data are first transformed to logs and the reference interval based on the logs. Several additional transformations can be found in the Clinical and Laboratory Standards Institute (formerly the National Committee of Clinical Laboratory Standards) document "How to Define and Determine Reference Intervals in the Clinical Laboratory."[2]

CLINICAL EFFICACY MEASUREMENTS

Diagnostic Sensitivity

Diagnostic sensitivity is the proportion of patients with the disease who have a positive test result. It is defined by the number of true positives (TP) divided by the sum of true positives and false negatives (FN), multiplied by 100: Sensitivity = (TP ÷ [TP + FN]) × 100. A diagnostically sensitive test should be used when a normal result serves to rule out a suspected disease. A distinction must be made between diagnostic sensitivity and analytical sensitivity. *Analytical sensitivity* describes the lowest amount of a substance that can be detected accurately by a test method.

Diagnostic Specificity

Diagnostic specificity is the proportion of patients who are identified correctly by the test as not having the disease. It is defined by the number of true negatives (TN) divided by the sum of true negatives and false positives (FP), multiplied by 100: Specificity = (TN ÷ [TN + FP]) × 100. A diagnostically specific test should be used when an abnormal result serves to confirm the presence of a disease. A distinction must be made here, too, between diagnostic specificity and analytical specificity. *Analytical specificity* describes how well a test method can detect a particular substance rather than similar ones.

Positive Predictive Value

Positive predictive value (PPV) is the proportion of patients with a disease who have a positive test result compared with all patients who have a positive test result. It is defined as the number of true positives (TP) divided by the sum of the true positives and false positives (FP): PPV = TP ÷ (TP + FP). A PPV for a test is used to assess the diagnostic reliability of a positive test result. It predicts the probability that an individual with a positive test result actually has the disease.

Negative Predictive Value

Negative predictive value (NPV) is the proportion of patients without a disease who have a negative test result compared with all patients who have a negative test result. It is defined as the number of true negatives (TN) divided by the sum of the true negatives and false negatives (FN): NPV = TN ÷ (TN + FN). An NPV for a test is used to assess the diagnostic reliability of a negative test result. It predicts the probability that an individual with a negative test result does not have the disease. Ideally a test method should have a high PPV and a high NPV.

TYPES OF ANALYTICAL ERRORS

Errors can occur at any stage of the testing process: before analysis (preanalytical), during analysis (analytical), and after analysis (postanalytical).

Systematic Errors

Systematic errors are errors within the test system or method. These may be caused by incorrect calibration procedures, malfunctioning components, or failure of some part of the testing process to perform accurately or precisely. This type of error affects the accuracy of a test method. Systematic errors are subdivided further into constant and proportional systematic errors. *Constant systematic errors* are errors in the test system in which the magnitude of an error remains constant throughout the range of the test measurement. This situation is also called a *constant bias* (e.g., all hemoglobin values read 2 g/dL higher than the true value). *Proportional systematic errors* are errors in the test system in which the magnitude of an error increases with the concentration of the substance being measured (e.g., at hemoglobin level of 8 g/dL, the error is 1 g; at 9 g/dL, it is 1.5 g/dL; at 10 g/dL, it is 2).

Random Errors

Random errors are mistakes that occur without prediction or regularity. These errors may be caused by instability of the instrument, change in temperature, or operator variability. This type of error affects the precision and accuracy of a test method.

SOURCES OF ERRORS

A laboratory test result is expected to reflect the concentration of analyte in the patient sample; however, errors may occur that can have an effect on the accuracy of the test result. In addition to errors that occur during analysis (systematic and random error), functions outside of the analytical activities (preanalytical and postanalytical) may have an effect on test results. All aspects of the testing process must be controlled to minimize errors because any error may have a direct effect on the well-being of the patient.

Preanalytical Errors

Preanalytical variables are those that occur before actual analysis takes place, yet still may affect test results. Some errors that may occur during preanalytical activities include misinterpreted physician test orders, patient misidentification, incorrect patient preparation for sample collection, incorrect sampling technique, improper collection container, and improper method of sample transport or handling.

Postanalytical Errors

Postanalytical variables are those that affect the handling of the test result after the analysis has taken place. Some errors that may occur during the postanalytical activities include incorrect result entry, failure to notify the physician of critical results, reports placed in the wrong patient chart, and miscommunication of results telephoned to nursing units or physicians.

INTERNAL QUALITY CONTROL

Internal quality control involves the analysis of control samples along with patients' samples and statistical evaluation of the results to determine the acceptability of the analytical run. In internal quality control, a test method's precision and analytical bias are monitored. A control sample is a specially prepared specimen inserted into the testing process that has the same matrix as patient samples and is treated as if it were a patient sample. The assayed value of the control sample should fall within a predetermined range, providing confidence that the assay is performing optimally.

A distinction must be made between controls and calibrators or standards. Calibrators and standards are used to adjust instrumentation or to define a standard curve from which patient results are read. Calibrators and standards have been assayed by a reference method and have an accurately assigned value. *Calibration and control materials are not interchangeable.* The control must be completely independent of the calibration process so that systematic errors caused by deterioration of the calibrator or a change in the analytical process are detected.

When selecting a control, it should have appropriate concentrations at medically significant levels (i.e., levels that the physician uses to make decisions concerning treatment). Control samples may be purchased from commercial suppliers or prepared by the laboratory from pooled patient samples. Attributes of the ideal hematology control material have been described by Bachner[3] and are listed in Box 5-1.

Levey-Jennings Control Charts

In 1950 Levey and Jennings[4] suggested the use of control charts in the clinical laboratory. This suggestion was based on the observation that, in a stable test environment, the distribution of the results of the same sample analyzed numerous times is gaussian. The Levey-Jennings control chart indicates the mean and the 1-, 2-, and 3–standard deviation ranges on both sides of the mean. Deviation from this distribution indicates the occurrence of an analytical systematic error. In a random distribution, approximately 65% of the repeated values are between the ± 1s ranges and are distributed evenly on either side of the mean. In a properly operating system, 95% of the

---

BOX 5-1 Ideal Hematology Control Substance

Inexpensive
Prolonged stability
Sampled directly
Suspends easily and does not agglutinate
Flow characteristics similar to those of blood
Optical and electrical properties similar to blood
Particle size and shape similar to blood
Assayable by independent methods

Modified from Bachner P: Quality assurance in hematology. In Howanitz JF, Howanitz JH (eds): Laboratory Quality Assurance, New York: McGraw-Hill, 1987:214-243.

values should fall between the ± 2*s* ranges and 99% between the ± 3*s* limits. This means that 1 data point in 20 should be located between either of the 2*s* and 3*s* limits, and 1 data point should occur outside of the 3*s* limits once in every 100 analyses. More than 1 point outside of the 3*s* limits per 100 analyses signifies that some form of error has occurred and that investigation is necessary. The ± 2*s* limits are considered warning limits. Values that exceed the 2*s* and 3*s* limits indicate that the analysis should be repeated. The ± 3*s* limits are rejection limits. When a point exceeds the limits expected, the analysis should stop, the patients' results should be held, and the system should be investigated. An example of a normal Levey-Jennings control plot is illustrated in Figure 5-3.

The pattern of the data points plotted over time is important for detecting shifts and trends in the calibration of the test method. A *shift* is a drift of values from one level of the control chart to another (Fig. 5-4). The shift may be sudden or gradual;

in the latter case, it is referred to as a *trend*. A trend is the continuous movement of values in one direction over six or more consecutive values (Fig. 5-5). In hematology, trends may be caused by deterioration of reagents or problems with pump tubing or light sources. Shifts occur with abrupt changes to the test system, such as introduction of new reagents or instrument components.

The occurrence of shifts or trends is the result of either proportional or constant systematic analytical error. Random error is evidenced by an increased number of values beyond the ± 2*s* limits. More than 1 in 20 values beyond this limit indicate increased random error.

Multirule (Westgard) Analysis

CLIA requires that a minimum of two levels of control be analyzed each day of testing. (There is an exception to this rule if the laboratory uses equivalent quality control methods, which are discussed later in this chapter.) One control should have a low concentration and the other a high concentration at medically significant levels or at the ends of the test method's linearity range. Westgard and associates[6] formulated a series of multirules to help evaluate paired control runs. Running and evaluating the results of two controls simultaneously allows shifts and trends to be detected earlier. These multirules are as follows:

1_{2s} *rule*—A control value is outside a 2*s* limit. This is a warning of a possible error of the instrument or method malfunction (Fig. 5-6).

1_{3s} *rule*—One value is outside a 3*s* limit. This may be the result of a random error and should be investigated (Fig. 5-7).

2_{2s} *rule*—Two consecutive values are outside the same 2*s* limits. This may be within the same control run involving both levels of control exceeding the same +2 or −2 limit or two consecutive analyses of the same control material exceeding the same 2*s* limit. This should be investigated as out of control.

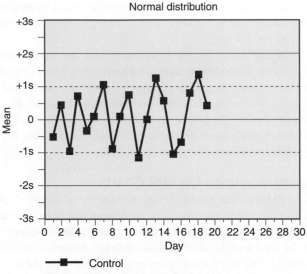

Figure 5-3 Normal Levey-Jennings control plot.

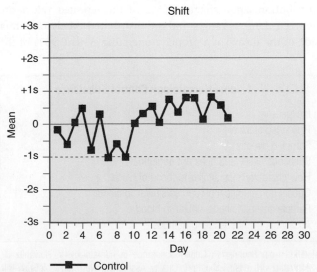

Figure 5-4 When a series of control values consistently falls on one side of the mean, a shift has occurred. A shift is a constant systematic error.

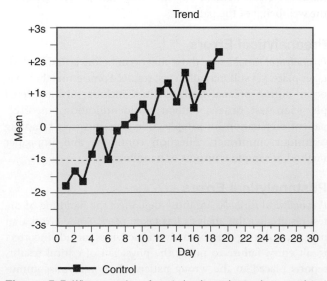

Figure 5-5 When a series of control values change in a consistent direction, a trend is occurring. A trend is a proportional systematic error.

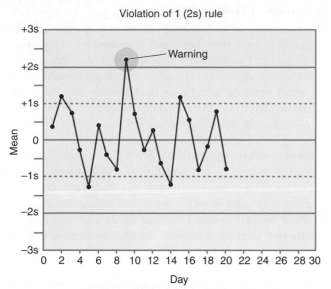

Figure 5-6 Violation of 1_{2s} rule. When one control value is more than 2 standard deviations away from the mean, this should serve as a *warning*, and laboratory staff should examine the quality control data carefully for a possible error.

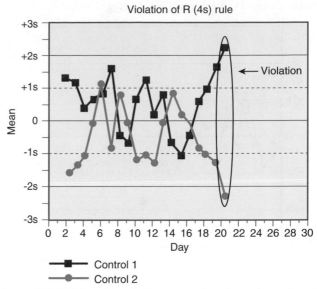

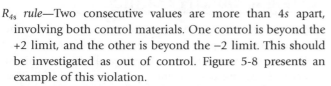

Figure 5-8 Violation of R_{4s} rule. Two consecutive values are more than 4s apart involving both control materials. This should be investigated as out of control.

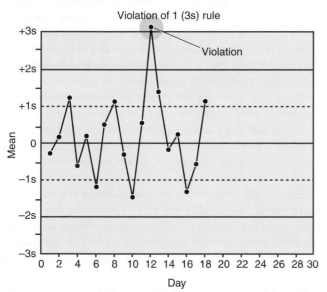

Figure 5-7 Violation of 1_{3s} rule. If there is a violation of this rule, the run should be rejected. This might be the result of a random error but should be investigated.

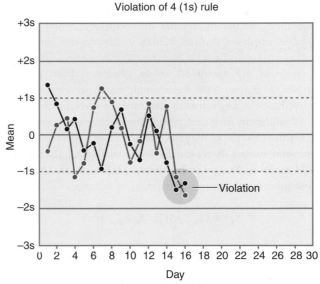

Figure 5-9 Violation of 4_{1s} rule. This example shows a violation of the rule across control levels. Violation of this rule indicates a shift or trend in the analytical process.

R_{4s} *rule*—Two consecutive values are more than *4s* apart, involving both control materials. One control is beyond the +2 limit, and the other is beyond the −2 limit. This should be investigated as out of control. Figure 5-8 presents an example of this violation.

4_{1s} *rule*—Four consecutive values have been plotted on the same side of the *1s* range. This may be within or across control materials. Violation of this rule indicates a shift or trend in the analytical process (Fig. 5-9).

10_x *rule*—Violation occurs when 10 consecutive values fall on the same side of the mean, either within the same control or across both controls. This indicates a shift in the analytical process (Fig. 5-10).

These rules can be adapted to a control chart similar to the Levey-Jennings chart; violation of the rules indicates the type of error that occurs. Rejection by the 1_{3s} and R_{4s} rules suggests random error. Rejection by the 2_{2s}, 4_{1s}, and 10_x rules, either by themselves or in combination with others, suggests that systematic errors have occurred in the system.

Moving Averages of the Red Blood Cell Indices

Automated hematology analyzers employ the unique moving average formula, popularly called *"Bull's algorithm"* ($\bar{X}_B$), to control precision.[7] Used nowhere else in medicine, moving averages rely on the population-wide stability of the RBC

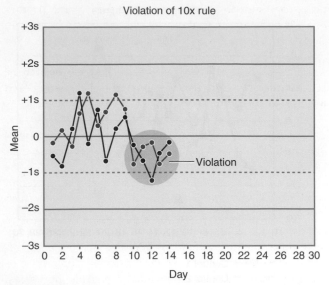

Violation of 10x rule

Figure 5-10 Violation of the 10$_x$ rule. This example shows a violation of the rule across both control levels. Violation of this rule indicates a shift in the analytical process.

indices; mean cell volume (MVC), mean cell hemoglobin (MCH), and mean cell hemoglobin concentration (MCHC). Even many forms of anemia are normocytic and normochromic, implying normal indices. Analyzers use circuitry to compute mean indices for each batch of 20 patient results and to compare the means to values generated from previous batches. A change ≥3% for a single batch or ≥2% each for consecutive batches warns of electronic or mechanical error.

At validation or recalibration, the instrument accumulates data from 15 to 50 batches (up to 1000 specimens) and computes means. A typical MCV mean is 89.5 fL, a typical MCH mean is 30.5 pg and a typical MCHC mean 34%. Each subsequent batch mean is computed as follows:

$$\bar{X}_{B,i} = \bar{X}_{B,i-1} + [(\Sigma \sqrt{\bar{X}_j - \bar{X}_{B,i-1}})/N]^2$$

Where
$\bar{X}_{B,i}$ = the mean of the current batch
$\bar{X}_{B,i-1}$ = the mean of the previous batch
X_j = the individual data point

The batch mean is compared to the previous mean, then assigned a weight of 60% and incorporated with the existing mean. Data are "smoothed" by incorporating the previous mean at the weight of 40%, thereby reducing shifts caused by coincidental series of similarly abnormal specimens. Data are "trimmed" as the square root function reduces the effects of outliers.

The use of actual patient specimens reduces need for preserved controls and eliminates matrix effect. Instrument drift is detected within 20 specimen assays. Moving averages has not been applied successfully to WBC or platelet parameters, although it is possible to cautiously generalize from the results of the indices. Obviously, the moving average function is only available on computerized instruments.

Automated Differential Counting

The imprecision and inaccuracy of the routine manual differential count have been well documented.[8] This imprecision is attributable to nonrandom cell distribution, cell identification errors, and statistical sampling errors caused by the small numbers of cells counted (usually 100-200).[9] The automated screening differential instruments count thousands of cells, greatly reducing the statistical sampling error and allowing for a high degree of precision. Quality control of the automated screening differential poses a new challenge, however, because cells are not as stable as other compounds, such as glucose in chemistry control material. Each laboratory must establish criteria for when the automated differential should be reviewed by performing a manual differential count. These criteria vary in accordance with the type of instrument being used and the population served.

EQUIVALENT QUALITY CONTROL

In 2003, a new quality control concept, called equivalent quality control (EQC) was introduced by the Centers for Medicare and Medicaid Services (CMS) in the "final rules" of CLIA. Many test systems now include internal monitoring systems or controls that check the analytic components of the test each time is it performed. Some test systems are able to maintain stable performance conditions and are only slightly influenced by environmental conditions, such as temperature or humidity. Additionally some minor variation in operator handling may have very little effect on some test systems. In these instances, CLIA regulations provide alternatives (EQC) to the traditional daily testing of two levels of quality control materials.[10] Depending on the test systems, EQC can reduce external QC frequency to once per week once per month. Three options are available.

CLIA specifies conditions for evaluation of test systems to determine if they quality for EQC. CMS does not offer a protocol for the evaluation of a test systems, but specifies that the laboratory director, in consult with the instrument manufacturer must determine whether EQC can be adopted for a particular instrument.[11]

Although this method of quality control is not currently widespread, it may become more commonplace as technology advances.

EXTERNAL QUALITY CONTROL

Internal quality control systems measure precision over time. External systems provide preserved specimens called proficiency surveys administered by national and international agencies. These are used to monitor accuracy, as individual laboratories analyze and report survey material results to the providing agency and receive a report comparing their results to the means of other participating laboratories and reference laboratories. The consensus mean is assigned reference status and a laboratory's performance is evaluated by how closely its results compare. Survey results may be qualitative or quantitative, continuous or discrete. The College of American

Pathologists provides an extensive proficiency survey, while state laboratories distribute surveys for legally required testing programs. Participation in external survey programs meets the requirements of JCAHO and CLIA. Esoteric tests for which no survey material exists may be tested for accuracy using interlaboratory exchange.

NEW ASSAY IMPLEMENTATION

Before a new test procedure can be implemented into routine testing in the laboratory, it must be validated that it consistently produces quality test results. This involves testing the equipment and procedures with samples with known values, such as calibrators, to ensure that expected results are obtained. The laboratory must verify or establish the performance characteristics for a test method before it can be used to produce patient test results. The performance characteristics of a test method include accuracy, precision, sensitivity, specificity, and reference intervals.

CONTINUING EDUCATION

Stewart and Koepke said, "The best prevention of errors is a well-trained and conscientious technologist."[1] A conscientious laboratory director hires only certified clinical laboratory scientists and technicians. To maintain staff skills, the manager implements a system of competency testing. To assure competency, a new employee is tested on knowledge and abilities at hiring, six months, and one year. For instance, the hematology supervisor may maintain a file of blood films that the applicant correctly analyzes at hiring. Continuing competency is assured through regularly scheduled re-testing. Results are maintained in personnel files. Competency assessments are available online from the University of Washington's Laboratory Training Library and several other sources.

The laboratory manager may also provide regular in-service continuing education, particularly as interesting cases or situations arise or when experts visit. Further, many institutions provide incentives for formal continuing educations in the form of time off, support for off-site meetings, and recording of continuing educations units. An ongoing education program raises professional staff awareness of unusual disease state or specimen anomalies. Personnel certified by the National Credentialing Agency for Laboratory Personnel or the Board of Registry of the American Society for Clinical Pathology accumulate continuing education units to maintain their credentials.

QUALITY ASSURANCE PLAN

The JCAHO requires that clinical laboratories participate in hospital-wide quality assurance programs to monitor and evaluate the appropriateness of medical services to correct problems and recognize clinical situations that require improvement.[12] A quality assurance plan helps to focus quality assurance activities. There should be a plan that identifies quality assurance issues, along with the mechanisms and people necessary to evaluate and report these issues. Features of a quality assurance plan vary for each laboratory, but certain central parameters should be identical. General features of any plan should include goals, objectives, sources of authority, definition of scope of services, selection of topics, a monitoring activity calendar, corrective action, periodic evaluation, and methods of communication.[13]

The goal of laboratory quality assurance is to verify that the quality of services contributes to the overall delivery of excellent medical care. Given this explicit goal of excellence, each laboratory should look at all aspects of care, from the preanalytical to postanalytical activities. These can be listed and considered as overall objectives for the laboratory. From these overall objectives, study topics should be selected and given priority according to potential impact on patient care. The key to a good quality assurance program is a focus on high-frequency problems, which can be identified by listening to or surveying the needs and complaints of patients, physicians, and staff on the units. Viewed in a positive manner, quality assurance should improve the laboratory's service, rather than hinder it.

There is no specific method to select topics for quality assurance review, but the selection should be based on whether the problem is clinically relevant. Topics to be avoided are so-called "safe topics"—those in which no problems are anticipated—because this serves no purpose. The following are examples of quality indicators that might be selected:

- Test requests

  Timeliness of preoperative orders

  Legibility of orders

  Stat orders, including the necessity for the order, whether the ordering physician was available to receive the results, and whether there was an appropriate response to the results

  Order accuracy—Do requisitions received in the laboratory accurately reflect the physician's orders in the chart?

  Order completeness—Are orders complete? Do they provide all the information needed (e.g., is it noted that a patient is taking anticoagulant medication when coagulation tests are ordered)?

- Specimen collection

  Success rate of phlebotomy draws—How often do unsuccessful attempts to draw blood occur?

  Patient availability—Is the patient on the unit when the phlebotomist arrives?

  Patient identification—How often does the patient have the correct identification (i.e., an armband)?

  Patient preparation—Was the patient's preparation for the testing appropriate?

  Timing of collection—How accurate were the timed phlebotomies? How much time elapsed between the drawing of a specimen for a therapeutic drug level and the actual time the patient was given medication?

  Labeling—The threshold for accurate specimen labeling should be 100%.

- Other indicators

  Delta check follow-ups

  Repeated testing—Why is the testing being repeated?

Turnaround time—How long is the time from order receipt to result reporting? Various times need to be defined for stat testing, emergency department or intensive care results, routine inpatient testing, and routine outpatient testing.

Critical test results—Are the results telephoned to the appropriate defined individuals? Were these individuals available to receive the critical results?

Charting—Are results entered into the patient's chart within an acceptable timeframe?

Telephone calls—Are clinicians or nurses calling the laboratory too often for results?

Computer errors—Are there errors in computer entries?

Patient satisfaction surveys—Were patients correctly identified? Was the conduct of the phlebotomist appropriate? Was there adequate explanation for specimen collection?

The previous list is not exhaustive and presents only examples of indicators that might be used. In 1988 Q Probes, a subscription program under the auspices of the College of American Pathologists, was developed.[14] The aim of this program was to provide a formatted quality assurance program for institutions that had not been able to develop programs of their own. Experts in quality assurance were assembled to develop a consensus of appropriate indicators of quality for pathology and laboratory medicine. The aim was also to provide a program that would document practice patterns, provide scientific evidence of areas in which improvement could occur, and improve the care of the patients served.

The quality assurance program must be comprehensive, including all sections and shifts, because effective quality assurance involves everyone. Involving staff at all levels in a quality assurance plan occurs most easily by giving each individual responsibility for monitoring some quality indicator; this also encourages increased awareness of quality assurance by the laboratory staff and makes quality assurance more of a team effort. Quality assurance must be ongoing, with evidence of continual quality assurance activity. Studies should be documented or summarized at least quarterly, with data generated throughout the year. The formation of a laboratory quality assurance team that defines and evaluates the selected indicators is crucial. Results and suggestions from the laboratory quality assurance team should be presented and discussed at the hospital quality assurance committee meeting, at which representatives from other areas and divisions of the hospital are included. Improvement in laboratory services and care of patients often can be implemented at this level as the important indicators and findings are discussed. The hospital quality assurance committee must disseminate the findings and suggestions to the various medical committees or departments as necessary.

CHAPTER at a GLANCE

- Quality assurance is the coordinated effort of staff to enhance care of patients through the monitoring, evaluation, and improvement of all aspects of laboratory service.
- The goal of quality assurance is to verify that the quality of services contributes to the overall delivery of excellent medical care.
- Quality control is the component of quality assurance that involves the process of monitoring the characteristics of the testing system, primarily by statistical analysis.
- Quality control includes internal and external components, necessary corrective actions, and continuing education to maintain technical performance.
- The distributions of many medical laboratory measurements in populations approximate a gaussian curve.
- Diagnostic sensitivity and specificity of tests influence how a test should be used when there is clinical suspicion of a disease.
- PPV and NPV provide measurements of the efficacy of a laboratory test.

- Analytical error in a test system or method may be constant systematic, proportional systematic, or random.
- Sources of error may come not only from analytical functions, but also from preanalytical and postanalytical activities.
- Levey-Jennings control charts allow a laboratory professional to detect shifts or trends in a testing system.
- Westgard rules can be used to determine the type of error that has occurred.
- Before a new assay may be implemented into the laboratory to obtain patient test results, it must be validated to ensure that it can produce quality test results.
- Staff competence can be maintained and controlled through participation in continuing education programs.

Now that you have completed this chapter, go back and read again the case study at the beginning and respond to the questions presented.

REVIEW QUESTIONS

1. The acceptable range for hemoglobin values on a control sample is 13 ± 0.4 g/dL. A hemoglobin determination is performed five times in succession on the same control sample. The results are (in g/dL) 12, 12.3, 12, 12.2, and 12.1. These results are:
   a. Precise, but not accurate
   b. Both accurate and precise
   c. Accurate, but not precise
   d. Neither accurate nor precise

2. A mean value of 6×10^9/L is determined for a leukocyte count. One standard deviation (s) is 0.3×10^9/L. The 95.5% confidence limits would be (as 10^9/L):
   a. 3.0-9.0
   b. 5.4-6.6
   c. 5.5-6.5
   d. 5.7-6.3

3. On a run of 20 hemoglobin samples, 95% are 0.4 g/dL more than known values. This type of error is known as:
   a. Random
   b. Proportional systematic
   c. Constant systematic
   d. Coefficient of variation

4. The following data for leukocyte counts are extracted from the last 10 control samples run on an automated instrument (in 10^9/L): 7.2, 7.6, 6.8, 7.2, 6.9, 6.8, 7.4, 7.5, 6.9, and 7.2. (The acceptable control range is 7.2 ± 0.4 × 10^9/L.) These data:
   a. Represent a random distribution
   b. Represent a trend
   c. Represent a shift
   d. Are impossible to interpret

5. Based on the data provided in question 4, how should the patient test results from day 10 (corresponding to the 7.2 value for the control value) be handled?
   a. Report them.
   b. Retest that run of samples with the control sample and if the control is within range, report them.
   c. Open a new bottle of control and run it. If the value is acceptable, report the patient results previously obtained.
   d. Recalibrate the instrument and rerun the original control sample and all patient values. If the control is acceptable, report the new patient results.

6. The control value for an erythrocyte count is 4.00 ± 0.4 × 10^{12}/L (2s). On 2 successive days, the laboratory professional obtains a value of 4.65 × 10^{12}/L. According to Levey-Jennings control charts, this value is:

   a. A warning limit
   b. Acceptable because it could be repeated
   c. A rejection limit
   d. Within normal random error

7. Given the following values for hemoglobin, calculate the mean (all values in g/dL): 7.3, 7.7, 7.3, 7.2, 7.5, 7.4, 7.5, 7.3, 7.6, and 7.2.

8. For the example in question 6, calculate the standard deviation.

9. The use of moving averages is most valuable in the hematology laboratory to detect:
   a. Random errors
   b. Systematic errors
   c. Imprecision and inaccuracy
   d. Interlaboratory variations

10. What is the relationship between quality control and quality assurance?
    a. *Quality control* and *quality assurance* are two names for the same process.
    b. *Quality control* is the name for the laboratory's quality practices, whereas *quality assurance* is the name used for the quality practices across the entire institution.
    c. *Quality control* is just one part of the larger array of *quality assurance* practices.
    d. *Quality assurance* is the name for use of external quality monitors, whereas *quality control* refers just to internal quality monitors.

REFERENCES

1. Stewart CE, Koepke JA: Basic Quality Assurance Practices for Clinical Laboratories. Philadelphia: JB Lippincott, 1987.
2. NCCLS: How to Define and Determine Reference Intervals in the Clinical Laboratory, 2nd ed. Document C28-A2. Wayne, PA: NCCLS, 2000.
3. Bachner P: Quality assurance in hematology. In Howanitz JF, Howanitz JH (eds): Laboratory Quality Assurance. New York: McGraw-Hill, 1987:214-243.
4. Levey S, Jennings ER: The use of control charts in the clinical laboratory. Am J Clin Pathol 1950;20:1059-1066.
5. Clinical Laboratory Improvement Amendments Brochure (CLIA) #1. Available at www.cms.hhs.gov/CLIA/downloads/6063bk.pdf. Accessed August 5, 2006.
6. Westgard JO, Barry PL, Hunt MR, et al: A multi-rule Shewhart chart for quality control in clinical chemistry. Clin Chem 1981;27:493-501.
7. Bull BS, Elashoff RM, Heilbron DC, et al: A study of various estimators for the derivation of quality control procedures from patient erythrocyte indices. Am J Clin Pathol 1974;61:473-481.
8. Koepke JA, Dotson MA, Shifman MA: A critical evaluation of the manual/visual differential leukocyte counting method. Blood Cells 1985;11:173-186.
9. Terrell JC: Laboratory evaluation of leukocytes. In Stiene-Martin EA, Lotspeich-Steininger CA, Koepke JA (eds): Clinical Hematology: Principles, Procedures, Correlations, 2nd ed. Philadelphia: Lippincott-Raven, 1998:331-345.
10. Clinical Laboratory Improvement Amendments (CLIA) Brochure #4 Available at: http://www.cms.hhs.gov/CLIA/downloads/6066bk.pdf. Accessed December 19, 2005.
11. Laessig RH, Ehrmeyer SS. CLIA 2003's new concept: equivalent quality control. MLO Med Lab Obs. 2005;37:32-4.
12. Comprehensive Accreditation Manual for Hospitals. Oakbrook Terrace, IL: Joint Commission on Accreditation of Healthcare Organizations, 2006.
13. Bozzo P: Implementing Quality Assurance. Chicago: ASCP Press, 1991.
14. Howanitz PJ, Schifman RB, Steindel SJ, et al: A nationwide quality assurance program can describe standards for the practice of pathology and laboratory medicine. Qual Assur Health Care 1992;3:245-256.

6

Morphology and Function of Cellular Components

Keila B. Poulsen

OBJECTIVES

After completion of this chapter, the reader will be able to:

1. Describe the general function and chemical composition of cellular membranes.
2. List and describe the components of the nucleus, including staining qualities visible by light microscopy.
3. Correlate the nuclear structures to the activities of the cell.
4. Name and describe the ultrastructural appearance of the cytoplasmic organelles found in the cell and staining qualities by light microscopy, if appropriate.
5. Correlate the cytoplasmic structures to the activities of the cell.

The numerous multichannel instruments that have become available for the clinical diagnostic process have revolutionized the study of hematology. The technologies of light scatter, electrical impedance, and conductivity have added parameters and scatterplots whose significance are yet to be fully realized and clinically applied, but morphologic examination of the peripheral blood smear with light microscopy remains the hallmark for clinical evaluation of hematologically abnormal patients. The study of cells under the microscope was greatly enhanced when Paul Ehrlich (1854-1915) developed staining techniques to better differentiate the various normal and abnormal cells present in human blood. The development of the electron microscope revolutionized the ability to study and understand the internal components of the cell.[1]

CELL ORGANIZATION

Cells are structural units that constitute living organisms (Figs. 6-1 and 6-2). Many cells have specialized functions and contain the components necessary to perform and perpetuate these functions. Regardless of shape, size, or function, most cells have three basic parts: unit membranes, the cytoplasm, and the nucleus. Each of these basic parts has components or subdivisions that assist in their varied functions. Table 6-1 summarizes the cellular components and functions, which are explained in more detail subsequently.

CELL MEMBRANE

The cell membrane serves as a semipermeable outer boundary separating the cellular components from their surrounding environments. The cell membrane serves three basic functions: (1) it restricts and facilitates the interchange of substances with the environment by selective permeability, endocytosis, exocytosis, and locomotion; (2) it detects hormonal signals facilitating cell-to-cell recognition; and (3) it is the location of surface markers for cell identity.[2] Monoclonal antibodies are used to identify a cell's surface markers. The nomenclature uses the letters *CD* (cluster designation) and a number following the CD. This common terminology assists in unifying classification in clinical practice, research efforts, and the literature (Chapter 33). Many components found within the cell (e.g., the mitochondria, Golgi apparatus, nucleus, and endoplasmic reticulum) have similarly constructed membrane systems. The red blood cell membrane has been widely studied and serves as an example of a cell membrane (see Fig. 9-2).

To accomplish its many requirements, this cell membrane must be resilient and elastic; it achieves these qualities by being a fluid structure of globular proteins floating in lipids. The lipids comprise phospholipids and cholesterol arranged in two layers. The phosphate end of the phospholipid and the hydroxyl radical of cholesterol are polar-charged hydrophilic (water-soluble) lipids oriented toward the inner and outer surfaces of the cell membrane. The fatty acid portion of the

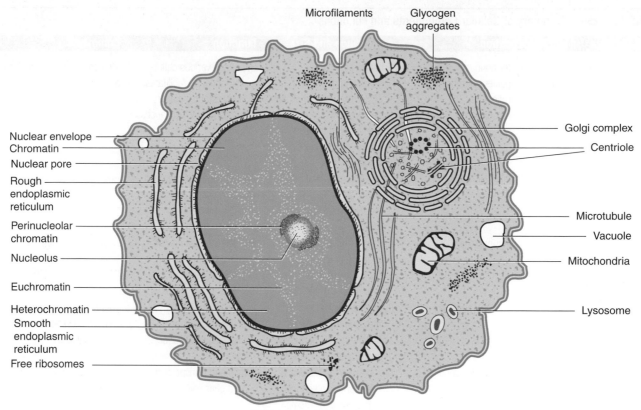

Figure 6-1 Cell organization.

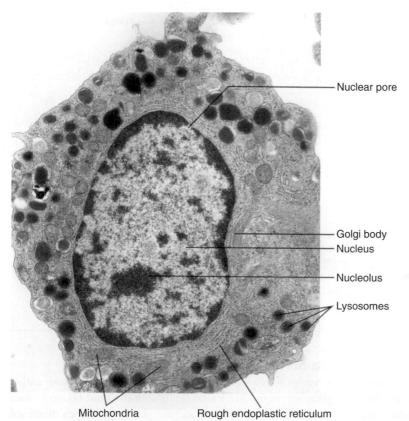

Figure 6-2 Electron micrograph with labeled organelles. (From Carr JH, Rodak BF: Clinical Hematology Atlas, 2nd ed. Philadelphia: Saunders, 2004.)

TABLE 6-1 Summary of Cellular Components and Functions

Organelle	Location	Appearance and Size	Function	Comments
Membranes: plasma, nuclear, mitochondrial, endoplasmic reticulum	Outer boundary of cell, nucleus, endoplasmic reticulum, mitochondria, and other organelles	Usually a lipid bilayer consisting of proteins, cholesterol, phospholipids, and polysaccharides; membrane thickness varies with the cell or organelle	Separates various cellular components; facilitates and restricts cellular exchange of substances	Membrane must be resilient and flexible
Nucleus	Within cell	Usually round or oval but varies depending on cell; varies in size; composed of DNA	Control center of the cell and contains the genetic blueprint	Governs the cellular activity and transmits information for cellular control
Nucleolus	Within nucleus	Usually round or irregular in shape; 2-4 μm in size; composed of RNA; there may be 1-4 within nucleus	Site of synthesis and procession of ribosomal RNA	Appearance varies with activity of the cells; larger when cell is actively involved in protein synthesis
Golgi body	Next to the nucleus	System of stacked, membrane-bound, flattened sacs; horseshoe shaped; varies in size	Involved in modifying and packaging macromolecules for secretion	Well developed in cells with large secretion responsibilities
Endoplasmic reticulum	Randomly throughout cytoplasm	Membrane-lined tubules that branch and connect to nucleus and plasma membrane	Stores and transports fluids and chemicals	Two types: smooth with no ribosomes; rough with ribosomes on surface
Ribosomes	Free in cytoplasm; outer surface of rough endoplasmic reticulum	Small granule (100-300 Å); composed of protein and nucleic acid	Protein production, such as enzymes and blood proteins	Large proteins are synthesized from polyribosomes (chains of ribosomes)
Mitochondria	Randomly in cytoplasm	Round or oval structures; 3-14 ηm in length, 2-10 ηm in width; membrane has 2 layers; inner layer has folds called *cristae*	Cell's "powerhouse"; make ATP, the energy source for the cell	Active cells have more present than do inactive cells
Lysosomes	Randomly in cytoplasm	Membrane-bound sacs; size varies	Contain hydrolytic enzymes for cellular digestive system	If membrane breaks, the hydrolytic enzymes can destroy the cell
Microfilaments	Near nuclear envelope and within proximity of mitotic process	Small, solid structure approximately 5 ηm in diameter	Support of cytoskeleton and motility	Consists of actin and myosin (contractile proteins)
Microtubules	Cytoskeleton, near nuclear envelope and component part of centriole near Golgi body	Hollow cylinder with protofilaments surrounding the outside tube; 20-25 ηm in diameter, variable length	Maintenance of cell shape, motility, and mitotic process	Produced from tubulin polymerization; make up mitotic spindles and part of the structure of centriole
Centriole	In centrosome near nucleus	Cylinders; 150 nm in diameter, 300-500 ηm in length	Serve as insertion points for mitotic spindle fibers	Nine sets of triplet microtubules

phospholipid and the steroid nucleus of cholesterol are non–polar-charged hydrophobic (water-insoluble) lipids directed toward each other in the center of the cell membrane. Other lipids, such as lipoproteins and lipopolysaccharides, contribute to the membrane structure.

Membrane Proteins

Most proteins found in the cell membrane are called *glycoproteins* and are found floating in the lipid bilayers.[3] Two types of proteins, integral and peripheral, have been described in the cell membrane. *Integral proteins* may traverse the entirety of the lipid bilayers and penetrate the outside of the membrane or only the cytoplasmic side of the membrane. These transmembrane proteins are thought to serve as a communication and transport system between the cell's interior and the external environment. *Peripheral proteins* are found only on the inner cytoplasmic side of the membrane and form the cell's cytoskeleton. Peripheral proteins also are attached to the cytoplasmic ends of integral proteins to form a reticular network for maintaining structural integrity and holding the integral proteins in a fixed position.

Membrane Carbohydrates

Membrane carbohydrates occur in combination with proteins (glycoproteins) and lipids (glycolipids). The carbohydrate portion usually extends beyond the outer cell surface, giving the cell a carbohydrate coat often called the *glycocalyx*. These carbohydrate moieties function in cell-to-cell recognition and provide a negative surface charge, surface receptor sites, and cell adhesion capabilities.[4] The function of the red blood cell membrane is discussed in detail in Chapter 9.

NUCLEUS

The nucleus is composed of three components: the chromatin, the nuclear envelope, and the nucleoli. It is the control center of the cell and the largest organelle within the cell. The nucleus is composed largely of deoxyribonucleic acid (DNA) and is the site of DNA replication and transcription. It is responsible for the chemical reactions within the cell and the cell's reproductive process. The nucleus has an affinity to the basic dyes because of the nucleic acids contained within it.

Chromatin

The chromatin consists of nucleic acids and proteins. The proteins are the histones, which are negatively charged, and the nonhistones, which are positively charged. Chromatin has been divided into two types: (1) the *heterochromatin*, which is represented by the more darkly stained, condensed clumping pattern and is the genetically inactive area of the nucleus, and (2) the *euchromatin*, which has diffuse, uncondensed chromatin and is the genetically active portion of the nucleus where ribonucleic acid (RNA) transcription occurs. This genetic material is loosely coiled and turns a pale blue when stained.

Nuclear Envelope

Surrounding the nucleus is a nuclear envelope consisting of an inner and an outer membrane. The outer membrane is continuous with an extension of the endoplasmic reticulum. Between the two membranes is a diaphragm approximately 50 nm in thickness that is continuous with the lumen of endoplasmic reticulum. Nuclear pores penetrate the nuclear envelope, allowing communication between the nucleus and the cytoplasm. The number of these pores decreases as the cell matures.

Nucleoli

The nucleus contains one to several nucleoli. The number is directly proportional to the amount of protein synthesis that occurs in the cell. These organelles contain a large amount of ribosomal RNA, DNA, and other proteins in a loose fibrillar form. The nucleolus is the site for the synthesis of the cell's ribosomes. Ribosomes consist of two subunits, a large and a small one. The subunits are produced in the nucleolus and are transported through the nuclear pores for ribosomal assembly and protein synthesis.

CYTOPLASM

The cytoplasmic matrix is a homogeneous, continuous, aqueous solution called *cytosol*. It is the environment in which the organelles join and function. These organelles are discussed individually.

Golgi Complex

The Golgi complex is a system of stacked, membrane-bound, flattened sacs referred to as *cisternae* that are involved in modifying, sorting, and packaging macromolecules for secretion or delivery to other organelles. The number of stacked cisternae ranges from 6 to 30 per cell, depending on the cell type. The Golgi complex is normally located next to the nucleus. The Golgi complex is horseshoe shaped and usually located in close proximity to the endoplasmic reticulum. The concave aspect has numerous enzymes for synthetic activities. The convex side is the "maturing surface" and is where the various products are packaged.[4]

Membrane-bound vesicles are closely associated with the stacks of cisternae. Some of the vesicles are coated and bud off for transport to other areas of the cell. The Golgi complex directs traffic in the cell. The exact mechanism of macromolecule modification and sorting is still being defined, although it is clearly a responsibility of the Golgi complex.

Endoplasmic Reticulum

The endoplasmic reticulum (Fig. 6-3) is a lacelike network found throughout the cytoplasm of cells and appears as flattened sheets, sacs, and tubes of membrane. The endoplasmic reticulum subdivides the cytoplasm into various compartments. The outer membrane of the nuclear envelope is in continuity with the endoplasmic reticulum membrane and specializes in making and transporting lipid and membrane proteins.

Rough endoplasmic reticulum has a studded look on its outer surface caused by the presence of ribosomes engaged in synthesis of proteins. The amount of endoplasmic reticulum found within a cell is proportional to the protein production required by the cell. More endoplasmic reticulum is necessary for increased protein synthesis. Smooth endoplasmic reticulum does not contain ribosomes and may serve as storage sites for the newly synthesized protein. Also, it has been suggested as a site for steroid hormone production and synthesis of lipid substances. Its function varies with the type of cell.

Ribosomes

Ribosomes are small particles composed of near-equal amounts of protein and ribosomal RNA. Ribosomes are found free in the cytoplasm, on the surface of rough endoplasmic

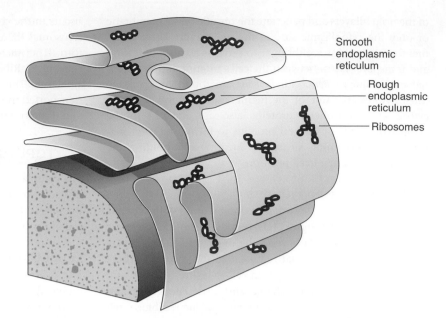

Figure 6-3 Endoplasmic reticulum.

reticulum, and in the nucleus and nucleoli of a cell. These bodies may exist singly (monoribosome) or form chains (polyribosomes). The more ribosomes present within the cell, the more protein production and the more basophilia observed with Wright stain. Ribosomes serve as the site of protein synthesis. This is accomplished with the assistance of transfer RNA, for amino acid transport to the ribosome, and messenger RNA, which provides the necessary information for the sequencing order of the amino acids for each protein.[5]

Mitochondria

The existence of mitochondria (Fig. 6-4) within the cell has been known since the 19th century, and their function is now clearly defined. Structurally, the mitochondrion has a continuous outer membrane. Running parallel to the outer membrane is an inner membrane that invaginates at various intervals, giving the interior a shelf- or ridgelike appearance. These internal ridges, termed *cristae mitochondriales*, are where

oxidative enzymes are attached. The two membranes differ chemically; the inner membrane has a higher protein content and a lower lipid content. The convoluted inner membrane increases the surface area to enhance the respiratory capability of the cell. The interior of the mitochondrion consists of a homogeneous material known as the *mitochondrial matrix*, which contains many enzymes for the extraction of energy from nutrients.

The mitochondria are responsible for the metabolic processes of energy-producing reactions and electron transfer–oxidative reactions. The oxidative systems described within the mitochondria are the Krebs cycle, the fatty acid cycle, and the respiratory chain.[6] Also present in the mitochondria are proteins, phosphorylase, ribosomes, and DNA.[7]

The mitochondria are capable of self-replication. It has been documented that this organelle has its own DNA and RNA for the mitochondrial division cycle. There may be fewer than 100 or several thousand mitochondria per cell. The

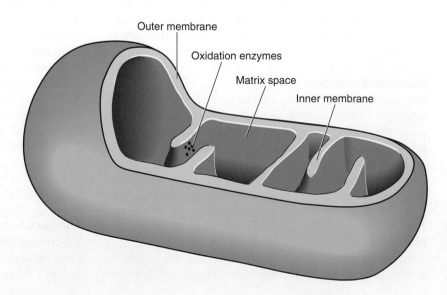

Figure 6-4 Mitochondrion.

number is directly related to the amount of energy required by the cell.

Mitochondria do not stain with Wright stain, but instead give a negative image or clear impression against the stained cytoplasm. When in a hyperactive state, these organelles become so swollen that they appear as short white rods against a blue cytoplasmic background.

Lysosomes

Lysosomes contain hydrolytic enzymes bound within a membrane and are involved in the cell's intracellular digestive process. The membrane prevents the enzymes from attacking the protein, nucleic acids, mucopolysaccharides, lipids, and glycogen within the cell.[8] The enzymes become active when lysosomes bind to the phagocytic vacuole, and the membrane ruptures, allowing the escape of the hydrolytic enzymes into the phagosome.

With Wright stain, lysosomes are visualized as granules. When stained, many of the granules appear azurophilic, unless they are too small to be visualized under the light microscope. Special staining techniques are required to indicate the presence of the smaller granules.

Microfilaments

Microfilaments are solid structures approximately 5 ηm in diameter and consist of actin and myosin proteins. These fibrils or groups of fibrils are located near the nuclear envelope or in the proximity of the nucleus and assist in cell division. They also are present near the membrane for cytoskeletal support and motility. Intermediate filaments are the most durable element of the cytoskeleton and provide structural stability for the cell, especially during stress.[9] Intermediate filaments also are detectable and identifiable as cancer markers.[10]

Microtubules

Microtubules are approximately 25 nm in diameter and vary in length. These organelles are organized from tubulin through self-assembly. The tubulin polypeptides form protofilaments. Usually 13 protofilaments are lined up in parallel rows of hollow spheres.[9,11] This arrangement gives the microtubules structural strength. A variety of conditions cause microtubules to become disorganized and disappear, especially after mitosis. Tubulin can polymerize and reform the microtubule as needed.

Microtubules have several functions. Their contribution to the cytoskeleton helps maintain the cell's shape and the movement of some intracellular organelles. The microtubule makes up the mitotic spindle fibers and the centrioles during mitosis.[12] In the peripheral smear, the microtubules and microfilaments are not visible, but in special conditions the mitotic spindles may cluster and form Cabot rings.[7]

Centrioles

Centrioles are paired structures consisting of nine bundles of three microtubules within each bundle. They are shaped like cylinders and serve as insertion points for the mitotic spindle fibers during metaphase and anaphase of mitosis. The cylinders are 150 nm in diameter and 300 to 500 nm in length. The long axes are typically at right angles to one another.

CHAPTER at a GLANCE

- Cells are building blocks of the living organism and provide the basis for all life processes.
- The nucleus serves as a control center: it directs, educates, and maintains the cell.
- The nucleolus is the site of synthesis and processing of ribosomal RNA.
- The Golgi complex modifies and packages macromolecules for secretion.
- Mitochondria make adenosine triphosphate to supply energy for the cell.
- Lysosomes contain hydrolytic enzymes involved in the cell's intracellular digestive process.

REVIEW QUESTIONS

1. The organelle involved in packaging and trafficking of cellular products is the:
   a. Nucleus
   b. Golgi complex
   c. Mitochondria
   d. Rough endoplasmic reticulum

2. The most common type of protein found in the cell membrane is:
   a. Lipoprotein
   b. Mucoprotein
   c. Glycoprotein
   d. Nucleoprotein

3. The "control center" of the cell is the:
   a. Nucleus
   b. Cytoplasm
   c. Membrane
   d. Microtubular system

4. The nucleus is composed largely of:
   a. RNA
   b. DNA
   c. Ribosomes
   d. Glycoproteins

5. Protein synthesis occurs in the:
   a. Nucleus
   b. Mitochondria
   c. Ribosomes
   d. Golgi complex

6. The shape of a cell is maintained by which of the following?
   a. Microtubules
   b. Spindle fibers
   c. Ribosomes
   d. Centrioles

7. Functions of the cell membrane include all of the following *except*:
   a. Interchange of substances
   b. Cell-to-cell recognition
   c. Receptors for cellular identity
   d. Lipid production

8. The energy source for cells is the:
   a. Golgi complex
   b. Endoplasmic reticulum
   c. Nucleolus
   d. Mitochondrion

9. Ribosomes are synthesized by the:
   a. Endoplasmic reticulum
   b. Mitochondrion
   c. Nucleolus
   d. Golgi apparatus

10. Euchromatin functions as the:
    a. Site of microtubule production
    b. Genetically active DNA
    c. Support structure for nucleoli
    d. Attachment site for centrioles

REFERENCES

1. Wintrobe MM: Blood, Pure and Eloquent. New York: McGraw-Hill, 1980.
2. Bennington JL: Dictionary and Encyclopedia of Laboratory Medicine and Technology. Philadelphia: Saunders, 1984.
3. Gallagher PG, Lux SE: Disorders of the erythrocyte membrane. In Nathan DG, Orkin SH, Ginsburg D, et al (eds): Hematology of Infancy and Childhood, 6th ed. Philadelphia: Saunders, 2003:560-684.
4. Guyton AC: Textbook of Medical Physiology, 10th ed. Philadelphia: Saunders, 2000.
5. Koss LG: Diagnostic Cytology and Its Histopathologic Bases, Vol 1, 4th ed. Philadelphia: JB Lippincott, 1992.
6. Prebble JN: Mitochondria, Chloroplasts and Bacterial Membranes. New York: Longman, 1981.
7. Bessis M: Blood Smears Reinterpreted. Berlin: Springer International, 1977.
8. De Duve C, Wattiaux R: Functions of lysosomes. Annu Rev Physiol 1966;28:435-492.
9. Alberts B, Johnson A, Lewis J, et al: Molecular Biology of the Cell, 4th ed. New York: Garland, 2002.
10. Becker WM, Kleinsmith LJ, Hardin J: World of the Cell, 6th ed. Menlo Park, CA: Benjamin Cummings, 2005.
11. Alberts B, Bray D, Hopkin K, et al: Essential Cell Biology, 2nd ed. New York: Garland, 2003.
12. Stephens RE, Edds KT: Microtubules: structure, chemistry and function. Physiol Rev 1976;56:709-777.

ADDITIONAL RESOURCE

Lodish H, Berk A, Zipursky L, et al: Molecular Cell Biology, 5th ed. New York: WH Freeman, 2004.

Hematopoietic Theory

7

Larry Smith

OBJECTIVES

After completion of this chapter, the reader will be able to:

1. Define *hematopoiesis*.
2. Discuss the evolution and formation of blood cells from embryo to fetus to adult including anatomic sites and cells produced.
3. Predict the likelihood of encountering active marrow from biopsy sites when given the patient's age.
4. Relate normal and abnormal hematopoiesis to the various organs involved in the hematopoietic process.
5. Explain the stem cell theory of hematopoiesis, including the names of various stem cells and progenitor cells and their lineage associations.
6. Discuss the roles of hematopoietic growth factors in differentiation and maturation sequences of hematopoietic progenitor cells, including differentiating nonspecific and lineage-specific factors.
7. Describe general morphologic changes that occur during cell maturation.
8. Define *apoptosis*, and discuss the relationship between apoptosis, growth factors, and stem cell differentiation.
9. Discuss the roles of various cytokines and hematopoietic growth factors in the process of hematopoiesis.
10. Discuss therapeutic applications of cytokines and hematopoietic growth factors.

HEMATOPOIETIC DEVELOPMENT

Hematopoiesis is a continuous, regulated process of blood cell production that includes cell renewal, proliferation, differentiation, and maturation. These processes result in the formation, development, and specialization of all of the functional blood cells that are released from the bone marrow to the circulation. In adults, all of these processes are restricted primarily to the bone marrow. During fetal development, hematopoiesis occurs in different areas of the developing fetus. This process has been divided into three phases: the mesoblastic phase, the hepatic phase, and the medullary phase.

Mesoblastic Phase (Yolk Sac Phase)

Hematopoiesis generally is considered to begin around the 19th day of embryologic development after fertilization. Progenitor cells of mesenchymal origin migrate from the aorta-gonad-mesonephros region of the developing aorta-splanchnopleura to the yolk sac.[1] The cells arising from the aorta-gonad-mesonephros region give rise to hematopoietic stem cells (HSCs), but not to primitive erythroblasts. The primitive erythroblasts found in the yolk sac arise from mesodermal cells, which initially line the cavity of the yolk sac. These primitive cells migrate from the periphery into the central cavity of the yolk sac, where they develop into primitive erythroblasts.[2-5] The remaining cells surrounding the cavity of the yolk sac are called *angioblasts* and form the future blood vessels.[2-5] The yolk sac phase of hematopoiesis is characterized by the development of primitive erythroblasts that produce measurable amounts of hemoglobins, including Portland, Gower I, and Gower II (Chapter 10). Yolk-sac hematopoiesis does not contribute significantly to definitive hematopoiesis.[4] This phase of hematopoiesis occurs intravascularly, or within a developing blood vessel.

Hepatic Phase

The hepatic phase of hematopoiesis begins around 4 to 5 gestational weeks and is characterized by recognizable clusters of developing erythroblasts, granulocytes, and monocytes.[5] The developing erythroblasts in this phase signal the beginning of definitive hematopoiesis with a decline in primitive hematopoiesis of the yolk sac. In addition, lymphoid cells begin to appear.[6,7] Hematopoiesis during this phase occurs extravascularly, with the liver remaining the major site of hematopoiesis during fetal life and retaining activity until 1 to 2 weeks after birth. Hematopoiesis in the aorta-gonad-mesonephros region and the yolk sac disappears during this stage. Hematopoiesis in the fetal liver reaches its peak by the third month of development (Fig. 7-1). The developing spleen, kidney, thymus, and lymph nodes contribute to the hematopoietic process during this phase. The thymus, the first fully developed organ in the fetus, becomes the major site of T cell production, whereas the kidney and spleen produce B cells.

Production of megakaryocytes also begins during the hepatic phase. The spleen gradually decreases granulocytic production and involves itself solely in lymphopoiesis. During the hepatic phase, detectable levels of hemoglobin (Hb) F, Hb A, and Hb A$_2$ may be shown.[8]

Medullary (Myeloid) Phase

During the fifth month of fetal development, hematopoiesis begins in the developing bone marrow cavity. This transition is called *medullary hematopoiesis* because it occurs in the medulla or inner part of the bone marrow. During this phase, mesenchymal cells, which are a type of embryonic tissue, migrate into the core of the bone and differentiate into skeletal and hematopoietic blood cells.[9,10] Hematopoietic activity, especially myeloid activity, is apparent during this stage of development, and the myeloid-to-erythroid ratio approaches the adult level of 3:1 by 21 weeks of gestation.[11] By the end of the sixth month, the bone marrow becomes the primary site of hematopoiesis. Measurable levels of erythropoietin (EPO), granulocyte colony-stimulating factor (G-CSF), granulocyte/monocyte colony-stimulating factor (GM-CSF), fetal Hb, Hb A$_2$, and adult Hb

can be determined. In addition, various stages of maturation can be seen in all three lineages.

ADULT HEMATOPOIETIC TISSUE

In adults, hematopoietic tissue is involved in the proliferation and maturation of blood cells. Numerous organs and tissues contribute to this process, including the bone marrow, lymph nodes, spleen, liver, and thymus. The bone marrow contains developing erythroid, myeloid, megakaryocytic, and lymphoid cells. The tissues where lymphoid development occurs are divided into primary and secondary lymphoid tissue. Primary lymphoid tissue consists of the bone marrow and thymus and is where T and B cells are derived. Secondary lymphoid tissue, where lymphoid cells become competent, consists of the spleen and lymph nodes and gut-associated lymphoid tissue.

Bone Marrow

Bone marrow, one of the largest organs in the body, is defined as the tissue located within the cavities of the cortical bones. These cavities consist of trabecular bone resembling a honeycomb-like structure. Normal bone marrow located within these cavities consists of two types of marrow: (1) red marrow, which is hematopoietically active marrow, and (2) yellow marrow, representing hematopoietically inactive marrow composed primarily of adipocytes (fat cells). Red marrow in adults is found in the sternum, skull, scapulae, vertebrae, ribs, pelvic bones, and proximal ends of the long bones. Normal adult bone marrow has approximately equal amounts of red and yellow marrow.

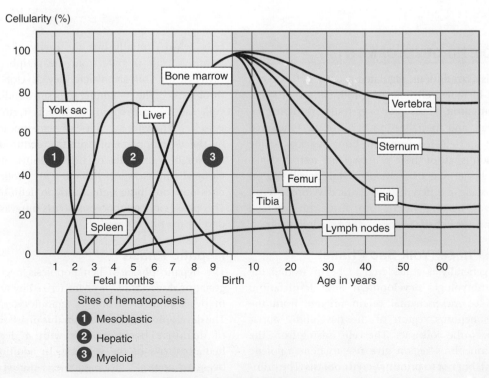

Figure 7-1 Sites of hematopoiesis.

A central space is created within the cavities of these bones by resorption of cartilage and endosteal bone. Mesenchymal cells migrate into the space and eventually differentiate into three cell types, which give rise to the blood and bone marrow matrix cells (reticular cells and adipose tissue). Reticular cells are formed on the exterior surface of the venous sinuses and extend long narrow branches into the perivascular space, creating a meshlike network; this provides a supportive skeletal network for developing hematopoietic cells, macrophages, and mast cells.[10] During infancy and early childhood, the bone marrow consists primarily of red active marrow. Between 5 and 7 years of age, adipose tissue becomes more abundant and begins to occupy the spaces in the long bones previously dominated by active marrow. The process of replacing the active marrow by adipose tissue during development is called *retrogression* and results in the active marrow becoming restricted to the flat bones, sternum, vertebrae, pelvis, ribs, skull, and proximal portion of the long bones (Fig. 7-2). Areas located within the bone marrow cavity where red marrow has been replaced by yellow marrow consist of an mixture of adipose cells, undifferentiated mesenchymal cells, and macrophages. The inactive yellow marrow is scattered throughout active red marrow and is capable of reverting back to the active marrow in cases of increased demand on the bone marrow.[8] Such cases might be due to excessive blood loss or increased erythrocyte destruction in the bone marrow by toxic chemicals or irradiation.

Red Marrow

The red marrow is composed of extravascular cords that contain all of the developing blood cell lineages, stem and progenitor cells, adventitial cells, and macrophages (Figs. 7-3 and 7-4). The cords are separated from the lumen of the sinusoids by endothelial and adventitial cells and are located between the trabeculae of spongy bone. The trabeculae are projections of calcified bone radiating out from the cortical bone into the marrow space and provide support for the developing marrow. The hematopoietic cells tend to develop in specific niches within the cords. Normoblasts develop in small clusters adjacent to the outer surfaces of the vascular sinuses (Fig. 7-5); in addition, some normoblasts are found surrounding iron-laden macrophages (Fig. 7-6). Megakaryocytes are located close to the vascular walls of the sinuses, which

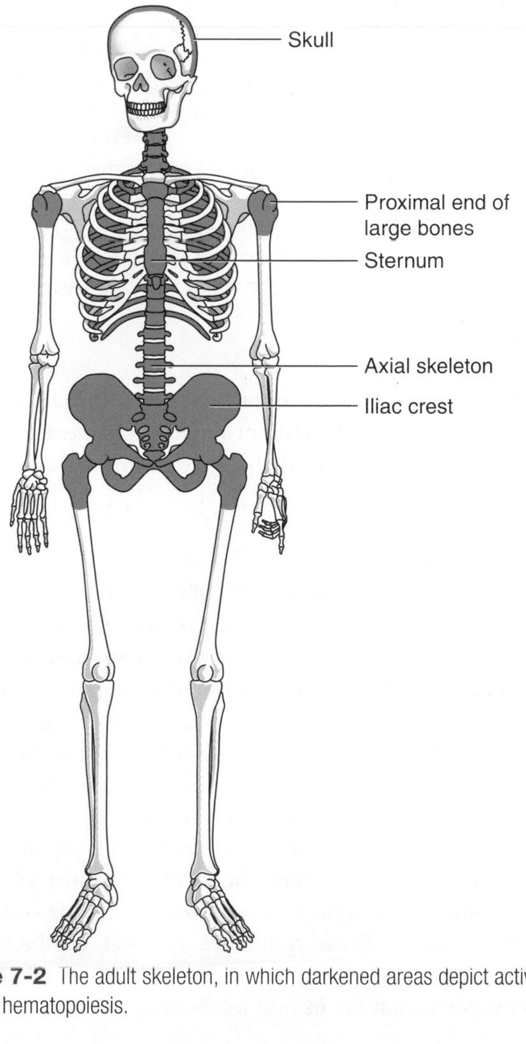

Figure 7-2 The adult skeleton, in which darkened areas depict active red marrow hematopoiesis.

Skull

Proximal end of large bones

Sternum

Axial skeleton

Iliac crest

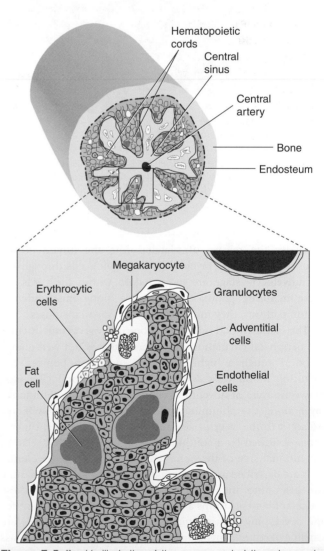

Figure 7-3 Graphic illustration of the arrangement of the extravascular area in hematopoietic tissue.

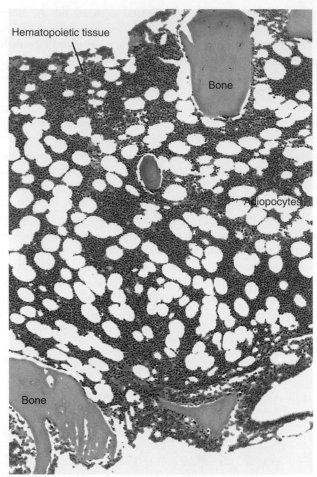

Figure 7-4 Fixed and stained bone marrow biopsy (hematoxylin and eosin, ×100). The extravascular tissue consists of blood cell precursors and various tissue cells with scattered fat tissue. A normal adult bone marrow displays 50% tissue and 50% fat.

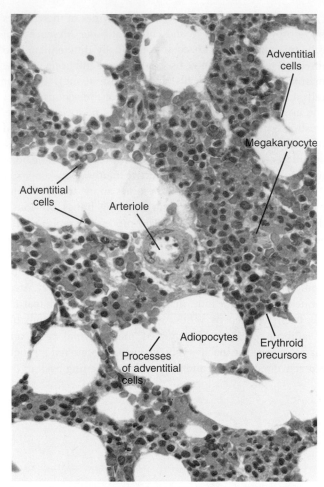

Figure 7-5 Fixed and stained bone marrow biopsy (hematoxylin and eosin, ×400). Hematopoietic tissue reveals areas of granulopoiesis (lighter-staining cells) and erythropoiesis (darker-staining nuclei). One megakaryocyte can be seen. Adventitial cells and their processes give support to the hematopoietic cells; they also guard apertures of the basement membrane.

facilitates the release of platelets into the lumen of the sinusoids. Immature myeloid (granulocytic) cells through the metamyelocyte stage are located deep within the cords. As these maturing granulocytes proceed along their differentiation pathway, they move closer to the vascular sinuses.[9]

The mature blood cells of the bone marrow eventually enter the peripheral circulation by a process that is not well understood. Through a highly complex interaction between the maturing blood cells and the sinus wall, blood cells pass between layers of adventitial cells that form a discontinuous layer along the abluminal side of the bone marrow sinus. Adjacent to the layer of adventitial cells is a basement membrane followed by a continuous layer of endothelial cells on the luminal side of the bone marrow sinus. These adventitial cells are described as *reticular cells* and extend long cytoplasmic processes into the marrow cords. The extension of these reticular filaments forms a meshwork that provides support for the developing hematopoietic cells. The adventitial cells are capable of contracting, which allows mature blood cells to pass through the basement membrane and interact with the endothelial layer.

As blood cells come in contact with endothelial cells, they bind to the surface via a receptor-mediated process. Cells pass through pores in the endothelial cytoplasm and are released into circulation.[12]

Marrow Circulation
The nutrient and gas requirements of the marrow are supplied by the nutrient and periosteal arteries, which enter the bone via the bone foramina. The nutrient artery supplies blood only to the marrow.[10] It coils around the central longitudinal vein, which passes along the bone canal. In the marrow cavity, it divides into ascending and descending branches that also coil around the central longitudinal brain. The arteriole branches that enter the inner lining of the cortical bone (endosteum) form sinusoids (endosteal beds), which connect to periosteal capillaries that extend from the periosteal artery.[13] The periosteal arteries provide nutrients for the osseous bone and the marrow. These capillaries connect to the venous sinuses located in the endosteal bed, which empty into a larger collecting sinus that opens into the central longitudinal vein.[14]

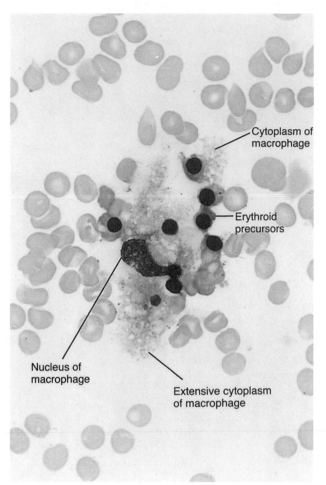

Figure 7-6 Bone marrow aspirate smear (Wright-Giemsa, ×100). Macrophage with extensive iron-laden cytoplasm, surrounded by developing erythroid precursors.

Blood exits the marrow via the central longitudinal vein, which runs the entire length of the marrow. The central longitudinal vein exits the marrow through the same foramen where the nutrient artery enters. Hematopoietic cells located in the endosteal bed receive their nutrients from the nutrient artery.

Hematopoietic Microenvironment

The hematopoietic inductive microenvironment plays an important role in stem cell differentiation and proliferation.[15,16] It is responsible for supplying semifluid matrix, which serves as an anchor for the developing hematopoietic cells. The matrix is responsible for maintaining differentiation and proliferation and provides a supporting tissue in the hematopoietic inductive microenvironment. Stromal cells in the matrix include several types: (1) endothelial cells, (2) adipocytes, (3) macrophages, (4) osteoblasts, (5) osteoclasts, and (6) reticular cells (fibroblasts). Endothelial cells are broad flat cells that form a single continuous layer along the inner surface of the bone marrow sinus.[15] They regulate the flow of particles entering and leaving hematopoietic spaces. Adipocytes are large cells with a single fat vacuole; they secrete various steroids that influence erythropoiesis and maintain bone

integrity.[14] They also play a role in regulating the volume of the marrow in which active hematopoiesis occurs.[14] Macrophages function in phagocytosis and secretion of various cytokines that regulate hematopoiesis and are located throughout the marrow space.[17] Other cells involved in cytokine production include endothelial cells, adipocytes, and fibroblasts. Osteoblasts are bone-forming cells, and osteoclasts are bone-resorbing cells. Reticular cells are associated with the formation of reticular fibers that form a lattice, which supports the vascular sinuses and developing hematopoietic cells. Stromal cells also are present, which are believed to be derived from fibroblasts. They play a role in support and regulation of hematopoietic stem/progenitor cell survival and differentiation.[15]

The extracellular matrix of the bone marrow contains proteoglycans or glycosaminoglycans, fibronectin, collagen, laminin, hemonectin, and thrombospondin.[15] Proteoglycans are expressed on the endothelial cell surface and mediate progenitor binding to the stroma. Fibronectin, collagen, laminin, hemonectin, and thrombospondin function as adhesion molecules, promoting the adhesion of HSCs to the extracellular matrix.

Liver

The liver plays a significant role in hematopoiesis beginning around the second trimester and serves as the major site of blood cell production during the hepatic stage of hematopoiesis. In adults, the liver has many cellular production functions, including synthesizing various transport proteins, storing essential minerals and vitamins that are used in DNA and RNA synthesis, conjugating bilirubin from Hb degradation, and transporting bilirubin to the small intestine for eventual excretion.

The liver consists of two lobes situated beneath the diaphragm in the abdominal cavity. The position of the liver with regard to the circulatory system is optimal for gathering, transferring, and eliminating substances via the bile.[18] Anatomically, the liver cells are arranged in radiating hepatic lobules emanating from a central vein (Fig.7-7). Adjacent to the longitudinal lobes of the liver and separated only by a small space are sinusoids, which are lined by two types of cells: Kupffer cells and epithelial cells. The Kupffer cells are macrophages, removing cellular and foreign debris from the blood that circulates through the liver; they also are responsible for protein synthesis.[20] The epithelial cells are arranged in the lining so as to be separated from one another by a noncellular area; this arrangement allows plasma to have direct access to the hepatocytes. This unusual organization of the liver and its location in the body enables it to be involved in many varied functions.

Pathophysiology

The liver is often involved in blood-related diseases. In porphyrias, the liver exhibits enzymatic deficiencies that result in the accumulation of the various intermediary porphyrins. In severe hemolytic anemias and red blood cell (RBC) dysplasias, the conjugation of bilirubin and the storage of iron are increased. The liver sequesters membrane-damaged RBCs

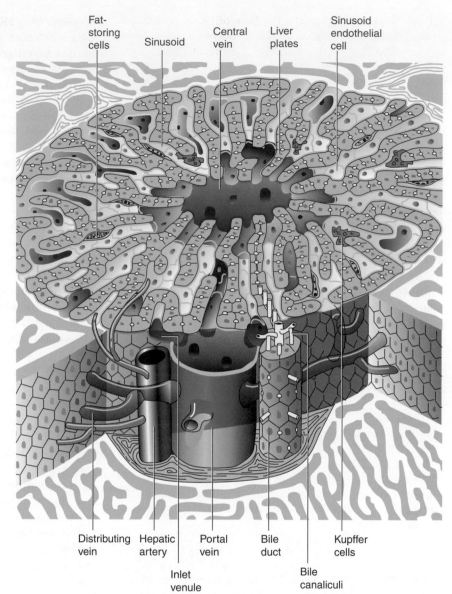

Figure 7-7 Three-dimensional schematic of the normal liver.

and removes them from the circulation. The liver is capable of extramedullary hematopoietic production in case of bone marrow shutdown.[14] It is directly affected by storage diseases of the monocyte/macrophage (Kupffer) cells as a result of enzymatic deficiencies that cause hepatomegaly with ultimate dysfunction of the liver (Gaucher, Niemann-Pick, Tay-Sachs diseases) (Chapter 28).

Spleen

The spleen is the largest lymphoid organ in the body. The spleen is located directly beneath the diaphragm behind the fundus of the stomach in the upper left quadrant of the abdomen. It is vital but not essential for life and functions as an indiscriminate filter of the circulating blood. In a healthy individual, the spleen contains about 350 mL of blood.[18]

The exterior surface of the spleen is surrounded by a layer of peritoneum and inwardly by a connective tissue capsule. The capsule projects inwardly, forming trabeculae that divide the

spleen into discrete regions. Located within these regions are three types of splenic tissue: (1) white pulp, (2) red pulp, and (3) a marginal zone. The white pulp consists of scattered follicles with germinal centers containing lymphocytes, macrophages, and dendritic cells. Aggregates of lymphocytes surround splenic arteries that pass through these germinal centers. Adjacent to the splenic arteries is a region called the *periarteriolar lymphatic sheath*. This area consists of lymphoid nodules containing primarily B lymphocytes. Activated B lymphocytes are found in the germinal centers.[20]

The marginal zone surrounds the white pulp and forms a reticular meshwork containing blood vessels, macrophages, and specialized B cells. The red pulp is composed primarily of vascular sinusoids and sinuses separated by cords of tissue (cords of Billroth) containing specialized macrophages that are loosely connected to the dendritic process, creating a spongelike region that functions as a filter for blood passing through the region.[20] As RBCs pass through the cords of

Billroth, there is a decrease in the flow of blood leading to stagnation and depletion of the RBCs' glucose supply. These cells are subject to increased damage and stress that may lead to their removal from the spleen. The spleen uses two methods for removing senescent RBCs from the circulation: (1) culling, whereby the cells are phagocytosed with subsequent degradation of cell organelles, and (2) pitting, whereby splenic macrophages remove inclusions or damaged surface membrane from the circulating RBCs. The spleen synthesizes immunoglobulin M (IgM) in the germinal centers, and it serves as a storage site for platelets. In a healthy individual, approximately 30% of the total platelet count is sequestered in the spleen.[21]

The spleen has a rich blood supply, receiving approximately 350 mL/min. Blood enters the spleen through the central splenic artery located at the hilum and branches outward through the trabeculae. The branches enter all three regions of the spleen: the white pulp with its dense accumulation of lymphocytes, the marginal zone, and the red pulp. The venous sinuses, which are located in the red pulp, unite and leave the spleen as splenic veins (Figs. 7-8 and 7-9).[22]

Pathophysiology

As blood enters the spleen, it may follow one of two routes. The first is a slow transit pathway through the red pulp in which the RBCs pass via a circuitous route through the macrophage-lined cords before reaching the sinuses. Plasma freely reaches the sinuses, but the RBCs have a more difficult time passing through the tiny openings created by the interendothelial junction of adjacent endothelial cells. The combination of the slow passage and the continued RBC metabolism creates an environment that is acidic, hypoglycemic, and hypoxic. The increased environmental stress on the RBCs circulating through the spleen leads to possible hemolysis of the erythrocytes. In the rapid transit pathway, blood cells enter the splenic artery and pass directly to the sinuses in the red pulp and continue to the venous system to exit the spleen. When splenomegaly occurs, the spleen becomes enlarged and is palpable. This occurs as a result of many conditions, such as chronic leukemias, genetically defective RBCs, hemoglobinopathies, Hodgkin disease, thalassemia, malaria, and the myeloproliferative disorders. Often splenectomy is beneficial in these cases of excessive destruction of

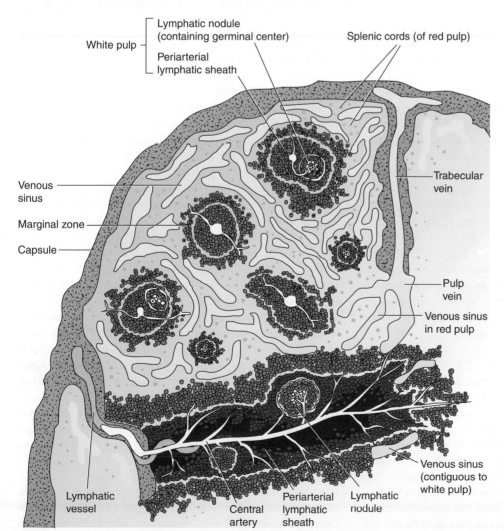

Figure **7-8** Schematic of normal spleen. (From Weiss L, Tavossoli M: Anatomical hazards to the passage of erythrocytes through the spleen. Semin Hematol 1970;7:372-380.)

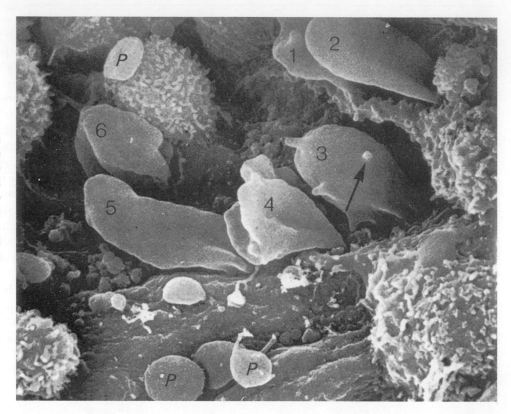

Figure 7-9 Scanning electron micrograph of spleen shows erythrocytes (numbered *1-6*) squeezing through the fenestrated wall in transit from the splenic cord to the sinus. The view shows the endothelial lining of the sinus wall, to which platelets *(P)* adhere, along with "hairy" white cells, probably macrophages. The *arrow* shows a protrusion on an RBC (×5000). (From Weiss L: A scanning electron microscopic study of the spleen. Blood 1974;43:665.)

RBCs, severe hereditary spherocytosis, storage disorders, and autoimmune hemolytic anemias when treatment with corticosteroids does not effectively suppress hemolysis.[23,24] Splenectomy also may be indicated in severe cases of agnogenic myeloid metaplasia associated with splenomegaly, severe refractory hemolytic anemia, thrombocytopenia, or qualitative platelet function defect syndromes.[23,24] After splenectomy, platelet and leukocyte counts increase transiently.[23] Repeated splenic infarcts caused by sickled RBCs trapped in the small vessel circulation of the spleen cause tissue damage and necrosis, often resulting in autosplenectomy (Chapter 26).

Hypersplenism is an enlargement of the spleen resulting in some degree of pancytopenia despite the presence of a hyperactive bone marrow. The most common cause is congestive splenomegaly secondary to cirrhosis of the liver and portal hypertension. Other causes include thrombosis, vascular stenosis, other vascular deformities such as aneurysm of the splenic artery, and cysts.[25]

Lymph Nodes

Lymph nodes are members of the lymphatic system located along the lymphatic capillaries that parallel, but are not part of, the circulatory system. They are bean-shaped structures (1-5 mm in diameter) and occur in groups or chains at various intervals along the lymphatic vessels. They may be superficially located (inguinal, axillary, cervical, supratrochlear) or deep (mesenteric, retroperitoneal). The afferent lymphatic vessels carry lymph to the lymph nodes. Lymph is the fluid portion resulting from blood that escapes into the connective tissue and is characterized by a low protein concentration and the absence of RBCs. Lymph circulates and is filtered by the lymph nodes and exits via the efferent lymphatic vessels located in the hilus of the lymph node.[26]

Similar in structure to the spleen, lymph nodes consist of an outer capsule that forms trabeculae and provides support for macrophages and the predominant population of lymphocytes. Lymph nodes can be divided into two basic regions: an outer region called the *cortex* and an inner region called the *medulla*. The trabeculae radiate through the cortex and the medulla, dividing the interior of the lymph node into specific areas (Fig. 7-10). In the cortical region, these areas are known as *cortical nodules* and contain follicles. These follicles contain foci of B cell proliferation termed *germinal centers*.[9,18] The cortical nodules are arranged in circles along the outer cortex region of the lymph node. Located between the cortex and the medulla is a region called the *paracortex*, which contains predominantly T cells and numerous macrophages. The medullary cords lie toward the interior of the lymph node. These cords consist primarily of B lymphocytes and plasma cells.[24] Lymph nodes have three main functions: (1) they play a role in the formation of new lymphocytes from the germinal centers; (2) they are involved in the processing of specific immunoglobulins; and (3) they are involved in the filtration of particulate matter, debris, and bacteria entering the lymph node via the lymph.

Pathophysiology

Lymph nodes, by their nature, are vulnerable to the same organisms that circulate through the tissue. Sometimes increased numbers of microorganisms enter the nodes, over-

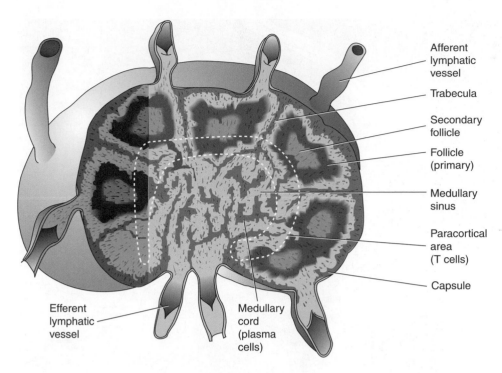

Afferent
lymphatic
vessel

Trabecula

Secondary
follicle

Follicle
(primary)

Medullary
sinus

Paracortical
area
(T cells)

Capsule

Efferent
lymphatic
vessel

Medullary
cord
(plasma
cells)

Figure 7-10 Histologic structure of a normal lymph node. The cortical layer is composed mainly of lymphatic nodules, whose germinal centers can be clearly seen.

whelming the macrophages and causing adenitis (infection of the lymph node). More serious is the frequent entry into the lymph nodes of malignant cells that have broken loose from malignant tumors. These malignant cells may establish new growths, which metastasize to other lymph nodes in the same group.

Thymus

To understand the role of the thymus in adults, certain formative intrauterine processes that affect function must be considered. First, the thymus tissue originates from endodermal and mesenchymal tissue. Second, the thymus is populated initially by lymphocytes from the yolk sac and the liver. This increased population of lymphoid cells physically pushes the epithelial cells of the thymus apart; however, their long processes remain attached to each other by desmosomes.

At birth, the thymus is an efficient, well-developed organ. It consists of two lobules, each measuring 0.5 to 2 cm in diameter. It is located in the upper part of the anterior mediastinum at about the level of the great vessels of the heart.[9,18] It resembles other lymphoid tissue in that the lobules are subdivided into two areas: the cortex (a peripheral zone) and the medulla (a central zone). Both areas are populated with the same cellular components—lymphocytes, mesenchymal cells, reticular cells, and many macrophages—although in different proportions. The cortex is characterized by a blood supply system that is unique in that it consists only of capillaries. Its function seems to be that of a "waiting zone," which is densely populated with progenitor lymphoid cells that migrated from the bone marrow. These cells have no identifiable surface markers when they enter the thymus but give rise to T cells that later express surface antigens and move

toward the medulla. Eventually, they leave the thymus to populate specific regions of other lymphoid tissue, such as the T cell–dependent areas of the spleen, lymph nodes, and other lymphoid tissues that are deficient in immunocompetent T lymphocytes (Fig. 7-11). It is theorized that the cytoplasmic processes of the epithelial reticular cells contain secretory products, thymic hormones, thymic factor, and thymic humoral hormones (protein/peptides extracted from the thymus), which promote differentiation of pre-T (nonmarked) from mature T lymphocytes. The cells that are not marked die in the cortex as a result of apoptosis and are phagocytosed by macrophages before release. The medulla contains only 5% mature T lymphocytes and seems to be a holding zone for conditioned cells until the cells are needed by the peripheral lymphoid tissues.[27] The thymus also contains myriad cell types, including B cells, dendritic cells, eosinophils, neutrophils, and myeloid cells.[20]

According to gross examination, the size of the thymus is related to age. At birth, the thymus weighs 12 to 15 g, increases at puberty to 30 to 40 g, and decreases at later ages to 10 to 15 g. It is hardly recognizable at old age, having atrophied (Fig. 7-12). The thymus retains the ability to produce new T cells, however, as has been shown after irradiation treatment that may accompany bone marrow transplantation.

Pathophysiology

Nondevelopment of the thymus during gestation results in the lack of formation of T lymphocytes. Related manifestations seen in patients with this condition involve failure to thrive, uncontrollable infections, and death in infancy. Adults with thymic disturbance are not affected because they have developed and maintained a pool of T lymphocytes for life.

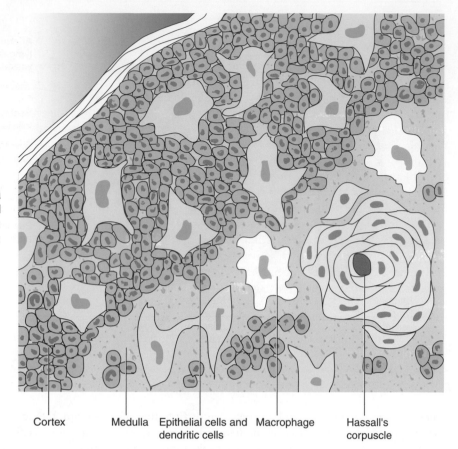

Figure 7-11 Schematic diagram of the edge of a lobule of the thymus, showing cells of the cortex and medulla. (From Abbas AK, Lichtman AH, Pober JS: Cellular and Molecular Immunology. Philadelphia: Saunders, 1991:25.)

Cortex   Medulla   Epithelial cells and dendritic cells   Macrophage   Hassall's corpuscle

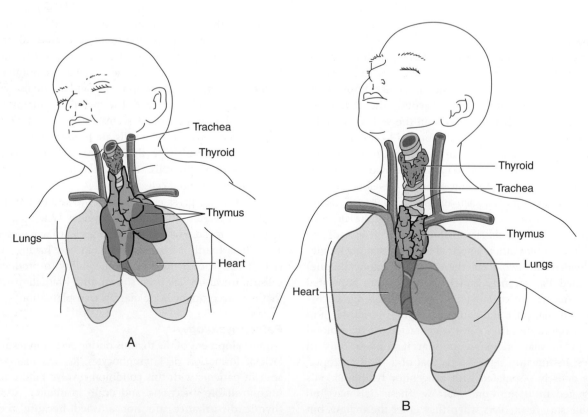

Figure 7-12 Differences in size of thymus of the infant **(A)** and the adult **(B)**.

STEM CELLS AND CYTOKINES

Stem Cell Theory

Hematopoiesis is a dynamic and complex developmental process of blood cell production. Blood cell production that occurs during the mesoblastic stage of development is referred to as *primitive hematopoiesis*, whereas *definitive hematopoiesis* begins during the fetal liver stage and continues through adult life.

In 1961 Till and McCulloch[25] conducted a series of experiments in which they irradiated spleens and bone marrows of mice, creating a state of aplasia. These aplastic mice were given an intravenous injection of marrow cells. Colonies of HSCs were seen 7 to 8 days later on the spleens of the irradiated (recipient) mice. These colonies were called *colony-forming unit spleen* (CFU-S). These investigators later showed that these colonies were capable of self-renewal and the production of differentiated progeny. The CFU-S represents what we now refer to as *committed myeloid progenitors* or CFU-GEMM.[28,29] These cells are capable of giving rise to multiple lineages of blood cells.

Morphologically unrecognizable hematopoietic progenitor cells can be divided into two major types: (1) noncommitted or undifferentiated stem cells and (2) multipotential and committed progenitor cells. These two groups give rise to all of the mature blood cells in the body. Originally there were two theories to the origin of hematopoietic progenitor cells. The monophyletic theory suggests that all blood cells are derived from a single progenitor stem cell called a *pluripotential stem cell*. The polyphyletic theory suggests that each of the blood cell lineages is derived from its own unique stem cell. The monophyletic theory is the most widely accepted theory among experimental hematologists today.

Stem cells by definition can be characterized as follows: (1) they are capable of self-renewal, (2) they give rise to differentiated progeny, and (3) they are able to reconstitute the hematopoietic system of a lethally irradiated host. The undifferentiated stem cells (HSCs) can differentiate into progenitor cells committed to either lymphoid or myeloid lineages. These lineage-specific progenitor cells consist of (1) the common lymphoid progenitor, which proliferates and differentiates into lymphocytes of T, B, and natural killer lineages, and (2) the common myeloid progenitor, which proliferates and differentiates into individual granulocytic, erythrocytic, monocytic, and megakaryocytic lineages. The resulting limited lineage-specific precursors give rise to morphologically recognizable, lineage-specific precursor cells (Fig. 7-13 and Table 7-1). Despite the limited numbers of HSCs in the bone marrow,

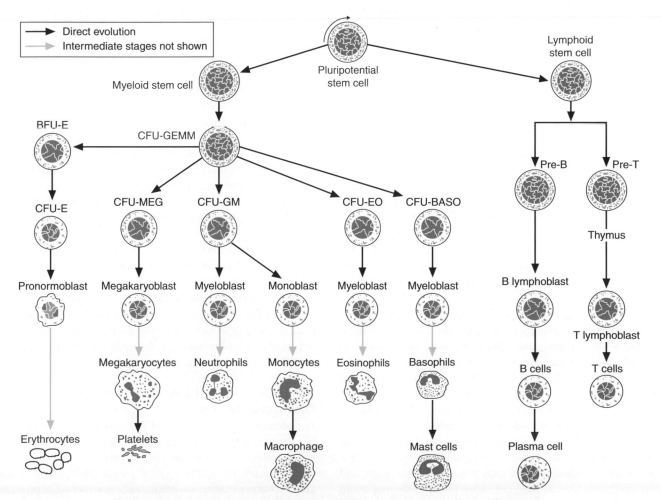

Figure 7-13 Diagram of hematopoiesis shows derivation of cells from the pluripotential stem cell.

TABLE 7-1 Culture-Derived Colony-Forming Units

Abbreviation	Cell Line
CFU-GEMM	Granulocyte, erythrocyte, megakaryocyte, monocyte
CFU-E	Erythrocyte
CFU-Meg	Megakaryocyte
CFU-M	Monocyte
CFU-GM	Granulocyte/monocyte
CFU-BASO	Myeloid to basophil
CFU-EO	Myeloid to eosinophil
CFU-G	Myeloid to neutrophil
CFU-pre-T	T lymphocyte
CFU-pre-B	B lymphocyte

more than 1 to 5×10^9 each of erythrocytes and leukocytes are produced each hour for the entire life span of an individual.[15] Most of the cells in normal bone marrow are precursor cells representing various stages of maturation.

HSCs are directed along one of three possible fates: (1) self-renewal, (2) differentiation, or (3) apoptosis.[30] When the HSC divides, it gives rise to two identical daughter cells. Both daughter cells may follow the path of differentiation leaving the stem cell pool (symmetric division), or one daughter cell may return to the stem cell pool and the other daughter cell may follow the path of differentiation (asymmetric division) or undergo apoptosis. Many theories have been proposed to describe the mechanisms that determine the fate of the stem cell. Till and McCulloch proposed that hematopoiesis was a random process whereby the HSCs randomly would commit to self-renewal or differentiation.[30] This model is also called the *stochastic* model of hematopoiesis. Later studies suggested that the microenvironment in the bone marrow determines whether the stem cell will self-renew or differentiate (*instructive* model of hematopoiesis).[30] Current thinking is that the ultimate decision made by the stem cell draws from the stochastic and instructive models of hematopoiesis. The initial decision to self-renew or differentiate is probably stochastic, whereas lineage differentiation that occurs later is determined by various signals from the hematopoietic inductive microenvironment in response to specific requirements from the body.

The multilineage priming model suggests that HSCs receive signals from the hematopoietic inductive microenvironment to amplify or repress genes associated with commitment to multiple lineages that are expressed only at low levels. The implication is that the cell's fate is determined by intrinsic and extrinsic factors. Extrinsic regulation involves proliferation and differentiation signals from specialized niches located in the hematopoietic inductive microenvironment via direct cell-to-cell or cell-extracellular signaling molecules.[30] Some of the cytokines released from the hematopoietic inductive microenvironment include factors that regulate proliferation and differentiation, such as stem cell factor (SCF), thrombopoietin (TPO), and Flt3 ligand. Intrinsic regulation involves genes such

as *SCL (TAL1)*, which is expressed in cells in the hemangioblast, a bipotential progenitor cell of mesodermal origin that gives rise to hematopoietic and endothelial lineages, and *GATA2*, which is expressed in later-appearing HSCs. Both of these genes are essential for primitive and definitive hematopoiesis.[30] In addition to factors involved in differentiation and regulation, there are regulatory signaling factors, such as Notch-1 and Notch-2, which allow HSCs to respond to hematopoietic inductive microenvironment factors, altering cell fate.[31]

As hematopoietic cells differentiate, they take on various morphologic features associated with maturation. These include an overall decrease in cell size and a decrease in the nuclear-to-cytoplasmic ratio. Additional changes that occur during maturation occur in the cytoplasm and nucleus. Changes occurring in the nucleus include (1) loss of nucleoli, (2) decrease in size of nucleus, (3) condensation of chromatin, (4) possible change in shape of the nucleus, and (5) possible loss of the nucleus. Changes occurring in the cytoplasm include (1) decrease in basophilia, (2) increase in the proportion of cytoplasm, and (3) possible appearance of granules in the cytoplasm. Specific changes of each lineage are discussed in subsequent chapters.

Stem Cell Cycle Kinetics

It has been estimated that the bone marrow is capable of producing approximately 3 billion erythrocytes, 2.5 billion platelets, and 1.5 billion granulocytes per kilogram of body weight daily. The determining factor controlling the rate of production is physiologic need. Stem cells exist in the marrow in the ratio of 1:1000 nucleated blood cells. Stem cells are capable of many mitotic divisions when stimulated by appropriate cytokines. When mitosis has occurred, the cell may reenter the cycle or go into a resting phase, termed G_0. Some cells from the resting phase reenter the active cell cycle and divide one additional time, whereas other cells are directed to terminal differentiation (Fig. 7-14).

From these data, a mitotic index can be calculated to establish the percentage of cells in mitosis in relation to the total number of cells. Factors affecting the mitotic index include the duration of mitosis and the length of the resting state. Normally, the mitotic index is approximately 1% to 2%. An increased mitotic index implies increased proliferation. An exception to this rule is in the case of megaloblastic anemia, when mitosis is prolonged.[32] An understanding of the mechanism of the generative cycle aids in understanding the mode of action of specific drugs used in the treatment and maintenance of proliferative disorders.

Stem Cell Phenotypic and Functional Characterization

The identification and origin of stem cells can be determined by immunophenotypic analysis using flow cytometry. The earliest identifiable human HSC capable of initiating long-term cultures are CD34+, CD38−, HLA-DR^{low}, Thy$_1$^{low}, and Lin−.[31] This population of marrow cells is enriched in primitive progenitors. The expression of CD38 and HLA-DR is associated

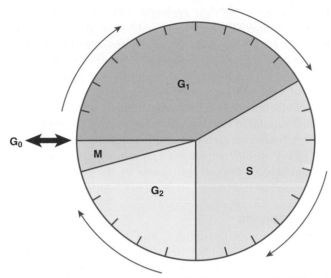

Figure 7-14 Cell cycle schematic. *G0*, Resting stage; *G1*, RNA and protein synthesis; *S*, DNA synthesis; *G2*, premitotic phase; *M*, mitosis.

with a loss of "stemness." The acquisition of CD33 and CD38 is seen on committed myeloid progenitors,[31] and the expression of CD10 and CD38 is seen on committed lymphoid progenitors.[31] The expression of CD7 is seen on T lymphoid progenitor cells and natural killer cells, and the expression of CD19 is seen on B lymphoid progenitors[31] (Chapter 33).

Functional characterization of HSC can be accomplished through in vitro techniques using long-term culture assays. These involve the enumeration of colony-forming units (e.g., CFU-GEMM, CFU-GM, BFU-E) on semisolid media, such as methylcellulose. Primitive progenitor cells, such as the high proliferative potential colony-forming cell and the long-term colony initiating cell, also have been identified. These hematopoietic precursor cells give rise to colonies that can survive for 5 to 8 weeks and be replated.[31] In vivo functional assays also are available and require transplanting cells into syngeneic, lethally irradiated animals followed by transferring the engrafted bone marrow cells to a secondary recipient.[31] These systems allow for the characterization of the ability of the stem cells to proliferate and differentiate and may serve as models for developing clinically applicable techniques for gene therapy and stem cell transplantation.

Cytokines and Growth Factors

A group of specific glycoproteins called *hematopoietic growth factors* or *cytokines* regulates the proliferation, differentiation, and maturation of hematopoietic precursor cells. Cytokines are a diverse group of soluble proteins that have direct and indirect effects on hematopoietic cells. Classification of cytokines has been difficult because of overlapping and redundant properties that they share. The terms *cytokines* and *growth factors* are often used synonymously; cytokines include interleukins (ILs), lymphokines, monokines, interferons, chemokines, and colony-stimulating factors (CSFs).[33] Cytokines are responsible for stimulation or inhibition of production, differentiation, and

trafficking of mature blood cells and their precursors.[34] Many of these cytokines exert a positive influence on stem cells and progenitor cells with multilineage potential (e.g., IL-1, IL-3, IL-6, IL-9, IL-11, GM-CSF, and kit ligand).[34] Cytokines that exert a negative influence on hematopoiesis include transforming growth factor-β, tumor necrosis factor-α, and the interferons.[31]

Hematopoietic precursor cells require growth factors on a continual basis for their growth and survival. Growth factors prevent hematopoietic precursor cells from dying by inhibiting apoptosis (or programmed cell death); they stimulate them to divide by decreasing the transit time from G_0 to G_1 of the cell cycle; and they regulate cell differentiation into the various cell lineages. *Apoptosis* refers to programmed cell death, a normal physiologic process that eliminates unwanted, abnormal, or harmful cells. Apoptosis differs from necrosis, which is accidental death from trauma. When cells do not receive the appropriate cytokines necessary to prevent cell death, apoptosis is initiated. In some disease states, apoptosis is "turned on," resulting in early cell death, or the mechanisms involved in apoptosis fail to initiate this process, allowing uncontrolled proliferation of cells.[34,35]

Research has accomplished the purification of many of these cytokines and the cloning of pure recombinant growth factors, some of which are discussed in detail in the appropriate section of this chapter. The number of growth factors recognized has expanded greatly in recent years and will further increase as research continues. This chapter focuses primarily on CSFs, kit ligand, Flt3 ligand, IL-3, and IL-6. A detailed discussion is beyond the scope of this text, and the reader is encouraged to consult current literature for further details.

Colony-Stimulating Factors

CSFs are produced by many different cells. They have a high specificity for their target cells and are active at low concentrations.[33] The names of the individual factors indicate the predominant cell lines that respond to their presence: The primary target of G-CSF is the granulocyte, and GM-CSF targets the granulocyte/monocyte cell line. The biologic activity of CSFs was first identified by their ability to induce hematopoietic colony formation in semisolid media. In addition, it was shown in cell culture experiments that although a particular CSF may show specificity for one cell lineage, it is often capable of influencing other cell lineages as well. This is particularly true when multiple growth factors are combined.[36] Although G-CSF stimulates the proliferation of granulocyte progenitors, it also works synergistically with IL-3 to enhance megakaryocyte colony formation.[36]

Stem Cell Factor, Flt3 Ligand, Granulocyte/Monocyte Colony-Stimulating Factor, Interleukin-3, and Interleukin-6

Ogawa[37] described early-acting growth factors (multilineage), intermediate-acting growth factors (multilineage), and late-acting growth factors (lineage-restricted). Kit ligand, also known as *SCF*, is an early-acting growth factor; its cell surface receptor is the product of the *c-kit* gene. *c-kit* is a type I tyrosine kinase receptor that is expressed on HSCs and is down-regulated with differentiation. The binding of SCF to its receptor (*c-kit*) induces a series of signals that are sent via signal transduction pathways from the cytoplasmic receptor of the HSC to the nucleus of the HSC, stimulating the cell to proliferate. As HSCs differentiate and mature, the expression of c-kit decreases. Activation of kit ligand by SCF is essential in the early stages of hematopoiesis.[34,38] Flt3 seems to act at an even earlier stage of HSC development than SCF. Flt3 stands for *c-fms*–like tyrosine kinase.[39] SCF and Flt3 work synergistically with IL-3, G-CSF, and GM-CSF to promote early HSC proliferation.

Other early-acting CSFs that are multilineage include IL-3, GM-CSF, and IL-6. IL-3 regulates blood cell production by controlling the production, differentiation, and function of granulocytes and macrophages.[40] GM-CSF induces expression of specific genes and stimulates hematopoietic stem cell proliferation, differentiation, and functional activation.[41] IL-6 is a pleiotropic growth factor with stimulatory effects on myeloid and lymphoid cell lineages.[42]

Interleukins

Cytokines originally were named according to their specific function, such as lymphocyte-activating factor (now called *IL-1*), but continued research showed that a particular cytokine may have multiple activities. A group of scientists began calling some of the cytokines *interleukins*, numbering them in the order in which they were identified (e.g., IL-1, IL-2). Figure 7-15 illustrates the hematopoietic system and the sites of action of some of the cytokines. These factors are discussed in more detail in subsequent chapters. Characteristics shared by interleukins include the following:

1. Proteins that exhibit multiple biologic activities, such as the regulation of autoimmune and inflammatory reactions and hematopoiesis
2. Synergistic interactions with other cytokines and growth factors
3. Interacting systems with amplification potential
4. Effective at very low concentrations

Table 7-2 lists the sources of cytokines and sites of activity.

LINEAGE-SPECIFIC HEMATOPOIESIS

Erythropoiesis

Erythropoiesis occurs in the bone marrow and is a complex, regulated process for maintaining adequate numbers of erythrocytes in the peripheral blood. The CFU-GEMM gives rise to the earliest identifiable colony of RBCs, called the *burst-forming unit–erythroid* (BFU-E). The BFU-E produces a large multiclustered colony that resembles a cluster of grapes containing brightly colored Hb. These colonies range in size from a single large cluster to 16 or more clusters. BFU-Es contain only a few receptors for EPO, and their cell cycle activity is not influenced significantly by the presence of exogenous EPO. BFU-Es under the influence of IL-3, GM-CSF, TPO, and kit

ligand develop into CFU erythroid (CFU-E) colonies.[29] The CFU-E has many EPO receptors and has an absolute requirement for EPO. Some CFU-Es are responsive to low levels of EPO and do not have the proliferative capacity of the BFU-E.[43]

EPO is a lineage-specific glycoprotein that prevents apoptosis of erythroid precursors. EPO is produced in the renal peritubular interstitial cells or renal tubular cells.[43] In addition, a small amount of EPO is produced by the liver.[38] EPO induces Hb synthesis and serves as a differentiation factor causing the CFU-E to differentiate into pronormoblasts, the earliest recognizable erythrocyte precursors in the bone marrow.[44] Erythropoiesis is discussed in detail in Chapter 8.

Leukopoiesis

Leukopoiesis can be divided into two major categories: myelopoiesis and lymphopoiesis. Factors that promote differentiation from the CFU-GEMM into neutrophils, monocytes, eosinophils, and basophils include GM-CSF, G-CSF, monocyte CSF (M-CSF), IL-3, IL-5, IL-11, and kit ligand. GM-CSF stimulates the proliferation and differentiation of neutrophil and macrophage colonies from the CFU-GM. G-CSF and M-CSF stimulate neutrophil differentiation and monocyte differentiation from the CFU-G and CFU-M.[43] IL-3 is a multilineage stimulating factor that stimulates the growth of granulocytes, monocytes, megakaryocytes, and erythroid cells. Eosinophils require GM-CSF, IL-5, and IL-3 for differentiation. The requirements for basophil differentiation are less clear but seem to depend on the presence of IL-3 and kit ligand. Growth factors promoting lymphoid differentiation include IL-2, IL-7, IL-12, and IL-15 and to some extent IL-4, IL-10, IL-13, IL-14, and IL-16.[39] Leukopoiesis is discussed further in Chapter 12.

Megakaryopoiesis

Earlier influences on megakaryopoiesis include GM-CSF, IL-3, IL-6, IL-11, kit ligand, and EPO.[34] The stimulating hormonal factor, TPO (also known as *mpl ligand*), along with IL-11, controls the production and release of platelets. The liver is the main site of production of TPO.[45,46] Megakaryopoiesis is discussed in Chapter 13.

ANALYTICAL AND THERAPEUTIC APPLICATIONS

Clinical use of growth factors approved by the U.S. Food and Drug Administration has contributed numerous options in the treatment of hematologic malignancies and solid tumors. In addition, growth factors can be used as priming agents to increase the yield of HSCs during apheresis for transplantation protocols. Advances in molecular biology have resulted in cloning of the genes that are responsible for the synthesis of various growth factors and the recombinant production of large quantities of these proteins. Table 7-3 is a concise overview of some growth factors, physiologic roles, and applications. Many more examples can be found in the literature.

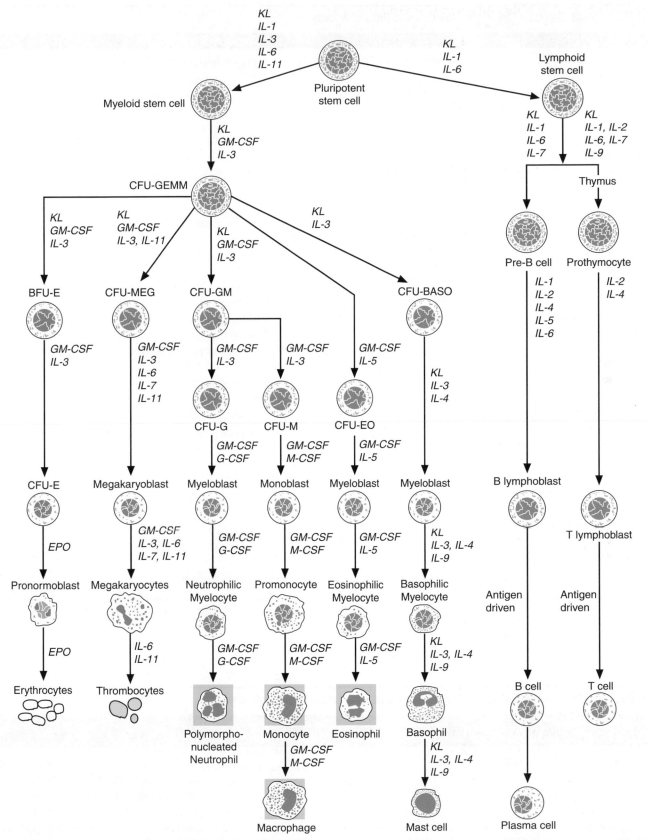

Figure 7-15 Diagram of derivation of hematopoietic cells, illustrating sites of activity of CSFs and ILs. (From Novartis Corporation, Summit, NJ, and Schering-Plough, Ltd., Lucerne, Switzerland.)

TABLE 7-2 Selected Cytokines, Sources, and Sites of Activity

Cytokine	Source	Target or Site of Activity
IL-1 (α and β)	Mono/macro, endothelial cells, fibroblasts, epithelial cells	Fibroblasts, endothelial cells, basophils
IL-2	T cells	T, B, and NK cells
IL-3	T cells, mono/macro, mast cells	Macrophages, neutrophils, eosinophils, basophils, mast cells, megakaryocytes, T and B cells
IL-4	T cells, B cells, macrophages, basophils, mast cells	Macrophages, myeloid progenitors, T and B cells, mast cells, fibroblasts
IL-5	T cells	T and B cells, eosinophils
IL-6	Mono/macro, endothelial, T cells, fibroblasts, osteoblasts	Fibroblasts, myeloid precursors, T and B cells, hepatocytes, megakaryocytes
IL-7	BM stromal cells, spleen, thymus	Pre-B cells, early T cells, CLL, Sézary cells, ALL
IL-8	Mono/macro, fibroblasts, neutrophils, endothelial cells, synovial cells, chondrocytes	Chemoattractant for neutrophils, T cells, eosinophils
IL-9	T cells	T cells, macrophages, mast cells
IL-10	T and B cells, macrophages	Lymphoid and myeloid cells
IL-11	BM stromal cells, fibroblasts	Progenitor cells and stromal cells
IL-12	Macrophages	T, NK cells
IL-13	T cells, basophils, stromal cells	Monocytes, B cells
IL-14	T cells, T and B lymphoma cells	Pre-B, T, NK cells
IL-15	Mono/macro, epithelial cells, skeletal muscle cells, BM and thymic stromal cells	T, B, and NK cells, mast cells
IL-16	CD8+ T cells, mast cells	T and B cells
IL-17	CD4+ cells	Macrophages
IL-18	Mono/macro, liver	Tumor cells, pathogens
G-CSF	Endothelial cells, placenta, mono/macro, fibroblasts	All granulocytes, macrophages, endothelial cells, fibroblasts, leukemic myeloblasts
M-CSF	B and T cells, endothelial cells, mono/macro, fibroblasts, epithelial cells, osteoblasts	Mono/macro, osteoblasts
GM-CSF	B, T, and NK cells, osteoblasts, endothelial cells, fibroblasts, mono/macro	All granulocytes, megakaryocytes, stem cells, BFU-E, mono/macro, leukemic myeloblasts
EPO (erythropoietin)	Kidney, liver	BFU-E, CFU-E
TPO (thrombopoietin; mpl ligand)	Kidney, liver, spleen, BM stroma, muscle, brain	Megakaryocytes, platelets, c-*mpl* +blasts
c-*kit* ligand	Fibroblasts, BM stroma, hepatocytes	Primitive progenitors

ALL, Acute lymphocytic leukemia; *BFU-E,* blast-forming units–erythroid; *BM,* bone marrow; *CFU-E,* colony-forming units–erythroid; *CLL,* chronic lymphocytic leukemia; *mono/macro,* monocytes/macrophages; *NK,* natural killer.
Compiled from a variety of sources, including references 33, 34, and 47.

TABLE 7-3 Selected Cytokines, Physiologic Roles, and Examples of Applications

Cytokine	Physiologic Roles			Example
	Autoimmunity	Inflammation	Hematopoiesis	
IL-1	X	X	X	Used in cases of inflammation, such as fever, and as a defense mechanism during infection[48]
IL-2	X	X	X	Enhances migration of cells with antitumor activity into tissues; induces release of IL-6, tumor necrosis factor, and interferon, which may have antitumor effects[49]
IL-3	X	X	X	Used in the treatment of refractory anemia with and without ringed sideroblasts; also used to stimulate megakaryopoiesis[50]

TABLE 7-3 Selected Cytokines, Physiologic Roles, and Examples of Applications—cont'd

Cytokine	Physiologic Roles			Example
	Autoimmunity	Inflammation	Hematopoiesis	
IL-4	X	X	X	Used to potentiate antitumor activity, especially in cases of gastric carcinoma[51]
IL-5	X	X	X	
IL-6	X	X	X	Used in the treatment of acute myeloid leukemia; has been found to initiate increases and suppression of blast cells[52]
IL-7	X	X	X	Enhances allocytolytic activity of lymphokine-activated killer cells[63]; is considered to be a promoter of thymopoiesis and immune recovery[54]
IL-8	X	X	X	Active in neutrophil chemotaxis and degranulation; acts as a principal mediator of inflammation that then can be acted on by IL-4[55]
IL-9		X	X	Potent lymphoid cell factor, stimulating growth of certain T cells and mast cells[56,57]
IL-10	X	X	X	Synergistic activity of IL-4 and IL-10 causes anti-inflammatory effect on human placental cells in vitro[58]
IL-11			X	Has shown activity in preclinical studies in association with myelosuppression, cancer therapy, neutropenia, and thrombocytopenia[59]; stimulates the growth and survivability of certain B and T cells[61]
IL-12	X	X	X	Used in stimulating proliferation of peripheral blood mononuclear cells and tumor-infiltrating lymphocytes in melanoma patients[61]; capable of reversing the immunosuppression mediated by the neoplastic agent paclitaxel[62]
IL-13	X		X	
IL-14	X			
IL-15	X		X	
IL-16	X			
IL-17	X	X	X	May be useful for further delineating mechanisms of G-CSF regulation[63]
IL-18	X			
G-CSF		X	X	
M-CSF		X	X	
GM-CSF		X	X	
EPO		X	X	
TPO			X	
c-*kit* ligand		X	X	

CHAPTER at a GLANCE

- Hematopoiesis is the formation, development, and specialization of all functional blood cells.
- Phases of hematopoiesis progress through mesoblastic, hepatic, and medullary.
- Organs that function at some point in hematopoiesis include the liver, spleen, lymph nodes, thymus, and bone marrow.

- The bone marrow is the primary site of hematopoiesis at birth and throughout life.
- In certain situations, blood cell production may occur outside the bone marrow; such production is termed *extramedullary*.
- The microenvironment in the bone marrow is essential for stem cell differentiation and proliferation.

CHAPTER at a GLANCE—cont'd

- Monophyletic theory suggests that all blood cells arise from a common progenitor.
- As cells mature, certain morphologic characteristics of maturation allow specific lineages to be recognized. General characteristics of maturation include decrease in cell size, decrease in nuclear size, loss of nucleoli, condensation of nuclear chromatin, and decreased basophilia in cytoplasm. Some morphologic changes are unique to specific lineages (e.g., loss of nucleus in RBCs).
- Cytokines and growth factors play a major role in determining differentiation of stem cells.

- Cytokines include ILs, CSFs, interferons, and others.
- Some cytokines exert influence on stem cells with multilineage potential, some are lineage specific, and some function only in combination with other cytokines.
- Cytokines are necessary to prevent premature apoptosis.
- Cytokines have contributed new options in the treatment of bone marrow malignancies, leukemias, and aplastic anemias.

REVIEW QUESTIONS

1. The process of formation and development of blood cells is termed:
   a. Hematopoiesis
   b. Hematemesis
   c. Hematocytometry
   d. Hematorrhea

2. During midfetal life, the primary source of blood cells is the:
   a. Bone marrow
   b. Spleen
   c. Lymph nodes
   d. Liver

3. Which of the following organs is responsible for the conditioning of T lymphocytes?
   a. Spleen
   b. Liver
   c. Thymus
   d. Bone marrow

4. The best source of active bone marrow from a 20-year-old would be:
   a. Iliac crest (hip)
   b. Femur (thigh)
   c. Distal radius (forearm)
   d. Tibia (shin)

5. Physiologic programmed cell death is termed:
   a. Angiogenesis
   b. Apoptosis
   c. Aneurysm
   d. Apohematics

6. Which organ is the site of sequestration of platelets?
   a. Liver
   b. Thymus
   c. Spleen
   d. Bone marrow

7. The earliest hematopoietic cell is termed a:
   a. Prehematopoietic blast
   b. Pluripotential stem cell
   c. CFU-GEMM
   d. Cytokinetic precursor

8. Which of the following cells is *not* a product of the CFU-GEMM?
   a. Megakaryocyte
   b. Lymphocyte
   c. Erythrocyte
   d. Granulocyte

9. Which of the following hematopoietic growth factors is produced in the kidney?
   a. EPO
   b. TPO
   c. GM-CSF
   d. M-CSF

10. A multilineage cytokine among the ILs is:
    a. IL-1
    b. IL-2
    c. IL-3
    d. IL-4

REFERENCES

1. Marcos MA, Godlin I, Cumano A, et al: Developmental events from hemopoietic stem cells to B-cell populations and Ig repertoires. Immunol Rev 1994;137:155-171.
2. Leung AYH, Verfaillie CM: Stem cell model of hematopoiesis. In Hoffman R, Benz EJ, Shattil SJ, et al (eds): Hematology Basic Principles and Practice, 4th ed. New York: Churchill Livingstone, 2005:200-213.
3. Peault B: Hematopoietic stem cell emergence in embryonic life: developmental hematology revisited. J Hematother 1996;5:369-378.
4. Tavian M, Coulombel L, Luton D, et al: Aorta-associated CD34+ hematopoietic cells in the early human embryo. Blood 1996;87:67-72.
5. Charbord P, Tavian M, Coulombel L, et al: Early ontogeny of the human hematopoietic system [abstract] (in French). C R Seances Soc Biol Fil 1995;189:601-609.
6. Dieterlen-Lievre F, Godin I, Pardanaud I: Where do hematopoietic stem cells come from? Arch Allergy Immunol 1997;112:3-8.
7. Chang Y, Paige CJ, Wu GE: Enumeration and characterization

of DJH structures in mouse fetal liver. EMBO J 1992;11:1891-1899.

8. Gallicchio VS: Hematopoiesis and review of genetics. In Steine-Martin EA, Lotspeich-Steininger CA, Koepke JA (eds): Clinical Hematology: Principles, Procedures, Correlations, 2nd ed. Philadelphia: JB Lippincott, 1998:46-56.

9. Junqueira LC, Cameiro J, Kelley RO: Basic Histology, 10th ed. Stamford, CT: Appleton & Lange, 2002.

10. Bevelander G, Ramaley JA: Essentials of Histology, 8th ed. St Louis: Mosby, 1979.

11. Segel G, Palis J: Hematology of the Newborn. In Beutler E, Lichtman M, Coller B, et al (eds): Williams Hematology, 6th ed. New York: McGraw-Hill, 2001:67-75.

12. Warren J, Ward P: The inflammatory response. In Beutler E, Lichtman M, Coller B, et al (eds): Williams Hematology, 6th ed. New York: McGraw-Hill, 2001:67-75.

13. Abboud C, Lichtman MA: Structure of the marrow and the hematopoietic environment. In Beutler E, Lichtman M, Coller B, et al (eds): Williams Hematology, 6th ed. New York: McGraw-Hill, 2001:29-58.

14. Schlueter AI: Structure and function of hematopoietic organs. In McKenzie SB (ed): Clinical Laboratory Hematology, 1st ed. Upper Saddle River, NJ: Prentice Hall, 2004:41-51.

15. Gupta P, Blazar B, Gupta K, et al: Human CD34+ bone marrow cells regulate stromal production of interleukin-6 and granulocyte colony-stimulating factor and increase the colony-stimulating activity of stroma. Blood 1998:91:3724-3733.

16. Klein G: The extracellular matrix of the hematopoietic microenvironment. Experientia 1995;51:914-926.

17. Sadahira Y, Mori M: Role of the macrophage in erythropoiesis. Pathol Int 1999;10:841-848.

18. Thibodeau GA, Patton KT: Anatomy and Physiology, 5th ed. St Louis: Mosby, 2003.

19. Aster JC: Diseases of white blood cells, lymph nodes, spleen, and thymus. In Kumar V, Abbas AK, Fausto N, (eds): Robbins and Cotran Pathologic Basis of Disease, 7th ed. Philadelphia: Elsevier, 2005:662-709.

20. Weinberg JB: Mononuclear phagocytes. In Greer JP, Foerster J, Lukens J, et al (eds): Wintrobe's Clinical Hematology, 11th ed. Philadelphia: Lippincott Williams & Wilkins, 2004:349-386.

21. Warkentin TE, Kelton JG: Thrombocytopenia due to platelet destruction and hypersplenism. In Hoffman R, Benz EJ, Shattil SJ, et al (eds): Hematology Basic Principles and Practice, 4th ed. New York: Churchill Livingstone, 2005:2305-2327.

22. Seeley RR, Stephens D, Tate P: Anatomy and Physiology, 3rd ed. St Louis: Mosby, 1995.

23. Shurin SB: The spleen and its disorders. In Hoffman R, Benz EJ, Shattil SJ, et al (eds): Hematology Basic Principles and Practice, 4th ed. New York: Churchill Livingstone, 2005:901-909.

24. Ware RE: The autoimmune hemolytic anemias. In Nathan DG, Orkin SH (eds): Nathan and Oski's Hematology of Infancy and Childhood, 6th ed. Philadelphia: Saunders, 2003:522-526.

25. Goodman J, Newman M, Chapman W: Disorders of the spleen. In Greer JP, Foerster J, Lukens J, et al (eds): Wintrobe's Clinical Hematology, 11th ed. Philadelphia: Lippincott Williams & Wilkins, 2004:1893-1909.

26. Kipps TJ: The lymphoid tissues. In Beutler E, Lichtman M, Coller B, et al (eds): Williams Hematology, 6th ed. New York: McGraw-Hill, 2001:59-66.

27. Paraskevas F: T lymphocytes and NK cells. In Greer JP, Foerster J, Lukens J, et al (eds): Wintrobe's Clinical Hematology, 11th ed. Philadelphia: Lippincott Williams & Wilkins, 2004:409-438.

28. Till TE, McCulloch EA: A direct measurement of the radiation sensitivity of normal mouse marrow cells. Radiat Res 1961;14:213.

29. Dessypris EN: Erythropoiesis. In Greer JP, Foerster J, Lukens J, et al (eds): Wintrobe's Clinical Hematology, 11th ed. Philadelphia: Lippincott Williams & Wilkins, 2004:195-216.

30. Dao M, Verfaillie CM: Bone marrow microenvironment. In Hoffman R, Benz EJ, Shattil SJ, et al (eds): Hematology Basic Principles and Practice, 4th ed. New York: Churchill Livingstone, 2005:215-231.

31. Verfaillie C: Regulation of hematopoiesis. In Wickramasinghe SN, McCullough J (eds): Blood and Bone Marrow Pathology. New York: Churchill Livingstone, 2003:71-85.

32. Antony A: Megaloblastic anemias. In Hoffman R, Benz EJ, Shattil SJ, et al (eds): Hematology Basic Principles and Practice, 4th ed. New York: Churchill Livingstone, 2005:519-556.

33. COPE: Cytokines Online Pathfinder Encyclopaedia, Horst Ibelfauft's Hypertext Information Universe of Cytokines, version 4.0 (August 1999). Available at: www.copewithcytokines.de. Accessed April 20, 2005.

34. Davey FR, Hutchinson RE: Hematopoiesis. In Henry JB (ed): Clinical Diagnosis and Management by Laboratory Methods, 20th ed. Philadelphia: Saunders, 2001:520-541.

35. Golub TR, Gillialand DG: The molecular biology of hematologic malignancies. In Nathan DG, Orkin SH (eds): Nathan and Oski's Hematology of Infancy and Childhood, 6th ed. Philadelphia: Saunders, 2003:1092-1146.

36. Clark S, Nathan DG, Sieff C: The anatomy and physiology of hematopoiesis. In Nathan DG, Orkin SH (eds): Nathan and Oski's Hematology of Infancy and Childhood, 6th ed. Philadelphia: Saunders, 2003:1219-1258.

37. Ogawa M: Differentiation and proliferation of hematopoietic stem cells. Blood 1993;81:2844-2853.

38. Bondurant MC, Koury MJ: Origin and development of blood cells. In Greer JP, Foerster J, Lukens J, et al (eds): Wintrobe's Clinical Hematology, 11th ed. Philadelphia: Lippincott Williams & Wilkins, 2004:169-193.

39. Shaheen M, Broxmeyer H: The humoral regulation of hematopoiesis. In Hoffman R, Benz EJ, Shattil SJ, et al (eds): Hematology Basic Principles and Practice, 4th ed. New York: Churchill Livingstone, 2005:233-265.

40. Dorssers L, Burger H, Bot F, et al: Characterization of a human multilineage–colony-stimulating factor cDNA clone identified by a conserved noncoding sequence in mouse interleukin-3. Gene 1987;55:115-124.

41. Lin EY, Orlofsky A, Berger MS, et al: Characterization of A1, a novel hemopoietic-specific early-response gene with sequence similarity to bcl-s. J Immunol 1993;151:1979-1988.

42. Kopf M, Ramsay A, Brombacher F, et al: Peliotropic defects of IL-6 deficient mice including early hematopoiesis, T and B cell function, and acute-phase responses. Ann NY Acad Sci 1995;762:308-318.

43. Quesenberry PJ, Colvin GA: Hematopoietic stem cells, progenitor cells, and cytokines. In Beutler E, Lichtman MA, Coller BS, et al (eds): Williams Hematology, 6th ed. New York: McGraw-Hill, 2001:153-174.

44. Sawada K, Krantz SB, Dai CH: Purification of human burst-forming units–erythroid and demonstration of the evolution of erythropoietin receptors. J Cell Physiol 1990;142:219-230.

45. Wolber EM, Ganschow R, Burdelski M, et al: Hepatic thrombopoietin mRNA levels in acute and chronic liver failure of childhood. Hepatology 1999;29:1739-1742.

46. Wolber EM, Dame C, Fahnenstich H, et al: Expression of the thrombopoietin gene in human fetal and neonatal tissues. Blood 1999;94:97-105.

47. Dinauer MC: The phagocyte system and disorders of granulopoiesis and granulocyte function. In Nathan DG, Orkin SH (eds): Nathan and Oski's Hematology of Infancy and Childhood, 6th ed. Philadelphia: Saunders, 2003:923-1010.

48. Scales WE: Structure and function of interleukin-1. In Kunkel SL, Remick DG (eds): Cytokines in Health and Disease. New York: Marcel Dekker, 1992:15-26.

49. Rosenberg SA, Lotze MT, Muul LM, et al: A progress report of the treatment of 157 patients with advanced cancer using lymphokine-activated cells and IL-2 or high dose IL-2 alone. N Engl J Med 1987;316:889-987.

50. Vrhovac R, Kusee R, Jaksic B: Myeloid hematopoietic growth factor. Int J Clin Pharmacol 1988;31:241-252.

51. Morisake T, Yuzuki D, Lin R, et al: Interleukin-4 receptor expression and growth inhibition of gastric carcinoma cells by interleukin-4. Cancer Res 1991;52:6059-6060.

52. Susuki T, Morio T, Tohida S, et al: Effects of interleukin-6 and granulocytic colony-stimulating factor on the proliferation of leukemia blast progenitors from acute myeloblastic leukemia patients. Jpn J Cancer Res 1990;81:979-986.

53. Lotze MT: T-cell growth factors and the treatment of patients with cancer. Clin Immunol Immunopathol 1992;62:2663-2670.

54. Malave I, Vethencourt MA, Chacon R, et al: Production of interleukin-6 in cultures of peripheral blood mononuclear cells from children with primary protein-calorie malnutrition and from eutrophic controls. Ann Nutr Metab 1998;42:266-273.

55. Schroder IM: Peptides and cytokines. Arch Dematol Res 1992;284(suppl 1):S22-S26.

56. Michaels LA, Ohene-Fremepong K, Zhao H, et al: Serum levels of substance P are elevated in patients with sickle cell disease and increase further during vaso-occlusive crisis. Blood 1998;92:3148-3151.

57. Modi WS, Pollack DD, Mock BA, et al: Regional localization of the human glutaminase (GLS) and interleukin-9 (IL-9) genes by in situ hybridization. Cytogenet Cell Genet 1991;57:114-116.

58. Goodwin VJ, Sato TA, Mitchell MD, et al: Anti-inflammatory effects of IL-4 and IL-10 and transforming growth factor-beta on human placental cells in vitro. Am J Reprod Immunol 1998;40:319-325.

59. Neben S, Tumer K: The biology of interleukin-11. Stem Cells 1993;11(suppl 2):156-162.

60. PeproTech, Inc: Product index: human growth factors and cytokines: recombinant human interleukin-11. Available at: www.peprotech.com. Accessed April 20, 2005.

61. Zeh HJ, Hurd S, Strojus WJ, et al: Interleukin-12 promotes the proliferation and cytolytic maturation of immune effectors: implications for the immunotherapy of cancer. J Immunother 1993;14:155-161.

62. Mullins DW, Koci MD, Burger CJ, et al: Interleukin-12 overcomes paclitaxel-mediated suppression of T-cell proliferation. Immunopharmacol Immunotoxicol 1998;20:473-492.

63. Javanovic DV, DiBattista JA, Martel-Pellitier J, et al: IL-17 stimulates the production and expression of proinflammatory cytokines IL-beta and TNF-alpha by human macrophages. J Immunol 1998;160:3513-3521.

Erythrocyte Production and Destruction

8

Kathryn Doig

OBJECTIVES

After completion of this chapter, the reader will be able to:

1. List the erythroid precursors in order of maturity, including the morphologic characteristics, cellular activities, normal location, and length of time in the stage for each.
2. Name the stage of erythroid development when given a written description of the morphology of a cell in a Wright-stained smear.
3. List and compare the cellular organelles of immature and mature erythrocytes and describe their specific functions.
4. Name the erythrocyte progenitors and distinguish them from precursors.
5. Explain the nucleus-to-cytoplasm ratio (N:C) and describe the appearance of a cell when given the N:C.
6. Explain how reticulocytes can be identified in a peripheral blood specimen.
7. Define and differentiate the terms *polychromasia, diffuse basophilia, punctate basophilia,* and *basophilic stippling.*
8. Discuss the difference between the reticulum of reticulocytes and punctate basophilic stippling in composition and conditions for viewing.
9. Define and differentiate *erythron* and *red blood cell (RBC)* mass.
10. Explain how hypoxia stimulates RBC production.
11. Describe the general chemical composition of erythropoietin (EPO) and name the site of production.
12. Discuss the various mechanisms by which EPO contributes to erythropoiesis.
13. Define and explain *apoptosis* resulting from Fas/FasL interactions and how this regulatory mechanism applies to erythropoiesis.
14. Describe the features of the bone marrow that contribute to establishing the microenvironment necessary for the proliferation of RBCs, including location and arrangement relative to other cells.
15. Discuss the role of macrophages in RBC development.
16. Explain how RBCs enter the bloodstream, how premature entry is prevented, and, when appropriate, promoted.
17. Describe the characteristics of senescent RBCs and explain why RBCs age.
18. Explain and differentiate the two normal mechanisms of erythrocyte destruction including location and process.

The red blood cell (RBC), or erythrocyte, provides a classic example of the biologic principle that cells have specialized functions and their structures are specific for those functions. The erythrocyte has one true function: to carry oxygen from the lung to the tissues where the oxygen is released. This is accomplished by the attachment of the oxygen to hemoglobin (Hb), the major cytoplasmic component of mature RBCs. The role of the RBC in returning carbon dioxide to the lungs and buffering the pH of the blood is important but quite secondary to its oxygen-carrying function. To provide this essential life function, the mechanisms controlling development, production, and normal destruction are fine-tuned to avoid interruptions in oxygen delivery, even under adverse conditions such as blood loss with hemorrhage. This chapter and subsequent chapters discussing iron, RBC metabolism, membrane structure, and Hb constitute the foundation for understanding the body's response to diminished oxygen-carrying capacity of the blood, called *anemia.*

Although in some ways a simple cell, and thus highly studied, the mammalian erythrocyte is quite unique among animal cells, having no nucleus in its mature, functional state. Although amphibians and birds possess RBCs highly similar to those of mammals, the nonmammalian cells retain their nuclei throughout the cells' lives. The implications of this unique mammalian adaptation are significant for cell function and life span.

NORMOBLASTIC MATURATION

Terminology

RBCs are formally called *erythrocytes*. The nucleated precursors in the bone marrow are called *erythroblasts*. They also may be called *normoblasts,* referring to developing nucleated cells (i.e., blasts) with normal appearance. This is in contrast to the abnormal appearance of the developing nucleated cells in megaloblastic anemia, where the erythroblasts are called *megaloblasts* because of their large size.

Three nomenclatures are used for naming the erythroid precursors (Table 8-1). The erythroblast terminology is used primarily in Europe. Similar to the normoblastic terminology used more often in the United States, it has the advantage of being descriptive of the appearance of the cells. Some prefer the rubriblast terminology because it parallels the nomenclature used for white blood cell development. Normoblastic terminology is used in this chapter.

Maturation Process
Erythroid Progenitors

As described in Chapter 7, the morphologically identifiable erythrocyte precursors develop from two functionally identifiable progenitors, burst-forming unit–erythroid (BFU-E) and colony-forming unit–erythroid (CFU-E), committed to the erythroid cell line. Estimates of time spent at each stage suggest that it takes about 1 week for the BFU-E to mature to the CFU-E and another week for the CFU-E to become a pronormoblast,[1] which is the first morphologically identifiable RBC precursor. While at the CFU-E stage, the cell completes approximately three to five divisions before maturing further.[1] As seen later, it takes approximately another 6 days for the precursors to become mature cells ready to enter the circulation, so it takes approximately 18 to 21 days to produce a mature RBC from the BFU-E.

Erythroid Precursors

Normoblastic proliferation, similar to proliferation of other cell lines, is a process encompassing replication (i.e., division)

to increase cell numbers and development from immature to mature cell stages (Fig. 8-1). The earliest morphologically recognizable erythrocyte precursor, the pronormoblast, is derived via the BFU-E and CFU-E from the multipotential stem cells as discussed in Chapter 7. The pronormoblast is able to divide, with each daughter cell maturing to the next stage of development, the basophilic normoblast. Each of these cells can divide, with each of its daughter cells maturing to the next stage, the polychromatophilic normoblast. Each of these cells also can divide and mature. In the erythrocyte cell line, there are typically three and occasionally as many as five divisions[2] with subsequent nuclear and cytoplasmic maturation of the daughter cells so that from a single pronormoblast, eight mature RBCs usually result. The conditions in which the number of divisions can be increased or reduced are discussed subsequently.

Criteria Used in the Identification of the Erythroid Precursors

Morphologic identification of blood cells depends on a well-stained blood smear. In hematology, a modified Romanowsky stain, such as Wright or Wright-Giemsa, is commonly used. The descriptions that follow are based on the use of these types of stains.

The stage of maturation of any blood cell is determined by careful examination of the nucleus and the cytoplasm. The qualities of greatest importance in identification of RBCs are the nuclear chromatin pattern (texture, density, homogeneity), nuclear size, nucleus-to-cytoplasm (N:C) ratio (Box 8-1), presence or absence of nucleoli, and cytoplasmic color.

As RBCs mature, several general trends affect their appearance. Figure 8-2 graphically represents these trends.
1. The overall size of the cell decreases.
2. The size of the nucleus decreases more significantly than does the size of the cell. As a result, the N:C also decreases.
3. The nuclear chromatin pattern becomes coarser, clumped, and condensed. The nuclear chromatin of RBCs is inherently coarser than that of myeloid precursors, as if it is made of rope rather than yarn. It becomes even coarser and clumpier as the cell matures, developing a raspberry-like appearance, where the dark staining of the chromatin is distinct from the almost white appearance of the parachromatin. This chromatin/parachromatin distinction is more dramatic than in myeloid cells. Ultimately, the nucleus

TABLE 8-1 Nomenclature for Erythroid Precursors

Normoblastic	Rubriblastic	Erythroblastic
Pronormoblast	Rubriblast	Proerythroblast
Basophilic normoblast	Prorubricyte	Basophilic erythroblast
Polychromatic normoblast (polychromatophilic)	Rubricyte	Polychromic erythroblast
Orthochromic normoblast	Metarubricyte	Orthochromic erythroblast
Reticulocyte	Reticulocyte	Reticulocyte
Erythrocyte	Erythrocyte	Erythrocyte

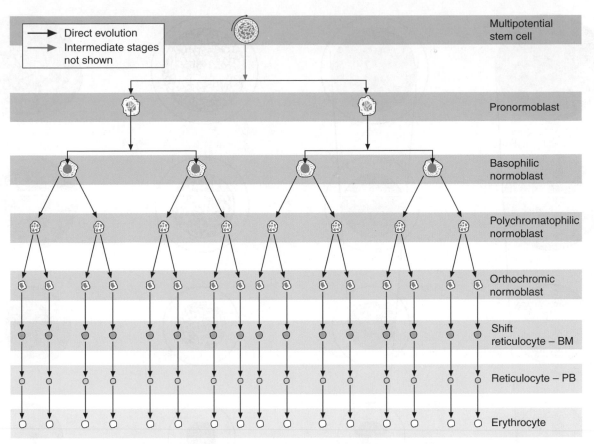

Figure 8-1 Typical production of erythrocytes from two pronormoblasts.

BOX 8-1

The N:C is one morphologic feature used to identify blood cells—not only the RBC precursors, but also white blood cells. The ratio is a visual estimate of how much of the cell is composed of nucleus compared with how much is composed of cytoplasm. If the amounts of each are estimated to be about equal, the N:C is 1:1. Although not mathematically proper, it is common for ratios other than 1:1 to be referred to as if they are fractions. If the nucleus takes up less than 50% of the area of the cell, the proportion of nucleus is lower, and the ratio is lower (e.g., 1:5 or <1). If the nucleus takes up more than 50% of the area of the cell, the ratio is higher (e.g., 3:1 or 3). As cells of the RBC line age, the proportion of nucleus shrinks, the cytoplasmic proportion increases, and the N:C decreases.

---

becomes quite condensed, with no parachromatin evident at all, and the nucleus is said to be pyknotic.

4. Nucleoli disappear. Nucleoli represent areas where the deoxyribonucleic acid (DNA) is unwound for ribonucleic acid (RNA) transcription and are seen early as cells begin actively synthesizing proteins. As RBCs mature, the nucleoli disappear, preceding the ultimate cessation of protein synthesis.

5. The cytoplasm changes from blue to gray to pink. Blueness or basophilia is due to acidic components that attract the basic stain such as methylene blue. The degree of cyto-

plasmic basophilia correlates with the amount of RNA and the number of organelles (mitochondria, rough endoplasmic reticulum, polyribosomes, and ribosomes). These organelles decline over the life of the developing RBC and the blueness fades. Pinkness or eosinophilia is due to more basic components that attract the acid stain, eosin. Eosinophilia of erythrocyte cytoplasm correlates with the accumulation of Hb as the cell matures. Thus the cell starts out being active in protein production on the organelles that make the cytoplasm quite basophilic, transitioning through a period where the red of Hb begins to mix with that blue, and ultimately ending with a thoroughly pink-red color when the organelles are gone and only Hb remains.

Maturation Sequence

Table 8-2 lists the stages of RBC development in order and provides a convenient comparison. The listing makes it appear that these stages are clearly distinct and easily identifiable. Similar to the maturing of human children into adults, the process of cell maturation is a gradual process with changes occurring in a generally predictable sequence but with some variation for each individual. The identification of a given cell's stage depends on the preponderance of characteristics, although it may not possess all the features of the archetypal descriptions that follow. Essential features of each stage are in italics in the following description. The cellular functions described subsequently also are summarized in Figure 8-3.

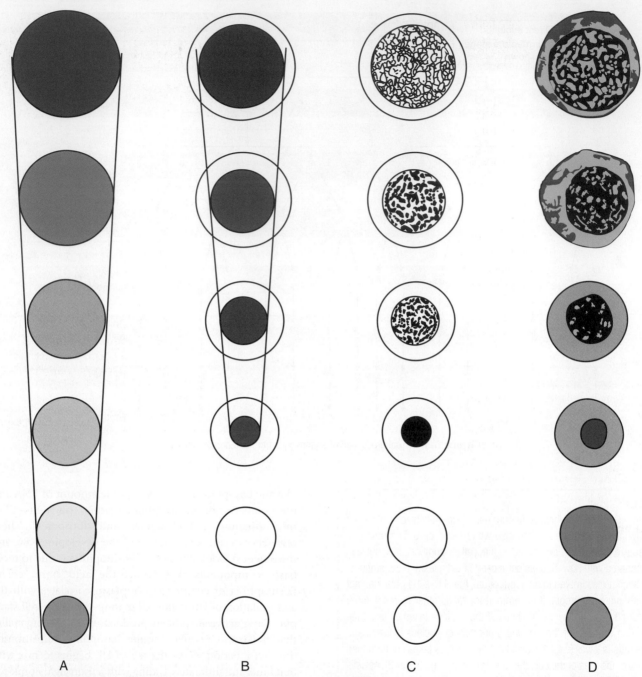

A   B   C   D

Figure 8-2 General trends affecting the morphology of RBCs during the developmental process. **A,** Cell size decreases and cytoplasm goes from blue to salmon; **B,** Nucleus decreases and color changes from purplish-red to dark blue; **C,** Nuclear chromatin becomes coarser, clumped, and condensed; **D,** Composite of changes during developmental process. (Modified from Diggs LW, Sturm D, Bell A: The Morphology of Human Blood Cells, 5th ed., Abbott Park, IL, Abbott Laboratories, 1985.)

Pronormoblast

Figures 8-4 and 8-5 show the pronormoblast.

Nucleus. The nucleus takes up much of the cell (high N:C). The nucleus is round to oval, *containing one or two nucleoli. The chromatin is open* and contains few, if any, fine clumps.

Cytoplasm. *The cytoplasm is quite blue* because of the concentration of organelles, especially the endoplasmic reticulum. The Golgi complex may be visible next to the nucleus as

a pale, unstained area. Pronormoblasts may show small tufts of irregular cytoplasm along the periphery of the membrane.

Division. The pronormoblast undergoes mitosis and gives rise to two daughter pronormoblasts. These mature into basophilic normoblasts before the next division.

Location. The pronormoblast is typically present only in the bone marrow.

TABLE 8-2 Normoblastic Series: Comparative Factual Information

Cell	Size (μm)	Nucleus-to-Cytoplasm Ratio	Nucleoli	% in Bone Marrow	Transit Time (hr in Bone Marrow)
Pronormoblast	12-20	8:1	1-2	1	24
Basophilic normoblast	10-15	6:1	0-1	1-4	24
Polychromatic normoblast	10-12	4:1	0	10-20	30
Orthochromic normoblast	8-10	1:2	0	5-10	48
Reticulocyte, shift	8-10	—	0	1	48-72*
Reticulocyte	8-8.5	—	0	—	24-48*

*Transit time in peripheral blood.

Cellular Activity. The pronormoblast is beginning to accumulate the components necessary for Hb production. The proteins and enzymes necessary for iron uptake and protoporphyrin synthesis are produced. Globin production begins.[3]

Length of Time in This Stage. This stage lasts slightly more than 24 hours.[3]

Basophilic Normoblast

Figures 8-6 and 8-7 show the basophilic normoblast.

Nucleus. *The chromatin begins to condense,* revealing clumps along the periphery of the nuclear membrane and a few in the interior. As the chromatin condenses, the parachromatin areas become larger and sharper, and the N:C decreases to about 6:1. The staining reaction is one of a deep purple-red. Nucleoli may be present early in the stage but disappear later.

Cytoplasm. When stained, *the cytoplasm may be a deeper, richer blue* than the pronormoblast—hence the name *basophilic* for this stage.

Division. The basophilic normoblast undergoes mitosis, giving rise to two daughter cells that mature into two polychromatic normoblasts.

Location. The basophilic normoblast is typically present only in the bone marrow.

Cellular Activity. Detectable Hb synthesis occurs,[3] but the large number of cytoplasmic organelles, including ribosomes and a substantial amount of messenger RNA (chiefly for Hb production), completely mask the minute amount of Hb pigmentation.

Length of Time in This Stage. This stage lasts slightly more than 24 hours.[3]

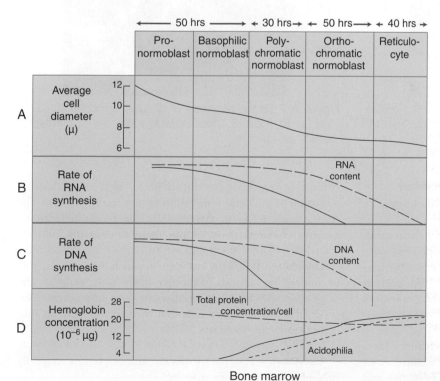

Figure 8-3 Timeline of cellular processes during erythropoiesis. (Modified from Granick S, Levere RD: Heme synthesis in erythroid cells. In Moore CV, Brown EB [eds]: Progress in Hematology. New York: Grune & Stratton, 1964.)

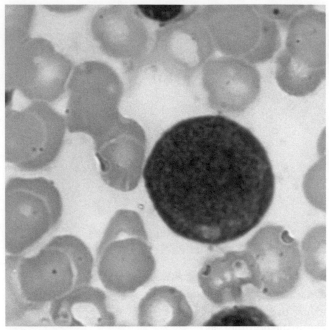

Figure 8-4 Pronormoblast (rubriblast), bone marrow (Wright stain, ×1000).

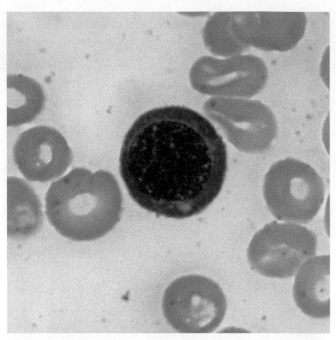

Figure 8-6 Basophilic normoblast (prorubricyte), bone marrow (Wright stain, ×1000).

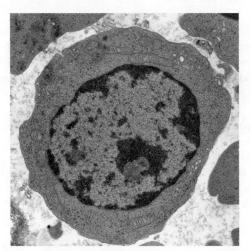

Figure 8-5 Electron micrograph of pronormoblast (×15,575). (From Carr JH, Rodak BF: Clinical Hematology Atlas, 2nd ed. Philadelphia: Saunders, 2004.)

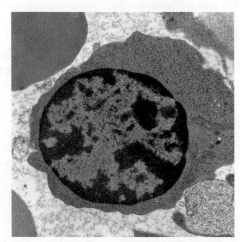

Figure 8-7 Electron micrograph of basophilic normoblast (×15,575). (From Carr JH, Rodak BF: Clinical Hematology Atlas, 2nd ed. Philadelphia: Saunders, 2004.)

Polychromatic (Polychromatophilic) Normoblast

Figures 8-8 and 8-9 show the polychromatic normoblast.

Nucleus.   The appearance of the chromatin pattern varies during this stage of development, from some openness early in the stage to becoming condensed by the end. *The condensation of chromatin* reduces the size of the nucleus considerably so that the N:C is about 4:1. Notably, *no nucleoli* are present.

Cytoplasm.   This is the first stage in which the redness associated with stained Hb can be seen. The stained color reflects the accumulation of Hb pigmentation over time and concurrent decreasing amounts of RNA. The color produced is a mixture of pink and blue resulting in a *murky gray-blue.* The stage's name refers to this combination of multiple colors because *polychromatophilic* means "many color loving."

Division.   This is the last stage in which the cell is capable of undergoing mitosis, although likely only early in the stage. The polychromatic normoblast goes through mitosis, producing two daughter cells that mature and develop into orthochromic normoblasts.

Location.   The polychromatic normoblast is typically present only in the bone marrow.

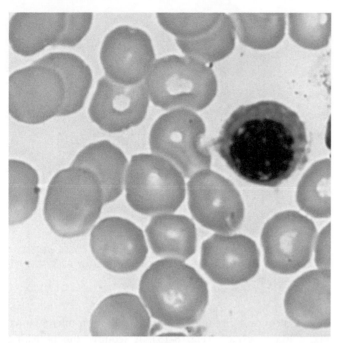

Figure 8-8 Polychromatic normoblast (rubricyte), bone marrow (Wright stain, ×1000).

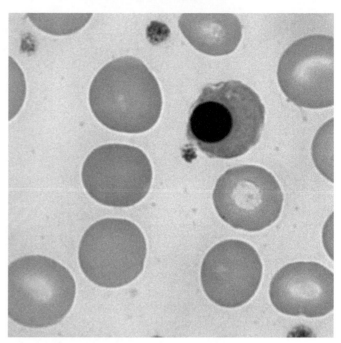

Figure 8-10 Orthochromic normoblast (metarubricyte), bone marrow (Wright stain, ×1000).

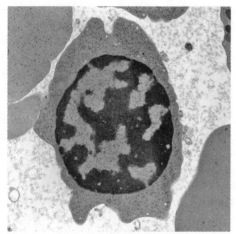

Figure 8-9 Electron micrograph of polychromatic normoblast (×15,575). (From Carr JH, Rodak BF: Clinical Hematology Atlas, 2nd ed. Philadelphia: Saunders, 2004.)

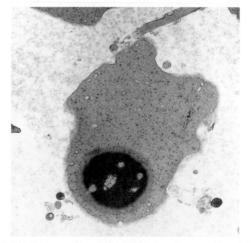

Figure 8-11 Electron micrograph of orthochromic normoblast (×20,125). (From Carr JH, Rodak BF: Clinical Hematology Atlas, 2nd ed. Philadelphia: Saunders, 2004.)

Cellular Activities. Hb synthesis is increasing and the accumulation begins to be visible in the color of the cytoplasm. Cellular organelles are still present, providing some blue aspect to the cytoplasm. The condensation of the nucleus and disappearance of nucleoli are evidence of cessation of DNA transcription.

Length of Time in This Stage. This stage lasts approximately 24 hours.[3]

Orthochromic Normoblast

Figures 8-10 and 8-11 show the orthochromic normoblast.

Nucleus. *The nucleus is completely condensed* (i.e., pyknotic) or nearly so. As a result, the N:C ratio is quite low.

Cytoplasm. The cytoplasm reflects nearly complete Hb production with a *pink-orange color.* The residual organelles, such as mitochondria, rough endoplasmic reticulum, and polyribosomes, react with the basic component of the stain and contribute a slightly bluish hue to the cell, but that fades toward the end of the stage as the organelles are degraded. The prefix *ortho* means "the same" and refers to the cell color being the same as the eosin stain, which is red.

Division. The orthochromic normoblast is not capable of division owing to the condensation of the chromatin.

Location. The orthochromic normoblast is typically present only in the bone marrow.

Cellular Activities. Hb production continues on the ribosomes with messenger RNA produced earlier. Late in this stage, the nucleus is ejected from the cell. The cell experiences apparent contractions that extrude the nucleus. Often, small fragments of nucleus are left behind. They are called Howell-*Jolly bodies* (see Table 18-3) when seen in peripheral blood cells and are typically removed from the circulating cells by the splenic pitting process when the cell enters the circulation.

Length of Time in This Stage. This stage lasts approximately 48 hours.[3]

Reticulocyte (Polychromatic erythrocyte)

Figure 8-12 shows the reticulocyte.

Nucleus. Beginning at the reticulocyte stage, there is *no nucleus.* The reticulocyte is a good example of the previous statement that a cell may not have all the classic features described but may be staged by the preponderance of features. In particular, when a cell loses its nucleus, regardless of cytoplasmic appearance, it is a reticulocyte.

Cytoplasm. The cytoplasm can be compared easily with that of the orthochromic normoblast in that the predominant color is that of Hb. By the end of the reticulocyte stage, the cell is the *same color as a mature RBC, salmon pink.* It remains *larger than a mature cell,* however. The shape of the cell is not the

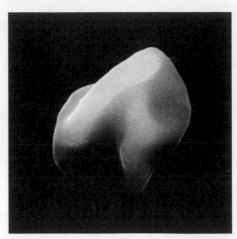

Figure 8-13 Scanning electron micrograph of polychromatic erythrocyte (×5000). (From Carr JH, Rodak BF: Clinical Hematology Atlas, 2nd ed. Philadelphia: Saunders, 2004.)

mature biconcave disc but is *irregular* in electron micrographs, like a lumpy potato (Fig. 8-13). It requires the polishing activity of the spleen to assist the RBC into its final discoid shape.

Division. Lacking a nucleus, the reticulocyte cannot divide.

Location. The reticulocyte resides in the marrow for 1 day and moves into the peripheral blood for 1 day. During the first several days after exiting the marrow, the reticulocyte is retained in the spleen for pitting and polishing by splenic macrophages.[4]

Activity. The reticulocyte completes production of Hb from residual messenger RNA using the remaining ribosomes. The cytoplasmic protein production machinery is simultaneously being dismantled. Endoribonuclease, in particular, digests the ribosomes. The acidic components that attract the basophilic stain decline over the stage to the point that the polychromatophilia of reticulocytes is not readily evident in the reticulocytes on a normal peripheral blood smear stained with Wright stain. A small amount of residual ribosomal RNA is present, however, and can be visualized with a vital stain such as new methylene blue, so called because the cells are stained while alive (i.e., vital), before the smear is made (Box 8-2). The residual organelles appear as a mesh of small blue strands, a reticulum, or, when more fully digested, merely blue dots (Fig. 8-14). This appearance is the origin of the name *reticulocyte.*

A second important functional change for reticulocytes is the reduced production of receptors for the adhesive molecules that hold developing RBCs in the marrow (see details later).[5,6] As these receptors decline, the cells are freed to egress the marrow.

Length of Time in This Stage. The cell typically remains a reticulocyte for about 2 days,[3] with the first day spent in the marrow and the second spent in the peripheral blood, although possibly sequestered in the spleen.

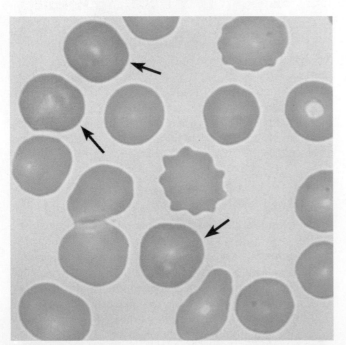

Figure 8-12 Polychromatic erythrocyte (shift reticulocyte), peripheral blood (Wright stain, ×1000).

BOX 8-2

The actual reticulum of a reticulocyte cannot be seen with typical Romanowsky stains; a vital stain is needed. With Wright stain, the residual organelles, in sufficient quantity, impart the bluish tinge to the cytoplasm seen in Figure 8-12. Based on the Wright-stained appearance, the reticulocyte can be called a *polychromatic erythrocyte* because it lacks a nucleus and is no longer an erythroblast but still has a bluish tinge and is polychromatic. When such cells are seen in a noticeable number on a blood smear, it is called *polychromasia* or *polychromatophilia*. Reticulocytes also can be called *diffusely basophilic erythrocytes,* referring to the bluish tinge that is throughout the cytoplasm in Wright-stained cells. This is to distinguish the reticulocyte basophilia from punctate basophilia of Wright-stained cells, where the blue appears in distinct dots throughout the cytoplasm. Also known as *basophilic stippling* (see Table 18-3), punctate basophilia is associated with some anemias. Similar to the basophilia of reticulocytes, it is due to residual ribosomal RNA, but it is degenerate, changing the chemical composition so that it stains deeply and can be seen with Wright stain.

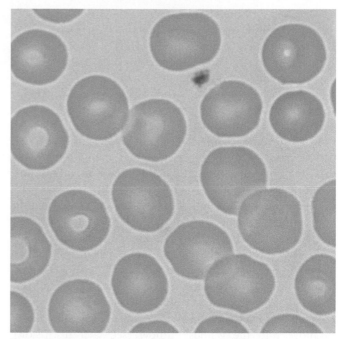

Figure 8-15 Mature erythrocytes, peripheral blood (Wright stain, ×1000).

Erythrocyte

Figures 8-15 and 8-16 show the erythrocyte.

Nucleus.   *No nucleus* is present in mature RBCs.

Cytoplasm.   The mature circulating erythrocyte is a biconcave disc measuring 7 to 8 μm in diameter with a thickness of about 1.5 to 2.5 μm. On a stained blood smear, it appears as a *salmon pink- or red-staining cell* with a central *pale area* that corresponds to the concavity. The pallor is about one third the diameter of the cell.

Division.   The erythrocyte cannot divide.

Location and Length of Time in This Stage.   Mature RBCs remain active in the circulation for approximately 120 days.[7] Aging leads to their removal by the spleen as described subsequently.

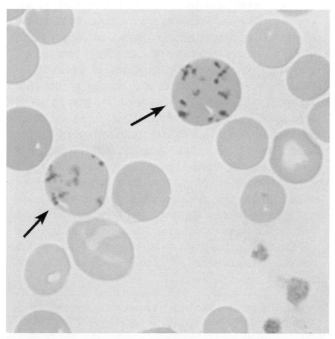

Figure 8-14 Reticulocyte, peripheral blood (new methylene blue stain, ×1000).

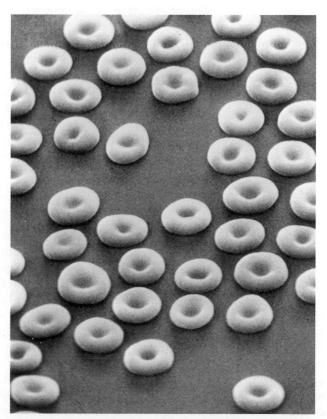

Figure 8-16 Scanning electron micrograph of mature erythrocytes.

Activity. The mature erythrocyte delivers oxygen to tissues, releases it, and returns to the lung to be reoxygenated. The dynamics of this process are discussed in detail in Chapter 10. The interior of the erythrocyte contains mostly Hb, the oxygen-carrying component, and a small proportion of water. It has a surface-to-volume ratio and shape that enable optimal gas exchange to occur. If the cell were to be spherical, it would have Hb at the center of the cell that would be relatively distant from the membrane and would not be readily oxygenated and deoxygenated. With the biconcave shape, even Hb molecules that are toward the center of the cell are not distant from the membrane and are able to exchange oxygen.

The cell's main function of oxygen delivery throughout the body requires a membrane that is flexible and deformable. The interaction of various membrane components described in Chapter 9 provides these functions. Deformability is an important feature worth mentioning here because RBCs must squeeze through small spaces such as the basement membrane of the marrow venous sinus. Similarly, when a cell enters the red pulp of the spleen, it must squeeze between epithelial cells to move into the venous outflow (see later discussion). Flexibility is crucial for RBCs to enter and remain in the circulation.

ERYTHROKINETICS

Erythrokinetics is the dynamics of RBC production and destruction. To understand erythrokinetics, it is helpful also to appreciate the concept of the erythron. *Erythron* is the name given to the collection of all stages of erythrocytes throughout the body: (1) the developing precursors in the bone marrow and (2) the circulating mature erythrocytes in the peripheral blood and the vascular spaces within specific organs such as the spleen. When the term *erythron* is used, the concept of a unified functional tissue is implied. The erythron must be distinguished from the *RBC mass*. Although the erythron is the entirety of erythroid cells in the body, the RBC mass refers only to the cells in circulation. This discussion of erythrokinetics begins by looking at the erythrocytes in the bone marrow and the factors that affect their numbers, their progressive development, and ultimate release into the blood.

Hypoxia—the Stimulus to Red Blood Cell Production

As mentioned previously, the role of RBCs is to carry oxygen. To regulate the production of RBCs for that purpose, the body requires a mechanism for sensing whether there is enough oxygen being carried to the tissues. If not, RBC production and functional efficiency of existing cells must be enhanced. Thus a second feature of the oxygen-sensing system must be a mechanism for influencing the production of RBCs.

The primary oxygen-sensing system of the body is located in peritubular interstitial cells of the kidney.[8,9] Hypoxia, too little oxygen in the tissue, is detected by the peritubular cells, which produce erythropoietin (EPO), the major stimulatory cytokine for RBCs. Under normal circumstances, the amount of EPO produced is fairly consistent, maintaining a level of RBC production that is sufficient to replace the approximately 1% of RBCs that normally die each day (see section on erythrocyte destruction). When there is hemorrhage, increased RBC destruction, or other factors that diminish the oxygen tension in the blood (Box 8-3), the production of EPO can be increased.

The mechanism by which hypoxia increases EPO production in peritubular cells is mainly via transcriptional regulation. There is a hypoxia-sensitive region of the 3' regulatory portion of the EPO gene that promotes gene transcription.[10] A hypoxia inducible factor, a transcription factor, is assembled in the cytoplasm when oxygen tension in the cells is decreased.[11] It migrates to the nucleus and interacts with the 3' enhancer for the EPO gene and upregulates the gene expression. With hypoxia, more messenger RNA molecules are produced, resulting in more EPO production.

Erythropoietin

Structure. Biochemically, EPO is a thermostable, non-dialyzable, glycoprotein hormone with a molecular weight of 34 kD.[12] It consists of a carbohydrate unit that is believed to convey specificity in recognizing target cell receptor sites and a terminal sialic acid unit, which is necessary for biologic activity in vivo.[13] On desialation, this activity ceases totally.[14]

BOX 8-3

Teleologically speaking, the location of the body's hypoxia sensor in the kidney is practical[1] because the kidney receives approximately 20% of the cardiac output[2] with little loss of oxygen between the lung and the kidney. This location provides an early indication when oxygen levels decline. Making the hypoxia sensor the cell that is able to stimulate RBC production also is practical because regardless of the cause of hypoxia, having more RBCs should help to overcome it. The hypoxia might result from decreased RBC numbers, as with hemorrhage. Decreased RBC numbers is only one cause for hypoxia, however. Another is when each RBC carries less oxygen than it should. This could be because the Hb is defective or because there is not enough Hb in each cell. The hypoxia may be unrelated to the RBCs in any way; poor lung function resulting in diminished oxygenation of existing RBCs is an example. The kidney's hypoxia sensor cannot know why there is hypoxia, but it does not matter. Even when there are plenty of RBCs compared with normal reference values, if there is still hypoxia, stimulation of RBC production is warranted because the numbers present are not meeting the oxygen need. An elevation of RBC numbers above the normal reference values, erythrocytosis, is seen in conditions such as lung disease and cardiac disease in which the blood is not being well oxygenated. Newborns have higher numbers of RBCs because the fetal Hb in their cells does not unload oxygen to the tissues readily, and so newborns are slightly hypoxic compared with adults. To compensate, they make more RBCs.

[1]Donnelly S: Why is erythropoietin made in the kidney? The kidney functions as a "critmeter" to regulate the hematocrit. Adv Exp Med Biol 2003;543:73-87.
[2]Stewart P: Physiology of the kidney. Update in Anaesthesia 1998;9. Available at: http://www.nda.ox.ac.uk/wfsa/html/u09/u09_016.htm. Accessed August 15, 2005.

Action.   EPO is a true hormone, being produced at one location (the kidney) and acting at a distant location (the bone marrow). It is a growth factor (or cytokine) that initiates an intracellular message to the developing RBCs, referred to as *signal transduction*. EPO must bind to its receptor on the surface of cells to initiate the message. Relatively few receptors require binding to initiate intracellular signaling.[15] The EPO-responsive cells vary in their sensitivity to EPO.[12] Some are able to respond to low levels of EPO, whereas others require higher levels. In healthy circumstances when RBC production needs to proceed at a modest but regular rate because hypoxia is not present, the cells requiring only low levels of EPO respond. If EPO levels rise secondary to hypoxia, however, a larger population of EPO-sensitive cells are able to respond.

The binding of EPO, the ligand, to its receptor on erythrocyte precursors and progenitors initiates a cascade of intracellular events that ultimately leads to more RBCs entering the circulation in a given time. It accomplishes this in two ways: by allowing early release of reticulocytes from the bone marrow and allowing more cells to mature into eythrocytes. In addition, EPO can reduce the time needed for cells to mature in the bone marrow. These processes are described in detail subsequently. The essence is that EPO puts more RBCs into the circulation at a faster rate than occurs without its stimulation.

Early Release of Reticulocytes.   EPO promotes early release of developing erythroid precursors from the marrow. Part of that results from EPO-induced changes in the adventitial cell layer of the marrow/sinus membrane.[16] Merely increasing the spaces through which cells might move is insufficient for cells to leave the marrow because RBCs are held in the marrow by possessing membrane receptors for adhesive molecules. EPO downregulates the production of the receptors on the RBC surface so that cells can exit the marrow earlier than they normally would.[5,6] The result is the presence in the circulation of reticulocytes that are still basophilic, having not spent the full day in the marrow that they normally would. These may be called *shift reticulocytes* because they have been shifted from the bone marrow early (see Fig. 8-12). Early release can even affect nucleated RBCs (i.e., normoblasts) in cases of extreme anemia where the demand for RBCs in the peripheral circulation is great. Releasing cells from the marrow early is a quick fix, so to speak; it is limited in effectiveness because the available precursors in the marrow are depleted within several days and still may not be enough to meet the need for more cells. A more sustained response is required in times of increased need for RBCs in the circulation.

Inhibition of Apoptosis.   A second, and probably more important, mechanism by which EPO increases the number of circulating RBCs is by increasing the number of cells that will be able to mature into circulating erythrocytes. It does this by decreasing apoptosis, the programmed death of RBC progenitors.[17,18] To understand this, an overview of apoptosis in general is appropriate.

Programmed Cell Death: Apoptosis.   As noted previously, it takes about 18 days to produce an RBC from stimulation of the earliest erythroid progenitor to release from the bone marrow. In times of increased need for RBCs, such as when

there is loss from the circulation owing to hemorrhage, this time lag would be a significant problem by delaying an effective compensatory response. One way to prepare for such a need would be to maintain a store of mature RBCs somewhere in the body for emergencies. RBCs cannot be stored in the body for this sort of eventuality, however, because they have a limited life span. The body uses a different mechanism to produce cells rapidly when needed. It does so by overproduction of RBC progenitors at all times. If they are not needed, which is normal, the extra progenitors are allowed to die. If they are needed, however, they have about an 8- to 10-day head start in the production process. It is like a fast food restaurant preparing extra hamburger patties for the lunch rush just to be sure they have plenty. If they are not sold, they are tossed in the garbage, but if they are needed, they just need the condiments and buns added, and they are ready to sell, significantly reducing the time needed to meet the demand. The process of intentional wastage of cells occurs by apoptosis, and it is part of the cell's genetic program.

Process of Apoptosis.   Apoptosis is a sequential process characterized by, among other things, the degradation of chromatin into large fragments of 5 to 300 kb that are degraded further into smaller monomers of 200 bases, protein clustering, and activation of transglutamase. In contrast to necrosis, in which cell injury causes swelling and lysing with release of cytoplasmic contents that stimulate an inflammatory response, apoptosis is not associated with inflammation.[19]

During the sequential process of apoptosis, the following morphologic changes can be seen: (1) condensation of the nucleus causing increased basophilic staining of the chromatin, (2) nucleolar disintegration, and (3) shrinkage of cell volume with concomitant increase in cell density and compaction of cytoplasmic organelles while mitochondria remain normal.[20] This is followed by a partition of cytoplasm and nucleus into membrane-bound apoptotic bodies that contain varying amounts of ribosomes, organelles, and nuclear material. The last stage of degradation produces nuclear DNA consisting of multimers of 180 base pairs. Characteristic blebbing of the plasma membrane is observed. The apoptotic cell contents remain membrane bound and are ingested by macrophages, avoiding an inflammatory reaction.

Erythroid Progenitors and Precursors Evade Apoptosis. Apoptosis of RBCs is a cellular process that depends on a signal from either the inside or outside of the cell. The crucial molecules in the messaging system are the death receptor on the earliest RBC precursors, Fas, and its ligand, FasL, which is expressed by more mature RBCs.[20,21]

When EPO levels are low, it means cell production should be at a low rate because hypoxia is not present. The excess early erythroid precursors should undergo apoptosis. This occurs when the older FasL-bearing erythroid precursors, such as polychromatic normoblasts, cross-link with Fas-marked immature erythroid precursors, such as pronormoblasts, which are stimulated to undergo apoptosis.[20] As long as the more mature cells with FasL are present in the marrow, erythropoiesis is subdued. If the FasL-bearing cells are depleted, as with EPO-stimulated early release, the younger Fas-positive precursors are allowed to develop, increasing the overall output of RBCs from the marrow.

A second mechanism for escaping apoptosis exists for young RBCs—by EPO rescue. This is the major way in which EPO is able to increase RBC production. When EPO binds to its receptor, one of the effects is to stimulate antiapoptotic molecules, allowing the cell to survive and mature.[22] The cells that have the most EPO receptors and are most sensitive to EPO are the CFU-E and pronormoblasts.[23] Without EPO, the CFU-E would not survive.[24]

The particular antiapoptotic molecules through which EPO exerts its influence have yet to be identified clearly. Bcl-X_L has been a promising candidate,[22] but more recent studies suggest that Bcl-X_L may act later in maturation, on cells that are actively producing Hb, rather than on the CFU-E.[25] Whatever the actual proteins may be, EPO-stimulated cells develop antiapoptotic molecules on their mitochondrial membranes and are able to resist the FasL activation of apoptosis.

Reduced Marrow Transit Time.   Apoptosis rescue is the major way in which EPO increases RBC mass, by increasing the number of erythroid cells that survive and mature to enter the circulation. The other effects of EPO are to increase the rate at which the surviving cells can enter the circulation. It is like a military recruiter that first recruits more young people to service but then puts them through a shortened boot camp training so that they are on the battlefield sooner. This is accomplished by two effects: increased rate of cellular processes and decreased cell cycle times.

EPO stimulates the synthesis of RBC RNA and effectively increases the rate of many processes, especially Hb production.[26] The accumulation of Hb is a factor that may control other cellular processes.[27] The cells continue to cycle through division and maturation, until the critical concentration of Hb is achieved,[27] typically after three divisions. Under the influence of EPO, if the messenger RNA increases and the critical concentration of Hb is achieved in two, rather than three, divisions, the cell can be released from the marrow earlier than usual, reducing the transit time in the marrow. Such cells are larger, due to a lost division, and do not have time before entering the circulation to dismantle the protein production machinery that gives the bluish tinge to the cytoplasm. These cells are true shift reticulocytes similar to those in Figure 8-12, recognizable in the stained peripheral blood as especially large, bluish cells lacking central pallor. They also are called "stress" reticulocytes because they exit the marrow early during conditions of bone marrow stress, such as certain anemias. Conversely, if Hb accumulates slowly, a cell may divide more times before achieving the critical Hb concentration to shut off division (Box 8-4).

The process by which Hb exerts this influence is probably as a transcription factor. The presence of Hb in the nucleus has been recognized for decades,[28] and its role as a transcription factor was hypothesized even before the concept of such influential molecules had been fully deduced.[27] It seems that Hb is transferred to the nucleus in proportion to its accumulation in the cytoplasm,[28] and there it influences other cellular processes.

> **BOX 8-4**
>
> The small size of erythrocytes seen in anemias of diminished Hb production, such as iron deficiency or the thalassemias, can be explained by the role of Hb in controlling cellular processes. If the cell continues the process of division and maturation until a critical concentration of Hb is accumulated within the cell,[1] in those anemias where Hb production is impaired and Hb accumulates more slowly, there is time for more divisions to occur before reaching the critical concentration. More divisions result in smaller cells. Such anemias include iron deficiency that prevents the production of the heme component of Hb and thalassemias where globin production is impaired. The converse also would be true—when cells undergo fewer than three divisions, as is the case under the influence of increased EPO, larger cells result. This is consistent with what is seen as patients recover from hemorrhage and larger cells (shift reticulocytes) emerge from the bone marrow.

[1]Stohlman F: Kinetics of erythropoiesis. In Gordon AS (ed): Regulation of Hematopoiesis, Vol 1. New York: Appleton Century Croft, 1970:318-326.

EPO also can reduce the time it takes for cells to mature in the marrow by reducing individual cell cycle time, specifically the length of time that cells spend between mitoses.[29] This effect is only about a 20% reduction, however, so that the normal transit time in the marrow of approximately 6 days from pronormoblast to erythrocyte can be shortened by about 1 day by this effect.

With the shortened cell cycle time and fewer mitotic divisions, the time it takes from pronormoblast to reticulocyte can be shortened by about 2 days. If the reticulocyte leaves the marrow early, another day can be saved, and the typical 6-day transit time is shortened to less than 4 days under the influence of increased EPO.

Measuring Erythropoietin.   Quantitative measurements of EPO are performed on plasma and other body fluids. EPO can be measured by immunoassays of various types, including radioimmunoassay or chemiluminescence. The reference range is approximately 5 to 30 mU/mL.[1] Increased amounts of EPO are expected in the urine of most patients with anemia with the exception of patients with anemia caused by renal disease.

Other Stimuli to Erythropoiesis

In addition to tissue hypoxia, other factors influence RBC production to a modest extent. It is well documented that testosterone directly stimulates erythropoiesis, which partially explains the higher Hb concentration in men compared with women.[30] Also, pituitary[31] and thyroid[32] hormones have been shown to affect the production of EPO, having indirect effects on erythropoiesis.

Microenvironment of the Bone Marrow

The general microenvironment of the bone marrow is described in Chapter 7, and the cytokines essential to hematopoiesis are discussed there. Here, the details pertinent to erythropoiesis (i.e., the erythropoietic inductive micro-environment) are emphasized, including the locale and arrangement of erythroid cells and the anchoring molecules involved.

Hematopoiesis occurs in marrow cords, essentially a loose arrangement of cells in a dilated sinus area between the arterioles that feed the bone and the venous sinus that returns blood to efferent veins. Erythropoiesis typically occurs close to the venous sinus in what are called *erythroid islands* (see Figs 7-5 and 7-6). These are macrophages surrounded by erythroid precursors in various stages of development. It was previously believed that these macrophages provided iron directly to the normoblasts for the synthesis of Hb. It was termed the "suckling pig" phenomenon. It is now clear, however, that developing RBCs acquire iron via transferrin (see Chapter 11), and so no direct contact with macrophages is needed for this. Because macrophages do release iron, it is logical that the iron would be in higher concentration near them. It could be bound to transferrin recycled from RBCs, providing a relatively high concentration of transferrin-bound iron in the area immediately surrounding the macrophage. The original notion that this arrangement facilitates iron uptake by normoblasts still may have some validity due to proximity. A more credible explanation of the cellular arrangement has been established, however, because the macrophages are now known to elabo-rate cytokines that are vital to the maturation process of the RBCs.[33,34] RBC precursors would not survive without macrophage support via such stimulation.

A second role for the macrophages in erythropoiesis also has been identified. Although movement of cells through the marrow cords is sluggish, developing cells would exit the mar-row prematurely in the outflow were it not for an anchoring system within the marrow that holds them there until devel-opment is complete. There are three components to the anchoring system: (1) a stable matrix of stromal cells to which normoblasts can attach, (2) bridging (adhesive) molecules for that attachment, and (3) receptors on the erythrocyte mem-brane. The system is analogous to anchoring a ship with the anchor corresponding with the matrix, the anchor cable cor-responding with the adhesive molecules, and the cable post on the ship corresponding with the receptor.

The major anchor for the RBCs is the macrophage. The adhesive molecule that is most important for normoblasts is fibronectin.[5] It is elaborated by the macrophages and other cells in the marrow and provides a connection between the macrophage and the developing RBC.

When it comes time for the RBCs to leave the marrow, they cease production of the receptors for the adhesive molecules.[6] Without the receptor, the cells are free to move with the effluent of the marrow into the venous sinus. Entering the venous sinus requires the RBC to traverse the barrier created by the adventitial cells on the cord side, the basement membrane, and the epithelial cells lining the sinus. There is evidence that egress through this barrier occurs between the adventitial cells[16] but through a pore in the endothelial cells, rather than between them (Fig. 8-17).[35,36]

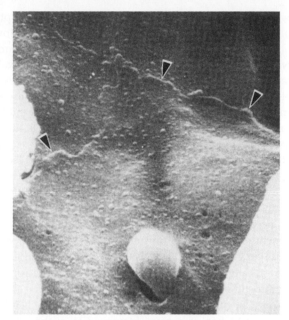

Figure 8-17 Egress of an RBC through a pore in an endothelial cell of the bone marrow venous sinus. *Arrowheads* indicate the endothelial cell junc-tions. (From DeBruyn PPH: Structural substrates of bone marrow function. Semin Hematol 1981;18:182.)

Erythrocyte Destruction

All cells experience the deterioration over time of their enzymes due to natural catabolism. Most cells are able to replenish needed enzymes and continue their cellular processes. As a non-nucleated cell, however, the mature ery-throcyte is unable to generate new proteins, such as enzymes, so as its cellular functions decline, the cell ultimately approaches death. The average RBC has sufficient enzyme capacity to live for 120 days. Because RBCs lack mitochondria, they rely on glycolysis for adenosine triphosphate (ATP) production. The loss of the glycolytic enzymes is central to this process of cellular aging, called *senescence*, which results in phagocytosis by macrophages. This is the major manner in which RBCs die normally.

Macrophage-Mediated Hemolysis (Extravascular Hemolysis)

At any given time, a substantial volume of blood is in the spleen. The environment is inherently stressful on cells. Movement through the red pulp is sluggish. The available glucose in the surrounding plasma is depleted quickly as the cell flow stagnates, so glycolysis slows. The pH is low, pro-moting iron oxidation. Maintaining reduced iron is an energy-dependent process, so factors that promote iron oxidation cause the RBC to expend more energy and speed the catab-olism of enzymes.

In this hostile environment, aged RBCs succumb to the various stresses. Their deteriorating glycolytic processes lead to reduced ATP production, which is complicated further by diminished amounts of available glucose. The membrane systems that rely on ATP begin to fail. Among these are enzymes that maintain the location and reduction of phospholipids of the membrane. Lack of ATP leads to oxidation of the membrane lipids and proteins. Other ATP-dependent enzymes are responsible for maintaining the high level of intracellular potassium while pumping sodium out of the cells. As this system fails, intracellular sodium increases and potassium decreases. The effect is that the selective permeability of the membrane is lost and water enters the cell. The discoid shape is lost and the cell becomes a sphere.

RBCs must remain highly flexible to exit the spleen by squeezing through the so-called *splenic sieve* formed by the endothelial cells lining the venous sinuses. Sphered RBCs are rigid and are not able to squeeze through the narrow spaces; they become trapped against the endothelial cells and basement membrane that form the sieve. In this situation, the RBC is like a fleeing thief who is trapped against a fence at the end of an alley. There, it is readily ingested by macrophages that patrol along the sinusoidal lining (Fig. 8-18).

Band 3, a membrane protein (see Chapter 9), begins to cluster[37] and when aggregated is referred to as the *senescence antigen*. The macrophages recognize the senescent RBCs by small amounts of autologous IgG molecules that attach to the clustered band 3 proteins.[38] The antibody may activate complement on the cell surface as well. Splenic macrophages possess receptors for the Fc fragment of IgG. They surround and ingest the RBC into a phagosome, where it bursts as a result of strong digestive enzymes. The RBC contents are degraded. This is hemolysis, destruction of RBCs, and it is occurring outside the vascular system, technically inside a macrophage, but generally in an organ, not the bloodstream. It is called *extravascular hemolysis*. The spleen is the major site for normal hemolysis of senescent cells; however, the macrophages of the liver (Kupffer cells) also can contribute to extravascular hemolysis of RBCs, especially those with complement on their membranes.

When an RBC lyses within a macrophage, the major components are catabolized. The iron is removed from the heme. It can be stored in the macrophage as ferritin until transported out. When outside the cell, the iron is picked up by the plasma transport protein, transferrin, which carries it to cells that require iron, especially developing RBCs in the bone marrow. The globin of Hb is degraded and returned to the metabolic amino acid pool. The protoporphyrin component of heme is degraded through several intermediaries to bilirubin, which is released into the plasma and ultimately excreted by the liver in bile. The details of bilirubin metabolism are discussed in Chapter 22.

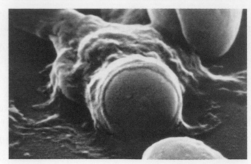

Figure 8-18 Macrophage ingesting a sphered erythrocyte. (From Bessis M: Corpuscles, Atlas of RBC Shapes. New York: Springer-Verlag, 1974.)

Mechanical Hemolysis (Intravascular Hemolysis)

Although most natural RBC death occurs in the spleen, a small portion of RBC hemolysis normally occurs *intravascularly* (within the lumen of blood vessels). An RBC's trip around the vascular system can be traumatic, with turbulence occurring in the chambers of the heart or at points of bifurcation of vessels. Small breaks in blood vessels and resulting clots can trap and lyse cells. A few cells lyse in the blood vessels from purely mechanical or traumatic causes; this is called *intravascular hemolysis*.

When the membrane of the RBC has been breached, regardless of where the cell is located when it happens, the cell contents enter the surrounding plasma. Although mechanical lysis is a relatively small contributor to RBC demise under normal circumstances, the body still has a system of plasma proteins, including haptoglobin and hemopexin, to salvage the released Hb so that its iron is not lost. These are discussed in detail in Chapter 22.

SUMMARY

RBCs can live only about 120 days because they lack a nucleus and the protein production machinery to replenish catabolized enzymes, such as those in the glycolytic pathway. They typically die in the spleen owing to its stresses, forming spherocytes that are ingested by resident macrophages. RBC production is balanced against this normal destruction to maintain a relatively stable number of circulating cells. That level is maintained not by the rate of production, but rather by the rate of apoptosis of overproduced progenitors and precursors. In times of increased need for cells, inhibition of apoptosis, chiefly by the effects of EPO, allows rapid increased output of RBCs from the marrow.

CHAPTER at a GLANCE

- RBCs develop from committed erythroid progenitor cells in the bone marrow, the BFU-E and CFU-E.
- The precursors of RBCs, in order from youngest to oldest, are the pronormoblast, basophilic normoblast, polychromatic normoblast, orthochromic normoblast, and reticulocyte.

- As erythroid precursors age, the nucleus becomes condensed and ultimately ejected from the cell, producing the reticulocyte stage. The cytoplasm changes color from blue, representing numerous organelles, to pink as Hb accumulates and organelles are degraded. Each stage can be identified by the extent of these nuclear and cytoplasmic changes.

CHAPTER at a GLANCE—cont'd

- It takes approximately 18 days for the BFU-E to mature to a RBC, of which about 6 days are spent as identifiable precursors in the bone marrow. The mature erythrocyte has a life span of 120 days in the circulation.
- Hypoxia of peripheral blood is detected by the peritubular cells of the kidney, which then produce EPO.
- EPO, the primary hormone that stimulates the production of erythrocytes, is able to (1) rescue the CFU-E from apoptosis, (2) shorten the duration between mitoses of precursors, (3) release reticulocytes from the marrow early, and (4) reduce the number of mitoses of precursors.
- Apoptosis is the mechanism by which excessive production of cells is controlled. Fas, the death receptor, is on young normoblasts, and FasL, the ligand, is on older normoblasts. As long as older cells mature slowly in the marrow, they suppress younger cells.
- EPO rescues cells by stimulating the production of antiapoptotic molecules that counteract the effects of Fas and FasL.
- Survival of RBC precursors in the bone marrow depends on cytokines and adhesive molecules, such as fibronectin, which are elaborated by macrophages. RBCs are found in erythroid islands, near the sinus membrane, where various stages of erythroblasts surround a macrophage.
- As RBC precursors mature, they lose fibronectin receptors and can leave the bone marrow. Egress occurs through pores in the endothelial cells of the venous sinus.
- Aged RBCs, or senescent cells, lacking a nucleus cannot regenerate catabolized enzymes. The semipermeable membrane becomes more permeable to water, so the cell swells and becomes spherocytic and rigid. It becomes trapped in the splenic sieve. Band 3 in the membrane of senescent cells clusters and attracts autologous IgG. When bound, the antibody is recognized by macrophages that engulf and lyse the cell. This is the mechanism of extravascular or macrophage-mediated hemolysis that accounts for most normal RBC death.
- Intravascular hemolysis results when mechanical factors breach the cell membrane while it is in the peripheral circulation. This pathway accounts for a minor component of normal destruction of RBCs.

REVIEW QUESTIONS

1. Which of the following is an erythrocyte progenitor?
   a. Pronormoblast
   b. Reticulocyte
   c. CFU-E
   d. Orthochromic normoblast

2. Which of the following is the most mature normoblast?
   a. Orthochromic normoblast
   b. Basophilic normoblast
   c. Pronormoblast
   d. Polychromatic normoblast

3. What erythroid precursor is described as follows: The cell is of medium size compared with other normoblasts, with an N:C of nearly 1:1. The nuclear chromatin is condensed and chunky throughout the nucleus. No nucleoli are seen. The cytoplasm is a muddy, blue-pink color.
   a. Reticulocyte
   b. Pronormoblast
   c. Orthochromic normoblast
   d. Polychromatic normoblast

4. Which of the following is *not* related to the effects of erythropoietin?
   a. The number of divisions of a normoblast
   b. The formation of pores in sinusoidal endothelial cells for marrow egress
   c. The time between mitoses of normoblasts
   d. The production of antiapoptotic molecules by erythroid progenitors

5. Hypoxia stimulates RBC production by:
   a. Inducing more pluripotent stem cells into the erythroid lineage
   b. Stimulating EPO production by the kidney
   c. Increasing the number of RBC mitoses
   d. Stimulating production of fibronectin by macrophages of the bone marrow

6. In the bone marrow, RBC precursors are located:
   a. In the center of the hematopoietic cords
   b. Adjacent to megakaryocytes along the adventitial cell lining
   c. Surrounding fat cells in apoptotic islands
   d. Surrounding macrophages near the sinus membrane

7. Which of the following determines the timing of egress of RBCs from the bone marrow?
   a. Maturing normoblasts slowly lose receptors for adhesive molecules that bind them to stromal cells.
   b. Stromal cells decrease production of adhesive molecules over time as RBCs mature.
   c. Endothelial cells of the venous sinus form pores at specified intervals of time, allowing egress of free cells.
   d. Periodic apoptosis of pronormoblasts in the marrow cords.

8. What single feature of normal RBCs is most responsible for limiting their life span?
   a. Loss of mitochondria
   b. Increased flexibility of the cell membrane
   c. Reduction of Hb iron
   d. Loss of nucleus

9. Intravascular hemolysis is the result of trauma to RBCs while in the circulation.
   a. True
   b. False

10. Extravascular hemolysis occurs when:
    a. RBCs are mechanically ruptured.
    b. RBCs extravasate from the blood vessels into the tissues.
    c. Splenic macrophages ingest senescent cells bearing autologous IgG.
    d. Erythrocytes are trapped in blood clots outside the blood vessels.

11. A pronormoblast belongs to the RBC mass of the body, but not the erythron.
    a. True
    b. False

12. A cell has an N:C of 4:1. Which of the following would describe it?
    a. The bulk of the cell is composed of cytoplasm.
    b. The bulk of the cell is composed of nucleus.
    c. The proportions of cytoplasm and nucleus are roughly equal.

REFERENCES

1. Dessypris EN, Sawyer ST: Erythropoiesis. In Greer JP, Foerster J, Lukens JN, et al (eds): Wintrobe's Clinical Hematology, 11th ed. Philadelphia: Lippincott Williams & Wilkins, 2004:195-216.

2. Shumacher HR, Erslev AJ: Bone marrow kinetics. In Szirmani E (ed): Nuclear Hematology. New York: Academic Press, 1956:89-132.

3. Granick S, Levere RD: Heme synthesis in erythroid cells. In Moore CV, Brown EB (eds): Progress in Hematology, Vol 4. New York: Grune & Stratton, 1964:1-47.

4. Song SH, Groom AC: Sequestration and possible maturation of reticulocytes in the normal spleen. Can J Physiol Pharmacol 1972;50:400-406.

5. Patel VP, Lodish HF: The fibronectin receptor on mammalian erythroid precursor cells: characterization and developmental regulation. J Cell Biol 1986;102:449-456.

6. Vuillet-Gaugler MH, Breton-Gorius J, Vainchenker W, et al: Loss of attachment to fibronectin with terminal human erythroid differentiation. Blood 1990;75:865-873.

7. Ashby W: The determination of the length of life of transfused blood corpuscles in man. J Exp Med 1919;29:268-282.

8. Jacobson LO, Goldwasser E, Fried W, et al: Role of the kidney in erythropoiesis. Nature 1957;179:633-634.

9. Lacombe C, DaSilva JL, Bruneval P, et al: Peritubular cells are the site of erythropoietin synthesis in the murine hypoxic kidney. J Clin Invest 1988;81:620-623.

10. Semenza GL, Nejfelt MK, Chi SM, et al: Hypoxia-inducible nuclear factors bind to the enhancer element located 3' to the human erythropoietin gene. Proc Natl Acad Sci USA 1991;88:5680-5684.

11. Wang GL, Semenza GL: Characterization of hypoxia inducible factor 1 and regulation of DNA binding by hypoxia. J Biol Chem 1993;268:21513-21518.

12. Kaushansky K: Hematopoietic growth factors and receptors. In Stamatoyannopoulos G, Majerus PW, Perlmutter RM, et al (eds): The Molecular Basis of Blood Diseases, 3rd ed. Philadelphia: Saunders, 2001:25-79.

13. Dordal MS, Wang FF, Goldwasser E: The role of carbohydrate in erythropoietin action. Endocrinology 1985;116:2293-2299.

14. Goldwasser E: On the mechanism of erythropoietin-induced differentiation: XIII. The role of sialic acid in erythropoietin action. J Biol Chem 1974;249:4202-4206.

15. Broudy VC, Lin N, Brice M, et al: Erythropoietin receptor characteristics on primary human erythroid cells. Blood 1991;77:2583-2590.

16. Chamberlain JK, Leblond PF, Weed RI: Reduction of adventitial cell cover: an early direct effect of erythropoietin on bone marrow ultrastructure. Blood Cells 1975;1:655-674.

17. Sieff CA, Emerson SG, Mufson A, et al: Dependence of highly enriched human bone marrow progenitors on hemopoietic growth factors and their response to recombinant erythropoietin. J Clin Invest 1986;77:74-81.

18. Eaves CJ, Eaves AC: Erythropoietin (Ep) dose-response curves for three classes of erythroid progenitors in normal human marrow and in patients with polycythemia vera. Blood 1978;52:1196-1210.

19. Allen PD, Bustin SA, Newland AC: The role of apoptosis (programmed cell death) in haemopoiesis and the immune system. Blood Rev 1993;7:63-73.

20. DeMaria R, Testa U, Luchetti L, et al: Apoptotic role of Fas/Fas ligand system in the regulation of erythropoiesis. Blood 1999;93:796-803.

21. Zamai L, Burattini S, Luchetti F, et al: In vitro apoptotic cell death during erythroid differentiation. Apoptosis 2004;9:235-246.

22. Dolznig H, Habermann B, Stangl K, et al: Apoptosis protection by the Epo target Bcl-X(L) allows factor-independent differentiation of primary erythroblasts. Curr Biol 2002;12:1076-1085.

23. Sawada K, Krantz SB, Dai CH, et al: Purification of human blood burst-forming units—erythroid and demonstration of the evolution of erythropoietin receptors. J Cell Physiol 1990;142:219-230.

24. Koury MJ, Bondurant MC: Maintenance by erythropoietin of viability and maturation of murine erythroid precursor cells. J Cell Biol 1988;137:65-74.

25. Rhodes MM, Kopsombut P, Bondurant M, et al: Bcl-X(L) prevents apoptosis of late-stage erythroblasts but does not mediate the anti-apoptotic effect of erythropoietin. Blood prepublished online May 17 2005. Available at: http://www.bloodjournal.org/cgi/content/abstract/2004-11-4344v1.

26. Gross M, Goldwasser E: On the mechanism of erythropoietin-induced differentiation: V. Characterization of the ribonucleic acid formed as a result of erythropoietin action. Biochem 1969;8:1795-1805.

27. Stohlman F, Lucarelli G, Howard D, et al: Regulation of erythropoiesis: XVI. Cytokinetic patterns in disorders of erythropoiesis. Medicine 1964;43:651-660.

28. Tooze J, Davies HG: The occurrence and possible significance of hemoglobin in the chromosomal regions of mature erythrocyte nuclei of the newt Triturus cristatus cristatus. J Cell Biol 1963;16:501-511.

29. Hanna IR, Tarbutt RO, Lamerton LF: Shortening of the cell-cycle time of erythroid precursors in response to anaemia. Br J Haematol 1969;16:381-387.

30. Jacobson W, Siegman RL, Diamond LK: Effect of testosterone on the uptake of tritiated thymidine in bone marrow of children. Ann NY Acad Sci 1968;149:389-405.

31. Golde DW, Bersch N, Li CH: Growth hormone: species-specific stimulation of in vitro erythropoiesis. Science 1977;196:1112-1113.

32. Popovic WJ, Brown JE, Adamson JW: The influence of thyroid hormones on in vitro erythropoiesis: mediation by a receptor with beta adrenergic properties. J Clin Invest 1977;60:908-913.

33. Sadahira Y, Mori M: Role of the macrophage in erythropoiesis. Pathol Int 1999;49:841-848.

34. Obinata M, Yanai N: Cellular and molecular regulation of an erythropoietic inductive microenvironment (EIM). Cell Struct Funct 1999;24:171-179.

35. Chamberlain JK, Lichtman MA: Marrow cell egress: specificity of the site of penetration into the sinus. Blood 1978;52:959-968.

36. DeBruyn PPH: Structural substrates of bone marrow function. Semin Hematol 1981;18:179-193.

37. Kay MM, Bosman GJ, Johnson GJ, et al: Band 3 polymers and aggregates and hemoglobin precipitates in red cell aging. Blood Cells 1988;14:275-295.

38. Turrini F, Arese P, Yuan J, et al: Clustering of integral membrane proteins of the human erythrocyte membrane stimulates autologous IgG binding, complement deposition and phagocytosis. J Biol Chem 1991;266:23611-23617.

9

Metabolism of the Erythrocyte

John Griep and Kathryn Doig

OBJECTIVES

After completion of this chapter, the reader will be able to:

1. List the red blood cell (RBC) processes that require energy.
2. Discuss the Embden-Meyerhof anaerobic glycolytic pathway (EMP) in the erythrocyte, including adenosine triphosphate (ATP) generation and consumption.
3. Identify the enzyme deficiency in the EMP responsible for most cases of hereditary nonspherocytic hemolytic anemia.
4. Identify the glycolytic enzyme involved in reduced nicotinamide adenine dinucleotide (NADH)–linked methemoglobin reductase.
5. Describe the role of 2,3-bisphosphoglycerate (2,3-BPG) in erythrocyte metabolism.
6. Explain the main function of the hexose monophosphate pathway (HMP).
7. Identify the enzyme deficiency in the HMP that causes erythrocytes to be vulnerable to oxidative damage.
8. Explain the importance of semipermeability of biologic membranes.
9. Discuss the arrangement of lipids in the RBC membrane.

10. Discuss the function of glycolipids in the RBC membrane.
11. Explain the concept of lipid exchange between the RBC membrane and the plasma, including factors that affect the exchange.
12. Explain the numbering system used for RBC membrane proteins, correlating protein size to relative number.
13. Define, locate, and provide examples of integral versus peripheral membrane proteins of RBCs.
14. Discuss the general structure of spectrin and its function and arrangement in the membrane.
15. Discuss how ankyrin, protein 4.1, and actin interact with spectrin and the lipid bilayer.
16. Describe the functions that band 3 provides for RBCs.
17. Cite the relative concentrations of sodium and potassium inside RBCs, and name the structure that maintains those concentrations.
18. Name conditions that develop from abnormalities of RBC membrane constituents.

After its release from the bone marrow as a reticulocyte, the erythrocyte survives about 120 days. The most important function of the erythrocyte is to deliver oxygen to body tissues and organs. This function, which involves oxygen and carbon dioxide transport and exchange, does not require consumption of energy.[1] Metabolic processes in the erythrocyte that do require energy are listed in Box 9-1. The mature erythrocyte, lacking a nucleus, mitochondria, and other organelles, is unable to synthesize proteins and lipids or to perform oxidative phosphorylation. When energy is no longer available for these common metabolic needs, the erythrocyte is destroyed prematurely. Necessary systems for sustenance of the

---

BOX 9-1 Erythrocyte Metabolic Processes Requiring Energy

Maintenance of intracellular cationic electrochemical gradients
Maintenance of membrane phospholipid
Maintenance of skeletal protein plasticity
Maintenance of functional ferrous hemoglobin
Protection of cell proteins from oxidative denaturation
Initiation and maintenance of glycolysis
Synthesis of glutathione
Mediation of nucleotide salvage reactions

---

erythrocyte include an intact erythrocyte membrane, a functioning glycolytic pathway, and nucleotide metabolism. This chapter reviews the important functions and roles that erythrocyte membranes contribute to the 120-day expected survival and presents the glycolytic pathways that provide for functional ferrous hemoglobin, protection from oxidative denaturation, synthesis of glutathione, and nucleotide metabolism. The regulations of erythrocyte metabolism, particularly of the energy-requiring processes, also are discussed.

Energy is stored and available as adenosine triphosphate (ATP), adenosine diphosphate (ADP), and adenosine monophosphate (AMP). Glycolysis serves to generate ATP from ADP. ATP, a high-energy phosphate source, represents the greatest reservoir of energy in the red blood cell (RBC).

Membrane exchange pathways allow maintenance of an intracellular cationic composition of high levels of potassium and low levels of sodium and calcium against extracellular gradients of low levels of potassium and high levels of sodium and calcium. These pump mechanisms prevent adverse accumulations of intracellular sodium and calcium. They consume approximately 15% of erythrocyte ATP production. When deprived of this ATP-derived energy, the erythrocyte swells and is destroyed.

Plasma glucose enters the erythrocyte glucose catabolic process through a facilitated membrane transport system.[2] It is metabolized anaerobically and aerobically. Anaerobic glycolysis, responsible for approximately 90% to 95% of the steady-state erythrocyte's glucose consumption, occurs in the Embden-Meyerhof pathway (EMP). By means of this pathway, glucose is metabolized to lactic acid, using two molecules of ATP per molecule of glucose and maximally providing four molecules of ATP per molecule of glucose, for a net gain of two molecules of ATP. In addition, a diversion metabolic shunt off this pathway provides 2,3-bisphosphoglycerate (2,3-BPG; also called *2,3-diphosphoglycerate* or *2,3-DPG*), and reduced nicotinamide adenine dinucleotide (NADH) is derived as a cofactor from the reaction. 2,3-BPG regulates oxygen delivery to tissues, and NADH is a cofactor in the methemoglobin reductase reaction, which maintains hemoglobin in its functionally reduced state. In aerobic glycolysis, which is responsible for 5% to 10% of glucose consumption, glucose is diverted into the hexose monophosphate pathway, which provides a pool of reduced glutathione to combat potential oxidant injury to the erythrocyte.

ANAEROBIC GLYCOLYSIS

The sequential list of biochemical intermediates involved in glucose metabolism, with corresponding enzymes, is summarized in Figure 9-1, but it does not indicate which enzyme reactions control glycolysis by functioning as rate-limiting enzymes. Tables 9-1 through 9-3 organize this information for better understanding and comprehension.

The first phase of glucose catabolism involves glucose phosphorylation, isomerization, and diphosphorylation to yield fructose-1,6-bisphosphate (F-1,6-P). F-1,6-P serves as the substrate for aldolase cleavage for the final product of phase 1

glycolysis: glyceraldehyde-3-phosphate (G3P) (see Fig. 9-1 and Table 9-1).

Hexokinase has the lowest activity of all the glycolytic enzymes. It requires magnesium and several other cofactors and exhibits increase in activity with increase in hydrogen ion concentration (pH). Phosphofructokinase requires magnesium, and its activity is modified by pH, inorganic phosphates, and ADP. Hexokinase and phosphofructokinase are rate limiting in steady-state anaerobic glycolysis. Deficiency of hexokinase is inherited as an autosomal recessive trait and is a rare cause of hereditary nonspherocytic hemolytic anemia (HNSHA).[3] Phosphofructokinase deficiency, inherited as an autosomal recessive trait, may be associated with severe muscle dysfunction (type VII glycogen storage disease). It may cause mild HNSHA.[4]

The second phase of glucose catabolism converts G3P to 3-phosphoglycerate (3-PG). The substrates, enzymes, and products for this phase of glycolytic metabolism are summarized in Table 9-2. During the first reaction step, G3P is phosphorylated with a high-energy phosphate and oxidized to 1,3-bisphosphoglycerate (1,3-BPG), through the action of glyceraldehyde-3-phosphate dehydrogenase (G3PD). This reaction is coupled to oxidized nicotinamide adenine dinucleotide (NAD^+) reduction to NADH, which is available as an essential cofactor for the reduction of methemoglobin to hemoglobin by methemoglobin reductase (methemoglobin reductase pathway).[5] 1,3-BPG may be dephosphorylated by phosphoglycerate kinase, generating ATP, or it may be shunted into the Luebering-Rapaport pathway, where it is isomerized to 2,3-BPG by bisphosphoglyceromutase. 2,3-BPG essentially competes with oxygen for hemoglobin, effectively enhancing release of oxygen from hemoglobin (Chapter 10). 2,3-BPG, the most concentrated organophosphate in the erythrocyte, forms 3-PG by the action of diphosphoglycerate phosphatase. Bisphosphoglyceromutase and bisphosphoglycerate phosphatase are activities of the same protein molecule.[6] The concentration of 2,3-BPG varies inversely with the pH, which is inhibitory to catalytic action of bisphosphoglyceromutase. Deficiency of phosphoglycerate kinase is X-linked and may be associated with neurologic disturbances and HNSHA.[7]

There is a delicate balance between the need to generate ATP to support energy requirements for cell metabolism and the need to maintain appropriate oxygenation/deoxygenation status of hemoglobin. This balance is maintained by dephosphorylation of 1,3-BPG to 3-PG with the generation of ATP or by mutation of 1,3-BPG to 2,3-BPG, which enhances the deoxygenation of hemoglobin. Low (acidic) pH inhibits the activity of bisphosphoglyceromutase and activates bisphosphoglycerate phosphatase, which favors generation of ATP.

The third phase of anaerobic glucose catabolism involves conversion of 3-PG to pyruvate with the generation of ATP. Substrates, enzymes, and products are listed in Table 9-3.

2,3-BPG is a cofactor in the monophosphoglyceromutase reaction. Pyruvate kinase activity is allosterically modulated by increased concentrations of F-1,6-P, which increases the affinity of pyruvate kinase for phosphoenolpyruvate.[8] Pyruvic acid may diffuse from the erythrocyte or may become a

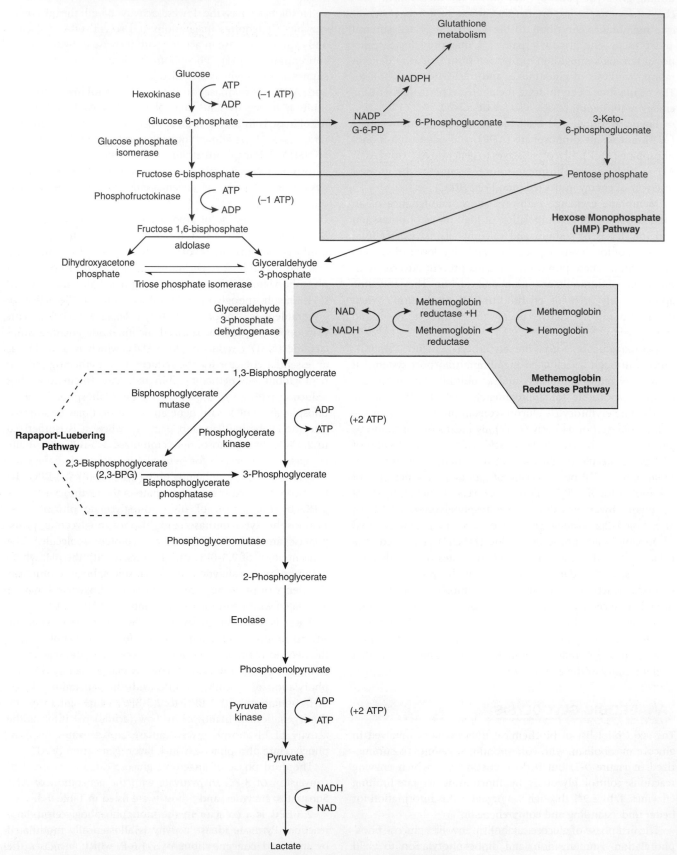

Figure 9-1 Glucose metabolism in the erythrocyte.

TABLE 9-1 Glucose Catabolism: First Phase

Substrates	Enzyme	Products
Glucose, ATP	Hexokinase	G6P, ADP
G6P	Glucose phosphate isomerase	F6P
F6P, ATP	Phosphofructokinase	F-1,6-P; ADP
F-1,6-P	Fructodiphosphate adolase	DHAP, G3P

DHAP, dihydroxyacetone phosphate.

TABLE 9-2 Glucose Catabolism: Second Phase

Substrates	Enzyme	Product
G3P	Glyceraldehyde-3-phosphate dehydrogenase	1,3-BPG
1,3-BPG, ADP	Phosphoglycerate kinase	3-PG, ATP
1,3-BPG	Bisphosphoglyceromutase	2,3-BPG
2,3-BPG	Bisphosphoglycerate phosphatase	3-PG

TABLE 9-3 Glucose Catabolism: Third Phase

Substrates	Enzyme	Product
3-PG	Monophosphoglyceromutase	2-PG
2-PG	Phosphopyruvate hydratase (enolase)	PEP
PEP, ADP	Pyruvate kinase	Pyruvate, ATP

PEP, phosphoenolpyruvate.

substrate for lactate dehydrogenase with regeneration of NAD^+. The ratio of NAD^+ to NADH may modify the activity of this enzyme. Pyruvate kinase deficiency is inherited as an autosomal recessive trait and is the most common cause of HNSHA. This deficiency is discussed in Chapter 23.

AEROBIC GLYCOLYSIS

Aerobic or oxidative glycolysis diverts glucose metabolism into the hexose monophosphate pathway (HMP), also known as the *pentose phosphate shunt,* for the purpose of maintaining reduced glutathione and reduced nicotinamide adenine dinucleotide phosphate (NADP) (see Fig. 9-1).[8] During steady-state glycolysis, approximately 5% to 10% of glucose-6-phosphate (G6P) is diverted into the HMP. After oxidative challenge, activity of the HMP may be increased 20-fold to 30-fold.[8] This pathway catabolizes G6P to ribulose-5-phosphate and carbon dioxide by oxidizing G6P at carbon 1. Ribulose-5-phosphate may be used during nucleotide metabolism or re-enter anaerobic glycolysis pathways as fructose-6-phosphate or G3P under enzymatic activity of pentose epimerase, isomerase, transketolase, and transaldolase. The substrates, enzymes, and products for the HMP are listed in Table 9-4.

During the conversion of glucose to pentose, reduced nicotinamide adenine dinucleotide phosphate (NADPH) is generated, which reduces oxidized glutathione via glutathione

TABLE 9-4 Glucose Catabolism: Hexose Monophosphate Pathway

Substrates	Enzyme	Product
G6P	Glucose-6-phosphate dehydrogenase	6-PG
6-PG	Phosphogluconolactonase	R5P
	Phosphogluconate dehydrogenase	

R5P, ribulose-5-phosphate.

reductase and, in the presence of glutathione peroxidase, can convert hydrogen peroxide to water. Hydrogen peroxide, regularly produced in small amounts, may be generated in large amounts by oxidant drugs.

The enzyme glucose-6-phosphate dehydrogenase (G6PD) functions to reduce NADP while oxidizing G6P. It governs the rate of reduction of NADP, which restores reduced glutathione through H^+ transfer by glutathione reductase.[9] G6PD provides the only means of generating NADPH, and in its absence erythrocytes are particularly vulnerable to oxidative damage.[10] Erythrocytes with normal G6PD activity are able to detoxify the oxidative compounds and safeguard the hemoglobin sulfhydryl-containing enzymes and membrane thiols, allowing normally functioning RBCs to carry enormous quantities of oxygen safely.[8] G6PD deficiency is the most common human enzyme deficiency worldwide (Chapter 23).

NUCLEOTIDE METABOLISM

Nucleotides, present in mature erythrocytes, cannot be synthesized de novo and must be maintained to preserve the energy requirements of the cell. The adenine nucleotide pool is the largest pool and is composed of approximately 88% ATP, 10% ADP, and 2% AMP. This relative proportion of nucleotides is maintained by the action of adenylate kinase and by the generation of ATP from ADP during glycolytic metabolism. AMP may be deaminated to inosine 5′-monophosphate or dephosphorylated to adenosine, which is diffusible across the erythrocyte membrane.

Nucleotide salvage may be possible through the relative activities of adenosine kinase and adenosine deaminase. Deficient activity of adenosine deaminase leads to accumulations of deoxyadenine nucleotides, whereas increased activity of adenosine deaminase leads to depletions of deoxyadenine nucleotides. A second potential salvage pathway is related to the activity of adenosine phosphoribosyl transferase, which converts adenine to AMP. This activity is likely limited by the availability of adenine.

REGULATION OF METABOLISM

As noted, the primary function of the RBC consists of transporting oxygen to the tissues from the lungs and carrying carbon dioxide from tissues to the lungs. Without a nucleus and with lack of translation to messenger ribonucleic acid (RNA), RBCs do not have coding for genetic control of RBC function. Control of metabolic functions within the RBC is intrinsic to the metabolic systems active within the cell.

Although it has a high capacity for phosphorylation of glucose, hexokinase activity is sensitive to the concentration of G6P, its product, and to 2,3-BPG.[11,12] Phosphofructokinase is inhibited by ATP and 2,3-BPG, and hexokinase and phosphofructokinase activity is inhibited by increases in hydrogen ion concentration. The reversible binding of G3PD to the cytoplasmic portion of membrane protein band 3 may represent a non–rate control process. In the HMP pathway, NADPH is an inhibitor of G6PD activity, and this enzyme activity increases only after oxidation of NADPH to NADP.[13]

2,3-BPG, which is important for proper oxygen delivery to tissue, is under a complex of factors for control of its concentration. Its synthesis rate is controlled by diphosphoglycerate mutase and degradation by diphosphoglycerate phosphatase. Its concentration reflects a balance between the relative activities of these enzymes. The mutase reaction rate is increased in the environment of low concentrations of H^+ and of high concentrations of 3-PG and 2-PG, whereas its activity is decreased in the presence of high concentrations of H^+, 2,3-BPG, and phosphate ion. The phosphatase reaction activity is increased under the conditions of high concentrations of H^+, pyrosulfite, sulfate, dithionite, phosphoglycerate (1000-fold),

phosphate, and chloride and reduced under the conditions of low H^+ concentration, low 3-PG levels, low phosphoenolpyruvate levels, and low ATP levels.

The regulation of ATP levels occurs through equilibrium with ADP and AMP catalyzed by adenylate kinase and through the deamination of AMP by adenylate kinase. ATP is synthesized from ADP during glycolytic metabolism, but is used by kinases in glycolytic and protein metabolism and by cationic related ATPase.

ERYTHROCYTE MEMBRANE

Functions

The biconcave shape of the RBC is crucial to its function, allowing for close to maximum surface-to-volume ratio[14] and optimal gaseous exchange.[15] The ability of the circulating erythrocyte to perform the function of gaseous exchange relies almost exclusively on the integral and structural composition and functional capabilities of the membrane components (Fig. 9-2) and sufficient generated ATP. The main physiologic functions of the RBC membrane are to (1) maintain cell shape and deformability, (2) maintain osmotic balance between plasma and the cell cytoplasm, (3) act as a supporting skeletal system for surface antigens and receptors, and (4) aid in the

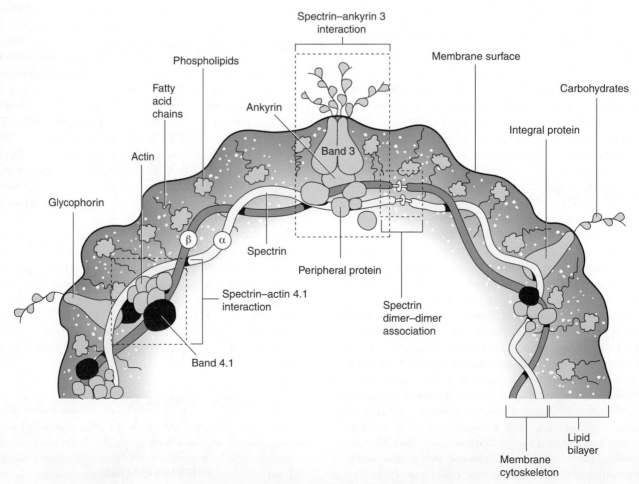

Figure 9-2 Schematic of erythrocyte membrane.

transportation of essential cellular ions and gases. The latter function involves *passive transportation* of some compounds such as gases and glucose, which move through the membrane by facilitated diffusion through cell pores. It also involves *active transportation* of substances such as sodium and potassium ions that move against an electrochemical gradient (Na^+, K^+).[16]

Composition

The RBC membrane can be studied after a hemolyzing process resulting in "ghosts," cells that have lost hemoglobin and appear empty microscopically so that only the membrane, or stroma, remains. Transmission electron microscopy has shown the membrane to be a typical biologic trilaminar structure that consists of approximately 40% lipid, 52% protein, and 8% carbohydrate.[17,18] The general structure of the membrane is a double matrix of phospholipids (lipid bilayer) in which specific proteins and phospholipids are embedded, with an underlying protein membrane skeleton.[17] The interplay of these components contributes to the fluidity of the membrane. This organization provides specialized domains for exchange of nutrients and transfer of information with other cells and their milieu. Any variability in this composition may alter the functional capabilities of the membrane and ultimately results in early cell death.

Lipid Layer

The RBC membrane consists of two interrelated parts: the outer bilayer of lipids with integral proteins embedded in it and the underlying protein membrane skeleton.[17,19] In the lipid bilayer, the hydrophilic ends of the molecules face the water-rich plasma and cytosol.[20] The hydrophobic ends of the molecules orient toward the interior of the membrane.[21] The insoluble lipid portion of the membrane serves as a barrier to separate the vastly different ion and metabolite concentrations of the interior of the RBC from its external environment, the blood plasma.[19]

The lipid bilayer, nearly 50% of the RBC membrane,[22] consists of almost equimolar quantities of nonesterified cholesterol and phospholipids, chiefly phosphatidylcholine, phosphatidylethanolamine, and sphingomyelin. The cholesterol reduces the fluidity of the membrane.[23] The remaining lipids are small quantities of free fatty acids and glycolipids.[20] There is an asymmetry of the distribution of the phospholipids with most of the phosphatidylethanolamine and phosphatidylserine in the cytosolic monolayer.[24] This asymmetry is important to RBC shape. Glycolipids also are embedded in the membrane and located entirely in the external half of the bilayer. Their carbohydrate moieties extend into the aqueous phase. They carry several important RBC antigens, including A, B, H, and Lewis.[25-29]

Lacking a membrane, the RBC cannot synthesize replacement phospholipids, so appropriate membrane phospholipid levels must be sustained by other phospholipid renewal pathways. There is an enzyme-facilitated exchange of lipids (especially cholesterol and lecithin) between the plasma and the cell membrane.[32] Deficiencies of the enzymes that affect this exchange can lead to hemolytic anemia.[33] The lipid

exchange also is affected by the bile salt composition of the plasma[34] so that in liver disease where bile salt composition changes, target cells appear (Chapter 18). The RBCs' membranes become more fluid and "loose" so that when they are spread on a slide, the extra membrane bulges into the center, forming a target appearance.

Membrane Proteins

The protein portion of the membrane is responsible for the shape and deformability of the RBC. The protein components of the membrane also include the pumps and channels for movement of ions and other material between the RBC's interior and the blood plasma. Various other proteins in the membrane act as receptors, RBC antigens, and enzymes. The lipid bilayer provides a fluid foundation into which proteins are inserted. Some proteins, particularly those that are on the exterior of the membrane, can move within the lipid matrix, floating like icebergs in the lipid sea.[35] Although some proteins span the membrane from plasma to cytosol, others are restricted to just the exterior or just the interior aspect (see Fig. 9-2).

Analogous to the connection of the body's skin to the skeleton, the lipid membrane bilayer is bound to a protein membrane skeleton that contains 10 to 12 major proteins and many minor proteins.[36] These skeletal proteins can be extracted from RBC membranes in sodium dodecyl sulfate, separated on polyacrylamide gel electrophoresis according to their size, and stained with Coomassie blue for membrane and skeletal proteins. Periodic acid–Schiff (PAS) that reacts with carbohydrates can be used to stain the sialoglycoproteins, also known as *glycophorins* (Fig. 9-3).[37-39] The electrophoretic

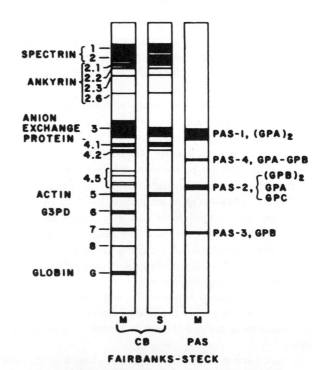

Figure 9-3 Bands of protein in erythrocyte membrane.

TABLE 9-5 Major Membrane Polypeptides

Electrophoretic Designation	Molecular Weight	Percent of Protein	Name	Relation to Membrane
1	240,000	15 }	Spectrin { α	Peripheral
2	225,000	15 }	β	
2.1	206,000	} 5	Ankyrin	Peripheral
2.2	190,000	}		
3	90,000-105,000	24	Anion channel	Integral
4.1	78,000	4.2		
4.2	72,000	5	Protein kinase	
4.5	45,000-75,000	5	Glucose transporter	Integral
5	43,000	4.5	Actin	Peripheral
6	35,000	5.5	G3PD	Peripheral
7	29,000	3.4		
PAS-1 } PAS-2 }	39,000	6.7	Glycophorin A	Integral

Modified from Steck TL: The organization of proteins in the human red blood cell membrane. J Cell Biol 1974;62:1.

bands are numbered 1 through 8 when stained with Coomassie blue or 1 through 4 when stained with PAS, beginning at the application point of the gel. The lower numbers correspond to the largest proteins that migrate the least. When PAS numbers are used, they typically are noted as PAS-1, for example, so that when just a number is given, it can be assumed to be a Coomassie staining number. Some of the bands have been given individual protein names. Table 9-5 lists these bands, their names, and their characteristics.

The membrane proteins are classified as integral or peripheral. The integral proteins penetrate or span the lipid bilayer and can interact with the hydrophobic lipid area. Integral proteins include the glycophorins (A, B, C, and D), which are rich in carbohydrates, give the RBC its overall negative charge due to abundant sialic acid residues, and carry membrane receptors and RBC antigens M and N.[40] These are the proteins that appear in the PAS-1, PAS-2, and PAS-3 bands as a result of their carbohydrate components.

Protein 3 (band 3 on Coomassie membrane proteins) also is an integral protein and functions as a transport or anion exchange channel in the membrane; more recently it has been called *AE1*. Chloride ions enter and leave the RBC through AE1 as the intracellular bicarbonate ion concentration varies with the carbon dioxide content of the blood (Chapter 10).[41] Band 3 is also a key site of attachment of the RBC membrane cytoskeleton to the lipid layer and may attach membrane hemoglobin and certain enzymes. The ABO and Ii RBC antigens are associated with band 3. During RBC senescence, band 3 clusters and binds autologous immunoglobulin (Ig), marking the cell for macrophage ingestion.[42]

The Rh blood group antigens also are integral proteins.[43] They are apparently important to RBC structure because lack of Rh antigens is associated with a hemolytic anemia (See Chapter 23).[44]

The peripheral proteins lie along the underside of the lipid bilayer but do not penetrate the bilayer area, thus the designation "peripheral". They line the inner membrane surface and interact to form a "membrane skeleton," or cytoskeleton. These fibrous proteins include the five major proteins: (1) spectin, (2) actin, (3) protein 4.1, (4) ankyrin, and (5) G3PD.[19] Several abnormalities in these proteins have been shown, however, to be related to morphologic disorders, such as spherocytosis and elliptocytosis, which clinically result in hemolytic processes.[45-47]

Spectrin comprises 50% to 70% of the skeletal mass and consists of two large polypeptide subunits that are structurally related but functionally distinct. These are the α chain, which is 267,000 D in length, and the β chain, which is 246,000 D in length. The strength of the skeleton is derived from lining up the chains side by side, but head to tail, and twisting them like rope, to form a long, fiber-like heterodimer[48] (Fig. 9-4). The two chains are weakly associated except at the ends, which makes the molecule flexible and contributes to RBC membrane pliancy.[47] This pliancy is important to allow the RBC to egress the bone marrow, pass the splenic sinus, and squeeze through capillaries. Each heterodimer joins with another heterodimer, this time head to head, to form heterotetramers

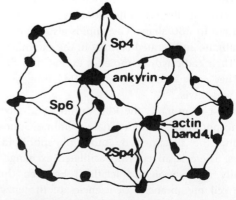

Figure 9-4 Schematic of spectrin structure.

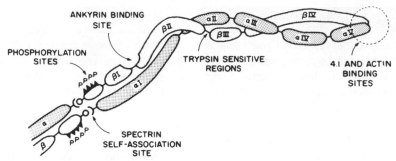

Figure 9-5 Hexagonal lattice of erythrocyte membrane. (From Becker PS, Lux SE: Disorders of the red cell membrane. In Nathan DG, Oski FA [eds]: Hematology of Infancy and Childhood, 4th ed. Philadelphia: Saunders, 1993:543.)

$(\alpha\beta)_2$, adding further strength to the molecule. The tetramers associate at their ends to form a two-dimensional radial arrangement that creates a hexagonal lattice on the underside of the lipid membrane that is analogous to a flexible chicken wire frame (Fig. 9-5).[50] The tetramers are held together by other peripheral proteins, including band 4.1 and actin (see Fig. 9-2).[51]

Similar to the bony skeleton of the body that attaches to the muscles via tendons, the spectrin cytoskeleton also must be connected to the lipid bilayer, in this case by specific proteins. As shown in Figure 9-2, protein 4.1, which already is attached to the spectrin tetramer at its end, can bind to glycophorin C.[50,52] Ankyrin, a large pyramid-shaped protein, binds to the spectrin β chain, linking it to band 3.[53] The result is a flexible but strong cytoskeleton that provides the physical integrity and morphologic shape of the normal RBC.

Osmotic Balance and Permeability

The selectively permeable membrane allows water and anions (HCO_3^-, Cl^-) to enter the cell freely. These substances enter through pores or channels formed by integral proteins, whose positive surface charges create a unidirectional flow. An active cation pump regulates the balance of Na^+ and K^+, maintaining intracellular and extracellular ratios of 1:12 and 25:1, respectively.[54,55] This mechanism enables the erythrocyte to maintain normal structure and function. Any slight deviation in the membrane's selective permeability causes an influx of Na^+, with water following osmotically. The cell swells, assumes a spheroid shape, and may rupture the membrane (lyse) with subsequent loss of hemoglobin. This is called *colloid osmotic hemolysis*. An example of increased cation permeability occurs in sickle cell disease. When sickle hemoglobin deforms the cells (Chapter 26), there is measurably increased cation permeability of Na^+, K^+, and Ca^{2+}, resulting in hemolysis.[56]

Calcium has been identified as also being necessary for maintenance of cell integrity. It is associated with the ATPase activity of spectrin. The energy-dependent calcium ATPase cationic pump maintains intracellular levels of 5 to 10 μmol/L RBCs.[57] Calmodulin, a cytoplasmic Ca^{2+}-binding protein, controls the calcium pumps.[58]

CHAPTER at a GLANCE

- The mature erythrocyte, lacking a nucleus and other organelles, must derive energy from other sources to survive its 120-day life span.
- The greatest reservoir of energy is ATP, which is generated by glycolysis. Glucose enters the erythrocyte by facilitated membrane transport.
- Glycolysis occurs aerobically and anaerobically.
- Through anaerobic glycolysis in the EMP, glucose is metabolized to lactic acid, using two molecules of ATP per molecule of glucose and providing four molecules of ATP per molecule of glucose, for a *net gain* of two molecules of ATP.
- By means of the Luebering-Rapaport pathway (a shunt off the EMP), 2,3-BPG necessary for the facilitation of oxygen delivery to the tissues is generated.
- The methemoglobin reductase pathway (also a bypass from the EMP) is responsible for maintaining iron in its reduced state.
- Aerobic glycolysis occurs in the hexose monophosphate pathway, which converts glucose into pentose with the generation of

- NADPH. NADPH reduces glutathione, which protects the cell from oxidative injury.
- The RBC membrane is a typical lipid bilayer with hydrophobic components oriented away from the water-rich plasma and cytosol. The membrane provides a semipermeable barrier separating the plasma constituents from the cytosol, allowing the cell to maintain necessary intracellular differences. The two lipid layers of the membrane differ in the composition of phospholipids.
- Lost membrane lipids are restored from the plasma by an enzyme-enhanced process of lipid exchange. Abnormalities in membrane lipids lead to abnormal cell shapes, such as the target cells that develop with liver disease, owing to the changes in plasma bile salts.
- The membrane proteins include the proteins that span from cytosol to plasma (integral proteins). These include ion channels and various receptors. The proteins that localize to the exterior or the interior surfaces of the membrane are called *peripheral proteins*. Proteins are able to move within the lipid matrix.

CHAPTER at a GLANCE—cont'd

- The membrane proteins can be extracted from RBC membranes in sodium dodecyl sulfate, separated on polyacrylamide gel electrophoresis, and stained for visualization. They are numbered from the point of application; lower numbers correlate to larger protein size. PAS staining correlates to proteins with high carbohydrate composition, designated as PAS-1, PAS-2, etc.
- The shape and flexibility of the RBC, which are essential to its function, are most strongly related to the cytoskeleton. The cytoskeleton is derived from a group of peripheral proteins on the interior side of the lipid membrane. The major structural protein is spectrin, which is held together and to the lipid membrane by ankyrin, actin, protein 4.1, and band 3.

- Abnormalities of the peripheral structural proteins such as spectrin and actin lead to abnormal RBC shapes. Hereditary spherocytosis and hereditary elliptocytosis are examples of diseases associated with abnormalities and deficiencies of structural proteins.
- The concentration of potassium inside the RBC is higher than that in the plasma, whereas its sodium concentration is lower than plasma. This disequilibrium is maintained by a Na^{2+}-K^+ pump in the membrane. Failure of the pump leads to an influx of sodium with water following by osmosis, leading to cell swelling and possible lysis.

REVIEW QUESTIONS

1. An RBC process that does *not* require energy is:
   a. Maintenance of intracellular cationic electrochemical gradients
   b. Oxygen transport
   c. Maintenance of skeletal protein plasticity
   d. Initiation and maintenance of glycolysis

2. ATP is generated by the:
   a. Embden-Meyerhof pathway
   b. Hexose monophosphate pathway
   c. Luebering-Rapaport pathway
   d. Aerobic glycolytic pathway

3. The enzyme deficiency in the Embden-Meyerhof pathway responsible for most cases of hereditary nonspherocytic hemolytic anemia is:
   a. Hexokinase
   b. Triose phosphate isomerase
   c. Glyceraldehyde-3-phosphate
   d. Pyruvate kinase

4. The glycolytic enzyme that catalyzes the formation of the cofactor NADH, which enhances methemoglobin reductase activity, is:
   a. Hexokinase
   b. Phosphotriptokinase
   c. Glyceraldehyde-3-phosphate dehydrogenase
   d. Pyruvate kinase

5. Which of the following is true concerning 2,3-BPG?
   a. It enhances the release of oxygen from hemoglobin.
   b. It provides a source of glucose for the RBC.
   c. It is unnecessary for RBC survival.
   d. It is the least of all organophosphates in the RBC.

6. The hexose monophosphate pathway activity increases the RBC source of:
   a. Glucose and lactic acid
   b. 2,3-BPG and methemoglobin
   c. NADPH and reduced glutathione
   d. ATP and other purine metabolites

7. The enzyme within the hexose monophosphate pathway that, when deficient, leaves cells vulnerable to oxidative damage is:
   a. Phosphogluconate dehydrogenase
   b. Pyruvate kinase
   c. Aldolase
   d. Glucose-6-phosphate dehydrogenase

8. The layer of the erythrocyte membrane that is largely responsible for the shape, structure, and deformability of the cell is the:
   a. Integral protein
   b. Exterior lipid
   c. Peripheral protein
   d. Interior lipid

9. The glycolipids of the RBC membrane:
   a. Provide flexibility to the membrane
   b. Constitute ion channels
   c. Carry RBC antigens
   d. Attach the cytoskeleton to the lipid layer

10. The lipids of the membrane are arranged:
   a. In chains beneath a protein exoskeleton
   b. So that the hydrophobic portions are facing the plasma
   c. In a hexagonal lattice
   d. In two layers that are not symmetric in composition

11. Lipid exchange between the RBC membrane and the plasma occurs:
   a. To replace lost lipids in the membrane
   b. To provide a mechanism for excretion of lipid-soluble RBC waste products
   c. To ensure symmetry between the composition of the interior and exterior lipid layers
   d. To provide lipid-soluble nutrients to the RBC

12. The numbering system for membrane proteins gives the lowest number to proteins that are:
    a. Smallest
    b. Most negatively charged
    c. Largest
    d. Most positively charged

13. Which of the following is an example of an integral membrane protein?
    a. Spectrin
    b. Glycophorin A
    c. Actin
    d. Ankyrin

14. Which of the following statements about spectrin structure is correct?
    a. Spectrin forms homodimers that twist into ropelike strands.
    b. Spectrin dimers associate into tetramers that are tightly bound to each other throughout their length.
    c. Seven spectrin tetramers join at their ends to create a lattice.
    d. The spectrin strands are connected to the lipid bilayer by ankyrin.

15. All of the following are functions of band 3 *except*:
    a. Provide a channel for anion movement through the membrane
    b. Contribute to membrane flexibility
    c. Attach spectrin to the lipid bilayer
    d. Identify senescent RBCs

16. Na$^+$K$^+$-ATPase maintains a concentration of ions in which:
    a. Potassium is in higher concentration inside the RBC than in the plasma, and sodium is in lower concentration in the RBC than in the plasma
    b. Sodium and potassium are in higher concentration inside the RBC than in the plasma
    c. Sodium is in higher concentration inside the RBC than in the plasma, and potassium is in equilibrium with the plasma
    d. Potassium and sodium are in lower concentration inside the RBC than in the plasma

REFERENCES

1. Beutler E: Disorders of red cells resulting from enzyme abnormalities. In Lichtman MA, Beutler E, Kipps TJ, et al (eds): Williams Hematology, 7th ed. New York: McGraw-Hill, 2006:603-631.
2. Kondo T, Beutler E: Developmental changes in glucose transport of guinea pig erythrocytes. J Clin Invest 1980;65:1-4.
3. Netzloff WL: Clinical consequences of enzyme deficiencies in the erythrocyte. Ann Clin Lab Sci 1980;10:414-424.
4. Vora S: Isoenzymes of human phosphofructokinase: biochemical and genetic aspects. In Rattazz MC, Scandalios JG, Whitt GS (eds): Isozymes: Current Topics in Biological and Medical Research, 2nd ed. New York: Alan R Liss, 1983:119-167.
5. Jaffé ER, Hultquist DE: Cytochrome b$_5$ reductase deficiency and enzymopenic hereditary methemoglobinemia. In Scriver CR, Beaudet AL, Sly WS, et al (eds): Metabolic and Molecular Bases of Inherited Disease, 8th ed. New York: McGraw-Hill, 2001:4555-4570.
6. Rosa R, Gaillardon J, Rosa J: Diphosphoglycerate mutase and 2,3-diphosphoglycerate phosphatase activities of red cells: comparative electrophoretic studies. Biochem Biophys Res Commun 1973;51:536-542.
7. Beutler E: Hemolytic Anemia in Disorders of Red Cell Metabolism. New York: Plenum, 1978.
8. Prchal JT, Gregg JT: Cell enzymopathies. In Hoffman R, Benz EJ, Shattil SJ, et al (eds): Hematology Principles and Practice, 3rd ed. New York: Churchill Livingstone, 2000:561-576.
9. Beutler E: Glucose-6-phosphate dehydrogenase deficiency. N Engl J Med 1991;324:169-174.
10. Beutler E: The genetics of glucose-6-phosphate dehydrogenase deficiency. Semin Hematol 1990;27:137-167.
11. Rijksen G, Staal GE: Regulation of human erythrocyte hexokinase: the influence of glycolytic intermediates and inorganic phosphate. Biochim Biophys Acta 1977;485:75-86.
12. Beutler E: 2,3-Diphosphoglycerate affects enzymes of glucose metabolism in the red blood cell. Nat New Biol 1971;232:20-21.
13. Messana I, Ferroni L, Misiti F: Blood bank conditions and RBCs: the progressive loss of metabolic modulation. Transfusion 2000;40:353-360.
14. Lenard JG: A note on the shape of the erythrocyte. Bull Math Biol 1974;36:55-58.
15. Schmid-Schönbein H: Erythrocyte rheology and the optimization of mass transport in the microcirculation. Blood Cell 1975;1:285-306.
16. Telen MH, Kaufman RE: The mature erythrocyte. In Greer JP, Foerster J, Lukens JN, et al (eds): Wintrobe's Clinical Hematology, 11th ed. Philadelphia: Lippincott, Williams & Wilkins, 2004:217-247.
17. Steck TL: The organization of proteins in the human red blood cell membrane. J Cell Biol 1974;62:1-19.
18. Cooper RA: Lipids of human red cell membrane: normal composition and variability in disease. Semin Hematol 1970;7:296-322.
19. Gallagher PG, Lux SE: Disorders of the erythrocyte membrane. In Nathan DG, Orkin SH (eds): Nathan and Oski's Hematology of Infancy and Childhood, 5th ed. Philadelphia: Saunders, 2003:560-684.
20. Danielli JF: The bilayer hypothesis of membrane structure. Hosp Pract 1973;8:63-71.
21. Stoeckenius W, Engelman DM: Current models for the structure of biological membranes. J Cell Biol 1969;42:613-646.
22. Parpart AK, Dzieman AJ: The chemical composition of the red cell membrane. Cold Spr Harb Symp Quant Biol 1940;8:17-24.
23. Cooper RA: Influence of the increased membrane cholesterol on membrane fluidity and cell function in human red blood cells. J Supramol Struct 1978;8:413-430.
24. Rothman JE, Lenard J: Membrane asymmetry. Science 1977;195:743-753.
25. Hakomori S, Jeanloz RW: Isolation and characterization of glycolipids from erythrocytes of human blood A (+) and B (+). J Biol Chem 1961;236:2827-2834.

26. Hakomori S, Strycharz GD: Investigations on cellular blood-group substances: I. Isolation and chemical composition of blood-group ABH and Le-b isoantigens of sphingoglycolipid nature. Biochemistry 1968;7:1279-1286.
27. Hakomori S, Andrews HD: Sphingoglycolipids with Le^b activity,and the co-presence of Le^a-, Le^b-glycolipids in human tumor tissue. Biochim Biophys Acta 1970;202:225-228.
28. Watkins WM: Blood group substances. Science 1966;152:172-181.
29. Watkins WM: Blood group substances: their nature and genetics. In Surgenor DM (ed): The Red Blood Cell, 2nd ed. New York: Academic Press, 1974:293-360.
30. Suyama K, Goldstein J: Enzymatic evidence for differences in the placement of Rh antigens. Blood 1991;75:225-260.
31. Agre P, Cartron JP: Molecular biology of the Rh antigens. Blood 1991;78:551-563.
32. Shohet SB: Hemolysis and changes in erythrocyte membrane lipids. N Engl J Med 1972;286:577-583.
33. Shohet SB, Livermore BM, Nathan DG, et al: Hereditary hemolytic anemia associated with abnormal membrane lipids: mechanism of accumulation of phosphatidylcholine. Blood 1971;38:445-456.
34. Cooper RA, Jandl JH: Bile salts and cholesterol in the pathogenesis of target cells in obstructive jaundice. J Clin Invest 1968;47:809-822.
35. Singer SJ, Nicholson GL: The fluid mosaic model of the structure of cell membranes. Science 1972;175:720-731.
36. Bennett V: The membrane skeleton of human erythrocytes and its implications for more complex cells. Annu Rev Biochem 1985;54:273-304.
37. Fairbanks G, Steck TL, Wallach DF: Electrophoretic analysis of the major polypeptides of the human erythrocyte membrane. Biochemistry 1971;10:2606-2617.
38. Gallagher PG: Disorders of the red cell membrane: Hereditary spherocytosis, elliptocytosis, and related disorders. In Lichtman MA, Beutler E, Kipps TJ, et al (eds): Williams Hematology, 7th ed. New York: McGraw-Hill, 2006:571-601.
39. Lux SE, Tse WT: Hereditary spherocytosis and hereditary elliptocytosis. In Scriver CR, Beaudet AL, Sly WS, et al (eds): The Metabolic and Molecular Bases of Inherited Disease, 8th ed. New York: McGraw-Hill, 2001:4665-4727.
40. Furthmayr H: Glycophorins A, B, and C: a family of sialoglycoproteins, isolation and preliminary characterization of trypsin derived peptides. In Lux SE, Marchesi VT, Fox CJ (eds): Normal and Abnormal Red Cell Membranes. New York: Alan R Liss, 1979:195-211.
41. Jennings ML: Topical review: oligometric structure and the anion transport function of human erythrocyte band 3 protein. J Membr Biol 1984;80:105-117.
42. Kay MM, Bosman GJ, Johnson GJ, et al: Band 3 polymers and aggregates and hemoglobin precipitates in red cell aging. Blood Cells 1988;14:275-295.
43. Cartron JP: Defining the Rh blood group antigens: biochemistry and molecular genetics. Blood Rev 1994;8:199-212.
44. Sturgeon P: Hematological observations on the anemia associated with blood type Rh null. Blood 1970;36:310-320.
45. Costa FF, Agre P, Watkins PC, et al: Linkage of dominant hereditary spherocytosis to the gene for the erythrocyte membrane-skeleton protein ankyrin. N Engl J Med 1990;323:1046-1050.
46. Gallagher PG, Forget BG: Hematologically important mutations: spectrin and ankyrin variants in hereditary spherocytosis. Blood Cells Mol Dis 1998;24:539-543.
47. Coetzer T, Zail S: Spectrin tetramer-dimer equilibrium in hereditary elliptocytosis. Blood 1982;59:900-905.
48. Shotton DM, Burke BE, Branton D: The molecular structure of human erythrocyte spectrin: biophysical and electron microscope studies. J Mol Biol 1979;131:303-329.
49. Speicher DW, Marchesi VT: Erythrocyte spectrin is composed of many homologous triple helical segments. Nature 1984;311:177-180.
50. Liu SC, Drick LH, Palek J: Visualization of the hexagonal lattice in the erythrocyte membrane skeleton. J Cell Biol 1987;104:527-536.
51. Shen BW, Josephs R, Steck TL: Ultrastructure of unit fragments of the skeleton of the human erythrocyte membrane. J Cell Biol 1984;99:810-821.
52. Anderson RA, Lovrien RE: Glycophorin is linked by band 4.1 protein to the human erythrocyte membrane skeleton. Nature 1984;307:655-658.
53. Bennett V, Stenbuck PJ: The membrane attachment protein for spectrin is associated with band 3 in human erythrocyte membranes. Nature 1979;280:468-473.
54. Harris EJ, Pressman BC: Obligate cation exchanges in red cells. Nature 1967;216:918-920.
55. Jorgensen PL: Mechanism of the Na$^+$, K$^+$ pump: protein structure and conformation of the pure (Na^{++} K$^+$)-ATPase. Biochim Biophys Acta 1982;694:27-68.
56. Rhoda MD, Aprovo N, Beuzard Y, et al: Ca^{++} permeability in deoxygenated sickle cells. Blood 1990;75:2453-2458.
57. James PH, Pruschy M, Vorherr TE, et al: Primary structure of the cAMP-dependent phosphorylation site of the plasma membrane calcium pump. Biochemistry 1989;28:4253-4258.
58. Takakuwa Y, Mohandas N: Modulation of erythrocyte membrane material properties by Ca^{2+} and calmodulin: implications for their role in skeletal protein interaction. J Clin Invest 1988;82:394-400.

Hemoglobin Metabolism

10

Mary Coleman

OBJECTIVES

After completion of this chapter, the reader will be able to:

1. Describe the primary structure of the globin chains found in hemoglobin (Hb).
2. Describe the quaternary structure of Hb.
3. Describe the biosynthesis of heme and globin.
4. Differentiate steps in heme synthesis that occur in the mitochondria and the cytoplasm.
5. Discuss the ontogeny of Hb with emphasis on the Hb of newborns and adults.
6. Name the three types of normal Hb in adults and their reference intervals.
7. Describe the regulatory effects of Hb metabolism.
8. Identify the important role that Hb plays in maintaining body functions.
9. Describe the mechanism by which Hb carries oxygen to the tissue.
10. Describe the Bohr effect.
11. Explain the significance of the sigmoid shape of the oxygen dissociation curve.
12. Correlate shifts in the oxygen dissociation curve with causes, predicting the impact on the curve.
13. Discuss the P_{50} value as it pertains to the oxygen dissociation curve.
14. Differentiate T and R forms of Hb.
15. Discuss 2,3-bisphosphoglycerate (2,3-BPG), including its source and impact on Hb oxygenation.
16. Discuss oxygen affinity of fetal Hb, including the cause of its relative oxygen binding ability and the impact it has on the molecule's function.
17. Describe the composition of the chemically modified Hbs—methemoglobin, carboxyhemoglobin, and sulfhemoglobin—and their affinity for oxygen.
18. Differentiate oxygenated versus oxidized Hb and ferric versus ferrous iron.
19. Describe how Hb is routinely measured in the laboratory.
20. Discuss the genetics of Hb, including the number of genes for each globin chain (for Hb A, A_2, and F) and their general arrangement on chromosomes.

CASE STUDY

After studying the material in this chapter, the reader should be able to respond to the following case study:

A mother and her newborn infant were seen in a clinic laboratory as part of a study group having Hb and Hb electrophoresis testing done. The testing was part of a screening program being done at the laboratory to establish reference values for these tests. The mother's Hb was 140 g/L (14 g/dL), and the infant's Hb was 200 g/L (20 g/dL). The mother's Hb electrophoresis results were 97% Hb A, 2% Hb A_2, and 1% Hb F. The newborn's Hb was 88% Hb F and 12% Hb A.

1. Were these Hb results within expected reference intervals?
2. Why were the mother's and the newborn's Hb results so different?
3. What is the difference between a Hb test and a Hb electrophoresis test?
4. Why were the mother's and newborn's Hb electrophoresis results so different?

STRUCTURE

The hemoglobin (Hb) molecule is a conjugated protein. It is the first protein whose structure was described by x-ray crystallography.[1-4] Each Hb molecule consists of four heme groups and two pairs of unlike polypeptide chains (Fig. 10-1).

Hb is the main component of erythrocytes/red blood cells (RBCs). Hb outside the RBCs (free Hb) does not survive long; it is rapidly salvaged and catabolized or excreted renally. The concentration of Hb within the erythrocytes/RBCs is approximately 34 g/dL, and its molecular weight is approximately 64,000 D. Hb's main function is as a vehicle for the transport of oxygen in the body.

Heme

The heme structure consists of a ring of carbon, hydrogen, and nitrogen atoms called *protoporphyrin IX* with an atom of divalent/ferrous iron (Fe^{2+}) attached (ferroprotoporphyrin) (Fig. 10-2). Each heme group is positioned in a pocket of the polypeptide chain near the surface of the Hb molecule. The heme component can combine reversibly with one molecule of oxygen. The heme component also renders blood red.

Globin

The globin in the Hb molecule consists of two pairs of polypeptide chains. These chains comprise 141 to 146 amino acids each. Variations in the amino acid sequences give rise to different types of polypeptide chains. Each polypeptide chain is designated by a Greek letter (Table 10-1).[5]

Each of the polypeptide chains is divided into eight helices and seven nonhelical segments. The helices, designated A to H, contain subgroup numberings for the sequence of the amino acids in each helix and are relatively rigid and linear. The nonhelical segments are more flexible and lie between the helical

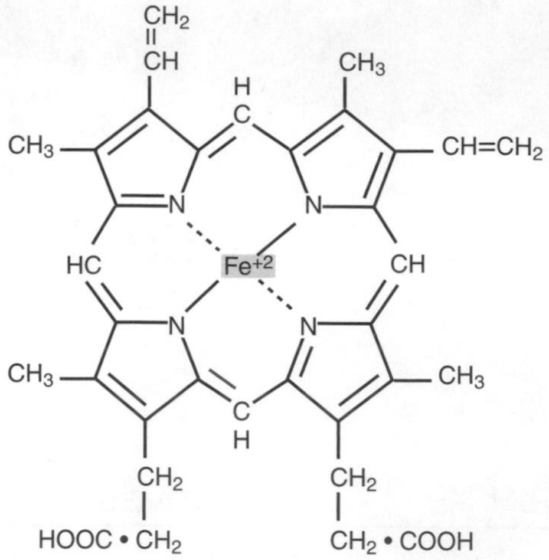

Figure 10-2 Protoporphyrin IX + Fe^{2+} = heme.

TABLE 10-1 Globin Chains

Symbol	Name	No. Amino Acids
α	Alpha	141
β	Beta	146
γ_A	Gamma A	146 (position 136: alanine)
γ_G	Gamma G	146 (position 136: glycine)
δ	Delta	146
ϵ	Epsilon	Unknown
ζ	Zeta	141
θ	Theta	Unknown

segments, as reflected by their designations: NA for the residues that lie between the N terminus and the A helix, AB for the residues between the A and B helices, and so forth with BC, CD, DE, EF, FG, GH, and HC (Fig. 10-3), and the carboxy terminus.

Complete Molecule

The Hb molecule can be described by its primary, secondary, tertiary, and quaternary protein structure. Its *primary structure* refers to the amino acids in the polypeptide chains. The *secondary structure* refers to the polypeptide chain arrangements in helices and nonhelices. The *tertiary structure* refers to the arrangement of the helices into a three-dimensional, pretzel-like structure. The globin chains are looped to form a cleft pocket for heme. Each chain contains a heme group that is suspended between the E and F helices of the polypeptide chain. The iron atom at the center of the protoporphyrin IX ring of heme is positioned between two histidine radicals, forming a bond with F8 (proximal histidine) and a close association with E7 (distal histidine residue). The distal histidine appears to swing in and out of its position to permit the passage of oxygen into and out of the Hb molecule. Amino acids in the cleft are hydrophobic, and amino acids on the outside are hydrophilic, rendering the molecule water soluble. The arrangement also helps iron stay in the divalent/ferrous form regardless of whether it is oxygenated (carrying oxygen molecules) or deoxygenated (not carrying oxygen molecules).

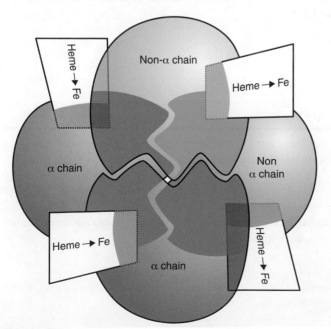

Figure 10-1 Hb molecule: a globular tetramer of four heme molecules each attached to a polypeptide chain.

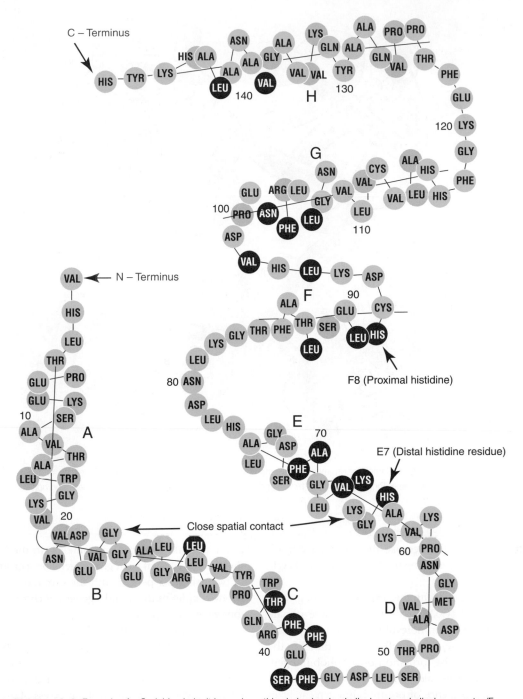

Figure 10-3 Example of a β globin chain. It is a polypeptide chain showing helical and nonhelical segments. (From Huisman TH, Schroder WA: New Aspects of the Structure, Function, and Synthesis of Hemoglobins. Boca Raton, Fla: CRC Press, 1971, modified from Stamatoyannopoulos G: The Molecular Basis of Blood Diseases, 2nd ed. Philadelphia: Saunders, 1994.)

The *quaternary structure* of Hb, also called a *tetrameric molecule,* is a complete Hb molecule. The complete Hb molecule is spherical, has four heme groups attached to four polypeptide chains, and may carry four molecules of oxygen. It is composed of two α globin chains and two non-α globin chains. Each globin chain has a heme group attached. Each heme molecule is capable of carrying one molecule of oxygen. Strong α 1, non-α 1 and α 2, non-α 2 dimeric bonds hold the molecule in a stable form. Tetrameric α 1, non-α 2 and α 2,

non-α 1 bonds also contribute to the stability of the structure (Fig. 10-4).[6,7]

BIOSYNTHESIS

Heme

Biosynthesis of heme occurs in the bone marrow in the mitochondria and cytoplasm of the erythrocyte precursors from the pronormoblast/proerythroblast to the reticulocyte. Mature

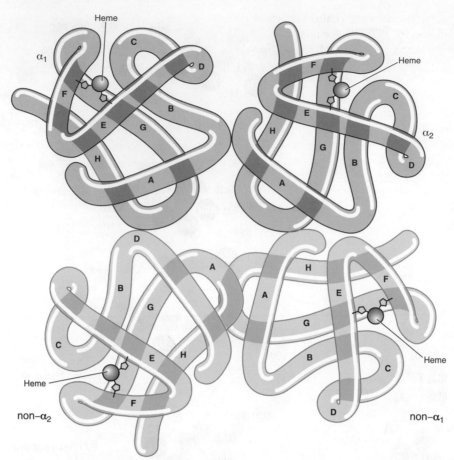

Figure 10-4 Complete Hb molecule. Heme is suspended between the E and F helices of the polypeptide chain. Pink represents α 1 (*left*) and α 2 (*right*); yellow represents non-α 2 (*left*) and non-α 1 (*right*).

erythrocytes cannot make Hb because they lose their mitochondria and the capability of using the tricarboxylic acid cycle necessary for Hb synthesis.

Heme biosynthesis begins with the condensation of glycine and succinyl coenzyme A (CoA) catalyzed by aminolevulinate synthase (ALAS) to form aminolevulinic acid (ALA). ALA dehydratase (ALA dehydrase/porphobilinogen synthase) in the presence of ALA catalyzes the formation of porphobilinogen. Porphobilinogen deaminase, also known as hydroxymethylbilane synthase, in the presence of porphobilinogen catalyzes the formation of hydroxyl methylbilane. This pathway continues until, in the final step of production of heme, Fe^{2+} combines with protoporphyrin IX in the presence of ferrochelatase/heme synthase to make heme (Fig. 10-5).[6]

Transferrin, a plasma protein, carries iron in the ferric (Fe^{3+}) form to developing RBCs. Iron goes through the RBC membrane to the mitochondria and is united with protoporphyrin IX to make heme. Heme leaves the mitochondria and is joined to the globin chains in the cytoplasm.

Globin

Six structural genes control the synthesis of the six globin chains. α and ζ genes are on chromosome 16; γ, β, δ, and ε genes are linked on chromosome 11. In the human genome, there is one copy of each globin gene per chromatid for a total of two genes per person with the exception of α and γ. There are two copies of the α and γ genes per chromatid for a total of four genes per person.

The production of the globin chains takes place from the pronormoblast to the reticulocyte.[8] The globin proteins are made via transcription of the genetic code to messenger ribonucleic acid (mRNA) and translation of mRNA to the globin polypeptide chain. A slight excess of α-globin mRNA is present in erythroblasts; however, β-globin mRNA is translated more efficiently than α-globin mRNA. This results in sets of single chains synthesized in approximately equal amounts. When synthesized, the chains are released from the ribosomes in the cytoplasm.[7]

Hemoglobin Assembly

After their release from ribosomes, each globin chain binds to a heme molecule and they pair off. An α chain and a non-α chain combine to form heterodimers. Two heterodimers spontaneously combine to form tetramers. The tetrameric $α_1β_2$ and $α_2β_1$ bonds also contribute to the stability of the structure. This completes the Hb molecule (Fig. 10-5).[6,7]

The combination of two α and two β chains along with the four heme molecules forms Hb A. This is the predominant Hb in postnatal life. Hb A$_2$ contains two α and two δ chains. δ chains are inefficiently expressed; only small amounts of Hb A$_2$ are found in the RBCs. Hb F contains two α and two γ chains. In adults, Hb F is not distributed evenly among the RBCs; it is present in a few RBCs called *F cells*.[7]

The various globin chains of Hb differ in the charge per molecule. In the procedure of Hb electrophoresis under the influence of an electric field, Hbs exhibit different mobilities, allowing differentiation of subtype. It may be necessary to use different assay procedures (support media, buffer, pH) for definitive identification (Chapter 26).

ONTOGENY

The Hb composition in the erythrocyte differs, depending on gestation or postnatal age. This change is due to changes in the activation and inactivation or switching of the globin genes, progressing from the ζ to the α gene on chromosome 16 and from the ε to the γ, δ, or β genes on chromosome 11. The ζ and ε genes normally appear only during the first 3 months of embryonic development. These two chains in addition to the α and γ chains are constituents of embryonic Hbs (Fig. 10-6). At birth, Hb F is the predominant Hb. Normal adult Hb is predominately Hb A ($\alpha_2\beta_2$) with small amounts of Hb A$_2$ ($\alpha_2\delta_2$) and Hb F ($\alpha_2\gamma_2$).[7] Table 10-2 presents adult reference intervals.

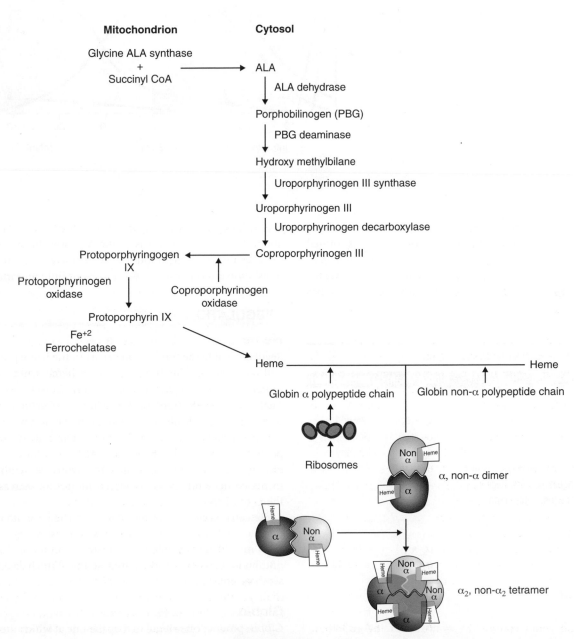

Figure 10-5 Hb assembly.

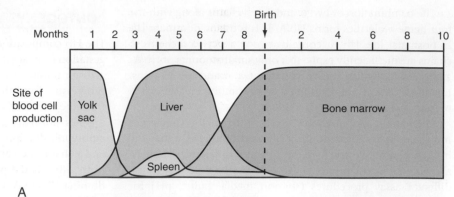

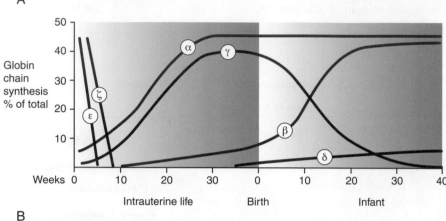

Figure 10-6 Timeline of globin chain production from intrauterine life to adulthood.

Hb A also has minor amounts of Hb that have been modified after translation (post-translation). Hb A_1 is formed by postsynthetic, nonenzymatic reactions of various sugars with amino groups of the globin chains, resulting in glycated Hb. The most common one is Hb A_{1c}, in which glucose has been added to the N terminal valine of the β chain. Normally, about 4% to 6% of Hb A is in the A_{1c} form. In uncontrolled diabetes mellitus, the amount of A_{1c} is increased. Other post-translational modifications seem to be of little importance.[7]

REGULATION

Heme

Regulation of heme production occurs in the heme production pathway. The key rate-limiting step in heme synthesis is the initial reaction of glycine and succinyl-CoA to form ALA, catalyzed by ALAS. Transcription of the ALAS gene is inhibited by heme, which leads to a decrease in heme production (a negative feedback mechanism). Other enzymes in the heme pathway inhibited by heme are ALA dehydrase and por-phobilinogen deaminase/hydroxymethylbilane synthase. An increased demand for heme would induce an increased synthesis of ALAS.[9]

Research suggests that ferrochelatase (heme synthase) also plays a regulatory role in heme biosynthesis. A negative feed-back mechanism by heme or substrate inhibition by proto-porphyrin IX is believed to inhibit the ferrochelatase/heme synthase enzyme.[9]

Globin

Globin production is regulated by the rate at which the DNA is transcribed to mRNA. The amount of the specific globins synthesized is proportional in general to the content of their

TABLE 10-2 Normal Hemoglobins

Time	Globin Chain	Hemoglobin
Intrauterine		
Early embryogenesis (product of the yolk sac erythroblasts)	$\zeta_2 + \varepsilon_2$	Gower-1
	$\alpha_2 + \varepsilon_2$	Gower-2
	$\zeta_2 + \gamma_2$	Portland
Begins in early embryogenesis; peaks during midgestation and begins rapid decline just before birth	$\alpha_2 + \gamma_2$	F
Birth		
	$\alpha_2 + \gamma_2$	F, 60-90%
	$\alpha_2 + \beta_2$	A, 10-40%
Adulthood		
	$\alpha_2 + \gamma_2$	F, <1-2%
	$\alpha_2 + \delta_2$	A_2, <3.5%
	$\alpha_2 + \beta_2$	A, >95%

individual globin mRNAs. Heme (in the form of hemin—the Fe^{3+} oxidation product of heme) is important in controlling the rate of globin synthesis in intact reticulocytes and various cell-free systems, and in its absence, polyribosomes disaggregate. A balanced globin chain and heme synthesis are important because excess components of Hb (unpaired chains, protoporphyrin, and iron) can decrease RBC survival. The end result is that normal mature RBCs contain only complete Hb molecules. Pools of free heme or globin chains are minute.[7,9]

Hemoglobin

Hb synthesis is normally stimulated by tissue hypoxia. Hypoxia causes the kidneys to produce increased amounts of erythropoietin, which stimulates the production of Hb and RBCs. Although each laboratory must establish its own reference ranges based on their instrumentation, methodology, and patient population, in general, reference intervals for Hb are as follows:

Men	14-18 g/dL (140-180 g/L)
Women	12-15 g/dL (120-150 g/L)
Newborns	16.5-21.5 g/dL (165-215 g/L)

Reference intervals for infants and children vary according to different age groups. Individuals living at high altitudes have slightly higher levels of Hb as a compensatory mechanism to provide more oxygen to the tissues in the oxygen-thin air. The tables on the inside front cover of this book show reference intervals for all age groups.

FUNCTION

The responsibility of Hb is to bind oxygen molecules readily in the lung (requiring a high affinity for oxygen), transport oxygen, and unload oxygen in the tissues (requiring a low oxygen affinity). Each of the four heme iron atoms in a Hb molecule can reversibly bind one oxygen molecule, resulting in oxygenation of Hb. Approximately 1.34 mL of oxygen is bound by each 1 g of Hb.

The affinity of Hb for oxygen depends on the partial pressure of oxygen (pO_2), often defined in terms of the amount of oxygen needed to saturate 50% of Hb, called the P_{50} value. The relationship is described by the oxygen dissociation curve of Hb, which plots the oxygen content of Hb (% oxygen saturation) versus the pO_2 (Fig. 10-7). The curve is sigmoidal and indicates a low Hb affinity for oxygen at low oxygen tension and a high affinity for oxygen at high oxygen tensions. Cooperation among the subunits of Hb within the tetramers contributes to the shape of the curve. Rather than undergo simultaneous oxygenation or deoxygenation, the state of each heme unit with regard to the number of other units influences further binding. That is, Hb that is completely deoxygenated has little affinity for oxygen, but with each oxygen molecule that is bound, the avidity increases, and the Hb molecule quickly becomes fully oxygenated.[7] Shifts of the curve to the left or right occur if there are changes in the pH of blood. This shift in the curve as a result of pH is termed the *Bohr effect*.

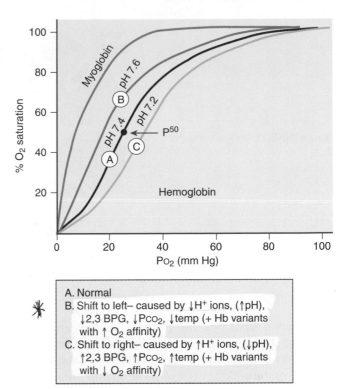

A. Normal
B. Shift to left– caused by ↓H^+ ions, (↑pH), ↓2,3 BPG, ↓Pco_2, ↓temp (+ Hb variants with ↑ O_2 affinity)
C. Shift to right– caused by ↑H^+ ions, (↓pH), ↑2,3 BPG, ↑Pco_2, ↑temp (+ Hb variants with ↓ O_2 affinity)

Figure 10-7 Oxygen dissociation curve.

Normally, a pO_2 of approximately 27 mm Hg results in 50% oxygen saturation of the Hb molecule. If there is a shift of the curve to the left, 50% oxygen saturation of Hb occurs at a Po_2 of less than 27 mm Hg. If there is a shift of the curve to the right, 50% oxygen saturation of Hb occurs at a pO_2 greater than 27 mm Hg.

The reference interval for arterial oxygen saturation is 96% to 100%. If the oxygen dissociation curve shifts to the left, a patient with arterial and venous pO_2 concentrations in the reference intervals (80-100 mm Hg arterial and 30-50 mm Hg venous) would have a higher oxygen saturation percent and a higher affinity for oxygen than a patient with a normal curve. With a shift to the right in the curve, a lower oxygen affinity is seen, and Hb does not pick up as much oxygen in the lungs but gives off more oxygen to the tissue than it normally would do, as in the presence of Hb S (Chapter 26).

Why and how 2,3-bisphosphoglycerate (2,3-BPG), formerly called 2,3-diphosphoglycerate, affects the oxygen affinity of Hb is a complex process. The Hb molecule is an allosteric molecule; that is, its function and structure are influenced by other molecules. In the presence of large amounts of 2,3-BPG, the Hb molecule changes from a relaxed (R) oxygenated molecule to a tense (T) deoxygenated molecule. Many conformational changes occur in the Hb molecule for it to bind to 2,3-BPG. The T structure is stabilized by salt bridges, which are broken as the molecule switches into the R structure. When the salt bridges are broken, the Hb molecule is able to bind to oxygen (Fig. 10-8). Carbon dioxide, hydrogen ions, and chloride ions all decrease the affinity of Hb for oxygen by strengthening the salt bridges that lock the molecule into its T

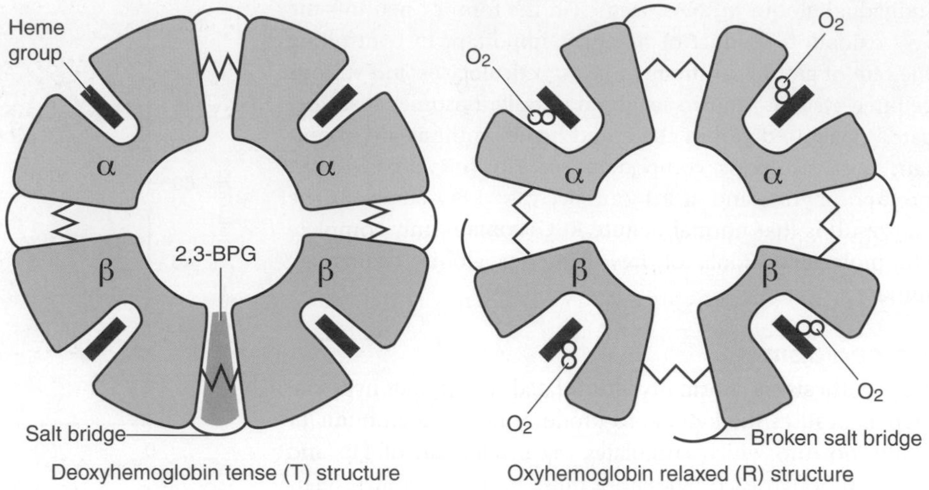

Figure 10-8 Hb molecular changes.

conformation. Some abnormal Hbs with a high oxygen affinity and low P_{50} occur as a result of amino acid substitutions that lead to loss of bonds that would have stabilized the tetramer in the T conformation. Without these binding sites, the Hb molecule holds on more tightly to oxygen—hence a higher oxygen affinity.[7]

Clinical conditions that produce a shift to the left include a lowered body temperature owing to external causes; multiple transfusions of stored blood with depleted 2,3-BPG; alkalosis; and the presence of methemoglobin, carboxyhemoglobin, or some other Hb variants. Conditions producing a shift of the curve to the right include increased body temperature, increased 2,3-BPG concentrations, increased H^+ concentration (decreased pH), and abnormal Hbs with low affinity for oxygen. Clinical conditions that produce a right shift include a high fever; acidosis; and conditions that produce hypoxia, such as high altitude, pulmonary insufficiency, congestive heart failure, severe anemia, and cardiac right-to-left shunt.[7]

Oxygen's sigmoidal curve is in contrast to myoglobin's hyperbolic curve (see Fig. 10-7). Myoglobin, which is present in cardiac and skeletal muscle, is an oxygen-binding heme protein. It has a molecular weight of 17,000 D. It exists in a monomer form and binds oxygen with greater affinity than does Hb. Its hyperbolic curve indicates that it releases oxygen only at very low partial pressures, which means it is not as effective as Hb in releasing oxygen to the tissues at physiologic tensions. It is released into the bloodstream when there is damage to the muscle in conditions such as a myocardial infarction, extensive trauma, or severe muscle damage, called *rhabdomyolysis*. Myoglobin normally is flushed out through the kidney, but in the presence of renal failure, it may be elevated. Testing for serum myoglobin may aid in detecting myocardial infarction but would be of no value in patients suspected to have myocardial infarction who also have extensive trauma, rhabdomyolysis, or renal failure. Elevated myoglobin levels give a positive result on the urine Hb dipstick and must be differentiated from Hb in the urine. Hemoglobinuria would be seen in intravascular hemolytic disorders, whereas myoglobinuria could be seen in the aforementioned disorders.[7]

Hb F (fetal Hb, the primary Hb in cord blood) has increased oxygen affinity relative to Hb A. Hb F has a P_{50} of 19 to 21 mm Hg, resulting in a left shift of the oxygen dissociation curve. The fetus has physiologic ability to extract oxygen from the maternal blood supply via Hb F. Hb F does not deliver oxygen to tissues as efficiently as adult Hb, however. To achieve adequate tissue oxygenation, the fetus must have more Hb, and the reference value of Hb for newborns is higher than in the postnatal period when adult Hb predominates.

A second crucial function of Hb is in transporting carbon dioxide in the blood. In the blood, carbon dioxide undergoes a pair of reactions in which carbon dioxide combines with water to form carbonic acid, and then carbonic acid disassociates to release H^+ and bicarbonate:

$$CO_2 + H_2O \rightarrow H_2CO_3$$

$$H_2CO_3 \rightarrow H^+ + HCO_3^-$$

The first of these reactions is RBC-facilitated by the enzyme carbonic anhydrase. The H^+ from the second reaction joins deoxygenated Hb. The bicarbonate diffuses across the RBC membrane, and a portion is exchanged with plasma Cl^-; this is called the *chloride shift*. The plasma bicarbonate travels to the lungs where it is expired. About 70% to 85% of tissue carbon dioxide is processed in this manner.[10] Approximately 10% to 20% of carbon dioxide binds to the N-terminal amino group of each globin chain as carbaminohemoglobin. Carbaminohemoglobin has a lower affinity for oxygen than does Hb in the absence of carbon dioxide.[11]

CHEMICALLY MODIFIED HEMOGLOBINS

Chemically modified Hbs are acquired Hb variants whose structure has been modified by drugs or environmental chemicals. Methemoglobin, sulfhemoglobin, and carboxyhemoglobin are chemically modified Hbs.

Methemoglobin

Methemoglobin is a form of Hb that contains iron in the ferric state (Fe^{3+}). Methemoglobin is continuously being formed within erythrocytes in small amounts because of spontaneous oxidation, but it is prevented from accumulating within the erythrocytes by the reduction of oxidized heme by numerous enzyme systems that restrict the normal concentration of methemoglobin to less than 1% of total Hb (Chapter 9).

Methemoglobin has a brownish to bluish color, and it does not revert to red on exposure to oxygen. Oxidized iron cannot bind oxygen, but when one or more iron atoms have been oxidized, the conformation of the Hb molecule changes, and the oxygen affinity of the remaining heme groups increases.[12,13] If increased in blood, methemoglobin produces a shift to the left in the oxygen dissociation curve, and oxygen is not delivered efficiently to the tissues. If methemoglobin is greater than 30% of total Hb, patients present with hypoxia and cyanosis.[5,14]

Elevated levels of methemoglobin are seen when there is excess production of methemoglobin as a result of presence of oxidants (e.g., nitrites) or if there is decreased activity of methemoglobin reductase (usually a genetic deficiency). It also is seen in patients who inherit Hb M disease, which is caused by an abnormality in the structure of the globin portion of the Hb molecule (Chapter 26).[15]

Methemoglobin levels can be detected by spectrum absorption instruments. Methemoglobin peaks in the range of 620 to 640 nm at pH 7.1. Treatment of acquired methemoglobinemia is removal of the offending substance or administration of ascorbic acid or methylene blue.[15]

Sulfhemoglobin

Sulfhemoglobin is a chemically modified Hb formed by the irreversible oxidation of Hb by certain drugs and chemicals, such as sulfonamides, phenacetin, acetanilide, and phenazopyridine. In vitro it is formed by the addition of hydrogen sulfide to Hb and has a greenish pigment. It is ineffective for oxygen transport (100 times less affinity for oxygen than unmodified Hb), and patients with elevated levels present with cyanosis. Sulfhemoglobin cannot be converted to unmodified Hb; it persists for the life of the cell. Treatment consists of avoidance of the offending agent.[5,11]

Sulfhemoglobin, similar to methemoglobin, peaks at 620 ηm on a spectral absorption instrument. The sulfhemoglobin spectral curve does not shift when cyanide is added, and that feature can be used to distinguish it from methemoglobin.[5]

Carboxyhemoglobin

Carboxyhemoglobin results from the binding of carbon monoxide to heme iron. Hb has about 200 times more affinity for carbon monoxide, and although carbon monoxide combines with Hb more slowly than oxygen, the union is much firmer and the release of carbon monoxide is 10,000 times slower than the release of oxygen from deoxyhemoglobin. Carbon monoxide has been termed the "silent killer" because it is an odorless and colorless gas, and victims may quickly become hypoxic.[5]

Some carboxyhemoglobin is produced endogenously. The reference interval is 0.2% to 0.8%. Exogenous carbon monoxide is derived from the exhaust of automobiles and from industrial pollutants, such as coal, gas, charcoal burning, and tobacco smoke. In smokers, levels may vary from 4% to 20%. Exposure to carbon monoxide may be coincidental, accidental, or intentional (suicidal). Many deaths from house fires are the result of inhaling smoke, fumes, or carbon monoxide.[16] Even when heating systems in the home are properly maintained, accidental poisoning with carbon monoxide does occur.[17] Toxic effects, such as headaches and dizziness, may be present at levels of 10% to 15%. Levels of more than 50% may cause coma and convulsions. Carboxyhemoglobin may be detected by spectral absorption instruments at 541 nm. It gives blood a cherry-red color, which is also imparted to the skin of poisoning victims. In severe carbon monoxide poisoning, hyperbaric oxygen treatments have been used.

HEMOGLOBIN MEASUREMENT

The reference method used to measure Hb is the cyanmethemoglobin method.[18] A lysing agent present in the cyanmethemoglobin reagent is used to free Hb from the RBCs. Hb combines with potassium ferricyanide, which is present in the cyanmethemoglobin reagent, converting the Hb iron from the ferrous state to the ferric state to form methemoglobin. Methemoglobin combines with potassium cyanide to form the stable pigment, cyanmethemoglobin. Cyanmethemoglobin is used to quantify Hb by reading the color change spectrophotometrically at 540 nm and comparing it with a standard (Chapter 14). This manual method has been adapted for use in automated instruments. Many instruments now use sodium lauryl sulfate (SLS) to convert Hb to SLS-methemoglobin. This method does not generate toxic wastes (Chapter 39).

CHAPTER at a GLANCE

- The Hb molecule is composed of four heme groups (protoporphyrin IX + Fe^{2+}) and two pairs of unlike polypeptide chains. Each heme molecule combines with one polypeptide chain.
- Hb, contained in RBCs, carries oxygen to the tissue bound to the ferrous iron in heme.
- Hb biosynthesis is regulated by hormones, oxygen tension in the kidneys, and enzymes in the heme synthesis pathway.

- 2,3-BPG produced by the glycolytic pathway facilitates the unloading of oxygen from Hb in the tissues.
- The oxygenation curve of Hb is sigmoid owing to cooperativity among its subunits.
- The Bohr effect explains the effect of pH on the oxygen release mechanism of Hb.
- The three normal adult Hbs are Hb A, Hb A_2, and Hb F. Hb A, composed of two $\alpha\beta$ heterodimers, is the predominant Hb of adults.

CHAPTER at a GLANCE—cont'd

- Hb ontogeny explains which Hbs are made in the fetus through birth to adulthood.
- Chemically modified Hbs do not transport oxygen to the tissues well, resulting in cyanosis.

Now that you have completed this chapter, go back and read again the case study at the beginning and respond to the questions presented.

REVIEW QUESTIONS

1 A Hb molecule is composed of:
   a. One heme molecule and four globin chains
   b. Ferrous iron, protoporphyrin IX, and a globin chain
   c. Protoporphyrin IX and four globin chains
   d. Four heme molecules and four globin chains

2. Normal adult Hb A contains the following polypeptide chains:
   a. α and β
   b. α and δ
   c. α and γ
   d. α and ϵ

3. A key rate-limiting step in heme synthesis is suppression of:
   a. Aminolevulinate synthase
   b. Transferrin mRNA synthesis
   c. Iron oxidase
   d. Protoporphyrin IX reductase

4. Which of the following forms of Hb molecule has the lowest affinity for oxygen?
   a. Tense
   b. Relaxed
   c. Arterial
   d. Venous

5. Using the normal Hb oxygenation curve in Fig. 10-7 for reference, predict the position of the oxygenation curve for methemoglobin.
   a. Shifted to the right of normal
   b. Shifted to the left of normal
   c. No change

6. The predominant Hb found in a normal newborn is:
   a. Gower 1
   b. Gower 2
   c. A
   d. F

7. What is the distribution of normal Hbs in adults?
   a. 80-90% Hb A, 5-10% Hb A_2, 1-5% Hb F
   b. 80-90% Hb A_2, 5-10% Hb A, 1-5% Hb F
   c. >95% Hb A, <3.5 % Hb A_2, <1-2% Hb F
   d. >90% Hb A, 5% Hb F, 1% Hb A_2

8. Which of the following is a description of the structure of oxidized Hb?
   a. Hb carrying oxygen on heme; synonymous with oxygenated Hb
   b. Hb with iron in the ferric state (methemoglobin) and not able to carry oxygen
   c. Hb with iron in the ferric state so that carbon dioxide replaces oxygen in the heme structure
   d. Hb carrying carbon monoxide, hence the "oxidized" refers to the single oxygen

9. In the quaternary structure of Hb, the globin chains associate into:
   a. α tetramers in some cells and β tetramers in others
   b. A mixture of α tetramers and β tetramers in each cell
   c. α dimers and β dimers
   d. Two $\alpha\beta$ dimers

10. How are the globin chain genes arranged?
   a. With α genes and β genes on the same chromosome including two α genes and two β genes
   b. With α genes and β genes on separate chromosomes; two α genes on one chromosome and one β gene on a different chromosome
   c. With α genes and β genes on the same chromosome including four α genes and four β genes
   d. With α genes and β genes on separate chromosomes; four α genes on one chromosome and two β genes on a different chromosome

11. The nature of the interaction between 2,3-BPG and Hb is that 2,3-BPG:
   a. Binds to the heme moiety blocking the binding of oxygen
   b. Binds simultaneously with oxygen to ensure it stays bound until it reaches the tissues when both molecules release from Hb
   c. Binds to amino acids of the globin chain, contributing to a conformational change that inhibits oxygen from binding to heme
   d. Oxidizes Hb iron, diminishing oxygen binding and promoting oxygen delivery to the tissues

REFERENCES

1. Perutz MF: Molecular anatomy, physiology and pathology of hemoglobin. In Stamatoyannopoulos G, Nienhuis AW, Leder P (eds): The Molecular Basis of Blood Diseases. Philadelphia: Saunders, 1987:127-173.

2. Perutz MF, Rossman MG, Cullis AP, et al: Structure of hemoglobin: a three dimensional fourier synthesis at 5.5A resolution obtained by x-ray analysis. Nature 1960;185:416-422.

3. Perutz MF, Kendrew JC, Watson HC: Structure and function of hemoglobin: II. Some relations between polypeptide chain configuration and amino acid sequence. J Mol Biol 1965;13:669-678.

4. Perutz MF, Muirhead H, Cox JM, et al: Three dimensional fourier synthesis of horse oxyhaemoglobin at 2.8A resolution: the atomic model. Nature 1968;219:131-139.

5. Schumacher HR, Alvares C, Mazzella FM: Hemoglobin. In Kaplan LA, Pesce AJ, Kazmierczak SC (eds): Clinical Chemistry Theory, Analysis, Correlation, 4th ed. St Louis: Mosby, 2003:675-694.

6. Deacon AC, Whatley SD, Elder GH: Porphyrins and disorders of porphyrin metabolism. In Burtis CA, Ashwood ER, Bruns DE (eds): Tietz Textbook of Clinical Chemistry and Molecular Diagnostics, 4th ed. Philadelphia: Saunders, 2006:1209-1235.

7. Steinberg MH, Benz EJ Jr, Adewoye HA, et al: Pathobiology of the human erythrocyte and its hemoglobins. In Hoffman R, Benz EJ Jr, Shattil SJ, et al (eds): Hematology Basic Principles and Practice, 4th ed. St Louis: Mosby, 2005:442-454.

8. Granick S, Levere RD: Heme synthesis in erythroid cells. In Moore CV, Brown EB (eds): Progress in Hematology, Vol IV. New York: Grune & Stratton, 1964:1-47.

9. Dessypris EN, Sawyer ST: Erythropoiesis. In Greer JP, Foerster J, Lukens JN, et al (eds): Wintrobe's Clinical Hematology, 11th ed. Philadelphia: Lippincott, Williams & Wilkins, 2004:195-216.

10. Hsia CCW: Respiratory function of hemoglobin. N Engl J Med 1998;338:239-248.

11. Telen MJ, Kaufman RE: The mature erythrocyte. In Greer JP, Foerster J, Lukens JN, et al (eds): Wintrobe's Clinical Hematology, 11th ed. Philadelphia: Lippincott, Williams & Wilkins, 2004:217-247.

12. Darling RC, Roughton FJW: The effect of methemoglobin on the equilibrium between oxygen and hemoglobin. Am J Physiol 1946;137:56-68.

13. Lukens J: Hemoglobins associated with cyanosis: methemoglobinemia and low-affinity hemoglobins. In Greer JP, Foerster J, Lukens JN, et al (eds): Wintrobe's Clinical Hematology, 11th ed. Philadelphia: Lippincott, Williams & Wilkins, 2004:1487-1493.

14. Benz EJ Jr: Hemoglobin variants associated with hemolytic anemia, altered oxygen affinity, and methemoglobinemias. In Hoffman R, Benz EJ Jr, Shattil SJ, et al (eds): Hematology Basic Principles and Practice, 4th ed. St Louis: Mosby, 2005:645-652.

15. Beutler E: Methemoglobinemia and other causes of cyanosis. In Williams WJ, Beutler E, Erslev, et al (eds): Hematology, 6th ed. New York: McGraw-Hill, 2001:611-618.

16. Runyan CW, Casteel C, Perkis D, et al: Unintentional injuries in the home in the United States: Part I. Mortality. Am J Prev Med 2005;28:73-79.

17. Krenzelok EP, Roth R, Full R: Carbon monoxide: the silent killer with an audible solution. Am J Emerg Med 1996;14:484-486.

18. Clinical and Laboratory Standards Institute: Reference and Selected Procedures for the Quantitative Determination of Hemoglobin in Blood: Approved Standard, 3rd ed (CLSI Document H15-A3). Wayne, PA: CLSI, 2000.

11

Iron Metabolism

Mary Coleman

OBJECTIVES

After completion of this chapter, the reader will be able to:

1. Discuss the role of iron as an essential nutrient for human survival.
2. List the sites in which iron is distributed in the body and state the approximate amount in each site.
3. State the minimum daily requirement of iron intake at various ages in men, women, and children.
4. Describe the mechanism of iron absorption and distinguish between the absorption of heme and nonheme iron.
5. State the site of iron absorption.
6. Describe transferrin, transferrin receptor, hepcidin, hemosiderin, and ferritin, including function and regulation.
7. Diagram the transport of iron from ingestion to incorporation into heme.
8. Define sideroblast, siderocyte, and siderosome.
9. Discuss regulation, excretion, transport, and storage of iron in the body.
10. Identify and discuss the laboratory tests currently used to assess iron status in the body.

CASE STUDY

After studying the material in this chapter, the reader should be able to respond to the following case study:

The efficacy of iron supplements in individuals with high iron requirements was studied in a group of blood donors age 64-71. Blood donors donated an average of 15 U of blood (485 mL blood/U) over 3.5 years without becoming anemic. Iron losses were determined from the amount of iron removed with each phlebotomy and estimated at a loss of approximately 1 mg iron/kg body weight daily. Dietary iron intake and the iron supplements each amounted to 20 mg of iron daily. As expected, a progressive decline in body iron stores occurred with each successive donation in all subjects. At the beginning of the study, the mean amount of iron stores in male and female donors was 12.5 mg/kg body weight. The mean amount in male donors at the end of the study was 9.5 mg/kg body weight in men who had taken an iron supplement and 11.3 mg/kg body weight in men who had not taken a supplement. In postmenopausal female donors, the mean amount was 10.6 mg/kg body weight for women who had taken a supplement and 13.1 mg/kg body weight for women who had not taken a supplement. At the end of the study, iron absorption was maximized to 4.1 mg/day in men and 3.6 mg/day in women.[1,2]

1. Why did these donors' iron stores decrease in the 3.5-year period?
2. What is an average iron absorption amount per day?
3. Why at the end of the study was the iron absorption maximized?
4. What laboratory tests on serum samples can be done to evaluate iron stores?
5. What are the general reference intervals for the iron study tests?
6. What does each iron study test indicate about a patient's iron stores?

Iron is essential for all living organisms.[3] Iron metabolism has been studied for more than 50 years, but the understanding of the molecular mechanisms involved in iron metabolism is currently being elucidated.[3,4] This chapter provides a general overview of iron metabolism.

Most functional iron in humans is in the form of hemoglobin (Hb) and myoglobin, heme proteins that are carriers of oxygen. In Hb, an atom of ferrous iron is incorporated into protoporphyrin IX, a ring of C, H, and N (Chapter 10). About one fourth of iron is in a storage form. Most nonheme iron is

TABLE 11-1 Iron Compartments in Normal Humans

Compartment	Total Body Iron (%)	Iron Content (mg/kg Body Weight)
Hb iron	~70	28.5
Storage iron (hemosiderin, ferritin)	~25	14.2
Myoglobin iron	~5	1.86
Other sources	<1	<1.3
Peroxidase, catalase		
Cytochromes		
Fiboflavin enzymes		
Transferrin		

stored in ferritin or hemosiderin in hepatocytes or macrophages. A very small amount is bound to transferrin, the plasma carrier protein (Table 11-1).

Iron is also a carrier of electrons and is used to bind with cofactors essential to basic metabolic oxidation and reduction reactions. It is a catalyst for oxygenation, hydroxylation, and other crucial metabolic processes, in part because of its ability to cycle reversibly and readily between the ferrous (Fe^{2+}) and the ferric (Fe^{3+}) forms. Iron must be regulated carefully because in its free form or in too-high amounts, it becomes toxic. Because of iron's catalytic action in one-electron redox reactions, it plays a key role in the formation of harmful oxygen radicals that can damage cellular structures. In living tissues, iron exists only transiently as a free cation; otherwise, it is bound by or incorporated into various proteins. The regulation of body iron is complex and is carefully controlled to preserve needed iron but not allow toxic levels.

In normal iron homeostasis, iron intake and loss are in balance. When the balance is disrupted, iron deficiency can occur from inadequate intake or excessive loss through bleeding, or iron overload can result when absorption is increased owing to genetic predisposition or repeated blood transfusions. Disorders of iron metabolism are discussed in Chapter 19.

If there is not enough iron in the body, cellular functions suffer. If too much iron accumulates (iron overload), iron toxicity may produce widespread organ damage and death. A person's iron status depends on iron intake, iron bioavailability, and iron losses. Evolution has given humans the mechanism for absorbing dietary iron efficiently but not for eliminating excess iron effectively.

DIETARY IRON

Many foods are good sources of iron, but it may not be bioavailable, or able to be used. The bioavailability of iron depends on its chemical form in the food and the presence of other food items that promote or inhibit the absorption. An average American diet may contain 10 to 20 mg of iron per day, but of that, only 1 to 2 mg is absorbed. Iron is absorbed in two forms: heme and nonheme iron. Heme iron (i.e., iron that is incorporated into the Hb molecule) is absorbed more effec-

tively than nonheme iron (inorganic iron) and in a different manner.[5] Heme iron is present in forms of Hb, myoglobin, and heme enzymes in meat sources. Approximately 5% to 35% of heme iron is absorbed from a serving of a meat source. Nonheme iron, found in nonmeat sources such as legumes and leafy vegetables, accounts for approximately 90% of dietary iron, but only 2% to 20% of it is absorbed, depending on the iron status of the individual and the ratio of enhancers and inhibitors in the diet.[3] The enhancer influence of ascorbate, citrate, and other organic acids and amino acids on nonheme iron is thought to be mediated by the formation of soluble chelates. Substances that form insoluble complexes with iron, such as phytates, tannates, phosphates, and oxalates, decrease iron absorption.[6] Calcium also may inhibit intestinal absorption of iron.[7] Cooking in iron pots and pans increases the amount of iron consumed. Iron can be supplemented in the diet with vitamin supplements or fortified foods. Iron has been fortified in some foods, including cereals and infant formula, in the United States since the 1940s. Iron supplementation should be targeted only to specific populations that are at risk for iron deficiency because the potential for iron overload exists in individuals with adequate iron status.

IRON ABSORPTION AND EXCRETION

The duodenum and upper jejunum are sites of maximal absorption of iron. For transport of oxygen in Hb, iron must be in the ferrous form (Fe^{2+}). To be absorbed, iron from food must be in the form of heme iron (Fe^{2+}) or converted from ferric nonheme iron to the soluble ferrous form by a duodenum-specific cytochrome b–like protein, DCYTB.[8] Heme iron binds to the enterocyte in the mucosal epithelium and is internalized (Fig. 11-1). The heme source of iron in the cell is degraded to ferrous iron, carbon monoxide, and bilirubin IXa by the enzyme heme oxygenase.

Ferrous iron is transported across the duodenal epithelium by the apical divalent metal transporter (DMT1). The ferrous iron is carried to the basolateral membrane (base and sides of membrane), where it is believed that ferrous iron is exported to the portal circulation and mediated by ferroportin, a basolateral transport protein. Ferroportin may work in conjunction with a copper-containing iron oxidase known as *hephaestin*. It is thought that hephaestin facilitates iron egress by reoxidation of ferrous iron to ferric iron.[8] Oxidized iron must be bound to transferrin to be transported into the circulation. Some absorbed iron remains in the enterocytes as ferritin, a storage form of iron while the cells are exfoliated. Some iron is stored only temporarily as ferritin to be released and absorbed over a few hours.

Hepcidin, an antimicrobial peptide produced in the liver, seems to act as a negative regulator of intestinal iron absorption and release from macrophages. Hepcidin binds to the ferroportin receptor causing degradation of ferroportin and resulting in trapping of iron in the intestinal cells. As a result, iron absorption and mobilization of storage iron from the liver and macrophages are lowered. Increased synthesis of hepcidin occurs when transferrin saturation is high (i.e., when

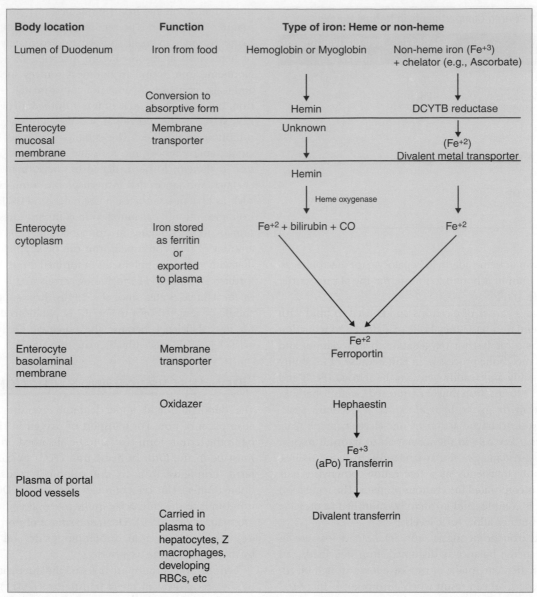

Figure 11-1 Simplified version of the mechanism for absorption of iron in the small intestine. CO, carbon monoxide; DCYTB, duodenum cytochrome *b*.

transferrin is carrying its maximum capacity of serum iron), and decreased synthesis occurs when iron saturation is low.[9-11] The role of hepcidin in anemia of chronic inflammation is discussed in Chapter 19.

Iron-loaded transferrin that is carried to hematopoietic and other tissues binds to a transferrin receptor on the cell membrane (Fig. 11-2). Transferrin receptors are expressed on all cells except highly differentiated ones. Transferrin receptor is expressed in larger amounts on immature erythroid cells and rapidly dividing cells, whether normal or malignant.[12] Transferrin is taken into the cell by endocytosis. An endosome forms containing the iron-loaded transferrin molecule. Iron is released from transferrin by acidification of the endosome to a pH of about 5.5. Iron is transported across the endosomal

membrane by DMT1 and used in the synthesis of iron-containing proteins. The excess iron is stored as ferritin or hemosiderin (see section on storage).[8]

Humans have no effective means to excrete iron. They regulate iron by controlling absorption. The amount of iron absorbed is inversely related to the amount of iron stores and the rate of erythropoiesis. As stated previously, normal absorption of iron is 1 to 2 mg/d. With decreased iron stores, iron absorption may be 3 to 4 mg/d. In iron overload, only 0.5 mg/d is absorbed.

The body conserves iron judiciously, losing only about $\frac{1}{1000}$ of its total body iron content. This amount is easily replaced if dietary sources are adequate. Normal iron losses occur mainly by way of the feces and amount to about 1 mg/d. Perspiration

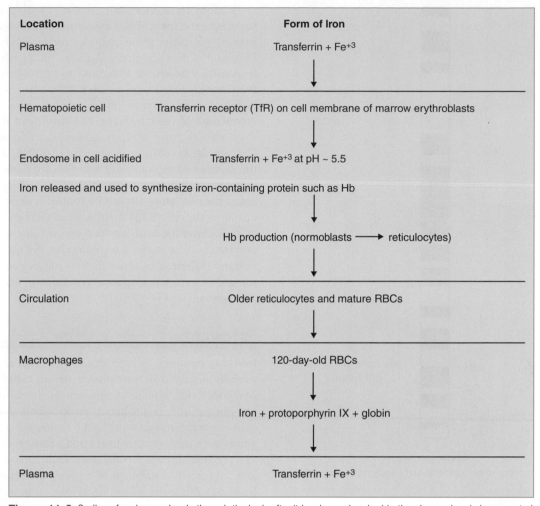

Location	Form of Iron
Plasma	Transferrin + Fe^{+3}
Hematopoietic cell	Transferrin receptor (TfR) on cell membrane of marrow erythroblasts
Endosome in cell acidified	Transferrin + Fe^{+3} at pH ~ 5.5
Iron released and used to synthesize iron-containing protein such as Hb	
	Hb production (normoblasts ⟶ reticulocytes)
Circulation	Older reticulocytes and mature RBCs
Macrophages	120-day-old RBCs
	Iron + protoporphyrin IX + globin
Plasma	Transferrin + Fe^{+3}

Figure 11-2 Cycling of an iron molecule through the body after it has been absorbed in the plasma. Iron is incorporated into marrow RBC precursors, released into the circulation for the life of the RBC, and sent back to the plasma, bound to transferrin.

and exfoliation of skin and dermal appendages result in minimal losses. Lactation and menstruation result in an additional loss of about 1 mg/d.[13]

CYCLE AND TRANSPORT

Iron cycles through the body, moving from absorption in the gastrointestinal tract via the circulation to the bone marrow, where it is incorporated with protoporphyrin IX in the mitochondria of the erythroid precursors to make heme (see Fig. 11-2). Hb synthesis is nearly completed by the reticulocyte stage. Iron circulates in red blood cells (RBCs) in the ferrous form in the Hb molecule. The iron in senescent RBCs is turned over to macrophages and reused.[8] Ferrokinetics involve these proteins: transferrin, transferrin receptor, and ferritin. They are regulated by an iron-responsive protein (IRP). The chromosomal locations of the corresponding genes and the amino acid sequences of each of these principal proteins have been identified.[14] Knowledge of the location of these genes may allow scientists to intervene someday in the treatment of hereditary iron disorders.

Most transferrin is produced by hepatocytes. The major function of the transferrin protein is to transport iron from the plasma to the normoblasts in the marrow. Transferrin binds to transferrin receptors on the normoblast membrane. The transferrin molecule has a half-life of 8 days and migrates in the β fraction in serum electrophoresis. It contains two terminal lobes, an N and a C, each of which can bind independently to a ferric (Fe^{3+}) ion. A bicarbonate ion locks the iron in place within the molecule by serving as a bridging ligand between the protein and iron. The transferrin molecule can exist as apoferritin, a single-chain glycoprotein with no iron attached, or in a monoferric or diferric form.[15] The transferrin gene is located on the long arm of chromosome 3, 3q21-qter (Fig. 11-3).[14]

The function of the transferrin receptor is to provide transferrin-bound iron access into the cell; it also plays a crucial role in the release of iron from transferrin within the cell. The transferrin receptor is a glycoprotein dimer, and it is located on virtually all cells (except mature RBCs). It is present in large numbers on erythroid precursors, the placenta, and the liver. The transferrin receptor can bind two molecules of transferrin.

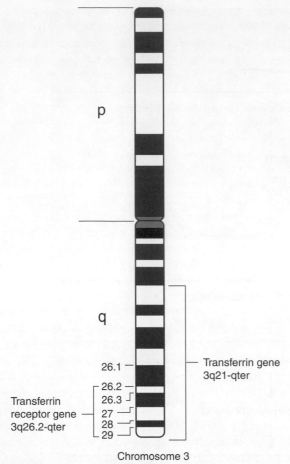

Figure 11-3 Location of the transferrin and transferrin receptor genes on chromosome 3.

The transferrin receptor's affinity for transferrin depends on the iron content and the physiologic pH. At a pH of 7.4 and with sufficient amounts of iron-bearing transferrin, the transferrin receptor has highest affinity for diferric transferrin, as opposed to monoferric transferrin or apotransferrin. The transferrin receptor gene is located near the transferrin gene at chromosome 3q26.2-qter (see Fig. 11-3).[14] Control of transferrin receptor biosynthesis is a major mechanism for regulation of iron metabolism. Synthesis of transferrin receptor is induced by iron deficiency. When transferrin is fully saturated, iron absorbed by the intestine is deposited in the liver. When transferrin is congenitally absent, iron is absorbed by the intestine and accumulates in the liver, pancreas, spleen, and other viscera; only a little makes its way to the marrow, and a severe hypochromic microcytic anemia results.[14]

Cellular uptake of iron is mediated largely by interaction of the transferrin receptor and the transferrin molecule. The ferric–transferrin receptor complex is endocytosed, iron is released into the cell, and the receptor-transferrin complex is returned to the cell surface, whereupon transferrin is released for reuse. Iron enters a "chelatable" soluble pool in the cell, where it is used for synthesis of essential cellular constituents or for deposition as ferritin, a nontoxic storage form of iron.

IRPs are messenger RNA (mRNA)-binding proteins that coordinate the intracellular expression of transferrin receptor, ferritin, and other proteins important for iron metabolism. IRPs bind to iron-responsive elements (IREs), which are stem-loop mRNA structures. IRPs bind to IREs when iron supply is decreased and dissociate from IREs when iron supply is increased. When there is little intracellular iron, IRPs regulate the increase of the translation and stability of the mRNA for transferrin receptor and aminolevulinic acid synthase and decrease the translation of apoferritin mRNA. This increases the number of molecules of transferrin receptor on the cell membrane, while decreasing the ferritin trapping of iron that enters the cell. More Hb can be formed if there is more iron uptake by the cell. At the same time, an increase in production of aminolevulinic acid synthase ensures that enough protoporphyrin can be made to accommodate the expected increase in iron.[8,13] There is evidence that, in addition to regulation at the mRNA level, transcriptional regulation of iron metabolism also occurs.[13]

STORAGE

Iron may be stored in accessible reserve form as ferritin or as partially degraded or precipitated ferritin called *hemosiderin*. Apoferritin, the protein component of the ferritin molecule without the iron, is a spherical protein shell about 12 nm in diameter and 1 nm in width and is composed of 24 subunits, which are a mixture of light (L) and heavy (H) subunits (Fig. 11-4). Within the apoferritin shell, ferric ions, hydroxyl ions, and oxygen are distributed in a lattice-like relationship. The liver and spleen, which function as major iron storage deposits, have a large amount of L subunits. Tissues such as heart tissue that do not act normally as iron storage sites have a higher proportion of H subunits. Genes for the H and L chains belong to multigene families with members of several chromosomes. The gene for two types of L chains is on chromosome 19; the gene for heavy chains is on chromosome 11.[14]

Hemosiderin is a degradation product of ferritin produced by the partial digestion of protein and release of iron micelles, which form insoluble ferritin aggregates. Normally, most of the stored iron is in the soluble ferritin form, but as iron stores increase, so does the proportion of hemosiderin in relation to ferritin.

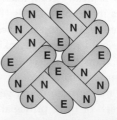

Figure 11-4 Ferritin structure. *N* and *E* designate the ends of the subunits.

Ferritin and hemosiderin stores are found in liver, bone marrow, and spleen, with most in the liver. When iron is needed from iron stores, it is returned to transferrin to be used by the cells that need the iron for metabolism.

LABORATORY ASSESSMENT OF IRON STORES

Reference intervals for laboratory tests of iron status are provided but are meant to be a guide only because values may differ among methodologies used (Table 11-2). Measuring iron status by only one type of test may not provide significant clinical information. An understanding of what the tests measure and what variations can occur because of diurnal variation and clinical status is helpful in interpreting the significance of the test result.

Serum iron concentration refers to the Fe^{3+} bound to serum transferrin and does not include any iron contained in serum as free Hb. Serum iron can be measured by chromogen-spectrophotometric methods. It exhibits diurnal variation, being highest in the morning and lowest in the evening. Serum iron is decreased not only in iron deficiency but also in inflammatory disorders, acute infection, certain immunizations, and myocardial infarction. Because normally only about one third of the iron-binding sites of transferrin are occupied by Fe^{3+}, two thirds of the iron-binding sites do not carry iron; this is known as the *serum unsaturated iron-binding capacity*. The total number of available sites is referred to as the *total iron-binding capacity*. Unsaturated iron-binding capacity can be measured by chromogen-spectrophotometric methods. Total iron-binding capacity can be measured in the laboratory indirectly by chemical means and directly by immunologic methods.[16,17] Measurement of serum iron concentration alone provides little useful clinical information; measuring the serum iron and total iron-binding capacity and calculating the percent saturation (the percentage of available sites that are carrying iron) provides more diagnostic information. Percent saturation is calculated by dividing the serum iron by the total iron-binding capacity and multiplying the result by 100.[8,13,14]

Ferritin can be measured by various immunologic methods. Plasma ferritin is present in the blood in low concentrations. It is in equilibrium with body stores, and variations in the quantity of iron in the storage compartment are reflected in the plasma ferritin concentration. The plasma ferritin concentration declines early in the development of iron deficiency. As an acute phase reactant, it is increased in many chronic diseases, regardless of the quantity of iron in storage.

Serum transferrin receptors can be measured by sensitive immunologic methods. The serum transferrin receptor appears to be a truncated form of the cellular receptor and circulates bound to transferrin. It seems to mirror the cellular form. The amount of circulating receptor increases when cells lack iron and is found to be lower in chronic diseases. Measurement of serum transferrin receptors may be useful in iron deficiency testing, although increases also have been seen with ineffective erythropoiesis.[8,13,18]

Erythrocyte protoporphyrin is an intermediate product of Hb production and may be seen in excess in conditions in which heme production is incomplete, such as iron deficiency or if iron use is blocked. Some excess protoporphyrin is produced and resides in the RBC and can be measured as "free" erythrocyte protoporphyrin. Free erythrocyte protoporphyrin combines with zinc when iron is unavailable and can be measured directly by measuring the fluorescence of zinc protoporphyrin in a hematofluorometer. The free protoporphyrin concentration of RBCs increases in disorders of heme synthesis, including iron deficiency, lead poisoning, sideroblastic anemias, and some other conditions (Chapter 19). Protoporphyrin levels are increased in chronic diseases, regardless of the iron status.[18]

Tissue iron concentrations can be assessed by a tissue biopsy of the bone marrow or liver. The amount of iron in macrophages, nucleated RBCs, and reticulocytes can be estimated visually using the Prussian blue reaction, which stains

TABLE 11-2 Assessment of Body Iron Status

Measurement	Reference Range (Adults)	Diagnostic Use
Serum ferritin	15-300 µg/L	Indicator of iron stores
Serum iron	10-30 µmol/L	Indicator of tissue iron supply
Serum TIBC/transferrin	47-70 µmol/L	Indicator of tissue iron supply
Saturation of transferrin	16-50% (female) 16-60% (male)	Indicator of tissue iron supply
Serum transferrin receptor	2.8-8.5 mg/L	Indicator of functional iron available
RBC zinc protoporphyrin	<80 µg/dL of RBCs	Indicator of functional iron available
Bone marrow or liver biopsy	Normal iron stores visualized qualitatively	Direct assessment of iron stores
Bone marrow sideroblast count	>10% sideroblasts	Direct assessment of functional iron available

TIBC, total iron-binding capacity.

the iron blue. Iron storage concentration can be estimated by reviewing the amount of iron in macrophages. This type of iron is hemosiderin, the degradative product of ferritin molecules that has been incorporated into lysosomes of the macrophages. The Prussian blue stain also can be used on peripheral blood and bone marrow aspirate smears to visualize iron in nucleated and non-nucleated RBCs. Normally in the

peripheral blood, no iron is detected in mature RBCs or reticulocytes. In the normal bone marrow smear, iron granules are found in 10% or more of the nucleated RBCs and contain one to three blue inclusions that represent iron. These cells are called *sideroblasts,* and the granules are called *siderosomes.* Reticulocytes in the bone marrow that contain iron are termed *siderocytes.*

CHAPTER at a GLANCE

- Iron is an essential nutrient for human survival. It plays a role in oxygen transport and basic metabolic oxidative and reductive reactions. Most of the iron in the body is in the form of Hb.
- Iron is obtained through dietary means via heme (Fe^{2+}) and nonheme (Fe^{3+}—inorganic) iron. More iron is absorbed from the heme form of iron than from the nonheme form.
- Iron is absorbed in the duodenum and jejunum enterocytes via a DMT1 transporter. Iron is carried to the basolateral membrane where it passes on to the plasma via a channel transporter, ferroportin. Hephaestin, a multicopper oxidase protein, aids in the transport process by reoxidation of ferrous iron to ferric iron. Hepcidin, an antimicrobial peptide, seems to regulate the basolateral iron export.
- Iron is transported in plasma bound to a carrier protein, transferrin. Transferrin receptors, located on all cells in the body except mature RBCs, aid in providing transferrin-bound iron access into cells and play a crucial role in the release of iron from transferrin

within the cell. The IRP regulates ALA sythetase, transferrin receptor, and ferritin in the cell by binding to the mRNA IREs.
- Ferritin and hemosiderin are storage forms of iron. Most storage iron is in the ferritin form, which is a water-soluble complex. Hemosiderin, a water-insoluble complex, is composed of ferritin aggregates and is found in macrophages in the bone marrow and liver.
- Laboratory tests that can assist in assessing the iron status in the body include serum ferritin, serum iron concentration, total iron-binding capacity, and percent iron saturation. Other tests include bone marrow or liver biopsy, serum transferrin receptor analysis, and the erythrocyte protoporphyrin test. Other tests are available but are done less frequently.

Now that you have completed this chapter, go back and read again the case study at the beginning and respond to the questions presented.

REVIEW QUESTIONS

1. Iron is transported in plasma via:
   a. Hemosiderin
   b. Ferritin
   c. Transferrin
   d. Hemoglobin

2. What is the major metabolically available storage form of iron in the body?
   a. Hemosiderin
   b. Ferritin
   c. Transferrin
   d. Hemoglobin

3. Approximately 70% of body iron is found in the form of:
   a. Hemosiderin
   b. Ferritin
   c. Transferrin
   d. Hemoglobin

4. Iron is incorporated into the heme molecule in which of the following forms?
   a. Ferro
   b. Ferrous
   c. Ferric
   d. Apoferritin

5. What protein associated with duodenum cells transports iron from the intestinal lumen into the intestinal cell?
   a. Transferrin
   b. Ferroportin
   c. Divalent metal transporter
   d. Ferrochelatase

6. Iron is transported out of cells such as macrophages and duodenal cells by what membrane protein?
   a. Transferrin
   b. Ferroportin
   c. Divalent metal transporter
   d. Ferrochelatase

7. Below are several of the many steps in the absorption and transport of iron to incorporation into heme. Place them in proper order.
   i. Transferrin picks up ferric iron.
   ii. Iron is transferred to the mitochondria.
   iii. Cytochrome *b*–like protein, DCYTB, converts ferric to ferrous iron.
   iv. Ferroportin transports iron across the cell membrane.
   v. The transferrin receptor transports iron into the cell.
   a. v, iv, i, ii, iii
   b. iii, ii, iv, i, v
   c. ii, i, v, iii, iv
   d. iii, iv, i, v, ii

8. In the iron cycle, the transferrin receptor carries
   a. iron into duodenal cells from the intestinal lumen
   b. iron out of duodenal cells into the plasma
   c. transferrin-bound iron in the plasma
   d. transferrin-bound iron into erythrocytes

9. What is the fate of the transferrin receptor when it has completed its role in the delivery of iron into a developing RBC?
   a. It is recycled to the plasma membrane and released into the plasma.
   b. It is recycled to the plasma membrane where it can bind its ligand again.
   c. It is catabolized and the amino acids are returned to the metabolic pool.

10. The transfer of iron from the duodenal cell into the plasma is regulated by:
    a. Transferrin
    b. Transferrin receptor
    c. Hephastin
    d. Hepcidin

REFERENCES

1. Baynes RD, Cook JD: Current issues in iron deficiency. Curr Opin Hematol 1996;3:145-149.
2. Garry PJ, Koehler KM, Simon TL: Iron stores and iron absorption: effects of repeated blood donations. Am J Clin Nutr 1995;62:611-620.
3. Beard JL, Dawson H, Pinero DJ: Iron metabolism: a comprehensive review. Nutr Rev 1996;54:295-317.
4. Sharma N, Butterworth J, Cooper BT, et al: The emerging role of the liver in iron metabolism. Am J Gastroenterol 2005;100:201-206.
5. Uzel C, Conrad ME: Absorption of heme iron. Semin Hematol 1998;5:27-34.
6. Conrad ME: Introduction: iron overloading and iron regulation. Semin Hematol 1998;35:1-4.
7. Andrews NC: Iron deficiency and related disorders. In Greer JP, Foerster J, Lukens JN, et al (eds): Wintrobe's Clinical Hematology, 11th ed. Philadelphia: Lippincott, Williams & Wilkins, 2004:980-1009.
8. Andrews NC: Pathology of iron metabolism. In Hoffman R, Benz EJ, Shattil SJ, et al (eds): Hematology, Basic Principles and Practice, 4th ed. New York: Elsevier, 2005:473-479.
9. Nemeth E, Tuttle MS, Powelson J, et al: Hepcidin regulates iron efflux by binding to ferroportin and inducing its internalization. Science 2004;306:2090-2093.
10. Knutson MD, Oukka M, Koss LM, et al: Iron release from macrophages after erythrophagocytosis is upregulated by ferroportin 1 overexpression and down regulated by hepcidin. Proc Natl Acad Sci USA 2005;102:1324-1328.
11. Vyoral D, Petrak J: Hepcidin: a direct link between iron metabolism and immunity. Int J Biochem Cell Biol 2005;37:1768-1773.
12. Ponka P, Lok CN: The transferrin receptor: role in health and disease. Int J Biochem Cell Biol 1999;31:1111-1137.
13. Beutler E: Disorders of iron metabolism. In Lichtman MA, Beutler E, Kipps, et al (eds): Williams Hematology, 7th ed. New York: McGraw-Hill, 2006:511-553.
14. Rouault TA, Klausner RD: Molecular basis of iron metabolism. In Stamatoyannopoulos G, Majerus PW, Perlmutter RM, et al (eds): Molecular Basis of Blood Diseases, 3rd ed. Philadelphia: Saunders, 2001:363-387.
15. Woods S, DeMarco T, Friedland M: Iron metabolism. Am J Gastroenterol 1990;85:1-8.
16. Worwood M: The laboratory assessment of iron status—an update. Clin Chim Acta 1997;259:3-23.
17. Higgins T, Beutler E, Doumas BT: Hemoglobin, iron and bilirubin. In Burtis CA, Ashwood ER, Bruns DE (eds): Tietz Textbook of Clinical Chemistry and Molecular Diagnostics, 4th ed. Philadelphia: Saunders, 2006:1165-1204.
18. Gardner LB, Benz EJ: Anemia of chronic disease. In Hoffman R, Benz EJ, Shattil SJ, et al (eds): Hematology, Basic Principles and Practice, 4th ed. New York: Elsevier, 2005:473-497.

12

Leukopoiesis

Susan J. Leclair

OBJECTIVES

After completion of this chapter, the reader will be able to:

1. Define categories of leukocytes based on site of origin, specific function, interrelationships, and morphology.
2. Explain the differentiation sequence required for producing neutrophilic/eosinophilic/basophilic granulocytes.
3. Explain the differentiation sequence required for producing monocytes/macrophages.
4. Explain the morphologic differentiation sequence required for producing lymphocytes.
5. List the important compounds synthesized or stored in the various leukocytes.
6. Correlate granulocytic function to morphology and maturation.
7. Compare and contrast the morphology of the peripheral blood lymphocyte with the various stages of immunologic activity.
8. Given written descriptions of the stages of granulocyte development or special staining characteristics, identify the cell stage.
9. Describe in general terms the processes involved in neutrophils' killing of bacteria.
10. Correlate leukocytes to the type of inflammatory reactions or microbe defense in which each is primarily involved.

Leukopoiesis, or the development of white blood cells (WBCs), with the exception of lymphocytes, occurs in the same locations as erythropoiesis.[1] These locations change during the life span starting with the yolk sac of the mesenchyme, followed by the spleen and liver, and finally the bone marrow (Chapter 7). This change should be considered a one-way process because other than in the neoplastic condition of myeloid metaplasia, the spleen and liver do not participate in blood cell formation after birth.

The term *erythron* defines the sum of erythrocytic development; there is no such term for leukocyte development and function. A term is lacking because of the complexity of the WBC populations and the different compartments that they occupy during their lives. In addition, control mechanisms that influence cellular behavior are more complex in leukocytes than the mechanisms seen in the erythrocyte because they seem also to include interrelations with adipose tissue, fibroblasts, and endothelial cells. There are many ways to evaluate the needs and functions of these cells throughout their lives. This chapter relates developmental needs and consequences to environmental constraints and controls.

At birth, all available marrow space is taken up by hematopoiesis. By the end of adolescence, active marrow typically is found only in the proximal ends of the long bones and in flat bones, such as the skull and sternum (see Fig. 7-2). Inactive, or "fatty," marrow can be converted to active marrow if the demands for a blood cell line increase.

LEUKOCYTES

Human blood leukocytes can be divided into various categories on the basis of their specific function, site of origin, or morphology. In essence, all leukocytes exist to defend the organism against nonself agents. This defense is accomplished through intricate cooperation among cells.[2] Independent of lymphocyte control, phagocytes attack and destroy a wide variety of matter. Through lymphokines (biologic response mediators released by B and T lymphocytes and by macrophages), lymphocytes direct and amplify phagocytic action.[3] For this discussion, leukocytes are divided into granulocytes and lymphocytes by virtue of the differentiation apparent at the primitive stem cell level (Fig. 12-1). Lymphocytes are produced in bone marrow and lymphoid tissue. They are under the control of environmental and hormonal stimuli different from the stimuli that control granulocytes and monocytes. Granulocytes, such as the neutrophils, function primarily as destroyers of pyogenic bacteria, whereas monocytes/macrophages are less discriminating in their phagocytic activities.

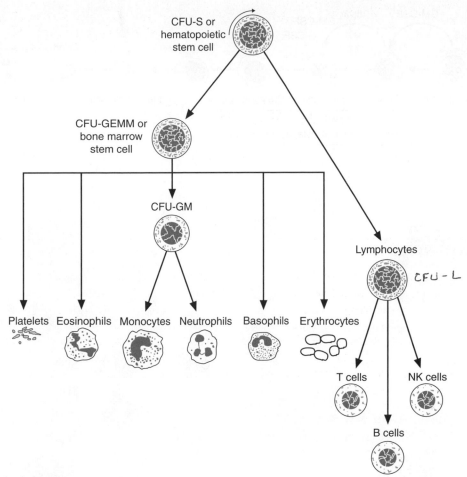

Figure 12-1 Representation of the division of human blood cells into major categories based on stem cell commitment.

Granulocytes contain visible granules and develop solely in the bone marrow. They are subdivided according to morphology and can be categorized as granulocytes containing large and easily visualized granules and granulocytes containing minute or barely visible granules. By convention, cells containing large visible granules usually are called granulocytes; these are subdivided further according to the type of reaction (neutrophilic, eosinophilic, basophilic) found in the granules when stained differentially with a Romanowsky-based stain. Monocytes contain minute granules, which, as a result of the resolution limitation of most bright-light microscopes, cause their cytoplasm to have a grainy appearance.

Flow cytometric analysis of receptor sites, antigenic labeling and functional studies are contributing increasing amounts of information. Lymphocytes and immature cells are commonly differentiated through the use of cellular markers that have been given an alphanumeric code (e.g., CD1), in which *CD* stands for *cluster designation* (Chapter 33).

GRANULOCYTES

As a group, granulocytes can be found in high concentrations in four locations: in bone marrow, circulating freely in the peripheral blood, marginating up against the endothelium of blood vessels, and in the tissues. These locations are called *granulocyte pools*. The bone marrow pool is quite large and has three functions: proliferation, maturation, and storage. Cells found in the proliferating component (i.e., myeloblasts, promyelocytes, and myelocytes) are capable of mitotic divisions. The maturation portion consists of metamyelocytes and bands (i.e., cells that are no longer capable of mitosis but are not yet fully functional). The storage component of the bone marrow, which consists of bands and polymorphonuclear leukocytes, contains approximately 25 times as many cells as are in the circulation. When a cell has fully matured and has been stimulated by chemotactic factors, it leaves the marrow and enters the peripheral blood, in which it can become part of the marginating pool or the circulating pool. The marginating pool consists of approximately 50% of total peripheral blood granulocyte levels. These cells adhere to the vessel endothelium or engage in egressing through vessel walls into the tissue. The circulating pool contains the remaining 50% of total peripheral blood granulocyte levels; these are the cells counted in a WBC count. Cells have freedom of movement between the marginating and circulating pools, and changes in the pool numbers can be reflected in changing WBC counts.

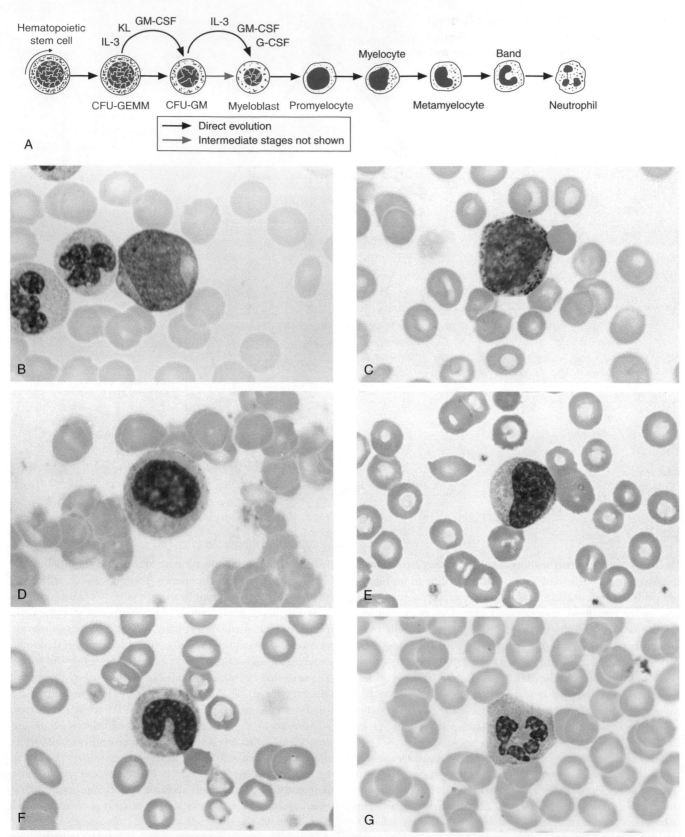

Figure 12-2 A, Schematic for the commitment and differentiation of granulocytes, showing the commitment and stimulation agents. **B,** Myeloblast showing delicate chromatin, multiple nucleoli, and nongranular cytoplasm. **C,** Promyelocyte showing the concentration of primary granules throughout the cytoplasm and over the nucleus. **D,** Neutrophilic myelocyte, so named because of the presence of secondary granules that, when stained, appear neutrophilic. Note the absence of nucleoli and the beginning condensation of chromatin in the nucleus. **E,** Metamyelocyte with the classic kidney bean–shaped nucleus. **F,** Band form with a nucleus whose indentation is greater than 50% of the width of the nucleus. The remaining primary granules are less apparent and when stained turn a lighter blue. **G,** Polymorphonuclear cell with a typically twisted and segmented nucleus.

Maturation: Stem Cell to Myeloblast

The earliest leukopoietic precursor was identified from mouse spleen cells and is referred to as either the *colony-forming unit spleen* (CFU-S) *hematopoietic stem cell* (HSC) (Chapter 7). Its identification with traditional Romanowsky-based stains is not possible. Flow cytometric analysis describes this cell as CD34+ thyl+ HLA-DR− Rh 123dull. CD34 antigen may be involved in signal transduction and is not present on granulocytes after the myelocyte stage.[4] Thy1 is a protein receptor that seems to be involved with cell cycling.[5] These cells do not possess the class II HLA-DR antigens. Rhodamine (Rh) 123 is a stain taken up by mitochondria in a cell undergoing cell cycle action. If the cell is not cycling, the uptake is dull. If the cell is cycling, the uptake is greatly enhanced.[6]

The HSC apparently can move among various activity sites and may look like a large, nongranular lymphocyte. It responds to circumstances as yet undefined and commits its progeny to cells of lymphoid or bone marrow (myeloid) origin through the action of growth factors that stimulate tyrosine kinase receptors or are cytokines.[7] For granulopoiesis, the HSC undergoes stimulation, mitosis, and maturation into a stem cell that is specific for bone marrow–derived or myeloid cells.[8] This cell is characterized by the presence of CD34 and CD33 antigens.[9] This common myeloid progenitor[10] (also called *CFU-GEMM*) matures into yet another progenitor cell called the *colony-forming unit granulocyte-monocyte/macrophage* (CFU-GM). This cell finally matures into the earliest recognizable cell of the neutrophilic series, the myeloblast. The stability of cell numbers and their functions is controlled by a complex interaction of humoral factors, such as interleukins (ILs) and various colony-stimulating factors (CSFs) (Fig. 12-2A).[11] CSFs are categorized by the type of cell stimulated. GM-CSF stimulates cells to form granulocytes and monocytes/macrophages, whereas G-CSF stimulates only granulocyte development and M-CSF stimulates only monocyte/macrophage development. Specificity for CSFs is mediated by receptor sites on precursors and mature cells. The structure of the receptor is thought to consist of a ligand-specific, low-affinity binding chain and a second chain for high-affinity binding and signal transduction. The second chain also interacts with IL-3 and IL-5 (Chapter 7).[12]

Neutrophil Maturation

Myeloblast

Myeloid stem cells expressing CD34 begin to downregulate CD34 as they mature and begin to express different antigens such as CD13 and CD33.[13] Cells in the bone marrow proliferation pool usually take 24 to 48 hours for a single cell cycle. Less than 1% of the normal bone marrow compartment is composed of myeloblasts. They vary in size but are usually large (15-20 μm). The nucleus is delicate, with prominent nucleoli. The meager cytoplasm contains rough endoplasmic reticulum, a developing Golgi apparatus, and, as it matures through its life cycle, the initial presence of primary or azurophilic granules. When stained with cytochemical methods, these granules color positively for the enzyme myeloperoxidase. Myeloperoxidase is required for intracellular kill, which means that the killing function is the first to be opera-

tional. The cell is incapable of motility, adhesion, and phagocytosis, so it is in essence a nonfunctional cell (Fig. 12-2B and 12-3A).

Promyelocyte (Progranulocyte)

After several days in the blast stage, the cell progresses to the promyelocyte stage. This cell is almost as rare as the myeloblast (1% to 5% in the bone marrow), and its size varies. It may exceed 20 μm, so it occasionally may be larger than the size of its precursor cell. The nuclear chromatin pattern may be as delicate as that of a myeloblast or may show slight clumping. Nucleoli begin to fade. The primary granules first noted in the myeloblast become a dominant characteristic of these cells. They are present throughout the larger cytoplasm and on top of the nucleus (see Figs. 12-2C and 12-3B). Some motility may be present toward the end of this stage of development.[14] Previously thought of as the mechanism for intracellular killing, myeloperoxidase and the peroxidase/superoxide burst are no longer considered to have a direct role in microbial killing. Instead, a complex interaction among reduced nicotinamide adenine dinucleotide phosphate oxidase and flavocytochrome B is believed to cause an increase of free electrons across the granule membrane. This activates neutral proteinases cathepsin G, elastase, and proteinases for killing to take place. These electrons are controlled and damage is limited by the presence of highly concentrated potassium.[15]

Neutrophilic Myelocyte

As the cell ceases to produce primary azurophilic granules, it begins to make a set of granules that are specific to the type of granulocyte. These are called *secondary* or *neutrophilic granules*. Accumulation of secondary granules is characteristic of the myelocyte, the last cell of the bone marrow compartment capable of mitosis. The myelocyte shows a good deal of morphologic variability because this stage of development is the longest, and the development of the granules over 4 to 5 days causes considerable alteration in the staining reaction of the cell. This cell is usually smaller than the promyelocyte and constitutes less than 10% of the total marrow cell population. The nucleus may be round to oval with a flattened side near the well-developed Golgi apparatus. The nuclear chromatin shows clumping, and nucleoli are usually no longer visible. During this stage, the second of the three major types of granules is synthesized.[16] The granules alter the staining reaction within the cytoplasm. They cause a "dawn of neutrophilia," or faint blush of pink first seen near the Golgi apparatus within the cytoplasm. Some important compounds contained within secondary granules are thrombospondin receptor, β2-microglobulin, apolactoferrin, lysozyme, and plasminogen activators. As the cell matures, secondary granule formation overshadows the primary granules. Alteration in the granule membrane causes the remaining primary granules to color less intensely with staining; they are light bluish and less noticeable. Additionally, the cell concentrates important compounds, such as alkaline phosphatase and decay-accelerating factor, in secretory vesicles. The cell also acquires some motility (see Figs. 12-2D and 12-3C).

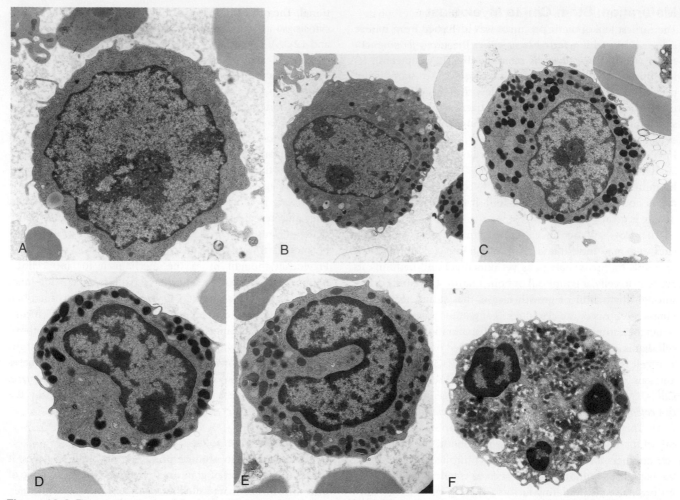

Figure 12-3 Electron micrographs of developmental stages of the neutrophil. **A,** Myeloblast (×16,500). **B,** Promyelocyte (×13,000). **C,** Myelocyte (×16,500). **D,** Metamyelocyte (×22,250). **E,** Band (×22,250). **F,** Polymorphonuclear neutrophil (×22,250). (From Carr JH, Rodak BF: Clinical Hematology Atlas, 2nd ed. Philadelphia: Saunders, 2004.)

Neutrophilic Metamyelocyte

After the cessation of all active deoxyribonucleic acid (DNA) synthesis, the myelocyte becomes a metamyelocyte. The traditional discriminator between myelocyte and metamyelocyte is the shape of the nucleus; that of the metamyelocyte becomes indented. It is far better to assess the relative maturity (nonclumped versus clumped chromatin pattern) of the nucleus, however, because microcinematography has shown that the shape of the myelocyte nucleus varies from round to deeply indented.[17] By this stage, the cytoplasm has a collection of primary and secondary granules with the secondary granule as the major feature of the cell's cytoplasm.[18] These granules constitute the major components necessary to kill and degrade toxic, infectious, or nonself agents. The cell is still incapable, however, of responding to chemotactic factors that draw it to the site of infection and initiate phagocytosis, the ingestion of bacteria. Metamyelocytes, which are not seen in the typical peripheral blood smear, constitute approximately 13% to 22% of the normal marrow differential.[19] Because this cell is still not fully functional, it is considered part of the maturation component of the marrow (see Figs. 12-2E and 12-3D). At the

end of this stage of development, the third type of neutrophilic granule, also known as the *gelatinase granule*, is made. These tertiary or gelatinase granules contain lysozyme and acetyltransferase among other compounds.

Neutrophilic Band (Nonsegmented Form)

After a time, the metamyelocyte assumes a band shape, a transitional form, so called because it is in the peripheral blood and the bone marrow and is considered to be part of the maturation and storage pools. Within the marrow, it constitutes one of the most common leukocytes, its numbers averaging 40% of the WBCs therein. The definition and name of this intermediate form have been debated extensively for more than 60 years. In one classification system, its discrimination is based on the presence or absence of nuclear segments composed of dense heterochromatin. The terms *segmented* and *nonsegmented* are used in this definition of these cells.[20] Another classification requires that the outer shape of the nucleus have uniform or parallel width (C or S shape) as its basis and identifies a cell whose nucleus is so described as a *band* and cells with all other nuclear forms as *polymorphonuclear neutrophils*. Finally, a third classification system defines a band as a cell whose nuclear indentation is less than half the width of the nucleus and a polymorphonuclear neutrophil as a cell whose nuclear indentation is more than half the width of the nucleus.[21] This third system reflects an appreciation of the role of change and maturity within the cell because chromatin maturity also is used as a criterion. Regardless of which classification is used, the band form is thought to represent the almost mature cell. It has been shown to possess full motility, active adhesion properties, and some phagocytic ability.[22] Membrane maturity is characterized by changes in the cytoskeleton, changes in surface charge, and the presence of receptors for complement (CRs), specifically for CR1 and CR3.[23] Although not connected, adhesion capabilities are found in parallel with the presence of certain secondary granules. When out in the peripheral blood, bands usually account for less than 6% of the WBCs. In the peripheral blood, they can be found in marginating and circulating pools (see Figs. 12-2F and 12-3E). In addition, a distinct, highly mobilizable intracellular compartment, the secretory vesicle, has now been recognized as an important store of surface membrane-bound receptors and may be functional in antigen presentation.[24] This compartment is formed in band cells and segmented cells by endocytosis (i.e., the cell forms this compartment from material already present in the cell), not by pinocytosis or phagocytosis.

Polymorphonuclear Neutrophil (Segmented Neutrophil)

The cell's nucleus continues its indentation until thin strands of membrane and heterochromatin form into segments and create a lobed nucleus. This nucleus is easily deformable because of the active motility of the cell. The name *polymorphonuclear* means "many-shaped nucleus" and accurately describes the nuclear shape. Most nuclei have visible segments, although some appear grossly twisted and folded.[25] A lesser amount of segmenting indicates immaturity or genetic anomaly; a greater amount suggests difficulty in maturation. Regardless of the number of nuclear segments, this cell is completely functional. These cells spend time in bone marrow (as part of the storage pool) and in the marginating and circulating pools of the peripheral blood, in which they constitute 50% to 70% of the total (see Figs. 12-2G and 12-3F).

Although neutrophils have long been regarded as a homogeneous population of cells, several studies[26] have indicated that there is a heterogeneous population of mature neutrophils, some with increased mobility, some with increased numbers of CD15 receptors involved in lymphocyte homing, and others with CD21 that binds to C3. As opposed to the immature cells, these mature cells are positive for CD62, which is an adhesion molecule active on neutrophils and epithelial cells, plus additional adhesion molecules, CD11a/CD18.[27] The functioning neutrophil spends its life performing phagocytosis and pinocytosis. These are essentially the same event at two sizes; phagocytosis usually involves larger material and can be seen at the light microscope level, whereas pinocytosis involves small material and can be seen adequately only with an elec-

tron microscope. These activities can be performed in the bloodstream, as in transient bacteremia, or in the tissues (Box 12-1).

Neutrophils are attracted to particles by several mechanisms. Chemotactic factors elaborated by damaged tissue and invading organisms, antibodies, or complement fixation cause the polymorphonuclear cell to migrate to the source. These chemical messengers interact with the neutrophil as it periodically determines whether the vessel endothelium is expressing surface molecules, which enhance a more firm contact (margination). Eventual egress of the neutrophils outside the blood circulation (diapedesis) occurs in response to a chemical gradient. Chemotactic recognition ability, mobility, and adhesion all are required for phagocytosis to occur. Cells deficient in any of these characteristics defend poorly against infections.[28] Normal cells adhere to particles whose presence has initiated the attraction. Pseudopods extend around the particle, engulfing it and forming a phagosome. Cytoplasmic granules surround the phagosome and, by fusing their membranes, dump their contents into it. Combined primary granule release of peroxide, myeloperoxidase, superoxide, and anions contributes to proteolysis. Secondary granules contain complement activators that increase complement fixation of the foreign material and the chemotactic response by the neutrophil. In addition, the secretion of collagenase, lysozyme, and proteases from the secondary granules causes degradation and detoxification of material. Granule release has been shown to be responsive to many different compounds that are endogenous to normal human plasma, suggesting a more complex homeostatic balance than previously thought.[29] The eventual degranulation of the neutrophil creates cytoplasts that function in anion generation and aggregation.[30] The release of proteases[15]

BOX 12-1 Phagocytosis/Pinocytosis

Recognition-Attachment Phase
Requires mediation by IgG or unknown factors
Stimulation of actin, myosin, and binding proteins

Ingestion Phase (Phagocytosis)
Pseudopod extension
Microfilament rearrangement
Engulfment

Intracellular Kill: Hypertonic Mechanism
Potassium influx

Digestion Phase: Degradation
Secondary lysosomal formation
Usually proteinases, hydrolases, arylsulfatases, and phosphatases

Exocytosis
Removal of indigestible elements
Reversal of phagocytosis

deleterious to the neutrophil itself, leading to its death. Cell content leakage or cell disruption can cause the release of cell contents into the surrounding area, creating the familiar appearance of pus.

Eosinophil Maturation

A close relative of the neutrophilic granulocyte is the eosinophil, whose prominent secondary granules are stained heavily with the eosin dye used in conventional Romanowsky-based stains. The control mechanisms for the selection and development of HSCs into eosinophils seems to be a bit more complex than that of the neutrophil, requiring IL-3, IL-5, and GM-CSF, and is inhibited by the presence of interferon.[31,32] The cell develops from the colony-forming unit specific for granulocytes, erythrocytes, megakaryocytes, and monocytes (CFU-GEMM) into a stem cell specific for eosinophils (CFU-Eo), then into a myeloblast stage similar to that seen in the neutrophils. The promyelocyte stage produces the same type of primary granules and is indistinguishable from other promyelocytes. In the myelocyte stage, the eosinophil is distinguished from the neutrophil by the presence of numerous large, round granules containing a crystalloid compound comprising major basic protein.[33] Major basic protein may be responsible for the staining qualities of the granules. The eosinophilic peroxidase is substantively different from neutrophilic myeloperoxidase and from an eosinophil-derived neurotoxin that is poorly understood. Eosinophil granules contain various proteolytic enzymes (Box 12-2) but do not contain secretory vesicles with lysozyme or alkaline phosphatase.

Eosinophils spend less than 1 week in the peripheral blood, but there is a large storage capacity in the marrow that allows for rapid mobilization on demand.[34] On stimulation by chemotactic factors, such as allergens or parasites, eosinophils leave the marrow and pass quickly through the peripheral blood into the tissues. They are actively motile and use the same migration as neutrophils. Because of the short time that eosinophils spend in transit in the peripheral blood, day-to-day variation in eosinophil numbers is quite high. In the absence of an allergic response, eosinophils should not number more than 5%.

The mature eosinophil typically contains a nucleus that is in band form or bilobed. Nuclei with higher lobe counts are seen rarely. The cell is slightly larger than the average neutrophil and may have an irregular border as a result of motility (Fig. 12-4).

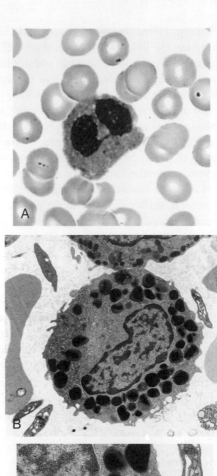

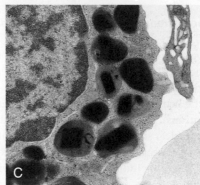

Figure 12-4 A, Eosinophil. **B,** Electron micrograph of eosinophil (×16,500). **C,** Electron micrograph of eosinophilic granule showing internal structures (×52,500). (From Carr JH, Rodak BF: Clinical Hematology Atlas, 2nd ed. Philadelphia: Saunders, 2004.)

Charcot-Leyden crystals are water-soluble, needle-shaped crystals that may be found in cells or in the tissue. They are the result of eosinophil disintegration. They may appear as empty areas or be completely washed out in cells that are poorly fixed.

Basophil Maturation

Similar to their eosinophilic counterparts, basophils are characterized by the presence of large, heavily staining granules. These granules differ from those of the eosinophil in that they are irregularly shaped, are unevenly distributed throughout the cell, and turn a deep purple to black with Romanowsky stains. The process of maturation of the basophil from the stem cell is not as well known as for the other peripheral blood

---

BOX 12-2 Eosinophilic Granule Contents

Acid phosphatase
Arylsulfatase
β-Glucuronidase
Cathepsin
Peroxidase
Phospholipase

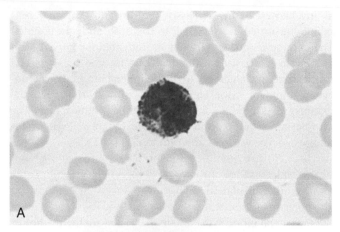

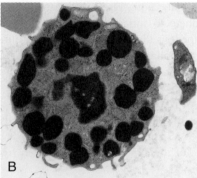

Figure 12-5 A, Basophil with obscured nucleus. **B,** Electron micrograph of basophil (×28,750). (**B** from Carr JH, Rodak BF: Clinical Hematology Atlas, 2nd ed. Philadelphia: Saunders, 2004.)

cells. It may parallel the development of eosinophils. Basophils can be differentiated into myelocytes, metamyelocytes, bands, and polymorphonuclear cells on the basis of nuclear development, although mature nuclei with more than two lobes are extremely rare. The granules contain heparin, chondroitin sulfate, histamine, and other vasoactive and immunomodulatory mediators, such as neutrophil chemotactic factor, the slow-reacting kallikrein found in anaphylaxis, and a platelet-activating factor.[35] Basophils are the least common cell in the peripheral blood; on average, they represent less than 1%. Human basophil membranes have specific high-affinity receptors for the Fc region of IgE. When IgE antibodies bound to the plasma membrane are connected to specific antigens, degranulation occurs (Fig. 12-5). Mast cells, the tissue equivalent of the circulating basophil, are also involved in allergic inflammation and initiate localized and system anaphylaxis.[36]

MONOCYTES

Monocyte/Macrophage Maturation
Stem Cell to Monoblast

Current theory holds that monocyte/macrophage cells are divided into monoblasts, promonocytes, blood monocytes, and free and fixed macrophages.[37] As stated in the section on granulocyte development, the commitment from HSC to common myeloid progenitor is poorly understood. By the action of IL-3, GM-CSF, and M-CSF, the monoblast is generated from the common myeloid progenitor and is found primarily in the bone marrow, although possible secondary sites include the spleen and other reticuloendothelial sites (Fig. 12-6). The same stimulating factors that are active for monoblast/macrophage maturation seem to be involved in osteoclast activity, suggesting additional links in certain malignant marrow diseases, such as multiple myeloma.[38] Monoblasts are distinguished from myeloblasts using flow cytometry because monoblasts are strongly positive for CD33 and only weakly positive for CD34. Monoblasts also are positive for CD4, a marker usually seen in T lymphocytes.[39] In addition to the morphogenesis into macrophages, monocyte precursors have been shown to mature into other cell forms, such as dendritic cells, through the action of such factors as interferon-β and IL-3 or GM-CSF and IL-4.[40,41]

Monoblasts are found in low numbers in the bone marrow, and their only function is in mitosis. They are large cells with an eccentrically placed nucleus containing one or two noticeable nucleoli. Their cytoplasm is nongranular, and when stained they may appear weakly positive for peroxidase (Fig. 12-7). Differentiation by light microscopy between the myeloblast and the monoblast may be difficult to impossible in certain neoplastic disorders.

Monoblast to Promonocyte

After mitosis and maturation, the blast becomes a promonocyte. Promonocytes are similar in size to the blast but have some granulation. They begin to assume a more monocytoid appearance with folded, twisted, or indented nuclei and irregularly shaped cytoplasm. They can be motile and participate in phagocytosis. As with other leukocytes, the nucleoli of the blast develop gradually and become less apparent as the cell matures into the promonocyte and monocyte forms. They are capable of phagocytizing opsonized bacteria and red blood cells coated with IgG, but they lack the range of activity seen in the more mature cells. Of major interest are the nonmorphologic changes present at this and subsequent stages.

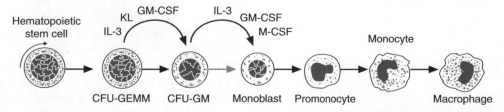

Figure 12-6 Schematic for the differentiation of monocytes, showing the appropriate commitment/stimulation agents.

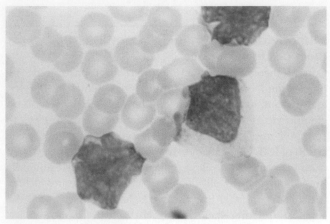

Figure 12-7 Although usually difficult to differentiate from a myeloblast, monoblasts can be identified by the presence of a single large nucleolus, an irregularly shaped nucleus, and delicate chromatin.

Promonocyte to Monocyte

Granule content and number vary considerably as the cell matures. More than 50 secretory compounds, such as transport proteins, nonspecific inflammatory agents, storage materials, and humoral-acting agents, have been identified (Box 12-3).[42] Peripheral blood monocytes have great morphologic vari-

---

BOX 12-3 Monocyte-Associated Compounds

Transport Proteins
Transferrin
Transcobalamin

Nonspecific Inflammatory Agents
Lysozyme
Endogenous pyrogens (IL-1)

Tissue Activators
Coagulation factors V, VII, IX, and X and tissue thromboplastin
Plasminogen activator
Complement (1-5)
Properdin

Specific/Humoral Agents
Colony-stimulating factors for CFU-GEMM, T and B cells, epithelial cells
Erythropoietin

Storage
Iron
Vitamin B$_{12}$

Self-Recognition/Nonself-Recognition/Defense Agents
Interferon
Tumor inhibitory factors such as tissue necrosis factor

---

ability. Because of their aggressive motility and adherence, cells may be distorted as they cling to the push and smear slides. The monocyte nucleus usually is indented or curved with chromatin that is lacy with small clumps, and it is typically described as the largest cell in the peripheral blood. The monocyte's abundant cytoplasm is filled with swirls of minute granules that produce a cloudy or turbid appearance. The cytoplasmic membrane may be quite irregular. Pseudopods and phagocytic vacuoles are common (Fig. 12-8).

This cell also may be thought of as a transitional cell because it leaves the bone marrow to enter the circulation, only to leave the circulation as it enters tissues in response to chemotactic factors. Monocytes account for less than 15% of the peripheral blood WBC differential. They are highly motile, tend to marginate along vessel walls, and have a strong tendency to adhere to surfaces. With appropriate stimuli, they undergo diapedesis through vessel walls and differentiate into larger free macrophages, which have greater phagocytic activity and a higher concentration of hydrolytic enzymes.

Monocyte to Macrophage

Macrophages are large, actively phagocytic cells with a size range of 15 to 85 μm in diameter. Their shape is pleomorphic, and because of their motility, they are seen frequently with

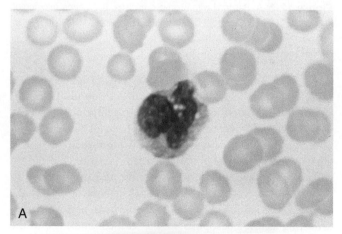

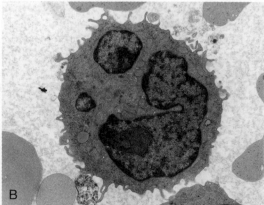

Figure 12-8 A, Typical monocyte showing vacuolated cytoplasm and cerebriform nucleus. **B,** Electron micrograph of monocyte (×16,500). (**B** from Carr JH, Rodak BF: Clinical Hematology Atlas, 2nd ed. Philadelphia: Saunders, 2004.)

pseudopods. The function of the monocyte/macrophage is phagocytosis, and the material ingested is more variable than the material ingested by the neutrophil. The process is similar to neutrophil phagocytosis, but much quicker. Monocytes require less opsonization (sensitization to phagocytosis) or complement, and phagocytosis can be initiated by simple contact. Pinocytosis occurs with items less than 2 µm in size and requires receptor mediation and some degree of protein synthesis. Both activities require the same multistep process found in neutrophils, including recognition/attachment, ingestion (phagocytosis), intracellular kill, digestion/degradation, and exocytosis. Through these mechanisms, monocytes kill any recognizable nonself agent: dead or dying cells, bacteria, fungi, and viruses.[43] They play a role in processing specific antigens for lymphocyte recognition and stimulation of lymphocyte transformation. They may function as an antitumor agent by phagocytic action of nonself cells through the elaboration of tumor necrosis factor and stimulation of lymphocyte activity.[44]

Macrophages

The terminal cell of the monocyte cell line is the macrophage. Macrophages can be divided into two categories: free and fixed. As the monocyte responds to chemotaxis, such as bacterial endotoxin, it enlarges and becomes highly motile. It leaves the peripheral blood and enters the tissue space. It elaborates additional chemotactic agents, such as tumor necrosis factor and decay accelerating factor, bringing additional macrophages and neutrophils into the space.

Free macrophages are found in varying concentrations in all sites of inflammation and repair, alveolar spaces, and peritoneal and synovial fluids, whereas fixed (tissue) macrophages are found in specific concentrations and in such specific sites as the nervous system (microglial cells), liver (Kupffer cells), spleen, bone marrow, and lymph nodes. They are large cells with ample cytoplasm filled with granules and frequently have multiple vacuoles. The nucleus is typically round to reniform and may contain one or two nucleoli (Fig. 12-9).

LYMPHOCYTES

Lymphocytes are human blood leukocytes whose site of development is not solely the bone marrow, but also tissues referred to as *primary* and *secondary lymphoid organs*. In humans, the primary organs are the thymus and the bone marrow, whereas secondary sites include the spleen, Peyer's patches in the gastrointestinal tract, the Waldeyer ring of the tonsils and adenoids, and lymph nodes and nodules scattered throughout the body.

The cells circulate throughout the body in peripheral blood and lymph, and these carrier streams bring them to sites of activity. Migrating lymphocytes travel from the thoracic duct through vessel endothelium to lymph nodes into the bloodstream and back again. The hand mirror shape of peripheral blood lymphocytes is a result of their characteristic form of locomotion. As with other cell lines that have subpopulations, lymphocytes can be categorized in a variety of ways: They may be short-lived or long-lived cells; they may produce antibodies or lymphokines (Table 12-1); and they have different surface charges, densities, and antigen receptors.[45]

Development

Probably as a result of specific hormone stimuli, the earliest maturation of the HSC results in a common lymphoid progenitor cell, which matures in several environments (Fig. 12-10).[46] The thymus and bone marrow give rise to lymphocytes, foster differentiation, and are independent of antigenic stimulation. Certain lymphokines and external proteins, such as G proteins, are thought to control the diversity found in the differentiation of T and B lymphocytes.[47] These environments determine to a great extent the functionality of the cell. Cells that develop under the influence of the thymus are called *T cells* and have a specific, unique set of receptors and responses. *B cells* are derived from the bone marrow and have a different set of functions and capabilities. The end cell of the B lymphocyte maturation is the plasma cell. When the

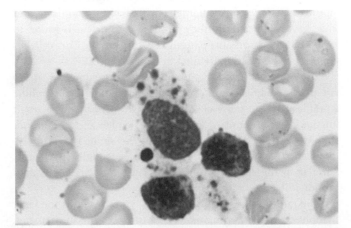

Figure 12-9 Bone marrow macrophage with an eccentrically placed nucleus and granulated cytoplasm.

TABLE 12-1 Some Important Lymphokines*

B cell growth factor	As a group, these three control
B cell differentiation factor	proliferation, growth rate, maturation,
B cell stimulatory factor	and stimulation of B cells
Colony-stimulating factors	Hematopoietic factors regulating proliferation and differentiation of myeloid cells
Macrophage inhibitory factor	Inhibits macrophages from migration
Histamine-producing cell-stimulating factor	Induces histamine synthesis by basophils and mast cells
T cell–activating factor	Influences the cytotoxic T cells and natural killer cells to become cytolytic

*Lymphokines are biologically active molecules elaborated by lymphocytes in response to specific needs. This table lists a selection of the more important lymphokines. The range of the activity can be appreciated by the variety of cell types influenced by these agents.

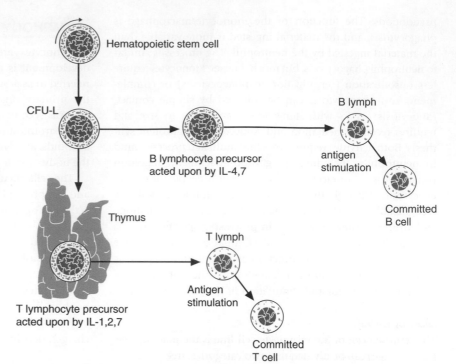

Figure 12-10 Schematic for the differentiation of T and B lymphocytes, showing the appropriate commitment/stimulation agents.

(figure labels: Hematopoietic stem cell; CFU-L; B lymphocyte precursor acted upon by IL-4,7; B lymph; antigen stimulation; Committed B cell; Thymus; T lymphocyte precursor acted upon by IL-1,2,7; T lymph; Antigen stimulation; Committed T cell)

environmental effects have been achieved, lymphocytes migrate to secondary lymphatic tissues, such as the spleen and tonsils, which act as the main repositories of already differentiated lymphocytes. Cellular interactions with dendritic cells and macrophages for the presentation of the antigen to the cells have a crucial role in priming cells for proliferation and affect cell maturation, especially T cells. These interactions are being elucidated at a rapid rate and are expected to result in additional testing modalities for lymphocyte discrimination.[48] This additional testing is needed because regardless of the environment, the cells cannot be differentiated into T or B cells by a routine examination. When seen through traditional Romanowsky-based staining methods, they can be divided into only three gross morphologic stages: lymphoblast, prolymphocyte, and mature lymphocyte.

Lymphocyte percentages in the peripheral blood vary depending on the age of the individual. Children younger than 4 years old have a much higher proportion of lymphocytes in the peripheral blood than do adults, although in adults lymphocytes are the second most common cell of the peripheral blood differential, accounting for approximately 20% to 40% of WBCs. Further differentiation into subpopulations reveals that approximately 20% to 35% of total circulating lymphocytes are B cells because they reside primarily in the lymph nodes. The T cell population is the dominant population in the bloodstream.

Lymphocyte Maturation
Lymphoblast to Prolymphocyte
The lymphoblast is a small to medium-sized cell (10-18 μm) with a round-to-oval nucleus containing loose chromatin and one or more active nucleoli. The cytoplasm is scanty and

has basophilia in proportion to the amount of RNA present (Fig. 12-11). The next stage, the prolymphocyte, may be difficult to distinguish from the blast stage because the prolymphocyte differs from the blast by subtle changes, such as slightly more clumped chromatin, a lessening of nucleolar prominence, and a change in the thickness of the nuclear membrane (Fig. 12-12). The prolymphocyte in leukemia has distinctive morphology and is discussed in Chapter 37.

Prolymphocyte to Lymphocyte
Morphology of lymphocytes, when seen with the aid of Wright stain, varies mostly by size. The size discrepancy may be due to the activity of the cell or the location in the smear in which it is found. Cells in thick areas of the smear tend to be rounded upward and to appear smaller and thicker than they actually are. The most common form is the small lymphocyte, which is approximately 9 μm in diameter with skimpy cytoplasm and may have a few azurophilic granules. The nucleus is round to oval, and its chromatin pattern is a block type. This cell has been described as nondividing or resting (Fig. 12-13).

The medium-sized lymphocyte is approximately 11 to 14 μm in diameter. Its cytoplasm may contain azurophilic granules that are more clearly discerned, probably as a result of the larger amount of cytoplasm in which they are found. Although these cells are larger than the small lymphocytes, their nucleus-to-cytoplasm ratios are essentially the same. Similar to the small lymphocytes, these cells are considered nondividing.

The rarest of the peripheral blood lymphocytes is the large lymphocyte. It is approximately 15 μm or more in diameter, and its more generous cytoplasm usually turns a deeper shade of blue when stained. The usual block-type DNA is spread

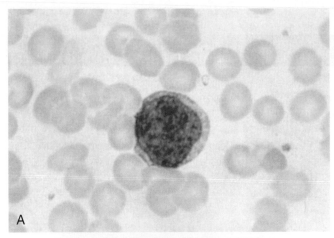

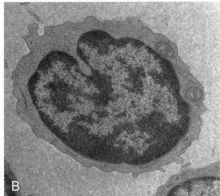

Figure 12-11 A, Lymphoblast. **B,** Electron micrograph of lymphoblast (×28,750). (**B** from Carr JH, Rodak BF: Clinical Hematology Atlas, 2nd ed. Philadelphia: Saunders, 2004.)

a little more loosely. The cell may be considered to be in transformation in association with active cell proliferation. According to examination by immunologic techniques, this cell, if it contains adequate granulation, may be part of a subpopulation of thymus-dependent cells called *natural killer cells*. Morphologic variants of lymphocytes are summarized in Table 12-2.

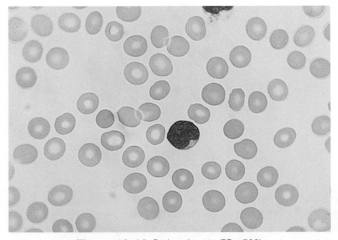

Figure 12-12 Prolymphocyte (PB ×500).

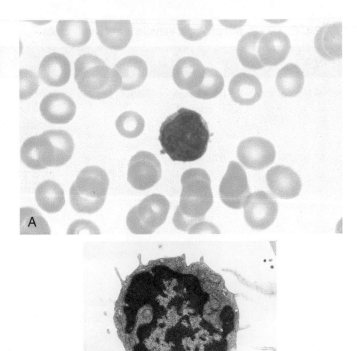

Figure 12-13 A, Lymphocyte. **B,** Electron micrograph of lymphocyte (×30,000). (**B** from Carr JH, Rodak BF: Clinical Hematology Atlas, 2nd ed. Philadelphia: Saunders, 2004.)

Immunologic Differentiation

Lymphocytes may be categorized by their immunologic function, and some connections to morphology may be made. The earliest cells show only the marker of a nuclear enzyme, terminal deoxynucleotidyl transferase (TdT), and may be the CFU-L.[35] Later stages show nonspecific immunoglobulin gene structures and TdT (morphologically, these may be *blasts*).

B Cells

B lymphocyte differentiation begins with the induction of immunoglobulin secretion and the activation of an intracellular signaling pathway called the *unfolded protein response*. This initiation requires inositol-requiring enzyme 1α, found in the endoplasmic reticulum. Inositol-requiring enzyme 1α also is required for immunoglobulin gene rearrangement, development of cytoplasmic immunoglobulin concentrations of mostly IgD and IgM, and production of B cell receptors; finally the enzyme plays a role in terminal differentiation of mature B cells into antibody-secreting plasma cells.[49] The fully committed B lymphocyte is the plasma cell (Fig. 12-14). Surface immunologic markers include receptors for the crystallizable fragment of IgG, complement, Epstein-Barr virus, class I and class II human leukocyte antigens (HLA-A, HLA-B, HLA-C, HLA-D, and HLA-DR), and pokeweed mitogens.

T Cells

T cells are harder to characterize because the receptors and markers appear, disappear, and reappear throughout the

TABLE 12-2 Morphologic Variations of Lymphocytes

	Nucleus				Cytoplasm		
Cell	Shape	Color	Chromatin	Nucleoli	Amount	Color	Granulation
Small lymphocyte	Round, oval; indented; stretched	Medium purple	Clumped, smudged, or streaked; not distinct	Not usually	Scanty to moderate	Colorless through shades of blue; clear	If present, few large azurophilic
Large lymphocyte	Round, oval; indented; stretched; usually not folded	Light to medium purple	Variable; clumped, smudged, or reticular	Variable	Moderate to abundant	Colorless through shades of azurophilic blue; clear	If present, few large; tend to localize
Basophilic lymphocyte	Round	Dense; medium to deep purple	Clumped	If present, indistinct; not in late stages	Moderate	Royal blue to deep purple	None or in blocks
Plasma cell	Round, eccentrically placed	Dense; medium to deep purple	Very coarse; clumping; sharp definition of parachromatin	None	Moderate to abundant	Deep blue; may have perinuclear halo	None

development of the cell, which indicates that these markers may serve some developmental or proliferative function.[50] The primitive T cell is the common lymphoid progenitor cell, which travels to the thymus for maturation and commitment. The earliest cell within the thymus is the pre-T cell, which shows the presence of TdT and common T cell marker (CD2), whereas the prothymocyte possesses TdT but loses CD2 and acquires a transferrin receptor that is apparently specific not to differentiation, but to cell proliferation. The common cortical thymocyte is characterized by the presence of TdT, CD1, CD2, and either CD4 (helper/inducer subset marker) or CD8 (cytotoxic/suppressor subset marker). Mature T cells lose all precursor markers and have an active helper or suppressor

function. T cells are differentiated further through the presence or absence of HLA-D class antigens. T cells also possess sheep erythrocyte rosetting receptor and receptors for phytohemagglutinin, concanavalin A, and class I antigens (HLA-A, HLA-B, HLA-C). (A further discussion of cell markers is presented in Chapter 33.)

Lymphocyte Activity: Regulation of Cellular Response

The main function of the lymphocyte is the regulation of immune function. If foreign material (exogenous antigenic matter or altered endogenous material, such as dead, dying, or malignant cells) is completely engulfed, degraded, and

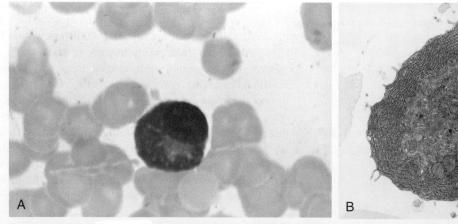

Figure 12-14 A, Plasma cell showing the typical abundant cytoplasm and perinuclear halo usually ascribed to the presence of the high lipid content of the Golgi apparatus. Notice the dense packing of the heterochromatin in the nucleus. **B,** Electron micrograph of plasma cell (×17,500). (**B** from Carr JH, Rodak BF: Clinical Hematology Atlas, 2nd ed. Philadelphia: Saunders, 2004.)

disposed of by phagocytes, no immune response occurs. If complete engulfment does not occur, antigenic fragments are transported to the subcapsular sinus of lymph nodes. In the medullary areas of the node, the antigen is fixed to the exterior surface and brought into the lysozymes of the macrophage. Dendritic cells also play a direct role with the stimulation of B lymphocytes. They deliver antigen to the B lymphocytes in a more intact form than the processed form essential for stimulating T lymphocytes and can release cytokines that assist the differentiation of the B lymphocytes into antibody-producing cells.[51] When this differentiation occurs, intense proliferation takes place for approximately 48 hours. The macrophage releases IL-1; T cells release factors that increase activation of antigen-specific CD8+ T cells, and the development of clones of antigen-specific B lymphocytes and cytotoxic T cells begins by the action of cytotoxic lymphocyte differentiation factor. Cytotoxic cells require prior activation and MHC class I antigens. T cells release numerous soluble factors that activate effector cells. Suppressor cells complete the feedback loop by dampening the specific response, not by immune responsiveness in general, and quench the activated T cells.[52]

If a B cell encounters a polysaccharide antigen, it does not need T-cell stimulation. Induction of a specific helper factor stimulates IgM secretion, and activated B cells expose surface receptors for the lymphokine B-cell growth factor, which, with IL-1, stimulates cell division. A second lymphokine, B-cell differentiation factor, promotes differentiation into plasma cells. Meanwhile, cytotoxic T cells have CD8+-like suppressors and lyse cells by surface-to-surface contact independent of antibody.

Morphology of Activation

The activity that accompanies clonal expansion necessary for successful removal of antigen can be seen to a certain degree in the morphology of the cells called *reactive, transformed,* or *variant* lymphocytes. An older term, "atypical", although inaccurate, is still used occasionally because the cells are atypical in appearance; however, they are responding to an antigen, so their function is not atypical. Cells must recognize the appropriate antigen (at times modified and presented by the macrophage), commit to producing the correct antibody or lymphokines necessary for the type of antigen attack, undergo clonal expansion to increase numbers of committed cells, and attempt to neutralize or eliminate the antigen in question. Doing all this requires frequent and significant amounts of morphologic change. These cells should not be confused with distinctly abnormal lymphocytes seen in such conditions as lymphoma (Chapter 37).

Causes of an increase in reactive lymphocytes are many. In essence, anything that is antigenic or material that is incompletely eliminated by phagocytes results in the presence of reactive lymphocytes. Causes of reactive lymphocytosis are discussed in Chapter 28.

As a result of antigen stimulation, lymphocytes may become quite large, sometimes more than 30 μm in diameter. The cells are highly pleomorphic. Compared with the nucleus of a common lymphocyte, the nucleus of the reactive lymphocyte is less clumped; faintly stained multiple nucleoli are more likely to be seen. Chromatin patterns are generally less striking in the reactive lymphocyte; some patterns appear similar to those of a blast. The shape of the common lymphocyte nucleus is round to oval; the shape of the reactive cell nucleus ranges from elliptic to cleaved to folded. The cytoplasm has greater variability in morphology than does the nucleus. The cytoplasm may range from large, deeply basophilic, and abundant to unevenly stained and granular. A Golgi apparatus is commonly seen. A variant of the reactive lymphocyte is the plasmacytoid lymphocyte, the appearance of which is somewhere between the appearance of the lymphocyte and plasma cell (Figs. 12-15 and 12-16).

The reporting protocol for reactive lymphocytes depends on individual facilities. Some institutions term all cells that are not small lymphocytes as *reactive;* others have more definitive criteria. However it is done, every clinical laboratory scientist within a given facility must use the same protocol to achieve reliability within the institution.

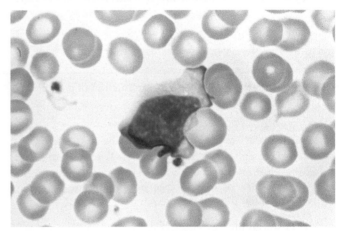

Figure 12-15 The typical reactive lymphocyte seen in most antigenic responses. This cell has a large, flared cytoplasm with a loose chromatin structure to its nucleus.

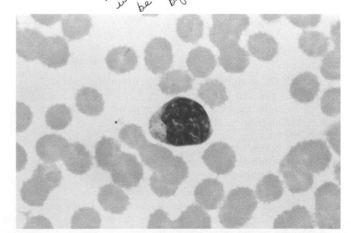

Figure 12-16 Quite different from the reactive lymphocyte shown in Fig. 12-15, this cell has a plasmacytoid appearance with a deeply basophilic cytoplasm, easily visualized Golgi apparatus, and dense nucleus.

CHAPTER at a GLANCE

- The locations of leukocyte production change throughout life, starting with the yolk sac of the mesenchyme, followed by the spleen and liver, and finally the bone marrow.
- Human blood leukocytes can be divided into various categories on the basis of their specific function, site of origin, or morphology. In essence, all leukocytes exist to defend the organism against nonself agents. This is accomplished through intricate cooperation among cells.
- Although traditional microscopic evaluation of cells continues to be the basic modality of clinical study, flow cytometric analysis of receptor sites, antigenic labeling, and functional studies contribute an increasing amount of information.
- Granulocytes contain visible granules and develop solely in the bone marrow. The function of neutrophils is primarily as destroyers of pyogenic bacteria, whereas eosinophils and basophils are active in allergic reactions. Monocytes/macrophages are less discriminating in their phagocytic activities.
- Lymphocytes are produced in bone marrow and lymphoid tissue. They are under the control of environmental and hormonal stimuli different from the stimuli that control granulocytes and monocytes.
- Granulocytes can be found in high concentrations in four locations: in bone marrow, circulating freely in the peripheral blood, marginating up against the endothelium of blood vessels, and in the tissues. These locations are called *granulocyte pools*.
- Granulocytes are subdivided further according to the type of reaction (neutrophilic, eosinophilic, basophilic) found in the granules when stained differentially with a Romanowsky-based stain.
- Monocytes contain minute granules, which, when viewed by light microscopy, cause their cytoplasm to have a grainy appearance.
- Lymphocytes that develop under the influence of the thymus are called *T cells* and have a specific, unique set of receptors and responses. B lymphocytes are derived from the bone marrow and have a different set of functions and capabilities. The end cell of the B lymphocyte maturation is the plasma cell.
- The main function of the lymphocyte is the regulation of immune function. Lymphocytes may be categorized by their immunologic function, and some connections to morphology may be made.

REVIEW QUESTIONS

1. The stem cell committed to the production of granulocytes is the:
   a. HSC
   b. CFU-S
   c. CFU-E
   d. CFU-G

2. The presence of major basic protein in the cytoplasm confirms that the cell is:
   a. Basophilic
   b. Eosinophilic
   c. Neutrophilic
   d. Monocytic

3. Vasoactive compounds are principal components of the granules of:
   a. Basophils
   b. Eosinophils
   c. Monocytes
   d. Neutrophils

4. Which cell is characterized by the following features?
   15 to 20 μm in diameter
   Delicate nucleus with prominent nucleoli
   Stains positive for myeloperoxidase
   a. Monocyte
   b. Myelocyte
   c. Myeloblast
   d. Lymphocyte

5. A cell with a round-to-oval nucleus, no visible nucleoli, evident Golgi apparatus, and the presence of secondary granules would be classified as a:
   a. Reactive lymphocyte
   b. Monoblast
   c. Myelocyte
   d. Promyelocyte

6. For neutrophils to defend against infection, they must be capable of all of the following *except*:
   a. Chemotaxis
   b. Mobility
   c. Adhesion
   d. Cell division

7. Allergic reactions frequently are associated with an increase in the presence of:
   a. Lymphocytes
   b. Neutrophils
   c. Monocytes
   d. Eosinophils

8. A cell that exhibits morphogenesis into one of several tissue cells, such as alveolar macrophages or dendritic cells, is a:
   a. Lymphocyte
   b. Neutrophil
   c. Monocyte
   d. Basophil

9. Which of the following cells may develop in sites other than bone marrow?
   a. Monocyte
   b. Lymphocyte
   c. Megakaryocyte
   d. Neutrophil

10. The final stage of B cell maturation is the:
    a. Large lymphocyte
    b. Atypical lymphocyte
    c. Plasma cell
    d. Vacuolated monocyte

REFERENCES

1. Davey FR, Hutchison RE: Hematopoiesis. In Henry JB (ed): Clinical Diagnosis and Management by Laboratory Methods, 20th ed. Philadelphia: Saunders, 2001:520.
2. Buitenhuis M, van Deutekom HW, Verhagen LP, et al: Differential regulation of granulopoiesis by the basic helix-loop-helix transcriptional inhibitors Id1 and Id2. Blood 2005;105:4272-4281.
3. Ueda Y, Kondo M, Kelsoe G: Inflammation and the reciprocal production of granulocytes and lymphocytes in bone marrow. J Exp Med 2005;201:1771-1780.
4. Krause DS, Fackler MJ, Civin CI, et al: CD34: structure, biology, and clinical utility. Blood 1996;87:1-13.
5. Takeda H, Yamamoto M, Morita N, et al: Relationship between Thy-1 expression and cell-cycle distribution in human bone marrow hematopoietic progenitors. Am J Hematol 2005; 79:187-193.
6. Darzynkiewicz Z, Staiano-Coico L, Melamed MR: Increased mitochondrial uptake of rhodamine 123 during lymphocyte stimulation. Proc Natl Acad Sci USA 1981;78:2383-2387.
7. Papayannopoulou T, Priestley GV, Rohde A, et al: Hemopoietic lineage commitment decisions: in vivo evidence from a transgenic mouse model harboring micro LCR-betapro-LacZ as a transgene. Blood 2000;95:1274-1282.
8. Nakahata T, Ogawa M: Identification in culture of a class of hemopoietic colony-forming units with extensive capability to self-renew and generate multipotential hemopoietic colonies. Proc Natl Acad Sci U S A 1982;79:3843-3847.
9. Lanza F, Castagnari B, Rigolin G, et al: Flow cytometry measurement of GM-CSF receptors in acute leukemic blasts and normal hemopoietic cells. Leukemia 1997;11:1700-1710.
10. Akashi K, Traver E, Miyamoto T, et al: A clonogenic common myeloid progenitor that gives rise to all myeloid lineages. Nature 2000;404:193-197.
11. Schwabe M, Hartert AM, Bertz H, et al: Treatment with granulocyte colony-stimulating factor increases interleukin-1 receptor antagonist levels during engraftment following allogeneic stem-cell transplantation. Eur J Clin Invest 2004;34:759-765.
12. Nicola NA, Smith A, Robb L, et al: The structural basis of the biological actions of the GM-CSF receptor. CIBA Found Symp 1997;204:19-27.
13. Freedman AS: Cell surface antigens in leukemias and lymphomas. Cancer Invest 1996;14:252-276.
14. Lichtman MA: Cellular deformability during maturation of the myeloblast: possible role in marrow egress. N Engl J Med 1970;283:943-948.
15. Segal AW: How neutrophils kill microbes. Ann Rev Immunol 2005;23:197-223.
16. Borregaard N, Lollike K, Kjeldsen L, et al: Human neutrophil granules and secretory vesicles. Eur J Haematol 1993;51:187-198.
17. Boll I, Kuhn A: Granulocytopoiesis in human bone marrow culture studies by means of kinematography. Blood 1965;26:449-470.
18. Ogawa M: Hemopoietic stem cells: stochastic differentiation and humoral control of proliferation. Environ Health Perspect 1989;80:199-207.
19. Carr JH, Rodak BF: Clinical Hematology Atlas, 2nd ed. Philadelphia: Saunders, 2004.
20. Ponder E, Mineola LI: The polycyte. J Lab Clin Med 1942;27:866-874.
21. 2004 Surveys and Anatomic Pathology Education Programs: Hematology, Clinical Microscopy and Body Fluids Glossary. Chicago: College of American Pathologists, 2004.
22. Scott RE, Horn RG: Ultrastructural aspects of neutrophil granulocyte development in humans. Lab Invest 1970;23:202.
23. Wallace PJ, Packman CH, Lichtman MA: Maturation-associated changes in the peripheral cytoplasm of human neutrophil: a review. Exp Hematol 1987;15:34-45.
24. Sandilands GP, Ahmed Z, Perry N, et al: Cross-linking of neutrophil CD11b results in rapid cell surface expression of molecules required for antigen presentation and T-cell activation. Immunology 2005;114:354-368.
25. Arneth J: Die Neutrophilen Wiessen Blutkoorperchen bei Infectious-Krankheiten. Jena, Germany: Fischer, 1904.
26. Krause PJ, Malech HL, Kristie J: Polymorphonuclear leukocyte heterogeneity in neonates and adults. Blood 1986;68:200-204.
27. Vermot Desroches C, Rigal D, Andreoni C: Regulation and functional involvement of distinct determinants of leucocyte function-associated antigen 1 (LFA-1) in T-cell activation in vitro. Scand J Immunol 1991;33:277-286.
28. Carstanjen D, Yamauchi A, Koornneef A, et al: Rac2 regulates neutrophil chemotaxis, superoxide production, and myeloid colony formation through multiple distinct effector pathways. J Immunol 2005;174:4613-4620.
29. Tuluc F, Garcia A, Bredetean O, et al: Primary granule release from human neutrophils is potentiated by soluble fibrinogen through a mechanism depending on multiple intracellular signaling pathways. Am J Physiol Cell Physiol 2004; 287:C1264-C1272.
30. Korchak HM, Roos D, Giedd KN, et al: Granulocytes without degranulation: neutrophil function in granule-depleted cytoplasts. Proc Natl Acad Sci USA 1983;8091:4968-4972.
31. Khanna-Gupta A, Berliner N: Granulocytopoieses and monocytopoiesis. In Hoffman R, Benz EJ, Shatil SJ, et al, eds. In Hematology: Basic Principles and Practice, 4th ed. Philadelphia: Elsevier, 2005:289-301.
32. Lundahl J, Sehmi R, Moshfegh A, et al: Distinct phenotypic adhesion molecule expression on human cord blood progenitors during early eosinophilic commitment: upregulation of beta(7) integrins. Scand J Immunol 2002;56:161-167.
33. Bainton DF: Morphology of neutrophils, eosinophils, basophils. In Beutler E, Lichtman MA, Williams WJ, et al (eds): Williams Hematology, 6th ed. New York: McGraw-Hill, 2001:729-743.
34. Galli SJ, Dvorak AM, Dvorak HF: Basophils and mast cells: morphologic insights into their biology, secretory patterns, and functions. Prog Allergy 1984;34:1-141.
35. Schwartz LB: Effector cells of anaphylaxis: mast cells and basophils. Novartis Found Symp 2004;257:65-74.
36. Pawankar R: Mast cells in allergic airway disease and chronic rhinosinusitis. Chem Immunol Allergy 2005;87:111-129.
37. Henkel GW, McKercher SR, Leenen PJ, et al: Commitment to the monocytic lineage occurs in the absence of the transcription factor PU.1. Blood 1999;93:2849-2858.
38. Hayashi S, Yamane T, Miyamoto A, et al: Commitment and differentiation of stem cells to the osteoclast lineage. Biochem Cell Biol 1998;76:911-922.
39. Gengenbacher D, Salm H, Vogt A, et al: Detection of cell surface determinants for anti-Leu M3 (CD14), MY9 (CD33) and MY4 (CD14) and phagocytic function of cord blood monocytes in the course of gestational age. Bone Marrow Transplant 1998;22(Suppl 1):S48-S51.
40. Buisson S, Triebel F: LAG-3 (CD223) reduces macrophage and dendritic cell differentiation from monocyte precursors. Immunology 2005;114:369-374.
41. Detournay O, Mazouz N, Goldman M, et al: IL-6 produced by type I IFN DC controls IFN-gamma production by regulating the suppressive effect of CD4+ CD25+ regulatory T cells. Hum Immunol 2005;66:460-468.
42. Logan MR, Odemuyiwa SO, Moqbel R: Understanding exocytosis in immune and inflammatory cells: the molecular basis of mediator secretion. J Allergy Clin Immunol 2003;111:923-932.

43. van Furth E (ed): Mononuclear Phagocytes: Characteristics, Physiology and Function. Dordrecht, The Netherlands: Martinus Nijhoff, 1985.

44. Balazs M, Martin F, Zhou T, et al: Blood dendritic cells interact with splenic marginal zone B cells to initiate T-independent immune responses. Immunity 2002;17:341-352.

45. Tough DF, Sprent J: Lifespan of lymphocytes. Immunol Res 1995;14:1-12.

46. Kondo M, Weissman IL, Akashi K: Identification of clonogenic common lymphoid progenitors in mouse bone marrow. Cell 1997;91:661-672.

47. Han SB, Moratz C, Huang NN, et al: Rgs1 and Gnai2 regulate the entrance of B lymphocytes into lymph nodes and B cell motility within lymph node follicles. Immunity 2005;22:343-354.

48. Molon B, Gri G, Bettella M, et al: T cell costimulation by chemokine receptors. Nat Immunol 2005;6:465-471.

49. Zhang K, Wong HN, Song B, et al: The unfolded protein response sensor IRE1alpha is required at 2 distinct steps in B cell lymphopoiesis. J Clin Invest 2005;115:268-281.

50. Kojima H, Kanno Y, Hase H, et al: CD4+CD25+ regulatory T cells attenuate the phosphatidylinositol 3-kinase/Akt pathway in antigen-primed immature CD8+ CTLs during functional maturation. J Immunol 2005;174:5959-5967.

51. McCullough KC, Summerfield A: Basic concepts of immune response and defense development. ILAR J 2005;46:230-240.

52. Mackey MF, Barth RJ Jr, Noelle RJ: The role of CD40/CD154 interactions in the priming, differentiation, and effector function of helper and cytotoxic T cells. J Leukoc Biol 1998;63:418-428.

Platelet Production, Structure, and Function

13

George A. Fritsma

OBJECTIVES

After completion of this chapter, the reader will be able to:

1. Diagram megakaryocytopoiesis, including megakaryocyte localization, growth factor control, endomitosis, and platelet shedding.
2. Describe the ultrastructure of resting platelets in the circulation, including the plasma membrane, tubules, microfibrils, and granules.
3. Discuss the value of counting reticulated platelets in peripheral blood.
4. List the important platelet receptors and their ligands.
5. Recount platelet function, including adhesion, aggregation, and secretion.
6. Reproduce the biochemical pathways of platelet activation, including integrins, G proteins, the eicosanoid, and the diacylglycerol-inositol triphosphate pathway.

CASE STUDY

After studying the material in this chapter, the reader should be able to respond to the following case study:

A 35-year-old woman noticed multiple pinpoint red spots and bruises on her arms and legs. The hematologist confirmed the presence of petechiae, purpura, and ecchymoses on her extremities and ordered a complete blood count, prothrombin time, and partial thromboplastin time. The platelet count was 35×10^9/L, the mean platelet volume was 13.2 fL, and the platelets appeared large on the Wright-stained peripheral blood film. Other complete blood count parameters and the coagulation parameters were within normal limits. A Wright-stained bone marrow aspirate revealed 10 to 12 small unlobulated megakaryocytes per low-power field.

1. What type of bleeding is indicated by these signs and symptoms?
2. What is the probable cause for the bleeding?
3. Is the thrombocytopenia the result of inadequate bone marrow production?
4. List the growth factors involved in recruiting megakaryocyte progenitors.

MEGAKARYOCYTOPOIESIS

Platelets are anucleate blood cells that circulate at 150 to 400×10^9/L, with mean counts slightly higher in women than in men.[1] Platelets trigger primary hemostasis on exposure to physical and fluid stimulants that are associated with blood vessel injury. On a Wright-stained wedge preparation blood film, platelets are distributed through a monolayer at 7 to 21 per 1000× field and have an average diameter of 2.5 μm, corresponding to a mean platelet volume (MPV) of 8 to 10 fL in a wet preparation, as determined using laboratory profiling instruments.[2] Their internal structure, although complex, is scarcely visible using light microscopy.

Platelets arise from unique bone marrow cells called *megakaryocytes*. Megakaryocytes are among the largest cells in the body (30-50 μm in diameter on a Wright-stained bone marrow aspirate film) and are polyploid. In healthy intact bone marrow tissue, megakaryocytes cluster in the extravascular compartment adjacent to the abluminal face of venous sinusoid endothelial cells (Fig. 13-1).[3] Other hematopoietic cells may cross the megakaryocyte cytoplasm to reach the sinusoid lumen, a faux phagocytosis known as "emperopolesis."[4] Megakaryocytes also are harvested from the lungs.[5] In a normal Wright-stained bone marrow aspirate, the microscopist may identify two to four megakaryocytes per 10× low-power field.

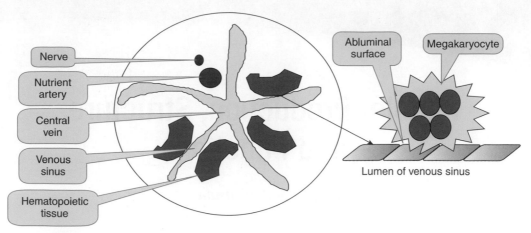

Figure 13-1 Megakaryocytes localize to the abluminal surface of sinusoid-lining endothelial cells.

Megakaryocyte Progenitors

The hematopoietic stem cell named the *colony-forming unit granulocyte, erythrocyte, megakaryocyte, monocyte* (CFU-GEMM) (Chapter 7) differentiates to the megakaryocyte lineage under the influence of the hormone thrombopoietin (TPO) and a series of cytokines. There are three megakaryocyte lineage–committed progenitor stages, defined by their culture colony characteristics. In order of differentiation, these are the *burst-forming unit* (BFU-Meg), *colony-forming unit* (CFU-Meg), and the *light-density CFU* (LD-CFU-Meg).[6] All three resemble small lymphocytes and cannot be distinguished by Wright-stained light microscopy. The BFU-Meg and CFU-Meg are diploid and participate in normal mitosis, maintaining a pool of megakaryocyte progenitors. Their proliferative properties are reflected in their ability to form colonies of hundreds (BFU) or scores (CFU) of progeny in culture (Fig. 13-2). In contrast to the BFU-Meg and CFU-Meg, the LD-CFU-Meg has little proliferative capacity and produces few cells but progresses to increased nuclear ploidy.

The LD-CFU-Meg may be a transitional, or promegakaryoblast, stage, in which polyploidy is established, but the morphology is indistinguishable from small lymphocytes. Megakaryocyte progenitors enter a second developmental compartment, terminal differentiation, as they lose their proliferative capacity.

In specialty laboratories, immunologic probes and flow cytometry are employed to identify megakaryocyte progenitors. Useful megakaryocyte-specific and platelet-specific immunologic markers are platelet factor 4 (PF4), von Willebrand factor (VWF), and platelet glycoproteins Ib (GP Ib, CD42b) and IIb/IIIa (GP IIb/IIIa, CD41).[7] Platelet peroxidase, localized in the endoplasmic reticulum of progenitors and megakaryoblasts, also may be identified by cytochemical stain in transmission electron microscopy. Identical peroxidase activity is localized to the dense tubular system of mature platelets.[8]

Terminal Megakaryocyte Differentiation

Megakaryocyte progenitors leave the proliferative phase and enter terminal differentiation, where they are identified and staged using Wright-stained morphology in bone marrow aspirate films (Fig. 13-3) or hematoxylin and eosin stain in bone marrow biopsy sections (Table 13-1). Past the LD-CFU-Meg,

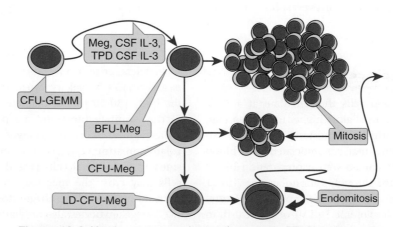

Figure 13-2 Megakaryocyte progenitors at three stages. BFU-Meg clones many daughter cells, CFU-Meg clones a few daughter cells, and LD-CFU-Meg undergoes the first stage of endomitosis.

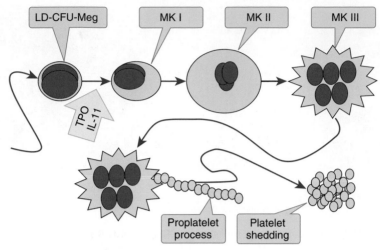

Figure 13-3 Morphologically identifiable megakaryocytes.

TABLE 13-1 Features of Terminal Megakaryocyte Differentiation

	MK I	MK II	MK III
% Precursors	19	25	56
Diameter	14-18 μm	15-40 μm	30-50 μm
Nucleus	Round	Indented	Multilobed
Nucleoli	2-6	Variable	Variable
Chromatin	Homogeneous	Condensed	Deeply condensed
N:C ratio	3:1	1:2	1:4
Mitosis	Present	Absent	Absent
Cytoplasm	Basophilic	Basophilic and granular	Eosinophilic and granular
α-granules	Present	Present	Present
δ-granules	Present	Present	Present
DMS	Present	Present	Present

there is no further mitosis, but three to four morphologically identifiable stages. Most microscopists use the terms *MK I* for megakaryoblast, *MK II* for promegakaryocyte, and *MK III* for megakaryocyte. A few add a postmature *MK IV* stage characterized by a multilobed, highly condensed nucleus.

The MK I cannot be reliably distinguished from the myeloblast or pronormoblast on the basis of Wright-stained morphology of bone marrow aspirates with light microscopy (Fig. 13-4). The morphologist may see plasma membrane blebs, blunt projections that resemble platelets, or nuclear lobulation that reflects polyploidy; megakaryoblasts have a greater diameter than the other two blasts on average. Immunologic probes are often necessary for definitive identification. In addition to progenitor markers listed previously, the MK I may be identified using immunologic probes for the more differentiated membrane structures GP Ib/IX/V (CD42), GP IV (CD36), or mpl, which is the TPO receptor site. Probes also may label cytoplasmic fibrinogen and VWF in α-granules.

Light microscopy aside, the MK I possesses most of the ultrastructure associated with the MK II and III stages and with platelets. The nucleus, although essentially round, reaches its full ploidy at the MK I stage. The cytoplasm possesses α-

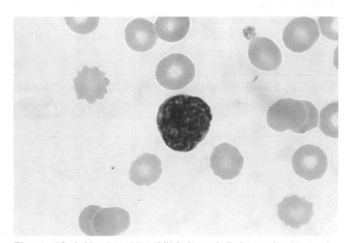

Figure 13-4 Megakaryoblast (MK I). Note similarity to other blast cells, which makes identification by morphology alone inadvisable.

granules and the demarcation system (DMS). The upcoming section on mature platelet ultrastructure discusses α-granules and their contents and membrane systems.

The DMS, a series of membrane-lined channels, invades from the plasma membrane and grows over the course of

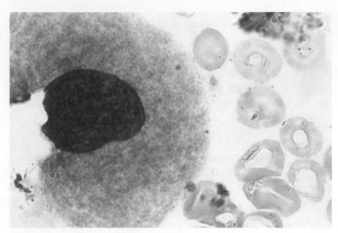

Figure 13-5 Promegakaryocyte (MK II). Large cell with no nuclear lobes.

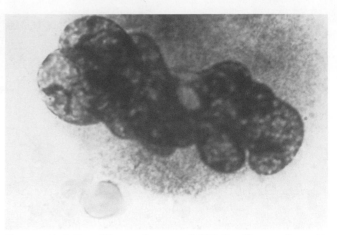

Figure 13-6 Basophilic megakaryocyte (MK III). Very blue cytoplasm with evidence of lines of demarcation.

terminal differentiation to subdivide the entire cytoplasm. The DMS is biologically identical to the plasma membrane and ultimately delineates the individual platelets during thrombopoiesis.

Despite intense cytoplasmic basophilia, the MK II is easily recognized as megakaryocytic on the basis of its 15- to 40-μm diameter (Fig. 13-5). The nucleus is indented or lobulated, although the degree of lobulation is only imprecisely proportional to ploidy.

MK III is the largest cell in the bone marrow, easily detected with the 10× objective (Fig. 13-6). The nucleus is intensely lobulated, and the chromatin is variably condensed. The cytoplasm is eosinophilic, granular, and platelet-like, owing to the thorough spread of the DMS and α-granules. The MK III is the stage from which platelet shedding, or thrombopoiesis, proceeds (Table 13-2).

Endomitosis

Megakaryocyte maturation is marked by a mysterious form of mitosis that lacks telophase and cytokinesis. Called

endoreduplication or *endomitosis,* DNA synthesis proceeds to the production of 8N, 16N, or 32N ploidy with completely duplicated sets of chromosomes but no cell division. Some megakaryocytes reach 128N, although this level of ploidy may signal hematologic disease. It is tempting to contemplate an evolutionary advantage for the production of extremely large cells in this unique fashion. A single megakaryocyte may shed 2000 to 4000 platelets. The search is ongoing for the molecular basis of endomitosis, a cell-cycle adaptation found in no other human cell. Just as mitosis ends at the progenitor stage, endomitosis is complete at MK I. The segmentation of the MK II and MK III nucleus probably reflects endomitosis in general, but the degree of duplication is not proportional to lobularity. Ploidy levels are measured easily using mepacrine, a nucleic acid dye, in megakaryocyte flow cytometry.[9]

Thrombopoiesis

Figure 13-7 appears to show platelet shedding. One cannot find reliable evidence for platelet budding or shedding by examining megakaryocytes in situ, even in well-structured bone

TABLE 13-2 Immunologic Probe or Cytochemical Markers at Each Stage of Megakaryocyte and Platelet Maturation

BFU-Meg	CFU-Meg	LD-CFU-Meg	MK I	MK II	MK III	Platelets
	CD34; stem cell marker					
		HLA-DR				
	Peroxidase by cytochemical stain in transmission electron microscopy (CD41; glycoprotein IIIa; part of fibrinogen receptor, by flow cytometry)					
			VWF by immunostaining CD42; glycoprotein Ib, part of VWF receptor Thrombospondin PF4 Mpl (TPO receptor site)			
					CD36; glycoprotein IV	
						Fibrinogen

BFU-Meg, burst-forming unit-megakaryocyte; CFU-Meg, colony forming unit-megakaryocyte; LD-CFU-Meg, low density colony-forming unit-megakaryocyte; MK I, megakaryoblast; MK II, promegakaryocyte; MK III, megakaryocyte, CD: Cluster of differentiation; HLA-DR, human leukocyte antigen-DR; VWF, von Willebrand factor.

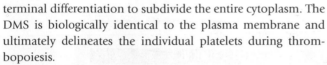

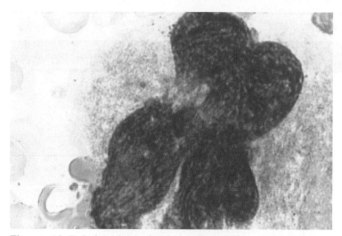

Figure 13-7 Active (platelet-forming) megakaryocyte. Note initial phase of platelet budding.

marrow biopsy preparations. In cultured megakaryocytes examined by transmission electron microscopy, the DMS dilates, longitudinal bundles of tubules form, cytoplasmic extensions called *proplatelet processes* extend, and transverse constrictions appear throughout the processes.[10] The proplatelet processes pierce through or between sinusoid-lining endothelial cells, extend into the venous blood, and release platelets (Fig. 13-8). Sometimes whole megakaryocytes escape the marrow in this fashion to lodge in other organs, such as the lungs. Morphologists presume that thrombopoiesis leaves behind naked megakaryocyte nuclei to be consumed by marrow macrophages, although these are rarely seen in bone marrow aspirate films.

Their absence leads a few morphologists to speculate that the lung is the primary site of thrombopoiesis.[11]

Hormones and Cytokines of Megakaryocytopoiesis

TPO is a 70-kD molecule with 23% homology to erythropoietin.[12] The messenger RNA for TPO has been found in the kidney, liver, and smooth muscle cells. TPO is primarily produced in the liver and is the ligand that binds to a megakaryocyte and platelet membrane receptor protein, mpl, named for v-mpl, a viral oncogene associated with murine myeloproliferative leukemia. TPO is produced remote from its active site and transported by plasma. TPO's concentration is inversely proportional to platelet and megakaryocyte mass, implying that binding and disposal of TPO by platelets is the primary control mechanism.[13] Investigators have used in vitro and in vivo experiments to show that TPO induces stem cells to differentiate into megakaryocyte progenitors in synergy with cytokines, further induces differentiation of megakaryocyte progenitors to megakaryocytes, and induces the proliferation and maturation of megakaryocytes (Table 13-3).[14,15] Recombinant TPO in several forms elevates the platelet counts in healthy donors and in patients treated for a variety of neoplasms, including acute leukemia, and has shown some promise in clinical trials.[16]

Cell-derived stimulators of megakaryocytopoiesis include interleukin (IL)-3, IL-6, and IL-11. IL-3 seems to act in synergy with TPO to induce early differentiation of stem cells, whereas IL-6 and IL-11 act in the presence of TPO to enhance the later phenomena of endomitosis, megakaryocyte maturation, and platelet release. IL-11 has been synthesized and used to

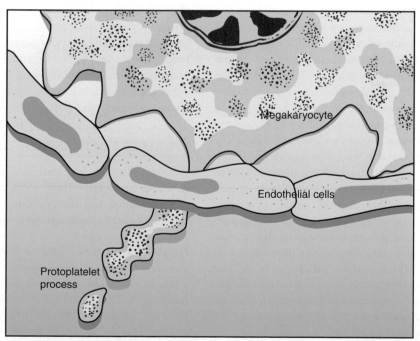

Figure 13-8 Protoplatelet process extends through sinusoidal lining into vascular sinus. (Modified from Powers LW: Diagnostic Hematology, Clinical and Technical Principles. St Louis: Mosby, 1989.)

TABLE 13-3 Hormones and Cytokines That Control Megakaryocytopoiesis

Cytokine/Hormone	Differentiation to Progenitors	Differentiation to Megakaryocytes	Late Maturation	Thrombopoiesis	Clinical Use
TPO	+	+	+	0	Trials
IL-11	0	+	+	+	Trials
IL-3	+	+	0	—	—
IL-6	0	0	+	+	—

Cytokines and hormones shown to interact synergistically with TPO and IL-3, IL-6, and IL-11: stem cell factor, also called *kit ligand* or *mast cell growth factor*, granulocyte-macrophage colony-stimulating factor, granulocyte colony-stimulating factor, and erythropoietin.
Megakaryocyte inhibition: PF4, β-thromboglobulin, neutrophil-activating peptide 2, IL-8.

stimulate platelet production in chemotherapy-induced thrombocytopenia.[17] Other cytokines and hormones that participate synergistically with TPO and the interleukins are stem cell factor, also called *kit ligand* or *mast cell growth factor;* granulocyte macrophage colony-stimulating factor; granulocyte colony-stimulating factor; and erythropoietin. The list continues to grow.

PF-4, β-thromboglobulin, neutrophil-activating peptide 2, IL-8, and other factors inhibit in vitro megakaryocyte growth, which indicates they may have a role in the control of megakaryocytopoiesis in vivo. Internally, reduction in the transcription factors FOG, GATA-1, and NF-E2 diminish megakaryocytopoiesis at the progenitor, endomitosis, and terminal maturation phases.[18]

PLATELETS

The proplatelet process sheds platelets, cells consisting of granular cytoplasm with a membrane but no nuclear material, into the venous sinus. Their diameter in the monolayer of a Wright-stained peripheral blood wedge film averages 2.5 µm. MPV as measured in an isotonic suspension flowing through the detector cell of a clinical profiling instrument ranges from 8 to 10 fL. A frequency distribution of platelet volume is log-normal, however, indicating a subpopulation of large platelets (see Fig. 40-15). *Volume heterogeneity in normal healthy humans reflects variation in platelet release volume and is not a function of platelet age or vitality, as many authors have previously assumed.*[5]

Circulating, resting platelets are biconvex, although collection of blood using the anticoagulant ethylenediamine tetraacetic acid induces them to round up. On a Wright-stained wedge preparation blood film, platelets appear circular to irregular, lavender, and granular, although their diminutiveness makes them hard to scrutinize. In the blood, their surface is even, and they flow smoothly through the blood vessel. In contrast to leukocytes, which tend to roll along the vascular endothelium, platelets cluster with the erythrocytes near the center of the blood vessel. In contrast to erythrocytes, platelets move laterally with the leukocytes into the white pulp of the spleen, where both become sequestered.

The normal peripheral blood platelet count is 150 to 400 × 10^9/L. This count represents only two thirds of available platelets, however, because the spleen sequesters an additional one third. Sequestered platelets are immediately available in times of demand; for example, in acute inflammation or after an injury or major surgery. In hypersplenism or splenomegaly, increased sequestration may cause a relative thrombocytopenia. Under conditions of hemostatic need, platelets answer cellular and humoral stimuli by becoming irregular and sticky, extending pseudopods, and adhering to neighboring structures or aggregating with each other.

Reticulated platelets, sometimes known as *stress platelets,* appear in compensation for thrombocytopenia.[19] Reticulated platelets are markedly larger than ordinary mature circulating platelets, their diameter in blood films exceeding 6 µm and their MPV reaching 12 to 14 fL.[20] Similar to ordinary platelets, they round up in ethylenediamine tetraacetic acid, but in *citrated* whole blood, reticulated platelets are cylindrical and beaded, resembling megakaryocyte proplatelet processes. Reticulated platelets carry free ribosomes and fragments of rough endoplasmic reticulum, analogous to reticulocytes, triggering speculation that they arise from early and rapid proplatelet extension and release. Nucleic acid dyes such as thiazole orange bind RNA of the endoplasmic reticulum, a property exploited by profiling instruments to provide a quantitative evaluation of platelet production under stress, a measurement that may be more useful than the MPV.[21] Regrettably, dense granules falsely increase the reticulated platelet count by taking up nucleic acid dyes.

PLATELET ULTRASTRUCTURE

Platelets, although anucleate, are strikingly complex and are metabolically active. Their ultrastructure has been studied using scanning and transmission electron microscopy, flow cytometry, and molecular sequencing techniques.

Resting Platelet Plasma Membrane

The platelet *plasma membrane* resembles any biologic membrane: a bilayer composed of proteins and lipids, as diagrammed in Figure 13-9. The predominant lipids are phospholipid, which form the basic structure, and cholesterol, which distributes asymmetrically throughout the phospholipids. The phospholipids form a bilayer with their polar heads oriented toward aqueous environments: toward the plasma externally and the cytoplasm internally. Their fatty acid chains, esterified to

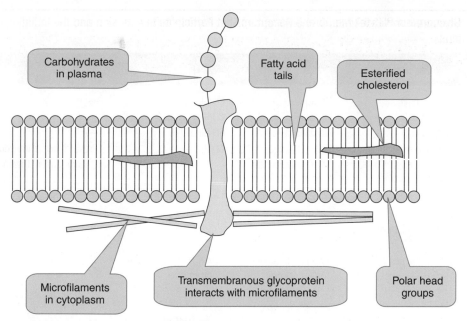

Figure 13-9 Biologic membrane.

carbons 1 and 2 of the phospholipid triglyceride backbone, orient toward each other, perpendicular to the plane of the membrane, to form a hydrophobic barrier sandwiched within the hydrophilic layers.

The neutral phospholipids phosphatidylcholine and sphingomyelin predominate in the plasma layer; the anionic or polar phospholipids phosphatidylinositol, phosphatidylethanolamine, and phosphatidylserine predominate in the inner, cytoplasmic layer. These phospholipids, especially phosphatidylinositol, support platelet activation by supplying arachidonic acid, an unsaturated fatty acid that becomes converted to the eicosanoids prostaglandin and thromboxane during platelet activation. Phosphatidylethanolamine flips to the outer surface on activation and is the phospholipid surface on which coagulation enzymes assemble.[22]

Esterified cholesterol moves freely throughout the hydrophobic layer, exchanging with unesterified plasma cholesterol. Cholesterol stabilizes the membrane, maintains fluidity, and helps control the transmembranous passage of materials.

Anchored within the membrane are glycoproteins and proteoglycans; these support surface glycosaminoglycans, oligosaccharides, and glycolipids. The platelet membrane surface, called the *glycocalyx*, also absorbs albumin, fibrinogen, and other plasma proteins, in many instances transporting them to storage organelles within, a process called *endocytosis*.

At 20 to 30 ηm, the platelet glycocalyx is thicker than the surface layer of leukocytes or erythrocytes. This thick layer is adhesive and responds readily to hemostatic requirements. The platelet literally carries its functional environment with it, meanwhile maintaining a negative surface charge that repels other platelets, other blood cells, and the endothelial cells that line the blood vessels.

The plasma membrane is selectively permeable, and the membrane bilayer provides phospholipids that support platelet activation internally and plasma coagulation exter-

nally. The anchored glycoproteins support essential plasma surface–oriented glycosylated receptors that respond to cellular and humoral stimuli, integrating their stimulus with internal organelles.

Surface-Connected Canalicular System

The plasma membrane invades the platelet interior, producing its unique surface-connected canalicular system (SCCS). The SCCS twists spongelike throughout the platelet, enabling the platelet to store additional quantities of the hemostatic proteins of the glycocalyx, increasing its capacity many-fold. The glycocalyx is less developed in the SCCS and lacks some of the glycoprotein receptors present on the surface. The SCCS is the route for endocytosis and for secretion of granular contents on activation.

Dense Tubular System

Parallel and closely aligned to the SCCS is the dense tubular system (DTS), a condensed remnant of the rough endoplasmic reticulum. Having abandoned its usual protein production function on platelet release, the DTS sequesters Ca^{2+} and bears a series of enzymes that support platelet activation. These enzymes include phospholipase A_2, cyclooxygenase, and thromboxane synthase, which support prostaglandin synthesis, and phospholipase C, which supports production of inositol triphosphate (IP_3) and diacylglycerol (DAG). The DTS is the control center for platelet activation.

Platelet Plasma Membrane Receptors That Provide for Adhesion

The platelet membrane supports more than 50 categories of receptors, including members of the cellular adhesion molecule (CAM) *integrin* family, the CAM *leucine-rich repeat* family, the CAM *immunoglobulin gene* family, the CAM *selectin* family, the *seven-transmembrane receptor* (STR) family, and some

TABLE 13-4 Glycoprotein Platelet Membrane Receptors That Participate in Adhesion and the Initiation of Aggregation by Binding Specific Ligands

Electrophoresis Nomenclature	Nomenclature	Ligand	Cluster Designation	Comment
GP Ia/IIa	Integrin: $\alpha_2\beta_1$	Collagen	CD49b, CD29	—
GP Ic/IIa	Integrin: $\alpha_5\beta_1$	Laminin	CD49e, CD29	—
GP Ic/IIa	Integrin: $\alpha_6\beta_1$	Fibronectin	CD49f, CD29	—
GP IV	Miscellaneous platelet receptor	Collagen II and thrombospondin	CD36	Provides signal transduction to trigger platelet aggregation. Distributed on plasma membrane, SCCS, and α-granule membranes (20%)
GP VI	CAM of the immunoglobulin gene family	Collagen	—	—
GP Ib/IX/V	CAM of the leucine-rich-repeat family	VWF and thrombin bind GP Ib$_\alpha$; thrombin cleaves a site on GP V	CD42b, CD42c, CD42a, CD42d	This CAM is a 2:2:2:1 complex of GP Ib$_\alpha$ and Ib$_\beta$, GP IX, and GP V. There are 25,000 copies on the resting platelet membrane surface, 5-10% on the α-granule membrane, but few on the SCCS membrane. GP Ib$_\alpha$ is the VWF-specific site. 50% of GP Ib is cleared from the membrane on activation. Bernard-Soulier syndrome mutations are identified for all but GP V. Bound to subsurface actin-binding protein
GP IIb/IIIa	Integrin: $\alpha_{IIb}\beta_3$	Fibrinogen, VWF	CD41, CD61	GP IIb and IIIa are distributed on the surface membrane, SCCS, and α-granule membranes (30%). Heterodimer forms on activation

CAM: cellular adhesion molecule.
SCCS: surface connected canalicular system.

miscellaneous receptors.[23] Table 13-4 lists the receptors that support the initial phases of platelet adhesion and aggregation.

Several integrins bind collagen to enable the platelet to adhere to the injured blood vessel lining. Integrins are heterodimeric (composed of two dissimilar proteins) CAMs that integrate their ligands, which they bind on the outside of the cell, with the internal cytoskeleton, triggering activation. GP Ia/IIa, or $\alpha_2\beta_1$, is an integrin that binds subendothelial collagen to promote platelet to vessel wall adhesion in regions of low blood flow. Likewise, $\alpha_5\beta_1$ and $\alpha_6\beta_1$ bind the adhesive proteins laminin and fibronectin, further promoting platelet adhesion. Another collagen-binding receptor is GP VI, a member of the immunoglobulin gene family, so named because members have multiple immunoglobulin-like domains. The unclassified platelet receptor, GP IV, also binds collagen and the adhesive protein thrombospondin.[24]

Perhaps the most important adhesion receptor is GP Ib/IX/V, a *leucine-rich-repeat* family CAM, named for its members' multiple leucine-rich domains. GP Ib/IX/V consists of seven noncovalently bound molecules in ratios of 2:2:2:1. The complex starts with two copies of the GP Ib subunit GP Ibα that account for VWF binding, necessary in regions with blood flow shear rates greater than 1000 s^{-1}, such as in capillaries and arterioles. Additional sites on the GP Ibα molecule bind

thrombin; thrombin digests a site within GP V. Two accompanying GP Ibβ molecules are noncovalently linked to the GP Ibα molecules. GP Ibβ molecules cross the membrane and interact with actin binding protein to provide "outside-in" signaling. Two molecules of GP IX and one of GP V hold the four GP Ib molecules together. Mutations in GP Ibα, GP Ibβ, or GP IX (but not GP V) are associated with a moderate-to-severe mucocutaneous bleeding disorder, Bernard-Soulier syndrome. VWF deficiency is the basis for the most common inherited bleeding disorder, von Willebrand disease. von Willebrand disease is also associated with mucocutaneous bleeding, although it is technically a plasma protein deficiency, not a platelet abnormality.

The two inactive subunits of GP IIb/IIIa, α_{IIb} and β_3, are distributed across the plasma membrane, the SCCS, and the internal layer of α-granule membranes. These form an active heterodimer, $\alpha_{IIb}\beta_3$, only when they encounter an "inside-out" signaling mechanism triggered by collagen binding GP VI or VWF binding GP Ib/IX/V. Although various agonists may activate the platelet, $\alpha_{IIb}\beta_3$ is a physiologic requisite because it binds fibrinogen, generating interplatelet aggregation. Mutations in α_{IIb} or β_3 cause a severe inherited mucocutaneous bleeding disorder, Glanzmann thrombasthenia. The $\alpha_{IIb}\beta_3$ integrin also binds VWF, vitronectin, and fibronectin, all adhesive proteins that share the target *arginine-glycine-aspartate* (RGD) amino acid sequence with fibrinogen.[25]

Platelet Plasma Membrane Receptors That Provide for Activation: the Seven-Transmembrane Receptors

Thrombin, adenosine diphosphate (ADP), epinephrine, and the prostaglandin (eicosanoid) pathway product thromboxane A_2 (TXA_2) all activate platelets. These platelet "agonists" are ligands for seven transmembrane repeat receptors (STRs), so named for their unique membrane-anchoring structure. The STRs have seven hydrophobic anchoring domains supporting an external binding site and an internal terminus that interacts with G proteins for outside-in signaling. The STRs are listed in Table 13-5.[26]

Thrombin cleaves two STRs, PAR1 and PAR4, that together total 1800 membrane copies. Thrombin cleavage activates the platelet through at least two internal physiologic pathways. Thrombin also interacts with platelets by binding or digesting two CAMs in the leucine-rich-repeat family, GP Ibα and GP V.

There are about 600 copies of the ADP receptors, $P2Y_1$ and $P2Y_{12}$. These STRs activate the platelet through the G protein signaling pathways. Platelets are partially inactivated by clopidogrel and ticlopidine, drugs that occupy $P2Y_{12}$. These drugs are standard antithrombotic treatments prescribed after acute myocardial infarctions, ischemic cerebrovascular accidents, and venous thromboembolic events.

TPα and TPβ bind TXA_2. This interaction produces more TXA_2 from the platelet, an autocrine (self-perpetuating) system that activates neighboring platelets. Epinephrine binds α2-adrenergic sites that couple G proteins and open membrane calcium channels. The α2-adrenergic sites function similar to those on heart tissue. Finally, the receptor site IP binds prostacyclin, a prostaglandin produced from endothelial cells. This interaction increases the internal cyclic adenosine monophosphate (cAMP) concentration and blocks activation. The platelet membrane also presents STRs for serotonin, platelet-activating factor, prostaglandin E_2, PF4 and β-thromboglobulin.

Additional Platelet Membrane Receptors

About 15 receptors were discussed in the preceding paragraphs. The platelet supports many additional receptors. The CAM immunoglobulin family includes the ICAMs (CD50, CD54, CD102), which play a role in inflammation and the immune reaction; PECAM (CD31), which mediates platelet to WBC and platelet to endothelial cell adhesion; and FcγRIIA (CD32), a low-affinity receptor for the immunoglobulin Fc portion that plays a role in heparin-induced thrombocytopenia.[27] P-selectin (CD62) is an integrin that encourages platelets to bind endothelial cells, leukocytes, and each other.[28] P-selectin is found on the α-granule membranes of the resting platelet but migrates via the SCCS to the surface of activated platelets. P-selectin or CD62 identification by flow cytometry is a successful clinical means for measuring in vivo platelet activation.

Platelet Cytoskeleton: Microfilaments and Microtubules

A thick circumferential bundle of microtubules maintains the platelet's shape. The *circumferential microtubules* parallel the plane of the disc and reside just within, although not touching, the plasma membrane. There are 8 to 20 tubules composed of multiple subunits of tubulin that disassemble at refrigerator temperature or when treated with colchicine. When microtubules disassemble, platelets become round, but on warming, they recover their original disc shape. On cross section, microtubules are cylindrical, with a diameter of 25 ηm, and hollow. The circumferential microtubules could be a single spiral tubule.[29] Besides maintaining platelet shape, microtubules contract on activation to encourage expression of α-granule contents. They also reassemble longitudinally to provide rigidity to pseudopods.

In the narrow area between the microtubules and membrane lies a thick meshwork of microfilaments composed of actin. Actin is contractile in platelets (as in muscle) and anchors the plasma membrane glycoproteins and proteoglycans. Actin also is present throughout the platelet cytoplasm,

---

TABLE 13-5 STRs for Thrombin, Adenosine Diphosphate, Epinephrine, and the Prostaglandins*

Receptor	Ligand	STR Receptor-Ligand Interaction Coupled to Signaling G-Proteins
PAR1	Thrombin	Coupled to G_1 protein that reduces cAMP; coupled to G_q and G_{12} proteins that increase IP_3 and DAG
PAR4	Thrombin	Coupled to G_q and G_{12} proteins that increase IP_3 and DAG
$P2Y_1$	ADP	Coupled to G_q protein that increases IP_3 and DAG
$P2Y_{12}$	ADP	Coupled to G_1 protein that reduces cAMP
TPα and TPβ	TXA_2	Coupled to G_q protein that increases IP_3 and DAG
α2-adrenergic	Epinephrine	Coupled to G_1 protein that reduces cAMP; potentiates effects of ADP, thrombin, and TXA_2
IP	PGI_2	Coupled to G_s protein that increases cAMP to inhibit activation

*Named for their peculiar membrane anchorage, these receptors mediate "outside-in" platelet activation through signaling G proteins.
PAR, protease activation receptor; PGI_2, prostaglandin I_2 (prostacyclin); prostacyclin receptor.

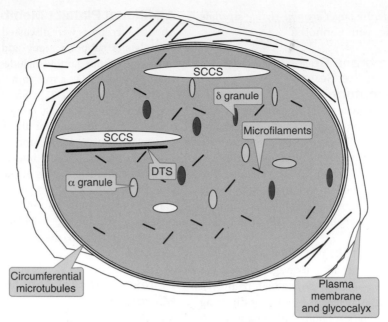

Figure 13-10 Platelet ultrastructure.

constituting 20% to 30% of platelet protein. In the resting platelet, actin is globular and amorphous; as the cytoplasmic calcium concentration increases, actin becomes filamentous and contractile.

The cytoplasm also contains intermediate filaments, ropelike polymers 8 to 12 ηm in diameter, of *desmin* and *vimentin*. The intermediate filaments connect with actin and the tubules, maintaining platelet shape. Microtubules, actin microfilaments, and intermediate microfilaments control platelet shape change, extension of pseudopods, and secretion of granule contents.

Platelet Granules: α-Granules, δ-Granules (Dense Bodies), and Lysosomes

There are 50 to 80 α-granules in each platelet. In contrast to the darker δ-granules, α-granules stain gray in osmium-dye transmission electron microscopy preparations (Fig. 13-10). The α-granules are filled with proteins, some endocytosed, some synthesized within the megakaryocyte and stored in released platelets (Table 13-6). Several α-granule proteins are membrane-bound. As the platelet becomes activated, α-granule membranes fuse with the SCCS. Their contents flow to the nearby microenvironment where they participate in adhesion and aggregation and support plasma coagulation.

Gray platelet syndrome is an inherited absence of α-granule contents. The granule membranes are present with their membrane-bound proteins, but the anticipated soluble proteins are missing. Platelets appear light gray in Wright-stained blood films. Platelet aggregation in response to ADP, collagen, epinephrine, and thrombin is diminished.

There are two to seven δ-granules per platelet. Also called *dense bodies*, these granules stain black when treated with osmium in transmission electron microscopy. Small molecules are probably endocytosed and are stored in the δ-granules;

these are listed in Table 13-7. In contrast to the α-granules, which employ the SCCS, δ-granules migrate to the plasma membrane and release their contents directly into the plasma on activation. Membranes of δ-granules support the same integral proteins as the α-granules—P-selectin, GP IIb/IIIa, and GP Ib/IX/V—implying a common source for the membranes. *Storage pool disorder* is the name given to diminished δ-granule contents. Most storage pool disorders occur in inherited diseases characterized by albinism, such as Hermansky-Pudlak syndrome, although some are not related to albinism and some are acquired, as in myelodysplastic syndromes. Storage pool disorder does not affect morphology, but platelets fail to secrete when treated with thrombin in aggregometry. Mepacrine, a quinidine-derived fluorescent dye, stains δ-granule phosphates, allowing for quantitation in flow cytometry.

Platelets also have a few lysosomes, 300-ηm diameter granules that stain positive for arylsulfatase, β-glucuronidase, acid phosphatase, and catalase. The lysosomes probably digest vessel wall matrix components during in vivo aggregation and digest autophagic debris.

PLATELET ACTIVATION

Although the following discussion implies a linear process, adhesion, aggregation, and secretion are often simultaneous.[30,31]

Adhesion: Platelets Reversibly Bind Elements of the Vascular Matrix

Platelets repair minor injuries to blood vessel linings, such as regular sloughing of senescent endothelial cells, through adhesion (Figs. 13-11 and 13-12).[32] Platelets may adhere directly to collagen of the vascular matrix in veins or venules through CAMs GP Ia/IIa, GP IV, and GP VI.

TABLE 13-6 Representative α-Granule Proteins

	Coagulation Proteins	Noncoagulation Proteins
Proteins Present in Plasma and α-Granules		
Endocytosed	Fibronectin	Albumin
	Fibrinogen	Immunoglobulins
Megakaryocyte-synthesized	Factor V	—
	Thrombospondin	—
	VWF	—
Present in α-Granules, but not Plasma (Megakaryocyte-Synthesized)		
	β-thromboglobulin	EGF
	HMWK	Multimerin
	PAI-1	PDC1
	Plasminogen	PDGF
	PF4	TGF-β
	Protein C inhibitor	VEGF/VPF
Membrane-Bound Proteins		
Restricted to α-granule membrane	P-selectin	GMP33
	—	Osteonectin
α-granule and plasma membrane	GP IIb/IIIa	cap1
	GP IV	CD9
	GP Ib/IX/V	PECAM-1

EGF, endothelial growth factor; GMP, guanidine monophosphate; HMWK, high-molecular-weight kininogen; PAI-1, plasminogen activator inhibitor-1; PECAM-1, platelet-endothelial cell adhesion molecule-1; PDCI, platelet-derived collagenase inhibitor; PDGF, platelet-derived growth factor; TGF-β, transforming growth factor-β; VEGF/VPF, vascular endothelial growth factor/vascular permeability factor.

TABLE 13-7 δ-Granule (Dense Body) Contents

Small Molecule	Comment
ADP	Nonmetabolic, supports neighboring platelet aggregation by binding to ADP receptors $P2Y_1$, $P2Y_{12}$
ATP	Function unknown, but ATP release is detected using firefly luciferase luminescence as an in vitro measure of platelet activation—a method called *lumiaggregometry*
Serotonin	Vasoconstrictor that binds endothelial cells and platelet membranes
Ca^{2+} and Mg^{2+}	Divalent cations support platelet activation and coagulation

In capillaries and arterioles, where the shear rate of blood exceeds 1000 s^{-1}, the site of injury is first "carpeted" by VWF. VWF circulates as a multimeric globulin with molecular weights between 800,000 D and 20 million D, one of the largest proteins in the plasma. The combination of injury and shear stress "unrolls" the globular molecule to form strands that coat injury sites and bind subendothelial collagen. A liver-secreted enzyme, VWF-cleaving protease, soon digests fibrillar VWF to inactive fragments.[33] Platelets adhere to fibrillar VWF through their GP Ib/IX/V receptor, and the VWF-platelet layer fills in the injury to await replacement by normal vascular cells (Fig. 13-13). Although seldom an isolated process, adhesion alone does not include the secretion of granule contents or the redistribution of CAMs such as GP IIb/IIIa or P-selectin. Adhesion does require actin contraction, however, and the formation of pseudopods.

Although history records several attempts, no one has devised a clinical laboratory method that isolates and measures platelet adhesion without simultaneously involving aggregation and secretion. Clinicians routinely employ laboratory instrumentation to measure VWF activity and concentration, however, and clinicians may quantitate several CAMs through flow cytometry in specialized laboratories.

Aggregation: Platelets Irreversibly Bind Each Other

When vessel damage is extensive, platelets adhere and aggregate (Figs. 13-14 and 13-15). Aggregation requires the active conformation of the GP IIb/IIIa integrin and includes

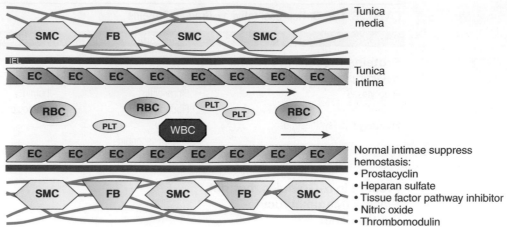

Figure 13-11 Normal blood flow in intact vessels. EC, endothelial cell; FB, fibroblast; IEL, internal elastic lamina; SMC, smooth muscle cell. *Lines* represent collagen.

Normal intimae suppress hemostasis:
• Prostacyclin
• Heparan sulfate
• Tissue factor pathway inhibitor
• Nitric oxide
• Thrombomodulin

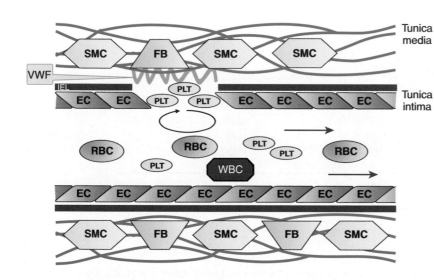

Figure 13-12 Platelet adhesion to collagen. VWF required in capillaries and arterioles. Vascular maintenance: platelets bind collagen; VWF required in arterioles and capillaries. EC, endothelial cell; FB, fibroblast; IEL, internal elastic lamina; SMC, smooth muscle cell. *Lines* represent collagen.

Figure 13-13 VIII/VWF interaction with platelets. EC, endothelial cell; FB, fibroblast; SMC, smooth muscle cell. *Lines* represent collagen.

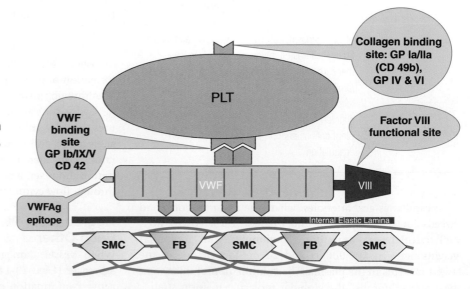

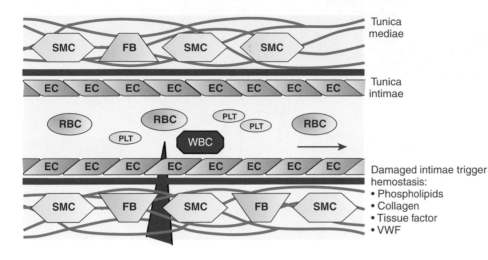

Figure 13-14 Trauma to vessel exposes collagen and tissue factor. EC, endothelial cell; FB, fibroblast; IEL, internal elastic lamina; SMC, smooth muscle cell. *Lines* represent collagen.

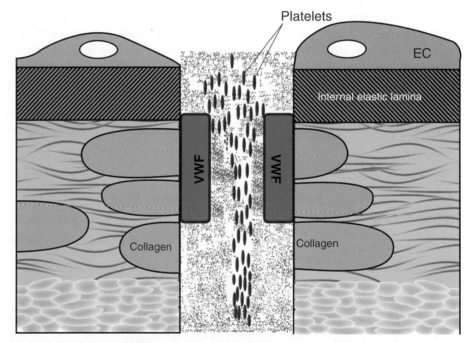

Figure 13-15 Blood enters wound, and platelets adhere directly to collagen or via VWF. *EC*, endothelial cell. (Courtesy of Kathy Jacobs, Chronolog, Inc., Havertown, PA.)

pseudopod formation and redistribution of P-selectin to the surface membrane (Fig. 13-16). Membrane phospholipids also redeploy, with the more polar molecules, such as phosphatidylserine, flipping to the outer layer. GP IIb/IIIa binds the RGD sequence of any plasma protein; the protein most readily available is fibrinogen, which is the major player. Membrane integrity is lost, and a syncytium of platelet cytoplasm forms as the platelet exhausts internal energy sources. Aggregation is part of primary hemostasis, and its irreversible end point is the "white clot" or platelet-VWF plug. Although a normal part of vessel repair, white clots imply inappropriate platelet activation in arterioles and arteries and are the pathologic basis for arterial thrombosis events, such as acute myocardial infarction,

peripheral vascular disease, and strokes. Except for VWF, coagulation proteins are excluded from white clots.

The combination of polar phospholipid exposure, platelet microparticle dispersion, and secretion of granule contents triggers secondary hemostasis, called *coagulation* (Chapter 40). Its product, fibrin, and red blood cells deposit around and within the platelet syncytium, forming a bulky "red clot." The red clot is essential to wound repair but is characteristic of inappropriate coagulation in venules and veins, resulting in deep vein thrombosis and pulmonary emboli.

Specialty coagulation laboratories provide in vitro whole blood or plasma platelet aggregometry and lumiaggregometry as a means for detecting and identifying aggregation abnormalities.

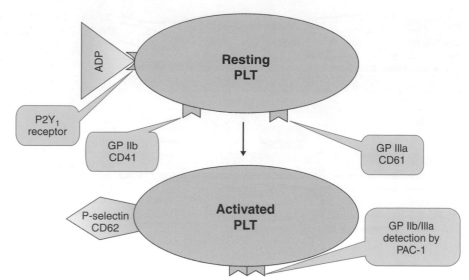

Figure 13-16 Inside-out activation. Formation of GP IIb/IIIa receptors and transfer of P-selectin to the surface.

The bleeding time test, although still used, has limited predictive value. Several physician office or near patient laboratory systems, such as the Dade-Behring PFA-100 and the Chronolog WBA, also are available to test for platelet function.

Secretion: Activated Platelets Release Granular Contents

"Outside-in" platelet activation through ligand binding to integrins and STRs triggers actin microfilament contraction.

Intermediate filaments and microtubules contract, compressing granules. Contents of α-granules and lysosomes flow through the SCCS; meanwhile, δ-granule contents are secreted through the plasma membrane (Fig. 13-17). The δ-granule contents are vasoconstrictors and platelet agonists that amplify primary hemostasis; several of the α-granule contents are coagulation proteins (Table 13-8).

By presenting polar phospholipids on their membrane surface, platelets provide a localized cellular milieu for coagu-

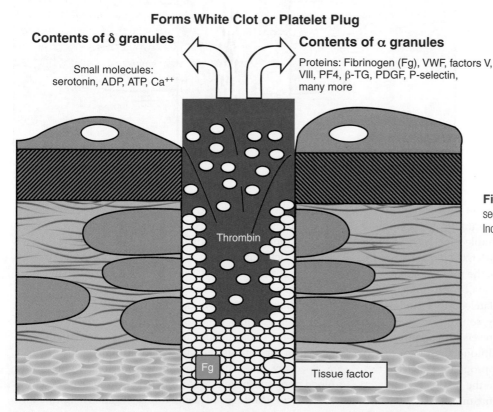

Figure 13-17 Platelet aggregation and secretion. (Courtesy of Kathy Jacobs, Chronolog, Inc., Havertown, PA.)

TABLE 13-8 Selected α-Granule Proteins and Their Properties

Platelet-derived growth factor	Supports mitosis of vascular fibroblasts and smooth muscle cells
Endothelial growth factor	Supports mitosis of vascular fibroblasts and smooth muscle cells
Transforming growth factor-β	Supports mitosis of vascular fibroblasts and smooth muscle cells
Fibronectin	Adhesion molecule
Thrombospondin	Adhesion molecule
PF4 ⎫ β-thromboglobulin ⎭	⎰ Heparin, heparin neutralization ⎱ Found nowhere but platelet α-granules
Plasminogen	Fibrinolysis promotion and control
Plasminogen activation inhibitor-1	Fibrinolysis promotion and control
α₂-antiplasmin	Fibrinolysis promotion and control
Protein C inhibitor	Coagulation control

lation. Phosphatidylserine is the phospholipid on which two coagulation pathway complexes, factor IX/VIII (tenase) and factor X/V (prothrombinase), form, supported by ionic calcium secreted by the δ-granules. α-granule fibrinogen, factors V and VIII, and VWF (which binds and carries factor VIII) are secreted and increase the localized concentrations of these essential coagulation proteins, further supporting the action of tenase and prothrombinase. Platelet secretions serve cell-based, controlled, localized coagulation. Table 13-8 lists some additional α-granule secretions that, although not proteins of the coagulation pathway, support hemostasis. Some proteins listed in Table 13-8 do not appear in Table 13-5. Neither list is exhaustive, as more α-granule contents are being identified.

There are several clinical laboratory assays of platelet secretion. The most successful is lumiaggregometry, which employs firefly luciferase to identify adenosine triphosphate (ATP) secreted from δ-granules. Assays of PF4 or β-thromboglobulin are confined to reference laboratories because uncontrolled ex vivo platelet activation factitiously elevates their levels in specimens that are collected and managed using routine processes.

PLATELET ACTIVATION PATHWAYS

G Proteins

G proteins control cellular activation for all cells (not just platelets) at the membrane (Fig. 13-18). G proteins are αβγ heterotrimers that bind guanosine diphosphate (GDP) when inactive. Membrane receptor-ligand binding promotes GDP release and its replacement with guanosine triphosphate (GTP). The Gα monomer briefly disassociates, exerts GTPase activity, and hydrolyzes the bound GTP to GDP, and the G protein resumes the resting state. The hydrolysis step provides the necessary phosphorylation trigger for zymogen activation such as in the eicosanoid synthesis or the IP₃-DAG pathway (Table 13-9).

Eicosanoid Synthesis

The eicosanoid synthesis pathway, alternatively named the *prostaglandin, cyclooxygenase,* or *thromboxane pathway,* is one of two essential platelet activation pathways triggered by G protein (Fig. 13-19). The membrane inner leaflet is rich in phosphatidylinositol, a phospholipid whose number 2 carbon binds numerous unsaturated fatty acids, including 5,8,11, 14-eicosatetraenoic acid, commonly named *arachidonic acid.* Membrane receptor-ligand binding through G protein activation triggers phospholipase A₂, a membrane enzyme that cleaves the ester bond connecting carbon 2 of the triglyceride backbone with arachidonic acid. Cleavage releases arachidonic acid to the cytoplasm, where it becomes the substrate for

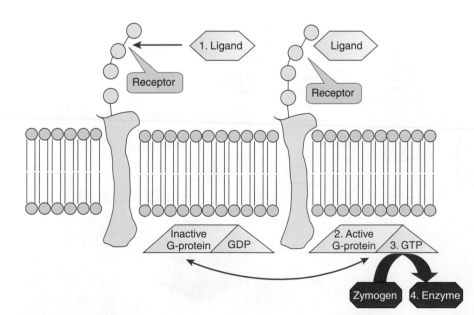

Figure 13-18 G protein function. (1) A ligand binds its receptor; (2) G-protein adds GTP (3) and becomes active; (4) the G-protein-GTP complex donates a phosphate and activates an internal enzyme. The G-protein returns to the resting state with GDP in place.

TABLE 13-9 G Proteins in Platelets and Their Functions

G Protein	Coupled to Receptor	Agonist (Ligand)	Action	Outcome
G_1	PAR1	Thrombin	Decelerate adenylate cyclase	Reduce cAMP concentration
	P2Y$_{12}$	ADP		
	α_2-adrenergic	Epinephrine		
G_q	PAR1	Thrombin	Activate phospholipase C	Increase IP$_3$/DAG
	PAR4	Thrombin		
	P2Y$_1$	ADP		
	TPα and TPβ	TXA$_2$		
G_{12}	PAR1	Thrombin	Activate protein kinase C	Activate pleckstrin, actin microfilaments
	PAR4	Thrombin		
	P2Y$_1$	ADP		
	Tpα and TPβ	TXA$_2$		
G_s	IP	Prostacyclin	Accelerate adenylate cyclase	Increase cAMP concentration

cyclooxygenase, anchored in the DTS. Cyclooxygenase converts arachidonic acid to prostaglandin G_2 and prostaglandin H_2, then thromboxane synthase acts on prostaglandin H_2 to produce TXA$_2$. TXA$_2$ binds membrane receptors TPα or TPβ, decelerating adenylate cyclase activity and reducing cAMP concentrations, which mobilizes ionic calcium from the DTS (Fig. 13-20). Increasing cytoplasmic calcium causes contraction of actin microfilaments and platelet activation.

The cyclooxygenase pathway in endothelial cells incorporates the enzyme prostacyclin synthase in place of the thromboxane synthase in platelets. The eicosanoid pathway end point for the endothelial cell is prostaglandin I_2, or prostacyclin, which binds the platelet IP receptor site. Prostacyclin binding accelerates adenylate cyclase, increasing cAMP, and moves ionic calcium to DTS sequestration. The endothelial cell pathway controls platelet activation in the intact blood vessel through this mechanism.

Deficiencies in calcium mobilization, cyclooxygenase, and thromboxane synthase activity reduce TXA$_2$ production and platelet activation, an inherited set of conditions identified collectively as *platelet release disorder* or *aspirin-like disorder*, associated with mucocutaneous bleeding and intracranial hemorrhages. Aggregometry patterns in these disorders mimic the effect of aspirin, which causes a reduced response to ADP, arachidonic acid, and epinephrine. Aspirin also reduces the response to low concentration (1 mg/mL) collagen, whereas aspirin-like disorders reduce aggregation response to low and high (5 mg/mL) collagen concentration.

TXA$_2$ has a half-life of 30 seconds, diffuses from the platelet, and spontaneously reduces to thromboxane B_2, a stable, measurable plasma metabolite. Efforts to produce a clinical plasma assay for thromboxane B_2 have been unsuccessful because special specimen management is required to prevent ex vivo platelet activation with factitious unregulated release of

Figure 13-19 Eicosanoid synthesis. ADP, thrombin, collagen, and epinephrine bind their respective receptors, activating phospholipase A$_2$ through the G-protein mechanism. Phospholipase A$_2$ releases arachidonic acid from membrane phosphatidyl inositol to activate the eicosanoid synthesis pathway. Reagent arachidonic acid bypasses the membrane and directly enters the eicosanoid synthesis pathway. Enzymes of the pathway are located in the dense tubular system and mediate thromboxane A$_2$ production, activating the platelet.

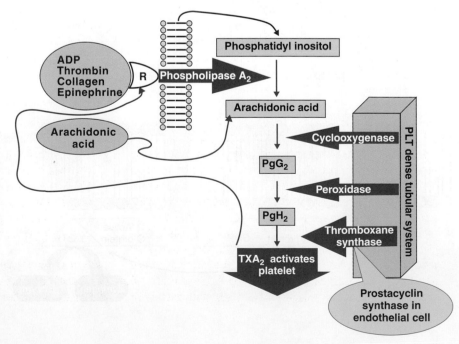

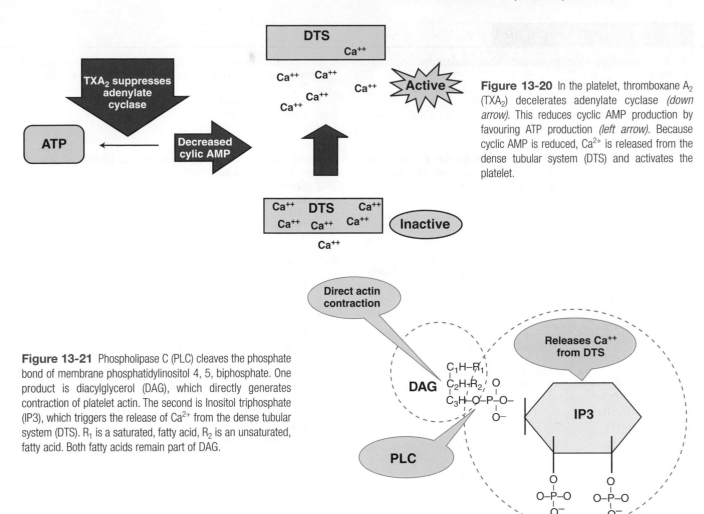

Figure 13-20 In the platelet, thromboxane A_2 (TXA$_2$) decelerates adenylate cyclase *(down arrow)*. This reduces cyclic AMP production by favouring ATP production *(left arrow)*. Because cyclic AMP is reduced, Ca^{2+} is released from the dense tubular system (DTS) and activates the platelet.

Figure 13-21 Phospholipase C (PLC) cleaves the phosphate bond of membrane phosphatidylinositol 4, 5, biphosphate. One product is diacylglycerol (DAG), which directly generates contraction of platelet actin. The second is Inositol triphosphate (IP3), which triggers the release of Ca^{2+} from the dense tubular system (DTS). R_1 is a saturated, fatty acid, R_2 is an unsaturated, fatty acid. Both fatty acids remain part of DAG.

thromboxane B_2. Thromboxane B_2 is acted on by a variety of liver enzymes to produce an array of soluble urine metabolites, including 11-dehydrothromboxane B_2, which is stable and measurable.[34] Immunoassays of urine 11-dehydrothromboxane B_2 are used to characterize in vivo platelet activation.[35]

Inositol Triphosphate and Diacylglycerol

The IP$_3$ and DAG pathway is the second G protein–dependent platelet activation pathway (Fig. 13-21). G protein activation triggers the enzyme phospholipase C. Phospholipase C cleaves membrane phosphatidylinositol 4,5-bisphosphate to form IP$_3$ and DAG, both second messengers for intracellular activation. IP$_3$ promotes release of ionic calcium from the DTS, triggering actin microfilament contraction. IP$_3$ also may activate phospholipase A_2. DAG triggers a multistep process: activation of phosphokinase C, which triggers phosphorylation of the protein pleckstrin, which regulates actin microfilament contraction.

CHAPTER at a GLANCE

- Platelets arise from bone marrow megakaryocytes, which reside near the venous sinusoid. Megakaryocyte progenitors are recruited by IL-3, IL-6, IL-11, and thrombopoietin and mature via endomitosis. Platelets are released from the bone marrow via shedding from proplatelet processes, a process called *thrombopoiesis*.
- Circulating platelets are complex anucleate cells with a thick glycocalyx bearing a potpourri of coagulation factors, extended by the SCCS. Inside is a system of microfibrils and microtubules that accomplish platelet contraction and pseudopod extension and the granules that provide coagulation factors and vasoactive chemicals.

- The platelet membrane supports many receptor sites that control platelet activation upon binding their respective ligands.
- Platelets adhere to foreign surfaces, aggregate with each other, and secrete the substances stored within their granules.
- Platelet activation is internally managed through G proteins, the eicosanoid synthesis pathway, and the DAG-IP$_3$ pathway.

Now that you have completed this chapter, go back and read again the case study at the beginning and respond to the questions presented.

REVIEW QUESTIONS

1. The megakaryocyte progenitor that undergoes endomitosis is:
   a. MK I
   b. BFU-Megakaryocyte
   c. CFU-Megakaryocyte
   d. LD-CFU-Megakaryocyte

2. The growth factor that is produced in the kidney and induces growth and differentiation of committed megakaryocyte progenitors is:
   a. IL-3
   b. IL-6
   c. IL-11
   d. Thrombopoietin

3. What platelet organelle sequesters ionic calcium and binds a series of enzymes of the eicosanoid pathway?
   a. G protein
   b. Dense granules
   c. Dense tubular system
   d. SCCS

4. What platelet membrane receptor binds fibrinogen and supports platelet aggregation?
   a. GP Ib/IX/V
   b. GP IIb/IIIa
   c. GP Ia/IIa
   d. $P2Y_1$

5. What platelet membrane phospholipid flips from the inner surface to the plasma surface on activation and serves as the assembly point for coagulation factors?
   a. Phosphatidyl ethanolamine
   b. Phosphatidyl inositol
   c. Phosphatidyl choline
   d. Phosphatidyl serine

6. What is the name of the eicosanoid metabolite produced from endothelial cells that suppresses platelet activity?
   a. TXA_2
   b. Arachidonic acid
   c. Cyclooxygenase
   d. Prostacyclin

7. Which of the following molecules is stored in platelet δ-granules (dense bodies)?
   a. Serotonin
   b. Fibrinogen
   c. PF4
   d. Platelet-derived growth factor

8. What plasma protein is essential to platelet adhesion?
   a. VWF
   b. Factor VIII
   c. Fibrinogen
   d. P-selectin

9. Reticulated platelets can be enumerated in peripheral blood to detect:
   a. Impaired production during disease states
   b. Abnormal organelles associated with diseases such as leukemia
   c. Increased platelet production in response to need
   d. Inadequate rates of membrane cholesterol exchange with the plasma

10. *Platelet adhesion* refers to platelets:
    a. Sticking to other platelets
    b. Releasing platelet granule constituents
    c. Providing the surface for assembly of coagulation factors
    d. Sticking to surfaces such as subendothelial collagen

REFERENCES

1. Butkiewicz AM, Kemona H, Dymicka-Piekarska V, et al: Platelet count, mean platelet volume and thrombocytopoietic indices in healthy women and men. Thromb Res 2005,118:199-204.
2. Tsiara S, Elisaf M, Jagroop IA, et al: Platelets as predictors of vascular risk: is there a practical index of platelet activity? Clin Appl Thromb Hemost 2003;9:177-190.
3. Lichtman MA, Chamberlain JK, Simon W, et al: Parasinusoid allocation of megakaryocytes in marrow. Am J Hematol 1978;4:303.
4. Breton-Gorius J: On the alleged phagocytosis by megakaryocytes. Br J Haematol 1981;47:635-636.
5. Pedersen NT: The pulmonary vessels as a filter for circulating megakaryocytes. Scand J Haematol 1974;13:225.
6. Cramer EM, Vainchenker W: Platelet production: cellular and molecular regulation. In Colman RW, Marder VJ, Clowes AM, et al (eds): Hemostasis and Thrombosis, 5th ed. Philadelphia: Lippincott, Williams & Wilkins, 2006:443-462.
7. Cramer EM, Fontenay M: Platelets: structure related to function. In Colman RW, Marder VJ, Clowes AM, et al (eds): Hemostasis and Thrombosis, 5th ed. Philadelphia: Lippincott, Williams & Wilkins, 2006:463-482.
8. George JN, Colman RW: Overview of platelet structure and function. In Colman RW, Marder VJ, Clowes AM, et al (eds): Hemostasis and Thrombosis, 5th ed. Philadelphia: Lippincott, Williams & Wilkins, 2006:437-442.
9. Choi ES, Hokom M, Bartley T, et al: Recombinant human megakaryocyte growth and development factor (rHuMGDF), a ligand for c-Mpl, produces functional human platelets in vitro. Stem Cells 1995;13:317-322.
10. Patel SR, Richardson JL, Schulze H, et al: Differential roles of microtubule assembly and sliding in proplatelet formation by megakaryocytes. Blood 2005;106:4076-4085.
11. Levine RF, Eldor A, Shoff PK, et al: Circulating megakaryocytes: delivery of large numbers of intact, mature megakaryocytes to the lung. Eur J Haematol 1993;51:233-246.
12. Kunicki TJ: Platelet glycoprotein polymorphisms and relationship to function, immunogenecity, and disease. In Colman RW, Marder VJ, Clowes AM, et al (eds): Hemostasis and Thrombosis, 5th ed. Philadelphia: Lippincott, Williams & Wilkins, 2006:493-506.
13. Emmons RVB, Reid DM, Cohen R, et al: Human thrombopoietin levels are high when thrombocytopenia is due to megakaryocyte deficiency and low when due to platelet destruction. Blood 1996;87:4068-4071.
14. McDonald TP: Thrombopoietin: its biology, clinical aspects, and possibilities. Am J Pediatr Hematol Oncol 1992;14:8-21.

15. Kaushansky K: Thrombopoietin: a tool for understanding thrombopoiesis. J Thromb Haemost 2003;1:1587-1592.
16. Kuter DJ, Begley CG: Recombinant human thrombopoietin: basic biology and evaluation of clinical studies. Blood 2002;100:3457-3469.
17. Demetri GD: Targeted approaches for the treatment of thrombocytopenia. Oncologist 2001; 6 (suppl) 5:15-23.
18. Chang M, Nakagawa PA, Williams SA, et al: Immune thrombocytopenic purpura (ITP) plasma and purified ITP monoclonal autoantibodies inhibit megakaryocytopoiesis in vitro. Blood 2003;102:887-895.
19. Ault KA: Flow cytometric measurement of platelet function and reticulated platelets. Ann NY Acad Sci 1993;677:293-308.
20. Abe Y, Wada H, Sakakura M, et al: Usefulness of fully automated measurement of reticulated platelets using whole blood. Clin Appl Thromb Hemost 2005;11:263-270.
21. Briggs C, Kunka S, Hart D, et al: Assessment of an immature platelet fraction (IPF) in peripheral thrombocytopenia. Br J Haematol 2004;126:93-99.
22. Zieseniss S, Zahler S, Muller I, et al: Modified phosphatidylethanolamine as the active component of oxidized low density lipoprotein promoting platelet prothrombinase activity. J Biol Chem 2001;276:19828-19835.
23. Kunapuli SP: Platelet adenosine 5'-diphosphate receptors. In Colman RW, Marder VJ, Clowes AM, et al (eds): Hemostasis and Thrombosis, 5th ed. Philadelphia: Lippincott, Williams & Wilkins, 2006:547-554.
24. Tandon NN, Kraslisz U, Jamieson GA: Identification of glycoprotein IV (CD36) as a primary receptor for platelet-collagen adhesion. J Biol Chem 1989;264:7576-7583.
25. Rao AK: Disorders of platelet function. In Kitchens CS, Alving BM, Kessler CM (eds): Consultative Hemostasis and Thrombosis. Philadelphia: Saunders, 2002:133-148.
26. Jackson SP, Nesbitt WS, Kulkarni S: Signaling events underlying thrombus formation. J Thromb Haemost 2003;1:1602-1612.
27. Walenga JM, Jeske WP, Prechel MM, et al: Newer insights on the mechanism of heparin-induced thrombocytopenia. Semin Thromb Hemost 2004;30(Suppl 1):57-67.
28. Keating FK, Dauerman HL, Whitaker DA, et al: Increased expression of platelet P-selectin and formation of platelet-leukocyte aggregates in blood from patients treated with unfractionated heparin plus eptifibatide compared with bivalirudin. Thromb Res 2005. Aug 31; [Epub ahead of print]
29. White JG, Rao GH: Microtubule coils versus the surface membrane cytoskeleton in maintenance and restoration of platelet discoid shape. Am J Pathol 1998;152:597-609.
30. Abrams CS, Brass LF: Platelet signal transduction. In Colman RW, Marder VJ, Clowes AM, et al (eds): Hemostasis and Thrombosis, 5th ed. Philadelphia: Lippincott, Williams & Wilkins, 2006:617-631.
31. Abrams CS: Intracellular signaling in platelets. Curr Opin Hematol 2005;12:401-405.
32. Tailor A, Cooper D, Granger DN: Platelet-vessel wall interactions in the microcirculation. Microcirculation 2005;12:275-285.
33. Levy GG, Motto DG, Ginsburg D: ADAMTS13 turns 3. Blood 2005;106:11-17.
34. Fritsma GA, Ens GE, Alvord MA, et al: Monitoring the antiplatelet action of aspirin. JAAPA 2001;14:57-62.
35. Eikelboom JW, Hankey GJ: Failure of aspirin to prevent atherothrombosis: potential mechanisms and implications for clinical practice. Am J Cardiovasc Drugs 2004;4:57-67.

14 Routine Testing in Hematology

Teresa G. Hippel

OUTLINE

Manual Cell Counts
Hemoglobin
 Determination
Microhematocrit
Rule of Three
Red Blood Cell Indices
Reticulocyte Count
Erythrocyte
 Sedimentation Rate

OBJECTIVES

After completion of this chapter, the reader will be able to:

1. State the dimensions of the counting area of a Neubauer ruled hemacytometer.
2. Describe the performance of manual cell counts for leukocytes, erythrocytes, and platelets, including types of diluting fluids, typical dilutions, and typical areas counted in the hemacytometer.
3. Calculate dilutions for cell counts when given appropriate data.
4. Calculate hemacytometer cell counts when given numbers of cells, area counted, and dilution.
5. Describe the principle of cyanmethemoglobin assay for determination of hemoglobin (Hb).
6. Calculate the values for a standard curve for cyanmethemoglobin determination when given the appropriate data. Plot values and use the standard curve to determine Hb values.
7. Describe the procedure for performing a microhematocrit.
8. Identify sources of error in routine manual procedures discussed in this chapter, and recognize written scenarios describing such.

9. Calculate the rule of three, mean cell volume (MCV), mean cell hemoglobin (MCH), and mean cell hemoglobin concentration (MCHC; erythrocyte indices) when given appropriate data.
10. Classify erythrocytes according to size and Hb content, using results of red blood cell (RBC) indices.
11. Describe the principle and procedure for performing a manual reticulocyte count and the clinical value of the test.
12. Recognize when it is necessary to calculate the relative, absolute, and corrected reticulocyte values and a reticulocyte production index, and then do so.
13. Interpret the results of reticulocyte calculations to evaluate the degree of bone marrow erythropoiesis.
14. Describe the procedure for performance of Westergren erythrocyte sedimentation rates (ESRs).
15. State the diagnostic value of ESRs.
16. Correct white blood cell counts for the presence of nucleated RBCs.

CASE STUDIES

After studying the material in this chapter, the reader should be able to respond to the following case studies:

Case 1

The following results are obtained from a patient:
 RBC—4.63×10^{12}/L
 Hb—15 g/dL
 Hct—0.40 L/L (40%)

1. Using the "rule of three" for Hb/Hct, what would be the expected value for the Hb?
2. What could cause the Hb to be falsely elevated?
3. What would you do to correct for the above interferences?

Case 2

From another patient, the following results are obtained:
 RBC—3.20×10^{12}/L
 Hb—5.8 g/dL
 Hct—0.189 L/L (18.9%)

1. Calculate the RBC indices
2. How would you describe the RBCs consistent with these indices?
3. How should you verify this?

Although most routine testing procedures in the hematology laboratory are automated, it may be necessary to use manual methods for counts that exceed the linearity of an instrument, when an instrument is nonfunctional and there is no backup, or in remote laboratories in Third World countries. Although the discussion in this chapter is directed toward whole blood, body fluid cell counts also generally are performed using manual methods. Chapter 17 discusses the specific diluents and dilutions for body fluid counts.

MANUAL CELL COUNTS

Manual cell counts are performed with the use of a hemacytometer, or counting chamber, and manual dilutions, made with self-contained diluting devices, such as Unopettes (Becton-Dickinson, Franklin Lakes, N.J.). The principle for performance of cell counts is essentially the same for leukocytes, erythrocytes, and platelets; only the dilution, diluting fluid, and area counted vary. Any particle (e.g., sperm) can be counted through the use of this system.

Equipment
Hemacytometer

The "heart" of the manual cell count is the hemacytometer, or counting chamber. The most common one is the Levy chamber with improved Neubauer ruling. It is composed of two raised surfaces, each in the shape of a 3-mm × 3-mm square (total area 9 mm²) separated by an H-shaped moat. As shown in Figure 14-1, this large square is made up of nine 1-mm × 1-mm squares, and each of the WBC squares is divided further into 16 squares with the center square subdivided into 25 smaller squares. Each of these smallest squares is $\frac{1}{25}$ or 0.04 mm². A coverslip is placed on top of the counting surfaces. The distance between each counting surface and the coverslip is 0.1 mm; the total *volume* is 9 mm³. Hemacytometers and coverslips must meet specifications of the National Bureau of Standards, as indicated by the initials "NBS" on the chamber. When the dimensions of the hemacytometer are thoroughly understood, the area counted can be changed to facilitate the counting of specimens with extremely low or high counts.

Unopette System

Unopettes were developed in the late 1950s. They have virtually replaced Thoma pipettes, which were the standard diluting devices for cell counting. The Unopette is a commercially available, self-contained diluting device that has eliminated many of the pipetting errors and makes the manual methods easier and more accurate. Unopettes are available for white blood cell (WBC), red blood cell (RBC), platelet, and eosinophil counts; for hemoglobin (Hb) determinations; and for reticulocyte counts.

The reservoir of the Unopette (Fig. 14-2) contains the appropriate diluting fluid and is covered at the top by a thin plastic diaphragm. The pipette varies in volume, depending on the dilution required. An overflow chamber is located at the

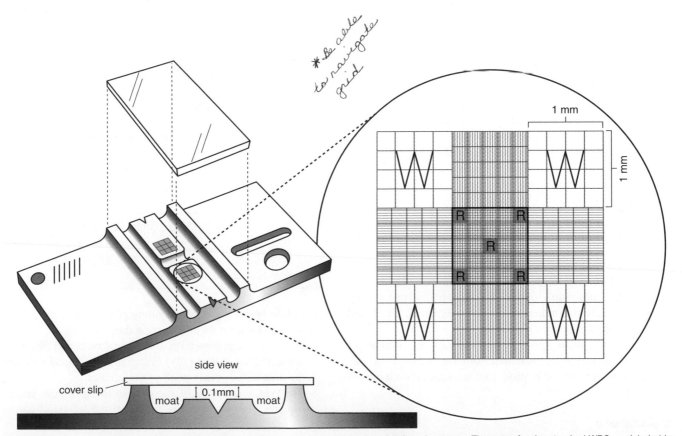

Figure 14-1 A hemacytometer and a close-up view of the counting areas as seen under the microscope. The areas for the standard WBC are labeled by *W*, and the areas for the standard RBC are labeled by *R*. The entire center square, outlined in blue, is used for counting platelets.

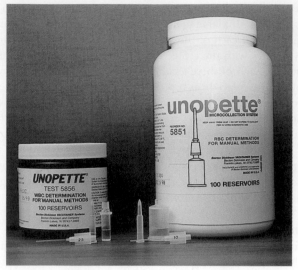

Figure 14-2 Unopette system, showing the 1:20 dilution for WBCs and the 1:200 dilution for RBC counts.

end of the pipette tip. The pipette shield is used to protect the pipette and to puncture the reservoir diaphragm.

Procedure

1. To open the reservoir, puncture the diaphragm, using the pointed end of the pipette shield. The hole should be large enough to insert the pipette easily into the reservoir.
2. Remove the pipette from the shield with a twisting motion.
3. Fill the pipette by capillary action from ethylenediamine tetraacetic acid (EDTA)–anticoagulated blood or capillary puncture. Wipe excess blood from the outside of the pipette.
4. Place a gloved index finger over the top of the overflow chamber. With the other hand, squeeze the reservoir enough to expel air without allowing liquid out.
5. Seat the pipette into the reservoir and release the finger from the top of pipette, while simultaneously releasing pressure on the reservoir. The sample is drawn into the diluting fluid.
6. Squeeze and release the reservoir several times to rinse pipette, allowing fluid to enter the overflow chamber without spilling out.
7. With a gloved finger covering the overflow chamber, invert the unit several times to mix.
8. After the incubation period (if required for procedure), convert the unit to a dropper assembly. Mix well, invert, and expel a few drops onto a tissue.
9. Maintaining steady pressure on the unit to prevent air bubbles, charge (fill) the hemacytometer, and proceed with the count, as directed in procedure sections for each type of count.

Calculations

The general formula for manual cell counts is as follows and can be used to calculate any type of cell count:

$$\text{Total count} = \frac{\text{cells counted} \times \text{dilution factor}}{\text{area } (\text{mm}^2) \times \text{depth } (0.1)}$$

or

$$\text{Total count} = \frac{\text{cells counted} \times \text{dilution factor} \times 10^*}{\text{area } (\text{mm}^2)}$$

White Blood Cell Count

The leukocyte, or WBC, count represents the number of WBCs in 1 L of whole blood. Whole blood from a capillary puncture or anticoagulated with EDTA is mixed with a diluting fluid that contains a weak acid (acetic or hydrochloric) to lyse the non-nucleated erythrocytes. In general, a 1:20 dilution is made; however, Unopettes for WBC and platelet counts also are available for a 1:100 dilution. A hemacytometer is charged (filled) with the dilution and placed under a microscope to count the number of cells.

Procedure

1. Clean the hemacytometer and coverslip with alcohol and dry thoroughly.
2. Make a 1:20 dilution in a Unopette containing 3% glacial acetic acid. (Alternatively, the Unopette containing ammonium oxalate and resulting in a 1:100 dilution may be used.)
3. Allow the Unopette to sit for 10 minutes to ensure RBC lysis.
4. Discard a few drops from the Unopette reservoir to expel any undiluted diluent. Charge both sides of the hemacytometer by holding the Unopette pipette at a 45-degree angle, and touch the tip of the pipette to the coverslip edge where it meets the chamber floor. Often there is a V-shaped indentation (see Fig. 14-1). The hemacytometer fills by capillary action. The chamber should be filled with a steady flow of fluid and be completely filled without overflowing.
5. After charging the counting chamber, place it in a moist chamber (Box 14-1) for 1 to 2 minutes before counting the cells to give them time to settle. Care should be taken not to disturb the coverslip.

BOX 14-1 How to Make a Moist Chamber

A moist chamber may be made by placing a piece of damp filter paper in the bottom of a Petri dish. An applicator stick broken in half can serve as a support for the chamber.

---

6. While keeping the hemacytometer in a horizontal position, place it on the microscope stage.
7. Lower the condenser on the microscope, and focus by using the low-power (10×) objective lens. The cells should be distributed evenly in all of the squares.
8. For WBCs, count all of the cells in the four large corner squares, starting with the square in the left-hand corner

---

*Reciprocal of depth

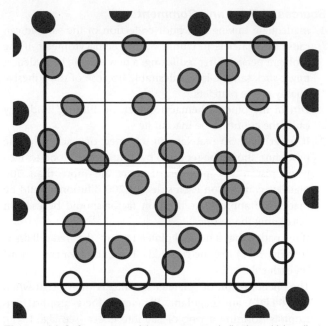

Figure 14-3 One square of hemacytometer indicating which cells to count. Cells touching the left and top lines *(solid circles)* are counted. Cells touching bottom and right *(open circles)* are not counted.

(see Fig. 14-1). Cells that touch the top and left lines should be counted; cells that touch the bottom and right lines should be ignored (Fig. 14-3). See Figure 14-4 for appearance of WBCs in the hemacytometer under the microscope.

9. Repeat the count on the other side of the counting chamber. The difference between the lowest and the highest count in the eight squares should not differ by more than 15 cells.

10. Average the two sides. Using the average, calculate the WBC count using the first equation (see earlier).

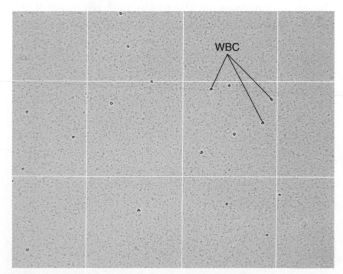

Figure 14-4 WBCs as seen in the hemacytometer under the 40× objective.

Example. The four large squares on one side of the chamber yielded counts of 23, 26, 22, and 21. The total count is 92.

The four large squares on the other side of the chamber yielded counts of 30, 24, 23, and 27. The difference between the lowest [21] and the highest [30] of the eight squares counted is <15). The total count is 104.

The average of the two sides of the chamber is 98. Using the average in the formula:

$$\text{WBC count} = \frac{\text{cells counted} \times \text{factor dilution}}{\text{area counted (mm}^2) \times \text{depth}}$$

$$= \frac{98 \times 20}{4 \times 0.1}$$

$$= 4900/\text{mm}^3 \text{ or } 4.9 \times 10^9/\text{L}$$

General reference ranges for males and females in different age groups can be found on the inside front cover of this text. *Laboratory values may vary slightly according to the population tested and should be established for each institution.*

Sources of Error and Comments

1. The hemacytometer and coverslip should be cleaned properly before they are used. Dust and fingerprints may cause difficulty in distinguishing the cells.

2. The diluting fluid should be free of contaminants.

3. If the count is less than $3 \times 10^9/\text{L}$, a greater area may be counted (e.g., 9 mm^2) to improve accuracy.

4. If the count is greater than $30 \times 10^9/\text{L}$, more dilution is needed. A dilution of 1:100 can be made using piston-type pipettes or the Unopettes for the 1:100 dilution.

5. The chamber must be charged properly to ensure an accurate count. Uneven flow of the diluted blood into the chamber results in an irregular distribution of cells. If the chamber is overfilled or underfilled, the chamber must be cleaned and recharged.

6. After the chamber is filled, allow the cells to settle for 1 to 2 minutes before counting. A pause much longer than that allows fluid to start evaporating and causes inaccuracies in the count.

7. Any nucleated erythrocytes (NRBCs) present in the sample are not lysed by the diluting fluid. The NRBCs are counted as WBCs because they are indistinguishable when seen on the hemacytometer. If five or more NRBCs per 100 WBCs on the differential are discovered, the WBC count must be corrected for these cells. This is accomplished by using the following formula:

$$\frac{\text{uncorrected WBC count} \times 100}{\text{number of NRBCs per 100 WBCs} + 100}$$

Report the result as the "corrected" WBC count.

8. The accuracy of the manual WBC count can be assessed by performing a WBC estimate on the peripheral blood smear (see Chapter 15). Box 14-2 shows another method of WBC estimation.

9. The C.V. in the manual WBC count with Unopettes is 5.6%.[1]

BOX 14-2 How to Perform a White Blood Cell Estimate

1. Scan thin area, using the 50× oil immersion lens
2. Observe 10 fields, counting all WBCs in each field
3. Average the number of WBCs seen per oil-immersion field
4. Multiply the number of WBC/oil-immersion field × 3000, and compare with WBC count

---

From US Army Medical Department Center and School Standard Operating Procedure, Fort Sam Houston, Texas, November 1, 2001. Other methods of WBC estimation are discussed in Chapter 15.

Platelet Count

A phase-contrast microscope is used in the reference method for performing a manual platelet count. Platelets are adhesive to foreign objects and to each other, which makes it difficult to count them. They also are small and could be confused easily with dirt. In this procedure, whole blood, with EDTA as the anticoagulant, is diluted with 1% ammonium oxalate, which lyses the non-nucleated erythrocytes. The platelets can be counted with the use of a phase-contrast microscope as described by Brecher and Cronkite.[2]

Procedure

1. Using a Unopette containing ammonium oxalate, make a 1:100 dilution.
2. Mix the dilution thoroughly and charge the chamber. (*Note:* A special thin flat-bottom counting chamber is used for phase platelet counts.)
3. Place the charged hemacytometer in a moist chamber for 15 minutes to allow the platelets to settle.
4. Platelets are counted with the use of the 40× objective lens. The platelets have a diameter of 2 to 4 μm and appear round or oval, displaying a light-purple sheen when phase-contrast microscopy is used. The shape and color help distinguish the platelets from highly refractile dirt and debris. "Ghost" RBCs often are seen in the background.
5. Count the 25 small squares in the center square of the grid (see Fig. 14-1). The area of this center square is 1 mm². Each side of the hemacytometer should be counted, and the counts should not differ by more than 10%.
6. Calculate the number of platelets per liter by using the first equation (see earlier). For example, if 200 platelets were counted in the entire center square,

$$\frac{200 \times 100}{1 \times 0.1}$$

$$= 200{,}000/\text{mm}^3 \text{ or } 200 \times 10^9/\text{L}$$

7. Platelet counts should be verified by performing an estimate on the Wright-stained peripheral blood smear (Chapter 15).

General reference ranges for males and females according to age groups can be found on the inside front cover, of this text.

Sources of Error and Comments

1. Inadequate mixing and poor collection of the sample can cause the platelets to clump on the hemacytometer. If the problem persists after rediluting, a new sample is needed. A finger-stick sample is less desirable because of the adhesive quality of the platelets.
2. Dirt in the pipette, hemacytometer, or diluting fluid may cause the counts to be inaccurate.
3. If fewer than 50 platelets are counted on each side, the procedure should be repeated by diluting the blood to 1:20 using piston-type pipettes. If there are more than 500 platelets counted on each side, a 1:200 dilution should be made. The appropriate dilution factor should be used in calculating the results.
4. If the patient has a normal platelet count, the "red cell area" (see Fig. 14-1) may be counted. Then, the area is 0.2 mm² on each side.
5. The phenomenon of "platelet satellitosis" may occur when using EDTA anticoagulant. Platelets adhere around neutrophils, forming a ring or satellite effect (see Fig. 15-1). Using sodium citrate as the anticoagulant should correct this problem. Because of the dilution in the citrate tubes, it is necessary to multiply the obtained platelet count by 1.1 for accuracy (Chapter 15).

Manual Erythrocyte Counts

Manual erythrocyte counts are rarely performed because of the inaccuracy of the count and questionable necessity. Other, more accurate manual RBC parameters, such as the microhematocrit and Hb, are desirable. Table 14-1 contains information on the performance of manual erythrocyte counts.

Body Fluid Cell Counts

Body fluid cell counts are discussed in detail in Chapter 17. Manual cell counts are summarized in Table 14-1.

HEMOGLOBIN DETERMINATION

The primary function of Hb within the erythrocyte is the carrying of oxygen to and carbon dioxide from the tissues. The cyanmethemoglobin (Hemiglobincyanide) method for Hb determination is the standard approved by the Clinical and Laboratory Standards Institute.[3]

Principle

In the cyanmethemoglobin method, blood is diluted in a solution of potassium ferricyanide and potassium cyanide. The Hb is oxidized to methemoglobin (Fe^{3+}) by the potassium ferricyanide, $K_3Fe(CN)_6$. The potassium cyanide (KCN) then converts the methemoglobin to cyanmethemoglobin:

$$\text{Hb}(Fe^{2+}) \xrightarrow{K_3Fe(CN)_6} \text{methemoglobin } (Fe^{3+}) \xrightarrow{KCN} \text{cyanmethemoglobin}$$

The absorbance of the cyanmethemoglobin at 540 nm is directly proportional to the Hb concentration. Sulfhemoglobin

TABLE 14-1 Manual Cell Counts with Most Common Dilutions, Counting Areas, and Reference Ranges

Cell Counted	Diluting Fluid	Dilution	Objective	Area Counted	Adult Reference Range*
Leukocyte	Weak acid	1:20	10×	4 mm²	$5\text{-}10 \times 10^9/\text{L}$
Erythrocyte	Isotonic saline	1:100	40×	0.2 mm² (5 small squares of center mm²)	Males: $4.30\text{-}5.70 \times 10^{12}/\text{L}$
					Females: $4.10\text{-}5.40 \times 10^{12}/\text{L}$
Platelet	Ammonium oxalate	1:100	40× phase	1 mm²	$150\text{-}500 \times 10^9/\text{L}$
Eosinophil	Propylene glycol, phloxine, and sodium carbonate	1:32	10×	9 mm²	$0.05\text{-}0.5 \times 10^9/\text{L}$

*From Baptist Memorial Health Care Corporation, Memphis, TN.

is not converted to cyanmethemoglobin; it cannot be measured by this method. Sulfhemoglobin fractions of more than 0.05 are seldom encountered in clinical practice, however.[4]

Procedure

Hemoglobin Reagent

1. Create a standard curve, using a commercially available cyanmethemoglobin standard.
   a. When a standard containing 80 mg/dL of Hb is used, the following dilutions should be made:

Hemoglobin Concentration (g/dL)	Blank	5	10	15	20
Cyanmethemoglobin standard	0	1.5	3	4.5	6
Cyanmethemoglobin reagent	6	4.5	3	1.5	0

   b. Transfer the dilutions to cuettes. Starting with the blank, measure the absorbance on a spectrophotometer (Fig. 14-5) at 540 nm.
   c. Using semilogarithmic paper, plot percentage transmittance on the *y*-axis and the Hb concentration on the *x*-axis. The Hb concentrations of the control and patient samples can be read from this standard curve (Fig. 14-6).

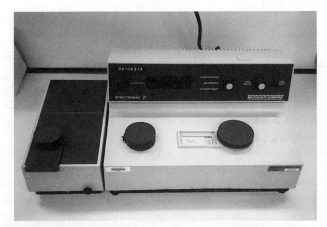

Figure 14-5 A spectrophotometer, used to measure transmittance or absorbance.

d. A standard curve should be set up with each new lot of reagents. It also should be checked when alterations (e.g., bulb change) are made to the instrument.
2. Controls should be run with each batch of specimens. Commercial controls are available.
3. Using the patient's whole blood anticoagulated with EDTA or heparin or from a capillary puncture, make a 1:251 dilution by adding 0.02 mL (20 µL) of blood to 5 mL of cyanmethemoglobin reagent. The pipette should be rinsed thoroughly with the reagent to ensure that no blood remains. Follow the same procedure for the control samples.
4. Cover and mix well by inversion or using a vortex mixer. Let stand for 10 minutes at room temperature to allow full conversion of Hb to cyanmethemoglobin.
5. Transfer all of the solutions to cuettes. Set the spectrophotometer to 100% transmittance at the wavelength of 540 nm, using cyanmethemoglobin reagent as a blank.
6. Using a matched cuette, continue reading the patient samples, and record the percentage transmittance.
7. Determine the Hb values of the control samples and the patient samples from the standard curve.

General reference ranges can be found on the inside cover of this text.

Sources of Error and Comments

1. Cyanmethemoglobin reagent is sensitive to light. It should be stored in a brown bottle or in a dark place.
2. A high leukocyte count ($>20 \times 10^9/\text{L}$) or a high platelet count ($>700 \times 10^9/\text{L}$) can cause turbidity and a falsely high result. In this case, the solution can be centrifuged and the supernatant measured.
3. Lipemia also can interfere, and a false result can be corrected by adding 0.01 mL of the patient's plasma to 5 mL of the cyanmethemoglobin reagent, this solution being used as the reagent blank.
4. Cells containing Hb S and Hb C may be resistant to hemolysis, causing turbidity; this can be corrected by making a 1:2 dilution with distilled water (1 part diluted sample plus 1 part water) and multiplying the results from the standard curve by 2.

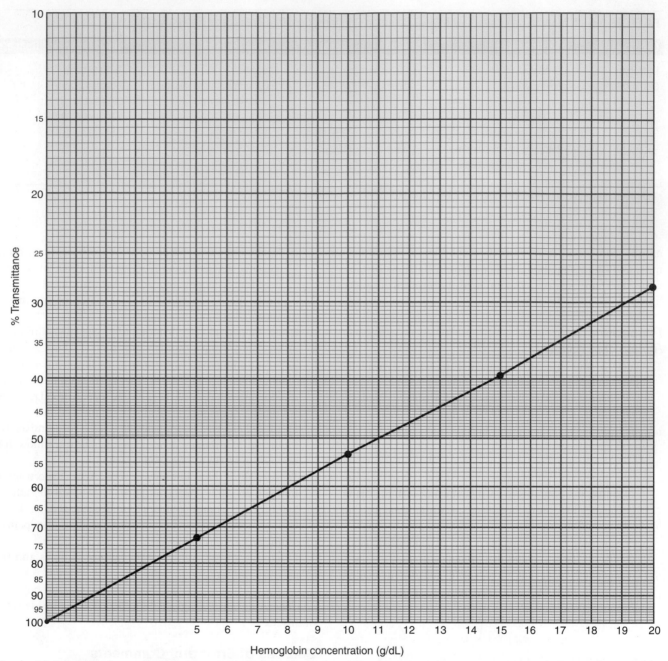

Figure 14-6 A standard curve obtained when a cyanmethemoglobin standard of 80 mg/dL is used. A blank (100% transmittance) and four dilutions were made: 5 g/dL (72.9% transmittance), 10 g/dL (53.2% transmittance), 15 g/dL (39.1% transmittance), and 20 g/dL (28.7% transmittance).

5. Abnormal globulins, such as those found in patients with multiple myeloma or Waldenström macroglobulinemia, may precipitate. If this occurs, add 0.1 g of potassium carbonate to the cyanmethemoglobin reagent. Commercially available cyanmethemoglobin reagent has been modified to contain KH_2PO_4 salt, so this problem is not likely to occur.

6. Carboxyhemoglobin takes 1 hour to convert to cyanmethemoglobin and theoretically could cause erroneous results in samples from heavy smokers. The degree of error is probably not clinically significant, however.

7. Because Hb reagent contains cyanide, it must be used cautiously; a minimum of 4 L of reagent is lethal. Acid-free sinks should be used for disposal of reagent and samples because acidification of cyanide releases hydrogen cyanide gas. Copious amounts of water should be used to flush the sink after disposal.

8. Commercial absorbance standards kits are available to calibrate spectrophotometers.

There also is a hand-held system that converts Hb to azide methemoglobin, which is read photometrically at two wavelengths (570 nm and 880 nm). This method avoids the necessity of sample dilution and interference from turbidity. An example is the HemoCue (HemoCue, Inc. Lake Forest, Calif).[5,6] Another method that has been used in some automated instruments involves the use of sodium lauryl sulfate (SLS) to convert Hb to SLS-methemoglobin. This method does not generate toxic wastes.[7-10]

MICROHEMATOCRIT

The hematocrit (Hct) is the volume of packed RBCs that occupies a given volume of whole blood. This is often referred to as the *packed cell volume* (PCV). It is reported either as a percentage (e.g., 36%) or in L/L (0.36 L/L).

Procedure

1. Fill two plain capillary tubes approximately three-quarters full with blood anticoagulated with EDTA or heparin. Mylar-wrapped tubes are recommended by the National Institute of Occupational Safety and Health to reduce the risks of capillary tube injuries.[11] Alternatively, blood for heparinized capillary tubes may be collected by capillary puncture. Wipe any excess blood from the outside of the tube.
2. Seal the end of the tube with the colored ring with nonabsorbent clay. Hold the filled tube horizontally and seal by placing the dry end into the tray with sealing compound at a 90-degree angle. Rotate the tube slightly and remove it from the tray. The plug should be at least 4 mm long.[11]
3. Balance the tubes in the centrifuge with the clay ends facing the outside away from the center, touching the rubber gasket.
4. Tighten the head cover on the centrifuge and close the top. Centrifuge the tubes at between 10,000G and 15,000G for the time that has been determined to obtain maximum packing of RBCs, as detailed in Box 14-3. Do not use the brake to stop the centrifuge.
5. Determine the Hct by using a microhematocrit reading device (Fig. 14-7). Read the level of RBC packing; do not include the buffy coat (leukocytes and platelets) when reading (Fig. 14-8).
6. The values of the two Hcts should agree within 1% (0.01).[11]

General reference ranges according to gender and age can be found on the inside front cover of this text.

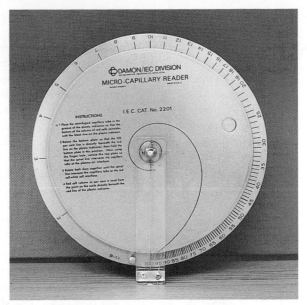

Figure 14-7 Microhematocrit reader.

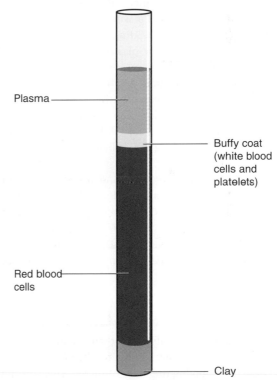

Plasma

Buffy coat (white blood cells and platelets)

Red blood cells

Clay

Figure 14-8 Representation of a capillary tube after it has been centrifuged. Notice the layers containing plasma, the buffy coat (leukocytes and platelets), and the erythrocytes.

Sources of Error and Comments

1. Improper sealing of the capillary tube causes a decreased Hct reading as a result of loss of blood during centrifugation. A higher number of erythrocytes are lost in relation to the plasma.
2. An increased concentration of anticoagulant decreases the Hct reading as a result of erythrocyte shrinkage.

BOX 14-3 **Determining Maximum Packing Time for Microhematocrit**

The time to obtain maximum packing of RBCs should be determined for each centrifuge. Duplicate microhematocrit determinations should be made using fresh, well-mixed, EDTA-anticoagulated blood. Two specimens should be used, with one of the specimens having a known Hct of 50% or greater. Starting at 2 minutes, spin duplicates at 30-second intervals and record results. When the Hct has remained at the same value for two consecutive times, optimum packing has been achieved, and the second time interval should be used for microhematocrit determinations.[11]

3. A decreased or increased result may occur if the specimen was not mixed properly.

4. The time and speed of the centrifugation and the time when the results are read are important. Insufficient centrifugation or a delay in reading results after centrifugation causes Hct readings to increase. Time for complete packing should be determined for each centrifuge and rechecked at regular intervals. When calibrating the microhematocrit centrifuge, one of the specimens used must have an Hct of 50% or greater.[11]

5. The buffy coat of the specimen should not be included in the Hct reading because its inclusion falsely elevates the result.

6. A decrease or increase in the readings may be seen if the microhematocrit reader is not used properly.

7. Many disorders, such as sickle cell anemia, macrocytic anemias, hypochromic anemias, spherocytosis, and thalassemia, may cause plasma to be trapped in the erythrocytes layer even if the procedure was performed properly. The trapping of the plasma causes the microhematocrit to be 1% to 3% (0.01-0.03 L/L) higher than that obtained on automated instruments that calculate the Hct and are unaffected by the trapped plasma.

8. A temporarily low Hct reading may result immediately after a blood loss because plasma is replaced faster than are erythrocytes.

9. The fluid loss of dehydration causes a decrease in plasma volume and falsely increases the Hct reading.

10. Proper specimen collection is an important consideration. The introduction of interstitial fluid from a skin puncture or the improper flushing of a catheter causes decreased Hct readings.

The READACRIT centrifuge (Clay Adams Becton Dickinson, Parsippany, N.J.) uses precalibrated capillary tubes and has built-in Hct scales, which eliminates the need for separate reading devices (Fig. 14-9). SUREPREP Capillary Tubes (Becton Dickinson) eliminate the use of sealants. They have a factory-inserted plug that seals automatically when the blood touches the plug.[12]

RULE OF THREE

When specimens are analyzed by automated or manual methods, a quick visual check of the results of the Hb and Hct can be done by applying the "rule of three." This rule applies only to specimens that have normocytic normochromic erythrocytes. The value of the Hct should be three times the value of the Hb plus or minus 3: Hb $\times$ 3 = Hct $\pm$ 3(0.03 L/L). It should become habit for the analyst to multiply the Hb by 3 mentally for every specimen; a discrepancy in this rule may indicate abnormal RBCs, or it may be the first indication of error.

For example, the following results are obtained from patients:

Case 1
Hb = 12 g/dL
Hct = 36% (0.36 L/L)

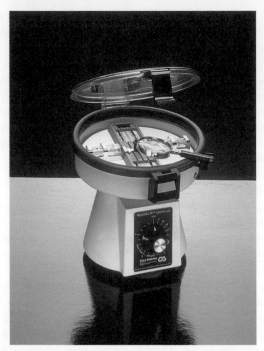

Figure 14-9 READACRIT centrifuge with built-in capillary tube compartments and Hct scales. (Courtesy of a division of Becton Dickinson, Parsippany, N.J.)

According to the rule of three,

$$\text{Hb } (12) \times 3 = \text{Hct } (36)$$

An acceptable range for the Hct would be 33% to 39%. These values conform to the rule of three.

Case 2
Hb = 9 g/dL
Hct = 32%
According to the rule of three,

$$\text{Hb } (9.0) \times 3 = \text{Hct } (27 \text{ versus actual value of } 32)$$

An acceptable range for Hct would be 24% to 30%, so these values do *not* conform to the rule of three.

Case 3
Hb = 15 g/dL
Hct = 36%
According to the rule of three,

$$\text{Hb } (15) \times 3 = \text{Hct } (45 \text{ versus obtained value of } 36)$$

An acceptable range for Hct would be 42% to 48%, so these values do *not* conform to the rule of three.

If values do not agree, the blood smear should be examined for abnormal erythrocytes. In the second example, the blood smear reveals erythrocytes that are abnormal in Hb content (hypochromic), so the values obtained are accurate. If erythrocytes do appear normal, the problem should be investigated. In the third example, the specimen is determined to have lipemic plasma, and a correction to the Hb must be made to obtain an accurate Hb value. (See Hemoglobin Determination in this chapter.)

When an unexplained discrepancy is found, the specimen before and after the specimen in question should be checked to determine whether they conform to the rule. If they do not conform, further investigation should be done to find the problem. A control specimen should be run when such a discrepancy is found. If the instrument is in control, random error may have occurred (Chapter 5).

RED BLOOD CELL INDICES

The mean cell volume (MCV), mean cell Hb (MCH), and mean cell Hb concentration (MCHC) are RBC indices. These are calculated to determine the size and Hb content of the average RBC. In addition to serving as a quality control check, the indices may be used to differentiate anemias. Table 14-2 provides a summary of the RBC indices, morphology, and correlation with anemias. The morphologic classification of anemia on the basis of MCV is discussed in detail in Chapter 18.

Mean Cell Volume

The MCV is the average volume of the RBC, expressed in femtoliters (fL), or 10^{-15} L:

$$MCV = Hct\ (\%) \times 10/RBC\ count\ (\times 10^{12}/L)$$

For example, if the Hct = 45%, and the RBC count = $5 \times 10^{12}/L$,

$$MCV = \frac{45 \times 10}{5} = 90\ fL$$

Mean Cell Hemoglobin

The MCH is the average weight of Hb in an RBC, expressed in picograms (pg), or 10^{-12} g:

$$MCH = Hb\ (g/dL) \times 10/RBC\ count\ (\times 10^{12}/L)$$

For example, if the Hb = 16 g/dL, and the RBC count = $5 \times 10^{12}/L$,

$$MCH = \frac{16 \times 10}{5} = 32\ pg$$

The reference range for adults is 28 to 32 pg. The MCH generally is not considered in the classification of anemias.

Mean Cell Hemoglobin Concentration

The MCHC is the average concentration of Hb in each individual erythrocyte. The units used are grams per deciliter (formerly referred to as a percentage):

$$MCHC = Hb\ (g/dL) \times 100/Hct\ (\%)$$

For example, if the Hb = 16 g/dL and the Hct = 48%,

$$MCHC = \frac{16 \times 100}{48} = 33.3\ g/dL$$

Values of normochromic cells range from 32 to 37 g/dL; values of hypochromic cells are less than 32 g/dL, and values of "hyperchromic" cells are greater than 37 g/dL. Hypochromic erythrocytes occur in thalassemias and iron deficiency. The term *hyperchromic* is a misnomer: a cell does not really contain more than 37 g/dL of Hb, but its shape may have become spherocytic, making the cell appear full. An MCHC greater than 37 g/dL should be scrutinized carefully for an error in Hb value (see Sources of Error and Comments in the section on Hb determination). Another cause for a markedly increased MCHC could be the presence of a cold agglutinin. Incubating the specimen in a 37° C water bath for 15 minutes before analysis usually produces accurate results. Cold agglutinin disease is discussed in more detail in Chapter 25.

RETICULOCYTE COUNT

The reticulocyte is the last immature erythrocyte stage. Normally, a reticulocyte spends 2 to 3 days in the bone marrow and 1 day in the peripheral blood before developing into a mature erythrocyte. The reticulocyte contains remnant cytoplasmic RNA and organelles such as the mitochondria and ribosomes. The reticulocyte count is used to assess erythropoietic activity of the bone marrow.

Principle

Whole blood, anticoagulated with EDTA, is stained with a supravital stain, such as new methylene blue. Any nonnucleated erythrocyte that contains two or more particles of

---

TABLE 14-2 Red Blood Cell Indices and Correlating Red Blood Cell Morphology and Disease States

MCV (fL)	MCHC (g/dL)	Red Blood Cell Morphology	Found in
<80	<32	Microcytic; hypochromic	Iron deficiency anemia, thalassemia, sideroblastic anemia, other conditions of defective iron use, chronic infection or inflammation, unstable hemoglobins, chronic diseases
80-100	32-36	Normocytic; normochromic	Hemolytic anemia, leukemia, metastatic malignancy, bone marrow failure, chronic renal disease
>100	32-36	Macrocytic; normochromic	Liver disease, myelodysplasias, megaloblastic anemias

blue-stained, granulofilamentous material after new methylene blue staining is defined as a *reticulocyte* (Fig. 14-10).

Procedure

1. Mix equal amounts of blood and new methylene blue stain (2-3 drops, or 50 μL each), and allow to incubate at room temperature for 3 to 10 minutes.[13]
2. Remix the preparation.
3. Prepare two wedge smears (Chapter 15).
4. In an area in which cells are close together but not touching, count 1000 RBCs under the oil-immersion objective lens. Reticulocytes are included in the total RBC count (i.e., a reticulocyte counts as an RBC and a reticulocyte).
5. To improve accuracy, have another laboratorian count the other smear; values should agree within 20%.
6. Calculate the reticulocyte count:

$$\text{Number of reticulocytes/1000 (RBCs observed)} \times 100 = \text{percentage reticulocytes}$$

For example, if 15 reticulocytes are counted,

$$\text{Reticulocyte (\%)} = 15/1000 \times 100 = 1.5\%$$

or the number of reticulocytes counted can be multiplied by 0.1 (100/1000) to obtain the result.

Reference Range

The following reticulocyte count reference values for male and female patients were developed at Baptist Memorial Health Care Corporation, Memphis, Tenn.:

Age	Reticulocyte Count (%)	Absolute Reticulocyte Count ($\times 10^9$/L)
Birth-1 day	2.00-6.00	70-330
1 day-2 weeks	0.30-1.50	10.5-82.5
2 weeks-adult	0.50-2.20	20-120

Sources of Error and Comments

1. If a patient is very anemic or polycythemic, the proportion of dye to blood should be adjusted accordingly.

2. An error may occur if the blood and stain are not mixed before the smears are made. The specific gravity of the reticulocytes is lower than that of the mature erythrocytes, and reticulocytes settle at the top of the mixture during incubation.
3. Moisture in the air, poor drying of the slide, or both may cause areas of the slide to appear refractile and could be confused for reticulocytes. The RNA remnants in a reticulocyte are not refractile.
4. Other RBC inclusions that stain supravitally include Heinz, Howell-Jolly, and Pappenheimer bodies. Heinz bodies represent precipitated Hb, usually appear round or oval, and tend to cling to the cell membrane (Fig. 14-11). Howell-Jolly bodies are round nuclear fragments and are usually singular. Pappenheimer bodies are hemosiderin in the mitochondria whose presence can be confirmed with an iron stain, such as Prussian blue. This stain is discussed in Chapter 16.

Absolute Reticulocyte Count

Principle

The absolute reticulocyte count (ARC) is the actual number of reticulocytes in 1 L of whole blood.

Calculations

$$\text{ARC} = \frac{\text{reticulocytes (\%)} \times \text{RBC count } (\times 10^{12})}{100}$$

For example, if a patient's reticulocyte count is 2%, and the RBC count is 2.20×10^{12}/L, the ARC would be calculated as follows:

$$\text{ARC} = \frac{2 \times (2.20 \times 10^{12}/\text{L})}{100} = 44 \times 10^9/\text{L}$$

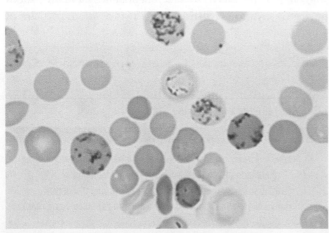

Figure 14-10 Reticulocytes under an oil immersion lens (peripheral blood ×1000).

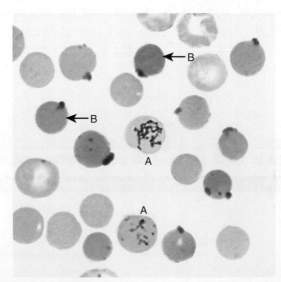

Figure 14-11 Reticulocytes *(A)* and Heinz bodies *(B)* in supravital stain (peripheral blood ×1000).

Reference Range

Values between $25 \times 10^9/L$ and $75 \times 10^9/L$ are within the reference range of most populations.[14]

Corrected Reticulocyte Count

Principle

In specimens with a low Hct, the percentage of reticulocytes may be falsely elevated because whole blood contains fewer RBCs. A correction factor is used, considering the average normal Hct to be 45%.

Calculation

Corrected reticulocyte count = reticulocytes (%) $\times \dfrac{\text{Hct (\%)}}{45}$

Reference Range

Patients with an Hct of 35% are expected to have a corrected reticulocyte count of 2% to 3%. In patients with an Hct less than 25%, the count should increase to 3% to 5% to compensate for anemia. The corrected reticulocyte count depends on the degree of anemia.

Reticulocyte Production Index

Principle

Reticulocytes that are released from the marrow prematurely are called *shift reticulocytes*. These reticulocytes are "shifted" from the bone marrow to the peripheral blood earlier than usual to compensate for anemia. Instead of losing their reticulum in 1 day, as do normal reticulocytes, these cells take 2-4 days to lose their reticulum. When erythropoiesis is evaluated, a correction should be made for the presence of shift reticulocytes if there is a report of polychromasia in the morphology. Normal (nonshift) reticulocytes become mature RBCs 1 day after entering the bloodstream, thus representing 1 day's production of RBCs in the bone marrow. Cells shifted to the peripheral blood prematurely stay as reticulocytes longer and would contribute to the reticulocyte count for more than 1 day. So, the reticulocyte count is falsely increased when polychromasia is present because the count no longer represents the cells maturing in just one day. On many automated instruments, this mathematical adjustment of the reticulocyte count has been replaced by the measurement of immature reticulocyte fraction.[13]

The patient's Hct is used to determine the appropriate correction factor (reticulocyte maturation time in days):

Patient's Hematocrit Value (%)	Correction Factor (Maturation) (days)
40-45	1
35-39	1.5
25-34	2
15-24	2.5
<15	3

Calculation

The reticulocyte production index (RPI) is calculated as follows:

$$RPI = \dfrac{\text{reticulocyte (\%)} \times \left[\dfrac{\text{Hct (\%)}}{45}\right]}{\text{maturation time}}$$

or

$$RPI = \dfrac{\text{corrected reticulocyte count}}{\text{maturation time}}$$

For example, for a patient with a reticulocyte count of 7.8%, Hct of 30%, and polychromasia noted, the previous table indicates a maturation time of 2 days. Thus

$$RPI = \dfrac{7.8 \times \left[\dfrac{30}{45}\right]}{2}$$

$$RPI = 2.6$$

Reference Range

An adequate bone marrow response usually is indicated by an RPI that is greater than 3. An inadequate response is seen when the RPI is less than 2.[14]

Reticulocyte Control

Several commercial controls are now available for monitoring the manual and automated reticulocyte counts (e.g., Retic-Chex, Streck Laboratories, Omaha, Neb.; Liquichek, Bio-Rad Laboratories, Hercules, Calif). Most of the controls are available at three levels. The control samples are treated in the same manner as the clinical specimens. The control can be used to verify the laboratorian's accuracy and precision when manual counts are performed.

Flow Cytometry

Most of the major instrument manufacturers offer analyzers that perform automated reticulocyte counts. All of the analyzers evaluate reticulocytes based on optical scatter or fluorescence after treating the RBCs with fluorescent dyes or nucleic acid stains to stain residual RNA in the reticulocytes. The percentage and the absolute count are provided. These results are statistically more valid because of the large number of cells counted. Other reticulocyte parameters that are offered on some automated instruments include maturation index, immature reticulocyte fraction, and reticulocyte indices. These measurements may be especially useful in monitoring erythropoietic activity in patients undergoing chemotherapy or stem cell or bone marrow transplantation or in patients with chronic renal failure. Automated reticulocyte counting is discussed in Chapter 39.

ERYTHROCYTE SEDIMENTATION RATE

The erythrocyte sedimentation rate (ESR) is useful for monitoring the course of an existing inflammatory disease or for differentiating between similar diseases. The ESR is normal in patients with osteoarthritis but is elevated in patients with rheumatic fever, rheumatoid arthritis, or pyogenic arthritis. The ESR is elevated in the early stage of acute pelvic inflammatory disease or a ruptured ectopic pregnancy but normal in the first 24 hours of acute appendicitis. The ESR may be used to indicate the activity of pulmonary tuberculosis.

Principle

When anticoagulated blood is allowed to stand at room temperature undisturbed for a period of time, the RBCs settle toward the bottom of the tube. The ESR is the distance in millimeters at which the RBCs fall in 1 hour. The ESR is affected by erythrocytes, plasma, and mechanical and technical factors. Erythrocytes have a net negative surface charge and tend to repel one another. The repulsive forces are partially or totally counteracted if there are increased quantities of positively charged plasma proteins; the erythrocytes settle more rapidly as a result of the formation of RBC aggregates or rouleaux. Examples of macromolecules that can produce this reaction are fibrinogen, β-globulins, and pathologic immunoglobulins.[15]

Normal erythrocytes have a relatively small mass and settle slowly. Certain diseases can cause rouleaux formation, in which the plasma fibrinogen and globulins are altered. This alteration changes the erythrocyte surface, leading to aggregation of the RBCs, increased RBC mass, and a more rapid ESR. The ESR is directly proportional to the RBC mass and inversely proportional to plasma viscosity.

Westergren Erythrocyte Sedimentation Rate
Procedure

1. Use blood collected in EDTA and dilute four parts blood and one part 3.8% sodium chloride (e.g. 2 mL blood and 0.5 mL sodium chloride). Alternatively, blood can be collected directly into special sedimentation test tubes containing sodium citrate. Standard coagulation test tubes are not acceptable, because the dilution is nine parts blood to one part sodium citrate.[16]
2. Place the pipette into the rack and allow to stand undisturbed for 60 minutes.
3. Record the number of millimeters the RBCs have fallen. The buffy coat should not be included in the reading. The ESR is reported as 1 hour = __ mm.

Reference ranges according to gender and age can be found on the inside front cover of this text.

Sources of Error and Comments

1. If the concentration of anticoagulant is increased, the ESR is falsely low as a result of sphering of the RBCS, inhibiting rouleaux.
2. The anticoagulants sodium or potassium oxalate and heparin cause the RBCs to shrink and falsely elevate the ESR.
3. A significant change in the temperature of the room alters the ESR.
4. Even a slight tilt of the pipette causes the ESR to increase.
5. If the specimen is allowed to sit at room temperature for more than 2 hours before being tested, the erythrocytes start to become spherical and may inhibit the formation of rouleaux.

6. Bubbles in the column of blood invalidate the test results.
7. The blood must be set properly to the zero mark at the beginning of the test.
8. A clotted specimen cannot be used.
9. Hematologic disorders that prevent the formation of rouleaux (e.g., sickle cells and spherocytes) decrease the ESR.
10. The ESR of patients with severe anemia is of little diagnostic value, as it will be falsely elevated.

Disposable Methods

Commercial kits are available for a disposable ESR test (Fig. 14-12). Several kits include safety caps for the pipettes that allow the blood to fill precisely to the zero mark. This safety cap makes the pipette a closed system and eliminates the error involved with manually setting the blood at the zero mark.

Automated Erythrocyte Sedimentation Rate

The Ves-Matic system (Diesse, Inc., Hialeah, Fla.) is a benchtop analyzer designed to determine ESR by use of an optoelectronic sensor, which measures the change in opacity of a column of blood as sedimentation of blood progresses. Blood is collected in special Ves-Tec or Vacu-Tec tubes, which contain sodium citrate and are compatible with the Vacutainer system. These tubes are used directly in the instrument (Fig. 14-13). Acceleration of sedimentation is achieved by positioning the tubes at an 18-degree angle in relation to the vertical axis. Results comparable with Westergren 1-hour values are obtained in 20 minutes.[17]

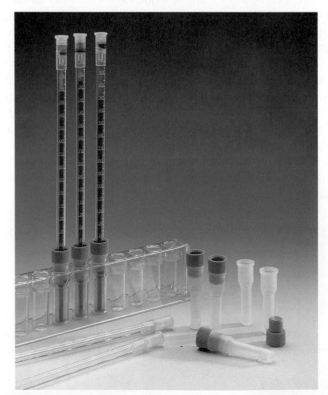

Figure 14-12 Sediplast (Polymedco) disposable sedimentation rate system. (Courtesy of Polymedco, Cortlandt Manor, N.Y.)

Another automated ESR analyzer is the Sedimat 15 (Polymedco, Cortlandt Manor, N.Y.), which uses the principle of infrared measurement. It has the capability of testing one to eight specimens randomly or simultaneously and provides results in 15 minutes (Fig. 14-14).

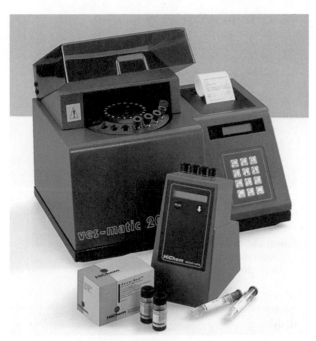

Figure 14-13 Two models of the Ves-Matic system: the Mini-Ves (for ≤4 samples) and the Ves-Matic 20 (for ≤20 samples simultaneously). Some Vacu-Tec primary sample collection tubes (black tops) and a quality control tube (orange top) are shown in the instruments. (Courtesy of ELAN Diagnostics, Smithfield, R.I.)

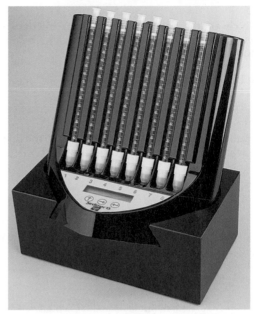

Figure 14-14 Sedimat 15 automated sedimentation rate system. (Courtesy of Polymedco, Cortlandt Manor, N.Y.)

CHAPTER at a GLANCE

- Although most laboratories are highly automated, the manual tests discussed in this chapter, such as the cyanmethemoglobin method of Hb determination and the microhematocrit, are used as a part of many laboratories' quality control and backup methods of analysis.
- The hemacytometer enables performance of counts of any type of cell or particle (e.g., WBCs, platelets, and eosinophils).
- The Unopette is a self-contained diluting system that simplifies dilutions for manual counts.
- Hb determination is based on the absorbance of cyanmethemoglobin at 540 nm. A standard curve is used to obtain the results.
- The microhematocrit is a measure of packed RBC volume.
- RBC indices—the MCV, MCH, and MCHC—are calculated to deter-

mine the size, Hb content, and Hb concentration of erythrocytes. The indices give an indication of the etiology of a patient's anemia.

- The reticulocyte count, which is used to assess the erythropoietic activity of the bone marrow, is accomplished through the use of supravital stains (e.g., new methylene blue) or by flow cytometric methods.
- The ESR, a measure of the settling of erythrocytes in a 1-hour period, depends on the erythrocytes' ability to form rouleaux. It is an indication of inflammation and may be used to differentiate various diseases or to monitor therapy for certain disorders.

Now that you have completed this chapter, go back and read again the case studies at the beginning and respond to the questions presented.

REVIEW QUESTIONS

1. A 1:20 dilution is made in a Unopette, with glacial acetic acid as the diluent. The four corner squares on *both* sides of the hemacytometer are counted for a total of 100 cells. What is the total WBC ($\times 10^9$/L)?
   a. 0.25
   b. 2.5
   c. 5
   d. 10

2. The total WBC count is 20×10^9/L. Twenty-five NRBCs per 100 WBCs are seen on the peripheral blood smear. What is the corrected WBC count ($\times 10^9$/L)?
   a. 0.8
   b. 8
   c. 16
   d. 19

3. If potassium cyanide and potassium ferricyanide are used in the manual method for Hb determination, the final product is:
   a. Methemoglobin
   b. Azide methemoglobin
   c. Cyanmethemoglobin
   d. Myoglobin

4. Which of the following would *not* interfere with Hb determination when performed by the cyanmethemoglobin method?
   a. Increased lipids
   b. Elevated WBC count
   c. Lyse-resistant RBCs
   d. Fetal Hb

5. A patient has a Hb of 8 g/dL. According to the rule of three, in what range would the Hct be expected?
   a. 21-24%
   b. 23.7-24.3%
   c. 24-27%
   d. 21-27%

6. Calculate the MCV and MCHC for the following values:
   RBC = 5.00×10^{12}/L
   Hb = 9 g/dL
   Hct = 30%

	MCV (fL)	MCHC (g/dL)
a.	30	18
b.	60	30
c.	65	33
d.	85	35

7. What does the reticulocyte count assess?
   a. Inflammation
   b. Response to infection
   c. Erythropoietic activity
   d. Ability of RBCs to form rouleaux

8. For the following patient, which index of bone marrow RBC production should be calculated?
   Observed reticulocyte count—5.3%
   Hct—35%
   Morphology—no polychromasia
   a. Absolute reticulocyte count
   b. Corrected WBC count
   c. Corrected reticulocyte count
   d. Reticulocyte production index

9. Given the following values, calculate the RPI:
   Observed reticulocyte count—6%
   Hct—30%
   a. 2
   b. 3
   c. 4
   d. 5

10. Which of the following would correlate with an elevated ESR value?
   a. Osteoarthritis
   b. Polycythemia
   c. Decreased globulins
   d. Inflammation

REFERENCES

1. Product circular for reorder #365856: WBC Unopette. Franklin Lakes, NJ: Becton Dickinson, 1998.
2. Brecher G, Cronkite EP: Morphology and enumeration of human blood platelets. J Appl Physiol 1950;3:365-377.
3. Clinical and Laboratory Standards Institute: Reference and Selected Procedures for the Quantitative Determination of Hemoglobin in Blood: Approved Standard, 3rd ed (CLSI Document H15-A3). Wayne, PA: CLSI, 2000.
4. International Council for Standardization in Haematology: Recommendations for reference method for haemoglobinometry in human blood (ICSH Standard 1995) and specifications for international haemiglobincyanide reference preparation (4th ed). J Clin Pathol 1996;49:271-274.
5. von Schenck H, Falkensson M, Lundberg B: Evaluation of "HemoCue," a new device for determining hemoglobin. Clin Chem 1986;32:526-529.
6. Hemoglobin test systems. Available at: at http://www.hemocue.com/hemocueus/isda_17.asp. Accessed February 11, 2006.
7. MacLaren IA, Conn DM, Wadsworth LD: Comparison of two automated hemoglobin methods using Sysmex SULFOLYSER and STROMATOLYSER. Sysmex J Int 1991;1:59-61.
8. Karsan A, MacLaren I, Conn D, et al: An evaluation of hemoglobin determination using sodium lauryl sulfate. Am J Clin Pathol 1993;100:123-126.
9. Matsubara T, Mimura T: Reaction mechanism of SLS-Hb Method. Sysmex J (Japan) 1990;13:206-211.
10. Fujiwara C, Hamaguchi Y, Toda S, et al: The reagent SULFOLYSER for hemoglobin measurement by hematology analyzers. Sysmex J (Japan) 1990;13:212-219.
11. Clinical and Laboratory Standards Institute: Procedure for Determining Packed Cell Volume by the Microhematocrit Method: Approved Standard, 3rd ed (NCCLS document H7-A3). Wayne, PA: CLSI, 2000.
12. Product Brochure: Clay Adams Brand SUREPREP capillary tubes. Sparks, MD: Becton Dickinson Primary Care Diagnostics, 1998.
13. Clinical and Laboratory Standards Institute: Methods for Reticulocyte Counting (Automated Blood Cell Counters, Flow Cytometry, and Supravital Dyes): Approved Guideline, 2nd ed (CLSI document H44-A2). Wayne, PA: CLSI, 2004.
14. Koepke JF, Koepke JA: Reticulocytes. Clin Lab Haematol 1986;8:169-179.
15. Perkins SL: Examination of the blood and bone marrow. In Greer JP, Foerster JL, Lukens JN, et al (eds): Wintrobe's Clinical Hematology, 11th ed. Philadelphia: Lippincott, Williams & Wilkins, 2004; 1-21.
16. Clinical and Laboratory Standards Institute: Reference and Selected Procedure for the Erythrocyte Sedimentation Rate (ESR) Test: Approved Standard, 4th ed (CLSI document H2-A4). Wayne, PA: CLSI, 2000.
17. VES-matic Line. Available at: http://www.diesse-usa.com/products/vesmatic/index.html. Accessed February 25, 2006.

Examination of the Peripheral Blood Smear and Correlation with the Complete Blood Count

15

Lynn B. Maedel and Kathryn Doig

OBJECTIVES

After completion of this chapter, the reader will be able to:

1. List the specimen sources and collection processes that are acceptable for blood smear preparation.
2. Describe the techniques for making peripheral blood smears.
3. Describe the qualities of a well-prepared peripheral blood smear, recognize a description of a slide that is consistent or inconsistent with that appearance, and troubleshoot problems with poorly prepared smears.
4. Explain the principle, purpose, and basic method of Wright staining of blood smears.
5. Identify and troubleshoot problems that cause poorly stained blood smears.
6. Describe the proper examination of a peripheral blood smear, including selection of "correct" area, sequence of examination, and observations to be made at each magnification. Recognize deviations from this protocol.
7. Given the number of cells observed per field and the magnification of the objective, apply formulas to estimate white blood cell (WBC) counts and platelet counts.
8. Explain the effect that platelet satellitosis and clumping may have on automated complete blood count (CBC) results. Recognize examples of results that would be consistent with these effects.
9. Follow the appropriate course of action to recognize and correct ethylenediamine tetraacetic acid (EDTA)–induced pseudothrombocytopenia and pseudoleukocytosis.
10. Apply a systematic approach to interpretation of CBC data that results in a verbal summary of the numerical data and communicates the blood picture succinctly.
11. Calculate absolute WBC differential counts.

CASE STUDY

After studying the material in this chapter, the reader should be able to respond to the following case study:

A healthy looking 56-year-old man had an automated CBC performed as part of a preoperative evaluation. Results are shown. Refer to reference ranges provided inside the front cover of this book.

WBC—15.8×10^9/L
RBC—4.93×10^{12}/L
Hb—14.8 g/dL
Hct—45.1%
MCV—91.5 fL
MCH—30 pg
MCHC—32.8 g/dL
RDW—14.2%
Platelets—34×10^9/L
MPV—6.6 fL

The peripheral blood smear was examined, and the only abnormal finding was "platelets in clumps."

1. What automated results should be questioned?
2. What is the best course of action to handle this problem?

A well-made, well-stained, and carefully examined peripheral blood smear can provide valuable information regarding a patient's health. More can be learned from this test than from many other routinely performed hematologic tests. White blood cell (WBC) and platelet estimates can be achieved, relative proportions of the different types of WBCs may be obtained, and the morphology of all three cell lines can be evaluated for abnormalities. Although routine work is now handled by the sophisticated automation found in most hematology laboratories, skilled and talented laboratory professionals are still essential to the reporting of reliable test results. Proper peripheral smear evaluation is most likely to be needed for some time.

The peripheral smear evaluation is the capstone on a panel of tests called the *complete blood count* (CBC) or hemogram. The CBC includes enumeration of cellular elements, quantitation of hemoglobin (Hb), and statistical analyses that provide a snapshot of cell appearances. These results can be derived from manual methods and calculations described in Chapter 14 or from the automated instruments described in Chapter 39. Regardless, the numerical values should be consistent with the assessment derived from examining the cells microscopically. Careful examination of the data in a systematic way ensures that all relevant results are noted and taken into consideration in the diagnosis.

This chapter begins with the preparation and assessment of the blood smear, followed by a systematic approach to review of the CBC, including blood smear evaluation. Such an evaluation can be applied to the hematology chapters that follow.

PERIPHERAL BLOOD SMEARS

Specimen Collection

Sources of Specimens

Essentially all specimens received for routine testing in the hematology section of the laboratory have been collected in lavender (purple)-top tubes. These tubes contain disodium or tripotassium ethylenediamine tetraacetic acid (EDTA), which anticoagulates the blood by chelating the calcium that is essential for coagulation. Liquid tripotassium EDTA is often preferred to the powdered form because it mixes more easily with blood. High-quality blood smears can be made from the EDTA tube, provided that they are made within 2 to 3 hours of drawing the specimen.[1] Smears from EDTA tubes that remain at room temperature for more than 5 hours often have unacceptable blood cell artifacts (echinocytic red blood cells [RBCs], spherocytes, necrobiotic leukocytes, and vacuolated neutrophils). Vacuolization of monocytes normally occurs almost immediately with EDTA but causes no evaluation problems.

The main advantages of making smears from the EDTA tube of blood are that multiple slides can be made if necessary and they do not have to be prepared immediately when the blood is drawn. In addition, EDTA generally prevents platelets from clumping on the glass slide, making the platelet estimate more accurate during smear evaluation. There are purists, however, who believe that anticoagulant-free blood is still the specimen of choice for evaluation of blood cell morphology.[2] Although some artifacts can be avoided, samples made from unanticoagulated blood pose other problems (see later).

Under certain conditions, a different anticoagulant or no anticoagulant may be helpful. Some patients' blood undergoes an in vitro phenomenon called *platelet satellitosis*[3] when anticoagulated with EDTA. The platelets surround or adhere to neutrophils, potentially causing pseudothrombocytopenia when counted by automated methods (Fig. 15-1).[3,4] In addition, spuriously low platelet counts and falsely increased WBC counts (pseudoleukocytosis) can result from EDTA-induced platelet clumping.[5] Pseudoleukocytosis occurs when platelet agglutinates are similar in size to WBCs and automated analyzers cannot distinguish the two. The platelet clumps are counted as WBCs instead of platelets. Platelet-specific autoantibodies that react best at room temperature are one of the mechanisms known to cause this phenomenon.[6] In these circumstances, the examination of a blood smear becomes an important quality control strategy, identifying these phenomena so that they can be corrected before the results are reported to the patient's chart.

Problems such as these can be eliminated by re-collecting specimens in sodium citrate tubes (light-blue top), ensuring that the proper ratio of 9 parts blood to 1 part anticoagulant is observed (a properly filled tube). These new specimens can be analyzed in the usual way by automated instrumentation. Platelet counts and WBC counts from sodium citrate specimens must be corrected for the dilution of blood with the anticoagulant, however. In a full draw tube, the blood is nine tenths of the total tube volume (2.7 mL blood and 0.3 mL sodium citrate). The "dilution factor" is the reciprocal of the dilution (i.e., $^{10}/_9$ or 1.1). The WBC and platelet counts are multiplied by 1.1 to obtain accurate counts. All other CBC parameters should be reported from the original EDTA tube and slide.

Another source of blood for smears is from finger and heel punctures. In general, the smears are made immediately at the patient's side. There are, however, a few limitations to this procedure. First, some platelet clumping must be expected if smears are made directly from a drop of finger-stick or heel-stick blood or if blood is collected in heparinized microhematocrit tubes. Generally, this clumping is not enough to interfere with platelet estimates if the smears are made

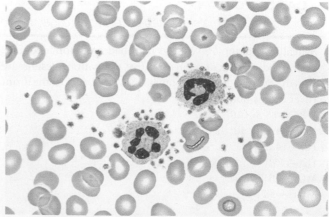

Figure 15-1 Photomicrograph of platelet satellitosis.

promptly before clotting begins in earnest. Second, only a few smears can be made directly from a skin puncture before the site stops bleeding. If slides are made quickly and correctly, however, cell distribution and morphology should be adequate. These problems with finger and heel sticks can be eliminated with the use of EDTA microcollection tubes, such as Microtainers (Becton Dickinson, Franklin Lakes, N.J.) (Chapter 3).

Peripheral Smear Preparation

Types of Smears

Manual Wedge Technique.   The wedge smear is probably the easiest to master. It is the most convenient and commonly used technique for making peripheral blood smears. This technique requires at least two 3 inch × 1 inch (75-mm × 25-mm) clean glass slides. High-quality, beveled-edge microscopic slides with chamfered (beveled) corners for good lateral borders are recommended. A few more slides may be kept handy in case a good-quality smear is not made immediately. One slide serves as the smear slide, and the other is the pusher or spreader slide. They can then be reversed. It also is possible to make good wedge smears by using a hemacytometer coverslip attached to a handle (pinch clip or tongue depressor) as the spreader.

A drop of blood (about 2-3 mm in diameter) from a finger, heel, or microhematocrit tube (nonheparinized for EDTA blood or heparinized for capillary blood) is placed at one end of the slide. The drop also may be delivered using a Diff-Safe dispenser (Alpha Scientific Corporation, Malvern, Penn.). The Diff-Safe dispenser is inserted through the rubber stopper of the EDTA tube, eliminating the need to remove the stopper.[7] The size of the drop of blood is important: Too large a drop creates a long or thick smear, and too small a drop often makes a short or thin blood smear. The pusher slide, held securely in the dominant hand at about a 30- to 45-degree angle (Fig. 15-2A), is drawn back into the drop of blood, allowing it to spread across the width of the slide (Fig. 15-2B). It is quickly and smoothly pushed forward to the end of the slide, creating a wedge smear (Fig. 15-2C). It is important that the whole drop is picked up and spread. Moving the pusher slide forward too slowly accentuates poor leukocyte distribution by pushing larger cells, such as monocytes and granulocytes, to the very end and sides of the smear. Maintaining an even, gentle pressure on the slide is essential. It also is crucial to keep the same angle all the way to the end of the smear. For higher than normal hematocrit (Hct), as found in patients with polycythemia or in newborns, the angle should be lowered (i.e., 25 degrees), so the smear is not too short and thick. For extremely low Hct, the angle may need to be raised. If two or three smears are made, the best one is chosen for staining, and the others are disposed of properly. Some laboratories make two good smears and save one unstained in case another slide is required.

The procedure just described is for a push-type wedge preparation. It is called *push* because the spreader slide is pulled into the drop of blood and the smear is made by pushing the blood along the slide. The same procedure can be modified to produce a *pulled* smear. In this procedure, the spreader slide is pushed into the drop of blood and pulled along the length of the slide to make the smear. Although less commonly used, it also provides a satisfactory wedge preparation and is easier for some individuals to perform. Other variations on the wedge technique include using the 3-inch side of the slide as the spreader slide or balancing the spreader slide on the fingers to avoid placing too much pressure on it. Learning to make consistently good blood smears takes a lot of practice but can be accomplished if one is patient and persistent.

Features of a Well-Made Wedge Peripheral Blood Smear.

1. Smear is two thirds to three fourths the length of the slide (Fig. 15-3).
2. Smear is finger-shaped, very slightly rounded at feather edge, not bullet-shaped; this allows for the widest area for examination.
3. Lateral edges of smear should be visible.
4. Smear is smooth without irregularities, holes, or streaks.
5. When slide is held up to light, the thin portion (feather edge) of the smear should have a "rainbow" appearance.
6. Whole drop is picked up and spread.

Figure 15-4 shows unacceptable smears.

Coverslip Technique.   The coverslip method of smear preparation is an older technique that is now only rarely used for peripheral blood smears, but it sometimes is still used for making bone marrow aspirate smears. The only advantage of this preparation is its excellent leukocyte distribution, which lends itself to more accurate differentials. For routine morphologic evaluation, however, this technique is neither convenient nor practical. Impeccably clean glass coverslips must be used.[2] Labeling, transport, staining, and storage of these small, breakable smears present many problems.

This technique requires that a small drop of blood or bone marrow be placed on one clean coverslip (22 × 22 mm), and another coverslip placed on top, allowing the blood to spread across the two coverslips. One is pulled across the other to create two thin smears, one smear on each coverslip (Fig. 15-5). The two smears can be stained and mounted on a 1-inch × 3-inch glass slide. When bone marrow smears are made by this technique, very slight pressure is applied to the coverslips between the index finger and thumb (sometimes called a *crush preparation*) to help spread the bone marrow spicule before the two smears are pulled apart. Refining the skills required to make high-quality crush preparation bone marrow smears takes practice. Too much pressure on the coverslips causes cell rupture, making morphologic evaluation impossible. Inadequate pressure prevents the spicule from spreading to a satisfactory monolayer. Bone marrow crush preparations similar to this can be made using regular glass slides instead of coverslips, and the smears are of equal quality.

Automated Slide Making and Staining.   The Sysmex SP-1000i (Sysmex Corporation of America, Mundelein, Ill.) is an automated slide making/staining system available to laboratorians. After the instrument has analyzed a CBC for a specimen, a conveyor moves the racked tube to the SP-1000i,

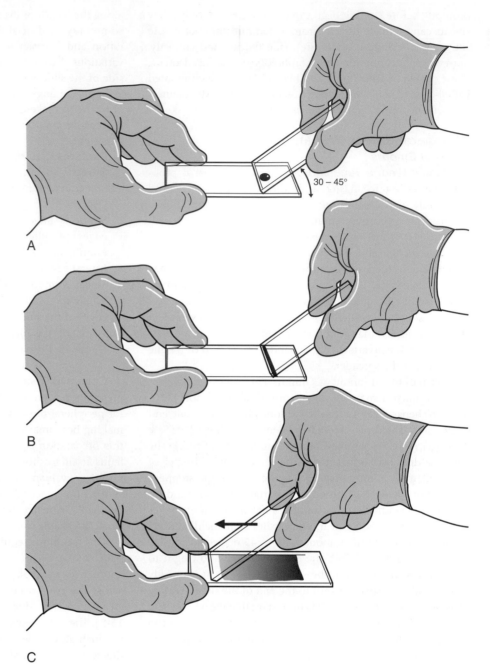

Figure 15-2 Wedge technique of making a peripheral blood smear.

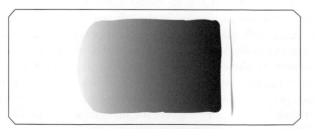

Figure 15-3 Well-made peripheral blood smear.

where the barcode is read. The computer already has determined from the automated results whether a slide is required. Criteria for a manual slide review are determined by each laboratory based on their patient population. Dependent on the Hct reading, the system adjusts the size of the drop of blood used and the angle and speed of the spreader slide in making a wedge preparation. After each blood smear is prepared, the spreader slide is automatically cleaned and ready for the next blood smear to be made. Smears can be made approximately every 30 seconds. Information such as specimen name, number, and date is printed on the slide. The slide is dried, loaded into a cassette, and moved to the stain position, where stain and then buffer and rinse are added at designated times. When staining is complete, the slide is moved to a dry position, then to a collection area where it can be picked up for microscopic evaluation. Smears made off-line, such as bone marrows and cytospin preparations, may be stained on this system as well. Other blood analyzer manufacturers, such as Beckman Coulter (Brea, Calif.), also have automated slide making/staining instrumentation (Fig. 15-6) (Chapter 39).

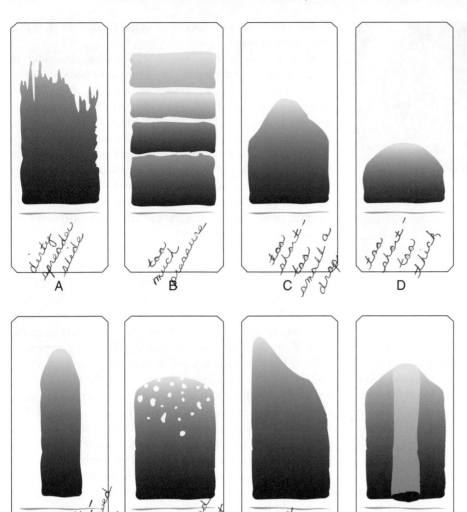

A — dirty spreader slide

B — too much pressure

C — too short — too small a drop

D — too short — too thick

E — bullet shaped — not allowed to spread

F — fat or not dried properly

G — pressure on one side

H — clotted

Figure 15-4   Unacceptable peripheral blood smears.

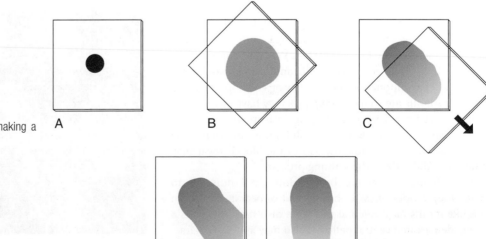

Figure 15-5   Coverslip method of making a peripheral blood smear.

A   B   C

D

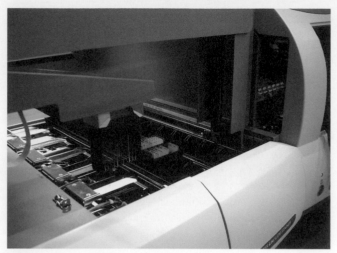

Figure 15-6 COULTER LH slide maker and stainer. (Courtesy of Beckman Coulter, Inc., Brea, Calif.)

Drying of Smears. Regardless of smear preparation method, before staining, all blood smears should be dried as quickly as possible to avoid drying artifact. In some laboratories, a small fan is used to facilitate drying. Blowing breath on a slide is counterproductive because the moisture in breath causes RBCs to become echinocytic (crenated) or develop water artifact (also called *drying artifact*) (see later).

Staining of Peripheral Blood Smears

Pure Wright stain or a Wright-Giemsa stain (Romanowsky stain)[8] is used for staining peripheral blood smears and bone marrow smears. These are considered polychrome stains because they contain both eosin and methylene blue. Giemsa stains additionally contain methylene blue azure. The purpose of staining blood smears is simply to see the cells and evaluate their morphology.

Methanol in the stain fixes the cells to the slide. Actual staining of cells or cellular components does not occur until the buffer is added. The oxidized methylene blue and eosin form a thiazine-eosinate complex, staining neutral components. The buffer that is added to the stain should be 0.05 M sodium phosphate (pH 6.4) or aged distilled water (distilled water placed in a glass bottle for at least 24 hours; pH 6.4-6.8). Staining reactions are pH dependent. Free methylene blue is basic and stains acidic (and basophilic) cellular components, such as RNA. Free eosin is acidic and stains basic (and eosinophilic) components, such as Hb or eosinophilic granules. Neutrophils are so named because they have cytoplasmic granules that have a neutral pH and pick up some staining characteristics from both stains. The slides must be completely dry before staining, or the thick part of the blood smear may come off of the slide in the staining process.

Water/drying artifact has been a long-lived nuisance to hematology laboratories. It has several appearances. It can look like moths have eaten at the RBCs or it may appear as a heavily demarcated central pallor. It also may appear as refractive (shiny) blotches on the RBCs. Other times, it is simply echinocytes (crenation) appearing in the areas of the slide that dried most slowly.

Multiple reasons contribute to this problem. Humidity in the air as the slide dries may add to the punched-out, moth-eaten, or echinocytic appearance of the RBCs. It is difficult to avoid drying artifact on extremely anemic patients' smears because of the very high ratio of plasma to RBCs. Water absorbed from the air into the alcohol-based stain also can contribute. Drying the slide as quickly as possible helps and keeping a stopper tightly on the stain bottle keeps moisture out. In some laboratories, slides are fixed in pure, anhydrous methanol before staining, to help alleviate water artifact. More recently, stain manufacturers use 10% v/v methanol to minimize water/drying artifact.

Wright Staining Methods

Manual Technique. Traditionally, Wright staining has been performed over a sink or pan with a staining rack. Slides are placed on the rack, smear side facing upward. The Wright stain may be filtered before use or poured directly from the bottle through a filter onto the slide (Fig. 15-7). It is important to flood the slide completely. The stain should remain on the slide at least 1 to 3 minutes to fix the cells to the glass. Then an approximately equal amount of buffer is added to the slide. Surface tension allows very little of the buffer to run off. The laboratory professional can blow gently on the slide to mix the aqueous buffer and the alcohol stain. A metallic sheen (or green "scum") should appear on the slide if mixing is correct. More buffer can be added if necessary. The mixture is allowed to remain on the slide for 3 minutes or more (bone marrow smears take longer to stain than peripheral blood smears). The timing may be adjusted to acquire the best staining characteristics. When staining is complete, the slide is rinsed with a steady but gentle stream of neutral-pH water, the back of the slide is wiped to remove any stain residue, and the slide is air dried in a vertical position. Coverslip-type blood smears must be stained by the manual method. These smears are placed on evacuated test tube rubber stoppers on the staining rack over a sink (Fig. 15-8).

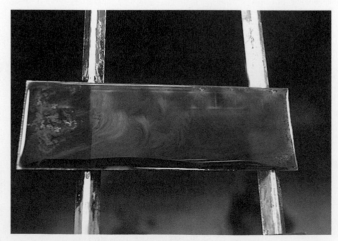

Figure 15-7 Manual Wright staining of slides.

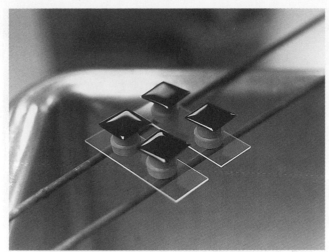

Figure 15-8 Manual Wright staining of coverslips.

The manual Wright staining technique is desirable for staining peripheral blood smears containing very high WBC counts, as in the smears from leukemic patients. As with bone marrow smears, the time can be lengthened easily to enhance the staining required by increased numbers of cells. Understaining is common when a leukemia slide is placed on an automated slide stainer. The main disadvantages of the manual technique are the increased risk of spilling the stain and the slower, more time-consuming procedure. This technique is best suited for low-volume laboratories.

Automated Slide Stainers.   Numerous automated slide stainers are commercially available. For high-volume laboratories, these instruments are essential. When set up and loaded with slides, they have walk-away capabilities. In general, it takes about 5 to 10 minutes to stain a batch of slides. The processes of fixing/staining and buffering are similar in practice to those of the manual method. The slides may be automatically dipped in stain and then in buffer and a series of rinses (Midas II [Fig. 15-9]) or propelled along a platen surface by two conveyor spirals (Hema-Tek [Fig. 15-10]). In the Hema-Tek, stain, buffer, and rinse are pumped through holes in the platen surface, flooding the slide at the appropriate time. Smear quality and color consistency are usually good with any of these instruments. Some commercially prepared stain, buffer, and rinse packages do vary from lot to lot or manufacturer to manufacturer, so testing is recommended. A couple of disadvantages of the batch, dip-type stainers are that (1) when the staining process has begun, stat slides cannot be added to the batch, and (2) working or aqueous solutions of stain are stable only 3 to 6 hours and need to be made often. Stats can be added any time to the Hema-Tek stainer and stain packages are stable for about 6 months.

Quick Stains.   Quick stains, as the name implies, are fast and easy. The whole process takes about 1 minute. The stain is purchased in a bottle as a modified Wright or Wright-Giemsa stain. The needed quantity can be filtered into a Coplin jar or a staining dish, depending on the quantity of slides to be stained. Aged distilled water is used as the buffer. Stained slides are finally rinsed under a gentle stream of tap water and allowed to air dry. It is helpful to wipe off the back of the slide with alcohol to remove any excess stain. Quick stains are convenient and cost-effective for low-volume laboratories, such as clinics and physicians' office laboratories, or whenever rapid turnaround time is essential. Quality of quick stains is often a concern. With a little time and patience for adjusting the staining and buffering times, however, color quality can be acceptable.

Features of a Well-Stained Peripheral Blood Smear. The proper staining of a peripheral blood smear is of equal importance to making a good smear. Macroscopically, a well-stained blood smear should be pink to purple. Microscopically, the RBCs should appear orange to salmon pink; WBC nuclei

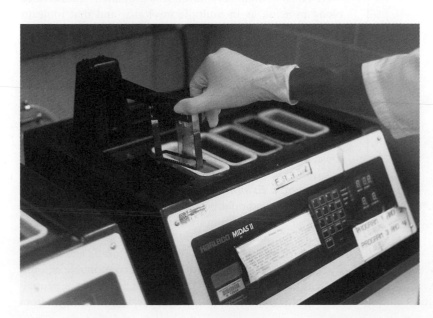

Figure 15-9 Midas II slide stainer (Courtesy of EM Science, Gibbstown, N.J.).

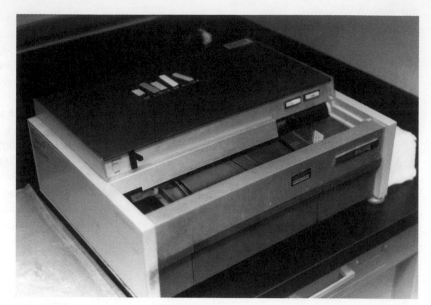

Figure 15-10 Hema-Tek slide stainer (Courtesy of Bayer, Pittsburgh, Penn.).

should be purple to blue. The cytoplasm of neutrophils should be pink to tan with violet or lilac granules. Eosinophils should have bright-orange refractile granules. Faulty staining can be troublesome for reading the smears, from causing minor shifts in color to causing the inability to identify cells and assess morphology. Trying to interpret a poorly prepared or poorly stained blood smear is extremely frustrating. If possible, a newly stained smear should be studied. Hints for troubleshooting poorly stained blood smears are provided in Box 15-1.

BOX 15-1 Troubleshooting Poorly Stained Blood Smears

First Scenario
Problems
RBCs appear gray
WBCs are too dark
Eosinophil granules are gray, not orange

Causes
Stain or buffer is too alkaline (most common)
Inadequate rinsing
Prolonged staining
Heparinized blood sample

Second Scenario
Problems
RBCs are too pale or are red color
WBCs barely visible

Causes
Stain or buffer is too acidic (most common)
Underbuffering (too short)
Over-rinsing

The best staining results are obtained on fresh slides because the blood itself acts as a buffer in the staining process. Slides stained after 1 week or more turn out too blue. In addition, specimens that have increased proteins (i.e., globulins) produce bluer-staining blood smears.

Peripheral Smear Examination

Microscopic blood smear review is essential whenever instrument analysis indicates specimen abnormalities exist. The laboratory professional evaluates the platelet and WBC count and differential, along with WBC, RBC, and platelet morphology.

Macroscopic Examination

Examining the smear before placing it on the microscope stage sometimes can give the evaluator an indication of abnormalities or tests that need rechecking. A smear that is bluer overall than normal may indicate that the patient has increased blood proteins, as in multiple myeloma, and that rouleaux may be seen on the smear. A grainy appearance to the smear may indicate RBC agglutination, as found in cold hemagglutinin diseases. In addition, holes all over the smear could mean the patient has increased lipids and some of the automated CBC parameters should be rechecked for interferences from lipemia. Markedly increased WBC counts and platelet counts can be detected from the blue specks out at the feather edge. Valuable information might be obtained before the evaluator looks through the microscope.

Microscopic Examination

The microscope should be adjusted correctly for blood smear evaluation. The light from the illuminator should be properly centered, the condenser should be almost all the way up and adjusted correctly for the magnification used, and the iris diaphragm should be opened to allow a comfortable amount of light to the eye. Many individuals prefer to use a neutral-density filter over the illuminator to create a whiter light from a tungsten light source. If the microscope has been adjusted for Koehler illumination, all these conditions should have been met (Chapter 4).

10× Objective Examination.　Blood smear evaluation begins with the 10× or low-power objective lens (total magnification = 100×). Not much time needs to be spent at this magnification. However, it is a common error to omit this step altogether and go directly to the higher-power oil-immersion lens. At the low-power magnification, overall smear quality, color, and distribution of cells can be assessed. The feather edge and lateral edges can be checked quickly for WBC distribution. More than four times the number of cells/field at the edges or feather as compared to the monolayer area of the smear indicates that the smear is unacceptable (i.e., a "snowplow" effect), and the smear should be remade. Under the 10× objective, it is possible to check for the presence of fibrin strands; if present, the sample should be rejected, and another one should be collected. RBC distribution can be noted as well. Rouleaux formation or RBC agglutination is easy to recognize at this power. The smear can be scanned quickly for any large abnormal cells, such as blasts, reactive lymphocytes, or even unexpected parasites. Finally, the area available for suitable examination can be assessed.

40× Objective Examination.　The next step is using the 40× high dry objective lens (total magnification = 400×). At this magnification, it is easy to select the correct area of the smear in which to begin the differential and to evaluate cellular morphology. The WBC estimate also can be performed at this power. To perform a WBC estimate, the evaluator selects an area in which two or three RBCs overlap, but most RBCs are separated from one another. The average number of WBCs per high-power field is multiplied by 2000 to get an adequate approximation of the WBC count. If after 8 to 10 fields are scanned, it is determined that there are four to five WBCs per field, this would be a WBC estimate of 8000 to 10,000/mm³ (8-10 × 10⁹/L). This technique can be helpful for internal quality control, although there are inherent errors with the process. Just being too deep (toward the heel) on the slide or too shallow (toward the feather) would affect the estimates. Additionally, field diameters may vary among microscope manufacturers. If a discrepancy exists between the estimate and the instrument WBC, a smear made on the wrong patient's blood sample or a mislabeled smear could be discovered more easily. In many laboratories, WBC estimates are performed on a routine basis; in others, these estimates are performed only as needed to confirm instrument values.

100× Objective Oil-Immersion Examination.　The 100× objective oil-immersion examination is the highest magnification for most standard binocular microscopes (10× eyepiece × 100× objective lens = 1000× magnification). The WBC differential generally is performed under 100× oil immersion. The differential normally includes counting and classifying 100 WBCs as WBC percentages. The RBC, WBC, and platelet morphology evaluation and the platelet estimate also

are performed under the 100× oil-immersion objective lens. At this magnification segmented neutrophils can be differentiated easily from bands. RBC inclusions, such as Howell-Jolly bodies, and WBC inclusions, such as Döhle bodies, can be seen easily if present. Reactive or abnormal cells are enumerated under the 100× lens as well. If present, nucleated RBCs (NRBCs) are counted and reported as NRBCs/100 WBCs (Chapter 14).

50× Objective Oil-Immersion Examination.　The performance of the WBC differential and morphology examinations described for the 100× oil-immersion objective also can be accomplished by experienced morphologists using a 50× oil-immersion objective. The larger field of view allows more cells to be evaluated faster. It is especially efficient for validating or verifying instrument values when a total microscopic assessment of the smear is not needed. Particular cell features that may require higher magnification can be assessed by moving the parfocal 100× objective into place, then returning to the 50× objective to continue the differential. The WBC estimate also can be performed with the 50× objective, but the multiplication factor would be higher than 3000. The observer should conform to the estimation protocol of the particular laboratory.

Optimal Assessment Area.　The tasks described especially for the 100×, 40×, and 50× objectives need to be performed in the best possible area of the peripheral blood smear. That occurs between the thick area, or "heel," where the drop of blood was initially placed and spread, and the very thin feather edge. Microscopically, the RBCs are uniformly and singly distributed, with few touching or overlapping, and have their normal biconcave appearance (central pallor) (Fig. 15-11). An area that is too thin, in which there are holes in the smear and the RBCs look flat, large, and distorted, is unacceptable. A too-thick area also distorts the RBCs by piling them on top of one another like rouleaux (Fig. 15-12). WBCs are similarly distorted, making morphologic evaluation more difficult and classification potentially incorrect. When viewing the correct area of a specimen from a patient with a normal RBC count, there are generally about 200 to 250 RBCs per 100× oil-immersion field.

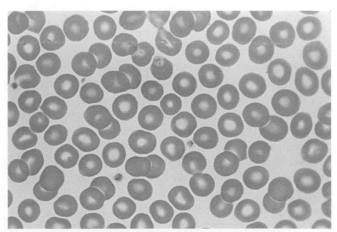

Figure 15-11 Photomicrograph of good area of smear.

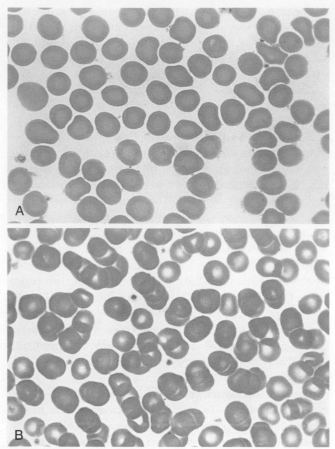

Figure 15-12 Photomicrograph of areas too thin **(A)** and too thick **(B)** to read.

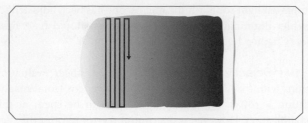

Figure 15-13 "Battlement" pattern for performing a differential.

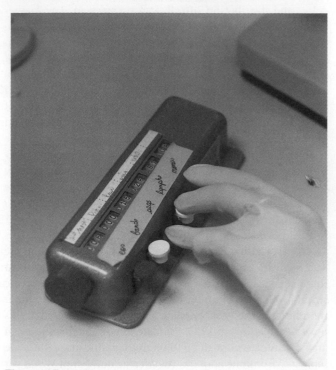

Figure 15-14 Clay Adams laboratory counter (Courtesy of Clay Adams, division of Beckman Coulter, Inc., Parsippany, N.J.).

Although mentioned in Chapter 4, a common "problem" encountered with the oil-immersion objective lens is worth mentioning again. If the blood smear was in focus under 10× and 40×, but is impossible to bring into focus under 100×, the slide is probably upside down. The 100× objective does not have sufficient depth of field to focus through the slide. The oil must be completely removed before the smear is put on the stage right side up.

Performance of White Blood Cell Differential. Fewer manual differentials are performed today because of the superior accuracy found in automated differentials and because of cost and time constraints. When indicated, however, the manual differential always should be performed in a systematic manner. When the correct area has been selected, a back-and-forth serpentine, or "battlement," track pattern is preferred for minimizing distribution errors (Fig. 15-13)[9] and ensuring that each cell is counted only once. One hundred WBCs are counted and classified through the use of push-down button counters (Fig. 15-14) or newer computer-interfaced touch pads (Fig. 15-15). To increase the accuracy, it is advisable to count at least 200 cells when the WBC count is greater than $40 \times 10^9/L$. The results are reported as percentages: for example, 54% seg-

mented neutrophils, 6% bands, 28% lymphocytes, 9% monocytes, 3% eosinophils. The evaluator always should check to ensure the sum of the percentages is 100%.

Performing 100 cell differentials on extremely low WBC counts can become tedious and time-consuming. This is one instance in which the 50× oil-immersion objective can be useful in simply helping to find the cells. In some laboratories, the WBCs are concentrated, and buffy coat smears are made. In others, evaluators perform a 25- or 50-cell differential, multiply the results by 4 or 2 to get a percentage, and document that this was done. The accuracy of this practice is questionable, however, and such counts should be avoided if possible. It is important to include the side margins of the blood smear in any differential so that the larger cells, such as monocytes, reactive lymphocytes, and immature cells, are not excluded.

In addition to counting the cells, their appearance is assessed. If present, WBC abnormalities such as toxic granulation, Döhle bodies, reactive lymphocytes, and Auer rods

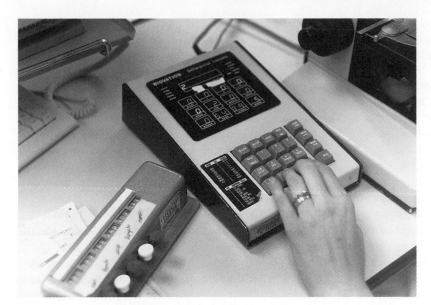

Figure 15-15 Biovation differential counter (ISYS/Biovation, Orlando, FL).

(Chapter 28) are evaluated and reported. The exact method in which these are reported varies from laboratory to laboratory. Reactive lymphocytes may be reported as a separate percentage of the 100 cells, as a percentage of the total number of lymphocytes that are reactive, or semiquantitatively (occasional to many). Toxic granulation generally is reported as present or semiquantitatively (slight to marked, or 1+ to 3+). Standardization of this process has been difficult. Regardless of reporting format, each laboratory should establish criteria for quantifying microscopic cell morphology.

Because the differential alone provides only partial information, the absolute cell counts are calculated for each cell type (see later) in some laboratories. Automated differentials already include this step.

Red Blood Cell Morphology.   RBC morphology is an important part of the blood smear evaluation, including an assessment of the cell size, variability in size (anisocytosis), cell color, cell shape (poikilocytosis), and cellular inclusions (Chapter 18). Some laboratories use specific terminology for reporting the degree of abnormal morphology, such as slight, moderate, or marked, or a scale from 1+ to 3+. Other laboratories have instituted a summary statement regarding the overall RBC morphology that is consistent with the RBC indices. The latter method is becoming more popular with the increased computer interfacing in most laboratories. Regardless of the reporting method, the microscopic RBC morphology should be congruent with the information given by the automated parameters. If not, further investigation is needed.

Platelet Estimate.   As previously mentioned, the platelet estimate is performed under the 100× oil-immersion objective lens. In an area of the smear where the RBCs barely touch, the number of platelets in 10 oil-immersion fields is counted. The average number of platelets per oil-immersion field × 20,000 approximates the platelet count. For example, 12 to 16 platelets per oil-immersion field would equal about 280,000 platelets/mm^3 (280 × 10^9/L) and would be considered adequate. A rougher estimate states that if there are 7 to 25 platelets per oil-immersion field, the platelet count is adequate, provided that there are approximately 200 RBCs per oil-immersion field. In situations in which the patient is anemic or has erythrocytosis, however, the relative proportion of platelets to RBCs is altered. In these instances, a more involved formula for platelet estimates may be used:

$$\frac{\text{Average no. of platelets/field} \times \text{total RBC count}}{200 \text{ RBCs/field}}$$

(200 is the average number of RBCs per oil-immersion field in the optimal assessment area.)

Regardless of whether an "official" estimate is done, verification of the instrument platelet count should be included in the overall examination. Blood smear examination also includes an assessment of the morphology of the platelets, including enlarged size and granularity/overall appearance.

As mentioned in Chapter 4, immersion oils with different viscosities do not mix well. If slides are taken to another microscope for review, oil should be wiped off first.

SUMMARIZING COMPLETE BLOOD COUNT RESULTS

To this point, this chapter has focused on slide preparation and performance of a differential cell count. The differential is only the capstone, however, on a panel of tests collectively called the *CBC* that includes many of the routine tests described in Chapter 14. Having completed the discussion of the testing for the component parts, interpretation of the results for the total panel can now be discussed.

The CBC has evolved over time to the typical test panel reported today including assessment of WBCs, RBCs, and platelets. The CBC provides information about the hematopoietic system, but because abnormalities of blood cells can be caused by diseases of other organ systems, the CBC also contributes to screening those organs for disease. The CBC provides such valuable information about a patient's health status that it is the most frequently ordered laboratory test performed by clinical laboratory scientists and laboratory technicians.

The process of interpreting the CBC test results has two phases. In phase 1, the numbers and description generated by the testing are summarized using appropriate terminology. This summary provides a verbal picture of the numbers that is easy to communicate to the physician or another laboratorian. It is so much more convenient to be able to say, "The patient has a microcytic anemia" than to say, "The Hb was low, and the MCV was also low." Phase 2 of interpretation is to recognize a pattern of results consistent with various diseases and be able to narrow the diagnosis for this patient or perhaps even pinpoint it so that appropriate follow-up testing can be recommended.

The following discussion focuses on phase 1 of CBC interpretation—how to collect the pertinent information and summarize. Phase 2 of the interpretation is the essence of the remaining chapters of this text on various hematologic conditions or other metabolic conditions that have an impact on the hematologic system.

Organization of Complete Blood Count Results

Today, most laboratorians perform CBCs on sophisticated, automated analyzers described in Chapter 39, but the component tests can be performed using manual methods described in Chapter 14. The blood smear assessment described in this chapter is also part of a CBC. The CBC "panel" is essentially divided into WBC, RBC, and platelet parameters.

For phase 2 interpretation, it is sometimes important to look at all three groupings of the CBC results; other times, only one or two may be of interest. If a patient has an infection, the WBC parameters may be the only ones of interest. If the patient presents with anemia, all three sets—WBCs, RBCs, and platelets—may require assessment. Generally, all the parameters interpreted together provide the best information, so a complete summary of the results should be generated.

Assessment of Hematology Results Relative to Reference Ranges

Proper performance of the phase 1 summarization of test results requires assessment of the patient values compared with the normal reference ranges. Examination of the table of reference values for the CBC on the inside cover of this text shows that there are different reference ranges for men and women, particularly for the RBC parameters. There also are different ranges for children of different ages, most notable in the WBC changes. It is important to select the appropriate set of reference values in hematology for the gender and age of the patient.

Several strategies can help in determining the significance of results. First, if the results are very far from the reference range, it is more likely that they are truly outside the range and represent a pathologic process. Second, if two or more diagnostically related parameters are slightly or moderately outside the range in the same direction (both high or both low), it suggests the results are clinically significant and associated with some pathologic process. Because some healthy individuals always have results outside the range, the best comparison for their results is not the reference range, but their own results from a prior time when they were known to be healthy.

Summarizing White Blood Cell Parameters

The WBC-related parameters of a routine CBC include the following:
1. Total WBC count (WBC $\times 10^9$/L)
2. WBC differential count expressed as percentages—relative counts
3. WBC differential count values expressed as the actual number of each type of cell (e.g., neutrophils $\times 10^9$/L)—absolute counts
4. WBC morphology

Step 1

Start by looking at the total WBC. When the count is elevated, it is called *leukocytosis*. If the WBC count is low, it is called *leukopenia*. As described later, increases and decreases of WBCs are associated with infections and conditions such as leukemias. Because there is more than one type of WBC, increases and decreases in the total count are usually due to changes in one of the subtypes. Determining which one is the next step.

Step 2

Step 2 is to examine the relative differential counts for a preliminary assessment of which cell lines are affected. The relative differential is reported in percentages. The proportion of each cell type can be described by its relative number (i.e., percent) and compared with its reference range. Then it is described using appropriate terminology, such as a relative neutrophilia, which is an increase of neutrophils, or a relative lymphopenia, which is a decrease of lymphocytes. The terms used for increases and decreases of each cell type are provided in Table 15-1.

TABLE 15-1 Terminology for Increases and Decreases of White Blood Cells

Cell Type	Increases	Decreases
Neutrophil	Neutrophilia	Neutropenia
Eosinophil	Eosinophilia	N/A
Basophil	Basophilia	N/A
Lymphocyte	Lymphocytosis	Lymphopenia (lymphocytopenia)
Monocyte	Monocytosis	Monocytopenia

TABLE 15-2 Comparison of Relative and Absolute White Blood Cell Counts

Complete Blood Count Parameter	Patient Value	Reference Range	Interpretation Relative to Reference Range	Summary
WBC	13.6	$4.3\text{-}10.8 \times 10^9/L$		Leukocytosis
Relative differential				
Neutrophils	67	48-70%	WRR	
Lymphocytes	26	18-42%	WRR	
Monocytes	3	1-10%	WRR	
Eosinophils	3	1-4%	WRR	
Basophils	1	0-2%	WRR	
Absolute differential				
Absolute neutrophils	9.1	$2.4\text{-}8.2 \times 10^9/L$	Elevated	Absolute neutrophilia
Absolute lymphocytes	3.5	$1.4\text{-}4 \times 10^9/L$	WRR	
Absolute monocytes	0.4	$0.1\text{-}1.2 \times 10^9/L$	WRR	

WRR, within reference range

If the total count is outside the range or if any of the relative values are outside the range, further analysis of the WBC differential is needed. If the proportion of one of the cell types increases, the others must decrease—that is, they are relative to one another. The second cell type may not have changed in actual number at all. The way to assess this accurately is with absolute differential counts.

Step 3

Absolute counts can be calculated easily using the total WBC count and the relative differential. Multiply each relative cell count (i.e., percentage) by the total WBC count and in so doing determine the absolute count for each.

Examine the set of WBC parameters from a CBC in Table 15-2. On first inspection, one may look at the WBC and recognize this is a leukocytosis, but it is important to determine what cell line is causing the increased count. In this case, the cells are all within normal reference ranges, relative to one another. There is no indication as to which cell line could be causing the increase in total numbers of WBCs.

When each relative number (e.g., neutrophils at 0.67 or 67%) is multiplied by the total WBC count ($13.6 \times 10^9/L$), the absolute numbers indicate that the neutrophils are elevated ($9.1 \times 10^9/L$ compared with the reference range provided). The absolute lymphocyte count ($3.5 \times 10^9/L$) is still normal. From this information, this blood picture is described as showing a leukocytosis with only an absolute neutrophilia, and the overall increase in the WBC count is due to an increase in only the neutrophils. This provides a concise summary of the WBC counts without the need to refer to every type of cell. Box 15-2 extends this concept to a convention used to describe the neutrophilic cells.

When the absolute numbers of each of the individual cells are totaled, it equals the WBC count (slight differences may

---

BOX 15-2 Summarizing Neutrophilia When Young Cells Are Present

A subtle convention in assessing the differential counts has to do with the presence of young cell types. The young cells of the granulocytic series (e.g., bands, metamyelocytes) typically are lumped together with the mature neutrophils to judge whether there is neutrophilia. For example, look at the following differential and the reference ranges provided:

Neutrophils (also called *granulocytes*)—65 (48-70%)

Bands—18 (0-10%)

Lymphocytes—13 (18-42%)

Monocytes—3 (1-10%)

Eosinophils—1 (1-4%)

Basophils—0 (0-2%)

Although the mature neutrophils are within the reference range, the bands exceed their range. The total of the two (65% + 18%) exceeds the upper limit of neutrophilic cells even when the two ranges are combined (70% + 10%), so this would be described as a *neutrophilia* (or granulocytosis) even though the neutrophils themselves are within range. See Step 4 of Summarizing White Blood Cell Parameters for how to communicate the increase in bands.

---

occur due to rounding, as in the example). This is a method for checking whether the absolute calculations are correct. Absolute counts may be obtained directly from automated analyzers which absolute counts and calculate relative values. Some laboratories do not report the absolute counts, so being able to calculate them is important.

As will be evident in later chapters, this particular example points toward a bacterial infection. Had there been an absolute lymphocytosis, a viral infection would be likely.

Step 4

Each cell line should be examined for immature cells. Young WBCs are not normally seen in the peripheral blood, and they may indicate infections or malignancies such as leukemia. For neutrophilic cells, there is a unique term that refers to having too many bands or having cells younger than bands present: *left shift* (Box 15-3).

The presence of young lymphocytic or monocytic cells could be reported in the differential as prolymphocytes, lymphoblasts, promonocytes, or monoblasts. Young eosinophils and basophils are typically just called *immature* and are not staged.

Because they possess a nucleus, NRBCs do not lyse during testing and can be counted as WBCs, falsely increasing the WBC count. Depending on the laboratory's instrumentation and protocol, a correction factor may need to be applied to obtain an accurate WBC when NRBCs are noted in the morphology (Chapter 14).

Step 5

Any abnormalities of appearance are reported in the morphology section of the report. For WBCs, abnormal morphologic features that would be noted may include changes in overall cellular appearance, such as reactive (atypical) lymphocytes or cytoplasmic inclusions. An example might be the presence of toxic granulation or vacuolization of the neutrophils or Döhle bodies. The clinical significance of these cytoplasmic changes is discussed in Chapter 28.

To summarize the WBC parameters, begin with the total WBC, followed by the relative differential, or preferably the absolute counts, noting whether any abnormal young cells are present in the blood. Finally, note the presence of any abnormal morphology or inclusions.

Summarizing Red Blood Cell Parameters

RBC parameters are as follows:
1. RBC count (RBC × 10^{12}/L)
2. Hb (g/dL)
3. Hct (% or L/L)
4. Mean cell volume (MCV, fL)
5. Mean cell Hb (MCH, pg)
6. Mean cell Hb concentration (MCHC, % or g/dL)
7. RBC distribution width (RDW, %)
8. Morphology

Step 1

Step 1 is to examine the Hb (or Hct) for anemia or polycythemia. Anemia is the more common condition. Together, these parameters sometimes are called the *H&H*. If the RBC morphology is relatively normal, three times the Hb approximates the Hct; this is "the rule of 3" (Chapter 14). If the rule of 3 holds, it creates the expectation that the following assessments would find normal RBC parameters. If the rule of 3 fails and all test results are reliable, further assessment should uncover some patient RBC abnormalities.

Step 2

When the Hb and Hct have been inspected and the rule of 3 applied, the next RBC parameter that should be evaluated is the MCV (Chapter 14). This value provides the average RBC volume. The MCV correlates to the morphologic appearance of the cells using the classification first introduced by Wintrobe a century ago (Table 15-3).

The MCV is expected to be within the established reference range (approximately 80-100 fL), and the RBC morphology is expected to be normal (normocytic). For a patient with anemia, classifying the anemia morphologically by the MCV narrows the range of possible causes to microcytic, normocytic, or macrocytic anemias.

Step 3

Step 3 is to examine the MCHC to evaluate how well the cells are filled with Hb. If the MCHC is below the reference range, the cells are called *hypochromic*, meaning too little color. This correlates to a larger central pallor (hypochromia) when examined on a Wright-stained smear. Otherwise, the cells are said to be *normochromic* and should show the typical pallor in the central third of the cells.

It is possible for the MCHC to be elevated in three conditions. A slight elevation may be seen when cells are spherocytic. They retain roughly normal volume but have decreased surface area, and the Hb is slightly more concentrated than usual. A more dramatic increase in MCHC can be due to interference from lipemia or icterus that falsely elevates the Hb and subsequently the calculation of the MCHC (Chapter 14).

Step 4

The RDW is determined from the histogram of the RBC. Briefly, when the volume of the RBCs is variable (more small cells, more large cells, or both), the histogram becomes wider.

BOX 15-3 Origin of the Phrase *Left Shift*

The origin of *left shift* came from a 1920s publication of Josef Arneth, in which neutrophil maturity was correlated to segment count. A graphical representation was made, and the fewer the segments, the further left was the median, hence *left shift*. This was called the Arneth Count or Arneth-Schilling Count and was abandoned around the time Arneth died in 1955, but the term *left shift* lived on as an indication of infection.

TABLE 15-3 Interpretation of Mean Cell Volume Values Using the Wintrobe Terminology

Mean Cell Volume Value	Wintrobe Description
Within reference range	Normocytic
Less than reference range	Microcytic
Greater than reference range	Macrocytic

The width of the histogram, the RDW, is reflected statistically as the coefficient of variation (CV) or the standard deviation (SD). Several analyzer manufacturers provide a CV and an SD, and the operator can select which to report.

The RDW provides information about the presence and degree of anisocytosis. What is important is increased values only, not decreased values. If a CV reference range is 10.5% to 14.5% and a patient has an RDW of 20.6%, the patient has a more heterogeneous RBC population with more variation in cell volume (anisocytosis).

If the RDW is elevated, a notation about anisocytosis is expected in the morphologic evaluation of the blood smear. Many individuals find that using the MCV along with the RDW provides the most helpful information (Chapters 18 and 39).

Step 5

Step 5 is to examine the morphology for pertinent abnormalities. Whenever anemia is indicated from the analyzer's RBC parameters, and potential abnormal RBC morphology is suggested by the indices and rule of 3, a Wright-stained peripheral blood smear must be examined. Abnormalities include (1) size, (2) shape, (3) inclusions, (4) young RBCs, (5) color, and (6) arrangement (Chapter 18). The blood smear also serves as quality control because the morphology seen through the microscope (e.g., microcytosis, anisocytosis) should be congruent with the results provided by the analyzer. When they do not agree, further investigation is necessary.

If everything is normal, there is no notation of morphology. Any notation in the morphology requires scrutiny. All RBC-related morphology should be noted, including poikilocytosis (abnormal shapes) and the presence of RBC inclusions, such as Howell-Jolly bodies.

When young RBCs are present, it suggests that the bone marrow is attempting to respond to an anemia. Polychromasia on the peripheral blood smear suggests bone marrow response. This is the bluer color of reticulocytes that have entered the bloodstream earlier than usual to try to improve oxygen-carrying capacity. If the anemia is quite severe, NRBCs also may be present. As noted earlier, it is also important to recognize NRBCs because they may falsely elevate the WBC count.

A better way to assess replacement erythropoiesis is with reticulocyte count and subsequent calculation of reticulocyte production index if appropriate. The reticulocyte count is not normally part of the CBC, although it is now performed on the same analyzers. If the reticulocyte count is available with the CBC, its interpretation can improve the assessment of young RBCs (Chapter 14).

Step 6

Step 6 is to examine the remaining RBC count and MCH.

On a practical level, the RBC count is not the parameter used to judge anemia because there are some instances of anemia, such as the thalassemias, when the RBC count is normal or even elevated. This inconsistency (low Hb and high RBC count) is helpful diagnostically.

The MCH follows the MCV, so for that reason it is less often used. In the instances when the MCH does *not* follow the MCV, the MCHC detects the discrepancy between size and Hb content of the cell. The MCH is not crucial to the assessment of anemia when the other parameters are provided.

In summary, when evaluating the RBC parameters of the CBC, examine the Hb first, then look at the MCV, RDW, and MCHC. Finally, take note of any abnormal morphology.

Summarizing Platelet Parameters

The platelet parameters of the CBC are as follows:
1. Platelet count ($\times 10^9$/L)
2. Mean platelet volume (MPV) (fL)
3. Morphology

Step 1

The platelets should be examined for increases (thrombocytosis) or decreases (thrombocytopenia) outside the established reference range. A patient who has presented with unexplained bruising or bleeding may have a decreased platelet count. The platelet count should be assessed along with the WBC and Hb to determine whether all three are decreased (pancytopenia) or increased (pancytosis). Pancytopenia is clinically significant in that it could indicate a possible developing acute leukemia or aplastic anemia. Pancytosis frequently is associated with a diagnosis of polycythemia vera.

Step 2

Step 2 is to examine the MPV to judge platelet size. The MPV is included on most automated analyzers. For interpretive purposes, this parameter, although analogous to platelets as MCV is to RBCs, is used only in certain situations, such as hematology-oncology practices. When there is thrombocytopenia and the bone marrow is responding by producing younger, larger platelets, the MPV may be elevated. There may be a connection between platelet diameter and consumptive coagulopathy; however, due to the fact that there is a wide physiologic variation in the MPV of normal subjects and that platelets swell in EDTA specimens, the MPV is of questionable significance.[10] Some instruments give a "large" platelet count, and others are developing a "reticulated platelet" count as an indication of thrombopoiesis.

Step 3

Step 3 is to examine the morphology and platelet arrangement. Although the MPV can recognize abnormally large platelets, the morphologic evaluation also notes this. Some laboratories distinguish between large/enlarged platelets (two times normal) and giant platelets (more than twice as large as normal) or by comparison to RBC size.

Additional morphologic descriptors include assessment of granularity, which is most important if missing and is described as "hypogranular" or "agranular." Sometimes the abnormalities are too variable to classify, and they are described simply as "bizarre." In some cases, platelets can be clumped or adherent to WBCs, and these arrangements should be noted. As described previously, corrective actions can be taken to derive accurate platelet and WBC counts when these arrangements are observed on the smear.

Summarizing the platelets includes assessment of total number, their size by either instrument MPV or morphology, and their appearance. Box 15-4 gives an example of how the entire CBC can be summarized using the steps described.

When a CBC is properly summarized, and no information has been overlooked, there is confidence that the phase 2 interpretation of the results will be reliable. A methodical approach to examining each parameter ensures that the myriad information available from the CBC can be used effectively and efficiently in patient care. Box 15-5 summarizes the systematic approach to CBC interpretation.

BOX 15-4 Applying a Systematic Process to Complete Blood Count Summarization

A man has the following CBC results (refer to the reference ranges inside the front cover of this book):

WBC—3.20×10^9/L
RBC—2.10×10^{12}/L
Hb—8.5 g/dL
Hct—26.3%
MCV—125.2 fL
MCH—40.5 pg
MCHC—32.3 g/dL
RDW—20.6%
Platelets—115×10^9/L
Differential in percentages:
   Neutrophils—43
   Bands—2
   Lymphocytes—45
   Monocytes—10
Morphology: hypersegmentation of neutrophils, anisocytosis, macrocytes, macro-ovalocytes, occasional teardrop, Howell-Jolly bodies, and basophilic stippling.

The step-by-step assessment of the WBCs indicates a leukopenia. Although the relative differential values are all within the reference range, calculation of absolute counts indicates an absolute neutropenia and lymphopenia. No unexpected young WBCs are noted, but the morphology indicates hypersegmentation of neutrophils. For the RBCs, a quick look at the Hb (8.5) indicates that this person is anemic. Inspection of the MCV indicates macrocytosis because the MCV is increased to greater than 100 fL, the upper limit of the reference range. A quick examination of the MCHC shows it is normal, so this blood picture would be described as *macrocytic, normochromic.* The elevated RDW indicates substantial anisocytosis. There is no mention of polychromasia, so no young RBCs are seen. The morphologic description supports the interpretation of the RDW with mention of anisocytosis due to macrocytosis and poikilocytosis characterized by macro-ovalocytes and occasional teardrop cells. Howell-Jolly bodies and basophilic stippling are RBC inclusions worth noting. The platelet count indicates thrombocytopenia. Although an MPV is not reported, the platelets are of normal size and show no morphologic abnormalities because there are no notations in the morphology.

BOX 15-5 Systematic Approach to Complete Blood Count Interpretation

White Blood Cells

Step 1. Examine the WBC for variations in total number of WBCs.
Steps 2 and 3. Examine the differential information (relative and absolute) on variations in the distribution of WBCs.
Step 4. Make note of immature cells in any cell line reported in the differential that should not appear in normal peripheral blood.
   • Nucleated RBCs may require correction of the WBC count
Step 5. Make note of any morphologic abnormalities and correlate smear findings to the numerical values.

Red Blood Cells

Step 1: Examine the Hb first to judge anemia.
Step 2: Examine the MCV to assess cell size.

Step 3: Examine the MCHC to assess cell Hb concentration.
Step 4: Examine the RDW to assess anisocytosis.
Step 5: Examine the morphology description and correlate with the numerical values.
Step 6: Review remaining information.

Platelets

Step 1. Examine the total platelet count.
Step 2. Examine MPV to assess platelet size.
Step 3. Examine platelet morphology and correlate with the numerical values.

CHAPTER at a GLANCE

- Although fewer manual peripheral blood smear evaluations are performed today, much valuable information still can be obtained from a well-made and well-stained smear.
- The specimen of choice for routine hematology testing is whole blood collected in a lavender (purple)-top evacuated tube. The tube additive is EDTA, which anticoagulates the blood by chelating plasma calcium.
- Only rarely does EDTA create analytical problems with certain individuals' blood. EDTA-induced platelet clumping or satellitosis causes automated analyzers to report falsely decreased platelet counts (pseudothrombocytopenia) and falsely increased WBC counts (pseudoleukocytosis). This problem must be recognized by blood smear examinations and the proper course of action followed to produce accurate results.
- Numerous methods exist for making peripheral blood smears; however, the manual wedge smear technique is used most frequently.
- Learning to make consistently good smears takes practice. The basic technique can be modified as needed to accommodate patients with very high or very low Hcts.

- The routine stain used in hematology is Wright or Wright-Giemsa. Staining of all cellular elements occurs when the pH-specific buffer is added to the stain already on the slide. Staining reactions depend on pH of the cells or cellular components.
- Wright staining is done manually, by larger automated techniques, or by quick stains, depending on venue and number of slides.
- Peripheral blood and bone marrow smears always should be evaluated in a systematic manner, beginning with the 10× objective lens and finishing with the 100× oil-immersion objective lens. Leukocyte differential and morphology evaluation, RBC and platelet morphology evaluation, and platelet number estimate all are included.
- Using a systematic approach to CBC interpretation ensures that all valuable information is assessed and nothing is overlooked. The systematic approach to CBC interpretation is summarized in Box 15-5.

Now that you have completed this chapter, go back and read again the case study at the beginning and respond to the questions presented.

REVIEW QUESTIONS

1. A laboratory science student consistently makes wedge technique blood smears that are too long and thin. What change in technique would improve the smears?
   a. Increasing the downward pressure on the pusher slide
   b. Decreasing the acute angle of the pusher slide
   c. Decreasing the size of the drop of blood used
   d. Increasing the acute angle of the pusher slide

2. When a blood smear is viewed through the microscope, the RBCs appear redder than normal, the neutrophils are barely visible, and the eosinophils are bright orange. What is the most likely cause?
   a. The slide was overstained.
   b. The stain was too alkaline.
   c. The buffer was too acidic.
   d. The slide was not rinsed adequately.

3. A stained blood smear is held up to the light and observed to be bluer than normal. What microscopic abnormality might be expected on this smear?
   a. Rouleaux
   b. Spherocytosis
   c. Reactive lymphocytosis
   d. Toxic granulation

4. A laboratorian using the 40× objective lens sees the following numbers of WBCs in 10 fields: 8, 4, 7, 5, 4, 7, 8, 6, 4, 6. Which of the following WBC counts most closely correlates with the estimate?
   a. 1.5×10^3 μL
   b. 5.9×10^3 μL
   c. 11.8×10^3 μL
   d. 24×10^3 μL

5. A very anemic patient with an RBC count of 1.25×10^6 μL has an average of seven platelets per oil-immersion field. Which of the following values most closely correlates with the estimate per cubic millimeter (or microliter)?
   a. 14,000
   b. 44,000
   c. 140,000
   d. 280,000

6. A patient with a normal RBC count has an average of 10 platelets per oil-immersion field. Which of the following values best correlates with the estimate per cubic millimeter?
   a. 20,000
   b. 100,000
   c. 200,000
   d. 400,000

7. What is the absolute count ($\times 10^9$/L) for the lymphocytes if the total WBC count is 9.5×10^9/L and there are 37% lymphocytes?
   a. 3.5
   b. 6.5
   c. 13
   d. 37

8. EDTA-induced pseudothrombocytopenia can be identified on a blood smear by:
   a. Finding the platelets pushed to the feathered end
   b. Finding the platelets adhering to WBCs
   c. Finding no platelets at all on the smear
   d. A bluish discoloration to the macroscopic appearance of the slide

9. Use a systematic approach to summarizing the WBC parameters of the CBC presented in the case study at the beginning of Chapter 34. Use the reference ranges provided inside the front cover of this text.

10. Use a systematic approach to summarizing RBC parameters of the CBC presented in the case study at the beginning of Chapter 19.

REFERENCES

1. Kennedy JB, Maehara KT, Baker AM: Cell and platelet stability in disodium and tripotassium EDTA. Am J Med Technol 1981;47:89-93.
2. Perkins SL: Examination of the blood and bone marrow. In Greer JP, Foerster J, Lukens J, et al (eds): Wintrobe's Clinical Hematology, 11th ed. Philadelphia: Lippincott, Williams & Wilkins, 2004:3-26.
3. Shahab N, Evans ML: Platelet satellitism. N Engl J Med 1998;338:591.
4. Bartels PC, Schoorl M, Lombarts AJ: Screening for EDTA-dependent deviations in platelet counts and abnormalities in platelet distribution histograms in pseudothrombocytopenia. Scand J Clin Lab Invest 1997;57:629-636.
5. Lombarts A, deKieviet W: Recognition and prevention of pseudothrombocytopenia and concomitant pseudoleukocytosis. Am J Clin Pathol 1988;89:634-639.
6. De Caterina M, Fratellanza G, Grimaldi E, et al: Evidence of a cold immunoglobulin M autoantibody against 78 kD platelet gp in a case of EDTA-dependent pseudothrombocytopenia. Am J Clin Pathol 1993;99:163-167.
7. Diff-safe. Available at: http://www.alpha-scientific.com/Diff-safe.html. Accessed March 9, 2006.
8. Power KT: The Romanowsky stains: a review. Am J Med Technol 1982;48:519-523.
9. MacGregor RG, Scott RW, Loh GL: The differential leukocyte count. J Pathol Bacteriol 1940;51:337-368.
10. Ryan DH: Examination of the blood. In Lichtman MA, Beutler E, Kipps TJ, et al (eds): Williams Hematology, 7th ed. New York: McGraw-Hill, 2006;14:11-19.

Bone Marrow Overview

16

John R. Krause

OBJECTIVES

After completion of this chapter, the reader will be able to:

1. Compare the location of red marrow at various age intervals.
2. Specify sites for bone marrow aspirate and biopsy in children and adults.
3. Discuss indications for bone marrow sampling.
4. Discuss advantages of bone marrow aspirate plus biopsy.
5. Describe the procedure for bone marrow aspirate and biopsy.
6. Summarize the purpose of examination of bone marrow under low-power and oil-immersion microscopy.
7. Describe in general the differences in cytologic features of hematopoietic cells found in the aspirate and core biopsy specimen.
8. Describe features of osteoblasts and osteoclasts, and differentiate them from similar cells found in bone marrow.
9. Characterize features of tumor cells.
10. List the three components of a bone marrow evaluation.
11. Discuss the importance of a systematic approach to bone marrow review in total patient assessment.
12. Calculate the myeloid-to-erythroid (M:E) ratio from the results of a cellular description of the bone marrow, and state the normal M:E ratio for an adult.
13. Describe the types of cells seen in normal bone marrow and their relative numbers.

CASE STUDY

After studying the material in this chapter, the reader should be able to respond to the following case study:

A patient presented with weakness, fatigue, and malaise. Hemoglobin was 7.5 g/dL, hematocrit was 21%, RBCs were 2.5×10^{12}/L, WBCs were 30×10^9/L, and platelets were 540×10^9/L. The WBC differential revealed 70% mature neutrophils, 20% immature neutrophils, 5% basophils, 1% eosinophils, and 4% lymphocytes. Bone marrow examination indicated 90% myeloid precursors and 10% erythroid precursors. There were 4 megakaryocytes per high-power field.

1. What aspect of the bone marrow provides information on normal blood cell production?
2. What is the M:E ratio in this patient and what does it indicate?
3. Are megakaryocytes normally seen in the bone marrow?

In adults, bone marrow occupies 3.4% to 5.9% of total body weight, which translates into roughly 1600 to 3700 g.[1] At birth, nearly all the bones in the body contain hematopoietic (red) marrow. In the fifth to seventh year, fat cells (yellow marrow) begin to replace the red marrow in the long bones of the extremities, and by adulthood the hematopoietic tissue becomes limited to the axial skeleton and the proximal portions of the extremities.[2] The site chosen for bone marrow sampling depends on the age of the patient. Most aspirates and biopsy samples of marrow are now obtained from the iliac crest (posterior superior iliac spine) (Fig. 16-1). In adults, the anterior iliac crest also can be used, and occasionally the ribs or vertebrae can be sampled, particularly if a suspicious lesion is seen on a radiograph. A good cellular aspirate can be obtained from the sternum at the second intercostal space, but obtaining a biopsy sample from this structure is not recommended because of the underlying heart and great vessels. In children younger than 1 year old, the anteromedial (front and middle) surface of the tibia is sometimes used.

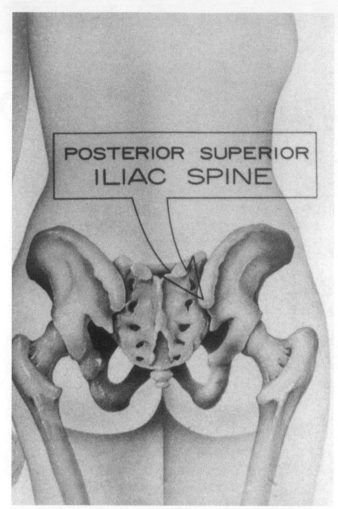

Figure 16-1 Bone marrow biopsy site. The posterior superior iliac spine is a good site for obtaining the aspirate smear and core biopsy specimen. (From Ellis LD, Jensen WJ, Westerman MP: Needle biopsy of bone and marrow. Arch Intern Med 1964;114:213. Copyright 1964, American Medical Association.)

BONE MARROW ASPIRATION AND BIOPSY

The arrangement of red marrow and its relationship to the central artery is illustrated in Fig. 7-3. Marrow fills the spaces between the trabeculae of bone in the marrow cavity and is soft and semifluid. It is amenable to sampling. A bone marrow sample usually consists of two parts: the aspirate and the core biopsy specimen. Aspiration provides a specimen that is useful for determining the cytologic types and proportions of hematopoietic cells in the marrow. The core biopsy provides another dimension and is extremely useful for determining cellularity and the anatomic relationship of cells to fat and connective tissue stroma. The core biopsy is particularly important for evaluating diseases that characteristically produce focal lesions, rather than diffuse involvement of the marrow, such as Hodgkin lymphoma, non-Hodgkin lymphoma, multiple myeloma, metastatic tumor, amyloid, and granulomas. It also allows evaluation of bone spicules, which may reveal changes in hyperparathyroidism or Paget disease.[3] A core biopsy is mandatory for the so-called dry tap on aspiration (no cells obtained), which may be the result of true hypocellularity (aplastic anemia), fibrosis, or the marrow cavity being too "tightly packed" with cells (leukemia) to yield a specimen.

Indications for Bone Marrow Exam

There are no hard and set rules that determine which patient would require a bone marrow examination. Each case must be evaluated in light of all clinical and laboratory information to determine whether this invasive procedure is necessary. A bone marrow examination is not required in cases of anemia when the etiology is apparent by red blood cell (RBC) indices and other laboratory tests, such as low serum iron and ferritin levels in iron deficiency anemia and low vitamin B_{12} and folate levels in megaloblastic anemia. When multilineage abnormalities are present in the peripheral blood, a bone marrow examination is generally necessary. Circulating blasts also generally necessitate a marrow examination except in newborns and infants with infection. Bone marrow examination is required for virtually all pancytopenic patients except those known to be receiving marrow-suppressive therapy. Likewise, a marrow examination is necessary for staging purposes in Hodgkin lymphoma, non-Hodgkin lymphoma, and carcinoma. The only major contraindication to bone marrow examination is failure to meet the appropriate indicative criteria. Bone marrow examination should be performed only when it is essential for diagnosis or patient management.

Bone Marrow Procedure

The most common and familiar needles used for marrow sampling include the Jamshidi (Kormed, Minneapolis, Minn.) and the Westerman-Jensen (Becton Dickinson, Franklin Lakes, N.J.). The use of these needles makes it possible to obtain a core of bone and its enclosed marrow. Then, by means of an attached syringe, the bone marrow aspirate can be obtained. The Jamshidi needle is shown in Figure 16-2. These needles are now disposable and are used only once before being properly discarded. The procedure using the Westerman-Jensen needle is illustrated in Figure 16-3. The procedure is similar using the Jamshidi needle. A Snarecoil biopsy needle also is available (Kendall Co., Mansfield, Mass.). The Snarecoil has a coil mechanism at the needle tip that allows for capture of the bone marrow specimen without redirection of the needle (Fig. 16-4).

For the biopsy procedure, the patient is placed in the right or left lateral decubitus position (lying on the right or left side). Universal [standard] precautions are observed throughout the procedure. The skin area to be penetrated is cleansed with a disinfectant and draped. The skin, dermis, and subcutaneous tissue are infiltrated with a local anesthetic solution, such as 1% or 2% lidocaine or procaine through a 25-gauge needle, producing a 5-mm to 1-cm papule (bubble). The 25-gauge needle is replaced with a 21-gauge needle, which is inserted through the papule to the periosteum. With the point of the needle on the periosteum, approximately 2 mL of anesthetic is injected over a dime-sized area as the needle is rotated, after which the anesthesia needle is withdrawn. Next, a 3-mm skin incision is made over the biopsy site with a No. 11 scalpel

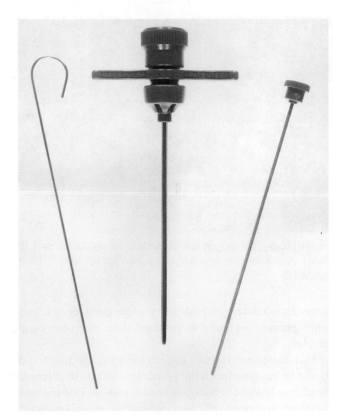

Figure 16-2 Jamshidi biopsy/aspiration needle. These needles are now disposable and come in a sterile package.

blade to facilitate insertion of the biopsy needle. Following this, the biopsy needle with the obturator locked in place is inserted through the skin and bone cortex. A rotating movement eases the anterior advancement of the needle.

A subtle decrease in resistance is felt as the medullary cavity of the bone is entered; the stylet is removed. A 10- to 20-mL syringe is attached, and 1 to 2 cc of marrow is aspirated. Aspirated particles are expelled from the syringe onto glass coverslips that have been washed previously in 70% ethanol. Each coverslip is quickly tilted, or the excess blood is removed with a small capillary tube, leaving pale gray-white marrow fragments and a small amount of blood. A second coverslip is placed on top of the first and a smear is made by pulling the coverslips apart in a sliding motion. Some practitioners prefer to use two alcohol-cleansed microscope slides in a manner similar to that described for coverslips (Chapter 15). Additional specimens may be taken at this time for flow cytometric analysis, cytogenetics, or other studies as deemed necessary. Marrow aspirates are stained with a polychrome dye, usually Wright or Wright-Giemsa stain.

When the aspirate has been taken, the cutting blades of the biopsy device are inserted into the outer cannula and are advanced until the medullary cavity is entered. The cutting blades are pressed into the medullary bone, with the outer cannula held firmly in a stationary position. After this, the outer cannula is advanced over the cutting blades with entrapment of the tissue, and the entire unit is withdrawn. The

Figure 16-3 Biopsy technique with the use of the Westerman-Jensen needle. (From Ellis LD, Jensen WJ, Westerman MP: Needle biopsy of bone and marrow. Arch Intern Med 1964;114:213. Copyright 1964, American Medical Association.)

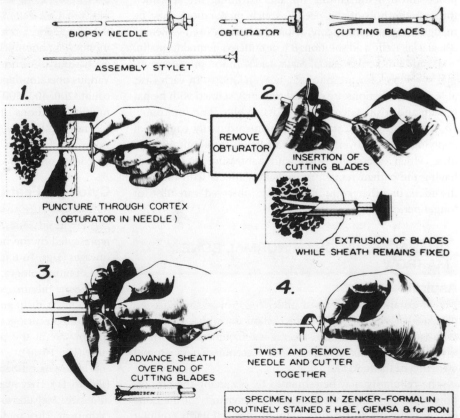

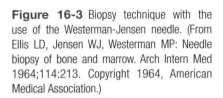

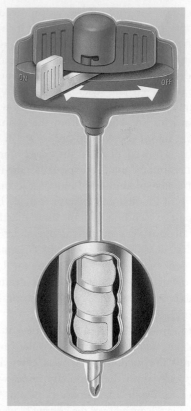

Figure 16-4 Snarecoil bone marrow biopsy needle. (Courtesy of Tyco Healthcare/Kendall, Mansfield, Mass.)

marrow core inside the needle is removed by inserting the probe through the cutting tip and extruding the specimen through the hub of the needle. Touch preparations may be made from the marrow core before the latter is fixed in Zenker 5% glacial acetic acid solution, B5, or buffered neutral formalin.

Fixation in Zenker glacial acetic acid solution provides optimal specimens for morphologic interpretations. In each case, at least three sections are cut and routinely stained with hematoxylin and eosin, Giemsa, and Prussian blue stain for iron.

After biopsy, the care of the patient ordinarily consists of applying pressure over the posterior ileum for about 60 minutes, which is accomplished with a pressure dressing and having the patient remain recumbent. Patients with bleeding disorders or other complications are observed carefully for longer periods.

CHARACTERISTICS OF NORMAL BONE MARROW

Aspirate

The preparation is examined under low power to detect the presence of bone spicules, which stain dark blue or purple (Fig. 16-5). A bone marrow spicule is a fragment of relatively intact marrow that consists of the hematopoietic and stromal elements of the marrow.

The cellularity may be estimated by observing the proportion of cells to empty fat vacuoles in the vicinity of the bone spicules. The smear is evaluated for relative cellularity (cellular

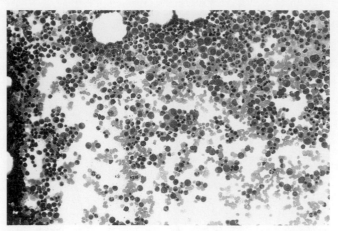

Figure 16-5 Bone marrow aspirate specimen shows cellular area that would provide a good site for cytologic evaluation and cell counting (Wright stain, ×100).

versus hypocellular) and adequacy of megakaryocytes, but a better estimate of both is obtained from the core biopsy sample.

After low-power microscopic examination, the preparation should be examined with the oil-immersion lens to determine the various types of hematopoietic cells present. Under normal situations, numerous cell types are usually present. Because the distribution pattern may be irregular, it is preferable to count 300 to 500 nucleated cells to obtain a reliable differential count and to determine the myeloid-to-erythroid (M:E) ratio, both of which are useful parameters in evaluating marrow function. The M:E ratio represents the number of granulocytic cells to erythroid precursors. All granulocytic cells, including blasts that are determined to be myeloid (by cytochemistry or flow cytometry), are included. Lymphocytes, plasma cells, monocytes, nonmyeloid blasts, and nonhematopoietic cells are excluded. All nucleated erythroid precursors are counted. Various operator-dependent factors include how many cells to count (200, 400, 500) and whether to count in one location or multiple locations of the preparation. For adults, the normal M:E range is 1.5:1 to 3.3:1 with a mean of 2.3:1.[4] Other normal values are found in the bone marrow report form (see Fig. 16-23 and on the inside cover of this text).

Cytologic Features

Most cells in the normal bone marrow consist of the myeloid and erythroid series. The myeloid (or granulocytic) series is represented by the neutrophilic, eosinophilic, and basophilic lineages (Figs. 16-6 to 16-9; see Chapters 8 and 12 for description of morphology). Although some laboratories differentiate erythrocyte precursors, others simply report nucleated erythroid cells. Others distinguish pronormoblasts and group all other erythroid precursors together. Most normoblasts in the normal marrow are at the polychromatophilic or the orthochromic stage (Fig. 16-10).

The largest cells in the normal marrow are megakaryocytes (Fig. 16-11). They may be pleomorphic in nuclear morphology and size. Megakaryoblasts have a single nucleus with blue cytoplasm. They undergo a process called *endomitosis* (nuclear

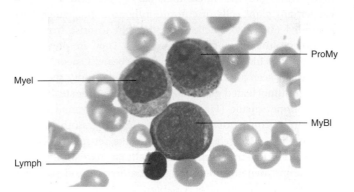

Figure 16-6 Bone marrow aspirate specimen. Cells present include a myeloblast (MyBl), promyelocyte (ProMy), myelocyte (Myel), and lymphocyte (Lymph) (Wright stain, ×1000).

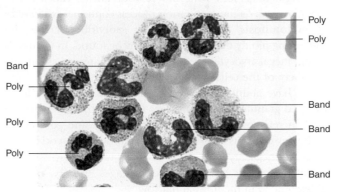

Figure 16-9 Bone marrow aspirate specimen. Cells present include bands and polymorphonuclear (Polys) granulocytes (Wright stain, ×1000).

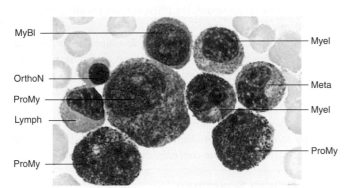

Figure 16-7 Bone marrow aspirate specimen. Cells present include a myeloblast (MyBl), promyelocytes (ProMy), two myelocytes (Myel), a metamyelocyte (Meta), an orthochromic normoblast (OrthoN), and a lymphocyte (Lymph) (Wright stain, ×1000).

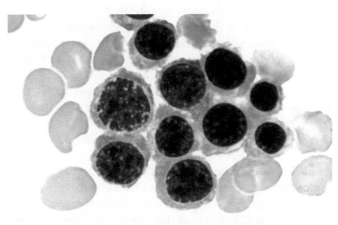

Figure 16-10 Bone marrow aspirate specimen shows a nest of nucleated RBC precursors with polychromatophilic and orthochromic normoblasts (Wright stain, ×1000).

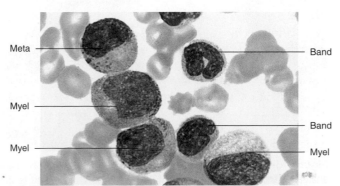

Figure 16-8 Bone marrow aspirate specimen. Cells present include myelocytes (Myel), a metamyelocyte (Meta), and bands (Wright stain, ×1000).

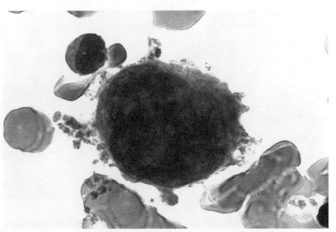

Figure 16-11 Bone marrow aspirate specimen shows a megakaryocyte with platelet budding (Wright stain, ×1000).

division without cytoplasmic division) one or two times, yielding a larger cell with two to four nuclei, called a *pro-megakaryocyte*. As the maturation process continues with cycles of endomitosis, large cells with polylobulated nuclei containing ploidy of 8, 16, and 32 may be found. In the developing megakaryocytes, red granules first appear about the periphery of the cells (platelets). The most mature megakaryocytes have abundant pink cytoplasm that is diffusely filled with red granules. The terms *stage I, II,* and *III* sometimes are used in reference to the degree of maturity and correspond to the designations of megakaryoblast, promegakaryocyte, and granular megakaryocyte. (See Chapter 13 for discussion of megakaryopoiesis.) Megakaryocyte stages usually are not differentiated in the normal marrow.

Abnormal megakaryocytes with small mononuclear, binuclear or bilobed nuclei, and abundant hypogranular cytoplasm are often seen in the bone marrow of individuals with myelodysplastic syndromes. Increased numbers of large polyploid megakaryocytes are more indicative of myeloproliferative disorders. Increased numbers of normal-appearing megakaryocytes are seen in idiopathic thrombocytopenic purpura. Megakaryocytes with multiple nonconnected nuclei (multinucleated cells) sometimes are found in individuals with megaloblastic anemias.

Osteoblasts and osteoclasts, occasionally seen in the bone marrow, are important to note because of their similarity to other cells. Osteoblasts are the cells responsible for the formation and remodeling of bone. They are derived from bone lining or endosteal cells. When dislodged from bone, they resemble plasma cells (Fig. 16-12). Osteoblasts have eccentric round-to-oval nuclei and abundant blue, mottled cytoplasm. They also may have a clear area within the cytoplasm, but not the well-defined "hof" seen in the plasma cell. Osteoblasts also lack secretory granules. Osteoblasts usually are found in a single cluster, and it would be unusual to find large numbers of these in the aspirate, in contrast to plasma cells, which would be diffusely present in the marrow. Osteoclasts are large cells

with multiple, evenly spaced nuclei, which should distinguish them from polylobulated megakaryocytes and from the Langerhans giant cells of chronic inflammation, which have palisaded nuclei. Osteoclasts are thought to arise from progenitor multilineage myeloid stem cells. They are physiologically responsible for the resorption of bone. Osteoclasts are most easily seen and recognized in the core biopsy specimen, being multinucleated giant cells close to the endosteal surface of the bone spicule (Fig. 16-13). The other stromal cells of the marrow consist of adipocytes (fat cells), endothelial cells that line blood vessels and fibroblast-like reticular cells. The stromal cells together with the extracellular matrix provide the suitable microenvironment for the maturation and proliferation of hematopoietic cells (Chapter 7).

A Prussian blue iron stain is commonly done on the aspirate smear, core biopsy, or both. Figure 16-14 illustrates normal iron, absent iron, and increased iron stores in aspirate smears. Caution in interpretation of iron stores in the core biopsy must be heeded because decalcifying agents used to soften the core biopsy during processing may leech iron stores from the biopsy, giving a false impression of decreased or absent iron stores. For this reason, the aspirate is favored for interpretation of iron stores if sufficient spicules are present for evaluation.

While scanning under the low-power objective, one should be alert for abnormal clusters of cells, such as metastatic tumor or lymphoid aggregates. In scanning for tumor cells, the observer should look for the presence of clusters of molded cells (syncytia) (Fig. 16-15). Tumor cell nuclei are usually darkly stained (hyperchromatic) and vacuoles are seen frequently in the cytoplasm. Tumor cell clusters are often found at or near the edge of the coverslip or glass slide.

Core Biopsy Specimen

The core biopsy specimen provides an intact portion of the bone marrow for examination. A typical specimen is approximately $\frac{3}{4}$ inch in length $\times$ $\frac{1}{16}$ to $\frac{1}{18}$ inch in diameter and

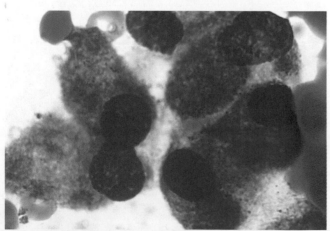

Figure 16-12 Bone marrow aspirate specimen shows a cluster of osteoblasts that superficially resemble plasma cells. Osteoblasts have round-to-oval eccentric nuclei and mottled blue cytoplasm that is devoid of secretory granules. They may have a clear area within the cytoplasm but lack the well-defined "hof" of the plasma cell (Wright stain, ×1000).

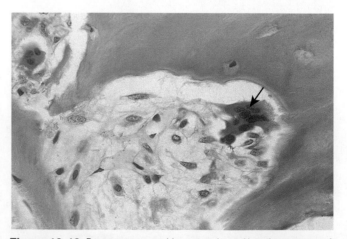

Figure 16-13 Bone marrow core biopsy specimen. Note the presence of a large multinucleated cell near the endosteal surface of bone. This is an osteoclast, which is a cell involved in resorption of bone. The spindle-shaped cells are fibroblasts. This specimen is from a patient with hyperparathyroidism (hematoxylin and eosin, ×400).

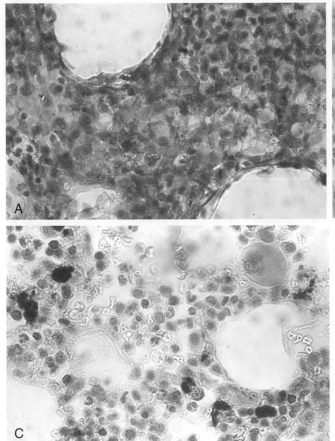

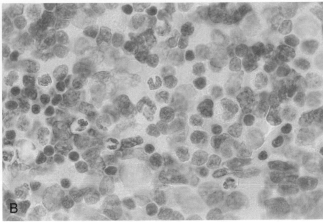

Figure 16-14 Prussian blue stain on bone marrow aspirates. **A,** Normal iron stores (Prussian blue, ×400). **B,** Absent iron stores (Prussian blue, ×400). **C,** Increased iron stores (Prussian blue, ×400).

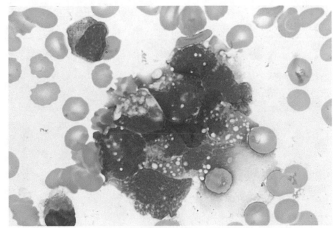

Figure 16-15 Bone marrow aspirate specimen shows a cluster or syncytia of tumor cells. Nuclei are irregular and hyperchromatic, and vacuoles are found within the cytoplasm of many cells. Cytoplasmic margins are not well delineated (Wright stain, ×400).

weighs about 150 mg; it represents only a minute fraction of the total body marrow. In most instances, however, the specimen is a representative sample of the total marrow picture as pertains to cellularity, the proportion of myeloid and erythroid cells present, and iron stores. There may be considerable variation within the sample, so the entire core should be examined.

Examples of hypocellular and hypercellular core biopsy specimens are illustrated for comparison with normocellular marrow in Figure 16-16. As described previously in the illustrations, the marrow is fixed in Zenker solution and sections are cut and stained with hematoxylin and eosin, Giemsa, and Prussian blue stain (for iron). The value of the Giemsa stain lies in its ability to stain differentially cells of the myeloid, lymphoid, and plasma cell series.[3]

Neutrophilic myelocytes and metamyelocytes are recognized in Giemsa-stained marrow by the light-pink appearance of the cytoplasm. Mature neutrophils and bands are recognized by their smaller size and darkly stained, C-shaped nuclei (bands) or multiple nuclear lobes (polys); the cytoplasm of these mature cells may be a very light pink or may not seem to stain at all (Fig. 16-17). Myeloblasts and promyelocytes have oval or round nuclei with cytoplasm that stains blue (Fig. 16-18). It may be difficult to differentiate these cells from pronormoblasts other than through the tendency of the latter to cluster with more mature normoblasts. The cytoplasm of eosinophils has a more intense red staining and these cells are easily recognized as the most brightly stained cells of the marrow (see Fig. 16-17). Basophils cannot be recognized on marrow specimens fixed with Zenker solution.

The more mature or older normoblasts have centrally placed, round nuclei that stain intensely, being so dark that light does not penetrate the nucleus to any extent (Fig. 16-19). The cytoplasm of these cells is not appreciably stained, but the

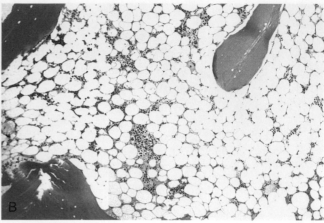

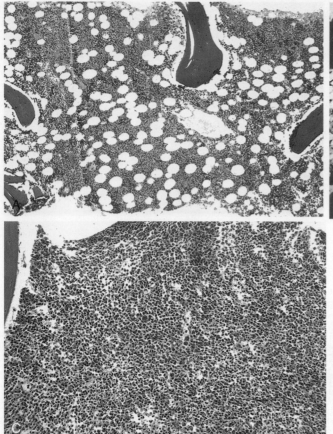

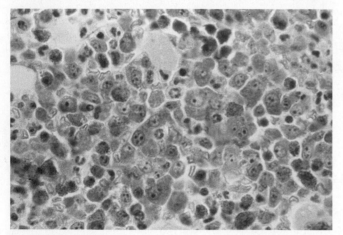

Figure 16-16 A, Representative sample of a core biopsy that may be obtained with biopsy needle. Cellularity is better estimated from the core biopsy specimen, which in this case is approximately 50% fat and 50% cellularity (hematoxylin and eosin, ×40). **B,** Hypocellular bone marrow core biopsy specimen from a patient with aplastic anemia. Only fat and connective tissue cells are found (hematoxylin and eosin, ×100). **C,** Hypercellular bone marrow specimen from a patient with chronic myelogenous leukemia. There is virtually 100% cellularity with no marrow fat visible (hematoxylin and eosin, ×100). (**B** Courtesy of Dennis P. O'Malley, MD, Medical Director, US LABS, Irvine, Calif.)

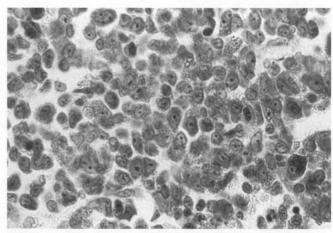

Figure 16-17 Bone marrow core biopsy specimen shows granulocytic area with myelocytes, metamyelocytes, bands, polymorphonuclear granulocytes, and eosinophils (dark red) (Giemsa, ×400).

Figure 16-18 Core biopsy specimen shows infiltration with blasts (blue cytoplasm) and a few myelocytes (pink cytoplasm) (Giemsa, ×400).

plasma membrane margin is often clearly discerned, giving the cells a "fried egg" appearance. Normoblasts have a tendency to cluster in small groups and are often recognized easily at lower power.

Lymphocytes are among the most difficult cells to recognize in the core biopsy specimen, other than when they occur in clusters. In the latter situation, the small, round, mature lymphocytes have a speckled nuclear chromatin in a small, round nucleus, along with a scant amount of blue cyto-

plasm (Fig. 16-20). More immature lymphocytes have larger round or lobulated nuclei but still only a small rim of blue cytoplasm.

Plasma cells can be difficult to distinguish from myelocytes in hematoxylin and eosin–stained sections but are recognized with Giemsa staining as cells with eccentric dark nuclei and blue cytoplasm with a pale, perinuclear Golgi zone ("hof") located next to the nucleus (Fig. 16-21). Plasma cells characteristically are located around blood vessels.

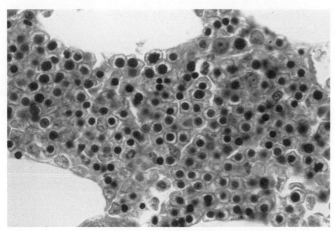

Figure 16-19 Erythroid island in bone marrow core biopsy specimen. Late-stage normoblasts often have a "fried egg" appearance (Giemsa, ×400).

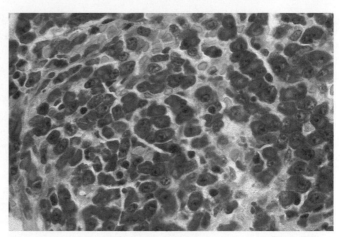

Figure 16-21 Collection of plasma cells in a core biopsy specimen. Nuclei are eccentric and a cytoplasmic clearing, or "hof," can be seen (Giemsa, ×400).

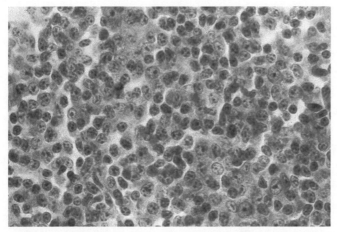

Figure 16-20 Bone marrow core biopsy specimen with lymphoid collection. Most lymphocytes are small and mature. A few lymphocytes are immature with a larger nucleus that contains a single prominent nucleolus (Giemsa, ×400).

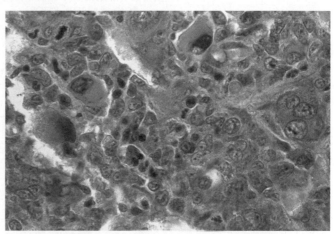

Figure 16-22 Bone marrow core biopsy specimen containing many large polylobated megakaryocytes and increased blasts (Giemsa, ×400).

Megakaryocytes are easily recognized as the largest cells of the marrow and have a characteristic polylobulated nucleus. The nucleus of older megakaryocytes becomes smaller and more darkly stained on hematoxylin and eosin staining. The cytoplasm varies from a light pink in younger cells to a dark pink in older cells (Fig. 16-22). Numbers of megakaryocytes are assessed more accurately by the biopsy. Under low power, there should be two to eight megakaryocytes per low-power field (10×). Using the 40× objective, there should be one to three megakaryocytes per high-power field.[3] Greater than 10 per low-power field would be considered increased.

BONE MARROW REPORTS

A bone marrow evaluation should include examination of the peripheral blood smear, the bone marrow aspirate, and the bone marrow core biopsy specimen. Each of these is important in the total assessment of the patient, and they complement one another. A systematic approach is recommended in eval-

uating each patient. This is especially useful in the training of clinical laboratory scientists, interns, residents, and fellows because it emphasizes the need to examine all facets of the bone marrow and not just to focus on a single abnormality, missing any associated or incidental findings.

The peripheral blood is examined first. The examination includes RBC morphology (e.g., size, shape, inclusions), white blood cell (WBC) numbers and morphology, and platelets (estimate and morphology). Examination of the peripheral blood often helps considerably in interpreting bone marrow findings. (See Chapter 15 for a discussion of the examination of peripheral blood smears.) The bone marrow aspirate smear is examined next. With recognition of the variability that occurs if only a small area of the aspirate is examined, a 300-cell (or more) differential count is done in a cellular area close to a bone spicule. The results of the differential count are related to the impression of the smear as a whole and then to the core biopsy specimen. Finally, the core biopsy specimen is examined. Because of the sample size obtained with the procedure discussed, the cellularity and M:E ratio of biopsy samples tend to be more representative than the aspirate smear and provide numerous other advantages that have been mentioned previously.[3] A systematic approach in examining the marrow smear or core biopsy includes evaluation of the following:

1. Cellularity
2. M:E ratio
3. Maturation of myeloid series
4. Maturation of erythroid series (normoblastic/megaloblastic)
5. Eosinophils/basophils, including mast cells
6. Megakaryocytes
7. Presence of other cells—lymphocytes, plasma cells, histiocytes, osteoclasts, fibroblasts

8. Stromal abnormalities (e.g., granulomas, fibrosis, necrosis, serous atrophy of fat)
9. Hemosiderin content
10. Vessel abnormalities (e.g., amyloid deposits)
11. Bone changes (e.g., Paget disease, osteodystrophy)

The final step is correlation of all results into a diagnosis, using morphologic features and supplementary laboratory and clinical material as available (Fig. 16-23). After the diagnosis, comments or notes may be added, especially if a differential diagnosis is involved or a definite diagnosis cannot be established. Finally, recommendations are offered for additional studies.

UNIVERSITY HEALTH CENTER OF PITTSBURGH
CENTRAL HEMATOLOGY LABORATORY
BONE MARROW REPORT

ASP. NO. H-92-000

NAME _____ LOCATION 11300-00   BX. NO. S-92-000

UNIT NO. 100-00-000   PHYSICIAN _____ DATE 02/01/92

CLIN. HX. 82 year old male with anemia.

MARROW DIFFERENTIAL: %

NEUTROPHIL SERIES:	MEAN	± 2 S.D.	PATIENT	ERYTHROID SERIES:	MEAN	± 2 S.D.	PATIENT
Blast	1	0-2	1	Total NRBC	26	15-37	24
Promyelocyte	3	2-5	2	Pronormoblast	1	0-2	29
Myelocyte	13	9-17	8				
Metamyelocyte	16	7-25	12	LYMPHOCYTE	16	8-24	1
Band	12	9-15	7	PLASMA CELL	1	0-4	1
PMN	7	3-11	9	MONOCYTE	1	0-2	1
				OTHER CELLS		1	
EOSINOPHIL SERIES:							
Myelocyte	1	0-2	1				
Band	1 ⟩3	0-2 ⟩1-7	1	M: E RATIO	2.3:1	1.5-3.3:1	0.8:1
Eosinophil	1	0-3	3				

PATIENT HEMATOLOGIC VALUES

HGB: 5.8   gms; HCT 15.8   %; MCV: 114.2 fL: MCH: 34.2 pq ; WBC: 3,160   /mm³;

Plts: 87,000   /mm³

IMPRESSION

PB: The RBC's are normochromic with prominent anisocytosis. Many macrocytes, microcytes, are present including oval forms. The WBC differential is: polys 66% (2086), bands 1% (32), lymphs 25% (790), monos 5% (158), eos 3% (95). Several multilobed (6 and 7 lobes) polys are seen. The platelets are reduced in number.

BMA: Cellular spicules are present. The M:E ratio is 0.8:1. Myeloid maturation is megaloblastic with giant bands and metamyelocytes present. Erythroid maturation is megaloblastic with numerous promegaloblasts. Megakaryocytes are present.

BMBX: The trabeculae are nomal. The cell to fat ratio is 40-60%. The M:E ratio is approximately 1:1. There is a preponderance of large round to polygonal cells (promegaloblasts) containing vesicular nuclei, 1-3 basophilic nucleoli and a small to moderate amount of amphophilic cytoplasm. Megakaryocytes are seen 0-1 per hpf. Iron stores are markedly increased.

DX: 1. Peripheral blood with macrocytic anemia, thrombocytopenia and mild leukopenia.
2. Bone marrow aspirate and bone marrow biopsy with erythroid predominance and marked megaloblastic changes.
3. Bone marrow biopsy with increased iron stores.

NOTE: There are striking megaloblastic features in this case. B12 and folate levels will be necessary to determine the type of megaloblastic anemia.

RESIDENT   PATHOLOGIST

Figure 16-23 Sample of bone marrow report, including normal values. HGB, hemoglobin; HCT, hematocrit; MCV, mean cell volume; MCH, mean cell hemoglobin; WBC, WBC count; Plts, platelet count; PB, peripheral blood; BMA, bone marrow aspirate; BMBX, bone marrow biopsy; DX, diagnosis.

CHAPTER at a GLANCE

- Bone marrow evaluation is a valuable adjunct to peripheral blood smear examination when hematologic diseases are suspected.
- The site chosen for bone marrow sampling depends on the age of the patient and whether both an aspirate and a biopsy specimen are desired.
- The necessity for a bone marrow examination should be evaluated in light of all clinical and laboratory information. In anemias in which the etiology is apparent from the RBC indices, a bone marrow examination is not required. Examples of indications for bone marrow examination include multilineage abnormalities in the peripheral blood, pancytopenia, circulating blasts, and for staging purposes in lymphomas and carcinomas.
- To determine a reliable differential count, 300 to 500 nucleated cells should be counted on the aspirate preparation. The normal M:E ratio in adults is 1.5:1 to 3.3:1.
- Most cells in the normal bone marrow are myeloid and erythroid. Other cells that may be observed are osteoblasts and osteoclasts, fat cells, and endothelial cells.

- A low-power scan of the aspirate should be performed, looking carefully for metastatic tumor cells or lymphoid aggregates. Tumor cell clusters are often found near the edge of the slide.
- The core biopsy provides a representative sample of total marrow cellularity, the proportion of myeloid to erythroid cells present, and iron stores. Because the process of decalcifying the biopsy specimen may leech iron stores, it is preferable to use the aspirate for this assessment if sufficient spicules are present.
- The bone marrow evaluation should include examination of the peripheral blood smear, bone marrow aspirate, and core biopsy, with correlation of all the results.

Now that you have completed this chapter, go back and read again the case study at the beginning and respond to the questions presented.

REVIEW QUESTIONS

1. The preferred site for bone marrow biopsy in an adult is the:
   a. Second intercostal space on the sternum
   b. Any of the thoracic vertebrae
   c. Anterior or posterior iliac crest
   d. Anterior head of the femur

2. The aspirate should be examined under low power to assess all of the following *except*:
   a. Number of megakaryocytes
   b. Cellularity
   c. Presence of tumor cells
   d. Morphology of abnormal cells

3. The normal M:E ratio range in adults is:
   a. 1.5:1 to 3.3:1
   b. 5.1:1 to 6.2:1
   c. 8.6:1 to 10.2:1
   d. 10:1 to 12:1

4. Most normoblasts in the normal marrow are:
   a. Pronormoblasts
   b. Pronormoblasts and basophilic normoblasts
   c. Basophilic and polychromatophilic normoblasts
   d. Polychromatophilic and orthochromic normoblasts

5. Cells occasionally seen in the bone marrow that are responsible for formation of bone are:
   a. Plasma cells
   b. Osteoblasts
   c. Osteoclasts
   d. Macrophages

6. The largest cell found in a normal bone marrow aspirate is the:
   a. Osteoblast
   b. Megakaryocyte
   c. Myeloblast
   d. Pronormoblast

7. All of the following are indications for a bone marrow evaluation *except*:
   a. Pancytopenia (reduced numbers of RBCs, WBCs, and platelets in the peripheral blood)
   b. Blasts detected in the peripheral blood differential count
   c. Anemia with RBC indices corresponding to a low serum iron and low ferritin
   d. Staging for Hodgkin lymphoma

8. In a bone marrow biopsy specimen, the RBC precursors were estimated to account for 40% of the cells in the marrow, and the other 60% were granuloctye precursors. The M:E ratio on this sample would be:
   a. 1:2
   b. 4:6
   c. 3:1
   d. 1.5:1

9. On a bone marrow biopsy sample several large cells with multiple nuclei were noted. They were located close to the endosteum and their nuclei were evenly spaced throughout the cell. These cells are:
   a. Osteoclasts
   b. Adipocytes
   c. Adventitial reticular cells
   d. Megakaryocytes

10. The advantage of a core biopsy sample of bone marrow compared with an aspirate is that the core sample:
   a. Can be acquired by a less invasive collection technique
   b. Permits assessment of the architecture and cellular arrangement
   c. Is better for the assessment of bone marrow iron stores with Prussian blue stain
   d. Retains the staining qualities of basophils owing to the use of Zenker fixative

REFERENCES

1. Mechanik N: Untersuchungen uber das Gewicht des Knochenmarkes des Menschen. Z Gesamte Anat 1926;79:58.
2. Kent DL, Larson EB: Magnetic resonance imaging of the brain and spine: is clinical efficacy established after the first decade? Ann Intern Med 1988;108:402-424.
3. Krause JR: Bone Marrow Biopsy. New York: Churchill Livingstone, 1981.
4. Perkins SL: Examination of the blood and bone marrow. In Greer JP, Foerster J, Lukens JN, et al (eds): Wintrobe's Clinical Hematology, 11th ed. Philadelphia: Lippincott, Williams & Wilkins, 2004:3-21.

ADDITIONAL RESOURCES

Farhi DC, Chai CC, Edelman AS, et al: Pathology of Bone Marrow and Blood Cells. Philadelphia: Lippincott, Williams & Wilkins, 2004.
Foucar K: Bone Marrow Pathology, 2nd ed. Chicago: ASCP Press, 2001.
Naeim F: Pathology of Bone Marrow, 2nd ed. Philadelphia: Lippincott, Williams & Wilkins, 1998.
Ryan DH, Cohen HJ: Bone marrow examination. In Hoffman R, Benz EJ, Shattil SJ, et al (eds): Hematology Basic Principles and Practice, 4th ed, Philadelphia: Churchill Livingstone, 2005:2656-2671.

Body Fluids in the Hematology Laboratory

17

Leilani Collins

OUTLINE

OBJECTIVES

After completion of this chapter, the reader will be able to:

1. Describe the method for performing cell counts on body fluids.
2. Given a description of a body fluid for cell counting, choose appropriate diluting fluid, select counting area, and calculate and correct counts (if necessary).
3. Discuss the gross appearance of body fluids, including proper terminology, its significance, and its practical use in determining cell count dilutions.
4. Discuss the advantages and disadvantages of cytocentrifuge preparations.
5. Differentiate between traumatic spinal tap and cerebral hemorrhage on the basis of cell counts and appearance of uncentrifuged and centrifuged specimens.
6. Identify from written descriptions normal cells found in cerebrospinal, serous, and synovial fluids.
7. Describe the characteristics of benign versus malignant cells in body fluids and recognize written descriptions of each.
8. Identify crystals in synovial fluids from written descriptions, including polarization.
9. Describe the process of obtaining bronchoalveolar lavage (BAL) samples, including safety precautions for analysis; state the purpose of BAL; and recognize types of cells that normally would be encountered.
10. Differentiate exudates and transudates based on formation (cause), specific gravity, protein concentration, appearance, and cell concentration.

CASE STUDY

After studying the material in this chapter, the reader should be able to respond to the following case study:

A 33-year-old semiconscious woman was brought to the emergency department by her husband. The previous day she had complained of a headache and had left work early, taken some aspirin and a nap, and felt better later in the evening. Her husband stated that the next morning "she couldn't talk," and he brought her to the emergency department. A spinal tap was performed. The fluid that arrived in the laboratory was cloudy. The white blood cell count was 10.6×10^9/L. Most of the cells seen on the cytocentrifuge slide were neutrophils.

1. What dilution should be made to obtain a satisfactory cytocentrifuge slide?
2. What should you look for on the cytocentrifuge slide?
3. What is the most likely diagnosis for this patient?

The examination of body fluids, including nucleated blood cell count and differential, can provide valuable diagnostic information. This chapter is not intended as a comprehensive study of all body fluids, but it covers cell counting and morphologic hematology. The fluids discussed in this chapter include cerebrospinal fluid (CSF), serous or body cavity fluids (pleural, pericardial, and peritoneal fluids), and synovial (joint) fluids. Bronchoalveolar lavage (BAL) specimens are discussed briefly.

PERFORMING CELL COUNTS ON BODY FLUIDS

Examination of all fluids should include color, turbidity, cell counts, and WBC examination. Blood cell counts should be performed and cytocentrifuge slides should be prepared as quickly as possible after collection of the specimen because white blood cells (WBCs) begin to deteriorate within 30 minutes after collection.[1] It is important to mix the specimen gently but thoroughly before every manipulation (i.e., cell counts, preparing any dilution, and preparing cytocentrifuge slides). Cell counts on fluids usually are performed on a hemacytometer (Chapter 14); however, some automated instruments now are capable of performing blood cell counts on fluids. Automated cell counts are limited by their poor sensitivity in specimens with low counts. Each instrument manufacturer should have a statement of intended use that defines which body fluids have been approved for testing by a regulatory agency.[2,3] Care should be taken to observe operating limits of these instruments and volume limits of the fluid received. Red blood cell (RBC) counts on serous and synovial fluids have little clinical value[4]; relevant clinical information is obtained merely from the appearance of the fluid (grossly bloody, bloody, slightly bloody).

Cell counts are performed with undiluted fluid if the fluid is clear. If the fluid is hazy or bloody, appropriate dilutions should be made to provide accurate counts of WBCs and RBCs. The smallest reasonable dilution should be made. The diluting fluid for RBCs is isotonic saline. Diluting fluids for WBCs include glacial acetic acid to lyse the RBCs, or Türk's solution, which contains glacial acetic acid and methylene blue to stain the nuclei of the WBCs. Acetic acid cannot be used for synovial fluids because mucin coagulates. Hypotonic saline solutions also lyse RBCs without coagulating with mucin, so it is a good alternative for synovial fluids.[5] Dilutions should be based on the turbidity of the fluid or on the number of cells seen on the hemacytometer when using an undiluted sample.

A WBC count of approximately 200/mm³ or an RBC count of approximately 400/mm³ causes a fluid to be slightly hazy. If the fluid is blood-tinged to slightly bloody, the RBCs can be counted using undiluted fluid, but it is advisable to use a small (1:2) dilution with Türk's solution (or similar) to lyse the RBCs and provide an accurate WBC or nucleated cell count. If the fluid is bloody, a 1:200 dilution for RBCs (standard dilution in

RBC Unopettes [Becton Dickinson, Rutherford, NJ]) and either a 1:2 dilution with Türk's solution or a 1:20 (standard dilution in WBC Unopettes) dilution to obtain an accurate nucleated cell count need to be used. A calibrated, handheld pipette or a Unopette pipette system should be used to prepare a body fluid suspension for cell counting.

The number of squares to be counted in the hemacytometer should be determined on the basis of the number of cells present. In general, all nine squares on both sides of the hemacytometer should be counted. If the number of cells is high, however, fewer squares may be counted.[5] Each square equals 1 mm². The formula (Chapter 14) for calculating the number of cells is:

$$\frac{\text{cells counted} \times \text{depth factor} \times \text{dilution factor}}{\text{area counted (mm}^2)}$$

Guidelines for counting are summarized in Table 17-1.

PREPARATION OF CYTOCENTRIFUGE SLIDES

The cytocentrifuge enhances the ability to identify the types of cells present in a fluid. This centrifuge spins at a low rate of speed, which minimizes distortion of the cellular elements and provides a "button" of cells that are concentrated into a small area. The cytocentrifuge assembly consists of a cytofunnel, filter paper to absorb excess fluid, and a glass slide. These three elements are clipped together in a clip assembly; a few drops of well-mixed specimen are dispensed into the cytofunnel, and the entire assembly is centrifuged slowly. The cells are deposited onto the slide, and excess fluid is absorbed into the filter paper, producing a monolayer of cells in a small button (Fig. 17-1).

Although there is some cell loss into the filter paper, this is not selective, and an accurate representation of the types of

TABLE 17-1 Guidelines for Counting Fluids

| | GROSS APPEARANCE | | | | |
Test	Clear	Hazy	Blood-tinged	Cloudy	Bloody
WBCs	0-200/mm³	>200/mm³	Unknown	High	Unknown
Dilution for counting cells	None	1:2 Türk's	1:2 Türk's	1:20 WBC Unopette	1:2 Türk's or WBC Unopette
No. squares to count on hemacytometer	9	9	9	9 or 4	9 or 4
RBCs	0-400/mm³	Unknown	>400/mm³	Unknown	>6000/mm³
Dilution for counting cells	None	None	None	None	1:200 RBC Unopette
No. squares to count on hemacytometer	9 large	9 large	9 or 4 large	4 large or 5 small	5 small
Cytospin dilution (0.25 mL [5 drops] of fluid)*	Undiluted	Dilute with saline to 100-200/mm³ nucleated cell count	Straight or by nucleated cell count	Dilute with saline to 100-200/mm³ nucleated cell count	Dilute by nucleated cell count; if RBC count >1 million/mm³, make a pushed smear and differentiate cells that are pushed out on the end

*Expected cell yield (WBC count for no. cells recovered on slide): 0/mm³ for 0-70, 1-2/mm³ for 12-100, >3/mm³ for >100.

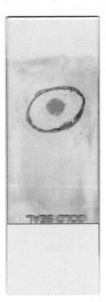

Figure 17-1 Wright-stained cytocentrifuge slide showing a concentrated button of cells within a marked circle. (From Carr JH, Rodak BF: Clinical Hematology Atlas, 2nd ed. Philadelphia: Saunders, 2004.)

cells present in a fluid is provided. There also may be some distortion of cells as a result of the centrifugation process or crowding of cells when high cell counts are present. To minimize distortion resulting from overcrowding of cells, appropriate dilutions should be made with normal saline before centrifugation. The basis for this dilution should be the WBC count or the nucleated cell count. A nucleated cell count of 200/mm³ or less provides a good preparation for the differential. If the RBC count is extremely elevated, a larger dilution may be necessary; however, an RBC count of 5000/mm³ would not cause significant nucleated cell distortion. If a fluid has a nucleated cell count of 2000/mm³ and an RBC count of 10,000/mm³, a 1:10 dilution should be made, producing a nucleated cell count of 200/mm³ and an RBC count of 1000/mm³ for the cytocentrifuge slide. If the RBC count of a fluid is greater than 1 million/mm³, it is best to make a "push" slide to perform the differential. In this case, the differential should be performed on the cells "pushed out" on the end of the smear instead of in the body of the smear because that is where the larger, and possibly more significant, cells would be deposited.

If a consistent amount of fluid is used when preparing cytocentrifuge slides, a consistent yield of cells can be expected; this can be used as a confirmation for the WBC or nucleated cell count. For example, if 5 drops of fluid (undiluted or diluted) is always used to prepare cytocentrifuge slides, a 100-cell differential should be obtainable if the WBC or nucleated cell count is equal to or greater than 3/mm³. In all cases, the entire cell button should be scanned before performing the differential to ensure that significant clumps of cells are not overlooked. The area of the cell button that is used for performing the differential is not important, but if the number of nucleated cells present is small, a "systematic meander" start-

ing at one side of the button and working toward the other side is best. In case the number of cells recovered is small, the area around the cell button should be marked on the back of the slide with a wax pencil, or premarked slides should be used to prepare cytocentrifuge slides (see Fig. 17-1).

CEREBROSPINAL FLUID

CSF is the only fluid that exists in quantities sufficient to sample in healthy individuals. CSF is present in volumes of 90 to 150 mL in adults and 10 to 60 mL in newborns.[6] This fluid bathes the brain and spinal column and serves as a cushion to protect the brain, as a circulating nutrient medium, as an excretory channel for nervous tissue metabolism, and as lubrication for the central nervous system.

Gross Examination

Normal CSF is non-viscous, clear, and colorless. A cloudy or hazy appearance may indicate the presence of WBCs (>200/mm³), RBCs (>400/mm³) or microorganisms.[6] A bloody fluid may be caused by a traumatic tap, in which blood is acquired as the puncture is performed, or by a pathologic hemorrhage within the central nervous system. If more than one tube is received, the tubes can be observed for clearing from tube to tube. If the first tube contains blood, but the remaining tubes are clear or progressively clearer, the blood is the result of a traumatic puncture. If all tubes are uniformly bloody, the probable cause is a subarachnoid hemorrhage. When a bloody sample is received, an aliquot should be centrifuged, and the color of the supernatant should be observed and reported. A clear, colorless supernatant indicates a traumatic tap, whereas a yellowish or pinkish yellow tinge may indicate a subarachnoid hemorrhage. This yellowish color sometimes is referred to as *xanthochromia*, but because not all xanthochromia is pathologic, the Clinical and Laboratory Standards Institute recommends avoiding the term and simply reporting the actual color of the supernatant (Fig. 17-2 and Table 17-2).[5]

Cell Counts

Normal cell counts in CSF are 0 to 5 WBC/mm³ and 0 RBC/mm³. If a high RBC count is obtained, one may determine whether the source of WBCs is peripheral blood contamination by using the peripheral blood ratio of 1 WBC per 500 to 900 RBCs. If peripheral blood cell counts are known, the number of blood WBCs added to the CSF sample can be calculated using the following formula (where B = blood):

$$WBC_B \times \frac{RBC_{CSF}}{RBC_B} = WBC \text{ added by traumatic puncture}$$

The corrected or true WBC count is calculated by:[5]

$$True \text{ } WBC_{CSF} = CSF_{WBC} - WBC \text{ added}$$

Some laboratories have questioned the value of an RBC count on CSF and report only the WBC count.

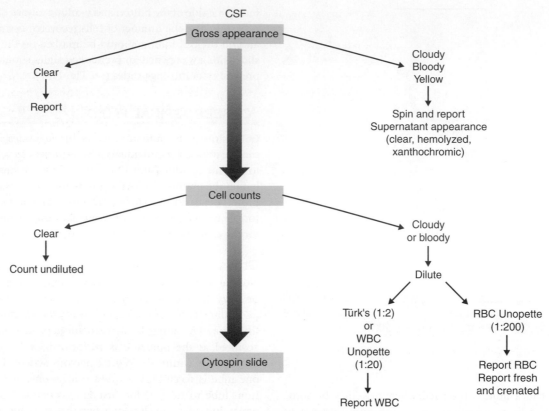

Figure 17-2 Flow chart for examination of CSF. (Modified from Kjeldsberg CR, Knight JA: Body Fluids, 3rd ed. Chicago: ASCP Press; reprinted with permission.)

TABLE 17-2 Characteristics of Cerebrospinal Fluid

Traumatic Tap	Pathologic Hemorrhage
Clear supernatant	Colored or hemolyzed supernatant
Clearing from tube to tube	Same appearance in all tubes
Fresh RBCs	Crenated RBCs
Bone marrow contamination	Erythrophages
Cartilage cells	Siderophages (may have bilirubin crystals)

A high WBC count may be found in fluid from patients with infective processes, such as meningitis. In general, WBC counts are much higher (in the thousands) in patients with bacterial meningitis than in patients with viral meningitis (in the hundreds).[7] The predominant cell type present on the cytocentrifuge slide—neutrophils or lymphocytes—is a better indicator, however, of the type of meningitis—bacterial or viral. Elevated WBCs or nucleated cell counts also may be obtained in patients with inflammatory processes and malignancies.

Differential

The normal cells seen in CSF are lymphocytes and monocytes (Fig. 17-3). In adults, the predominant cells are lymphocytes; in newborns, the predominant cells are monocytes.[6] Neutrophils are not normal in CSF but may be seen in small numbers because of concentration techniques. When the WBC count is elevated and large numbers of neutrophils are seen, a thorough and careful search should be made for bacteria because organisms may be present in very small numbers early in bacterial meningitis (Fig. 17-4). In viral meningitis, the predominant cells seen are lymphocytes, including reactive or viral lymphocytes and plasmacytoid lymphocytes (Fig. 17-5). Eosinophils and basophils may be seen as a reaction to foreign materials, such as shunts, or as a result of an allergic reaction (Fig. 17-6).[6] When nucleated RBCs are seen, bone marrow contamination resulting from accidental puncture of the vertebral body during spinal tap should be suspected and a comment should be made on the report. In the case of bone marrow contamination, other immature neutrophils and megakaryocytes also may be seen. When there is obvious bone marrow contamination, the WBC differential is likely to be equivalent to the bone marrow and not the CSF.

Ependymal and choroid plexus cells, lining cells of the central nervous system, may be seen. These are large cells with abundant cytoplasm that stains lavender with Wright stain. They most often appear in clumps, and although they are not diagnostically significant, it is important not to confuse them with malignant cells (Fig. 17-7).

Cartilage cells may be seen if the vertebral body is accidentally punctured. These cells usually occur singly, are medium to large, and have cytoplasm that stains wine red with a deep wine-red nucleus with Wright stain (Fig. 17-8).

Siderophages are macrophages (i.e., monocytes or histiocytes) that have ingested RBCs and, as a result of the

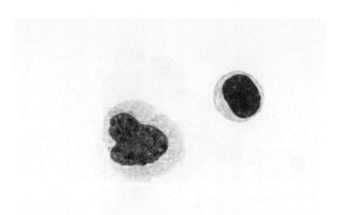

Figure 17-3 Monocyte *(left)* and lymphocyte *(right)* seen in normal CSF (×1000).

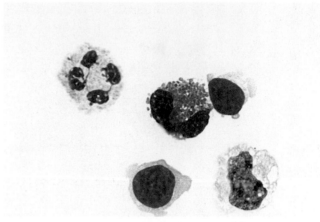

Figure 17-6 Eosinophil, lymphocytes, monocyte, and neutrophil in CSF from a patient with a shunt (×1000).

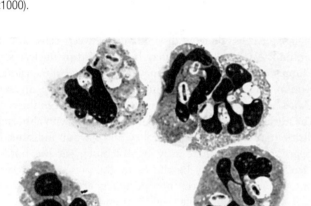

Figure 17-4 Neutrophil with bacteria in CSF from a patient with bacterial meningitis (Wright stain, ×1000). (From Carr JH, Rodak BF: Clinical Hematology Atlas, 2nd ed. Philadelphia: Saunders, 2004.)

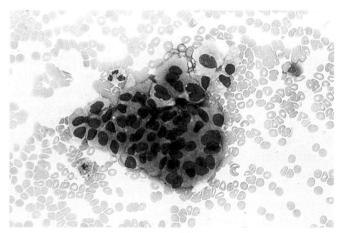

Figure 17-7 Clump of ependymal cells in CSF (×200).

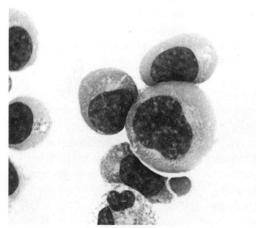

Figure 17-5 Reactive (viral) lymphocytes in CSF from a patient with viral meningitis (×1000).

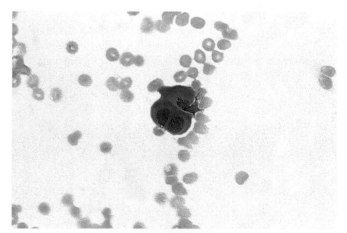

Figure 17-8 Cartilage cells in CSF (×400).

breakdown of the RBCs, contain hemosiderin. Hemosiderin appears as large, rough-shaped, dark-blue or black granules in the cytoplasm of the macrophage. These cells also may contain bilirubin or hematoidin crystals, which are golden yellow and are a result of further breakdown of the ingested RBCs. The presence of siderophages indicates a pathologic hemorrhage. Siderophages appear approximately 48 hours after hemorrhage and may persist for 2 to 8 weeks after the hemorrhage has occurred (Fig. 17-9).

A high percentage of patients with acute lymphoblastic leukemia or acute myelocytic leukemia have central nervous

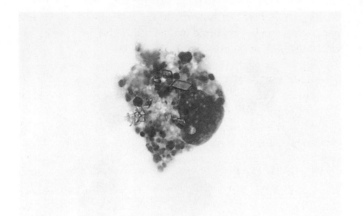

Figure 17-9 Siderophage with bilirubin crystals (hematoidin) in CSF (×400).

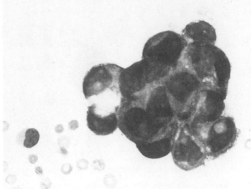

Figure 17-11 Clump of breast tumor cells in CSF (×400).

system involvement.[6] It is always important to look carefully for leukemic cells (i.e., blast forms) in the CSF of patients with leukemia. Patients with lymphoma, myeloma, and chronic myelocytic leukemia in blast crisis also may have blast cells in the CSF. These blast cells have the characteristics of blast forms in the peripheral blood, including a high nuclear-to-cytoplasmic ratio, a fine "stippled" nuclear chromatin pattern, and prominent nucleoli. They are usually large cells that stain basophilic with Wright stain and have a fairly uniform appearance (Fig. 17-10). If a traumatic tap has occurred and the patient has a high blast count in the peripheral blood, the blasts seen in the CSF may by the result of peripheral blood contamination and not central nervous system involvement. The possibility of peripheral blood contamination should be reported and the tap should be repeated in a few days.

Malignant cells resulting from metastases to the central nervous system may be found. The most common primary tumors that metastasize to the central nervous system are breast, lung, and gastrointestinal tract tumors and melanoma.[6] Malignant cells are usually large with a high nuclear-to-cytoplasmic ratio and are often basophilic or hyperchromic. They often occur in clumps but may occur singly. Within clumps of

malignant cells, there is dissimilarity between cells, and in multinucleated cells, there may be variation in nuclear size. Clumps of malignant cells may appear three-dimensional, requiring up-and-down focusing to see the cells on different planes, and there are usually no "windows" between the cells. The nuclei of these cells are usually large, often with abnormal distribution of chromatin, and they may have an indistinct or jagged border, or there may be "blebbing" at the border. Increased mitosis may be shown by the presence of several mitotic figures in the cell button. Malignant cells frequently have a bizarre appearance (Fig. 17-11 and Table 17-3).[8]

TABLE 17-3 Characteristics of Benign and Malignant Cells

Benign	Malignant
Occasional large cells	Many cells may be very large
Light-to-dark staining	May be very basophilic
Rare mitotic figures	May have several mitotic figures
Round-to-oval nucleus; nuclei are uniform in size with varying amounts of cytoplasm	May have irregular or bizarre nuclear shape
Smooth nuclear edge	Edges of nucleus may be indistinct and irregular
Nucleus intact	Nucleus may be disintegrated at edges
Nucleoli are small, if present	Nucleoli may be large and prominent
In multinuclear cells (mesothelial), all nuclei have similar appearance (size and shape)	Multinuclear cells have varying sizes and shapes of nuclei
Moderate-to-small N:C ratio	May have high N:C ratio
Clumps of cells have similar appearance among cells, are on the same plane of focus, and may have "windows" between cells	Clumps of cells contain cells of varying sizes and shapes, are "three-dimensional" (have to focus up and down to see all cells), and have dark-staining borders

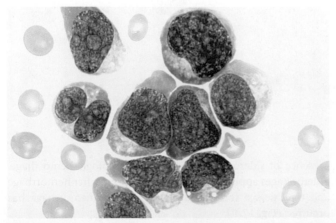

Figure 17-10 Lymphoblasts in CSF (×1000). (From Carr JH, Rodak BF: Clinical Hematology Atlas, 2nd ed. Philadelphia: Saunders, 2004.)

N:C ratio, nuclear-to-cytoplasmic ratio.

SEROUS FLUID

Serous fluids, including pleural, pericardial, and peritoneal fluids, normally exist in very small quantities and serve as lubricant between the membranes of an organ and the sac in which it is housed. Pleural fluid is found in the space between the lungs and the pleural sac; pericardial fluid, in the space between the heart and the pericardial sac; and peritoneal fluid, between the intestine and the peritoneal sac (Fig. 17-12). An accumulation of fluid in a cavity is termed *effusion*. When an effusion is in the peritoneal cavity, it also may be referred to as *ascites* or *ascitic fluid*.[4] It would be difficult to remove these fluids from a healthy individual; the presence of these fluids in detectable amounts indicates a disease state.

Transudates versus Exudates

The accumulation of a large amount of fluid in a cavity is called an *effusion*. Effusions are subdivided further into *transudates* and *exudates* to distinguish whether disease is present within or outside the body cavity. In general, transudates develop as part of systemic disease processes, such as congestive heart failure, whereas exudates indicate disorders associated with bacterial or viral infections, malignancy, pulmonary embolism, or systemic lupus erythematosus. Several parameters can be measured to determine whether an effusion is a transudate or an exudate (Table 17-4).

Gross Examination

Transudates should appear straw-colored and clear. A cloudy or hazy fluid may indicate an exudate from an infectious process; a bloody fluid, trauma or malignancy; and a milky fluid, effused chyle in the pleural cavity.

Differential Cell Counts

The cells found in normal serous fluid are lymphocytes, mono-histiocytes (macrophages), and mesothelial cells. Neutrophils commonly are seen in the fluid sent to the laboratory for analysis but would not be present in normal fluid. When neutrophils are seen, they have more segments and longer filaments than in peripheral blood (Fig. 17-13).

Mesothelial cells are the lining cells of body cavities and are shed into these cavities constantly. These are large (12-30 μm) cells and have a "fried egg" appearance with basophilic cytoplasm, oval nucleus with smooth nuclear borders, stippled nuclear chromatin pattern, and one to three nucleoli.[6] Mesothelial cells may vary in size, may be multinucleated

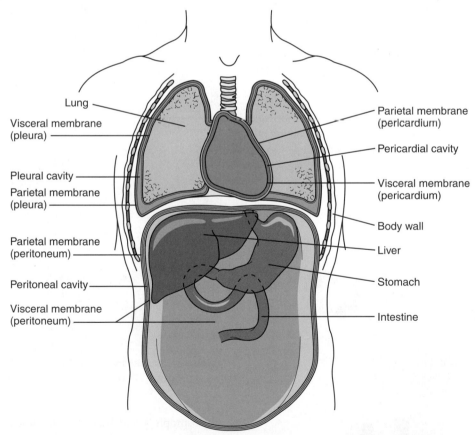

Figure 17-12 Parietal and visceral membranes of the pleural, pericardial, and peritoneal cavities. Parietal membranes line the body wall, whereas visceral membranes enclose organs. The two membranes are actually one continuous membrane. The space between opposing surfaces is identified as the body cavity (i.e., pleural, pericardial, and peritoneal cavities). (From Brunzel NA: Fundamentals of Urine and Body Fluid Analysis, 2 ed. Philadelphia: Saunders, 2004.)

TABLE 17-4 Serous Fluid: Transudates versus Exudates

Characteristic	Transudates	Exudates
Specific gravity	<1.016	>1.016
Protein	<3 g/dL	>3 g/dL
Lactate dehydrogenase	<200 IU	>200 IU
WBCs	<1000/mm³ (predominant cell type mononuclear)	>1000/mm³
Protein: fluid-to-serum ratio	<0.5	>0.5
Lactate dehydrogenase: fluid-to-serum ratio	<0.6	>0.6
Color	Clear/straw	Cloudy/yellow, amber, or grossly bloody
Volume	—	Extremely large

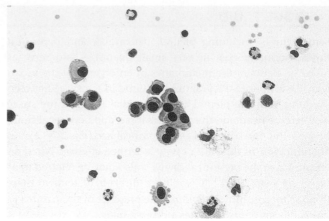

Figure 17-14 Mesothelial cells in peritoneal fluid (×200). Note "fried egg" appearance.

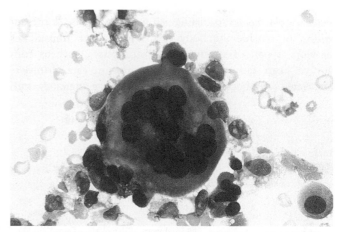

Figure 17-15 Mesothelial cell with 21 nuclei in pleural fluid (×400).

(including giant cells with 20-25 nuclei), and may have frayed cytoplasmic borders, cytoplasmic vacuoles, or both. They may occur singly, in small or large clumps, or in sheets. When they occur in clumps, there are usually "windows" between the cells. The nuclear-to-cytoplasmic ratio is 1:2 to 1:3, and this is generally consistent despite the variability in cell size.[6] They tend to have a similar appearance to each other on a slide. Mesothelial cells are seen in most effusions and are increased in sterile inflammations and decreased in tuberculous pleurisy and bacterial infections (Figs. 17-14 and 17-15).[6]

Macrophages appear as monocytes or histiocytes in serous fluids and may contain RBCs (erythrophages) or siderotic granules (siderophages), or they may appear as signet ring cells when lipid has been ingested and the resulting large vacuole pushes the nucleus to the periphery of the cell (Figs. 17-16 and 17-17).

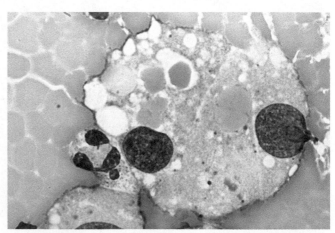

Figure 17-16 Erythrophage in peritoneal fluid (×1000).

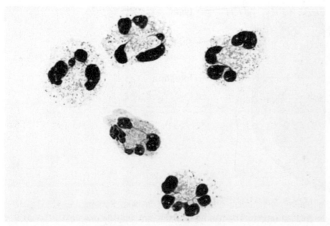

Figure 17-13 Hypersegmented neutrophil with prominent filaments. Normal appearance of neutrophils in body fluids. (From Carr JH, Rodak BF: Clinical Hematology Atlas, 2nd ed. Philadelphia: Saunders, 2004.)

Eosinophils and basophils are not normally seen. These may be present in large numbers, however, as a result of allergic reaction or sensitivity to foreign material.

When large numbers of neutrophils are seen, a thorough search should be made for bacteria. If possible, a Gram stain should be performed on a second cytocentrifuge slide to aid in

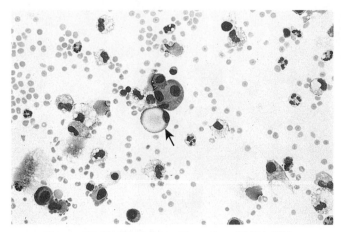

Figure 17-17 Signet ring cell in peritoneal fluid (×200).

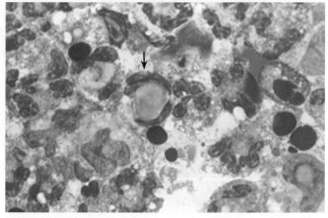

Figure 17-18 Lupus erythematosus cell *(arrow)* in pleural fluid (×1000).

rapid identification if bacteria are found. Table 17-5 lists Gram-stained organisms most commonly seen in body fluids.

Lupus erythematosus cells may be seen in serous fluids of patients with systemic lupus erythematosus because all the factors necessary for the formation of these cells—presence of the lupus erythematosus factor, incubation, and trauma to the cells—exist in vivo. A lupus erythematosus cell is an intact neutrophil that has engulfed a homogeneous mass of degenerated nuclear material, displacing the normal nucleus. Lupus erythematosus cells can form in vivo and in vitro in serous and synovial fluids and should be reported (Fig. 17-18).

Malignant cells are seen in serous fluids from primary or metastatic tumors. They have the characteristics of malignant cells found in CSF (Figs. 17-19 through 17-22). Figure 17-23 presents a flow chart for examination of serous fluids.

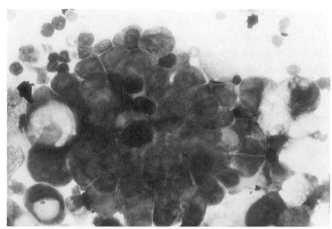

Figure 17-19 Clump of tumor cells in pleural fluid (×200).

TABLE 17-5 Gram-Stained Organisms Most Commonly Seen in Body Fluids

Fluid	Organism
Cerebrospinal	Gram-negative diplococci
	Gram-positive cocci
	Gram-negative coccobacilli
	Yeast—stains gram-positive
	Cryptococcus—look for capsule
Serous (peritoneal, pleural, or pericardial)	Gram-positive cocci
	Gram-negative bacilli
	Gram-positive bacilli
	Yeast—stains gram-positive
Synovial (joint)	Gram-positive cocci
	Gram-negative bacilli
	Gram-negative diplococci
	Gram-negative coccobacilli

Note: If the Gram-stained organisms seen on a fluid are not listed above for that fluid, do *not* report Gram stain results. Save the slide for review.

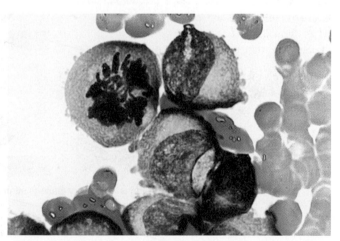

Figure 17-20 Tumor cells and mitotic figure in pleural fluid (×1000).

SYNOVIAL FLUID

Gross Examination

Synovial fluid is normally present in very small amounts in the synovial cavity surrounding joints. When fluid is present in amounts large enough to aspirate, there is a disease process in the joint. Normally this fluid is straw-colored and clear.

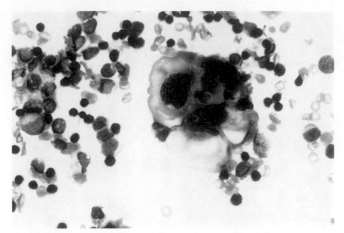

Figure 17-21 Adenocarcinoma cells in pleural fluid (×200).

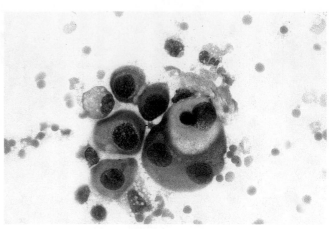

Figure 17-22 Tumor cells in peritoneal fluid (×200). Note cannibalism.

Synovial fluid contains hyaluronic acid, which makes it very viscous. A small amount of hyaluronidase powder should be added to all joint fluids to liquefy them before cell counts are performed or cytocentrifuge slides are prepared. If a crystal analysis is to be performed, an aliquot of fluid should be removed for this purpose *before* the hyaluronidase is added.

Differential Cell Counts

Cells that are normal in synovial fluid are lymphocytes, monocytes/histiocytes, and synovial cells. Synovial cells line the synovial cavity and are shed into the cavity. They resemble mesothelial cells but are usually present in smaller numbers (Fig. 17-24).

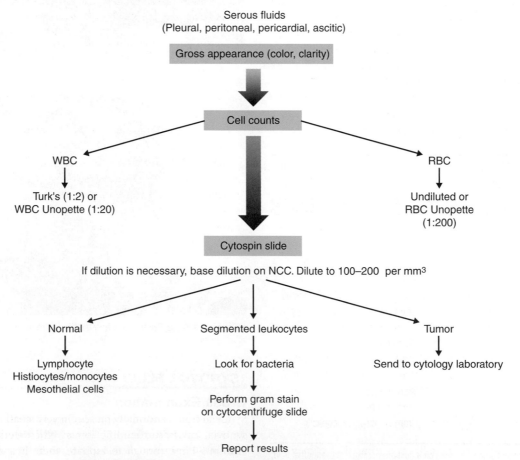

Figure 17-23 Flow chart for examination of serous fluid. NCC, nucleated cell count.

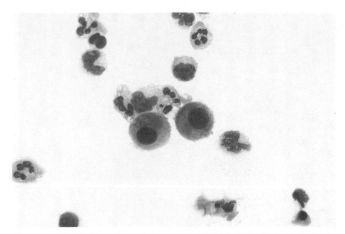

Figure 17-24 Synovial cells in synovial fluid (×400). Note similarity to mesothelial cells.

Lupus erythematosus cells may be present in synovial fluid just as in serous fluid. Malignant cells are rarely seen in synovial fluid, but when present resemble tumor cells seen in serous fluids or CSF.

Many neutrophils are present in acute inflammation of joints. As always, a careful search should be made for bacteria when many neutrophils are seen.

Crystals

Intracellular and extracellular crystals may be present in synovial fluid. Crystal examination may be performed by placing a drop of fluid on a slide and adding a coverslip, or by examination of a cytocentrifuged preparation. However, the specimen should be fresh, without hyaluronidase added. All synovial fluids should be examined carefully for crystals using a polarizing microscope with a red compensator. The most common crystals seen in synovial fluids are cholesterol, calcium pyrophosphate, and monosodium urate.

Cholesterol crystals are large, flat, extracellular crystals with a notched corner.[9] They are seen in patients with chronic effusions, particularly patients with rheumatoid arthritis.

Calcium pyrophosphate crystals are seen in pseudogout. These crystals are intracellular and are small rhomboid, platelike, or rodlike crystals.[9] These crystals are weakly birefringent when polarized (i.e., they do not appear bright when polarized). When the red compensator is used, calcium pyrophosphate crystals appear blue when the longitudinal axis of the crystal is parallel to the y axis (Fig. 17-25).[9]

Monosodium urate crystals are seen in gout. They are large, needle-like crystals that may be intracellular or extracellular. These crystals are strongly birefringent when polarized. When the red compensator is used, monosodium urate crystals appear yellow when the longitudinal axis of the crystal is parallel to the y axis (Fig. 17-26).[9] Figure 17-27 presents a flow chart for synovial fluid analysis.

BRONCHOALVEOLAR LAVAGE SPECIMENS

BAL specimens are not naturally occurring fluids; they are produced when the BAL procedure is performed. The pro-

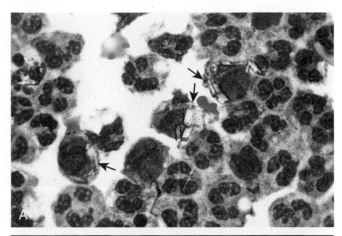

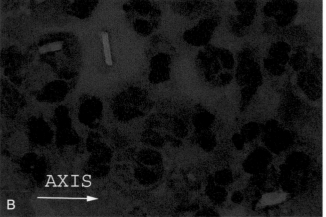

AXIS →

Figure 17-25 Intracellular calcium pyrophosphate crystals in synovial fluid (×1000). **A,** Wright stain. **B,** Polarized with red compensator. (**B** courtesy of George Girgis, MT (ASCP), Indiana University Medical Center, Indianapolis, IN.)

cedure consists of introducing warmed saline into the lungs in 50-mL aliquots and then withdrawing it. The specimen received in the laboratory is the withdrawn fluid. The purpose of the procedure is to determine types of organisms and cells that are present in areas of the lung that are otherwise inaccessible. This procedure is performed on patients with severe lung dysfunction. The specimen should always have an extensive microbiologic workup and often cytologic examination. It is common to see bacteria, yeast or both on cytocentrifuge slides prepared on these specimens. Because samples are obtained from the interior of the lung and may contain airborne organisms, care should be taken to avoid aerosol production. Samples should be mixed and containers opened under a biologic safety hood and a mask should be worn when performing cell counts. Because the risk of performing cell counts and preparing cytocentrifuge slides on BAL specimens outweighs the clinical relevance of the information obtained, some hematology laboratories no longer perform this procedure and defer to information reported from the microbiology laboratory.

Cell counts and cytocentrifuge preparations are performed as with any body fluid. Significant cell deterioration occurs within 30 minutes of collection, with the neutrophils disintegrating most rapidly.

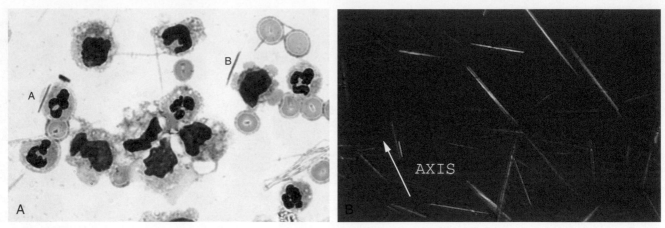

Figure 17-26 Intracellular (**A**) and extracellular (**B**) monosodium urate crystals in synovial fluid (×1000). **A,** Wright stain. **B,** Polarized with red compensator. (**A** from Carr JH, Rodak BF: Clinical Hematology Atlas, 2nd ed. Philadelphia: Saunders, 2004. **B** courtesy of George Girgis, MT (ASCP), Indiana University Medical Center, Indianapolis, IN).

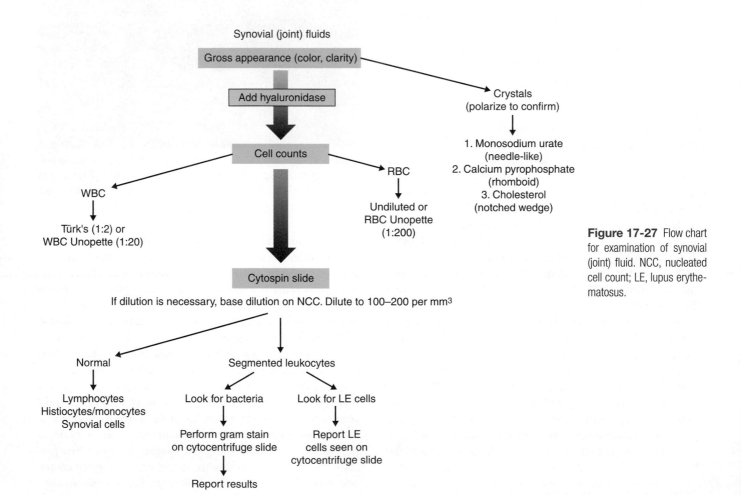

Figure 17-27 Flow chart for examination of synovial (joint) fluid. NCC, nucleated cell count; LE, lupus erythematosus.

Differential

The most common cell types seen in BAL specimens are neutrophils, monohistiocytes (macrophages), and lymphocytes. Mesothelial cells are not seen in BAL specimens because these cells line the body cavities and not the interior of the lung.

Pneumocytes, which can resemble mesothelial cells or adenocarcinoma, may be seen in patients with adult respiratory distress syndrome.

Ciliated epithelial cells can be seen and should be reported because they indicate that the sample was obtained from the

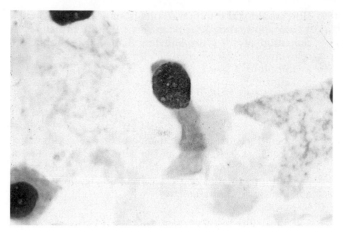

Figure 17-28 Ciliated epithelial cells in BAL fluid (×100).

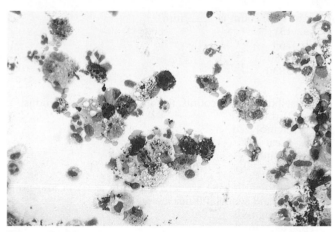

Figure 17-29 Histiocytes with carbonaceous material in BAL fluid (×40).

upper respiratory tract instead of deeper in the lung. These are columnar cells with the nucleus at one end of the cell, elongated cytoplasm, and cilia at the opposite end of the cell from the nucleus. They can occur in clusters. If the sample is not aged when the cell count is performed, these cells are in motion in the hemacytometer because they can be propelled by their cilia (Fig. 17-28).

Histiocytes laden with carbonaceous material are seen in patients who smoke tobacco. These cells resemble siderophages in other fluids, but the carbonaceous material is black, brown, or blue-black and is more droplet-like (Fig. 17-29).

Pneumocystis carinii may be seen in specimens from patients infected with human immunodeficiency virus. The *P. carinii* appear as clumps of amorphous material. Close examination of the clumps may reveal cysts (Fig. 17-30).

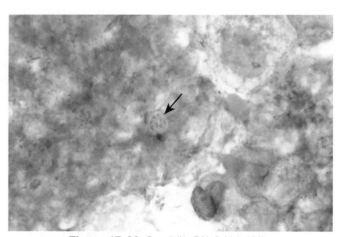

Figure 17-30 *P. carinii* in BAL fluid (×100).

CHAPTER at a GLANCE

- Cell counts and differentials on body fluid specimens are valuable diagnostic tools.
- Calibrated methods must be used when performing cell counts to provide accurate counts.
- To optimize cell morphology, specimens should not be overdiluted or underdiluted when preparing cytocentrifuge slides.
- Normal cell types in any fluid are lymphocytes, macrophages (monocytes, histiocytes), and lining cells (ependymal cells in CSF, mesothelial cells in serous fluids, synovial cells in joint fluids).
- Bacteria and yeast may be seen in any fluid.

- Malignant cells may be seen in any fluid but are rare in synovial fluid.
- Synovial fluids should be examined for crystals using a polarizing microscope.
- BAL specimens are not a true body fluid, but examination of cells present may provide diagnostic information.

Now that you have completed this chapter, go back and read again the case study at the beginning and respond to the questions presented.

REVIEW QUESTIONS

Refer to the following scenario to answer questions 1 and 2: A spinal fluid specimen is diluted 1:2 with Türk's solution to perform the nucleated cell count. Six nucleated cells were counted on both sides of the hemacytometer, counting all nine squares on both sides. Undiluted fluid is used to perform the RBC count. A total of 105 RBCs were counted on both sides of the hema-cytometer, counting four large squares on both sides.

1. The nucleated cell count is _____/mm³.
   a. 3
   b. 7
   c. 13
   d. 66

2. The RBC count is ____/mm^3.
   a. 131
   b. 263
   c. 1050
   d. 5830

3. Based on the cell counts, the appearance of the fluid is:
   a. Turbid
   b. Hemolyzed
   c. Clear
   d. Cloudy

4. All of the following are cells normally seen in CSF, serous fluids, and synovial fluids *except*:
   a. Lining cells
   b. Neutrophils
   c. Lymphocytes
   d. Monocytes/histiocytes (macrophages)

5. Spinal fluid was obtained from a 56-year-old woman. On receipt in the laboratory, the fluid was noted to be slightly bloody. When a portion of the fluid was centrifuged, the supernatant was clear. The cell counts were RBC 5200/mm^3 and WBC 24/mm^3. On the cytocentrifuge preparation, several nucleated RBCs were seen. The differential was 52% lymphocytes, 20% neutrophils, 22% monocytes, 4% myelocytes, and 2% blasts. What is the most likely explanation for these results?
   a. Bone marrow contamination
   b. Bacterial meningitis
   c. Peripheral blood contamination
   d. Leukemic infiltration in central nervous system

6. A 34-year-old woman with a history of breast cancer developed a pleural effusion. The fluid obtained was bloody and had a nucleated cell count of 284/mm^3. On the cytocentrifuge preparation, there were several neutrophils and a few monocytes/histiocytes. There were also several clusters of large, dark-staining cells. These cell clumps appeared "three-dimensional" and contained some mitotic figures. What is the most likely identification of the cells in clusters?
   a. Mesothelial cells
   b. Metastatic tumor cells
   c. Cartilage cells
   d. Pneumocytes

7. How would you interpret results from a serous fluid with a clear appearance, specific gravity of 1.010, protein concentration of 1.5 g/dL, and less than 500 mononuclear cells/mm^3?
   a. Infectious
   b. Exudate
   c. Transudate
   d. Sterile

8. On the cytocentrifuge slide from a peritoneal fluid, many large cells are seen, singly and in clumps. The cells have a "fried egg" appearance, basophilic cytoplasm, and some are multinucleated. These cells should be reported as:
   a. Suspicious for malignancy
   b. Macrophages
   c. Large lymphocytes
   d. Mesothelial cells

Refer to the following scenario to answer questions 9 and 10: A 56-year-old man presented in his physician's office with complaints of pain and swelling in his left great toe. Fluid aspirated from the toe was straw-colored and cloudy. The WBC count was 2543/mm^3. The differential consisted mainly of neutrophils and monocytes/histiocytes. Intracellular and extracellular crystals were seen on the cytocentrifuge slide. The crystals were needle-shaped and, when polarized with the use of the red compensator, appeared yellow on the y axis.

9. The crystals are:
   a. Cholesterol
   b. Hyaluronidase
   c. Monosodium urate
   d. Calcium pyrophosphate

10. This patient's painful toe was caused by:
    a. Gout
    b. Infection
    c. Inflammation
    d. Pseudogout

REFERENCES

1. Glasser L: Cells in cerebrospinal fluid. Diagn Med 1981;4:33-50.
2. Barnes PW, Eby CS, Shiner AG: An evaluation of the utility of performing body fluid counts on the Coulter LH 750. Lab Hematol 2004;10:127-131.
3. Brown W, Keeney M, Chin-Yee I, et al: Validation of body fluid analysis on the Coulter LH 750. Lab Hematol 2003;9:155-159.
4. Brunzel N: Fundamentals of Urine and Body Fluid Analysis, 2nd ed. Philadelphia: Saunders, 2004.
5. Clinical and Laboratory Standards Institute: Body Fluid Analysis for Cellular Composition: Proposed Guideline. H56-P; vol 25, no. 20. Wayne, PA: CLSI, 2005.
6. Kjeldsberg C, Knight J: Body Fluids, 3rd ed. Chicago: ASCP Press, 1993.
7. Krueger R: Meningitis: a case study. Lab Med 1987;18:677-681.
8. Cornbleet J: Microscopy of CSF and body fluids. Workshop material presented before the National Meeting of the American Society of Clinical Pathologists, 1991.
9. Strasinger SK, DiLorenzo MS: Urinalysis and Body Fluids, 4th ed. Philadelphia: Davis, 2001.

Anemias: Red Blood Cell Morphology and Approach to Diagnosis

18

Rakesh Mehta

OUTLINE

Definition of Anemia
Clinical Findings
Physiologic Adaptations
Laboratory Procedures
Mechanisms of Anemia
Approach to Evaluating
 Anemias

OBJECTIVES

After completion of this chapter, the reader will be able to:

1. Define anemia and recognize anemic patients given complete blood count results and appropriate reference ranges.
2. Discuss the importance of the history and the physical examination in the diagnosis of anemia.
3. Describe clinical signs and symptoms of anemia, and recognize them in written clinical scenarios.
4. List procedures that are commonly performed for the detection and diagnosis of anemia.
5. Distinguish among effective, ineffective, and insufficient erythropoiesis when given examples.
6. Discuss the importance of the reticulocyte count in the evaluation of anemia.
7. Characterize the three groups of decreased production anemias that are based on the mean cell volume (MCV) and give one example of each.

8. Recognize the importance of reviewing the peripheral smear when assessing anemias and distinguish the important findings.
9. Describe the use of the red blood cell distribution width (RDW) in the diagnosis of anemias.
10. Briefly explain how the body adapts to anemia over time and the impact on the patient's experience of the anemia.
11. Use an algorithm for differential diagnosis of anemia incorporating the MCV, reticulocyte count, and RDW to narrow the differential diagnosis.
12. Classify given examples of variations in red blood cell morphology as inclusions, shape changes, volume changes, and color changes.

CASE STUDY

After studying the material in this chapter, the reader should be able to respond to the following case study:

A 45-year-old woman phoned her physician and complained of fatigue, shortness of breath on exertion, and general malaise. She requested some "B_{12} shots" to make her feel better. The physician asked the patient to schedule an appointment so that she could determine the cause of the symptoms before offering treatment. A finger-stick hematocrit done in the office determined that the patient's hematocrit was 20% (0.20 L/L). The physician requested additional laboratory tests, including complete blood count with a peripheral smear and a reticulocyte count.

1. Why did the physician want the patient to come into the office before she prescribed B_{12} shots?
2. How do the mean cell volume (MCV) and reticulocyte count help determine the classification of the anemia?
3. Why is the examination of the peripheral blood smear important in the workup of anemia?

Red blood cells (RBCs) perform the vital physiologic function of oxygen delivery to the tissues. The hemoglobin (Hb) within the erythrocyte has the incredible capacity to bind oxygen in the lungs and to release it appropriately in the tissues.[1] A decrease in the number of RBCs or amount of Hb results in decreased oxygen delivery and subsequent tissue hypoxia. Anemia, derived from the Greek word *anaimia*, meaning "without blood,"[2] indicates a reduced number of RBCs, which results in decreased oxygen delivery. Anemia should not be thought of as a disease in itself, but rather a manifestation of numerous other underlying disease processes.[3,4] Anemia is the most common manifestation of disease worldwide. This chapter provides an overview of the diagnosis, mechanism, and classification of anemia. In the following chapters, each type of anemia is discussed in detail.

DEFINITION OF ANEMIA

A functional definition of anemia is a decrease in the oxygen-carrying capacity of the blood. It can arise if there is too little Hb or the Hb is nonfunctional. The former is the more frequent cause.

Anemia is defined operationally as a reduction from the baseline value for the total number of RBCs, amount of circulating Hb, and RBC mass for a particular patient. Practically, this definition is not applicable because a patient's baseline value is rarely known.[4] A more conventional definition is a decrease in RBCs, Hb, and hematocrit (Hct) below the previously established reference values for healthy individuals of the same age, gender, and race and under similar environmental conditions.[1,3-7] Problems with this conventional definition may occur for several reasons. The blood values of nonanemic individuals may fall just below the "normal" level. Likewise, the blood values of mildly anemic individuals may fall within the low-normal range. This latter group usually is not recognized unless the blood smear is evaluated, or the reticulocyte count, RBC indices, and RBC distribution width (RDW) are calculated.

Hematologic reference values for adults are listed on the inside cover of this text. The values may vary in different areas according to age, gender, race, and environment, but are given for the purpose of discussion in the approach to anemias. Each laboratory should determine its reference ranges in accordance with the patient population because numerous factors, such as geographic elevation, can influence Hb levels. A patient whose values fall below those listed in these tables is considered most likely to be anemic.

CLINICAL FINDINGS

The clinical diagnosis of anemia includes assessment of the history, physical examination, signs, symptoms, hematologic values, and other laboratory procedures.

History and Physical Examination

The approach to a patient with anemia begins with a complete history and physical examination,[1,3,4,6,7] which can yield information that often helps to identify and narrow the possible cause or causes of anemia. This knowledge leads to a more rational approach to ordering the helpful diagnostic tests. The classic symptoms associated with anemia are fatigue and shortness of breath. Understandably, if oxygen delivery is decreased, patients do not have enough energy to perform their daily functions. Obtaining a good history requires questioning of the patient, particularly in regard to diet, drug ingestion, exposure to chemicals, occupation, hobbies, travel, bleeding history, ethnic group, family history of disease, neurologic symptoms, previous medication, jaundice, and various underlying diseases that produce anemia.[1,3,4,6,7] Iron deficiency causes a fascinating set of symptoms called *pica*.[8] Patients with pica have strange cravings for substances such as ice (pagophagia), clay, or cornstarch. A patient with anemia and these symptoms invariably has iron deficiency. Some patients may have no symptoms, which typically would indicate a congenital or slowly progressive anemia.

Certain features should be evaluated closely on the physical examination to provide clues to hematologic disorders, such as skin (e.g., pallor, jaundice, petechiae), eyes (hemorrhage), mouth (mucosal bleeding), sternal tenderness, lymphadenopathy, cardiac murmurs, splenomegaly, and hepatomegaly.[1,3,4,6,7] Jaundice is particularly important to the assessment of anemia because it may imply evidence of increased RBC destruction and suggest a hemolytic component to the anemia. The vital signs also are a crucial component of the physical evaluation. Patients with rapid falls in their Hb levels typically are tachycardic (fast heart rate), whereas if the anemia is long-standing, the heart rate may be normal, due to the body's ability to compensate for the low count.

Moderate anemias (Hb 7-10 g/dL) may not produce clinical signs or symptoms if the onset of anemia is slow.[3] Depending on the patient's age and cardiovascular state, however, moderate anemias may be associated with pallor of conjunctivae and of nail beds, dyspnea, vertigo, headache, muscle weakness, lethargy, and other symptoms.[1,3,6,7] Severe anemias (Hb <7 g/dL) usually produce tachycardia, hypotension, and other symptoms of volume loss, in addition to symptoms listed earlier. The severity of the anemia is gauged by the degree of reduction in RBC mass, cardiopulmonary adaptation, and rapidity of progression of the anemia.[3] The history and physical examination remain important components in making the clinical diagnosis of anemia.

PHYSIOLOGIC ADAPTATIONS

In anemia that develops slowly, the body adapts to anemia over time, leading to few symptoms. Reduced delivery of oxygen to tissue secondary to reduced Hb causes increased erythropoietin secretion by the kidneys. With persistent anemia, physiologic adaptations develop consisting of mechanisms that increase the oxygen-carrying capacity of a reduced amount of Hb. There is more rapid delivery of blood with reduced oxygen content. Heart rate and respiratory rate are increased. Cardiac output is increased. With tissue hypoxia, there is an increase in RBC 2,3-bisphosphoglycerate, which shifts the oxygen dissociation curve to the right (decreased oxygen affinity of Hb) and results in increased delivery of oxygen to tissues (Chapter 10).[3] This is a highly significant mechanism in chronic anemias: that a patient with anemia may be relatively asymptomatic at very low levels of Hb. With persistent and marked anemia, however, the strain on the heart ultimately can lead to heart failure.

LABORATORY PROCEDURES

Complete Blood Cell Count with Cell Indices

To detect the presence of anemia, the clinical laboratory professional performs a complete blood count on a hematology cell analyzer to determine the RBC count, Hb, Hct, RBC indices, white blood cell (WBC) count, and platelet count. The RBC indices determine mean corpuscular size or mean cell volume (MCV), mean cell Hb (MCH), and mean cell Hb concentration (MCHC) (Table 18-1) (Chapter 14).[9] The most important of these indices is the MCV, which measures the RBC volume in femtoliters (fL). Standard reference ranges for these determinations are listed on the inside cover of this text. Some electronic counters also provide for a RBC histogram, a calculated value for the RDW, or both. A relative and absolute reticulocyte count, described subsequently, should be performed for every patient when anemia is suspected or observed. Several automated analyzers are available to perform reticulocyte counts and increase the accuracy of the count.

Modern automated counters generate an RBC histogram (RBC size frequency distribution curve) with relative number of cells plotted on the ordinate and RBC volume in femtoliters plotted on the abscissa. The curve is approximately gaussian for normal RBCs. Abnormalities include a shift in the curve to the left (microcytosis) or to the right (macrocytosis), a widening caused by a greater variation about the mean, and two populations of cells. The histogram complements the blood smear in identifying variant RBC populations.[10] (Histograms are discussed further with examples in Chapter 39.)

The RDW is the mathematical expression of variability within the volume distribution of the RBC population expressed as a percentage. It indicates the variation of the RBC size within the population measured (anisocytosis). The RDW is the coefficient of variation of the ordinarily gaussian-shaped RBC volume distribution histogram. The RDW is determined by dividing the standard deviation of the MCV by the MCV and multiplying by 100 to convert to a percentage value. The RDW is a quantitative measure of the volume variation of circulating RBCs.[9] The usefulness of the RDW is discussed later.

Reticulocyte Count

The reticulocyte count serves as an important tool to indicate shortened RBC survival and the subsequent appropriate response by the bone marrow to increase the RBC production.

Reticulocytes are young RBCs that have just left the marrow but still contain residual RNA. Normally, they remain for only 1 to 1.5 days in the blood with a range of 0.5% to 2.5% for adults.[9] The normal newborn range is 1.8% to 5.8%, but these values change to approximately those of the normal adult range in a few weeks.[1,3,6,7] In addition to the percentage of reticulocytes present, an absolute reticulocyte count should be determined by multiplying the percent reticulocytes by the RBC count. The low-normal absolute reticulocyte count is 25×10^9/L; the upper range has been given as 75×10^9/L (although this reference range is for a normal RBC count).[3] A patient with a severe anemia may seem to be producing increased numbers of reticulocytes if only the percentage is considered. A patient with 1.5×10^{12}/L RBCs and 3% reticulocytes has an absolute reticulocyte count of 45×10^9/L. Although the percentage of reticulocytes is technically above the normal range, the absolute reticulocyte count is in the normal range. For the degree of anemia, however, these results are inappropriately low because these values should be much higher. In other words, production of reticulocytes within the predefined normal reference range is inadequate for an RBC count that is approximately one third of normal.

The reticulocyte count may be corrected for anemia if the absolute count is not performed. The corrected reticulocyte count is determined by multiplying the reticulocyte percentage by the patient's Hct and dividing the result by the normal Hct. If the reticulocytes are released prematurely from the bone marrow and remain in the circulation 2 to 3 days (instead of 1-1.5 days), the corrected reticulocyte count must be divided by maturation time to determine the reticulocyte production index, which is a better indication of the rate of RBC production.[3]

The reticulocyte count helps divide anemias into decreased production or shortened RBC survival. In hemolytic anemia, in which RBCs are destroyed shortly after release from the bone marrow, the reticulocyte count is appropriately elevated. In anemic states resulting from decreased RBC production, the reticulocyte count is often decreased (or inappropriately low). Reticulocytes and related calculations are discussed further in Chapter 14.

Blood Smear Examination

An important component in the evaluation of an anemia is examination of the peripheral blood smear, giving particular attention to the RBCs regarding variation in size, shape, color

TABLE 18-1 Formulas for Reticulocyte Counts and Red Cell Indices

Test	Formula	Reference Range
Absolute reticulocyte count	$= \%$ reticulocytes $\times$ RBC count (10^{12}/L)	$25\text{-}75 \times 10^9$/L
Corrected reticulocyte count	$= \dfrac{\% \text{ reticulocytes} \times \text{patient's hematocrit }\%}{45}$	—
Reticulocyte Production Index	$= \dfrac{\text{Corrected Reticulocyte Count}}{\text{maturation time}}$	In the anemic patient, the RPI should be greater, than two, depending on the severity of the anemia.
MCV (fL)	$=$ Hematocrit (L/L) $\times$ 1000/RBC count (10^{12}/L)	80-94 fL
MCH (pg)	$=$ Hemoglobin (g/L)/RBC count (10^{12}/L)	26-32 pg
MCHC (g/L or %)	$=$ Hemoglobin (g/L)/hematocrit (L/L)	320-360 g/L

content, and inclusions. The peripheral blood smear also serves as quality control to verify the results from automated analyzers. Normal RBCs on a Wright-stained blood film are nearly uniform in size, being 7 to 7.9 μm in diameter. Small or microcytic cells are less than 6 μm in diameter, and large or macrocytic RBCs are greater than 9 μm in diameter. Certain abnormalities of diagnostic value, such as sickle cells, spherocytes, fragments, target cells, hypochromic microcytes, oval macrocytes, malarial parasites, and other RBC inclusions (Tables 18-2 and 18-3), can be detected only by studying the RBCs on a peripheral blood smear carefully. Some examples of abnormal shapes are seen in Figure 18-1.

TABLE 18-2 Description of Red Blood Cell Abnormalities and Association with Disease States

RBC Abnormality	Cell Description	Associated Disease State
Anisocytosis	Abnormal size variation	Severe anemia (e.g., megaloblastic, iron deficiency)
Macrocytes	Large cells (>8 μm), MCV >100 fL	Megaloblastic anemia (B_{12} or folate deficiency)
		Liver disease
		Hemolytic anemia: increased reticulocytes
		Myeloma
		Macrocytosis: newborn
		Myelophthisic anemia
Oval macrocytes	Large oval cells	Megaloblastic anemia
Microcytes	Smaller than normal cell (<6 μm)	Iron deficiency anemia
	MCV <80 fL	Sideroblastic anemia
		Thalassemia
		Lead poisoning
Poikilocytosis	Abnormal shape variation	Severe anemia
		Certain shapes helpful diagnostically
Spherocytes	Small, round, dense cells with lack of central pallor; usually microcytic	Hereditary spherocytosis
		DAT-positive hemolytic anemia
		Other hemolytic anemias (e.g., Heinz body hemolytic anemia)
		After transfusion
		Fragmentation hemolysis
Ovalocytes (elliptocytes)	Oval or elliptical-shaped cells	Hereditary elliptocytosis
		Iron deficiency
		Megaloblastic anemia
		Thalassemia
		Myelophthisic anemia
Stomatocytes	RBCs with slit-like area of central pallor	Hereditary stomatocytosis
		Obstructive liver disease
		Alcoholism; cirrhosis
		Artifact
Sickle cells (drepanocytes)	Thin, elongated RBCs pointed at each end (no central pallor)	Sickle cell anemia
		Hb SC
		Hb S thalassemia
		Hb O-Arab
Hb CC crystals	Tetragonal crystals, well filled with hemoglobin, formed within cell membrane	Hb CC
Hb SC crystals	Finger-like or quartz crystal–like projections protruding from cell membrane	Hb SC
Target cells (codocytes)	Hypochromic cell with central area of hemoglobin pigment; thin cell	Liver disease (obstructive)
		Hb SS, SC, S thalassemia
		Thalassemia
		Iron deficiency
		Postsplenectomy

TABLE 18-2 Description of Red Blood Cell Abnormalities and Association with Disease States—cont'd

RBC Abnormality	Cell Description	Associated Disease State
Poikilocytosis—cont'd		
Schistocytes (schizocytes, fragments)	Fragmented cells, irregularly contracted cells	MAHA, TTP, DIC
		HUS
		Uremia; carcinoma; severe burns
		Heart valve hemolysis
		March hemoglobinuria
Folded cells (pocketbook roll)	Membrane of cell folded over	Hb SC
		Hb CC
Helmet cells (Keratocytes)	Cell fragment in shape of football helmet	TTP, DIC
		HUS
		MAHA
Acanthocytes (thorns, spicules, spur cells)	Small cell with few, irregularly spaced spicules of varying length	MAHA
		Alcoholic liver diseases
		Hereditary acanthocytosis
		Abetalipoproteinemia
Burr cells	Cells with irregularly spaced blunt processes	Liver disease
		Uremia
		Hemolytic anemia
		MAHA
		TTP, DIC
		Carcinoma (stomach)
		Pyruvate kinase deficiency
Teardrop cells (dacryocytes)	Cell with one pointed extremity (in shape of drop)	Myelofibrosis with myeloid metaplasia
		Ineffective erythropoiesis
		Myelophthisic anemia
		Thalassemia
		Megaloblastic anemia
Pear-shaped cells (pointed)	Cell with one blunt projection similar to a pear	Megaloblastic anemia
		Ineffective erythropoiesis
Leptocytes	Thin, flat cell with hemoglobin at periphery, increased central pallor	Thalassemia
		Obstructive liver disease with iron deficiency
Crenated (echinocytes)	Equally spaced, short projections (10-30)	Renal disease
Dessicocyte ("puddled" RBCs)	Shrunken, dehydrated, spiculated cell (extensive loss of K^+, gain in Na^+ with loss in cell water)	Pyruvate kinase deficiency
		Familial potassium deficiency (hereditary xerocytosis)
Triangular cells	Cells with three sides	Hb SS, SC
		MAHA, TTP, DIC
Marginal achromia (blister)	Raised portion of membrane appearing free of hemoglobin	MAHA, TTP, HUS
		Hb SS with pulmonary emboli
Pinched cells	Small, raised portion appearing to be squeezed from cell	MAHA, TTP, HUS
Poikilospherocytes	Small, dark, irregular spherocyte	MAHA
		Unstable hemoglobin

DAT, direct antiglobulin test; DIC, disseminated intravascular coagulation; HUS, hemolytic-uremic syndrome; MAHA, microangiopathic hemolytic anemia; TTP, thrombotic thrombocytopenic purpura.

The types of WBCs should be differentiated, and any WBC abnormalities, such as hypersegmented neutrophils, blast cells, early or abnormal granulocytes, and reactive lymphocytes, should be noted. The number of platelets per oil-immersion field must be determined by counting 10 consecutive oil-immersion fields in an area of the smear in which the RBCs are separated or gently touch one another. (See Chapter 15 for a complete discussion of the peripheral blood film.) Additional information from the blood smear examination always complements the helpful analytic information from the cell counter.

Bone Marrow Examination

The cause of many anemias can be determined from the history and results of laboratory tests. When the cause cannot be determined, however, or the differential diagnosis remains

TABLE 18-3 Erythrocyte Inclusions

Inclusion	Appearance in Supravital Stain	Appearance in Wright Stain	Inclusion Composed of	Associated Disease State
Diffuse basophilia	Granules and filaments (reticulum)	Bluish tinge throughout red cell; polychromasia	RNA	Hemolytic anemia After treatment for iron deficiency or megaloblastic anemia
Basophilic stippling (punctuate basophilia)	Granules and filaments (reticulum)	Blue-black specks distributed throughout the cytoplasm	Precipitated RNA	Lead or heavy metal intoxication Thalassemia After treatment for iron deficiency or megaloblastic anemia
Howell-Jolly body	Dense, round, blue granule	Dense, round, bluish-red granule	DNA (nuclear fragment–aberrant chromosome)	Megaloblastic anemia Hyposplenism
Heinz body	Round, blue granule	Not visible (visible in phase contrast)	Denatured hemoglobin	Glucose-6-phosphate dehydrogenase deficiency Hb Zurich, Hb Ube, other hereditary hemolytic anemias
Siderotic granules	Bluish green–staining in Prussian blue reaction	Dark-blue granule, often near periphery (Pappenheimer body)	Ferric iron	Sideroblastic anemia Hemolytic anemia Hyposplenism
Cabot ring	Blue ring or figure-eight strand	Reddish ring or figure-eight strand	Remnant of mitotic spindle of nucleus	Pernicious anemia Lead intoxication
Hb H	Bluish-green granules in suprarital stain	Not visible	Precipitate of β chains	Hb H disease

broad, a bone marrow aspiration and biopsy may help in determining the cause of anemia.[3,7] A bone marrow examination may be indicated in a patient with an unexplained anemia associated with other cytopenias, fever of unknown origin, or suspected hematologic malignancies. A bone marrow examination reveals the maturation patterns of RBCs and WBCs, the presence of megakaryocytes or any abnormalities of the megakaryocytes, the myeloid-to-erythroid ratio, results of stains for iron and of any other stains that may be needed, and the presence of granuloma and tumor cells in hematoxylin and eosin–stained marrow sections. (Chapter 16 discusses the bone marrow procedure and examination in detail.)

Other Laboratory Tests

Other laboratory tests that can assist in establishing the cause of anemia include a complete urinalysis (including microscopic examination) and a fecal analysis with occult blood test and microscopic examination for parasites. Also, certain chemistry tests are important, such as the renal function and hepatic function studies.

After the hematologic laboratory studies are completed, the anemia may be classified based on reticulocyte count, MCV, and peripheral smear. After it has been classified, particular tests may be performed to finalize the diagnosis. Iron studies (including a serum iron, iron-binding capacity, and serum ferritin) are valuable if a low-reticulocyte-count (indicating decreased production), microcytic hypochromic anemia is present. The physician eventually determines the pathophysiologic cause of the anemia and makes the final diagnosis after

the results from all the procedures are available. Because of the numerous potential etiologies for the anemia, the cause needs to be determined before therapy can begin.[1,11]

MECHANISMS OF ANEMIA

The life span of the RBC in the circulation is about 120 days. In a healthy individual with no anemia, approximately 1% of the senescent circulating RBCs are lost daily, and the bone marrow normally continues to produce RBCs to replace those lost. Hematopoietic stem cells must function satisfactorily by maturing the erythroid precursor cells and releasing mature RBCs into the peripheral blood. Adequate RBC production requires several nutritional factors, such as iron, vitamin B_{12}, and folic acid. Hemoglobin synthesis also must function normally. The maintenance of a stable Hct requires the production of an amount of blood equaling the amount normally lost.[1,3,7]

Erythropoiesis

Erythropoiesis is the term used to refer to marrow erythroid proliferative activity. Normal erythropoiesis occurs only in the bone marrow with the formation of an adequate total number of RBCs (Chapter 8).[3] When the bone marrow is able to produce functional cells that leave the marrow and supply the blood with adequate numbers of cells, the process is termed *effective erythropoiesis.*

Ineffective erythropoiesis refers to the production of progenitor cells that are defective and thus are destroyed before leaving the marrow. Several conditions, such as megaloblastic

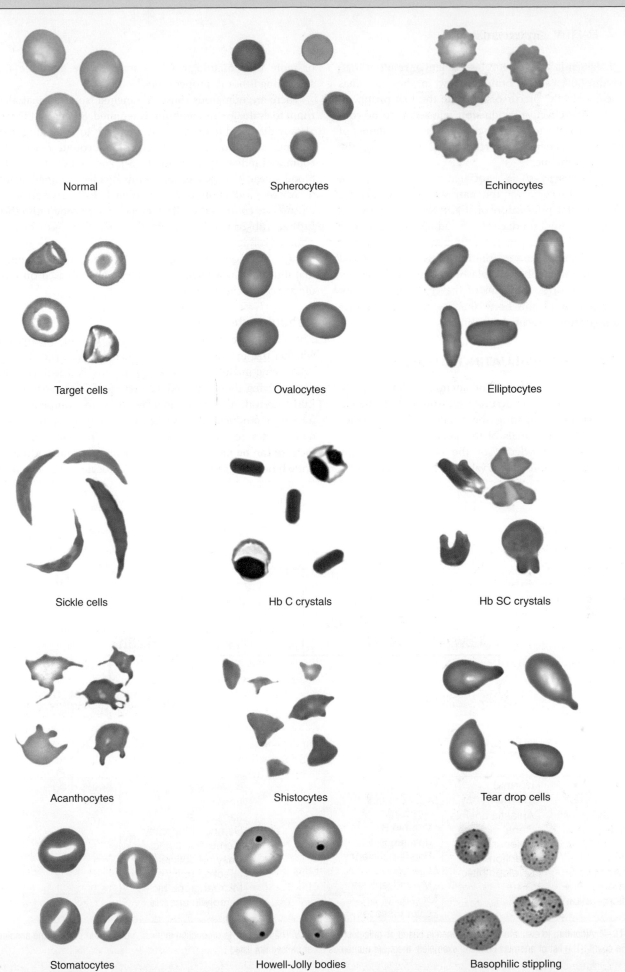

Normal

Spherocytes

Echinocytes

Target cells

Ovalocytes

Elliptocytes

Sickle cells

Hb C crystals

Hb SC crystals

Acanthocytes

Shistocytes

Tear drop cells

Stomatocytes

Howell-Jolly bodies

Basophilic stippling

Figure 18-1 RBCs: varied RBC shapes and inclusions. (Modified from Carr JH, Rodak BF: Clinical Hematology Atlas, 2nd ed. Philadelphia: Saunders, 2004.)

anemia, thalassemia, and sideroblastic anemia, result in ineffective erythropoiesis. The bone marrow in these anemias reveals increased RBC precursors, despite the low peripheral blood count. The effective production rate seems to be considerably less than the total production rate so that number of functional RBCs generated is reduced. Consequently, the patient becomes anemic.[11]

Insufficient erythropoiesis is associated with a quantitative lack of erythroid precursors in the marrow. The anemia is due to decrease in total production of RBCs. Several factors can lead to decreased RBC production, including lack of iron or erythropoietin (the cytokine that stimulates erythroid precursor cell proliferation and maturation), loss of the erythroid precursor to an autoantibody (aplastic anemia) or infection (parvovirus B19), or suppression of the erythroid precursor due to infiltration of the bone marrow with granulomas (sarcoidosis) or tumor (acute leukemia).[11]

APPROACH TO EVALUATING ANEMIAS

The first step in the diagnosis of anemia is detecting the presence of anemia by the accurate measurement of hematologic values and comparing these values with reference values for healthy individuals of the same age, gender, race, and environment. Knowledge of the results of previous hematologic examination often is valuable. A reduction of 10%

or more in hematologic values may be the first clue that something is not in proper order.[3-5]

There are numerous causes of anemia, so a rational algorithm to evaluate this condition is required. Several of the tests already discussed help guide the approach to evaluating these patients, including the complete blood count, reticulocyte count, cell indices (particularly MCV), and examination of the blood smear. The reticulocyte count divides the anemia into decreased production versus shortened RBC survival. If the reticulocyte count is low, the anemia can be divided into three further subgroups based on the MCV: (1) normocytic, normochromic anemia; (2) microcytic, hypochromic anemia; and (3) macrocytic anemia. Figure 18-2 presents a schematic that illustrates how anemias can be evaluated based on reticulocyte count and MCV.

Reticulocyte Count

The reticulocyte count plays a crucial role in determining whether the anemia is due to production defect (not enough RBCs being made) or to increased or early destruction (RBCs not surviving their expected 120 days). If there is shortened RBC survival, the bone marrow tries to compensate by increasing production. This increased production causes more reticulocytes to be released into the circulation, and the increase can be measured by the reticulocyte count. Although acute blood loss can increase the reticulocyte count, it is most

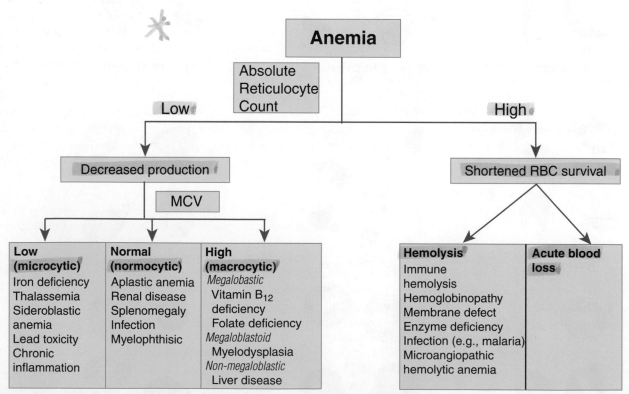

Figure 18-2 Algorithm to evaluate causes of anemia based on reticulocyte and MCV. The reticulocyte production index can be used in place of the absolute reticulocyte count. (The list of anemias contains examples; there are numerous other causes not listed.)

often elevated in hemolytic anemias.[3,6,11] Chronic blood loss *does not* increase the reticulocyte count. Chronic blood loss leads to iron deficiency and subsequently a low reticulocyte count. An inappropriately low reticulocyte count results from decreased production of the RBCs, whether it is insufficient or ineffective erythropoiesis.

Mean Corpuscular Volume and Anemia Subtypes

Microcytic, hypochromic anemia is present when the MCV is less than 80 fL and the MCHC is less than 32 g/dL, with small cells that have increased central pallor on the smear. Microcytic anemias generally are caused by conditions that result in reduced Hb synthesis: iron deficiency, deficiency of heme synthesis (sideroblastic anemia), deficiency of globin synthesis (thalassemia), and inability to use iron (chronic disease states or lead poisoning). The most common microcytic anemia results from an iron level insufficient for maintaining normal erythropoiesis and is characterized by abnormal results of iron studies. Early development of a microcytic anemia may reveal reduced iron stores, but an obvious anemia has not developed. The causes of iron deficiency vary in infants, children, adolescents, and adults, and it is imperative to find the cause before treatment begins (see Chapter 19).

Macrocytic, normochromic anemias typically are characterized by an MCV greater than 100 fL and MCHC greater than 32 g/dL. RBCs appear macrocytic. Macrocytic anemias may be megaloblastic or nonmegaloblastic. Megaloblastic anemias are caused by conditions that interfere with DNA synthesis, such as vitamin B_{12} deficiency, folate deficiency, or myelodysplasia. (In myelodysplasia, the morphology is megaloblastoid.) Nuclear maturation lags behind cytoplasmic development as a result of lack of DNA synthesis. This dyssynchrony between nuclear and cytoplasmic development results in the large cells. All cells of the body ultimately are affected by the deficiency in the production of DNA (Chapter 20). Pernicious anemia is one cause of vitamin B_{12} deficiency, whereas malabsorption secondary to inflammatory bowel disease is one known cause of folate deficiency. A megaloblastic anemia is characterized by oval macrocytes and teardrop-shaped cells in blood and by megaloblasts or large nucleated RBC precursors in bone marrow. The megaloblastic anemias can result in a markedly elevated MCV (>115 fL), although modest elevations (100-115 fL) occur as well.

Nonmegaloblastic forms of anemia also are characterized by large RBCs, but in contrast to megaloblastic anemias, they are typically related to membrane changes owing to disruption of the cholesterol-to-phospholipids ratio. These macrocytic cells are mostly round and the marrow nucleated RBCs do not display the megaloblastic maturation changes. Macrocytic anemias are often seen in patients with chronic liver disease and thyroid disease. It is rare for these nonmegaloblastic anemias to have an MCV greater than 115 fL.

Normocytic, normochromic anemia has an MCV of 80-100 fL, an MCH of 27-32 pg, and an MCHC of 32-36 g/dL. (The RBCs on the smear must be examined to rule out a dimorphic population of microcytes and macrocytes, which also would yield a normal MCV.) Most of the other conditions that lead to anemia result in normocytic anemias. Renal disease (due to reduced production of erythropoietin), aplastic anemia, splenomegaly, and infections (e.g., parvovirus B19) all are etiologies for normocytic anemias.[5] Figure 18-3 presents a schematic illustrating evaluation of anemias based on MCV alone.

Red Blood Cell Distribution Width

The RDW also often can help determine the cause of an anemia, especially when used in conjunction with the MCV (Table 18-4). Each of the three morphologic categories (normocytic, microcytic, macrocytic) mentioned earlier also can be subclassified by the automated RDW as homogeneous (normal RDW) or heterogeneous (increased or high RDW), according to Bessman et al.[12,13] Four examples are given:

- MCV low, RDW normal: heterozygous thalassemia
- MCV low, RDW high: iron deficiency
- MCV high, RDW high: vitamin B_{12} or folate deficiency
- MCV normal, RDW high: anemic hemoglobinopathy

The classification described by Bessman et al[12,13] can help narrow the diagnostic possibilities of the underlying cause of anemia. It is based first on the orderly approach of classifying anemia by the MCV followed by the subclassification with the RDW (see Table 18-4).

Hemolytic Anemias

In cases of an elevated reticulocyte count caused by a shortened RBC survival, an evaluation of a hemolytic anemia is required. Numerous causes of hemolysis exist, including immune-mediated destruction, RBC membrane defects, hemoglobinopathies, RBC enzyme deficiencies, infections, and intravascular destruction (microangiopathic hemolytic anemias).[3,7,11] A direct antiglobulin test (DAT; Coombs' test) helps differentiate immune-mediated destruction from the other causes. In the other hemolytic anemias, reviewing the peripheral smear is vital in determining the cause of hemolysis (see Table 18-2 and Fig. 18-2). Hemolytic anemias are discussed in Chapters 22 to 26.

Pathophysiologic Classification

A pathophysiologic classification of anemias relates disease processes to associated causes and currently described mechanisms. It is based on concepts that may be changed later, but at present they serve as an aid to physicians in the clinical investigation of anemia. In the pathophysiologic classification, the anemias caused by decreased RBC production (e.g., disorders of DNA synthesis) are distinguished from the anemias caused by increased RBC destruction or loss (intracorpuscular or extracorpuscular abnormalities of RBCs). Box 18-1 presents the pathophysiologic classification of anemia, lists the causes of the abnormality, and gives one or more examples of a type of anemia.

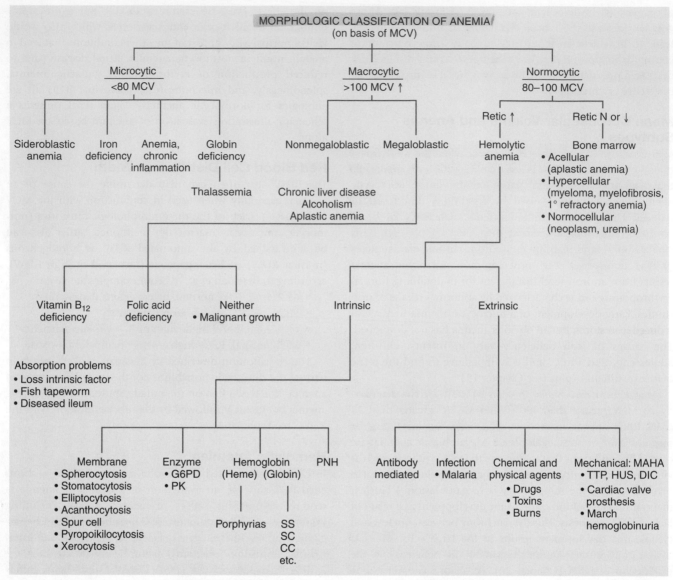

Figure 18-3 Morphologic classification of anemia on the basis of MCV only.

TABLE 18-4   Classification of Anemic Disorders Based on Red Blood Cell Mean Volume (MCV) and Heterogeneity (RDW)

MCV Low, RDW Normal (Microcytic Homogeneous)	MCV Low, RDW High (Microcytic Heterogeneous)	MCV Normal, RDW Normal (Normocytic Homogeneous)	MCV Normal, RDW High (Normocytic Heterogeneous)	MCV High, RDW Normal (Macrocytic Homogeneous)	MCV High, RDW High (Macrocytic Heterogeneous)
Heterozygous thalassemia	Iron deficiency	Normal	Mixed deficiency	Aplastic anemia	Folate deficiency
Chronic inflammation	S-β-thalassemia	Chronic inflammation (e.g., rheumatoid arthritis)	Early iron or folate deficiency		Vitamin B$_{12}$ deficiency
	Hb H	Nonanemic hemoglobinopathy (e.g., AS, AC)	Anemic hemoglobinopathy (e.g., SS, SC)		Reticulocytosis
	RBC fragmentation	Transfusion	Myelofibrosis		Cold agglutinins
		Chemotherapy	Sideroblastic		Myelodysplastic syndrome
		Hemorrhage			
		Hereditary spherocytosis			

Modified from Bessman JD, Gilmer PR, Gardner FH: Improved classification of anemias by MCV and RDW. Am J Clin Pathol 1983;80:324.

BOX 18-1 Pathophysiologic Classification of Anemias

Anemia Caused by Decreased Production of Red Blood Cells

Disturbance of hematopoietic stem cell proliferation and differentiation: aplastic anemia

Disturbance of DNA synthesis: megaloblastic anemia

Disturbance of Hb synthesis: iron deficiency anemia, thalassemia

Disturbance of proliferation and differentiation of precursor erythroid cells: anemia of chronic renal failure, anemia of endocrine disorders

Unknown or multiple mechanisms: anemia of chronic disease, anemia associated with marrow infiltration, sideroblastic anemia

Anemia Caused by Increased Destruction or Loss

Intracorpuscular Abnormality

Membrane defect: hereditary spherocytosis, hereditary elliptocytosis, pyropoikilocytosis

Enzyme deficiency: glucose-6-phosphate dehydrogenase, pyruvate kinase, porphyria

Globin abnormality: hemoglobinopathies (e.g., Hb SS, CC, SC)

Paroxysmal nocturnal hemoglobinuria

Extracorpuscular Abnormality

Mechanical: microangiopathic hemolytic anemia (thrombotic thrombocytopenic purpura, hemolytic uremic syndrome), traumatic cardiac hemolytic anemia

Infection: hemolytic anemia secondary to infection with malaria, *Babesia, Bartonella, Ehrlichia*

Chemical and physical agents: drugs, toxins, burns

Antibody-mediated: acquired hemolytic anemia secondary to warm reacting antibodies

Blood loss: acute blood loss anemia

Modified from Erslev AJ: Clinical manifestations and classification of erythrocyte disorders. In Beutler E, Lichtman MA, Coller BS, et al (eds): Williams Hematology, 5th ed. New York: McGraw-Hill, 1995:444.

CHAPTER at a GLANCE

- *Anemia* is defined conventionally as a decrease in RBCs, Hb, and Hct below the previously established normal values for healthy individuals of the same age, gender, and race under similar environmental conditions.
- Clinical diagnosis of anemia should include history, physical examination, signs, symptoms, and laboratory values.
- Many anemias have common manifestations. Careful questioning of the patient may reveal contributing factors, such as diet, medications, occupational hazards, bleeding history, and ethnicity.
- A thorough physical examination is valuable in determining the cause of anemia. Some features that should be evaluated are skin, nail beds, eyes, mucosa, lymph nodes, size of spleen and liver, and heart.
- Moderate anemias may not manifest clinical symptoms if onset is slow. Severe anemias (Hb <7 g/dL) usually produce pallor, dyspnea, vertigo, headache, muscle weakness, lethargy, hypotension, and tachycardia.
- Laboratory procedures helpful in the diagnosis of anemia include:
  Complete blood count with indices, including RDW
  Reticulocyte count
  Careful examination of the peripheral blood smear, with emphasis on RBC morphology

Bone marrow examination, if indicated

Other tests as indicated by the RBC indices, history, and physical examination (e.g., serum iron, iron-binding capacity, ferritin, folate, vitamin B_{12}, direct antiglobulin test, Hb electrophoresis)

- The cause of anemia should be determined before treatment is begun.
- The reticulocyte count and MCV play crucial roles in determining the cause of an anemia.
- Subclassification based on MCV includes:
  Normocytic, normochromic
  Microcytic, hypochromic
  Macrocytic
- The MCV when combined with the RDW also can aid in diagnosing anemia.
- The peripheral smear plays an important role in diagnosing hemolytic anemias.
- Some anemias may have more than one pathophysiologic cause.

Now that you have completed this chapter, go back and read again the case study at the beginning and respond to the questions presented.

REVIEW QUESTIONS

1. All of the following are clinical signs or symptoms of anemia *except*:
   a. Fatigue
   b. Jaundice
   c. Lymph node swelling
   d. Eating unusual things such as ice

2. The RBC index that is used to describe average RBC volume is the:
   a. RDW
   b. MCV
   c. MCH
   d. MCHC

3. Variation in RBC volume is expressed by the:
   a. RDW
   b. MCV
   c. MCH
   d. MCHC

4. There is an anemia that develops because the bone marrow becomes scarred. As a result, the amount of active bone marrow is diminished, including RBC precursors. The cells that are present are normal, but there are too few to meet the demand for blood cells, and anemia develops. The reticulocyte count is low. This anemia would be described as:
   a. Effective erythropoiesis
   b. Ineffective erythropoiesis
   c. Insufficient erythropoiesis

5. An elevation of which of the following points to reduced RBC life span and a hemolytic anemia?
   a. Reticulocyte count
   b. RDW
   c. Hemoglobin
   d. Hct

6. Refer to Table 18-4. An elevated MCV, along with a high RDW, suggests
   a. Iron deficiency anemia
   b. Vitamin B_{12} or folate deficiency
   c. Sickle cell anemia
   d. Normal blood picture

7. Which of the following is detectable only by examination of a peripheral blood smear?
   a. Microcytosis
   b. Anisocytosis
   c. Poikilocytosis
   d. Hypochromia

8. Refer to Fig. 18-2 and Table 18-4. Which of the following would be within the differential diagnosis of a patient with an MCV of 115 fL and an RDW of 20% (reference range 11.5-14.5)?
   a. Myelofibrosis
   b. Sideroblastic anemia
   c. Porphyria
   d. Folate deficiency

9. When anemia is long-standing, which of the following is among the adaptations of the body?
   a. Reduced respiratory rate
   b. Reduced oxygen affinity of Hb
   c. Lower heart rate
   d. Reduced volume of blood ejected from the heart with each contraction

10. Which of the following patients would be considered anemic with a Hb value of 14.5 g/dL? Refer to reference ranges inside the front cover of this text.
    a. A newborn boy
    b. An adult woman
    c. An adult man
    d. A 10-year-old girl

ACKNOWLEDGMENT

The foundation for this chapter is based on the work of Ann Bell. The author expresses his gratitude for the opportunity to amend her fine endeavor.

REFERENCES

1. Berliner N: Disorders of red blood cells. In Andreoli TE, Carpenter CCJ, Griggs RC, et al (eds): Cecil Essentials of Medicine, 6th ed. Philadelphia: Saunders, 2004:449-460.
2. Pickett JP (ed): The American Heritage Dictionary of the English Language, 4th ed. Boston: Houghton Mifflin, 2000.
3. Glader B: Anemia: General considerations. In Greer JP, Foerster J, Lukens JN, et al (eds): Wintrobe's Clinical Hematology, 11th ed. Philadelphia: Lippincott, Williams & Wilkins, 2004:947-978.
4. Tefferi A: Anemia in adults: a contemporary approach to diagnosis. Mayo Clin Proc 2003;78:1274-1280.
5. Brill JR, Baumgardner DJ: Normocytic anemia. Am Fam Physician 2000;62:2255-2263.
6. Aird WC: Anemia. In Furie B, Cassileth PA, Atkins MB, et al (eds): Clinical Hematology and Oncology: Presentation, Diagnosis, and Treatment. Philadelphia: Churchill Livingstone, 2003:232-240.
7. Marks PW, Glader B: Approach to anemia in the child and adult. In Hoffman R, Benz EJ Jr, Shattil SJ, et al (eds): Hematology: Basic Principles and Practice, 4th ed. Philadelphia: Churchill Livingstone, 2005:455-464.
8. Andrews NC: Iron deficiency and related disorders. In Greer JP, Foerster J, Lukens JN, et al (eds): Wintrobe's Clinical Hematology, 11th ed. Philadelphia: Lippincott, Williams & Wilkins, 2004:980-1087.
9. Perkins SL: Examination of the blood and bone marrow. In

Greer JP, Foerster J, Lukens JN, et al (eds): Wintrobe's Clinical Hematology, 11th ed. Philadelphia: Lippincott, Williams & Wilkins, 2004:1-25.

10. Jandl JH: Blood: Textbook of Hematology. Boston: Little, Brown, 1996.

11. Adamson JW, Longo DL: Anemia and polycythemia. In Kasper DL, Fauci AS, Longo DL, et al (eds): Harrison's Principles of Internal Medicine, 16th ed. New York: McGraw-Hill, 2005: Chapter 52.

12. Bessman JD, Gilmer PR, Gardner FH: Improved classification of anemia by MCV and RDW. Am J Clin Pathol 1983;80:322-326.

13. Bessman JD, Gilmer PR, Gardner FH: Education program of American Society of Hematology, 25th Annual Meeting, 1983:54-56.

19

Disorders of Iron and Heme Metabolism

Kathryn Doig

OBJECTIVES

After completion of this chapter, the reader should be able to:

1. Recognize complete blood count (CBC) results consistent with iron deficiency anemia, anemia of chronic inflammation, and sideroblastic anemias.

2. Given results of iron studies, free erythrocyte protoporphyrin (FEP), and serum transferrin receptors, distinguish results consistent with iron deficiency anemia, anemia of chronic inflammation, sideroblastic anemias, thalassemias, and iron overload conditions.

3. Recognize individuals at risk for iron deficiency anemia by virtue of age, gender, diet, physiologic circumstance such as pregnancy and menstruation, or pathologic conditions such as gastric ulcers.

4. Given a description of the appearance of the Prussian blue stain of bone marrow, recognize results consistent with iron deficiency anemia, anemia of chronic inflammation, or a sideroblastic anemia.

5. Recognize a bone marrow description consistent with iron deficiency anemia, anemia of chronic inflammation, or a sideroblastic anemia.

6. Recognize conditions in which anemia of chronic inflammation may develop.

7. Recognize predisposing factors for sideroblastic anemias or conditions in which sideroblastic anemias may develop.

8. Discuss the clinical significance of increased levels of FEP.

9. Discuss the differences in disease etiology, diagnosis, and treatment between iron overload resulting from hereditary hemochromatosis and transfusion-related hemosiderosis.

10. Discuss the pathogenesis of iron deficiency anemia, anemia of chronic inflammation, sideroblastic anemia secondary to lead poisoning, and hemochromatosis.

CASE STUDY

After studying the material in this chapter, the reader should be able to respond to the following case study:

An 85-year-old slender, frail Caucasian woman was hospitalized for diagnosis and treatment of anemia suspected during a routine examination by her physician. The physician noted that she appeared pale and inquired about fatigue and tiredness. Although she generally felt well, the patient admitted to feeling slightly tired when climbing stairs. A hematocrit (Hct) performed in the physician's office showed a dangerously low value, so she was hospitalized for further evaluation. Her CBC results are as follows:

	Patient	Reference Range
WBC ($\times 10^9$/L)	8.5	4.5-11
RBC ($\times 10^{12}$/L)	1.66	4.3-5.9
Hb (g/dL)	3	13.9-16.3

	Patient	Reference Range
Hct (L/L)	0.11	0.39-0.55
MCV (fL)	63	80-100
MCH (pg)	18.1	25.4-34.6
MCHC (g/dL)	28	31-37
RDW (%)	20	11.5-14.5
Platelet count ($\times 10^9$/L)	165	150-400
WBC differential	Unremarkable	
RBC morphology	Marked anisocytosis, marked poikilocytosis, marked hypochromia, marked microcytosis	

GENERAL CONCEPTS IN ANEMIA

Anemia may result whenever red blood cell (RBC) production is impaired, RBC life span is shortened, or there is frank loss of cells. The anemias associated with iron typically are categorized as anemias of impaired production. The formation of RBCs requires many constituents, chief among them being the components for the production of hemoglobin (Hb): iron, heme, and globin. Depending on the cause, lack of available iron results in iron deficiency anemia or the anemia of chronic inflammation. Inadequate availability of heme results in a relative excess of iron manifested in sideroblastic anemias. These causes are discussed in this chapter. Inadequate globin production results in the thalassemias, which are discussed separately in Chapter 27.

As discussed more extensively in Chapter 11, iron is absorbed from the diet in the small intestine, carried by transferrin to a cell in need, and incorporated into the cell where it is held as ferritin until incorporated into its final functional molecule. That functional molecule may be a heme-based cytochrome, muscle myoglobin, or, in the case of developing RBCs, Hb. Iron may be unavailable for incorporation into heme because of inadequate stores of body iron or merely because of impaired mobilization. The anemia associated with inadequate stores is termed *iron deficiency*, whereas the anemia resulting from impaired mobilization is *anemia of chronic inflammation* due to its association with chronic inflammatory conditions, such as rheumatoid arthritis. When the iron supply is adequate and mobilization is unimpaired, but an intrinsic RBC defect prevents incorporation of iron into heme, the resulting anemia is termed *sideroblastic*, referring to the presence of iron in the developing RBCs.

IRON DEFICIENCY ANEMIA

Etiology

Iron deficiency anemia develops when the intake of iron is inadequate to meet a standard level of demand, when the need for iron expands, or when there is chronic loss of Hb from the body.

Inadequate Intake

Iron deficiency anemia can develop as the erythron is slowly starved for iron. Each day, approximately 1 mg of iron is lost

from the body mainly in the mitochondria of desquamated skin and sloughed intestinal epithelium.[1] Because the body tenaciously conserves all other iron from senescent cells, including RBCs, replacing 1 mg of iron in the diet daily maintains iron balance and supplies the body's need for RBC production. When the diet is consistently inadequate in iron, over time the body's stores of iron become depleted. Ultimately, RBC production slows as a result of the inability to produce Hb. With approximately 1% of cells naturally dying each day, the anemia becomes apparent when the production rate cannot replace lost cells.

Increased Need

Iron deficiency also can develop when the level of iron intake becomes inadequate to meet the needs of an expanding erythron. This is the case in periods of rapid growth, such as infancy, childhood, and adolescence. Pregnancy and nursing place similar demands on the mother's body to provide iron for the developing fetus or nursing infant and herself. In each of these instances, what had previously been an adequate intake of iron for the individual becomes inadequate as the need for iron increases.

Chronic Blood Loss

A third way iron deficiency develops is with excessive loss of Hb from the body. This loss occurs with slow hemorrhage or hemolysis. Any condition in which there is a slow, low-level loss of RBCs may result in iron deficiency. For women, heavy menstrual bleeding can constitute a chronic loss of blood leading to iron deficiency, as can bleeding associated with fibroid tumors. For women or men, gastrointestinal bleeding from ulcers or tumors can be the cause. Loss of blood via the urinary tract with kidney stones or tumors also can lead to iron deficiency. Individuals with chronic intravascular hemolytic processes, such as paroxysmal nocturnal hemoglobinuria, can develop iron deficiency due to the loss of iron in Hb passed into the urine.

Pathogenesis

Iron deficiency anemia develops slowly, progressing through stages that physiologically blend one into the other but are useful delineations for understanding disease progression.[2] As shown in Figure 19-1, iron is distributed among three compartments: (1) the storage compartment, principally as ferritin in

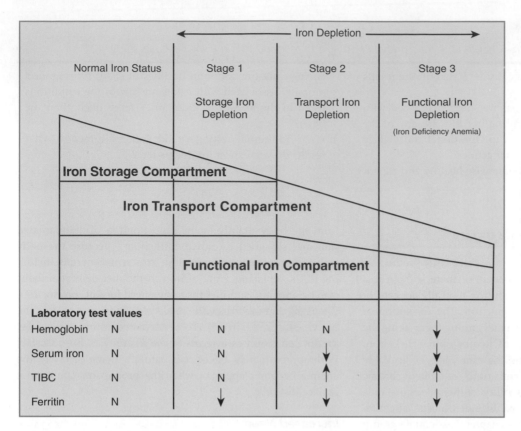

Figure 19-1 The development of iron deficiency anemia. (Adapted from Suominen P, Punnonen K, Rajamäki A, et al: Serum transferrin receptor and transferrin receptor–ferritin index identify healthy subjects with subclinical iron deficits. Blood 1998;92:2934-2939; reprinted with permission.)

the bone marrow macrophages and liver cells; (2) the transport compartment of serum transferrin; and (3) the functional compartment of Hb, myoglobin, and cytochromes. Hb and intracellular ferritin constitute nearly 95% of the total distribution of iron.[3]

For a period of time as iron intake lags behind loss, essentially normal iron status continues. Absorption of iron through the intestine is accelerated in an attempt to meet the relative increased demand for iron, but this is not apparent in laboratory tests or patient symptoms. The individual appears healthy. As the negative iron balance continues, however, a stage of iron depletion develops.

Stage 1

Stage 1 of iron deficiency is characterized by a progressive loss of storage iron. The body's reserve of iron is sufficient to maintain the transport and functional compartments through this phase, so RBC development is normal. There is no evidence of iron deficiency in the peripheral blood picture and the patient experiences no symptoms of anemia. If ferritin levels are measured, however, they are low, indicating the decline in stored iron, which also could be detected in an iron stain of the marrow. Without evidence of anemia, however, neither of these tests would be performed, and individuals appear healthy. It is estimated that nearly 50% of U.S. infants are in this phase of iron deficiency at any given time.[4]

Stage 2

Stage 2 of iron deficiency is defined by the exhaustion of the storage pool of iron. For a time, RBC production continues as

normal, relying on the iron available in the transport compartment. Anemia, as measured relative to the reference range of Hb, is still not evident, although an individual's Hb may begin dropping. Other iron-dependent tissues, such as muscles, may begin to be affected, although the symptoms may be nonspecific. If measured, ferritin levels and serum iron are still low, whereas total iron-binding capacity (TIBC) (i.e., transferrin) increases (see section on iron studies). Free erythrocyte protoporphyrin (FEP), the porphyrin into which iron is inserted to form heme, begins to accumulate. Transferrin receptors increase on the surface of iron-starved cells as they try to capture as much available iron as possible. They also are shed into the plasma, and levels increase measurably in stage 2. Prussian blue stain of the marrow in stage 2 would show essentially no stored iron and iron deficient erythropoiesis would be evident (see subsequent description). As in stage 1, iron deficiency in stage 2 is subclinical, and testing is not likely to be undertaken.

Stage 3

Stage 3 of iron deficiency is frank anemia. The Hb and hematocrit (Hct) are low relative to the reference ranges. Having thoroughly depleted storage iron and diminished transport iron, developing RBCs are unable to develop normally. The number of cell divisions per precursor increases because hemoglobin accumulation in the developing cells is slowed, allowing more time for divisions. The result is first smaller cells with adequate Hb concentration, although ultimately even these cannot be filled with Hb. These cells become microcytic and hypochromic (Fig. 19-2). As would be expected, ferritin

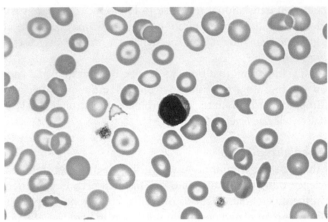

Figure 19-2 Hypochromic, microcytic anemia with increased RDW. Note small lymphocyte in field for comparison of RBC size (peripheral blood, ×1000).

levels are exceedingly low. Other iron studies (see later) also are abnormal, and the FEP and transferrin receptor levels increase.

In this phase, the patient experiences the nonspecific symptoms of anemia, typically fatigue and weakness, especially with exertion. Pallor is evident in light-skinned individuals but also can be noted in the conjunctivae, mucous membranes, or palmar creases of dark-skinned individuals.[3] More severe signs are not seen as often in the United States[3] but include a sore tongue (glossitis) due to iron deficiency in the rapidly proliferating cells of the alimentary tract and inflamed cracks at the corners of the mouth (angular chelosis). Koilonychia (spooning of the fingernails) may be seen if the deficiency is long-standing. Patients also may experience cravings for nonfood items, which is called *pica*. The cravings may include things such as dirt, clay, laundry starch, or most commonly ice, specifically called *pagophagia*.[3]

As should be evident from this discussion, numerous individuals may be iron deficient while appearing healthy. Until late in stage 2, they may experience no symptoms at all and are unlikely to come to medical attention. Even in stage 3, frankly anemic patients may not seek medical care because the body is able to compensate remarkably for slowly developing anemia (Chapter 18) as in the case study at the beginning of this chapter. Because routine screening tests included in the CBC do not become abnormal until late in stage 2 or early in stage 3, most patients are not diagnosed until relatively late in the progress of the iron depletion.

Epidemiology

From the previous discussion, it is apparent that certain groups of individuals are more prone to the development of iron deficiency anemia. Menstruating women are at especially high risk. Their monthly loss of blood increases their routine need for iron, which is often not met with the standard U.S. diet.[3] For adolescent girls, this is compounded by increased need with growth. If women of childbearing age are not properly supplemented, pregnancy and nursing can lead to a loss of nearly 900 mg of iron, further depleting iron stores. Succeeding

pregnancies can exacerbate the problem, leading to iron deficient fetuses.[5]

Growing children also are at high risk.[5] The increasing need for iron as the child grows can be coupled with dietary inadequacies. Cow's milk is not a good source of iron, and infants need to be placed on supplemented formula by about age 6 months when their fetal stores of iron become depleted.[3] This assumes infants were able to establish adequate stores from their mothers in utero. Even though breast milk is a better source of iron than cow's milk,[6] it is not a consistent source.[7] Iron supplementation also is recommended for breastfed infants after 6 months of age.[3]

Iron deficiency is relatively rare in men and postmenopausal women because the body conserves iron so tenaciously and these individuals lose only about 1 mg/d. Gastrointestinal disease, such as ulcers, tumors, or hemorrhoids, should be suspected for iron deficient patients in either of these groups if the diet is known to be adequate in iron. Regular aspirin ingestion can lead to gastritis and chronic bleeding, as can alcohol. Elderly individuals, particularly those living alone, may not eat a balanced diet, however, and pure dietary deficiency is seen among these individuals. In some elderly individuals, the loss of gastric acidity with age can impair iron absorption.

Iron deficiency is associated with infection by hookworms, *Necator americanus* and *Ancylostoma duodenale*. The worm attaches to the intestinal wall and literally sucks blood from the gastric vessels.

Soldiers and long-distance runners also can develop iron deficiency. "Marching anemia" develops when RBCs are hemolyzed by foot-pounding trauma and iron is lost as Hb in the urine.[8] The amount lost in the urine can be so little that it is not apparent on visual inspection.

Laboratory Diagnosis

The early stages of iron deficiency can be detected by sophisticated tests. Individuals are unlikely to be referred for such studies, however, because there is virtually no physiologic evidence of the declining iron state. Nevertheless, iron deficiency might be suspected in an individual in a high-risk group, and appropriate testing can be ordered.[8] The tests can be grouped into three general categories: screening, diagnostic, and specialized.

Screening for Iron Deficiency Anemia

When iron deficient erythropoiesis is under way, the CBC begins to show evidence of microcytosis and hypochromia (see Fig. 19-2). The classic picture of iron deficiency anemia in stage 3 includes a decreased Hb. An RBC distribution width (RDW) greater than 15% would be expected and may precede the decrease in Hb.[9] For patients in high-risk groups, the elevated RDW can be an early and sensitive indicator of iron deficiency.[10] As the Hb continues to fall, microcytosis and hypochromia become more prominent with progressively declining values for mean cell volume (MCV), mean cell hemoglobin (MCH), and mean cell hemoglobin concentration (MCHC). The RBC count ultimately becomes decreased, as does the Hct. Polychromasia may be apparent early, although not a prominent finding. An absolute reticulocyte count confirms a diminished rate of effective erythropoiesis.[11] In addition to anisocytosis, poikilocytosis, including occasional target cells and elliptocytes, may be present, although no particular shape is characteristic or predominant. Thrombocytosis may be present, particularly if the iron deficiency results from a chronic bleed, but this is not a diagnostic parameter. White blood cells typically are normal in number and appearance. Iron deficiency should be suspected when the CBC findings show a hypochromic, microcytic anemia with elevated RDW but no consistent morphologic changes to the RBCs.

Diagnosis of Iron Deficiency

Iron studies remain the backbone for diagnosis of iron deficiency (Chapter 11). They include assay of serum iron, TIBC, transferrin saturation, and ferritin. Serum iron is a measure of the amount of iron bound to transferrin (transport protein) in the serum. TIBC is an indirect measure of transferrin and the available binding sites for iron in the plasma. The percent of transferrin saturated with iron can be calculated from the total iron and the TIBC:

$$\text{Transferrin saturation (\%sat)} = \frac{\text{serum iron (}\mu\text{g/dL)} \times 100}{\text{TIBC (}\mu\text{g/dL)}}$$

Ferritin is not truly an extracellular protein, since it provides an intracellular storage repository for metabolically active iron. However, ferritin is present in serum with serum levels reflecting the levels of iron stored within cells. Serum ferritin is an easily accessible surrogate for stainable bone marrow iron.

The iron studies are used collectively to assess the iron status of an individual. Table 19-1 shows that, as expected, ferritin and serum iron values are decreased in iron deficiency anemia. Transferrin levels increase when the hepatocyte detects low iron, with research showing that this is a transcriptional and post-translational response to low iron.[12] The result is a decline in the iron saturation of transferrin that is more dramatic than might be expected just from the decrease in serum iron.

It is important that iron studies are drawn fasting and early in the morning. Iron shows a diurnal variation with levels dropping throughout the day.[13] Iron absorbed from a meal can falsely elevate levels.[14]

Specialized Tests

Although not commonly used for the diagnosis of iron deficiency, other tests show abnormalities that become important in the differential diagnosis of similar conditions. Test results for the accumulated porphyrin precursors to heme are elevated (see Table 19-1). FEP accumulates when iron is unavailable. In the absence of iron, FEP may be preferentially chelated with zinc to form zinc protoporphyrin (ZPP).[15] The FEP and the zinc chelate can be assayed fluorometrically. Serum transferrin receptors (STfR) also can be assayed using immunoassay. Levels increase as the disease progresses, and individual cells seek to absorb as much iron as possible.[16]

A bone marrow assessment is not indicated for suspected uncomplicated iron deficiency. A therapeutic trial of iron provides a less invasive and less expensive diagnostic assessment. Marrow examination may be performed, however, if the diagnosis is complicated or if other tests are equivocal. With routine stains, the iron deficient bone marrow appears hyperplastic early in the progression of the disease, with a decreased myeloid-to-erythroid ratio as a result of increased erythropoiesis.[3] As the disease progresses, hyperplasia subsides, and the profound deficiency of iron leads to slowed RBC production. Polychromatophilic normoblasts (i.e., rubricytes) show the most dramatic morphologic changes (Fig. 19-3). Nuclear cytoplasmic asynchrony with the cytoplasm lagging behind the nucleus becomes evident. Without the pink provided by Hb,

TABLE 19-1 Iron Studies in Microcytic, Hypochromic Anemias

	Iron Deficiency	Thalassemia Minor	Anemia of Chronic Inflammation	Sideroblastic Anemia	Lead Poisoning
Serum ferritin	↓	↑/N	↑/N	↑	N
Serum iron	↓/N	↑/N	↓	↑	Variable
TIBC	↑	N	↓	↓/N	N
Transferrin saturation	↓	↑/N	↓	↑	↑
FEP/ZPP	↑	N	↑	↑	↑ (marked)
BM iron (Prussian blue reaction)	No stainable iron	↑/N	↑/N	↑	N
Sideroblasts in BM	None	N	None/very few	↑ (ringed)	N (ringed)
Other special tests		↑ Hb A₂ (β-thalassemia minor)	Specific tests for inflammatory disorders, or cancer		↑ ALA in urine ↑ whole-blood lead levels

N, normal; ↑, increased; ↓, decreased.
ALA, aminolevulinic acid; BM, bone marrow; FEP/ZPP, free erythrocyte protoporphyrin or zinc protoporphyrin.

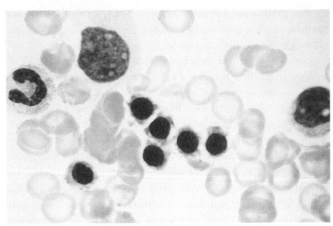

Figure 19-3 Bone marrow smear of iron deficiency anemia. The late-nucleated RBCs show the characteristic "shaggy blue" cytoplasm owing to asynchronism in maturation. (Courtesy of Ann Bell, University of Tennessee, Memphis.)

the cytoplasm remains bluish after the nucleus has begun to condense. The cell membranes appear irregular, usually described as "shaggy."

Treatment and Its Effects
Treatment
The first therapy for iron deficiency is to treat any underlying contributing cause, such as hookworms, tumors, or ulcers. As with simple nutritional deficiencies or increased need, dietary supplementation is necessary to replenish the body's iron stores. Oral supplements of ferrous sulfate (3 tablets/d containing 60 mg elemental iron) are the standard prescription.[3] The supplements should be taken on an empty stomach to maximize absorption. Many patients experience side effects, however, such as nausea and constipation, which lead to poor patient compliance. Vigilance on the part of the health care provider is important to ensure that patients complete the course of iron replacement, which usually lasts 6 months or more.[17] In rare cases in which intestinal absorption of iron is impaired, as with gastric achlorhydria, parenteral administration of iron dextrans can be used, although the side effects of this therapy are notable.[3] The risks of blood transfusions are rarely warranted for the correction of uncomplicated iron deficiency, unless the patient's Hb has become dangerously low.

Response to Treatment
Assuming optimal treatment with iron, the effects are quickly evident. Reticulocyte counts (relative and absolute) begin to increase within 5 to 10 days.[18] The anticipated increase in Hb appears in 2 to 3 weeks and should return to normal for the individual by about 2 months after the initiation of adequate treatment.[18] The blood smear and indices still reflect the iron deficient population of cells for several months, but the normal cell population slowly predominates. Iron therapy must continue for another 3 to 4 months to replenish the storage pool and prevent a relapse.

Assuming the patient has been compliant, the failure to respond to iron treatment points to the need for further investigation. The patient may be iron deficient but experiencing continued occult loss of blood or inadequate absorption. Alternatively, causes of hypochromic, microcytic anemia unrelated to iron deficiency, such as thalassemia, should be examined.

ANEMIA OF CHRONIC INFLAMMATION

Anemia commonly is associated with systemic diseases, including chronic inflammatory conditions such as arthritis, chronic infections such as tuberculosis or human immunodeficiency virus (HIV) infection, and malignancies. Cartwright[19] was the first to suggest that although the underlying diseases seem quite disparate, the associated anemia may be from a single cause, proposing the concept of anemia of chronic disease. This anemia represents the most common anemia among hospitalized patients.[20]

Etiology
Although originally called *anemia of chronic disease*, chronic blood loss is not among the conditions leading to the anemia of chronic disease. Chronic blood loss leads to clear-cut iron deficiency. Anemia of chronic disease is more correctly termed *anemia of chronic inflammation* because inflammation seems to be the unifying factor among the three above-mentioned general types of conditions in which this anemia is seen. The central feature of anemia of chronic inflammation is sideropenia in the face of abundant iron stores. The etiology is now understood to be largely due to impaired ferrokinetics.

The apparent inconsistency of decreased serum iron but abundant iron stores has been explained by the discovery of the role of hepcidin in regulation of body iron. Hepcidin is a hormone produced by hepatocytes to regulate body iron levels, particularly absorption of iron in the intestine and release of iron from macrophages. Hepcidin seems to interact with the protein ferroportin that exports iron from enterocytes into the plasma, reducing the amount of iron absorbed into the blood from the intestine.[21] Macrophages also use ferroportin to export iron into plasma and are affected by hepcidin.[21] When body iron levels decrease, hepcidin production by hepatocytes decreases,[22] and enterocyte iron export to plasma increases. Macrophage release of iron also increases. Iron accumulates in hepatocytes.[23] When iron levels are high, hepcidin increases, enterocyte iron release decreases, and macrophages retain iron.

Hepcidin is an acute-phase reactant,[24] so levels increase during inflammation, unrelated to iron levels in the body. As a result, during inflammation, intestinal iron absorption is decreased and release from macrophages declines. Although there is plenty of iron in the body, it is unavailable to developing RBCs by virtue of being sequestered in the macrophages and hepatocytes.

This response of hepcidin during inflammation would seem to be a nonspecific defense against invading bacteria. If the body can sequester iron, it reduces the amount of iron available to bacteria and contributes to their demise. Although this response of hepcidin is fine for conditions of short duration, causing no ill effects for the host, chronically high levels of hepcidin mean that iron is embargoed for long periods, leading to diminished production of RBCs.

A second acute-phase reactant seems to contribute to anemia of chronic inflammation, although probably to a much smaller extent than hepcidin. Lactoferrin is an iron-binding protein in the granules of neutrophils. Its avidity for iron is greater than that of transferrin. It has been suggested that lactoferrin is important intracellularly for phagocytes to prevent phagocytized bacteria from using intracellular iron for their metabolic processes.[25] During infection and inflammation, however, neutrophil lactoferrin also is released into the plasma. There it scavenges available iron, at the expense of transferrin. When it is carrying iron, the lactoferrin is bound to macrophages and liver cells that salvage the iron. RBCs are deprived of this iron, however, because they do not have lactoferrin receptors.

Finally, a third acute-phase reactant, ferritin, contributes to the etiology of anemia of chronic inflammation. Increased levels of ferritin in the plasma also bind some iron. Because developing RBCs do not have a ferritin receptor, this iron is unavailable for incorporation into Hb.

The result of these effects is that although iron is present in abundance in bone marrow macrophages, its release to developing erythrocytes is slowed. This can be seen histologically with iron stains that show iron in macrophages but not in erythroblasts.[26] The effect on the RBCs is essentially no different than in mild iron deficiency because they are effectively deprived of the iron.

Diminished erythropoiesis and a blunted response to erythropoietin also may contribute to the anemia of chronic inflammation.[27] The impaired ferrokinetics likely are the more significant cause of the anemia, however.

Laboratory Diagnosis

The peripheral blood picture in anemia of chronic inflammation is that of a mild anemia with Hb usually 9 to 11 g/dL without reticulocytosis. The cells are usually normocytic and normochromic, although a microcytic and hypochromic picture may develop in about one third of patients and may represent coexistent iron deficiency.[3] The inflammatory condition leading to the anemia also may cause leukocytosis, thrombocytosis, or both. Iron studies (see Table 19-1) show a low serum iron and TIBC. Because hepatocyte production of transferrin is regulated by iron levels,[12] the low TIBC (an indirect measurement of transferrin) reflects the abundant body iron stores. The transferrin saturation may be normal or low. Ferritin usually is increased beyond what would be expected for the same patient without the inflammatory condition. It may not be outside the reference range, but it is nevertheless increased. The failure to incorporate iron into heme results in elevation of FEP, although this test typically is not used diagnostically. The bone marrow shows hypoproliferation of the RBCs, consistent with the lack of reticulocytes

in the peripheral blood. Prussian blue stain of the bone marrow confirms abundant stores of iron in macrophages, although not in RBC precursors.

Patients with iron deficiency anemia who have an inflammatory condition present a special diagnostic dilemma. The iron deficiency may be missed because of the increase in ferritin associated with the inflammation, although the inflammatory condition may not induce anemia of chronic inflammation. Iron deficiency anemia and anemia of chronic inflammation can be distinguished in such situations by measuring serum (soluble) transferrin receptors (STfRs).[28] These receptors are sloughed from cells into the plasma. As noted earlier, levels increase during iron deficiency anemia but remain essentially normal during anemia of chronic inflammation. Another automated assay that may be useful is the reticulocyte Hb (CHr).[29] This is analogous to the MCH but for reticulocytes. The MCH is the average weight of Hb/cell across the entire RBC population. Some of the cells are nearly 120 days old, whereas others are just 1 to 2 days old. If iron deficiency is developing, the MCH does not change until a substantial proportion of the cells are iron deficient, and the diagnosis is effectively delayed for several months after iron deficient erythropoiesis begins. The reticulocyte Hb is able to assess iron deficient erythropoiesis within days as the first iron deficient cells leave the marrow. It is a sensitive indicator of iron deficiency and can assist in distinguishing iron deficiency anemia and anemia of chronic inflammation.

Treatment

Therapeutic erythropoietin can correct anemia of chronic inflammation,[30] but iron must be administered concurrently, because stored body iron remains sequestered and unavailable.[31] The anemia is typically not severe, however, and this costly treatment is warranted only in select patients. The best course of treatment is effective control or removal of the underlying condition.

SIDEROBLASTIC ANEMIAS

As with anemia resulting from inadequate supplies of iron for production of Hb, diseases that interfere with the production of adequate amounts of heme also can produce anemia. (See Chapter 10 for heme synthesis.) Similar to iron deficiency, the anemia may be microcytic and hypochromic. In contrast to iron deficiency, however, iron is abundant in the marrow. A Prussian blue stain of the marrow shows normoblasts with iron deposits in the mitochondria surrounding the nucleus. The location in the mitochondria shows that the iron is awaiting incorporation into heme. These *ringed sideroblasts* are the hallmark of the sideroblastic anemias (Fig. 19-4).

The sideroblastic anemias are a diverse group of diseases including hereditary and acquired conditions (Box 19-1). Among the hereditary forms, X-linked and autosomal varieties of this condition are known. Some patients experience at least modest improvement of anemia with pharmacologic doses of pyridoxine to stimulate heme synthesis.[32] Pyridoxine is a

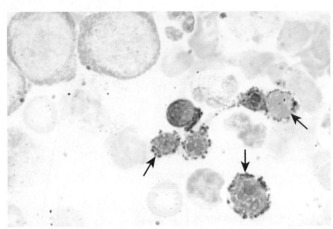

Figure 19-4 Ringed sideroblasts *(arrows)* shown with Prussian blue stain (bone marrow, ×1000).

BOX 19-1 Disorders Included in Sideroblastic Anemias

Hereditary
X-linked
Autosomal

Acquired
Primary sideroblastic anemia (refractory)
Secondary sideroblastic anemias
    Drugs and bone marrow toxins
    • Antitubercular therapy
    • Chloramphenicol
    • Alcohol
    • Lead
    • Chemotherapeutic agents

---

cofactor in the first step of porphyrin synthesis (Fig. 19-5) in which glycine is condensed with succinyl coenzyme A to form aminolevulinic acid.

Lead Poisoning

The acquired conditions leading to sideroblastic anemia constitute a diverse group in themselves. Certain drugs, such as chloramphenicol or isoniazid, can induce sideroblastic anemia.[33] Other toxins including heavy metals also have been identified. Among these, lead poisoning is a significant public health concern. Adults may be exposed at work with leaded compounds. Adults and children living in older homes can be exposed to lead from paints produced before the 1970s. They are at risk if dust is created during renovations. Toddlers and crawling infants are at special risk by getting dust on their hands and placing them in their mouths. Although anyone can experience lead poisoning, it is of special concern in children because the metal affects the central nervous system and the hematologic system, leading to impaired mental development.[34] In children and adults, a peripheral neuropathy[35] can be seen with abdominal cramping and vomiting or seizures.

Lead interferes with porphyrin synthesis at several steps. The most critical are as follows (see Fig. 19-5):

1. The conversion of aminolevulinic acid to porphobilinogen, resulting in the accumulation of aminolevulinic acid
2. Incorporation of iron into protoporphyrin IX by ferrochelatase (also called *heme synthetase*), resulting in accumulation of iron and protoporphyrin[36]

Of these, the impairment of ferrochelatase is probably the more significant of these inhibitions. Accumulated aminolevulinic acid is measurable in the urine, and protoporphyrin is measurable in an extract of RBCs as FEP or zinc protoporphyrin.

Anemia, when present in lead poisoning, is most often normocytic and normochromic; however, with chronic exposure to lead, a microcytic, hypochromic clinical picture may be seen. The degree of anemia in adults may not be dramatic, but in children it may be more profound. The reticulocyte count in acute poisoning may be quite elevated, suggesting that the anemia has a hemolytic component. The hemolytic component is supported by studies showing impairment of the pentose-phosphate shunt by lead,[37] making the cells sensitive to oxidant stress as in glucose-6-phosphate dehydrogenase deficiency (Chapter 23). In contrast, chronic poisoning results in hypoplasia of the marrow.[38] Basophilic stippling is a classic finding associated with lead toxicity. Lead interferes with the breakdown of pyrimidine 5'-nucleotides, which are believed to retard the breakdown of ribosomal RNA.[39] This causes undegraded ribosomes to aggregate, forming basophilic stippling. Because basophilic stippling also is seen in other anemias, this is not a pathognomonic finding. The size of the aggregates in lead poisoning is typically large, making the stippling heavier than what is seen in many anemias.

Removal of the drug or toxin is usually successful in the treatment for acquired sideroblastic anemias. In the case of lead, salts of ethylenediamine tetraacetic acid are often used to chelate the lead present in the body so that it can be excreted in the urine.[38]

Porphyrias

Lead poisoning is an example of not only an acquired sideroblastic anemia, but also an acquired porphyria. The porphyrias are diseases characterized by impaired production of heme. The impairments to heme synthesis may be acquired, as with lead poisoning, or hereditary. The term *porphyria* is most often used to refer to the hereditary conditions. Among the hereditary conditions, single deficiencies of most enzymes in the synthetic pathway for heme have been identified. When an enzyme is missing, the products from earlier stages in the pathway accumulate in the blood and may be excreted in urine or feces, allowing for their assay for diagnosis. The accumulated products also deposit in body tissues, contributing to the varied clinical pictures. Some of the accumulated products are fluorescent. Their deposition in skin can lead to severe photosensitivity and fluorescence of teeth and bones. Hematologic evidence of the diseases is usually minimal, with other clinical findings being more significant. Table 19-2 summarizes the deficient enzymes, accumulating compounds, clinical findings, and treatment.

Text continued on page 242

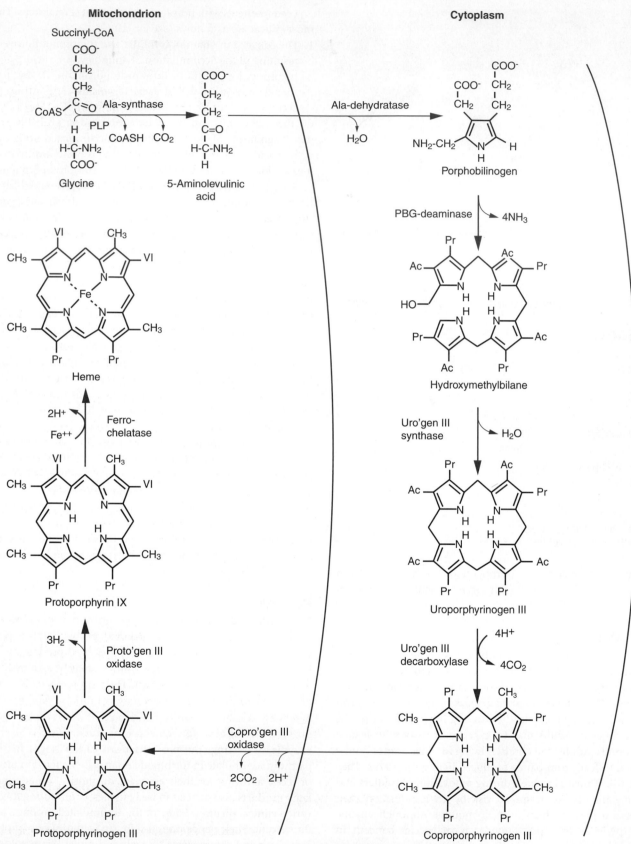

Figure 19-5 Heme synthesis. (From Bottomley SS, Muller-Eberhard UM: Pathophysiology of heme synthesis. Semin Hematol 1988;25:282-302; reprinted with permission.)

TABLE 19-2 Porphyrias

Disease	Missing Enzyme	Buildup	Cutaneous Signs	Systemic Manifestations	Treatment
Congenital erythropoietic porphyria (CEP)	Uroporphyrinogen III cosynthetase	Uroporphyrins II and III; coproporphyrin in marrow; uroporphyrin I in plasma, nucleated RBCs, excreta	Exposure to daylight incurs photo-oxidation, mutilating photosensitivity, erythrodontia, scarring, alopecia, hypertrichosis of face	Splenomegaly, hemolytic anemia; most nucleated RBCs, particularly metarubricytes, show intense red fluorescence in ultraviolet light; progressive disfigurement of exposed areas, leading to mutilation	Avoidance of sunlight; ingestion of beta carotene (antioxidant) to confer dermal tolerance to sunlight
Porphyria cutanea tarda (PCT)	Hepatic uroporphyrinogen decarboxylase	Hepatic accumulation and urinary excretion of uroporphyrin I and coproporphyrin	Photosensitivity of exposed skin, vesicles, bullae, erosions, moderate scarring, alopecia, milia formation, increased facial hair and periorbital pigmentation, hypertrichosis	Diabetes mellitus, occasional hepatic tumor, increased hepatic iron level; most common porphyria; occurs in alcoholic cirrhosis	Iron removal by phlebotomy or iron-chelating agents; decrease of alcohol consumption and estrogen hormones
Acute intermittent porphyria (AIP)	Porphobilinogen deaminase (impairs synthesis of uroporphyrinogen I synthetase)	Massive production of porphobilinogen aminolevulinic acid in urine	None	Muscle paralysis, acute abdominal colic, hypertension, insomnia, polyneuropathy, depression	Avoidance of barbiturates, anticonvulsants, sulfonamide derivatives, sedatives
Hereditary coproporphyria	Coproporphyrinogen III oxidase	Coproporphyrin	Symptomless (50% of patients); photosensitivity—less than in VP; abdominal colic—less than in VP; neurologic and mental manifestations	Similar to VP: abdominal colic, neurologic and mental manifestations	Aggravated by barbiturates, anticonvulsants, and variety of sedatives
Erythropoietic protoporphyria	Heme synthetase	Free protoporphyrin IX	"Burning," erythema, edema, moderate scarring, "waxy" thickening of light-exposed areas; mild epidermal photosensitivity	Cholelithiasis and occasional hepatic failure, protoporphyrin leaks out from erythroblasts into skin and tissues and is excreted in feces and urine; common porphyria	Avoidance of sunlight; ingestion of beta carotene to confer dermal tolerance to sunlight

Continued

TABLE 19-2 Porphyrias—cont'd

Disease	Missing Enzyme	Buildup	Cutaneous Signs	Systemic Manifestations	Treatment
Variegated porphyria (VP)	Protoporphyrinogen oxidase	Coproporphyrin III in feces (vast increase) and urine	Photosensitivity to sunlight; chronic cutaneous involvement; bullae, erosions, hyperpigmentation scarring, hypertrichosis (but not as unsightly as in CEP)	Combinations of systemic manifestations of AIP and PCT, excrete increased coproporphyrin in feces; episodic attacks of abdominal colic, neuropsychiatric malfunction	Avoidance of barbiturates, sulfonamides, excess alcohol consumption

IRON OVERLOAD

Chapter 11 describes the body's tenacity in conserving iron. For some individuals, this tenacity becomes the basis for disease related to excess iron accumulations in nearly all cells. Iron overload may be primary as in hereditary hemochromatosis or secondary to chronic anemias and their treatments. In both cases, the toxic effects of excess iron lead to serious health problems.

Etiology

Excess accumulation of iron results from acquired or hereditary conditions in which the body's rate of iron acquisition exceeds the rate of loss, which is usually about 1 mg/d. Regardless of the source of the iron, the body's first reaction is to store excess iron in the form of hemosiderin within cells. Eventually the storage system is overwhelmed, and, as described subsequently, parenchymal cells are damaged in organs including the liver, heart, and pancreas.

Accumulation of excess iron may be an acquired condition. It occurs when there is a need for repeated transfusions as treatment for anemias such as thalassemia. The iron present in the transfused RBCs exceeds the usual 1 mg/d of iron typically added to the body's stores by a healthy diet. This is called *transfusion-related hemochromatosis* or *hemosiderosis*.

Hemochromatosis also may develop as a result of mutations affecting the proteins of iron metabolism. An autosomal recessive disease had been known for many years; however, it was only more recently that advances in molecular biology allowed identification of mutant genes that contribute to the phenotype. Homozygous hereditary hemochromatosis affecting certain genes occurs in approximately 5 of 1000 northern Europeans.[40] Heterozygosity approaches 13%.[40] The first two known mutations to produce the hereditary hemochromatosis phenotype involve *Hfe*, a gene on the short arm of chromosome 6 that encodes for an HLA type I–like molecule that is closely linked to HLA-A.[41] The most common mutation substitutes tyrosine for cysteine at position 282 (Cys282Tyr), and the other substitutes aspartate for histidine at position 63

(His63Asp).[42] The normal HFE protein binds β_2-microglobulin intracellularly.[42] This binding is necessary for the HFE to appear on the cell surface, where it interacts with transferrin receptor 1 (TfR1). Interaction with transferrin receptor 1 reduces transferrin binding to the receptor, inhibiting cellular iron absorption.[43] The mutated HFE molecule either does not bind β_2-microglobulin and thus does not reach the cell surface, or does not bind the transferrin receptor 1 if it does reach the cell surface.[44] In either case, the result is that when HFE is mutated, the transferrin receptor 1 is inappropriately available for transferrin binding, even when the cell is replete with iron.

The above-described role of HFE in cellular iron uptake does not address a significant feature in the pathogenesis of hereditary hemochromatosis, which is the excess absorption of dietary iron. Enterocytes do not absorb iron from the diet through a transferrin-dependent mechanism[45]; rather it is absorbed by the divalent metal transporter 1 on the luminal side of enterocytes.[46] The active transport of iron into the plasma seems to be at the heart of the pathophysiology in hereditary hemochromatosis. This is accomplished by ferroportin on the basolaminal side of the enterocyte. In hereditary hemochromatosis, the enterocytes may absorb no more iron than normal from the diet, but they transport more of it into the plasma. Because hepcidin regulates this process, it plays a central role in the pathogenesis of hereditary hemochromatosis. How HFE interacts with hepcidin to produce the hereditary hemochromatosis phenotype has yet to be fully determined. Still, a central role for hepcidin is supported by the discovery that mutations in the hepcidin gene itself, *HAMP*, or another iron-regulating protein, hemojuvelin, can produce a disease picture affecting children that is identical to hereditary hemochromatosis.[46] Mutations of other genes affecting proteins in the iron regulatory process, such as ferroportin and transferrin receptor 2, also can produce a phenotype similar to hereditary hemochromatosis.[46] What is emerging is a picture of hereditary hemochromatosis as a general phenotype that can be produced by various genotypes when the gene for any of the iron regulatory proteins is mutated (Table 19-3). At this writing, the roles and interactions of all these proteins in

TABLE 19-3 Known Mutations Producing Phenotypes Similar to Hereditary Hemochromatosis Phenotypes

Feature	HFE-Related Hemochromatosis	Juvenile Hereditary Hemochromatosis		TfR2-Related Hereditary Hemochromatosis	Ferroportin-Related Iron Overload
Affected gene	*HFE*	*HAMP*	*HJV*	*TfR2*	*SLC40AI*
Mutated protein	HFE	Hepcidin	Hemojuvelin	Transferrin receptor 2	Ferroportin
Normal function of affected protein	Facilitates TfR1-mediated iron uptake; possibly modulation of hepcidin	Downregulation of ferroportin-mediated iron transport in macrophages and enterocytes	Regulator of hepcidin expression	Provides hepatocyte iron uptake	Transports iron out of enterocytes and macrophages
Age of onset of symptoms (yr.)	30-40	Teens-20	Teens-20	20-40, mild	30-40

*TfR1: transferrin Receptor-1.

normal iron regulation have not been fully elucidated, and a completely satisfactory explanation of the pathogenesis of hereditary hemochromatosis has yet to be established. Suffice it to say that because the biologic default is to absorb and store iron, and the regulatory mechanisms typically dampen that process, failure of normal regulation due to mutations leads to excessive absorption and storage.

Pathogenesis

The processes described previously lead to increased amounts of iron in parenchymal cells throughout the body. The cells' first reaction to excess iron is to form hemosiderin, essentially a degenerate and non–metabolically active form of ferritin. When cells exhaust the capacity to store iron as hemosiderin, free iron (ferrous) accumulates intracellularly. In the presence of oxygen, ferrous iron initiates the generation of superoxide and other free radicals, resulting in the peroxidation of membrane lipids.[3,47] The membranes affected include not only the cell membranes, but also mitochondrial, nuclear, and lysosomal membranes. Cell respiration is compromised and lysosomal enzymes are released intracellularly. Vitamins E and C can act to moderate the effects and interrupt the chain reaction, but in iron overload, even these protective mechanisms are overwhelmed. The ultimate result is cell death owing to irreversible membrane damage.

Because all cells except mature RBCs require iron and have the cellular machinery for iron acquisition, most cells have the potential for iron damage. The tissues most obviously affected include the skin, where deposition of hemosiderin gives the skin a golden color; the liver, where cirrhosis and subsequent cancer develop; and the pancreas, where damage results in diabetes mellitus. Hence the traditional characterization of hemochromatosis as "bronzed diabetes." The heart muscle also is especially vulnerable to excessive iron deposition, leading to congestive heart failure. Early diagnosis and treatment (see later) now can prevent the development of these secondary effects of iron overload. Hepatocellular carcinoma occurs more frequently in patients with hemochromatosis. Mutations of the *p53* tumor-suppressor gene seem to contribute to the

pathogenesis of the carcinoma,[48] with some evidence that the free radicals produced by the iron cause the mutations to the *p53* gene.[49]

The development of clinical disease associated with excess iron is heavily influenced by other physiologic conditions and environment. The phenotypic expression of the tissue damage described earlier in hereditary hemochromatosis is more common in men, although the gene frequency is not higher in men. This is because the blood loss associated with menstruation and childbirth forestalls the effects of excess iron in affected women, and they usually develop clinical symptoms later in life than affected men. In each gender, homozygous individuals develop disease faster than heterozygotes. The amount of iron available in the diet for absorption affects the rate at which disease can develop. Factors that can promote iron absorption even in normal individuals, such as ascorbic acid and alcohol, also affect absorption in individuals with hemochromatosis. Finally, time is an important factor in the development of disease. In classic hereditary hemochromatosis, individuals usually harbor 20 to 30 g of iron by the time their disease becomes clinically evident in the age range of 40 to 60 years.[50] This represents more than 10 times the stored iron of normal individuals and represents just 1 to 2 mg/d of excess iron absorbed over many years.[51] In the juvenile form of the disease associated with mutations to the hepcidin gene, the process of iron accumulation is accelerated so that these effects may appear as early as the teenage years.[46] In transfusion-related hemochromatosis, the frequency of transfusions over time affects the rate of development of clinical disease.

Laboratory Diagnosis

Laboratory testing in hemochromatosis serves three purposes. It can be used to screen for the condition, diagnose the cause of organ damage, and monitor treatment. The increase in transferrin saturation is the common screening test for hereditary hemochromatosis[51] and can be done cost-effectively in populations with a prevalence of at least 3 per 1000.[52] In a screening situation, repeated transferrin saturation of 60% or greater warrants further investigation.[51] Transferrin saturation also can be used to follow transfusion-dependent anemia patients and detect the development of hemochromatosis.

Undiagnosed individuals with hereditary hemochromatosis may come to medical attention because of organ function problems or may be discovered incidentally with routine laboratory testing. Abnormalities of common tests of liver function (e.g., elevated alanine transaminase) may be among the first laboratory findings that would lead a physician to further testing to identify the cause. Because inflammation is minimal, however, diminished levels of the liver's synthetic products, such as albumin, may be more helpful. If hereditary hemochromatosis is in the differential diagnosis being considered to explain organ dysfunction, serum iron, transferrin saturation, and plasma ferritin testing would be warranted. Elevations of these parameters are among the earliest findings in most forms of hemochromatosis. Genetic testing for known mutations provides confirmation of the diagnosis for most patients with hereditary hemochromatosis.

Whether hemochromatosis is acquired or hereditary, ferritin provides an assessment of the degree of iron overload and can be followed after treatment is initiated to reduce iron stores. Hb and Hct also can be used inexpensively to monitor treatment as described subsequently.

Actual determination of the extent of tissue damage is beyond the scope of the clinical laboratory for diagnosis. Liver biopsy with assessment of iron staining and degree of scarring is essential to determining the degree of organ damage.

Treatment

The treatment of secondary tissue damage, such as liver cirrhosis and heart failure, follows standard protocols. Treatment of the underlying condition leading to excess iron accumulation also is needed. Hereditary hemochromatosis and transfusion-related hemochromatosis require different treatment approaches. In forms of hereditary hemochromatosis, removing blood by phlebotomy provides a simple, inexpensive, and effective means for removing iron from the body. The regimen calls for weekly phlebotomy early in treatment, with maintenance phlebotomies about every 3 months for life.[3] Hb levels are monitored, and a mild anemia is sought and maintained. This is an easy and inexpensive substitute for iron studies because, as explained in the discussion of iron deficiency, iron stores must be exhausted before anemia develops.

Individuals who rely on transfusions to maintain Hb levels and prevent anemia cannot be treated with phlebotomy. Instead, iron-chelating drugs are used to bind excess iron in the body for excretion. Desferrioxamine is the treatment of choice, although it is not without side effects. The drug typically is injected subcutaneously to maximize exposure time for iron binding.[3] When absorbed into the bloodstream with its bound iron, it is readily excreted in the urine.

CHAPTER at a GLANCE

- Impaired iron or heme metabolism can result in microcytic, hypochromic anemias.
- Three conditions affecting iron metabolism can result in microcytic, hypochromic anemias: iron deficiency, anemia of chronic inflammation, and sideroblastic anemias, especially lead poisoning. The RBCs in thalassemias also may be microcytic, hypochromic and must be differentiated from the anemias of disordered iron metabolism.
- Iron deficiency results from inadequate iron intake, increased need, or excessive loss. All three of these situations create a relative deficit of body iron, which over time results in a microcytic, hypochromic anemia.
- Infants, children, and women in childbearing years are at greatest risk for iron deficiency anemia. If iron deficiency anemia is present in men and postmenopausal women, gastric bleeding should be investigated as the primary, although not only, cause of iron loss.
- Iron deficiency may be suspected when the CBC shows microcytic, hypochromic RBCs and elevated RDW, but no consistent morphologic abnormality. The diagnosis is confirmed with iron studies showing low total iron, elevated iron-binding capacity, decreased transferrin saturation, and low ferritin.
- Iron deficiency is treated by oral supplements, and with good patient compliance, the anemia should be corrected within 3 months. Gastrointestinal distress resulting from iron supplements can make patient compliance a significant concern.

- The anemia of chronic inflammation is associated with chronic infections such as tuberculosis, chronic inflammatory conditions such as rheumatoid arthritis, and tumors. It may be a microcytic, hypochromic anemia, but most often is normocytic, normochromic.
- Increased levels of hepcidin, an acute-phase reactant, decrease iron absorption in the intestines and sequester iron in macrophages and hepatocytes in the anemia of chronic inflammation. Bone marrow macrophages show abundant stainable iron, whereas developing RBCs show inadequate iron stores. Inflammatory cellular products also impair the production and action of erythropoietin.
- Iron studies in the anemia of chronic inflammation show decreased total serum iron, decreased iron-binding capacity, decreased transferrin saturation, and normal or increased ferritin.
- Sideroblastic anemias develop when the incorporation of iron into heme is blocked. The result is accumulation of iron in the mitochondria of developing RBCs. When stained using Prussian blue, the iron appears in deposits around the nucleus of the developing cells. These cells are called *ringed sideroblasts*.
- Iron incorporation into heme can be blocked when any of the enzymes of the heme synthetic pathway are deficient or impaired. Deficiencies of these enzymes may be hereditary, as in the porphyrias, or acquired, as in heavy metal poisoning. The most common of the latter conditions is lead poisoning.

CHAPTER at a GLANCE—cont'd

- Iron studies in sideroblastic anemias show elevated total iron, variable iron-binding capacity, normal to decreased transferrin saturation, and increased ferritin. Tests for the accumulating products of the heme synthetic pathway, such as zinc protoporphyrin or FEP, would be expected to be positive.

- Lead interferes at several steps in heme synthesis, preventing iron incorporation into heme and resulting in a microcytic, hypochromic anemia, although more often it is normocytic, normochromic. Lead also impairs glucose-6-phosphate dehydrogenase, producing a hemolytic component to the anemia.

- Children are especially vulnerable to the effects of lead on the central nervous system, which may result in irreversible brain damage. Treatment consists of removing the source of lead from the patient's environment and, if necessary, chelating drug therapy to facilitate excretion of lead in the urine.

- Because the body has no mechanism for iron excretion, iron overload can occur when transfusions are used to sustain patients with chronic anemias such as thalassemia (i.e., transfusion-related hemochromatosis).

- A defective *Hfe* gene can cause hereditary hemochromatosis by causing all body cells to bind transferrin inappropriately. Affected men develop symptoms earlier in life than women; homozygotes develop more severe disease than heterozygotes.

- Mutations of other genes affecting iron regulation can produce a phenotype similar to that of hereditary hemochromatosis. When the hepcidin gene is mutated, the disease develops early in life, affecting even teenagers.

- Free iron becomes available in cells when ferritin and hemosiderin become saturated. Free iron causes tissue damage by creating free radicals that cause cell membrane damage and perhaps mutations. Tissues damaged especially by excess iron deposition include the liver, pancreas, skin, and heart muscle.

- Elevated transferrin saturation is a good screening test for hemochromatosis. Hereditary hemochromatosis and the other known forms of the disease can be diagnosed using polymerase chain reaction to identify mutated genes.

- Hereditary hemochromatosis and similar diseases are treated by lifelong, periodic phlebotomy to induce a mild iron deficiency anemia and keep body iron levels low. Transfusion-related hemochromatosis must be treated with iron-chelating drugs, such as desferrioxamine.

Now that you have completed this chapter, go back and read again the case study at the beginning and respond to the questions presented.

REVIEW QUESTIONS

1. The mother of a 4-month-old infant who is being breast-fed sees her physician for a routine postpartum visit. She expresses concern that she may be experiencing postpartum depression because she does not seem to have any energy. Although the physician is sympathetic to the patient's concern, she orders a CBC and iron studies seeking an organic explanation for the patient's symptoms. The results are as follows:

   CBC: All results within reference range except RDW = 15%
   Total iron: decreased
   Iron-binding capacity: increased
   % saturation: decreased
   Ferritin: decreased

   Correlate the patient's laboratory and clinical findings. What can you conclude?
   a. The iron studies reveal thalassemic findings that were apparently previously undiagnosed.
   b. The patient is in stage 2 of iron deficiency, before frank anemia develops.
   c. The iron studies are inconsistent with the CBC results, and a laboratory error should be investigated.
   d. There is no evidence of a hematologic explanation for the patient's symptoms.

2. A bone marrow biopsy was performed as part of the cancer staging protocol for a patient with Hodgkin lymphoma. Although no evidence of spread of the tumor was apparent in the marrow, other abnormal findings were noted, including a slightly elevated myeloid-to-erythroid ratio. White blood cell and RBC morphology appeared normal, however. The Prussian blue stain showed abundant stainable iron in the marrow macrophages. The patient's CBC revealed a Hb of 10.8 g/dL, but RBC indices were within reference ranges. RBC morphology was unremarkable. These findings would be consistent with:
   a. Anemia of chronic inflammation
   b. Sideroblastic anemia
   c. Thalassemia
   d. Iron deficiency anemia

3. Predict the iron study results for the patient with Hodgkin disease described in Question 2.

	Total Iron	Iron Binding	% Saturation	Ferritin
a.	Decreased	Increased	Decreased	Decreased
b.	Increased	Normal	Increased	Normal
c.	Increased	Increased	Normal	Increased
d.	Decreased	Decreased	Decreased	Increased

4. A 35-year-old Caucasian woman saw her physician, complaining of headaches, dizziness, and nausea. The headaches had been increasing in severity over the last 6 months. This was coincident with her move into an older house built about 1900. She had been renovating the house, including stripping paint from the woodwork. Her CBC results showed a mild hypochromic, microcytic anemia with polychromasia and basophilic stippling noted. Which of the following tests would be most useful in confirming the cause of her anemia?
   a. Serum lead
   b. Total serum iron and iron binding
   c. Absolute reticulocyte count
   d. Finding iron stores in macrophages using a Prussian blue stain of the bone marrow

5. In men and postmenopausal women whose diets are adequate, iron deficiency anemia most often results from:
   a. Increased need associated with aging
   b. Impaired absorption in the gastric mucosa
   c. Chronic gastrointestinal bleeding
   d. Diminished resistance to hookworm infections

6. Which of the following individuals is at greatest risk for development of iron deficiency anemia?
   a. A 15-year-old boy who eats mainly fast food and junk food
   b. A 37-year-old woman who has never been pregnant and has amenorrhea
   c. A 63-year-old man with reactivation of tuberculosis from his childhood
   d. A 40-year-old man who lost blood during surgery to repair a fractured leg

7. Which of the following individuals is at the greatest risk for the development of anemia of chronic inflammation?
   a. A 15-year-old girl with asthma
   b. A 40-year-old woman with type 2 diabetes mellitus
   c. A 65-year-old man with hypertension
   d. A 30-year-old man with severe rheumatoid arthritis

8. Which of the following assays can be used cost-effectively in screening for hereditary hemochromatosis?
   a. Polymerase chain reaction
   b. Ferritin
   c. Transferrin saturation
   d. Total bilirubin

9. In the pathogenesis of the anemia of chronic inflammation, hepcidin levels:
   a. Decrease during inflammation and reduce iron absorption from enterocytes
   b. Increase during inflammation and reduce iron absorption from enterocytes
   c. Increase during inflammation and increase iron absorption from enterocytes
   d. Decrease during inflammation and increase iron absorption from enterocytes

10. Sideroblastic anemias are anemias that result from:
    a. The sequestration of iron in hepatocytes
    b. Inability to incorporate heme into apohemoglobin
    c. Sequestration of iron in myeloblasts
    d. Failure to incorporate iron into protoporphyrin IX

REFERENCES

1. Hallberg L: Bioavailability of dietary iron in man. Annu Rev Nutr 1981;1:123-147.
2. Suominen P, Punnonen K, Rajamaki A, et al: Serum transferrin receptor and transferrin receptor–ferritin index identify healthy subjects with subclinical iron deficits. Blood 1998;92:2934-2939.
3. Andrews N: Disorders of iron metabolism. In Handin RI, Lux SE, Stossel TP (eds): Blood: Principles and Practice of Hematology, 2nd ed. Philadelphia: Lippincott, Williams & Wilkins, 2003;1399-1434.
4. Dallman PR, Siimes MA, Stekel A: Iron deficiency in infancy and childhood. Am J Clin Nutr 1980;33:86-118.
5. Green R, Charlton R, Seftel H, et al: Body iron excretion in man: a collaborative study. Am J Med 1968;45:336-353.
6. Saarinen UM, Siimes MA, Dallman PR: Iron absorption in infants: high bioavailability of breast milk iron as indicated by the extrinsic tag method of iron absorption and by the concentration of serum ferritin. J Pediatr 1977;91:36-39.
7. Siimes MA, Vuori E, Kuitunen P: Breast milk iron: a declining concentration during the course of lactation. Acta Paediatr Scand 1979;68:29-31.
8. Beutler E, Larsh SE, Gurney CW: Iron therapy in chronically fatigued, non-anemic women: a double blind study. Ann Intern Med 1960;52:378-394.
9. Thompson WG, Meola T, Lipkin M Jr, et al: Red cell distribution width, mean corpuscular volume, and transferrin saturation in the diagnosis of iron deficiency. Arch Intern Med 1988;148:2128-2130.
10. McClure S, Custer E, Bessman JD: Improved detection of early iron deficiency in nonanemic subjects. JAMA 1985;253:1021-1023.
11. Charlton RW, Bothwell TH: Definition, prevalence and prevention of iron deficiency. Clin Haematol 1982;11:309-325.
12. Cox LA, Adrian GS: Postranscriptional regulation of chimeric human transferrin genes by iron. Biochemistry 1993;32:4738-4745.
13. Sinniah R, Doggart JR, Neill DW: Diurnal variations of the serum iron in normal subjects and in patients with haemochromatosis. Br J Haematol 1969;17:351-358.
14. Crosby WH, O'Neil-Cutting MA: A small-dose iron tolerance test as an indicator of mild iron deficiency. Clin Invest 1984;251:1986-1987.
15. Lamola AA, Joselow M, Yamane T: Zinc protoporphyrin (ZPP): a simple, sensitive fluorometric screening test for lead poisoning. Clin Chem 1975;21:93-97.
16. Huebers HA, Beguin Y, Pootrakul P, et al: Intact transferrin receptors in human plasma and their relation to erythropoiesis. Blood 1990;75:102-107.
17. O'Sullivan DJ, Higgins PG, Wilkinson JF: Oral iron compounds: a therapeutic comparison. Lancet 1955;2:482-485.
18. Swan HT, Jowett GH: Treatment of iron deficiency with ferrous fumarate: assessment by a statistically accurate method. BMJ 1959;2:782-787.
19. Cartwright GE: The anemia of chronic disorders. Semin Hematol 1966;3:351-375.
20. Sears DA: Anemia of chronic disease. Med Clin North Am 1992;76:567-579.
21. Nemeth E, Tuttle MS, Powelson J, et al: Hepcidin regulates iron efflux by binding to ferroportin and inducing its internalization. Science 2004;306:2090-2093.
22. Nicolas G, Bennoun M, Devaux I, et al: Lack of hepcidin gene expression and severe tissue iron overload in upstream stimulatory factor 2 (USF2) knockout mice. Proc Natl Acad Sci USA 2001;98:8780-8785.
23. Rivera S, Liu L, Nemeth E, et al: Hepcidin excess induces the sequestration of iron and exacerbates tumor-associated anemia. Blood 2005;105:1797-1802.
24. Nicolas G, Chauvet C, Viatte L, et al: The gene encoding the iron reulatory peptide hepcidin is regulated by anemia, hypoxia, and inflammation. J Clin Invest 2002;110:1037-1044.
25. Masson PL, Heremans JF, Schonne E: Lactoferrin: an iron binding protein in neutrophilic leukocytes. J Exp Med 1969;130:643-658.
26. Ganz T: Hepcidin, a key regulator of iron metabolism and mediator of anemia in inflammation. Blood 2003;102:783-788.
27. Means RT Jr, Krantz SB: Progress in understanding the pathogenesis of the anemia of chronic disease. Blood 1992;80:1639-1647.

28. Mast AE, Blinder MA, Gronowski AM, et al: Clinical utility of the soluble transferrin receptor and comparison with serum ferritin in several populations. Clin Chem 1998;44:45-51.

29. Mast A: The clinical utility of peripheral blood tests in the diagnosis of iron deficiency anemia. Bloodline Reviews. Available at: http://www.bloodline.net/stories/storyReader-$2820. Accessed June 11, 2006.

30. Pincus T, Olsen NJ, Russell, IJ, et al: Multicenter study of recombinant human erythropoietin in correction of anemia in rheumatoid arthritis. Am J Med 1990;89:161-168.

31. Arndt U, Kaltwasser JP, Gottschalk R, et al: Correction of iron-deficient erythropoiesis in the treatment of anemia of chronic disease with recombinant human erythropoietin. Ann Hematol 2005;84:159-166.

32. Horrigan DL, Harris JW: Pyridoxine responsive anemia: analysis of 62 cases. Adv Intern Med 1964;12:103-174.

33. Verwilghen R, Reybrouck G, Callens L, et al: Antituberculosis drugs and sideroblastic anemia. Br J Haematol 1965;11:92-98.

34. Benson P: Lead poisoning in children. Dev Med Child Neurol 1965;7:569-571.

35. Campbell AM, Williams ER: Chronic lead intoxication mimicking motor neurone disease. BMJ 1968;4:582.

36. Granick S, Sassa S, Granick JL, et al: Assays for porphyrins, delta-aminolevulinic acid dehydratase, and porphyrinogen synthetase in microliter samples of blood: application to metabolic defects involving the heme pathway. Proc Natl Acad Sci USA 1972;69:2381-2385.

37. Lachant NA, Tomoda A, Tanaka KR: Inhibition of the pentose phosphate shunt by lead: a potential mechanism for hemolysis in lead poisoning. Blood 1984;63:518-524.

38. Sassa S, Shibahara S: Disorders of heme production and catabolism. In Handin RI, Lux SE, Stossel TP (eds): Blood: Principles and Practice of Hematology. Philadelphia: Lippincott, Williams & Wilkins, 2003:1435-1502.

39. Valentine WN, Fink K, Paglia DE, et al: Hereditary hemolytic anemia with human erythrocyte pyrimidine 5'-nucleotidase deficiency. J Clin Invest 1974;54:866-879.

40. Edwards CQ, Griffen LM, Ajioka RS, et al: Screening for hemochromatosis: phenotype versus genotype. Semin Hematol 1998;35:72-76.

41. Feder JN, Gnirke A, Thomas W, et al: A novel MHC class I-like gene is mutated in patients with hereditary haemochromatosis. Nat Genet 1996;13:399-408.

42. Waheed A, Parkkila S, Zhou XY, et al: Hereditary hemochromatosis: effect of C282Y and H63D mutations on association with β2-microglobulin, intracellular processing, and cell surface expression of the HFE protein in COS-7 cells. Proc Natl Acad Sci USA 1997;94:12384-12389.

43. Salter-Cid L, Brunmark A, Li Y, et al: Transferrin receptor is negatively modulated by the hemochromatosis protein HFE: implications for cellular iron homeostasis. Proc Natl Acad Sci USA 1999;96:5435-5439.

44. Lebron JA, Bjorkman PJ: The transferrin receptor binding site on HFE, the class I MHC-related protein mutated in hereditary hemochromatosis. J Mol Biol 1999;289:1109-1118.

45. Andrews NC, Levy JE: Iron is hot: an update on the pathophysiology of hemochromatosis. Blood 1998;92:1845-1851.

46. Pietrangelo A: Herediary hemochromatosis—a new look at an old disease. N Engl J Med 2004;350:2383-2398.

47. McCord JM: Iron, free radicals, and oxidative injury. Semin Hematol 1998;35:5-12.

48. Vautier G, Bomford AB, Portmann BC, et al: p53 mutations in British patients with hepatocellular carcinoma: clustering in genetic hemochromatosis. Gastroenterology 1999;117:154-160.

49. Hussain SP, Raja K, Amstad PA, et al: Increased p53 mutation load in nontumorous human liver of Wilson disease and hemochromatosis: oxyradical overload diseases. Proc Natl Acad Sci USA 2000;97:12770-12775.

50. Niederau C, Strohmeyer G, Stremmel W: Long term survival in patients with hereditary hemochromatosis. Gastroenterology 1996;110:1107-1119.

51. Bothwell TH, MacPhail AP: Hereditary hemochromatosis: etiologic, pathologic, and clinical aspects. Semin Hematol 1998;35:55-71.

52. Phatak PD, Guzman G, Woll JE, et al: Cost effectiveness of screening for hemochromatosis. Arch Intern Med 1994;154:769-776.

20

Anemias Caused by Defects of DNA Metabolism

Kathryn Doig

OBJECTIVES

After completion of this chapter, the reader will be able to:

1. Discuss the relationships among macrocytic anemia, megaloblastic anemia, and pernicious anemia, and classify anemias appropriately within these categories.
2. Discuss the roles of folic acid and vitamin B_{12} in DNA production and the general metabolic pathways in which they act.
3. Describe the absorption and distribution of vitamin B_{12}, including carrier proteins and the biologic activity of various vitamin-carrier complexes.
4. Describe the biochemical basis for development of anemia with deficiencies of vitamin B_{12} and folic acid, and explain the etiology of the accompanying macrocytosis.
5. Recognize individuals at risk for megaloblastic anemia by virtue of age, race/ethnicity, dietary habits, physiologic circumstance such as pregnancy, drug regimens, or pathologic conditions.
6. Recognize complete blood count, reticulocyte count, and bone marrow findings consistent with megaloblastic anemia.
7. Given results of tests for vitamin B_{12}, methymalonic acid, folic acid, and antibodies to intrinsic factor and parietal cells, determine the likely cause of a patient's deficiency.
8. Recognize results of bilirubin and lactate dehydrogenase tests that are consistent with megaloblastic anemia and explain why these results are elevated in this condition.

CASE STUDY

After studying the material in this chapter, the reader should be able to respond to the following case study:

During a holiday visit, the children of a 76-year-old Scandinavian man noticed that he seemed more forgetful than usual and that he had difficulty walking. Concerned that he had had a mild stroke, the children insisted that he see his physician. The physician diagnosed a peripheral neuropathy affecting his ability to walk. Additionally, the physician noted that he was quite pale and slightly jaundiced and ordered routine hematologic studies. The results were as follows:

	Patient	Reference Range
WBC ($\times 10^9$/L)	3.20	4.5-11
RBC ($\times 10^{12}$/L)	2.22	4.3-5.9
Hb (g/L)	85	139-163
Hct (L/L)	0.27	0.39-0.55
MCV (fL)	120	80-100
MCH (pg)	38.3	25.4-34.6
MCHC (g/dL)	32	31-37
RDW (%)	18	11.5-13.5
Platelet count ($\times 10^9$/L)	115	250-400
Reticulocyte count (%)	1.8	0.5-1.5

	Patient
WBC differential	Unremarkable with the exception of hypersegmentation of neutrophils
RBC morphology	Moderate anisocytosis, moderate poikilocytosis, macrocytes, oval macrocytes, few dacryocytes

As a result of these findings and in light of the patient's ethnic background, the following tests were ordered:

Vitamin B_{12}: decreased

Folic acid: within reference range

Methymalonic acid: increased

1. Which of the complete blood count findings led the physician to order the vitamin assays?

Impaired deoxyribonucleic acid (DNA) metabolism has systemic effects by impairing production of all readily dividing cells of the body. These are chiefly the skin, the epithelium of the gastrointestinal tract, and the hematopoietic tissues. Because these all must be replenished throughout life, any impairment of cell production is evident in these tissues first. Patients may experience symptoms in any of these systems, but the blood provides a ready tissue for analysis. The hematologic effects, especially megaloblastic anemia, have come to be recognized as the hallmark of the diseases affecting DNA metabolism.

ETIOLOGY

The root cause of megaloblastic anemia is impaired DNA synthesis. The anemia is named for the very large cells of the bone marrow that develop a distinctive morphology (see section on laboratory diagnosis), due to reduced numbers of divisions. Megaloblastic anemia is one example of a macrocytic anemia. Box 20-1 shows the relationship among the causes of macrocytosis and the various underlying causes of megaloblastic anemia. Understanding the etiology of megaloblastic anemia requires a review of DNA synthesis with particular attention to the roles of folic acid (folate) and the cobalt-containing vitamin, vitamin B_{12} (cobalamin).

Roles of Folic Acid and Vitamin B_{12} in DNA Synthesis

As seen in Figure 20-1, deoxythymidylate monophosphate (dTMP) is a precursor to deoxythymidylate triphosphate (dTTP), which, similar to the other nucleotide triphosphates, is a building block of the DNA molecule. dTMP is produced by the action of thymidylate synthetase to add a methyl group ($-CH_3$) to deoxyuridylate monophosphate (dUMP). The donor of the methyl group is N^5,N^{10}-methylene tetrahydrofolate. This donor is replenished through a cycle in which tetrahydrofolate is methylated by serine. Folate in several forms is essential to the production of the thymidine nucleotides used in DNA production. This dependency on folate has been used effectively in cancer chemotherapy (Box 20-2).

The production of tetrahydrofolate is tied to vitamin B_{12}. Because some of the folate is catabolized, the cycle requires a source, which is 5-methyltetrahydrofolate. It releases its methyl group, forming tetrahydrofolate, and donates it to detoxify homocysteine by conversion to methionine. The cofactor in this reaction is vitamin B_{12}.

BOX 20-1 Causes of Macrocytic Anemias and Relationships Among the Underlying Causes of Megaloblastic Anemia

Reticulocytosis
Liver disease/alcoholism
Myelodysplastic syndromes
Erythroleukemia (FAB-M6)
Megaloblastic anemia
    Folate deficiency
        Dietary inadequacy
            Inadequate intake
            Increased need during growth
            Impaired absorption (e.g., inflammatory bowel disease)
        Impaired use due to drugs
        Excessive loss with renal dialysis
    Vitamin B_{12} deficiency
        Dietary deficiency
            Inadequate intake
            Increased need during growth
        Impaired absorption
            Failure to split from haptocorrin
            Lack of intrinsic factor
                Gastrectomy
                Pernicious anemia
                Malabsorption (e.g., inflammatory bowel disease)
            Competition for the vitamin
                Diphyllobothrium latum infestation
                Blind loop syndrome
    Impaired transport—transcobalambin II deficiency

Defect in Megaloblastic Anemia

When either folic acid or vitamin B_{12} is missing, thymidine nucleotide production for DNA synthesis is impaired. Folate deficiency has the more direct effect, ultimately preventing the methylation of dUMP. The deficiency of vitamin B_{12} is more indirect, preventing the production of tetrahydrofolate from 5-methyltetrahydrofolate. This constitutes what has been called the "folate trap" as 5-methyltetrahydrofolate is trapped and accumulates, unable to supply the folate cycle with tetrahydrofolate. Homocysteine also accumulates because vitamin B_{12} is unable to convert it to methionine (see Fig. 20-1).

In this state of diminished thymidine availability, DNA can unwind and replication can begin, but at any point where a

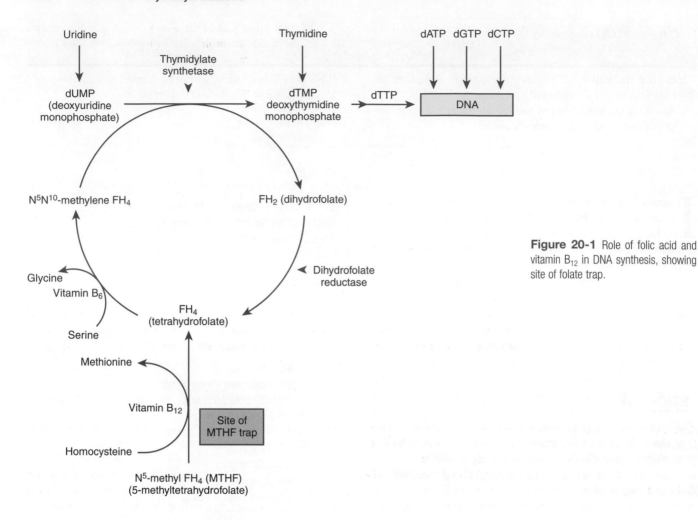

Figure 20-1 Role of folic acid and vitamin B_{12} in DNA synthesis, showing site of folate trap.

BOX 20-2 Disruption of the Folate Cycle in Cancer Chemotherapy

The central role of folic acid in cell division makes it a target for chemotherapeutic drugs used to treat cancer. Folate analogues can be used to compete for folic acid in DNA production and result in impaired cell division. The cells in cycle, such as cancer cells and normally dividing cells such as epithelium and blood cells, are most susceptible to the drug interference. Methotrexate, used in the treatment of leukemia, is an example of a folate antimetabolite drug. It has a higher affinity for dihydrofolate reductase than does tetrahydrofolate; methotrexate enters the folate cycle in preference to tetrahydrofolate. The folate cycle is blocked by the drug. Methotrexate treatment typically is followed by what is known as *leukovorin rescue*. Leukovorin is a folic acid derivative that can be administered to counteract the effects of methotrexate or other folic acid antagonists.

---

thymidine nucleotide is needed, there is essentially an empty space in the replicated DNA sequence. There is evidence that uridine nucleotides may be used as temporary replacements,[1] but ultimately they must be replaced during the repair process. Without available thymidine, repair is unsuccessful. The result-

ing DNA is nonfunctional, and the DNA replication process is incomplete. Cell division is halted, resulting in either cell lysis or apoptosis.[2]

CLINICAL FINDINGS

Anemia

When DNA synthesis and subsequent cell division is impaired by lack of folate or vitamin B_{12}, megaloblastic anemia and its systemic manifestations develop. In the case of developing red blood cells (RBCs), these deficiencies result in ineffective hematopoiesis with blood cells dying in the bone marrow. Pancytopenia is evident with certain distinctive cellular changes (see section on laboratory diagnosis). With either vitamin deficiency, patients may experience generic symptoms related to the anemia (fatigue, weakness, and shortness of breath) and symptoms related to the alimentary tract. The loss of epithelium on the tongue results in a smooth surface and soreness (glossitis). Loss of epithelium along the gastrointestinal tract can result in gastritis, nausea, or constipation.

Other Effects of Vitamin B_{12} and Folate Deficiencies

Although the anemias seen with the two vitamin deficiencies are indistinguishable, the clinical presentations vary. In vitamin

B$_{12}$ deficiency, neurologic symptoms may be pronounced. They include memory loss, numbness and tingling in toes and fingers, loss of balance, and further impairment of walking by loss of vibratory sense, especially in the lower limbs.[3] These symptoms seem to be the result of demyelinization of the spinal cord and peripheral nerves.[4]

At one time, folate deficiency was believed to be more benign clinically than vitamin B$_{12}$ deficiency. Later research suggested that low levels of folate and the resulting high homocysteine were risk factors for cardiovascular disease.[5] More recent research has not substantiated this association,[6-8] although some point to high folic acid providing a cardio-protective effect for diabetic patients or certain ethnic populations.[9,10] The evidence at this time is unclear as to whether persistent suboptimal folate status may have a significant long-term health impact. Additionally, although it was previously believed that neurologic symptoms did not accompany folate deficiency, evidence of depression, peripheral neuropathy, and psychosis related to folate deficiency has now emerged.[11,12] Folic acid levels seem to affect the effectiveness of treatments for depression.[13] Folate deficiency during pregnancy can result in impaired formation of the fetal nervous system, resulting in neural tube defects such as spina bifida,[14] despite the fact that the fetus accumulates folate at the expense of the mother.

CAUSES OF VITAMIN DEFICIENCIES

In general, vitamin deficiencies may be absolute in that the vitamin is in relatively short supply, or they may result from impaired use or excessive loss. Folate deficiency can occur by all of these mechanisms.

Folate Deficiency
Dietary Deficiency
Dietary deficiency of folic acid results when there is inadequate intake, increased need, or impaired absorption.

Inadequate Intake.   Folate is ubiquitous in foods, but a generally poor diet can result in deficiency. Good sources of folate include leafy green vegetables, dried beans, liver, beef, and some fruits, especially oranges.[15] Folic acid is heat labile, and overcooking foods can diminish their nutritional value.[15]

Increased Need.   Increased need for folate occurs during pregnancy and lactation when the mother must supply her own needs plus those of the fetus and infant. Infants and children also have increased need for folate during growth.[3]

Impaired Absorption.   Folic acid is absorbed from the diet in the small intestine; however, only 50% of what is ingested is available for absorption.[16] Once across the intestinal cell, most folic acid is transported in the plasma unbound to any specific carrier.[3] Its entry into cells is carrier mediated, however.[17]

Folate absorption may be impaired by intestinal disease, especially sprue. Sprue is characterized by weakness, weight loss, and steatorrhea (fat in the feces), which is evidence that the intestine is not absorbing food properly. It is seen in the tropics, where its cause generally is considered to be overgrowth of enteric pathogens.[18] Nontropical sprue has been traced to intolerance of gluten in the diet (gluten-induced enteropathy)[18] and can be corrected by eliminating wheat products. Surgical resection of the small intestine and inflammatory bowel disease also can impair folate absorption.

Impaired Use
Numerous drugs impair folic acid metabolism. Antiepileptic drugs are particularly known for this,[19] resulting in macrocytosis with frank megaloblastic anemia. In most instances, supplemental folic acid is sufficient to override the impairment and allow the patient to continue therapy.[20]

Excessive Loss
Physiologic loss of folate occurs through the kidney. The amount is small and not a cause of deficiency. Patients on renal dialysis do lose folate in the dialysate, however, so supplemental folic acid is routinely provided to these individuals to prevent megaloblastic anemia.[3]

Vitamin B$_{12}$ Deficiency
Dietary Deficiency
Dietary deficiencies of vitamin B$_{12}$ result from inadequate intake, increased need, and impaired absorption.

Inadequate Intake.   True dietary deficiency of vitamin B$_{12}$ is possible for strict vegetarians (vegans) who do not eat meat, eggs, or dairy products. Although it is an essential vitamin for animals, plants do not use it, and it is not available from vegetable sources. The best dietary sources are animal products, such as liver, milk, and eggs.[15]

Increased Need.   As with folate, increased need for vitamin B$_{12}$ occurs during pregnancy, lactation, and growth. What would otherwise be a diet adequate in vitamin B$_{12}$ can become inadequate during these periods, when the rate of cell replication is vigorous.

Impaired Absorption.   Vitamin B$_{12}$ in food is bound by a specific protein in saliva, haptocorrin. In the small intestine, it is released from haptocorrin by the action of trypsin. It is then bound by intrinsic factor produced by the gastric parietal cells (Fig. 20-2). Vitamin B$_{12}$ binding to intrinsic factor is required for absorption by the ileal cells (enterocyte), which possess a receptor for the intrinsic factor–vitamin B$_{12}$ complex. The receptor and its ligand are internalized by the ileal cell, and the vitamin B$_{12}$ is released to the plasma side of the cell. In the plasma, most vitamin B$_{12}$ is carried by transcobalamin I (haptocorrin).[3] This does not seem to be the metabolically active transport protein, however. The minority of the vitamin is bound to transcobalamin II. The ligand-bound protein is called holotranscobalamin II. Cells possess a membrane receptor for holotranscobalamin II,[21] making holotranscobalamin II the metabolically important transport protein. The

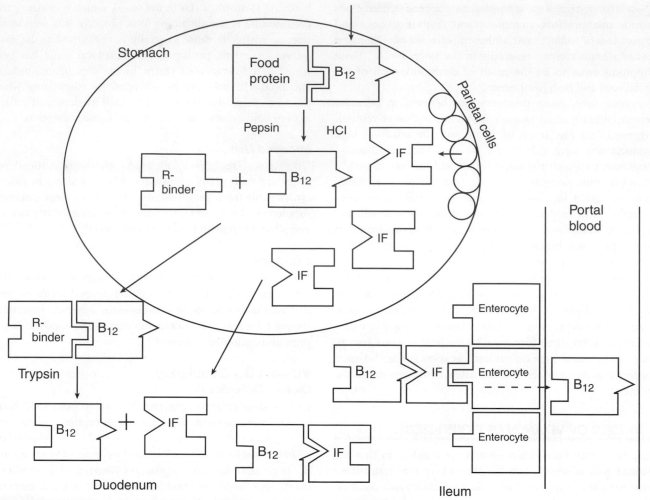

Figure 20-2 Vitamin B$_{12}$ in food is freed by pepsin and HCl to be taken up by R-binder that shuttles it to the small intestine. There it is freed by trypsin to bind to intrinsic factor (IF). IF is able to bind to the enterocytes of the ileum permitting Vitamin-B$_{12}$ absorption into the blood.

holotranscobalamin II enters the cell by endocytosis, with subsequent release of the vitamin B$_{12}$ from the carrier.[22] The body maintains a substantial reserve of absorbed vitamin B$_{12}$ in liver cells.

The absorption of vitamin B$_{12}$ can be impaired by (1) failure to separate vitamin B$_{12}$ from haptocorrin in the intestine for binding to intrinsic factor, (2) lack of intrinsic factor, (3) general malabsorption, and (4) competition for available vitamin.

Failure to Separate from Haptocorrin.   Lack of gastric acidity or lack of trypsin as a result of chronic pancreatic disease can prevent vitamin B$_{12}$ absorption because the vitamin remains bound to haptocorrin in the intestine and unavailable to intrinsic factor.[3]

Lack of Intrinsic Factor.   Lack of intrinsic factor constitutes a significant cause of impaired vitamin B$_{12}$ absorption. It can result from the loss of parietal cells with gastrectomy. A condition resulting from the autoimmune lymphocyte-mediated destruction of parietal cells also can cause a loss of intrinsic factor.[23] This condition is called *pernicious anemia* because the disease was fatal before its cause was discovered.

Pernicious anemia is seen most often in individuals older than age 50.[24] Although it may be seen in African-Americans, who may develop the disease at a younger age,[25] it is far more common in individuals of northern European descent.[23]

The impaired absorption of vitamin B$_{12}$ in pernicious anemia results from loss of intrinsic factor–secreting gastric cells as well as antibodies that block intrinsic factor action. Pathologic CD4 T cells recognize as an antigen the H$^+$,K$^+$-adenosine triphosphatase embedded in the membrane of gastric parietal cells.[26] These cells secrete H$^+$ and intrinsic factor. The T cell response to these cells initiates an autoimmune reaction. A chronic inflammatory infiltration follows, which extends into the wall of the stomach.[23] Over a period of years and even decades, there is progressive development of atrophic gastritis resulting from the loss of the parietal cells with their secretory products, H$^+$ and intrinsic factor. The loss of H$^+$ production in the stomach constitutes achlorhydria. Low gastric acidity was previously an important diagnostic criterion. The loss of intrinsic factor also can be detected using the Schilling test. Because the test requires the use of radioactive cobalt in vitamin B$_{12}$ to trace absorption, however, the test has fallen from favor with preference for safer diagnostic tests (see section on laboratory diagnosis).

Another feature of the autoimmune response in pernicious anemia is the production of antibodies to intrinsic factor[27] and gastric parietal cells[28] that are detectable in serum. The most common antibody to intrinsic factor blocks the site on intrinsic factor where vitamin B_{12} binds,[23] inhibiting the formation of the intrinsic factor–vitamin B_{12} complex and preventing the absorption of the vitamin. These blocking antibodies are present in about 70% of patients with pernicious anemia.[23] Parietal cell antibodies are detectable in about 90% of patients with pernicious anemia.[23]

Pernicious anemia is one example of impaired absorption of vitamin B_{12} that is due to an autoimmune process. Loss of gastric parietal cells causes loss of intrinsic factor and impaired vitamin B_{12} absorption. Even before the gastric cells are lost, antibodies to intrinsic factor can impair vitamin B_{12} absorption by preventing vitamin binding to intrinsic factor.

General Malabsorption. Malabsorption of vitamin B_{12} also can be caused by the same conditions interfering with folate absorption, such as inflammatory bowel disease.

Competition for Vitamin B_{12}. Competition for the vitamin B_{12} available in the intestine may come from intestinal organisms. The fish tapeworm *Diphyllobothrium latum* is able to split vitamin B_{12} from intrinsic factor,[29] rendering the vitamin unavailable for host absorption. Abnormalities of the intestinal anatomy or surgical sequelae that result in stenotic areas called *blind loops* can become overgrown with intestinal bacteria that compete effectively with the host for available vitamin B_{12}.[3] In both of these conditions, the host is unable to absorb sufficient vitamin B_{12}, and megaloblastic anemia results.

Hereditary Transcobalamin Deficiency

A hereditary recessive deficiency of transcobalamin has been described in multiple case reports since the 1970s.[30,31] This rare condition results in megaloblastic anemia in childhood. If unrecognized and untreated, permanent neurological damage may occur.[32]

LABORATORY DIAGNOSIS

The tests used in the diagnosis of megaloblastic anemia include screening tests and specific diagnostic tests to ascertain the specific vitamin deficiency and perhaps its cause.

Screening Tests

Four tests used to screen for megaloblastic anemia are the complete blood count (CBC), neutrophil lobe count, bilirubin, and lactate dehydrogenase.

Complete Blood Count

Patients with uncomplicated megaloblastic anemia are expected to have pancytopenia and decreased hemoglobin (Hb) and hematocrit (Hct). The MCV is usually 100 to 150 fL and commonly greater than 120 fL. The RBC distribution width (RDW) also is elevated. The MCH is elevated by the

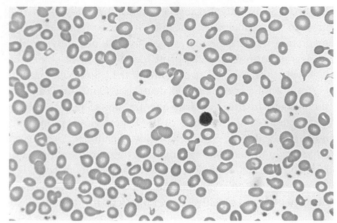

Figure 20-3 Oval macrocytes, dacryocytes, other RBC abnormalities, and a small lymphocyte for size comparison in megaloblastic anemia (peripheral blood, ×500).

increased size of the cells, but the mean cell Hb concentration (MCHC) is usually within reference range because Hb production is unaffected. The characteristic morphologic findings of megaloblastic anemia in the peripheral blood include oval macrocytes (enlarged, oval-shaped RBCs) (Fig. 20-3) and hypersegmented neutrophils with five or more lobes (Fig. 20-4).[33] Impaired cell production means the absolute reticulocyte count is low, especially in light of the anemia, and polychromasia is not seen on the blood smear. Additional morphologic changes include dacryocytes, fragments, and microspherocytes. These smaller cells further widen the RDW. Nucleated RBCs, Howell-Jolly bodies, and basophilic stippling may be observed. Cabot rings also may be seen.

Neutrophil Lobe Count

Hypersegmentation of the neutrophils is essentially pathognomonic for megaloblastic anemia. It appears early in the course of the disease[34] and persists throughout treatment.[35] Reporting hypersegmented neutrophils in the routine CBC is a significant finding and requires a reporting rule that can be

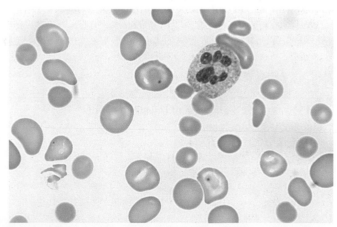

Figure 20-4 Hypersegmented neutrophil in megaloblastic anemia (peripheral blood, ×1000).

applied consistently because even healthy individuals may have an occasional one. One such rule is to report hypersegmentation when there are at least five 5-lobed polymorphonuclear neutrophils per 100 white blood cells (WBCs), or there is at least one 6-lobed neutrophil noted.[3] Some laboratories perform a lobe count on 100 neutrophils and then calculate the average. In megaloblastic anemia, the average should be greater than 3.4.[3] The cause of the hypersegmentation is not understood, despite considerable investigation.[36] More recent advances in understanding growth factors and their impact on transcription factors may yet solve this mystery. Nevertheless, its recognition on a peripheral blood smear constitutes an inexpensive yet sensitive screening test for megaloblastic anemia.

Bilirubin and Lactate Dehydrogenase

Although generally considered a nutritional anemia, megaloblastic anemia is in one sense a hemolytic anemia because the cells die during division in the marrow. This intramedullary cell death is known as *ineffective erythropoiesis* because many RBCs never enter the bloodstream—hence the lack of reticulocytes in the peripheral blood. The usual signs of hemolysis are evident in the serum, including an elevation of total and indirect bilirubin and lactate dehydrogenase, which, if fractionated, would be predominantly RBC derived.

The constellation of findings, including moderate-to-marked pancytopenia, macrocytosis with oval macrocytes and hypersegmented neutrophils, plus increased bilirubin and lactate dehydrogenase, would justify further testing to confirm a diagnosis of megaloblastic anemia and determine its cause. Occasionally, the classic findings may be obscured by coexisting conditions, such as iron deficiency, making the diagnosis more challenging. Most hematologic aberrations do not appear until vitamin deficiency is fairly well advanced (Box 20-3).[37]

Specific Diagnostic Tests

Bone Marrow Examination

Modern tests for vitamin deficiencies and autoimmune antibodies have made bone marrow examination an infrequently used diagnostic test for megaloblastic anemia. Nevertheless, it remains the reference confirmatory test to identify the megaloblastic appearance of the developing RBCs.

Megaloblastic, in contrast to *macrocytic*, refers to specific morphologic changes in the developing RBCs. The cells are characterized by a nuclear-cytoplasmic asynchrony in which the cytoplasm progresses as expected with increasing pinkness as Hb accumulates. The nucleus lags behind, however, appearing younger than expected for the degree of maturity of the cytoplasm (Fig. 20-5). This asynchrony is most striking at the stage of the polychromatophilic normoblast. The cytoplasm appears as expected for that stage. The nuclear chromatin remains more open than expected, more similar to the nucleus of a basophilic normoblast. Overall, the marrow is hypercellular, with a myeloid-to-erythroid ratio of about 1:1 by virtue of the increased erythropoietic activity. The hematopoiesis is ineffective, however, and although cell production in the bone marrow is increased, the death of cells in the marrow results in peripheral pancytopenia.

Megaloblastic RBCs may be seen in the congenital dyserythropoietic anemias (Chapter 21). These are rare conditions that are evident at birth and may be easily distinguished from the acquired causes of megaloblastosis. Another condition with a similar morphology that also must be distinguished from megaloblastosis is M6 acute myeloblastic leukemia, also called *erythroleukemia* (Chapter 36). In this condition, the cells are macrocytic, and the immature appearance of the nuclear chromatin is similar to the more open appearance of the chromatin in megaloblasts. There are usually other aberrant findings in erythroleukemia, however, and experienced morphologists can discern the subtle differences.

The WBCs also are affected in megaloblastic anemia and appear larger than normal. This is most evident in metamyelocytes and bands because, in the usual development of neutrophils, the cells should be getting smaller at these stages. The effect creates what are called "giant" metamyelocytes (Fig. 20-6) and bands.

Megakaryocytes do not show consistent changes in megaloblastic anemia. They may be either increased or decreased in number and may show diminished lobulation. The latter finding is not consistently seen and, even when present, is difficult to assess.

BOX 20-3 Sequence of Development of Megaloblastic Anemias

1. Vitamin levels decrease
2. Hypersegmentation of neutrophils
3. Oval macrocytosis in peripheral blood
4. Definite megaloblastic bone marrow
5. Anemia

Note: Hypersegmentation of neutrophils is the first sign to manifest in the peripheral blood and is the last sign to disappear.

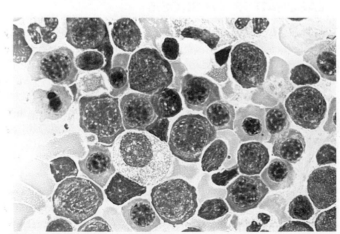

Figure 20-5 Erythroid precursors in megaloblastic anemia (bone marrow, ×1000).

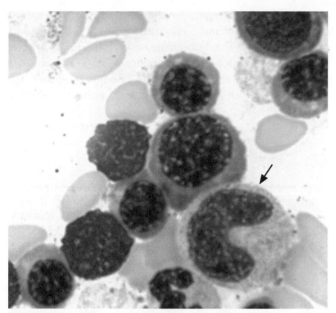

Figure 20-6 Giant metamyelocyte in megaloblastic anemia (bone marrow, original magnification ×1000).

Assays for Folate, Vitamin B₁₂, and Methylmalonic Acid

Although bone marrow aspiration is truly confirmatory for megaloblastosis, the invasiveness of the procedure and its expense mean that other testing is performed more often than a bone marrow examination. Furthermore, the confirmation of megaloblastic morphology in the marrow does not identify its cause. Assays for serum folate and vitamin B_{12} are readily available using radioimmunoassay. In equivocal circumstances, an RBC folate level may be performed. Folic acid is concentrated in tissues, and the RBC folate measurement may be a more accurate reflection of true folate status.

Some laboratories conduct a reflexive assay for methylmalonic acid if vitamin B_{12} levels are low. In addition to its role in folate metabolism, vitamin B_{12} is a cofactor in fatty acid oxidation. It is required for conversion of methylmalonyl CoA to succinyl CoA by the enzyme methylmalonylmutase (Fig. 20-7). If vitamin B_{12} is deficient, methylmalonyl CoA accumulates. Some of it hydrolyzes to methylmalonic acid, and the increase can be detected in serum and urine. Although there are reports that methylmalonic acid is an extremely sensitive marker for vitamin B_{12} deficiency,[38] more recent studies dispute this.[39] Methylmalonic acid is assayed by tandem mass spectrometry.

Gastric Analysis

Gastric analysis may be used to confirm achlorhydria, an expected finding in pernicious anemia. Achlorhydria occurs in other conditions, however, including natural aging. When other causes of vitamin B_{12} deficiency have been eliminated, achlorhydria is supportive, although not diagnostic, of pernicious anemia. It is determined by titrating gastric juice acidity after stimulation with compounds such as caffeine.

$$
\begin{array}{c}
\text{COOH} \\
| \\
\text{HC—CH}_3 \\
| \\
\text{C—S—CoA} \\
\| \\
\text{O} \qquad \text{Methylmalonyl CoA}
\end{array}
$$

Methylmalonyl mutase ↕ Vitamin B_{12}

$$
\begin{array}{c}
\text{COOH} \\
| \\
\text{CH}_2 \\
| \\
\text{CH}_2 \\
| \\
\text{C—S—CoA} \\
\| \\
\text{O} \qquad \text{Succinyl CoA}
\end{array}
$$

Figure 20-7 Role of vitamin B_{12} in fatty acid oxidation.

Antibody Assays

Antibodies to intrinsic factor and parietal cells can be detected in the serum of most patients with pernicious anemia, as mentioned earlier. Intrinsic factor–blocking antibodies are detected using enzyme-linked immunosorbent assays. Parietal cell antibodies are assayed using indirect immunofluorescence of mouse stomach cells.

Schilling Test

The Schilling test is used to distinguish malabsorption of vitamin B_{12} resulting from pernicious anemia from other causes of malabsorption discussed earlier. An oral dose of radioactive vitamin B_{12} is given. A 24-hour urine collection is completed and tested for the radioactive vitamin. The presence of radioactive vitamin B_{12} in the urine indicates that the patient is able to absorb vitamin B_{12}. If the radioactive vitamin does not appear in the urine, it means that there is a malabsorption problem. To determine whether it is due to pernicious anemia, the test is repeated. In the second phase, intrinsic factor is given orally along with the radioactive vitamin B_{12}. A 24-hour urine collection is completed and tested for the radioactive vitamin. If the radioactive vitamin now appears in the urine, it means that intrinsic factor corrected the problem, and the patient is diagnosed as having pernicious anemia. If the radioactive vitamin still fails to appear in the urine, another cause of malabsorption other than pernicious anemia must be pursued. Because of the availability of high-quality assays for the auto-antibodies of pernicious anemia, a Schilling test is rarely needed to establish the diagnosis.

Stool Analysis for Parasites

When vitamin B_{12} is found to be deficient, a stool analysis for eggs or proglottids of the fish tapeworm *D. latum* may be part of the diagnostic workup.

TREATMENT

Treatment should be directed at the specific vitamin deficiency established by the diagnostic tests. Although the blood picture can be corrected by cross-treatment (i.e., a folate-deficient patient treated with vitamin B$_{12}$), the neurologic deficits associated with vitamin B$_{12}$ deficiency would not be corrected by folate. Vitamin B$_{12}$ usually is administered intramuscularly to bypass the need for intrinsic factor. This is essential for patients with pernicious anemia, who depend on such injections for the remainder of their lives. Folate can be administered orally. Iron is often supplemented concurrently to support the rapid cell production that accompanies effective treatment.

When the proper treatment is initiated, the body's response is prompt and brisk and can be used to confirm the accuracy of the diagnosis. The bone marrow morphology will begin to revert to a normoblastic appearance within a few hours of treatment. A substantial reticulocyte response is apparent at about 1 week, with Hb increasing toward normal in about 3 weeks.[3]

CHAPTER at a GLANCE

- Impaired DNA synthesis affects all rapidly dividing cells of the body, including the skin, gastrointestinal tract, and bone marrow. The effect on hematologic cells results in megaloblastic anemia, so named for the very large RBCs that develop. Megaloblastic anemia is a type of macrocytic anemia.
- Vitamin B$_{12}$ and folic acid are needed in the production of thymidine nucleotides for DNA synthesis. Deficiencies of either vitamin impair DNA replication and halt cell division, resulting in megaloblastic anemia.
- Patients with vitamin B$_{12}$ or folate deficiency develop megaloblastic anemia and the generic symptoms of anemia. Patients with vitamin B$_{12}$ deficiency may develop impaired gait as a result of demyelinization of peripheral nerves. Folate deficiency, in particular, leads to elevation of homocysteine levels and possible risk of coronary artery disease. Peripheral neuropathy and depression also may accompany folate deficiency. Folate deficiency in pregnancy can lead to neural tube defects in the fetus.
- Folate deficiency may result from dietary deficiency, impaired use, or excessive loss. Dietary deficiency may result if intake is inadequate, need increases with growth or pregnancy, or absorption is impaired by disease. The action of folic acid can be impaired by drugs such as those used for epilepsy. Renal dialysis patients experience significant folate loss to the dialysate.
- Vitamin B$_{12}$ deficiency arises from dietary deficiencies—inadequate intake, increased need, or inadequate absorption. Inadequate intake of vitamin B$_{12}$, although possible, is uncommon because vitamin B$_{12}$ is ubiquitous in animal products. Pregnancy and growth create increased need for vitamin B$_{12}$.
- Absorption of vitamin B$_{12}$ depends on production of intrinsic factor by parietal cells of the stomach.
- Impaired absorption of vitamin B$_{12}$ can be caused by several mechanisms. Lack of trypsin in the intestine causes vitamin B$_{12}$ to be excreted in the stool rather than absorbed. Malabsorption can be caused by intestinal diseases, such as inflammatory bowel disease. Competition for vitamin B$_{12}$ can develop from intestinal

parasites or bacteria. Lack of intrinsic factor may result from loss of gastric parietal cells with gastrectomy or pernicious anemia.
- Pernicious anemia is vitamin B$_{12}$ deficiency resulting from an autoimmune disease causing atrophic loss of gastric parietal cells. H$^+$ secretion is lost, as is intrinsic factor secretion. Antibodies to parietal cells or intrinsic factor or both are detectable in the serum.
- Classic findings in the CBC in megaloblastic anemia include decreased Hb, Hct, and RBC count; elevated MCV (usually >120 fL); elevated RDW and MCH; MCHC within the reference range; oval macrocytes; hypersegmented neutrophils; leukopenia; and thrombocytopenia. Reticulocytes are decreased for the degree of anemia present. Additional abnormal laboratory test findings may include elevated total and indirect bilirubin and elevated lactate dehydrogenase due to the ineffective erythropoiesis and intramedullary hemolysis.
- The bone marrow in megaloblastic anemia is hyperplastic with increased erythropoiesis, but it is ineffective. RBC precursors show nuclear-cytoplasmic asynchrony, with the nucleus lagging behind the cytoplasm. Giant metamyelocytes or bands or both are evident.
- The cause of megaloblastic anemia is determined with specific radioimmunoassays for folate and vitamin B$_{12}$. Immunoassays for antibodies to intrinsic factor and parietal cells can diagnose pernicious anemia. Additional tests for gastrointestinal disease or parasites may be needed.
- Treatment of megaloblastic anemia is directed at removing the cause of the deficiency, supplementing the missing vitamin or both.
- For pernicious anemia, lifelong intramuscular injections of vitamin B$_{12}$ are necessary.

Now that you have completed this chapter, go back and read again the case study at the beginning and respond to the questions presented.

REVIEW QUESTIONS

1. Which of the following findings is *not* consistent with a diagnosis of megaloblastic anemia?
   a. Absolute decrease of neutrophils
   b. Increased RDW
   c. Increased serum lactate dehydrogenase
   d. Absolute increase in reticulocytes

2. A patient has a clinical picture of megaloblastic anemia. The folate level is decreased, and the vitamin B$_{12}$ is normal. What would be the expected value for the methylmalonic acid assay?
   a. Increased
   b. Decreased
   c. Normal

3. Which of the following statements does *not* correctly characterize the relationships among macrocytic anemia, megaloblastic anemia, and pernicious anemia?
   a. Megaloblastic anemia is macrocytic.
   b. Pernicious anemia is macrocytic.
   c. Macrocytic anemias are megaloblastic.
   d. Pernicious anemia is megaloblastic.

4. Which of the following CBC findings is most suggestive of a megaloblastic anemia?
   a. MCV of 103 fL
   b. Hypersegmentation of neutrophils
   c. RDW of 16%
   d. Hb of 9.1 g/dL (91 g/L)

5. In the following description of a bone marrow smear, find the statement that is *inconsistent* with the expected picture in megaloblastic anemia.

   The marrow appears hypercellular with a myeloid-to-erythroid ratio of 1:1 due to prominent erythroid hyperplasia. Megakaryocytes appear normal in number and appearance. The WBC elements appear larger than normal with especially large metamyelocytes, although they otherwise appear morphologically normal. The RBC precursors also appear large. There is nuclear-cytoplasmic asynchrony, with the nucleus appearing more mature than expected for the color of the cytoplasm.
   a. RBC nucleus more mature than cytoplasm
   b. Larger than normal WBC elements
   c. Larger than normal RBCs
   d. Normal appearance of megakaryocytes

6. Which of the following findings would be *inconsistent* with elevated levels of parietal cell antibodies?
   a. Hypersegmentation of neutrophils
   b. Low levels of methylmalonic acid
   c. Macrocytic RBCs
   d. Elevated levels of intrinsic factor blocking antibodies

7. Which of the following is the most metabolically active form of absorbed vitamin B_{12}?
   a. Transcobalamin
   b. Intrinsic factor–vitamin B_{12} complex
   c. Holotranscobalamin II
   d. Haptocorin–vitamin B_{12} complex

8. Folate and vitamin B_{12} work together in production of:
   a. Amino acids
   b. RNA
   c. Adenosine triphosphate
   d. DNA

9. The macrocytosis associated with megaloblastic anemia results from:
   a. Reduced numbers of cell divisions
   b. Activation of a gene that is typically active only in megakaryocytes
   c. Reduced concentration of Hb in the cells so that larger cells are needed to provide the same oxygen carrying capacity
   d. Reticulocytosis attempting to compensate for the anemia

10. Individuals descended from which of the following ethnic/racial groups are at highest risk for pernicious anemia?
    a. African
    b. Asian
    c. Northern European
    d. Southern European (Mediterranean)

REFERENCES

1. Blount BC, Mack MM, Wehr CM, et al: Folate deficiency causes uracil misincorporation into human DNA and chromosome breakage: implications for cancer and neuronal damage. Proc Natl Acad Sci USA 1997;94:3290-3295.
2. Koury MJ, Horne DW, Brown ZA, et al: Apoptosis of late-stage erythroblasts in megaloblastic anemia: association with DNA damage and macrocyte production. Blood 1997;89:4617-4623.
3. Carmel R, Rosenblatt DS: Disorders of cobalamin and folate metabolism. In Handin RI, Lux SE, Stossel TP (eds): Blood: Principles and Practice of Hematology, 2nd ed. Philadelphia: Lippincott, Williams & Wilkins, 2003;1361-1398.
4. Steiner I, Kidron D, Soffer D, et al: Sensory peripheral neuropathy of vitamin B12 deficiency: a primary demyelinating disease? J Neurol 1988;235:163-164.
5. Morrison HI, Schaubel D, Desmeules M, et al: Serum folate and risk of fatal coronary heart disease. JAMA 1996;275:1893-1896.
6. Voutilainen S, Virtanen JK, Rissanen TH, et al: Serum folate and homocysteine and the incidence of acute coronary events: the Kuopio Ischaemic Heart Disease Risk Factor Study. Am J Clin Nutr 2004;80:317-323.
7. de Bree A, Verschuren WM, Blom HJ, et al: Coronary heart disease mortality, plasma homocysteine, and B-vitamins: a prospective study. Atherosclerosis 2003;166:369-377.
8. Hung J, Beilby JP, Knuiman MW, et al: Folate and vitamin B12 and risk of fatal cardiovascular disease: cohort study from Busselton, Western Australia. BMJ 2003;326:131-137.
9. Soinio M, Marniemi J, Laakso M, et al: Elevated plasma homocysteine level is an independent predictor of coronary heart disease events in patients with type 2 diabetes mellitus. Ann Intern Med 2004;140:94-100.
10. Lindeman RD, Romero LJ, Yau CL, et al: Serum homocysteine concentrations and their relation to serum folate and vitamin B12 concentrations and coronary artery disease prevalence in an urban, bi-ethnic community. Ethn Dis 2003;13:178-185.
11. Alpert JE, Fava M: Nutrition and depression: the role of folate. Nutr Rev 1997;55:145-149.
12. Reynolds EH, Rothfeld P, Pincus JH: Neurological disease associated with folate deficiency. BMJ 1973;2:398-400.
13. Alpert JE, Mischoulon D, Nierenberg AA, et al: Nutrition and depression: focus on folate. Nutrition 2000;16:544-546.
14. Mulinsky A, Jick H, Jick SS, et al: Multivitamin/folic acid supplementation in early pregnancy reduces the prevalence of neural tube defects. JAMA 1989;262:2847-2852.
15. Gallagher ML: Vitamins. In Mahan LK, Escott-Stump S (eds): Krause's Food, Nutrition, and Diet Therapy, 11th ed. Philadelphia: Saunders, 2004:74-119.
16. Cooper BA: Reassessment of folic acid requirements. In White PL, Selvey N (eds): Nutrition in Transition: Proceedings of the

Western Hemisphere Nutrition Congress V. Monroe, WI: American Medical Association, 1978:281-288.

17. Henderson GB, Tsuji JM, Kumar HP: Mediated uptake of folate by a high-affinity binding protein in sublines of L1210 cells adapted to nanomolar concentrations of folate. J Membr Biol 1988;101:247-258.

18. Westergaard H: The sprue syndromes. Am J Med Sci 1985;290:249-262.

19. Kishi T, Fujita N, Eguchi T, et al: Mechanism for reduction of serum folate by antiepileptic drugs during prolonged therapy. J Neurol Sci 1997;145:109-112.

20. Froscher W, Maier V, Laage M, et al: Folate deficiency, anticonvulsant drugs, and psychiatric morbidity. Clin Neuropharmacol 1995;18:165-182.

21. Seligman PA, Allen RH: Characterization of the receptor for transcobalamin II isolated from human placenta. J Biol Chem 1978;253:1766-1772.

22. Sennett C, Rosenberg LE, Mellman IS: Transmembrane transport of cobalamin in prokaryotic and eukaryotic cells. Annu Rev Biochem 1981;50:1053-1086.

23. Toh BH, vanDriel IR, Gleeson PA: Pernicious anemia. N Engl J Med 1997;337:1441-1448.

24. Carmel R: Prevalence of undiagnosed pernicious anemia in the elderly. Arch Intern Med 1996;156:1097-1100.

25. Carmel R, Johnson CS: Racial patterns in pernicious anemia: early age at onset and increased frequency of intrinsic factor antibody in black women. N Engl J Med 1978;298:647-690.

26. Karlsson FA, Burman P, Loof L, et al: Major parietal cell antigen in autoimmune gastritis with pernicious anemia in the acid-producing H+,K+-adenosine triphosphatase of the stomach. J Clin Invest 1988;81:475-479.

27. Bardhan KD, Hall JR, Spray GH, et al: Blocking and binding autoantibody to intrinsic factor. Lancet 1968;1:62-64.

28. Strickland RG, Hooper B: The parietal cell heteroantibody in human sera: prevalence in a normal population and relationship to parietal cell autoantibody. Pathology 1972;4:259-263.

29. Nyberg W, Gräsbeck R, Saarni M, et al: Serum vitamin B12 levels and incidence of tape worm anemia in a population heavily infected with Diphyllobothrium latum. Am J Clin Nutr 1961;9:606-612.

30. Teplitsky V, Huminer D, Zoldan J, et al: Hereditary partial transcobalamin II deficiency with neurologic, mental and hematologic abnormalities in children and adults. Isr Med Assoc J 2003;5:868-872.

31. Monagle PT, Tauro GP: Long-term follow up of patients with transcobalamin II deficiency. Arch Dis Child 1995;72:237-238.

32. Hall CA: The neurologic aspects of transcobalamin II deficiency. Br J Haematol 1992;80:117-120.

33. Zittoun J, Zittoun R: Modern clinical testing strategies in cobalamin and folate deficiency. Semin Hematol 1999;36:35-46.

34. Herbert V: Experimental nutritional folate deficiency in man. Trans Assoc Am Physicians 1962;75:307-320.

35. Nath BJ, Lindenbaum J: Persistence of neutrophil hypersegmentation during recovery from megaloblastic granulopoiesis. Ann Intern Med 1979;90:757-760.

36. Wickramasinghe SN: The wide spectrum and unresolved issues in megaloblastic anemia. Semin Hematol 1999;36:3-18.

37. Carmel R: Introduction: beyond megaloblastic anemia. Semin Hematol 1999;36:1-2.

38. Moelby L, Rasmussen K, Jensen MK, et al: The relationship between clinically confirmed cobalamin deficiency and serum methylmalonic acid. J Intern Med 1990;228:373-378.

39. Solomon LR: Cobalamin-responsive disorders in ambulatory care setting: unreliability of cobalamin, methylmalonic acid, and homocysteine testing. Blood 2005;105:978-985.

Bone Marrow Failure

21

Elaine M. Keohane

OBJECTIVES

After completion of this chapter, the reader will be able to:

1. Describe the clinical consequences of bone marrow failure.
2. Describe the etiology of acquired and inherited aplastic anemias.
3. Discuss the pathophysiologic mechanisms of acquired and inherited aplastic anemias.
4. Describe the characteristic peripheral blood and bone marrow features in aplastic anemia.
5. Classify aplastic anemia as nonsevere, severe, or very severe based on laboratory tests.
6. Discuss treatment modalities for acquired and inherited aplastic anemia and the patients for whom each is most appropriate.
7. Differentiate among causes of pancytopenia based on laboratory tests and clinical findings.
8. Discuss the possible relationship between defects in the telomerase complex and bone marrow failure in acquired and inherited aplastic anemia.
9. Compare and contrast the pathophysiology, clinical picture, and laboratory findings in transient erythroblastopenia of childhood, Diamond-Blackfan anemia, and congenital dyserythropoietic anemia.
10. Describe the mechanisms causing cytopenia in myelophthisic anemia and anemia of chronic renal disease.

CASE STUDY

After studying the material in this chapter, the reader should be able to respond to the following case study:

A 52-year-old female data entry clerk complained of bilateral wrist pain. Her physician prescribed a nonsteroidal anti-inflammatory agent. Her wrist pain improved; however, over the next 3 months, she noted increasing fatigue and scattered bruises. Past medical history was unremarkable. She was on no other medications and had no recent chemical exposure. Physical examination revealed pallor and scattered ecchymoses with petechiae on chest and shoulders with no other abnormalities. Complete blood count results were as follows: hemoglobin, 8 g/dL; mean cell volume, 104 fL; reticulocytes, 0.6%; absolute reticulocytes 16×10^9/L; and WBC, 2×10^9/L, with absolute values of neutrophils 1.1×10^9/L and lymphocytes of 0.4×10^9/L. Platelet count was 27×10^9/L. Serum vitamin B_{12} and folate levels were normal. Bone marrow aspirate was normocellular with dyserythropoiesis,

normal myelopoiesis, and normal megakaryopoiesis. Iron stain revealed normal stores. Bone marrow biopsy was moderately hypocellular (30%) with reduced activity in all three cell lines. There was no increase in reticulin or blasts. Cytogenetics were normal and Ham test was negative.

1. What term is used to describe a decrease in all cell lines?
2. Which anemia of bone marrow failure should be considered?
3. How would an increase in either reticulin or blasts alter the preliminary diagnosis?
4. How would the severity of this patient's condition be classified?
5. What treatment modality would be considered for this patient?

PATHOPHYSIOLOGY OF BONE MARROW FAILURE

Bone marrow failure is the reduction or cessation of blood cell production affecting one or more cell lines. Pancytopenia, or decreased numbers of circulating red blood cells (RBCs), white blood cells (WBCs), and platelets, is seen in most cases of bone marrow failure, particularly in severe or advanced stages.

The pathophysiology of bone marrow failure includes the following mechanisms: (1) destruction of hematopoietic stem cells due to injury by drugs, chemicals, radiation, viruses, or autoimmune mechanisms; (2) premature senescence and apoptosis of stem cells due to inherited mutations; (3) ineffective hematopoiesis owing to stem cell mutations or vitamin B_{12} or folate deficiency; (4) disruption of the bone marrow microenvironment that supports hematopoiesis; (5) decreased production of hematopoietic growth factors or related hormones; or (6) loss of normal hematopoietic tissue due to infiltration of the marrow space with abnormal cells.

The clinical consequences of bone marrow failure vary depending on the extent and duration of the cytopenias. Severe pancytopenia can be rapidly fatal if untreated. Some patients may present initially with no symptoms and their cytopenia is inadvertently detected during a routine examination. Thrombocytopenia can result in clinically significant bleeding. The decrease in RBCs and hemoglobin (Hb) leads to symptoms of anemia, including fatigue, pallor, and cardiovascular complications. Sustained neutropenia increases the risk of bacterial or fungal infections that can be life-threatening.

This chapter focuses on aplastic anemia, a bone marrow failure syndrome resulting from damaged or defective stem cells (mechanisms 1 and 2). Bone marrow failure resulting from other mechanisms may have a presentation similar to aplastic anemia and differentiation is discussed later. Because there are many mechanisms involved in the various bone marrow failure syndromes, accurate diagnosis is essential so that the appropriate treatment can be instituted.

APLASTIC ANEMIA

Aplastic anemia is a rare but potentially fatal bone marrow failure syndrome. The first reported case of aplastic anemia is attributed to Ehrlich[1] in 1888, who described a patient with severe anemia and neutropenia exhibiting a yellow hypocellular marrow on postmortem examination. The name *aplastic anemia* was given to the disease by Chauffard in 1904.[2] The characteristic features of aplastic anemia include pancytopenia, reticulocytopenia, bone marrow hypocellularity, and depletion of hematopoietic stem cells (Box 21-1). Aplastic anemia may be acquired or inherited. In adults, the acquired type constitutes most cases. In infants and children, approximately 70% of aplastic anemias are acquired, and 30% are inherited. Box 21-2 provides an etiologic classification of aplastic anemia.

Acquired Aplastic Anemia

Acquired aplastic anemia is classified as idiopathic when the cause is unknown and secondary when the etiology can be identified. The idiopathic type accounts for approximately 70% to 80% of aplastic anemia cases.[3] Clinical and laboratory findings are similar for idiopathic and secondary aplastic anemia. Patients with aplastic anemia initially may present

---

BOX 21-1 Characteristic Features of Aplastic Anemia

Peripheral blood pancytopenia
Reticulocytopenia
Bone marrow hypocellularity
Depletion of hematopoietic stem cells

BOX 21-2 Etiologic Classification of Aplastic Anemia

Acquired
Idiopathic (70-80% of cases)
Secondary
    Dose dependent
        Cytotoxic drugs
        Benzene
        Radiation
    Idiosyncratic
        Drugs (see Box 21-3)
        Chemicals
            Pesticides
            Lubricating agents/cutting oils
    Viruses
        Epstein-Barr virus
        Hepatitis (some types)
        Human immunodeficiency virus (HIV)
    Miscellaneous conditions
        Paroxysmal nocturnal hemoglobinuria
        Autoimmune diseases
        Pregnancy

Inherited
Fanconi anemia
Dyskeratosis congenita

---

with a normocytic or macrocytic anemia without reticulocytosis. Depending on the progression of the bone marrow failure, pancytopenia may develop slowly. More than half of aplastic anemias progress at a rapid rate, however, with complete cessation of erythropoiesis.

Incidence

In North America and Europe, the incidence per year approximates 2 per 1 million.[4] In Asia and East Asia, the frequency is two to three times higher than in North America or Europe. Aplastic anemia can occur at any age but is more frequent in individuals 10 to 25 years old and individuals older than age 60.[4,5] There is no gender difference in incidence.[4]

Etiology

The cause of the bone marrow failure in idiopathic aplastic anemia is unknown. Secondary aplastic anemia is associated with exposure to certain drugs, chemicals, radiation, or infectious agents. Cytotoxic drugs, radiation, and chemicals, such as benzene, suppress the bone marrow in a predictable, dose-dependent manner.[6-8] Depending on the dose and exposure time, the bone marrow generally recovers after withdrawal of the agent. About 90% of secondary aplastic anemias occur secondary to idiosyncratic reactions to drugs or chemicals. In idiosyncratic reactions, the bone marrow failure is unpredictable and unrelated to dose, and the bone marrow does not usually recover when the agent is withdrawn.[6] Documentation of an identifiable factor or agent inducing aplastic anemia in these cases is difficult because evidence is primarily circumstantial and symptoms may occur months or years after exposure. Some drugs associated with idiosyncratic, acquired aplastic anemia are listed in Box 21-3.[5,6]

Aplastic anemia as an idiosyncratic, adverse reaction to a drug, chemical, or other agent is a rare event and is likely due to a combination of genetic and environmental factors in susceptible individuals. Currently no tests are available to predict individual susceptibility to these idiosyncratic reactions; however, genetic differences affecting metabolic and immune response pathways may play a role. There is a twofold higher incidence of HLA-DR2 and its major serologic split, HLA-DR15, in aplastic anemia patients compared with the general population, but the relationship of this finding to the disease pathophysiology has not been elucidated.[9,10] A deficiency in the enzyme glutathione S-transferase resulting from *GSTT1* and *GSTM1/GSTT1* gene deletions was found in 30% and 22% of Caucasians with acquired aplastic anemia.[11] This deficiency and other factors yet to be discovered may affect the biometabolism of certain drugs and chemicals leading to the bone marrow suppression.

Acquired aplastic anemia appears occasionally as a complication from infections. Viruses implicated in aplastic anemia include Epstein-Barr virus, human immunodeficiency virus (HIV), hepatitis virus, and human parvovirus B19. A history of acute non-A, non-B, or non-C hepatitis 1 to 3 months before onset is found in 2% to 10% of patients with acquired aplastic anemia.[12] Posthepatitis aplastic anemia syndrome has a poor prognosis.

Acquired aplastic anemia has been reported as a rare complication in pregnancy and autoimmune disorders.[6] Aplastic anemia also occurs as a complication in paroxysmal nocturnal hemoglobinuria. The distinction between these conditions is discussed later.

Pathophysiology

The primary lesion in acquired aplastic anemia is a quantitative and qualitative deficiency of hematopoietic stem cells, rather than a defect of the bone marrow stroma or a deficiency of growth factors. In culture, stem cells of patients with acquired aplastic anemia have diminished colony formation.[13] The hematopoietic stem and early progenitor cell compartment is identified by expression of CD34 surface antigens. When measured by flow cytometry, the CD34+ cell population in the bone marrow of patients with aplastic anemia can be 10 times lower compared with normal individuals.[13] There is an increase in apoptotic CD34+ cells in aplastic anemia, and they have an increased expression of Fas receptors that mediate apoptosis.[14,15] Bone marrow cells in aplastic anemia also have an increased expression of apoptotic genes determined by gene chip analysis.[16] The bone marrow stroma is functionally normal in acquired aplastic anemia. Stromal cells from patients with aplastic anemia produce normal or increased quantities of growth factors, and they are able to support the growth of CD34+ cells from normal donors in culture and in vivo after transplantation.[6,17] Individuals with aplastic anemia have elevated levels of growth factors in their serum, such as erythropoietin.[18] Additionally, the serum level of flt3 ligand, a growth factor that stimulates proliferation of stem and progenitor cells, is 200 times higher in patients with severe aplastic anemia compared with normal individuals.[19] Despite elevated levels, growth factors are generally unsuccessful in correcting the cytopenias found in acquired aplastic anemia secondary to the damage and depletion of the stem cells.

The pathophysiology of acquired a plastic anemia involves the severe depletion of hematopoietic stem and progenitor cells from the bone marrow by a direct or indirect mechanism. In the direct mechanism, a cytotoxic drug, chemical, radiation, or virus damages the DNA of the stem and progenitor cells

---

BOX 21-3 Drugs Reported to Have a Rare Association with Idiosyncratic Aplastic Anemia

Antiarthritics
Gold compounds
Penicillamine

Antibiotics
Chloramphenicol
Sulfonamides

Anticonvulsants
Carbamazepine
Phenytoin

Antidepressants
Dothiepin
Phenothiazine

Antidiabetes Agents
Chlorpropamide
Tolbutamide

Anti-inflammatories (Nonsteroidal)
Diclofenac
Fenoprofen
Ibuprofen
Indomethacin
Naproxen
Phenylbutazone
Piroxicam
Sulindac

Antiprotozoals
Chloroquine
Quinacrine

Antithyroidals
Carbimazole
Thiouracil

causing apoptosis and cytolysis.[6] In the indirect method, exposure to certain drugs or chemicals in susceptible individuals results in an autoimmune T cell attack that destroys the stem and progenitor cells.[20] The autoimmune pathophysiology was first suggested in the 1970s when aplastic anemia patients undergoing immunosuppressive conditioning before bone marrow transplant experienced an improvement in cell counts.[21] Evidence that supports the autoimmune pathophysiology is that in acquired aplastic anemia (1) there is an increase in cytotoxic (CD8⁺) T lymphocytes in the blood and bone marrow detected by flow cytometry; (2) these T cells produce increased amounts of cytokines that inhibit hematopoiesis and induce apoptosis, including interferon-γ and tumor necrosis factor-α[22-24]; (3) there is an increase in tumor necrosis factor-α receptors on CD34⁺ cells[25]; and (4) there is improvement in the cytopenia in most patients after immunosuppression therapy.[6,20] Possible mechanisms by which a drug, chemical, or virus may elicit an autoimmune response may be by altering self-proteins, inducing expression of abnormal proteins, exposing hidden antigens, inducing an immune response that cross-reacts with self-antigens, or disrupting immune regulation networks.[20,23] The antigens responsible for triggering and sustaining the autoimmune attack on the stem cells are unknown. Autoantibodies to kinectin, an intracellular protein found in hematopoietic cells, have been detected in aplastic anemia patients but not in normal controls; the relationship of the autoantibody to the pathophysiology of the disease is unknown.[26]

Blood cells in patients with aplastic anemia who do not respond to immunosuppression therapy have a progressive shortening of their telomeres and a decrease in telomerase activity.[27] In addition, mutations in the RNA component of the telomerase gene (*TERC*) and the telomerase reverse transcriptase gene (*TERT*) have been found in subsets of patients with aplastic anemia.[28,29] Telomerase is an enzyme that is important for the repair and maintenance of telomeres at the end of chromosomes. Cells with abnormally short telomeres are unable to proceed through the cell cycle and become senescent and apoptotic. The mechanism of stem cell depletion in a subset of patients with aplastic anemia may be linked to defective telomere maintenance imparting a susceptibility to bone marrow failure after environmental insult.[29]

Clinical Findings

Symptoms vary in acquired aplastic anemia from very severe to mild or asymptomatic. Patients usually present with symptoms typical of insidious-onset anemia: pallor, fatigue, and weakness. Severe anemia can result in serious cardiac complications or even cardiac failure and death. Petechiae, bruising, epistaxis, bleeding gums, menorrhagia, retinal hemorrhages, intestinal bleeding, and sometimes intracranial bleeding may occur secondary to thrombocytopenia. Fever and bacterial or fungal infections are unusual at initial presentation but may occur after prolonged periods of neutropenia. Splenomegaly and hepatomegaly are absent.

Laboratory Findings

Pancytopenia is typical, although initially only one or two cell lines may be decreased. The absolute neutrophil count is decreased, and the absolute lymphocyte count may be normal or decreased. The Hb is usually less than 10 g/dL, the mean cell volume (MCV) is normal or increased, and the percent and absolute reticulocytes and immature reticulocyte fraction are decreased. Table 21-1 contains the diagnostic criteria for aplastic anemia by degree of severity.[4,5,30,31] This classification is helpful in guiding treatment decisions.

On a peripheral blood film, neutrophils, monocytes, and platelets are decreased, and the RBCs are normocytic or macrocytic. Toxic granulation may be observed in the neutrophils, but the RBCs and platelets are normal in appearance. Blasts and other immature blood cells are characteristically absent.

Serum iron and percent transferrin saturation are increased reflecting the decreased use of iron for erythropoiesis. Liver function tests may be abnormal if the pancytopenia was preceded by hepatitis. Approximately one third of aplastic anemia patients develop paroxysmal nocturnal hemoglobinuria.[32] In paroxysmal nocturnal hemoglobinuria, an acquired stem cell mutation results in circulating blood cells that lack glyco-

TABLE 21-1 Diagnostic Criteria for Aplastic Anemia

	NSAA	SAA	VSAA
Bone marrow	Hypocellular bone marrow plus at least two of the following:	Bone marrow cellularity <25%* plus at least two of the following:	Same as SAA
Neutrophils (× 10⁹/L)	0.5-1.5	0.2-0.5	<0.2
Platelets (× 10⁹/L)	20-50	<20	Same as SAA
Other	Hb ≤10 g/dL plus reticulocytes <30 × 10⁹/L	Reticulocytes <20 × 10⁹/L or <1% corrected for Hct	Same as SAA

*Or 25% to 50% cellularity with <30% residual hematopoietic cells.
NSAA, nonsevere aplastic anemia; SAA, severe aplastic anemia; VSAA, very severe aplastic anemia; Hct, hematocrit.

sylphosphatidylinositol-linked proteins, such as CD55 and CD59. The absence of CD55 and CD59 on the surface of the RBCs renders them more susceptible to lysis by complement. The Ham test for complement-mediated hemolysis is positive if there are a sufficient number of paroxysmal nocturnal hemoglobinuria cells; however, flow cytometry is a more sensitive method to detect small numbers of circulating CD55 and CD59 negative paroxysmal nocturnal hemoglobinuria cells compared with the Ham test[5] (see Chapter 33). Flow cytometry has been able to detect small numbers of circulating paroxysmal nocturnal hemoglobinuria granulocytes in almost 90% of newly diagnosed aplastic anemia patients by concentrating the cells in the granulocyte gate.[33] The significance of this finding is unclear, but it may be related to the ability of glycosylphosphatidylinositol-deficient stem cells to escape the immune destruction in aplastic anemia.[33]

Bone marrow aspirates and biopsy specimens have prominent fat cells with areas of patchy cellularity. Biopsy samples are required for an accurate quantitative assessment of the marrow cellularity, and severe hypocellularity is a characteristic feature (Fig. 21-1). Erythroid, granulocytic, and megakaryocytic cells are decreased or absent. Dyserythropoiesis may be present, but there is no dysplasia of the granulocyte or platelet cell lines. Blasts and abnormal cell infiltrates are characteristically absent. Reticulin staining is normal.

An abnormal karyotype is infrequent at presentation, but approximately one fourth of aplastic anemia patients develop chromosome abnormalities over the course of the disease, particularly monosomy 7 and trisomy 8.[34] Conventional cytogenetics may underestimate the incidence of karyotype abnormalities. Detection of chromosome abnormalities with conventional culture techniques is difficult and insensitive in aplastic anemia owing to the hypocellularity of the bone marrow and scarcity of cells in metaphase. Newer methods that employ interphase fluorescent in situ hybridization using DNA probes for specific chromosomes have a greater sensitivity and have the ability to use nondividing cells.[5,34]

Treatment and Prognosis

Severe aplastic anemia requires immediate treatment to prevent the dire consequences of serious pancytopenia. If a potential causative agent is suspected, it should be discontinued. To keep blood counts at safe levels, platelets generally are administered when the platelet count decreases to less than 10×10^9/L, whereas RBCs are given when the patient becomes symptomatic.[5] One of the most important early decisions that must be made is whether a patient is a candidate for a hematopoietic stem cell transplant. Hematopoietic stem cell transplant is the treatment of choice for patients with severe aplastic anemia who are younger than age 40 and have an HLA-identical sibling.[3,5] For patients older than age 40 or of any age without an HLA-identical sibling, immunosuppressive therapy, consisting of antithymocyte globulin with cyclosporine is the preferred therapy.[3,5] The antithymocyte globulin decreases the number of activated T cells, and the cyclosporine inhibits their function, suppressing the autoimmune reaction against the stem cells. For patients with severe disease who are not responsive to immunosuppression, hematopoietic stem cell transplant from an HLA-matched unrelated donor may be an option, but survival is not as favorable compared with an HLA-identical sibling.[3,5] Recombinant humanized antibody to the interleukin-2 receptor is under evaluation as a possible therapy.[35]

Other supportive therapy includes antibiotic and antifungal prophylaxis in cases of prolonged neutropenia. Growth factors such as recombinant human erythropoietin are not recommended for primary treatment in that they are generally ineffective and can have serious side effects.[5] Patients with non-severe aplastic anemia may not require treatment but must be monitored periodically for cytopenia and abnormal cells.

Long-term survival is achieved in 80% to 90% of younger patients who receive a hematopoietic stem cell transplant from an identical sibling.[3] In patients treated with immunosuppression, 75% show an improvement in cytopenia, but 12% to 30% eventually relapse.[3] The presence of monosomy 7 denotes a poor prognosis, whereas trisomy 8 has a good prognosis.[34] Over the course of the disease, 10% to 25% of patients treated with immunosuppression develop paroxysmal nocturnal hemoglobinuria, and 10% to 20% progress to myelodysplastic syndrome or leukemia.[32,34]

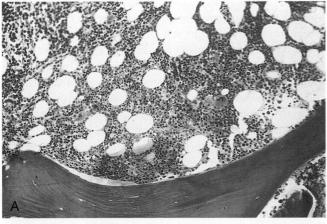
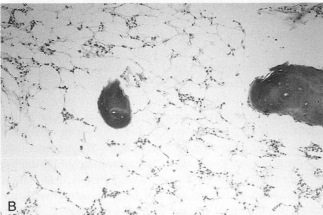

Figure 21-1 A, Normal bone marrow tissue section stained with hematoxylin and eosin. **B,** Hypoplastic bone marrow tissue section stained with hematoxylin and eosin from a patient with aplastic anemia. (Courtesy of Ann Bell, University of Tennessee, Memphis.)

Inherited Aplastic Anemia

Patients with inherited aplastic anemia usually present at an early age and may have associated congenital malformations. The two inherited diseases with bone marrow failure and pancytopenia as a consistent feature are Fanconi anemia and dyskeratosis congenita.

Fanconi Anemia

Fanconi anemia is an autosomal recessive chromosome instability disorder characterized by aplastic anemia, congenital abnormalities, and cancer susceptibility. It was first described by Fanconi in 1927 in three brothers with skin pigmentation, short stature, and hypogonadism.[36] Fanconi anemia occurs at a rate of 3 per 100,000. The carrier rate is 1 in 300 in the United States and Europe, 1 in 89 in Ashkenazi Jews, and 1 in 83 in Africans.[37] It is the most common of the inherited aplastic anemias.

Clinical Findings. There is no typical presentation for Fanconi anemia. Patients may present at birth with congenital malformations or may first present with hematologic abnormalities as children or adults. Approximately two thirds of patients with Fanconi anemia have congenital malformations. Congenital anomalies vary considerably, although there is a higher frequency of skeletal abnormalities (malformations of the thumbs, radial hypoplasia, microcephaly, hip dislocation, and scoliosis); skin pigmentation (hyperpigmentation or hypopigmentation and café-au-lait spots); short stature; and abnormalities of the eyes, kidneys, and genitals.[37,38] Low birth weight and developmental delays also are common.

The symptoms associated with pancytopenia usually become apparent at 5 to 10 years of age; however, some patients may be asymptomatic until adulthood.[37,38] Adults with Fanconi anemia have an increased risk of developing solid tumors, particularly oral, esophageal, anogenital, and hepatic tumors.

Genetics and Pathophysiology. Using cell fusion studies, 11 complementation groups have been identified for Fanconi anemia, and from those groups, eight different genes have been characterized: *FANCA, FANCC, BRCA2 (FANCD1), FANCD2, FANCE, FANCF, FANCG,* and *FANCL*.[38] Mutations in the *FANCA* gene occur with the highest frequency.[38] The relationship between mutations in the Fanconi anemia genes and disease pathology is not clear. At least five Fanconi anemia proteins form a core complex in the nucleus and possibly interact with other nuclear regulatory proteins in DNA repair processes, maintenance of chromosome stability, and cell cycle control, but the exact pathways and mechanisms are unknown. Other possible functions of Fanconi anemia proteins include involvement in cell oxygen sensitivity, apoptosis and telomere maintenance, and regulation of hematopoietic stem cells.[37,38]

Laboratory Findings. Laboratory results are similar to those in acquired aplastic anemia. Macrocytic RBCs are often the first detected abnormality, and thrombocytopenia usually precedes the development of the other cytopenias. The Hb F level may be strikingly elevated. Chromosomes show abnormal fragility in Fanconi anemia. The addition of a DNA cross-linking agent, such as diepoxybutane or mitomycin C, to Fanconi anemia cells in culture causes characteristic chromosome breakage and is the diagnostic test for this disorder.[37] Patients with Fanconi anemia also have cell cycle disturbances with a prolonged progression to, and arrest within, the G_2 phase. Flow cytometry can detect the accumulation of G_2 phase cells in culture, and this can be used as an adjunct diagnostic test for Fanconi anemia only if there is no concurrent leukemia or myelodysplastic syndrome.[39]

Treatment and Prognosis. More than 90% of patients with Fanconi anemia develop bone marrow failure by their 30s. In addition, patients with Fanconi anemia have a 33% risk of a developing a hematologic malignancy, particularly acute myeloid leukemia and myelodysplastic syndrome, and a 28% risk of developing other cancers by age 40.[40] Squamous cell carcinomas of the head and neck, anogenital region, and skin are the most common, followed by tumors of the liver, brain, and kidney.[38,40] Death by age 20 as a result of complications of bone marrow failure or leukemia is common. Patients with mutations in the *FANCC* gene have an earlier onset of bone marrow failure and the poorest survival.[40] An increased rate of telomere shortening in Fanconi anemia cells is associated with a greater severity of pancytopenia and higher risk of developing malignancies; however, the role of telomere shortening in the evolution of bone marrow failure and cancer is unclear.[41]

Supportive treatment for cytopenia includes transfusions, androgens, and cytokines (granulocyte colony-stimulating factor and granulocyte macrophage colony-stimulating factor).[37] Currently the only curative treatment for cytopenia is hematopoietic stem cell transplant, preferably from an HLA-identical sibling. Patients still have an increased risk of developing secondary malignancies even after successful transplantation.[40] Gene therapy clinical trials have been attempted but have not been successful.

Dyskeratosis Congenita

Dyskeratosis congenita is a rare, inherited bone marrow failure syndrome with only several hundred known cases worldwide.

Clinical Findings. Dyskeratosis congenita is characterized by mucocutaneous abnormalities, bone marrow failure, and pancytopenia. The typical clinical presentation includes abnormal skin pigmentation, dystrophic nails, and oral leukoplakia, with an onset between 5 and 10 years of age. Three fourths of patients develop bone marrow failure and pancytopenia before 20 years of age.[42] Approximately 15% to 25% of patients also present with developmental delay, short stature, prematurely gray hair and hair loss, extensive dental caries, or pulmonary disease. Patients with dyskeratosis congenita have a predisposition for developing acute myeloid leukemia, myelodysplastic syndrome, and epithelial malignancies.

Genetics and Pathophysiology. Inherited defects in the telomerase complex are implicated in the pathology of dyskeratosis congenita.[43] The telomerase complex synthesizes telomere repeats to elongate the ends of chromosomes, and maintaining the length of the telomeres is important for cell survival. Three inheritance patterns are recognized in dyskeratosis congenita: autosomal dominant, X-linked, and autosomal recessive.[43] The autosomal dominant form is due to a mutation in *TERC*, the gene that codes for the RNA component of telomerase. The X-linked recessive form is the most common and is due to a mutation in the *DKC1* gene that codes for dyskerin protein. Dyskerin is a ribonucleoprotein involved in RNA processing and it associates with *TERC* in the telomerase complex. The autosomal recessive type is not yet characterized. The exact pathophysiologic mechanisms of dyskeratosis congenita are unknown; however, mutations in dyskerin and *TERC* may disrupt telomerase function, resulting in shorter telomeres and premature death in rapidly dividing cells in the bone marrow and epithelium.[43]

Laboratory Findings. Pancytopenia and macrocytic RBCs are typical findings after onset. The Hb F level also may be increased. The autosomal dominant and X-linked forms of dyskeratosis congenita are diagnosed by detecting mutations in the *TERC* and *DKC1* genes by DNA sequencing. A subset of patients develop secondary immunodeficiency with decreased T and B cells and abnormal levels of immunoglobulin.[42]

Treatment and Prognosis. Approximately two thirds of dyskeratosis congenita patient deaths are due to the effects of bone marrow failure.[42] Typically, death occurs before patients reach their 20s as a result of complications of infections. Treatment with allogeneic stem cell transplantation has not been optimal because of the high incidence of fatal pulmonary complications in patients with dyskeratosis congenita. Although androgens and growth factors produce a transient response, they do not halt effectively the progression of the bone marrow failure. Approximately 10% of patients develop fatal pulmonary disease, and another 10% die because of complications of malignancies.[42]

Differential Diagnosis

A differential diagnosis must be made between acquired aplastic anemia, inherited aplastic anemia, and other causes of pancytopenia, including paroxysmal nocturnal hemoglobinuria, myelodysplastic syndrome, megaloblastic anemia, acute leukemia, and hairy cell leukemia. The key features that distinguish these conditions are listed in Table 21-2.[5] These conditions have different therapeutic regimens, so it is essential to distinguish them so that the patient receives the appropriate treatment. In addition, recognition of paroxysmal nocturnal hemoglobinuria is important because of the hemolysis and thrombosis associated with the disease (Chapter 42).

Lymphomas, Hodgkin disease, myelofibrosis, and mycobacterial infections occasionally may present with pancytopenia but can be distinguished through careful examination of the bone marrow and, in the case of lymphomas, molecular tests for chromosome abnormalities. Anorexia nervosa also may present with pancytopenia, but the bone marrow is hypocellular and has a decrease of fat cells.[5]

OTHER FORMS OF BONE MARROW FAILURE

Pure Red Cell Aplasia

Pure red cell aplasia (PRCA) is a rare disorder of erythroplasia characterized by a selective and severe decrease in erythrocyte precursors in an otherwise normal bone marrow. Patients present with severe anemia, reticulocytopenia, and a normal WBC and platelet count. PRCA may be acquired or congenital.[44]

Acquired Pure Red Cell Aplasia

Acquired PRCA may occur in children or adults and can be acute or chronic. Primary PRCA may be idiopathic or autoimmune related. Secondary PRCA may occur in association with an underlying hematologic malignancy, solid tumor, infection, chronic hemolytic anemia, collagen vascular disease, or exposure to drugs or chemicals.[44] Therapy involves treatment of the underlying condition and immunosuppression.

The acquired form of PRCA in children also is known as *transient erythroblastopenia of childhood*. A history of viral infection is found in half of patients and an immune mechanism is involved in its etiology. The anemia is normocytic and Hb F levels are normal. Transfusions are the initial therapy and restoration of normal erythropoiesis occurs in most patients.[45]

Congenital Pure Red Cell Aplasia: Diamond-Blackfan Anemia

Diamond-Blackfan anemia is a congenital erythroid hypoplastic disorder of early infancy occurring in 2 to 7 per 1 million live births.[46] Stem cells are defective, but the cause is unknown; they are diminished in number and are erythropoietin resistant. Approximately 25% of patients have a mutation in the *RPS19* gene located on chromosome 19, and approximately half of those are due to a sporadic mutation.[46,47] Patients present with severe normocytic or macrocytic anemia and reticulocytopenia during the first year of life. WBCs are normal or slightly decreased, and platelets are normal or slightly increased. Bone marrow examination distinguishes Diamond-Blackfan anemia from the hypocellular marrow in aplastic anemia because there is normal cellularity of myeloid cells and megakaryocytes and hypoplasia of erythroid cells. The karyotype in Diamond-Blackfan anemia is normal. Hb F and erythrocyte adenosine deaminase are increased, distinguishing it from transient erythroblastopenia of childhood, in which these levels are normal.[46] Approximately half of patients with Diamond-Blackfan anemia have anomalies such as craniofacial dysmorphism, growth retardation, neck malformations, and thumb malformations. Therapy includes transfusions and corticosteroids. Stem cell transplantation may be considered for patients with severe anemia and an HLA-identical sibling.

TABLE 21-2 Differentiation of Aplastic Anemia from Other Causes of Pancytopenia

Condition	Peripheral Blood	Bone Marrow	Laboratory Test Results	Clinical Findings
Failure of Bone Marrow to Produce Blood Cells				
Aplastic anemia	No immature WBCs or RBCs; ↓ reticulocytes; MCV normal or ↑	Hypocellular; blasts and abnormal cells absent; reticulin normal; RBC dyspoiesis ±; WBC and platelet dyspoiesis absent	PNH cells* ±; Ham test ±; chromosome abnormalities may be present; FA and DC: Hb F may be ↑; FA: chromosome breakage with DEB or MMC; DC: mutations in *DKC1* or *TERC*	Splenomegaly absent; FA and DC may have congenital malformations
Increased Destruction of Blood Cells				
PNH	Reticulocytes ↑; MCV normal or ↑; nucleated RBCs ±	Erythroid hyperplasia; may be hypocellular	PNH cells* +; Ham test +; chromosome abnormalities may be present	Splenomegaly absent; thrombosis may be present
Ineffective Hematopoiesis				
Myelodysplastic syndrome	Variable pancytopenia; reticulocytes ↓; MCV normal or ↑; blasts and abnormal WBCs, RBCs, and platelets may be present	Hypercellular; 20% hypocellular; dyspoiesis in one or more cell lines present; blasts and immature cells present; reticulin ↑	Chromosome abnormalities usually present	Splenomegaly uncommon
Megaloblastic anemias	MCV ↑; oval macrocytes; hypersegmented neutrophils	Hypercellular with megaloblastic features	Serum B_{12} or folate or both ↓	Splenomegaly absent
Bone Marrow Infiltration				
Acute leukemia	Blasts present	Hypercellular; blasts ↑; reticulin ↑	Chromosome abnormalities may be present	Splenomegaly may be present
Hairy cell leukemia	Hairy cells present; monocytes ↓	Hairy cells and fibrosis present; reticulin ↑	Hairy cells† +; TRAP +	Splenomegaly present 60-70%

*PNH cells are detected by flow cytometry by their lack of expression of CD55 and CD59.
†Hairy cells are detected by flow cytometry by their expression of CD20, CD11c, CD25, and FMC7.
↑, increased; ↓, decreased; ±, positive or negative; +, positive.
DEB, diepoxybutane; MMC, mitomycin C; TRAP, tartrate-resistant acid phosphatase; FA, Fanconi anemia; DC, dyskeratosis congenita; PNH, paroxysmal nocturnal hemoglobinuria.

Congenital Dyserythropoietic Anemia

The congenital dyserythropoietic anemias (CDAs) are a heterogeneous group of rare disorders characterized by refractory anemia, reticulocytopenia, hypercellular bone marrow with markedly ineffective erythropoiesis, and distinctive dysplastic changes in bone marrow erythroblasts, including giantism, multinuclearity, and karyorrhexis. The megaloblastoid features are not due to vitamin B_{12} or folate deficiency. The anemia varies from mild to moderate, even among affected siblings. Secondary hemosiderosis arises from the chronic intramedullary and extramedullary hemolysis of erythroblasts and circulating RBCs and the increase in iron absorption associated with the accelerated inefficient erythropoiesis. Iron overload develops even in the absence of blood transfusions. Jaundice and cholelithiasis (as a result of hyperbilirubinemia) and splenomegaly are common findings.

CDA usually manifests in childhood but may first be recognized in adulthood, depending on the severity of symptoms. CDA is grouped into three major types: CDA I, CDA II, and CDA III. There are variant types, however, that do not fall into any of these categories.[48] CDA I is autosomal recessive with a moderate-to-severe chronic anemia. It is caused by mutations in the *CDAN1* gene on chromosome 15.[49] *CDAN1* codes for codanin-1, a protein that may be important for nuclear envelope integrity.[49] Approximately 150 cases of CDA I have been reported.[48] Malformations of fingers or toes, brown skin pigmentation, and neurologic defects are found more frequently in CDA I compared with the other types. The Hb is usually 8 to 11 g/dL. Erythrocytes are macrocytic and may exhibit basophilic stippling and Cabot rings. The megaloblastoid erythroblasts characteristically include multinucleated forms and internuclear chromatin bridges or nuclear strands between two erythroblasts or between two nuclei in a single cell (Fig. 21-2). Ultrastructurally, the erythroblasts typically have spongy heterochromatin and nuclear membranes that are disrupted and invaginated, carrying cytoplasmic organelles into the nucleus. Treatment includes interferon-α and iron depletion.[48] CDA II is the most common type and is autosomal recessive. More than 300 cases have been reported.[48] The gene associated with CDA II maps to chromosome 20.[48] The anemia is mild to severe, and the late erythroblasts in the bone marrow include binuclear and multinuclear forms. The Hb is usually 8 to 11 g/dL, and erythrocytes are usually normocytic with anisocytosis, poikilocytosis, and basophilic stippling. Mature erythrocytes test positive in the acidified serum test (but not in the sucrose hemolysis test), giving it the name *HEMPAS* (hereditary erythroblastic multinuclearity with positive acidified serum).[45] They also are reactive with anti-i antisera.[48] Treatment includes splenectomy and iron depletion.[48]

CDA III is the least common of the CDAs. A familial, autosomal dominant form was found in three families and is mapped to chromosome 15; the nonfamilial or sporadic form is extremely rare with fewer than 20 cases reported.[48] The anemia is mild, and giant erythroblasts with 12 nuclei are a characteristic feature. Patients are transfusion independent, and clinical iron overload is not observed.

Myelophthisic Anemia

Myelophthisic anemia is the infiltration of abnormal cells into the bone marrow and subsequent destruction and replacement of the normal hematopoietic cells. Metastatic solid tumor cells (particularly lung, breast, and prostate), leukemic cells, fibroblasts, and inflammatory cells (found in miliary tuberculosis and fungal infections) are implicated.[50,51] Cytokines, growth factors, and other substances are released that suppress hematopoiesis or destroy stem, progenitor, or stromal cells, resulting in peripheral cytopenias.[51] If the infiltration and proliferation of the abnormal cells disrupts the normal bone marrow architecture, premature release of immature cells from the bone marrow occurs. In addition, because of the unfavorable bone marrow environment, stem and progenitor cells migrate to the spleen and liver and establish extramedullary hematopoietic sites.[51] Because blood cell production in these sites is less efficient, immature cells also may be released prematurely into the circulation from these organs.[50]

Myelophthisic anemia is typically mild to moderate with normocytic erythrocytes. The typical findings on the peripheral blood film are teardrop erythrocytes and nucleated RBCs, but immature myeloid cells (leukoerythroblastic blood picture), megakaryocyte fragments, and giant platelets also may be present.[50] Although myelophthisic anemia and aplastic anemia exhibit cytopenias, myelophthisic anemia is distinguished from aplastic anemia by the presence of normocytic RBCs with teardrop forms, a leukoerythroblastic blood picture, and abnormal cells in the bone marrow aspiration or biopsy.

Anemia of Chronic Renal Insufficiency

Anemia occurs in most patients with chronic renal insufficiency.[52-54] In the United States, more than 800,000 adults with chronic renal disease have a Hb less than 11 g/dL.[52] The major cause of the anemia in chronic renal disease is the inadequate production of erythropoietin by the kidneys.[53] Without erythropoietin, the bone marrow is unable to increase RBC production in response to tissue hypoxia, and anemia ensues. The anemia occurs even in moderate impairment of renal function.[53] Other factors also contribute to the anemia in renal disease. Patients on dialysis experience chronic blood loss (and iron loss) and folate depletion as a result of the dialysis procedure itself. Waste products accumulate secondary to renal excretory failure and shorten the life span of the erythrocytes, and chronic inflammatory conditions and poor diet may limit the iron available for erythropoiesis.[53,54] The anemia in chronic renal disease is normocytic and normochromic, with normal or decreased reticulocytes.

Because anemia can lead to cardiovascular complications and affect quality of life, the National Kidney Foundation K-DOQI clinical practice guidelines recommend laboratory investigation for other underlying conditions in premenopausal women and prepubertal children with a Hb less than 11 g/dL and in men and postmenopausal women with a Hb less than 12 g/dL.[54] Treatment of anemia resulting from chronic renal disease involves the administration of recombinant human erythropoietin with a goal to maintain the Hb between 11 g/dL and 12 g/dL.[54] Erythropoietin ameliorates the anemia in most patients with chronic renal disease. In addition, successful erythropoietin therapy requires adequate iron stores, so the plasma ferritin and percent transferrin saturation should be monitored. Iron therapy is initiated if the plasma ferritin level decreases to less than 100 ng/mL, with a goal to maintain the plasma ferritin level greater than 100 ng/mL but less than 800 ng/mL and the transferrin saturation between 20% and 50%.[54]

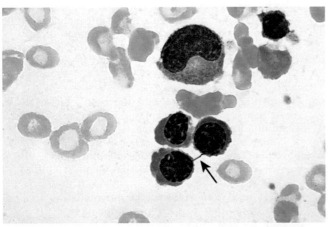

Figure 21-2 Erythrocyte precursors with nuclear bridging indicating dyserythropoiesis (bone marrow ×1000). (Modified from Carr JH, Rodak BF: Clinical Hematology Atlas, 2nd ed. Philadelphia: Saunders, 2004.)

CHAPTER at a GLANCE

- Bone marrow failure is the reduction or cessation of blood cell production affecting one or more cell lines. Pancytopenia, or a decrease in RBCs, WBCs, and platelets, is a common finding. Sequelae of pancytopenia include weakness and fatigue, infections, and bleeding.
- Aplastic anemia may be acquired or inherited. The acquired type may be idiopathic or secondary to drugs, chemicals, radiation, viruses, or miscellaneous conditions such as paroxysmal nocturnal hemoglobinuria, autoimmune diseases, and pregnancy. The inherited types include Fanconi anemia and dyskeratosis congenita.
- Bone marrow failure in acquired aplastic anemia is due to the destruction of hematopoietic stem cells by the direct toxic effects of a drug, chemical, or radiation or indirectly by an autoimmune T cell attack against the stem cells. The autoimmune reactions are a rare adverse event after exposure to a drug, chemical, or virus and are called *idiosyncratic* in that they are unpredictable and unrelated to the dose or amount of exposure.
- Aplastic anemia is classified as nonsevere, severe, or very severe based on bone marrow hypocellularity, absolute neutrophil count, platelet count, Hb, and reticulocyte count. The severity classification helps to guide treatment decisions.
- Treatment for severe and very severe acquired aplastic anemia is hematopoietic stem cell transplantation in younger patients with an HLA-identical sibling or immunosuppression with antithymocyte globulin and cyclosporine for patients who are not candidates for transplant.
- Fanconi anemia and dyskeratosis congenita are inherited forms of aplastic anemia with progressive bone marrow failure and pancytopenia that may present with or without congenital malformations. Fanconi anemia is autosomal recessive, and mutations in eight genes, *FANCA, FANCA-C, FANCA-D2, FANCA-E, FANCA-F, FANCA-G, FANCA-L,* and *BRCA2,* have been identified. Chromosome breakage with diepoxybutane or mitomycin C is diagnostic. Dyskeratosis congenita can be X-linked, autosomal dominant, or autosomal recessive, and mutations in two genes, *DKC1* and *TERT,* have been characterized.
- Defects in the telomerase complex may play a role in the pathology of inherited aplastic anemia and a subset of acquired aplastic anemia by the inability to elongate telomeres at the ends of chromosomes, leading to premature stem cell senescence and death.
- PRCA affects only the erythroid arm of hematopoiesis. Transient erythroblastopenia of childhood is the acquired form, and Diamond-Blackfan anemia is the inherited form.
- Patients with CDA exhibit refractory anemia, secondary hemosiderosis, and abnormalities of bone marrow cells, including giantism, multinuclearity, and karyorrhexis. Three major types are recognized.
- Myelophthisic anemia is the result of normal bone marrow replacement with abnormal cells. The anemia of chronic renal disease is due to the inadequate production and release of erythropoietin by the kidneys.

Now that you have completed this chapter, go back and read again the case study at the beginning and respond to the questions presented.

REVIEW QUESTIONS

1. The clinical consequences of pancytopenia include:
   a. Pallor and thrombosis
   b. Renal failure and fever
   c. Fatigue, infection, and bleeding
   d. Weakness, hemolysis, and infection

2. Idiopathic, acquired aplastic anemia is due to a(n):
   a. Drug reaction
   b. Benzene exposure
   c. Inherited mutation in stem cells
   d. Unknown cause

3. The pathophysiologic mechanism in acquired, idiosyncratic aplastic anemia is the:
   a. Replacement of bone marrow by abnormal cells
   b. Destruction of stem cells by autoimmune T cells
   c. Defective production of hematopoietic growth factors
   d. Inability of bone marrow stroma to support stem cells

4. What is the aplastic anemia classification of a patient with a bone marrow cellularity of 10%, a Hb of 7 g/dL, an absolute neutrophil count of 0.1×10^9/L, and a platelet count of 10×10^9/L?
   a. Nonsevere
   b. Moderate
   c. Severe
   d. Very severe

5. The most consistent peripheral blood findings in severe aplastic anemia are:
   a. Hairy cells, monocytopenia, and neutropenia
   b. Macrocytosis, thrombocytopenia, and neutropenia
   c. Blasts, immature granulocytes, and thrombocytopenia
   d. Polychromasia, nucleated RBCs, and hypersegmented neutrophils

6. The treatment that has shown the best success rate in young patients with severe aplastic anemia is:
   a. Immunosuppression therapy
   b. Long-term RBC and platelet transfusions
   c. Hematopoietic growth factors and androgens
   d. Stem cell transplant from an HLA-identical sibling

7. The test that is most useful in differentiating Fanconi anemia from other causes of pancytopenia is:
   a. Bone marrow biopsy
   b. Ham acidified serum test
   c. Diepoxybutane-induced chromosome breakage
   d. Flow cytometric analysis of CD55 and CD59 cells

8. Mutations in genes that code for the telomerase complex may induce bone marrow failure by:
   a. Resistance of stem cells to normal apoptosis
   b. Autoimmune reaction against telomeres in stem cells
   c. Decreased production of hematopoietic growth factors
   d. Premature death of stem cells

9. Diamond-Blackfan anemia differs from inherited aplastic anemia in that in the former:
   a. Reticulocytes are increased.
   b. Hb F is decreased.
   c. Only erythropoiesis is affected.
   d. Congenital malformations are absent.

10. What anemia should be suspected in a patient with refractory anemia, hemosiderosis, and multinuclearity of erythrocyte precursors in the bone marrow?
    a. Fanconi anemia
    b. Dyskeratosis congenita
    c. Acquired aplastic anemia
    d. CDA

11. The pathophysiology of anemia of chronic renal disease is mainly due to:
    a. Inadequate production of erythropoietin
    b. Excessive hemolysis
    c. Stem cell mutation
    d. Toxic destruction of stem cells

REFERENCES

1. Ehrlich P: Uber einen Fall von Anamie mit Bemerkungen uber regenerative Veranderungen des Knochenmarks. Charite Annal 1888;13:301.
2. Chauffard M: Un cas d'anemie pernicieuse aplastique. Bull Soc Med Hop Paris 1904;21:313.
3. Marsh JCW: Management of acquired aplastic anaemia. Blood Rev 2005;19:143-151.
4. International Agranulocytosis and Aplastic Anemia Study: Incidence of aplastic anemia: the relevance of diagnostic criteria. Blood 1987;70:1718-1721.
5. Marsh JCW, Ball SE, Darbyshire P, et al: Guidelines for the diagnosis and management of acquired aplastic anaemia. Br J Haematol 2003;123:782-801.
6. Young NS, Maciejewski JP: Aplastic anemia. In Hoffman R, Benz EJ, Shattil SJ, et al (eds): Hematology: Basic Principles and Practice, 4th ed. Philadelphia: Churchill Livingstone, 2005:318-417.
7. Muir KR, Chilvers CED, Harriss C, et al: The role of occupational and environmental exposures in the aetiology of acquired severe aplastic anaemia: a case control investigation. Br J Haematol 2003;123:906-914.
8. Smith MT: Overview of benzene induced aplastic anaemia. Eur J Haematol 1996;60(Suppl):107-110.
9. Nimer SD, Ireland P, Meshkinpour A, et al: An increased HLA DR2 frequency is seen in aplastic anemia patients. Blood 1994;84:923-927.
10. Saunthararajah Y, Nakamura R, Nam JM, et al: HLA-DR15 (DR2) is overrepresented in myelodysplastic syndrome and aplastic anemia and predicts a response to immunosuppression in myelodysplastic syndrome. Blood 2002;100:1570-1574.
11. Sutton JF, Stacey M, Kearns WG, et al: Increased risk for aplastic anemia and myelodysplastic syndrome in individuals lacking glutathione S-transferase genes. Pediatr Blood Cancer 2004;42:122-126.
12. Brown KE, Tisdale J, Barrett AJ, et al: Hepatitis-associated aplastic anemia. N Engl J Med 1997;336:1059-1064.
13. Maciejewski JP, Selleri C, Sato T, et al: A severe and consistent deficit in marrow and circulating primitive hematopoietic cells (long term culture-initiating cells) in acquired aplastic anemia. Blood 1996;88:1983-1991.
14. Philpott NJ, Scopes J, Marsh JCW, et al: Increased apoptosis in aplastic anemia bone marrow progenitor cells: possible pathophysiologic significance. Exp Hematol 1995;23:1642-1648.
15. Maciejewski JP, Selleri C, Sato T, et al: Increased expression of Fas antigen on bone marrow CD34+ cells of patients with aplastic anaemia. Br J Haematol 1995;91:245-252.
16. Zeng W, Chen G, Kajigaya S, et al: Gene expression profiling in CD34 cells to identify differences between aplastic anemia patients and healthy volunteers. Blood 2004;103:325-332.
17. Novitzky N, Jacobs P: Immunosuppressive therapy in bone marrow aplasia: the stroma functions normally to support hematopoiesis. Exp Hematol 1995;23:1472-1477.
18. Koijima S: Hematopoietic growth factors and marrow stroma in aplastic anemia. Int J Hematol 1998;68:19-28.
19. Wodnar-Filipowicz A, Lyman SD, Gratwohl A, et al: Flt3 ligand level reflects hematopoietic progenitor cell function in aplastic anemia and chemotherapy-induced bone marrow aplasia. Blood 1996;88:4493-4499.
20. Young NS, Maciejewski J: The pathophysiology of acquired aplastic anemia. N Engl J Med 1997;336:1365-1372.
21. Mathe G, Amiel JL, Schwarzenberg L, et al: Bone marrow graft in man after conditioning by antilymphocytic serum. BMJ 1970;2:131-136.
22. Hara T, Ando K, Tsurumi H, et al: Excessive production of tumor necrosis factor-alpha by bone marrow T lymphocytes is essential in causing bone marrow failure in patients with aplastic anemia. Eur J Haematol 2004;73:10-16.
23. Young NS: Hematopoietic cell destruction by immune mechanisms in acquired aplastic anemia. Semin Hematol 2000;37:3-14.
24. Selleri C, Sato T, Anderson S, et al: Interferon-gamma and tumor necrosis factor-alpha suppress both early and late stages of hematopoiesis and induce programmed cell death. J Cell Physiol 1995;165:538-546.
25. Kasahara S, Hara T, Itoh H, et al: Hypoplastic myelodysplastic syndromes can be distinguished from acquired aplastic anaemia by bone marrow stem cell expression of the tumour necrosis factor receptor. Br J Haematol 2002;118:181-188.
26. Hirano N, Butler MO, von Bergwelt-Baildon MS, et al: Autoantibodies frequently detected in patients with aplastic anemia. Blood 2003;102:4567-4575.
27. Brummendorf TH, Maciejewski JP, Mak J, et al: Telomere length in leukocyte subpopulations of patients with aplastic anemia. Blood 2001;97:895-900.
28. Vulliamy T, Marrone A, Dokal I, et al: Association between aplastic anaemia and mutations in telomerase RNA. Lancet 2002;359:2168-2170.
29. Yamaguchi H, Calado RT, Ly H, et al: Mutations in TERT, the gene for telomerase reverse transcriptase, in aplastic anemia. N Engl J Med 2005;352:1413-1424.
30. Camitta BM, Thomas ED, Nathan DG, et al: Severe aplastic anemia: a prospective study of the effect of early marrow transplantation on acute mortality. Blood 1976;48:63-70.
31. Bacigalupo A, Hows J, Gluckman E, et al: Bone marrow transplantation (BMT) versus immunosuppression for the treatment of severe aplastic anaemia (SAA): a report of the EMBT SAA working party. Br J Haematol 1988;70:177-182.

32. Socie G, Rosenfeld S, Frickhofen N, et al: Late clonal diseases of treated aplastic anemia. Semin Hematol 2000;37:91-101.

33. Wang H, Chuhjo T, Yamazaki H, et al: Relative increase of granulocytes with a paroxysmal nocturnal hemoglobinuria phenotype in aplastic anaemia patients: the high prevalence at diagnosis. Eur J Haematol 2001;66:200-205.

34. Kearns WG, Sutton JF, Maciejewski JP, et al: Genomic instability in bone marrow failure syndromes. Am J Hematol 2004;76:220-224.

35. Maciejewski JP, Sloand EM, Nunez O, et al: Recombinant humanized anti-IL-2 receptor antibody (daclizumab) produces responses in patients with moderate aplastic anemia. Blood 2003;102:3584-3586.

36. Fanconi G: Familiaere infantile perniziosaartige Anaemie (pernizioeses Blutbild und Konstitution). Jahrbuch Kinderheil 1927;117:257-280.

37. Tischkowitz MD, Hodgson SV: Fanconi anaemia. J Med Genet 2003;40:1-10.

38. Tischkowitz M, Dokal I: Fanconi anaemia and leukaemia—clinical and molecular aspects. Br J Haematol 2004;126:176-191.

39. Seyschab H, Friedl R, Sun Y, et al: Comparative evaluation of diepoxybutane sensitivity and cell cycle blockage in the diagnosis of Fanconi anemia. Blood 1995;85:2233-2237.

40. Kutler DI, Singh B, Satagopan J, et al: A 20-year perspective on the International Fanconi Anemia Registry (IFAR). Blood 2003;101:1249-1256.

41. Li X, Leteurtre F, Rocha V, et al: Abnormal telomere metabolism in Fanconi's anaemia correlates with genomic instability and the probability of developing severe aplastic anaemia. Br J Haematol 2003;120:836-845.

42. Dokal I: Dyskeratosis congenita in all its forms. Br J Haematol 2000;110:768-779.

43. Bessler M, Wilson DB, Mason PJ: Dyskeratosis congenita and telomerase. Curr Opin Pediatr 2004;16:23-28.

44. Dessypris EN: Pure red cell aplasia. In Hoffman R, Benz EJ, Shattil SJ, et al (eds): Hematology: Basic Principles and Practice, 4th ed. Philadelphia: Churchill Livingstone, 2005:429-436.

45. Freedman MH: Inherited forms of bone marrow failure. In Hoffman R, Benz EJ, Shattil SJ, et al (eds): Hematology: Basic Principles and Practice, 4th ed. Philadelphia: Churchill Livingstone, 2005:339-379.

46. Bagby GC, Lipton JM, Sloand EM, et al: Marrow failure. Hematology (Am Soc Hematol Educ Program) 2004;318-336.

47. Orfali KA, Ohene-Abuakwa Y, Ball SE: Diamond-Blackfan anaemia in the UK: clinical and genetic heterogeneity. Br J Haematol 2004;125:243-252.

48. Heimpel H: Congenital dyserythropoietic anemias: epidemiology, clinical significance, and progress in understanding their pathogenesis. Ann Hematol 2004;83:613-621.

49. Dgany O, Avidan N, Delaunay J, et al: Congenital dyserythropoietic anemia type I is caused by mutations in codanin-1. Am J Hum Genet 2002;71:1467-1474.

50. Prchal JT: Anemia associated with marrow infiltration. In Lichtman MA, Beutler E, Kipps TJ, et al (eds): Williams Hematology, 7th ed. New York: McGraw-Hill, 2006:561-563.

51. Makoni SN, Laber DA: Clinical spectrum of myelophthisis in cancer patients. Am J Hematol 2004;76:92-93.

52. Hsu C-Y, McCulloch CE, Curhan GC: Epidemiology of anemia associated with chronic renal insufficiency among adults in the United States: results from the Third National Health and Nutrition Examination Survey. J Am Soc Nephrol 2002;13:504-510.

53. Caro J: Anemia of chronic renal failure. In Lichtman MA, Beutler E, Kipps TJ, et al (eds): Williams Hematology, 7th ed. New York: McGraw-Hill, 2006:449-457.

54. National Kidney Foundation. K/DOQI clinical practice guidelines for anemia of chronic kidney disease. Am J Kidney Dis 2001;37(Suppl 1):S182-238.

22

Introduction to Increased Destruction of Erythrocytes

Kathryn Doig

OBJECTIVES

After completion of this chapter, the reader will be able to:

1. Define the hemolytic process and recognize its hallmark clinical findings.
2. Differentiate a hemolytic disorder from hemolytic anemia by definition and recognition of laboratory findings.
3. Discuss methods to classify hemolytic anemias, and apply the classification to an unfamiliar anemia.
4. Describe the processes of intravascular fragmentation and extravascular (macrophage-mediated) hemolysis, emphasizing sites of hemolysis for each and associating the clinical findings of each.
5. Differentiate intravascular and extravascular hemolysis when given clinical and laboratory findings.

6. Describe the process of normal red blood cell (RBC)/hemoglobin (Hb) catabolism, emphasizing the process for catabolism of protoporphyrin.
7. Identify laboratory tests that indicate accelerated RBC destruction, explain why the results do so, and interpret results of each.
8. Identify, explain, and interpret laboratory tests that indicate increased erythropoiesis.
9. Differentiate between hemolytic anemias and other causes of increased erythropoiesis given necessary laboratory or clinical information.
10. Describe the mechanisms that salvage Hb during intravascular hemolysis.
11. Explain the rationale for tests of the Hb salvage mechanisms and interpret the results of each.

CASE STUDY

After studying the material in this chapter, the reader should be able to respond to the following case study:

A 34-year-old woman was admitted to the hospital for a vaginal hysterectomy. Except for excessive menstrual bleeding, she was in otherwise good health, and all of her preoperative laboratory tests were within the normal reference range. There was no excessive blood loss during or after surgery, and recovery was uneventful except for some cramping, for which the patient received ibuprofen.

Three days postsurgery, a CBC revealed a Hb of 5.8 g/dL. Subsequently, the patient began to experience abdominal pain and passed "root beer"-colored urine.

1. What process is indicated by the "root beer"-colored urine?
2. What tests differentiate the cause of the hemolysis?
3. Based on the patient's clinical presentation, predict the results expected for each test in Question 2.

This chapter presents an overview of the hemolytic process and provides a foundation that is applicable in the following red blood cell (RBC) disorder chapters. The term *hemolysis* or *hemolytic disorder* refers to increased destruction (i.e., lysis) of RBCs, shortening their life span. The reduced number of cells results in reduced tissue oxygenation and increased erythropoietin production by the kidney. When the patient is otherwise healthy, the bone marrow responds by accelerating erythrocyte production (reticulocytosis). Hemolytic *anemia* occurs when RBC survival is so short that anemia develops despite a robust erythropoietic response. A hemolytic process is present without anemia if the bone marrow is able to compensate. A normal bone marrow can increase its production of RBCs by six to eight times normal; significant destruction must occur before an anemia develops.[1]

CLASSIFICATION

Many anemias have a hemolytic component, including the anemia associated with vitamin B_{12} or folate deficiency and the anemia of chronic inflammation, renal disease, and iron deficiency. In these, the hemolysis alone does not cause anemia, and so they are not considered hemolytic disorders. Rather, these anemias develop as a result of the inability of the bone marrow to increase production of RBCs. Because hemolysis is not the primary underlying cause, these are considered anemias with a secondary hemolytic component.

Hemolytic anemias are classified as:

- Acute versus chronic
- Inherited versus acquired
- Intrinsic versus extrinsic
- Intravascular (i.e., fragmentation that) versus extravascular (i.e., macrophage-mediated)

Every hemolytic condition can be classified according to each of these descriptors; Table 22-1 shows this with a noncomprehensive list of hemolytic anemias. This chapter focuses on the distinction between intravascular and extravascular hemolytic conditions. The other classifying schemes are summarized here briefly and are used to organize the chapters that follow.

Acute versus chronic hemolysis delineates its clinical presentation. Acute hemolysis has a rapid onset and is isolated (sudden), episodic, or paroxysmic, as in *paroxysmal cold hemoglobinuria* (PCH) or *paroxysmal nocturnal hemoglobinuria* (PNH)a. Whatever causes the hemolysis either disappears or subsides between episodes, during which time the patient's condition returns to normal. A hemolytic transfusion reaction is an example of a single acute incident. Patients with PCH experience hemolysis only after exposure to cold, and patients with PNH experience hemolysis while sleeping.

Compensated chronic hemolysis may not be evident but may be punctuated over time with hemolytic *crises*. Glucose-6-phosphate dehydrogenase deficiency is such a condition. RBC life span is chronically shortened, but bone marrow compensation prevents anemia. When the cells are challenged with oxidizing agents such as antimalarial drugs, a dramatic acute hemolytic event occurs. When the drug is withdrawn, compensation returns.

Inherited hemolytic conditions are passed to offspring by mutant genes from the parents. *Acquired* hemolytic disorders develop in individuals who were previously hematologically normal but acquire an agent that lyses RBCs. Infectious diseases such as malaria is an example.

The hemolytic conditions are also classified as *intrinsic* or *extrinsic* RBC defects, the latter caused by the action of external agents. This is the classification scheme used for subsequent chapters in this book. Examples of intrinsic hemolytic disorders include abnormalities of RBC membranes, enzymatic pathways, or the hemoglobin (Hb) molecule. With *intrinsic* defects, if the RBCs of the affected patient were to be transfused into a normal individual, they would still have a shortened life span because the defect is *in* the RBC. If normal RBCs are transfused into a patient who has an intrinsic defect, the transfused cells have a normal life span because the transfused cells are normal.

Extrinsic hemolytic conditions are conditions outside the RBC, typically substances in the plasma or conditions affecting the anatomy of the circulatory system. An antibody against RBC antigens and a prosthetic heart valve are examples of extrinsic agents. In extrinsic hemolysis, cross-transfusion studies have shown that the patient's RBCs have a normal life span in the bloodstream of a normal individual but normal cells are lysed more rapidly in the patient's circulation. These studies confirm that something outside the RBCs is causing the hemolysis. Most intrinsic defects are inherited; most extrinsic ones are acquired (see Table 22-1). A few exceptions exist, such as paroxysmal nocturnal hemoglobinuria, which is an acquired disorder involving an intrinsic defect (Chapter 23).

Intrinsic disorders are subclassified as membrane defects, enzyme defects, and hemoglobinopathies. Extrinsic hemolysis may be immunohemolytic, traumatic, or microangiopathic or anemias caused by infectious agents, chemical agents (drugs and venoms), and physical agents (see Table 22-1).

Another classification scheme is based on the site of hemolysis—*intravascular* (within the bloodstream) or *extravascular* (inside macrophages). This classification is useful because laboratory testing readily distinguishes the two. However, the cause of the hemolysis must still be determined for treatment.

HEMOLYSIS

Normal Bilirubin Metabolism

Detecting hemolysis depends partly on detection of RBC breakdown products. A prominent product is bilirubin. The process of normal bilirubin production is described to provide the relationship between hemolysis and increased bilirubin.

The story of bilirubin production is, in part, a story of iron salvage. The body salvages and recycles iron like a precious metal. If this were not true, there would perhaps be a Hb and iron excretion system. Because iron must be salvaged, however, there is a process for saving heme and globin. Bilirubin is the excretory product for protoporphyrin. Bilirubin and its derivatives provide physiologic functions during excretion.

RBCs live approximately 120 days. During this time, various metabolic and chemical changes occur, resulting in a loss of deformability. Under normal circumstances, macrophages of the mononuclear phagocyte system (or reticuloendothelial system) recognize these changes and phagocytize the aged erythrocytes (Chapter 8). The organs of this system include the spleen, bone marrow, liver, lymph nodes and circulating monocytes, but it is primarily the spleen and liver that process senescent RBCs. The macrophages in the spleen (littoral cells) are especially sensitive to subtle RBC changes, whereas the macrophages of the liver, called *Kupffer cells*, detect and destroy more severely damaged RBCs. This is an extravascular

TABLE 22-1 Classification of Selected Hemolytic Anemias by Primary Etiology and Presentation

	Intrinsic Red Cell Defects				Extrinsic Red Cell Defects			
	Inherited		Acquired		Inherited		Acquired	
	Intravascular Hemolysis	Extravascular Hemolysis	Intravascular Hemolysis	Extravascular Hemolysis	Intravascular Hemolysis	Extravascular Hemolysis	Intravascular Hemolysis	Extravascular Hemolysis
Acute (or episodic)			Paroxysmal nocturnal hemoglobinuria				Immune hemolytic anemia—cold-reacting antibody; Microangiopathic hemolytic anemias; Infectious agents like malaria; Thermal injury; Chemicals/drugs; Venoms	Immune hemolytic anemia—warm reacting antibody; Drug-induced hemolysis
Chronic	Enzyme defects: G6PD deficiency (with acute episodes); Globin structure and synthesis defects: Sickle cell anemia, Other hemoglobinpathies, Thalassemias	Enzyme defects: Pyruvate kinase deficiency, other glycolytic pathway enzyme deficiencies; Membrane defects: Hereditary spherocytosis, Hereditary elliptocytosis, Pyropoikilocytosis, Hereditary stomatocytois, Rh null phenotypes, Abetalipoproteinemia				Lecithin cholesterol acyltransferase deficiency	Prosthetic heart valves	Secondary to liver/renal disease

Some conditions may exhibit mixed presentations under certain circumstances. It is evident that most hereditary conditions lead to chronic hemolysis while acquired conditions are more often acute. Furthermore, the intrinsic red cell defects typically are due to hereditary conditions while extrinsic factors typically lead to acquired hemolytic disorders.

hemolytic process. Hemolysis occurs within macrophages; thus *macrophage-mediated hemolysis* is a more precise term.

Normal RBC degradation occurs extravascularly as enzymes of the macrophage lyse the phagocytized erythrocyte. Hb is hydrolyzed into heme and globin; the latter is further degraded into amino acids that return to the amino acid pool. Iron is released from the heme, returned to the plasma via ferroportin, bound to its protein carrier molecule (transferrin), and recycled to developing RBCs. The remaining protoporphyrin is degraded through a series of biochemical reactions in different tissues.

Figure 22-1 illustrates protoporphyrin catabolism. While inside the macrophage, protoporphyrin reacts with heme oxy-genase, breaking the porphyrin ring to yield a linear molecule, biliverdin. The lungs excrete a byproduct of that reaction, carbon monoxide. The green biliverdin is reduced to bilirubin, a nonpolar yellow molecule that is secreted into the plasma (Box 22-1). Because it is hydrophobic, bilirubin must attach to albumin to be transported in plasma to the liver. The bilirubin-albumin complex enters the liver parenchymal cells, where the bilirubin dissociates from the albumin and is joined (i.e., conjugated) with two molecules of glucuronic acid by the enzyme glucuronyl transferase to form bilirubin diglucuronide.[2] The addition of the two sugar acid molecules makes the molecule polar and water soluble. Bilirubin diglucuronide is also

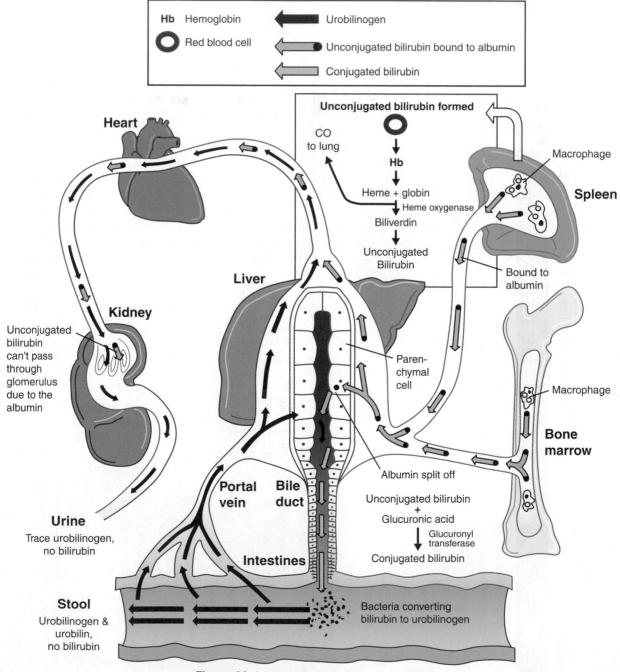

Figure 22-1 Normal catabolism of aged RBCs.

BOX 22-1 Visualizing the Color Changes of Hemoglobin Degradation

The degradation of heme can be seen in bruises in fair-skinned individuals or in the sclera of the eye after a vascular bleed. The same process that macrophages facilitate can occur in tissues. At first, the extravasated but deoxygenated blood gives the injury a purple-red appearance of hemoglobin. As the Hb is degraded, the color changes to a greenish hue owing to biliverdin, but ultimately it becomes yellow owing to bilirubin.

---

called *conjugated* bilirubin. The bilirubin originally released from macrophages that lacks these sugars is termed *unconjugated*.

When conjugated, bilirubin is excreted as bile acid into the intestines. There it assists with the emulsification of fats for absorption from the diet. Conjugated bilirubin is oxidized by gut bacteria into various water-soluble compounds, collectively called *urobilinogen*. Most urobilinogen is oxidized further to stercobilin and similar compounds that give the brown color to stool, the ultimate route for excretion of protoporphyrin.

Because they are water soluble, some conjugated bilirubin and urobilinogen are reabsorbed from the intestines and can be detected in the plasma. The portal circulation, the blood vessels that surround the intestines to absorb nutrients, also collect bile products by osmosis. The portal circulation carries blood directly to the liver, so most of the absorbed conjugated bilirubin and urobilinogen is recycled directly into the bile again. Some remains in the plasma and is filtered by the renal glomerulus and excreted in the urine. The direct bilirubin is virtually undetectable in urine, but a measurable amount of urobilinogen can be expected normally. The yellow of urine is due to urobilin, a derivative of urobilinogen that is itself colorless.

Normal Plasma Hemoglobin Salvage During Intravascular Hemolysis

Intravascular hemolysis is the destruction of circulating RBCs with release of RBC contents, chiefly Hb, directly into plasma (Box 22-2). Approximately 10% to 20% of normal RBC destruction is intravascular,[3] secondary to turbulence and anatomic restrictions in the vasculature. Intravascular hemolysis is trauma to the RBC membrane that causes a breach sufficient for the cell contents to spill into the plasma.

BOX 22-2 Laboratory Impact of Significant Hemoglobinemia

The routine hematology test results are unreliable for patients with significant hemoglobinemia. Under normal circumstances, the measured hemoglobin represents the hemoglobin present inside the RBCs. For individuals with hemoglobinemia, the intracellular hemoglobin and the plasma hemoglobin are measured. The hemoglobin value is falsely elevated. An unrealistically high MCHC may provide a clue to this problem, which can be remedied in several ways (Chapters 14 and 39).

Because Hb is filtered by the kidney, iron could be lost in normal intravascular hemolysis. Additionally, free Hb and iron can cause oxidative damage to cells. Several layers of backup exist to salvage Hb iron and prevent oxidation, the haptoglobin/hemopexin/methemalbumin system (Fig. 22-2).

When free in the plasma, Hb exists as α/β dimers bound to a liver-produced plasma protein called *haptoglobin*. By binding to haptoglobin, Hb avoids filtration at the glomerulus and is saved from urinary loss. The complex is carried to the liver, where the haptoglobin-Hb complex is bound to macrophage receptors and internalized into the macrophage.[4] Inside the macrophage, iron is salvaged, and the remaining protoporphyrin is converted to bilirubin just as though the RBC had been ingested by the macrophage. Haptoglobin is depleted by this process, however, the amount produced by the liver is sufficient for normal level intravascular hemolysis. If haptoglobin consumption increases, there is no compensatory increase in liver production of haptoglobin.

A second layer of iron salvage exists with hemopexin. In Hb that is not bound by haptoglobin, the iron becomes oxidized, forming methemoglobin. The heme molecule (actually metheme) dissociates from the globin and binds to another liver-produced plasma protein, hemopexin.[5,6] This binding saves the iron from urinary loss and prevents oxidation of cell membranes. Hemopexin-metheme binds to hepatocyte receptors and is internalized. There the iron is salvaged, and the protoporphyrin is converted to bilirubin, as in a macrophage. In contrast to haptoglobin, hemopexin is recycled to the plasma so that it collects and salvages more free metheme molecules. Although its production is constant, because it is recycled to the plasma, levels do not fall dramatically during periods when there is an increase in intravascular hemolysis.

A third layer of iron salvage is the metheme-albumin system. Albumin acts a carrier for many molecules. Metheme can bind to albumin, further reducing urinary loss. This is probably a temporary holding state for the metheme, which transfers to hemopexin because of its higher binding affinity for metheme than is observed in albumin.[7] It is then transported to the liver for processing.

If the previous systems are inadequate, iron still can be retained in the kidney.[8,9] Some Hb or (met)heme that enters the filtrate is reabsorbed, not by specific carriers but as part of the general filtrate in the proximal tubule. When inside the renal tubular cell, the iron is separated from the protoporphyrin. There it is stored as ferritin or hemosiderin. Currently, no mechanism is known for the renal tubular cell to export the iron into the plasma.

EXCESSIVE EXTRAVASCULAR HEMOLYSIS

Many hemolytic anemias are a result of increased extravascular hemolysis (Fig. 22-3). Macrophages ingest defective RBCs faster than normal. Under normal circumstances, senescent cells display markers, especially clustered band 3 with bound endogenous immunoglobulin, on their surface that identify them to the macrophages for ingestion and removal (Chapter 8).

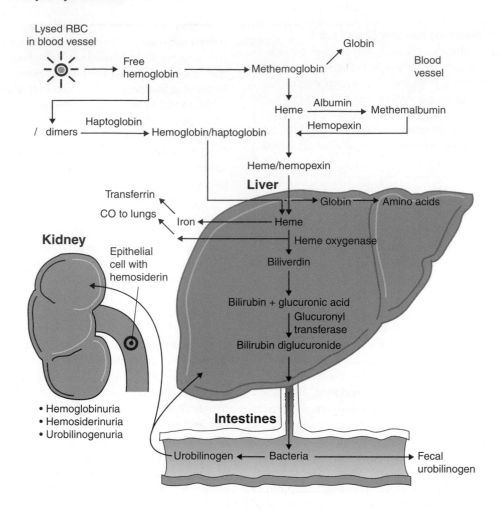

Figure 22-2 Removal of Hb from blood plasma after intravascular hemolysis.

Pathologic processes also lead to expression of these receptors, however, so that abnormal cells are identified and removed. As an example, Heinz bodies, aggregates of denatured Hb formed in various anemias, bind to the inner surface of the RBC membrane, leading to clustering of band 3 and initiating the same sequence of events that leads to RBC removal during senescence.[10] When something causes increased formation of Heinz bodies or other intracellular inclusions, the cells are removed from the circulation prematurely by macrophages. A similar process occurs with intracellular parasites or when complement or immunoglobulins are on the surface of the RBC.

When the RBC is ingested, it is lysed within a phagosome, and the contents are processed within the macrophage as described previously. The contents of the RBC are *not* detected in plasma because it is lysed inside the macrophage, and the contents are degraded there—hence the designation *extra-vascular* hemolysis. Another more descriptive term for extra-vascular hemolysis is *macrophage-mediated hemolysis*. It occurs most often in the spleen and liver, where the macrophages possess receptors for the markers that identify defective RBCs, principally immunoglobulins and complement.

Sometimes the macrophage ingests a portion of the membrane, leaving the remainder to reseal. Little, if any, cytoplasmic volume is lost, but with less membrane, the cell becomes a spherocyte, the characteristic shape change associated with extravascular hemolysis. Although the spherocyte reenters the circulation, its survival is shortened because of its rigidity and inability to traverse the splenic sieve during subsequent passages through the red pulp. It may become trapped against the basement membrane of the splenic sinus and be fully ingested by a macrophage, or it may lyse mechanically and in so doing contribute an intravascular component to what is otherwise an extravascular process.

In extravascular hemolytic anemias, the plasma bilirubin level rises. The bilirubin is largely unconjugated. As long as the liver is healthy, it processes the increased load of unconjugated bilirubin, producing conjugated bilirubin that enters the intestine. Increased urobilinogen forms in the intestines and is subsequently absorbed by the portal circulation and excreted by the kidney. As a result, increased urobilinogen is detectable in the urine. Although there is an increase in unconjugated bilirubin in the plasma, none of it appears in the urine because it is bound to albumin and cannot pass through the glomerulus.

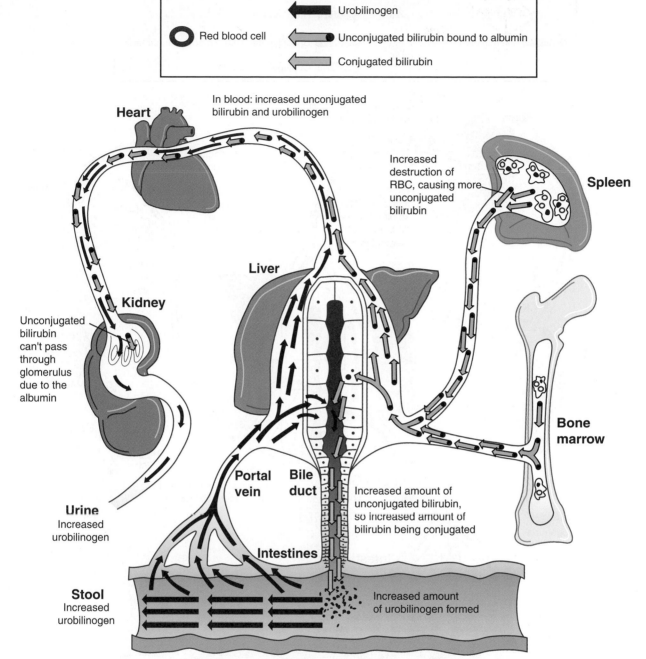

Figure 22-3 Increased extravascular hemolysis.

EXCESSIVE INTRAVASCULAR HEMOLYSIS

Although intravascular hemolysis is a minor component of normal RBC destruction, it can be a major feature of pathologic processes (Fig. 22-4). A dramatic example is the trauma caused by mechanical heart valves. Intracellular parasites such as malaria burst the cell from the inside out when they mature, similar to a bird hatching from an egg. In these instances, the intravascular destruction of RBCs causes profound anemias.

Intravascular hemolysis releases detectable plasma hemoglobin. Characteristic laboratory findings are hemoglobinemia, hemoglobinuria, and hemosiderinuria. In addition, methemal-

bumin and hemopexin-heme are detected in plasma, and haptoglobin is decreased. Plasma bilirubin (largely unconjugated) and elevated urinary urobilinogen are also measurable. The time course of these findings assists with the differential diagnosis.

In a properly collected specimen, normal intravascular hemolysis produces a plasma Hb level of less than 1 mg/dL.[11] Plasma becomes visibly red at 50 mg/dL, so hemoglobinemia may be invisible.[11] Typical values during hemolytic processes can range from 15 to 100 mg/dL.[12]

During excess *intravascular* hemolysis, plasma haptoglobin is depleted rapidly. Levels of hemopexin also decline, but not as significantly as haptoglobin, due to its recycling. Hemopexin

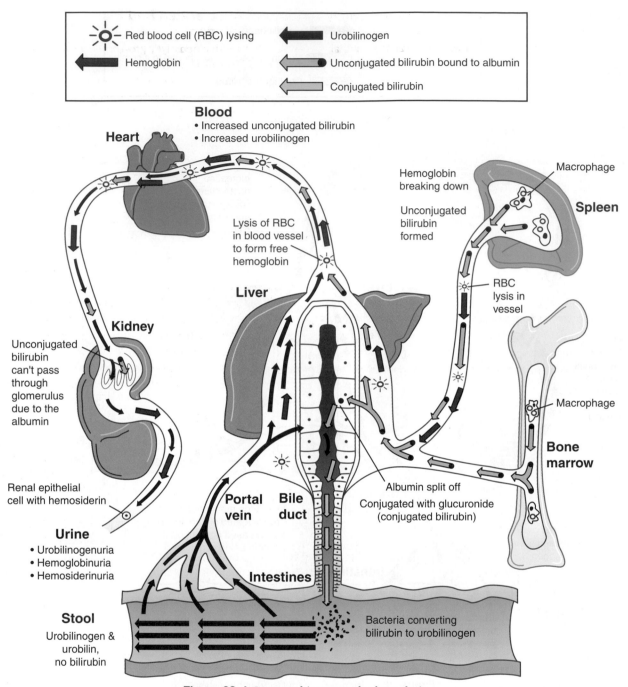

Figure 22-4 Increased intravascular hemolysis.

is not measured broadly, although hemopexin is decreased during severe hemolysis. The hemopexin-heme complex increases, however, and methemalbumin can also be detected. The presence of methemalbumin and hemopexin-heme, which impart a coffee-brown color to plasma, strongly suggests intravascular hemolysis.[13,14] These pigments can be observed in plasma spectrophotometrically at 620 to 630 nm and do not disappear with the addition of hydrogen peroxide, as does methemoglobin. If ammonium sulfide is added (Schumm test), the 620- to 630-nm band disappears, and a band at 558 nm forms.[15]

Additionally, if hemoglobinemia is sufficiently elevated, hemoglobin is detected in the urine (hemoglobinuria). When an acute intravascular hemolytic transfusion reaction is suspected, a urine sample is tested promptly for Hb using the urinalysis reagent strip. Hb may give a dark-red or brown color (owing to methemoglobin) to the urine if the amount is sufficiently high and thus may be described as looking like root beer or beer. In chronic intravascular hemolysis, iron absorbed into renal tubular epithelial cells may be visualized. As these cells slough into the urine and appear in the sediment, they can be stained with Prussian blue. This is an easy and inexpensive way to detect intravascular hemolysis.[12] Urinary iron can be measured spectrophotometrically after wet digestion of a measured urine specimen. The normal value is less than 0.1 mg/d, and in intravascular hemolysis it is 3 to 11 mg/d.[9]

CLINICAL FEATURES

The clinical findings typical of hemolysis may be prominent if the hemolytic process is the primary cause of anemia. For patients in whom hemolysis is secondary, however, other clinical features may be more noticeable. If hemolysis is sufficient to result in anemia, patients experience the general symptoms of fatigue, dyspnea, and dizziness to a degree that is consistent with the severity and rate of development of the anemia. The associated signs of pallor and tachycardia can be expected.

Increased bilirubin gives a yellow tinge to the plasma and body tissues. It is readily evident in the sclera of the eyes and the skin of fair-skinned individuals. *Jaundice* refers to the color of the skin and sclera, whereas *icterus* describes plasma. An increase in plasma bilirubin and subsequent jaundice can occur in other conditions besides hemolysis, but if the jaundice is the result of hemolysis, it is called *hemolytic jaundice*. It also may be called *prehepatic jaundice*, reflecting the predominance of unconjugated bilirubin.

The frequency or constancy of jaundice provides clues to the cause. In G6PD deficiency, for example, hemolysis is periodic, appearing during a crisis. In thalassemia, jaundice is chronic. Jaundice may not be evident if the level of hemolysis is minimal and the liver is able to process the added bilirubin, as is often the case in hereditary elliptocytosis.

Some signs differentiate chronic from acute hemolysis. Splenomegaly can develop, particularly with chronic extravascular hemolytic processes. Gallstones (cholelithiasis) can occur whenever hemolysis is chronic; the constantly increased amount of bilirubin in the bile leads to the formation of the stones.[16] When hemolysis is chronic in children, the persistent compensatory bone marrow hyperplasia can lead to bone deformities because the bones are still forming (see Fig. 27-3). For patients developing an acquired, acute hemolytic process, the associated malaise, aches, vomiting, and possible fever may be confused with an acute infectious process. Profound prostration and shock may develop, particularly with acute intravascular hemolysis. Flank pain, oliguria, or anuria develops as the RBC stroma clog the renal glomeruli, leading to acute renal failure.

Other clinical features may offer a clue as to whether hemolysis is intravascular or extravascular. In particular, brown urine, associated with (met)hemoglobinuria, points to an intravascular hemolytic process.

LABORATORY FINDINGS

In patients with the clinical features of hemolytic anemia, laboratory tests typically show evidence of increased erythrocyte destruction and the compensatory increase in the rate of erythropoiesis. Other tests that are specific to a particular diagnosis also may be indicated.

Tests of Accelerated Red Blood Cell Destruction

For a patient with a hemolytic process, a complete blood count (CBC) may provide clues to the etiology. Extravascular hemolysis can be expected to show spherocytes (see Table 22-2), whereas intravascular hemolysis shows ruptured cells, chiefly schistocytes. Clues to the particular etiology of the hemolysis also may be present in the morphology, such as malarial ring forms, sickle cells for sickle cell anemia, target cells in sickle cell anemia and thalassemia, or microspherocytes in hereditary spherocytosis.

In either intravascular or extravascular hemolysis, the increased rate of Hb catabolism results in increased amounts of the principal byproducts bile and carbon monoxide. Most bilirubinemia is unconjugated (Box 22-3). If liver function is normal, conjugated bilirubin is excreted, and the serum direct bilirubin remains within the normal reference range. No bilirubin is detected in the urine because unconjugated bilirubin is not filtered by the glomerulus. Urinary urobilinogen may be increased, however, because there is increased urobilinogen in the stool, and more than usual amounts are absorbed by the portal circulation. Serum bilirubin values can be misleadingly low because the amount of bilirubin in the blood depends on the rate of RBC catabolism and hepatic function. In some

---

BOX 22-3 Laboratory Testing for Serum Bilirubin

Because bilirubin occurs in two forms, conjugated and unconjugated, the total bilirubin in plasma/serum is the total of the two forms: Total serum bilirubin = unconjugated serum bilirubin + conjugated serum bilirubin.

Normally, there is relatively little total bilirubin, and most of it is composed of the unconjugated form in transit from the macrophages, where it was produced to the liver. The small amount of direct bilirubin in the plasma has been absorbed from the intestine by the portal circulation.

Typical reference ranges are as follows:

Total serum bilirubin = 0.5-1.0 mg/dL

Direct serum bilirubin = 0-0.2 mg/dL

Indirect serum bilirubin = 0-0.8 mg/dL

Conjugated bilirubin is a polar molecule and reacts well in the water-based assay that uses diazotized sulfanilic acid. Unconjugated bilirubin does not react well in this system unless alcohol is added to promote its solubility in water. Conjugated bilirubin also is called *direct* bilirubin because it reacts directly with the reagent, and unconjugated bilirubin is called *indirect* because it has to be solubilized first.[1,2] When alcohol is added to the test system, however, the direct and indirect forms react. In practice, the total bilirubin is measured by adding a solubilizing reagent. In a separate test, the direct bilirubin is measured alone. The indirect bilirubin is calculated by subtracting the direct from the total: Total serum bilirubin − direct serum bilirubin = indirect serum bilirubin.

[1]Van den Bergh AA, Muller P: Uber eine direkte und eine indirekte diazoreaktion aus bilirubin. Biochem Z 1916;77:90.

[2]Hutchinson DW, Johnson B, Knell AJ. The reaction between bilirubin and aromatic diazo compounds. Biochem J 1972;127:907.

TABLE 22-2 Comparison of Laboratory Findings Indicating Accelerated Red Blood Cell Destruction in Intravascular versus Extravascular Hemolysis

Test Sample	Result	Intravascular	Extravascular
Serum	Increased total bilirubin	X	X
	Increased unconjugated bilirubin	X	X
	Normal direct bilirubin	X	X
	Increased RBC fraction lactate dehydrogenase activity	X	x
	Decreased haptoglobin	X	x
	Increased free hemoglobin	X	x
	Decreased hemopexin	X	x
Urine	Increased urobilinogen	X	X
	Positive free hemoglobin	X	
	Positive methemoglobin	X	
	Positive Prussian blue reaction on urine sediment	X	
Anticoagulated whole blood	Decreased hemoglobin/hematocrit/RBC	X	X
	Schistocytes	X	
	Spherocytes		X
	Decreased glycated hemoglobin	X	X
Special tests	Increased endogenous carbon monoxide	X	X
	Decreased erythrocyte life span	X	X

X = typically expected; x = minor components.

patients with hemolytic anemia, if the rate of hemolysis is low and the liver is healthy, the total serum bilirubin is within normal range. Quantitative measurements of fecal urobilinogen excretion provide a sensitive indication of increased hemolysis but require accurate timed collection of fecal specimens and are rarely necessary.[17]

A decline in serum haptoglobin indicates intravascular hemolysis. To a smaller extent, it can be true in extravascular hemolysis as spherocytes lyse intravascularly. Whenever the level of Hb in the plasma increases, haptoglobin declines. In one study, a low haptoglobin level indicated an 87% probability of hemolytic disease.[18] Haptoglobin results are prone to false-positives and false-negatives, however. Low values suggest hemolysis but may be due instead to impaired synthesis from liver disease. Alternatively, a patient with hemolysis may have relatively normal haptoglobin if there is also a complicating infection or inflammation because haptoglobin is an acute-phase reactant.

Determinations of the rate of endogenous carbon monoxide production have been developed because carbon monoxide is produced in the first step of protoporphyrin breakdown. Values of 2 to 10 times the normal rate have been detected in some patients with hemolytic anemia, but the methods are too complex for the routine clinical laboratory.[19]

Other laboratory tests are incidentally abnormal. Serum lactate dehydrogenase activity is often increased in patients with intravascular hemolysis, but other conditions, such as myocardial infarction, also can cause increases.[20] Although fractionation points to the RBC origin of the increase, this is generally not needed. Rather, when other results point to hemolysis, one should expect an increase in lactate dehydrogenase and other RBC enzymes and not be misled to assume there is liver damage (Table 22-2).

General evidence of reduced RBC survival can be gleaned from measuring glycosylated (glycated) Hb.[21] Glycosylated Hb increases over the life of a cell as it is exposed to plasma glucose. Glycosylated Hb usually is reduced in hemolytic disease because the cells have less exposure to the plasma before lysis. Normal values average 6.7%; in a hemolytic process, the average value is 3.9%.[21] The magnitude of the decrease is related to the magnitude of the hemolytic process over the previous 4- to 8-week period. Glycosylated Hb is not a reliable indicator of shortened RBC survival in patients with diabetes mellitus because of the increased rate of glycosylation with elevated blood glucose levels.

A more exact RBC survival assay uses random labeling with chromium radioisotope. This is the reference method for RBC survival studies published by the International Committee for Standardization in Haematology.[22] A sample of blood is collected, mixed with the isotope, and returned to the patient. The labeled cells are of all ages, reflecting normal peripheral blood. This method differs from cohort labeling, in which RBCs are labeled as they are produced in the bone marrow. In cohort labeling the patient receives a dose of radioactive iron and the labeled cells are of roughly the same age. In both methods, the disappearance of the label from the blood is measured over time. As measured with the random chromium labeling technique, the normal half-time of chromium is 25 to 32 days.[22] A half-time of 20 to 25 days suggests mild hemolysis; 15 to 20 days, moderate hemolysis; and less than 15 days, severe hemolysis. Erythrocyte life span determinations are time-consuming and expensive and are rarely necessary for diagnosis except in a patient with difficult diagnostic problems.

Tests of Increased Erythropoiesis

If the bone marrow is healthy, the hypoxia associated with hemolysis leads to increased erythropoiesis. Recognition may be a first clue to the presence of a hemolytic process. Laboratory findings indicating increased erythropoiesis are listed in Table 22-3. These findings are persistently present in chronic hemolytic disease and are evident within 5-19 days after an acute hemolytic episode. Increased erythropoiesis is not unique to hemolytic anemias and is not diagnostic. Similar results are expected after hemorrhage and with successful specific therapy for anemia caused by iron, folate, or vitamin B_{12} deficiency. An assessment of erythropoiesis can determine the effectiveness of the bone marrow response, however, and should be factored into the differential diagnosis (see Differential Diagnosis).

Complete Blood Count and Morphologic Findings

Peripheral blood smear evaluation is crucial. Polychromatic RBCs (reticulocytosis) and nucleated RBCs represent bone marrow compensation for hemolysis or blood loss.

An increase in the mean cell volume usually is seen with *extreme* compensatory reticulocytosis resulting from the larger, prematurely released "shift" reticulocytes. The increase must be assessed by comparison with the value early in hemolysis, before the shift reticulocytes have emerged. The mean cell volume may not increase above the reference range but rather may be above what was normal for the patient. Exceptions occur if the hemolytic condition itself involves smaller cells that counter the increased volume of the reticulocytes. In

hereditary spherocytosis, microspherocytes are the cause of the anemia, and the mean cell volume may be within the reference range when larger shift reticulocytes are generated—hence the importance of a baseline value for comparison. In other circumstances, such as severe burns, numerous schistocytes or microspherocytes may outnumber the reticulocytes so that the mean cell volume remains low.

Reticulocytosis

The reticulocyte count is the most commonly used test to determine accelerated erythropoiesis and is useful for this purpose. An increased reticulocyte count and an increased reticulocyte production index (Chapter 14) support a diagnosis of anemia secondary to blood loss or destruction of RBCs. When hemolysis is severe enough to produce anemia, the reticulocyte count is expected to be substantially increased. The association is so strong that if a patient has an elevated reticulocyte count, a cause of hemolysis should be sought. The increase usually correlates well with severity of the hemolysis. Exceptions occur during aplastic crisis of hemolytic anemias and in some immunohemolytic anemias with hypoplastic marrow, which suggests that the autoantibodies were directed against the bone marrow RBC precursors and circulating erythrocytes.[11] Chapters 14 and 18 describe the interpretation of reticulocyte indices in patients with anemia.

Bone Marrow

Bone marrow examination is usually not necessary to diagnose hemolytic anemia. If conducted, however, bone marrow examination would reveal erythroid hyperplasia. The myeloid-to-erythroid ratio decreases in hemolytic disease from a normal of about 3:1 as the denominator (the erythroid component) increases. (The myeloid-to-erythroid ratio is defined in Chapter 16.) As always, the cellularity of the bone marrow should be determined on a core biopsy specimen, rather than an aspirated specimen, for a more accurate judgment.

Laboratory Tests to Determine Specific Hemolytic Processes

A well-made blood smear is helpful in determining the cause of hemolytic anemia. Certain abnormalities found on the smear, such as spherocytes, elliptocytes, acanthocytes, echinocytes, sickle cells, target cells, schistocytes, helmet cells, fragmented cells, agglutination, erythrophagocytosis, or parasites, may help reveal the disorder causing the hemolysis (Table 22-4).

Leukocytosis and thrombocytosis may accompany acute hemolytic anemia and are considered reactions to the hemolytic process. Conversely, conditions that cause leukocytosis, such as septicemia, also might cause hemolysis. When there is thrombocytosis, the platelets are generally large, resulting in an increased mean platelet volume. Low platelet counts in association with other signs of hemolysis may indicate a microangiopathic hemolysis, such as disseminated intravascular coagulopathy. Other tests dealing with specific entities are discussed in subsequent chapters, including the direct antiglobulin test, osmotic fragility, autohemolysis, Heinz body

TABLE 22-3 Hematologic Findings Indicating Accelerated Red Blood Cell Production

Specimen	Peripheral Blood
Anticoagulated blood	Increased reticulocyte count
	Rising MCV (compared with baseline)
	Polychromasia/nucleated RBCs
Bone marrow	Presence of erythroid hyperplasia
Special studies	Increased plasma iron turnover
	Increased erythrocyte iron turnover
	Increased activity of certain erythrocyte enzymes

TABLE 22-4 Morphologic Abnormalities Associated with Hemolytic Anemia

Red Blood Cell Morphology	Hemolytic Disorders
Spherocytes	Hereditary spherocytosis, warm hemolytic anemia, burns, chemical injury to RBC
Elliptocytes (ovalocyte)	Hereditary elliptocytosis
Acanthocytes	Abetalipoproteinemia
Echinocytes	Pyruvate kinase deficiency, phosphoglycerate kinase deficiency, uremia
Schistocytes	Microangiopathic anemia
Erythrophagocytosis	Damage to RBC surface, especially owing to complement-fixing antibodies
Autoagglutination	Cold agglutinins, immunohemolytic disease

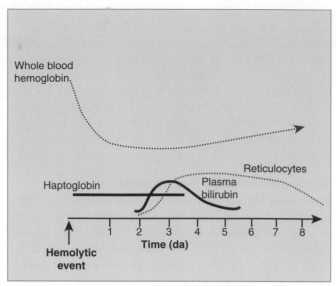

Figure 22-6 Extravascular (macrophage-mediated) hemolysis timeline.

test, RBC enzyme studies, serologic tests, and immunophenotyping.

DIFFERENTIAL DIAGNOSIS

The differential diagnosis of hemolytic anemias incorporates several intersecting lines of deduction. The first is to establish the hemolytic nature of the anemia. A rapid decrease in blood Hb concentration (e.g., 1 g/dL/wk) from previously normal levels can signal hemolysis when hemorrhage and hemodilution have been ruled out. Jaundice and reticulocytosis provide the additional confirmation of a hemolytic etiology for an anemia of at least several days' duration. When the indirect fraction of the total serum bilirubin is elevated, hemolytic

jaundice is confirmed. An elevated urinary urobilinogen strengthens the conclusion. The rapid decrease in Hb during an acute hemolytic episode usually presents before reticulocytosis and bilirubinemia develop, however. For acute hemolysis, hemoglobinemia and resulting hemoglobinuria are expected for intravascular causes; therefore their absence suggests an extravascular cause. RBC morphology and haptoglobin levels can assist with the differentiation of intravascular versus extravascular cause. Figures 22-5 and 22-6 present graphic representations of the general timeline of the events in acute intravascular or extravascular hemolysis. For chronic hemolysis, persistence of the findings of hemoglobinemia, hemoglobinuria, decreased serum haptoglobin, indirect bilirubinemia, and elevated reticulocytes is expected, depending on the etiology of the hemolysis.

Hemolytic anemias must be differentiated from other anemias associated with bilirubinemia, reticulocytosis, or both. Anemia with reticulocytosis but without bilirubinemia is expected during recovery from untransfused hemorrhage or with effective treatment of deficiencies, such as iron. Anemia that results from hemorrhage into a body cavity shows reticulocytosis during recovery and bilirubinemia due to catabolism of the Hb in the hemorrhaged cells. The RBC morphology should remain normal throughout the event. Anemias associated with ineffective erythropoiesis, such as megaloblastic anemia, are essentially hemolytic, with the cell death occurring in the bone marrow. Bilirubinemia and elevated serum lactate dehydrogenase are to be expected, but the reticulocyte count is low. Because the cells never reach the periphery, such anemias typically are classified as production anemias rather than hemolytic. As summarized in Table 22-5, the differential diagnosis in each of these instances may rely on negative tests for increased cell destruction or accelerated production.

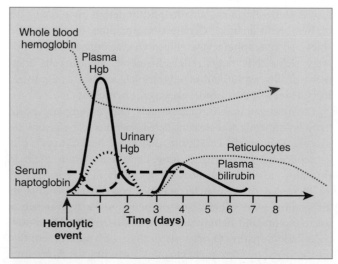

Figure 22-5 Intravascular (fragmentation) hemolysis timeline.

TABLE 22-5 Differential Diagnosis of Hemolytic Anemias versus Other Causes of Indirect Bilirubinemia and Reticulocytosis

	Hemoglobin	Indirect Bilirubinemia	Reticulocytosis	Spherocytes or Schistocytes
Hemolytic anemia—acute, intravascular	Rapidly dropping	Delayed	Delayed	Schistocytes
Hemolytic anemia—acute, extravascular	Rapidly dropping	Delayed	Delayed	Spherocytes
Hemolytic anemia—chronic, intravascular	Persistently low	Persistent	Persistent	Schistocytes
Hemolytic anemia—chronic, extravascular	Persistently low	Persistent	Persistent	Spherocytes
Hemorrhage	Rapidly dropping	Absent	Absent	Absent
Hemodilution	Rapidly dropping	Absent	Absent	Absent
Recovery from hemorrhage	Rising	Absent	Present	Absent
Treated anemia (iron deficiency)	Rising	Absent	Present	Absent
Hemorrhage into a body cavity	Rapidly dropping	Delayed	Delayed	Absent
Ineffective erythropoiesis (i.e., megaloblastic anemia)	Dropping	Persistent	Absent	Absent

CHAPTER at a GLANCE

- A hemolytic disorder is a condition in which there is increased destruction of erythrocytes and compensatory accelerated production of erythrocytes by the bone marrow.
- A hemolytic anemia develops when the bone marrow is unable to compensate for the shortened survival of the RBCs.
- Hemolytic anemias can be classified as acute or chronic, intravascular or extravascular, acquired or inherited, and intrinsic or extrinsic.
- Normally, the bulk of erythrocyte catabolism occurs extravascularly in the macrophages of the spleen, liver, and bone marrow. A small component occurs intravascularly secondary to mechanical trauma.
- Hb from the RBCs is converted to heme and globin within macrophages. Heme is further degraded to iron and unconjugated bilirubin. The bilirubin attaches to albumin and is transported to the liver. In the liver, the bilirubin is conjugated with glucuronic acid and excreted as bile into the intestines and converted to urobilinogen. Some urobilinogen is reabsorbed into the portal circulation and re-excreted through the liver. A small amount is carried in the plasma to the kidney, where it is excreted in the urine.
- In extravascular (macrophage-mediated) hemolytic anemia, there is an increased unconjugated bilirubin in the blood plasma and increased urobilinogen in the urine. Spherocytes may be seen on the blood smear.
- Signs of intravascular hemolysis include hemoglobinemia, (met)hemoglobinuria, and hemosiderinuria. Haptoglobin is decreased. Schistocytes may be seen on the blood smear.

- Jaundice resulting from increased plasma bilirubin is associated with all hemolytic anemias.
- The major clinical features in chronic inherited hemolytic anemia are varying degrees of anemia, jaundice, the occurrence of crises, splenomegaly, and the development of cholelithiasis. In children, bone abnormalities develop as a result of accelerated erythropoiesis.
- Laboratory findings in hemolytic anemia must show increased erythrocyte destruction and compensatory increase in the rate of erythropoiesis. The reticulocyte count is the most commonly used laboratory test to determine accelerated erythropoiesis. Elevated indirect bilirubin with normal direct bilirubin indicates accelerated RBC destruction. Other tests that are specific to a particular diagnosis also may be indicated.
- The peripheral blood smear evaluation can identify morphologic changes that point to intravascular or extravascular etiology and to specific anemias. It is a valuable assessment in the differential diagnosis of anemia.
- Hemolytic anemias must be differentiated from other anemias with reticulocytosis, including the posthemorrhage state and recovery from deficiencies of iron.

Now that you have completed this chapter, go back and read again the case study at the beginning and respond to the questions presented.

REVIEW QUESTIONS

1. The term *hemolytic disorder* in general refers to a disorder in which there is:
   a. Increased destruction of RBCs after entering the bloodstream
   b. Excessive loss of RBCs from the body
   c. Inadequate RBC production by the bone marrow

2. RBC destruction that occurs when macrophages ingest and destroy RBCs is termed:
   a. Extracellular
   b. Extravascular
   c. Intraorgan
   d. Extrahematopoietic

3. Signs of hemolysis that typically are associated with intravascular hemolysis (and not extravascular) include all of the following *except*:
   a. Hemoglobinuria
   b. Hemosiderinuria
   c. Hemoglobinemia
   d. Elevated urinary urobilinogen

4. An elderly Caucasian woman is evaluated for worsening anemia with a decrease of approximately 0.5 mg/dL of Hb each week. The patient is pale, and her skin and eyes are slightly yellow. She complains of extreme fatigue, being unable to complete the tasks of daily living without napping mid-morning and mid-afternoon. She also tires with exertion, finding it difficult to climb even five stairs. Which of the features of this description points to a hemolytic cause for her anemia?
   a. Pallor
   b. Yellow skin and eyes
   c. Rate of decline of Hb
   d. Tiredness on exertion

5. Which of the following tests is a good indication of accelerated erythropoiesis?
   a. Urine urobilinogen
   b. Hemosiderin
   c. Reticulocyte count
   d. Glycosylated Hb

6. A 5-year-old girl was seen by her physician several days ago and diagnosed with pneumonia. Her mother has brought her to the physician again because the girl's urine began to darken after the first visit and now is alarmingly dark. The girl has no history of anemia, and there is no family history. A CBC shows a mild anemia, polychromasia, and a few schistocytes. This anemia could be categorized as:
   a. Acquired, intravascular
   b. Acquired, extravascular
   c. Hereditary, intravascular
   d. Hereditary, extravascular

7. Which of the findings reported for the following patient is *inconsistent* with a diagnosis of intravascular hemolysis?
   The patient has a personal and family history of a mild hemolytic anemia. The patient has a consistently elevated total and indirect serum bilirubin and elevated urinary urobilinogen. The serum haptoglobin is consistently decreased, whereas reticulocytes are elevated. The latter can be seen as polychromasia on the patient's blood smear along with spherocytes as evidence of the hemolysis.
   a. Elevated total and indirect serum bilirubin
   b. Elevated urinary urobilinogen
   c. Decreased haptoglobin
   d. Spherocytes on the peripheral smear

8. Select the statement that is true about bilirubin metabolism.
   a. Indirect bilirubin is formed in the liver by addition of two sugar molecules to direct bilirubin.
   b. Macrophages of the spleen liberate bilirubin during Hb catabolism.
   c. Urobilinogen is not water soluble and is not excreted in urine.
   d. Normally, the major fraction of bilirubin in the blood is the direct (conjugated) form released from macrophages.

9. A patient is evaluated for anemia, and the conclusion is drawn that the anemia does *not* have a hemolytic component. Why was hemolysis ruled out as the cause of the anemia?
   The patient's anemia has been worsening over the last several months. The Hb has been declining slowly with a drop of 1.5 g/dL of Hb over about 6 weeks. Polychromasia and anisocytosis are seen on the blood smear, consistent with the elevated reticulocyte count and RDW. Serum total bilirubin and indirect fractions are normal. Urinary urobilinogen also is normal.
   a. The decline in Hb is too gradual to be hemolytic.
   b. The elevation of the reticulocyte count suggests a malignant cause.
   c. Evidence of increased protoporphyrin catabolism is lacking.
   d. Elevated RDW points to an anemia of decreased production.

10. Which of the following sets of results is expected with intravascular hemolysis?

	Serum Haptoglobin	Serum Methemalbumin	Serum Hemopexin-Heme
a	Increased	Increased	Increased
b	Decreased	Decreased	Decreased
c	Decreased	Increased	Increased
d	Increased	Increased	Decreased

REFERENCES

1. Crosby WH, Akeroyd JH: The limit of hemoglobin synthesis in hereditary hemolytic anemia. Am J Med 1952;13:273-283.
2. Cui Y, Konig J, Leier I, et al: Hepatic uptake of bilirubin and its conjugates by the human organic anion transporter SLC21A6. J Biol Chem 2001;276:9626-9630.
3. Glader B: Destruction of erythrocytes. In Greer JP, Foerster JL, Lukens JN, et al (eds): Wintrobe's Clinical Hematology, 11th ed. Philadelphia: Lippincott, Williams & Wilkins, 2004:249-265.
4. Kristiansen M, Graversen JH, Jacobsen C, et al: Identification of the haemoglobin scavenger receptor. Nature 2001;409:198-201.
5. Tolosano E, Altruda F: Hemopexin: structure, function, and regulation. DNA Cell Biol 2002;21:297-306.

6. Delanghe JR, Langlois MR: Hemopexin: a review of biological aspects and the role in laboratory medicine. Clin Chim Acta 2001;312:13-23.

7. Morgan WT, Liem HH, Sutor RP, et al: Transfer of heme from heme-albumin to hemopexin. Biochem Biophys Acta 1976;444:435-445.

8. Pimstone N: Renal degradation of hemoglobin. Semin Hematol 1972;9:31-42.

9. Sears DA, Anderson PR, Foy AL, et al: Urinary iron excretion and renal metabolism of hemoglobin in hemolytic disease. Blood 1966;28:708-725.

10. Waugh SM, Willardson BM, Kannan R, et al: Heinz bodies induce clustering of band 3, glycophorin, and ankyrin in sickle cell erythrocytes. J Clin Invest 1986;78:1155-1160.

11. Glader B: Anemia: general considerations. In Greer JP, Foerster JL, Lukens JN, et al (eds): Wintrobe's Clinical Hematology, 11th ed. Philadelphia: Lippincott, Williams & Wilkins, 2004:947-978.

12. Crosby WH, Dameshek W: The significance of hemoglobinemia and associated hemosiderinuria, with particular reference to various types of hemolytic anemia. J Lab Clin Med 1951;38:829-841.

13. Fairley NH: Methemalbumin: clinical aspects. QJM 1941; 10:115-138.

14. Muller-Eberhard U: Hemopexin. N Engl J Med 1970;283:1090-1094.

15. Rosen H, Sears DA, Meisenzahl D: Spectral properties of hemopexin-heme: the Schumm test. J Lab Clin Med 1969; 74:941-945.

16. Trotman BW: Pigment gallstone disease. Gastroenterol Clin North Am 1991;20:111.

17. Miller E, Singer K, Dameshek W: Use of the daily fecal output of urobilinogen and the hemolytic index in the measurement of hemolysis. Arch Intern Med 1942;70:722-737.

18. Marchand A, Galen RS, Van Lente F: The predictive value of serum haptoglobin in hemolytic disease. JAMA 1980; 243:1909-1911.

19. Coburn RF: Endogenous carbon monoxide production in man. N Engl J Med 1970;282:207-209.

20. Karliner JS: Clinical usefulness and limitations of serum lactic dehydrogenase determinations. In Griffiths JC (ed): Clinical Enzymology. New York: Masson, 1979:25-29.

21. Panzer S, Kronik G, Lechner K, et al: Glycosylated hemoglobin (GHb): an index of red cell survival. Blood 1982;59:1348-1350.

22. International Committee for Standardization in Haematology: Recommended method for radioisotope red cell survival studies. Br J Haematol 1980;45:659-666.

23

Intracorpuscular Defects Leading to Increased Erythrocyte Destruction

Vishnu V. B. Reddy

OBJECTIVES

After completion of this chapter, the reader will be able to:

1. Describe the membrane defects and membrane skeletal abnormalities associated with hereditary spherocytosis (HS).
2. Describe the hematologic and chemical laboratory results associated with the hemolytic process in HS.
3. Correlate the peripheral blood and bone marrow morphology that is characteristic of HS.
4. Explain the clinical findings, therapy, and prognosis of HS.
5. Explain the principle of and interpret results of the osmotic fragility test in HS.
6. Discuss the membrane defects and skeletal protein abnormalities associated with hereditary elliptocytosis (HE) and hereditary pyropoikilocytosis (HPP).
7. List laboratory results that are associated with HE.
8. List hematologic and chemical laboratory results that are associated with the hemolytic process of HPP.
9. Describe the morphology of red blood cells (RBCs) in the peripheral blood in the different types of HE.
10. Describe the peripheral blood and bone marrow morphology characteristic of HPP.
11. Explain the thermal sensitivity of RBCs in HPP and the testing procedure.
12. Explain the inherited disorders of RBC cation permeability and volume, and describe the expected morphologic variations.
13. Discuss the general genetic inheritance patterns and the pathophysiology of glucose-6-phosphate dehydrogenase (G6PD) deficiency.
14. List the clinical and laboratory findings associated with G6PD deficiency.
15. List the causes of hemolytic episodes in G6PD deficiency.
16. Describe Heinz bodies and explain their relevance to G6PD deficiency.
17. State the principle of the screening test for G6PD deficiency, and explain when it needs to be performed relative to hemolytic crises and why.
18. Name the most common enzyme deficiency in the glycolytic pathway.
19. List the clinical findings of an individual with pyruvate kinase (PK) deficiency.
20. State the principle of the screening test for PK deficiency.
21. Describe the main defect in paroxysmal nocturnal hemoglobinuria (PNH), and explain why it leads to hemolysis.
22. Classify the subpopulation of PNH erythrocytes according to their deficiency of immunologically attached surface proteins as measured by flow cytometry.
23. Describe the hemolytic anemia and nocturnal hemoglobinuria that may be associated with PNH.
24. State expected results of flow cytometric analysis of the RBCs in PNH.
25. Given appropriate hematologic data, recognize findings consistent with each of the anemias discussed in the chapter, and suggest additional tests to confirm the diagnosis.
26. Interpret the results of confirmatory tests for the anemias discussed in the chapter.

CASE STUDY

After studying the material in this chapter, the reader should be able to respond to the following case study:

A 55-year-old man sought medical attention for the onset of chest pain. Physical examination revealed slight jaundice and splenomegaly. The past medical history included gallstones, and there was a family history of anemia. A complete blood count (CBC) yielded the following results:

Laboratory Data	Patient	Reference Range
WBC ($\times 10^9$/L)	13.4	4.5-11
RBC ($\times 10^{12}$/L)	4.28	4.3-5.9
Hemoglobin (g/dL)	11.7	13.9-16.3
Hematocrit (%)	32.5	39-55
MCV (fL)	76	80-100
MCH (pg)	27.3	25.4-34.6
MCHC (g/dL)	36	31-37
RDW (%)	22.9	11.5-13.5

The peripheral blood smear revealed slight anisocytosis, slight polychromasia, and several dark, round microspherocytes lacking central pallor. The platelet count and platelet distribution on the smear were normal (Fig. 23-1).

1. From the data given, what is your initial diagnostic assessment of the anemia?
2. What additional laboratory tests would be of value in establishing the diagnosis, and what abnormalities in these tests would be expected in confirming your impression?
3. What is the cause of this type of anemia?

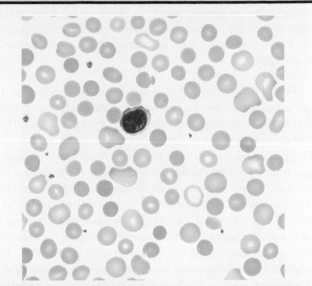

Figure 23-1 Peripheral blood smear of patient in case study (×1000). (From Carr JH, Rodak BF: Clinical Hematology Atlas, 2nd ed. Philadelphia: Saunders, 2004.)

HEREDITARY DEFECTS OF THE RED BLOOD CELL MEMBRANE

Biochemistry and Structure of the Normal Red Blood Cell Membrane

The red blood cell (RBC) membrane consists of two interrelated parts: the outer bilayer of lipids with embedded integral proteins and the underlying protein skeleton (see Fig. 9-2).[1,2] The insoluble lipid portion serves as a barrier to separate the vastly different ion and metabolite concentrations of the interior of the RBC from its external environment, the blood plasma. The protein portion is responsible for shape, structure, and deformability. It also contains the pumps and channels for movement of ions and other material between the RBC's interior and the blood plasma. Various membrane proteins also act as receptors, RBC antigens, and enzymes. The RBC membrane is discussed in more detail in Chapter 9; the reader is encouraged to review that chapter when studying defects in the membrane.

Classification of Hereditary Defects of the Red Blood Cell Membrane

Hereditary RBC membrane defects have historically been classified by morphologic features. The two major disorders are hereditary spherocytosis (HS), characterized by microsphero-cytes, and hereditary elliptocytosis (HE), characterized by elliptical RBCs. Other rare membrane disorders include hereditary stomatocytosis (hydrocytosis), characterized by stomatocytes, and hereditary xerocytosis (dessicocytosis), characterized by dehydrated, shrunken RBCs. Hereditary pyropoikilocytosis (HPP), now thought to be a variant of HE, involves bizarrely shaped, shrunken, and dehydrated cells that hemolyze when heated to temperatures 2° C to 3° C below that required for normal RBCs to hemolyze (49° C). Research has increased knowledge of specific defects in the membrane skeleton that are associated with these morphologic abnormalities and clinical syndromes.[1-3]

Hereditary Spherocytosis

History and Mode of Inheritance. HS is a hemolytic anemia characterized by numerous microspherocytes on the peripheral blood smear. It was first described in 1871 by Belgian physicians Vanlair and Masius.[4] In 1890 Wilson first identified the spleen as the cause of the anemia, and at the turn of the century, Minkowski and Chauffard defined increased osmotic fragility and reticulocytosis as the hallmarks of the disease.[5] Its incidence is worldwide but is highest in Northern Europeans, affecting 1 in 2500 individuals in the United States and England.[1] In 75% of families, it is inherited as an autosomal dominant trait expressed in heterozygotes who have one affected parent. No homozygotes for this form of HS have been identified, suggesting possible incompatibility with life. In approximately 25% of cases, neither parent has this abnormality, indicating that a recessive form of the disease apparently exists. A decreased penetrance of a dominant gene or a new mutation also has been suggested for some of these 25%.[6,7]

Pathophysiology.   The primary molecular defects in HS are in the membrane skeletal proteins, especially the proteins that connect the membrane skeleton to the lipid bilayer. These include spectrin, ankyrin, protein 4.2, and band 3. Almost all European and American HS patients have some degree of spectrin and ankyrin deficiencies, including the dominant and recessive forms, and only a small group are deficient in band 3 and protein 4.2.[8] The latter deficiencies are most common in Japan.[9] The degree of deficiency correlates with the severity of the disease and with the degree of spherocytosis measured by the osmotic fragility test.[10] As with most genetic disorders, when the molecular basis of many families with HS clinical disease is determined, it becomes apparent that the disorder is a heterogeneous group of defects.[8-10]

The mechanisms of spectrin deficiency are not completely understood. Heterozygous α-spectrin defects are usually asymptomatic because α- to β-spectrin synthesis is 3-4 to 1, and a deficiency of this chain must be great before a clinically detectable disease is noted.[11] The combination of two α-spectrin gene defects in *trans* leads to a significant α-spectrin deficiency and severe spherocytic anemia.[12] Several mutations have been identified for β-spectrin defects that cause dominant HS. Many of these patients have had acanthocytes and spherocytes on the peripheral blood smear.[11-15]

Biochemical analyses and genetic studies have implicated ankyrin defects in many cases of HS.[16] It has been hypothesized that ankyrin deficiency or dysfunction may lead to spectrin deficiency in HS. Screening of HS patients using polymerase chain reaction–based, single-stranded conformational polymorphism techniques suggests that ankyrin mutations are common in patients with dominant and recessive HS.[17] In about one third of patients with dominant HS, the primary protein defect is in band 3.[18,19] These patients probably have a combined deficiency of band 3 and protein 4.2 in the 20% to 40% range. They have a mild-to-moderate HS, and their RBC spectrin content is normal. Many of these patients have a few mushroom-shaped or "pincered" erythrocytes, a morphology not seen in other protein defects.[7] Several investigators have described families that lack RBC protein 4.2 and have clinically recessive HS.[16-20]

These membrane skeletal protein abnormalities cause RBCs progressively to lose unsupported lipid membrane because of local disconnection of the skeleton and bilayer. Essentially, small portions of the membrane peel off without loss of much volume. They acquire a decreased surface area–to–volume ratio and a spheroidal shape on the blood smear.[7] These cells are rigid and are not as deformable as normal biconcave disc RBCs, and their survival in the spleen is decreased.[21] The spleen selectively sequesters spherocytes from HS as they try to squeeze through spaces in the endothelial cells of the venous sinuses. As these spherocytes move more slowly through the narrow, elliptical fenestrations of the splenic sinusoids, which are smaller than RBCs, they are especially susceptible to even further membrane loss and become so damaged that they are selectively removed by the macrophages of the red pulp of the spleen.[3,7,21]

The mechanism of this *splenic conditioning* and HS RBC destruction is uncertain. Various ideas have been proposed to explain this phenomenon (Fig. 23-2). The longest-held theory is that because of the low glucose level in the spleen, less adenosine triphosphate (ATP) is produced for these already leaky, membrane-defective cells. The cation pumps cannot maintain their electrolyte balance; the cells take on water and lyse. Research has proved, however, that this phenomenon could occur only if the cells were repeatedly metabolically deprived as they went through the spleen several times. Other theories have suggested that HS RBCs have increased susceptibility to the acidic, oxidant-rich environment of the spleen because of their membrane abnormalities,[7] and when exposed to oxidants in vitro, they undergo remarkable blebbing.[22] Oxidation may be a part of splenic conditioning. Another possible factor in splenic conditioning is splenic macrophage processing of the HS cells that results from their abnormal membranes.[7,23] RBC lifespan is prolonged in corticosteroid therapy, and conditioned RBCs (spherocytes) are reduced. The steroids probably suppress macrophage-induced conditioning and phagocytosis. If steroids are unsuccessful, splenectomy is considered. While not correcting the basic lesion, splenectomy increases the RBC life span and reduces the spherocytosis.[1,23,24]

Clinical and Laboratory Findings.   The three key clinical manifestations with which typical HS patients usually present are anemia, jaundice, and splenomegaly along with spherocytes on the peripheral blood smear and a positive osmotic fragility test (Box 23-1).[7,25] HS may manifest in infancy or childhood or even in old age.[26] HS has been divided into the silent carrier, mild, moderate, moderately severe, and severe states (Table 23-1).[7] Silent carriers are parents of patients with "nondominant" or recessive HS and are clinically asymptomatic without anemia, splenomegaly, hyperbilirubinemia, or spherocytosis.[27] They may show subtle laboratory signs of HS with a slight reticulocytosis, low haptoglobin levels, and a slightly increased osmotic fragility. Mild HS occurs in 20% to 30% of patients who have a compensated hemolysis wherein RBC production and destruction are balanced.[10] Their reticulocyte count is usually less than 6%, and only 60% of patients have significant spherocytosis. Hemolysis may be more severe during illnesses that cause splenomegaly (e.g., infectious mononucleosis), pregnancy, and exercise.[27,28] Two thirds to three fourths of patients have mild-to-moderate HS with incompletely compensated hemolysis and mild-to-moderate anemia, which is usually asymptomatic except for fatigue and pallor.[7] Jaundice is seen at some time in about half of these patients, usually during viral infections. About 5% to 10% of HS patients have moderately severe to severe anemias.[10] In moderately severe disease, hemoglobin (Hb) values are 6 to

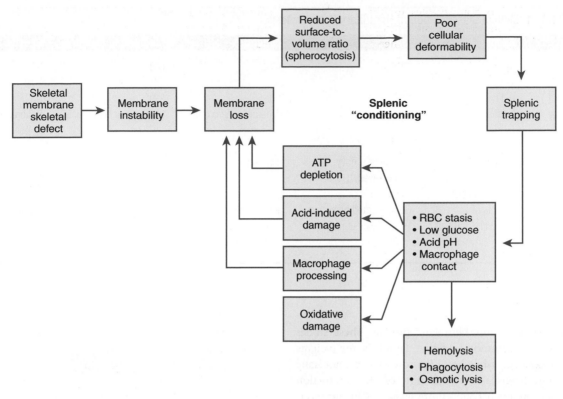

Figure 23-2 Pathophysiology of splenic trapping and destruction of spherocytes. (Modified from Becker PS, Lux SE: Disorders of the red cell membrane. In Nathan DG, Oski FA [eds]: Hematology of Infancy and Childhood, 4th ed. Philadelphia: Saunders, 1993;529-633.)

BOX 23-1 Clinical and Laboratory Findings in Spherocytosis

Clinical Manifestations
Anemia
Splenomegaly
Intermittent jaundice
Aplastic crises
Megaloblastic crises
Excellent response to splenectomy

Inheritance
Dominant 75%
Recessive 25%

Laboratory Characteristics
Reticulocytosis
Spherocytosis
Elevated MCHC
Increased osmotic fragility
Normal DAT

---

addition to typical spherocytes on their blood smear. Rare cases of concurrent glucose-6-phosphatase deficiency (G6PD) also are reported.[30]

Although most patients have a well-compensated hemolysis and are rarely symptomatic, complications may require medical intervention. Patients may experience various crises, classified as hemolytic, aplastic, and megaloblastic.[7] Hemolytic crises occur most frequently, but are usually not severe. They often are associated with viral syndromes, and children may develop transient jaundice. During viral infections, often caused by parvovirus B19 (commonly called *fifth disease of childhood*), which invades hematopoietic stem cells and inhibits their growth, the bone marrow function may decrease (*aplastic crises*), and the young patient may become rapidly and severely anemic.[31] These crises usually are observed in the first 6 years of life. Many HS patients also have a folic acid deficiency resulting from the increased needs for this vitamin during chronic increased cell production in the bone marrow. This phenomenon is termed *megaloblastic crisis* and is particularly acute during pregnancy and during recovery from an aplastic crisis. All HS patients with hemolytic anemia should receive folic acid supplements routinely.[7] Often the bone marrow compensates well for the increased destruction, however, and HS is detected in adult life only when splenic enlargement increases with increased hemolysis and less efficient bone marrow compensation occurs, resulting in jaundice or anemia. Adults may present with the sudden onset of more severe jaundice caused by pigment (bilirubinate) gallstones, a

8 g/dL, and reticulocyte counts are about 10%. Dominant and recessive HS are in this category. Patients with severe disease have by definition a life-threatening anemia and are transfusion dependent.[29] Almost all have recessive HS and often have some irregularly contoured or budding spherocytes in

TABLE 23-1 Clinical Classification of Hereditary Spherocytosis

	Silent Carrier	Mild	Moderate	Moderately Severe	Severe
Hemoglobin (g/dL)	Normal	11-15	8-12	6-8	≥8
Reticulocytes (%)	1-3	3-6	6-10	≥10	≥10
Bilirubin (mg/dL)	0-1	1-2	2-3	2-3	≥3
RBC morphology	Normal	Few spherocytes	Moderate spherocytosis	Moderate spherocytosis	Spherocytosis and poikilocytes
Osmotic fragility					
Fresh blood	Normal	Normal or slightly increased	Increased	Increased	Increased
Incubated blood	Slightly increased	Increased	Increased	Increased	Markedly increased
Other	Parents of mild HS patients	Compensated hemolysis increases during illness	Incompletely compensated hemolysis	Includes recessive and dominant HS	Transfusion-dependent, usually recessive HS

manifestation of a chronic hemolytic process. These stones tend to occlude the common bile duct. Finally, some patients may present in old age, when bone marrow function normally becomes more sluggish. Compensation of the destruction lessens, and the anemia becomes more severe.[26] Chronic ulceration of ankle skin may occur in 10% to 15% of adult patients.[32,33]

Blood Smear Morphology. The hallmark of HS is spherocytes on the blood smear. When present in patients with childhood hemolytic anemia and a family history of similar abnormalities, the uniform spherocytes are highly suggestive of HS. Some of these are microspherocytes—small, round, dense RBCs that are filled with hemoglobin and lack a central pallor (Fig. 23-3). When examined in wet preparation or by electron microscopy, many HS RBCs may appear more as stomatocytes or spherostomatocytes. Normal-appearing RBCs, along with diffusely basophilic (polychromatophilic) RBCs and varying degrees of anisocytosis and poikilocytosis, are present.[1,7]

Complete Blood Count. The most outstanding abnormality noted in the complete blood count (CBC) is the increased mean cell hemoglobin concentration (MCHC) (>36%) in about 50% of patients.[1] It may be 40% or greater in some patients. This abnormality probably results from dehydration of cells that have gone through the spleen and have low levels of water and potassium. Newer cell counters that provide RBC information by light scatter can provide a more accurate mean cell volume (MCV). The Technicon H1[34] (Bayer Corporation, Tarrytown, N.Y.) and its successors, such as the Bayer Advia (Bayer Corporation, Tarrytown, N.Y.), use light scatter to provide cellular Hb information, which is beneficial in identifying spherocytes as indicated in HS. This may be an inexpensive screen with which to diagnose family members of a known HS patient. This increased destruction in HS is usually compensated, and the anemia, if present, is mild. The Hb, hematocrit, and RBC counts reflect this balance of hemolysis and compensation. The hemoglobin usually ranges

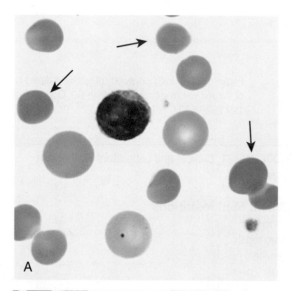

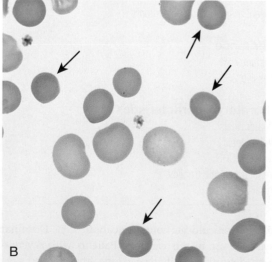

Figure 23-3 Spherocytes (peripheral blood, ×1000).

from 12 to 18 g/dL but varies among individuals. The MCV and MCH usually are normal but also can vary. Reticulocytes typically are 5% to 20% but may be higher, especially during recovery from aplastic crisis.[29] The RBC distribution width is increased.[35] During the aplastic crisis, the hemoglobin, hematocrit, reticulocyte values, and RBC count decrease dramatically.

Other Laboratory Values. The bone marrow in HS shows erythroid hyperplasia resulting from the increased demand to compensate for the decreased life span of the circulating HS RBCs. The RBC precursors are morphologically normal because the morphologic defect is acquired gradually in the circulation.[7]

Values of the chemistry profile reflect extravascular hemolysis. The unconjugated (indirect) bilirubin level is elevated from slight to moderate, fecal urobilinogen level is elevated, and haptoglobin levels are decreased.[1,7,21] The values associated with intravascular hemolysis (i.e., hemoglobinemia, hemoglobinuria, and hemosiderinuria) are not features of HS (Chapter 22).

Special Tests

Osmotic Fragility. The results of the osmotic fragility test are abnormal in blood samples whose cells have decreased surface area–to–volume ratios.[36] When RBCs are put in hypotonic solutions, water enters the cells until equilibrium is achieved. As this phenomenon occurs, the cells swell until the internal volume is too great, causing them to burst or lyse. Because spherocytes already have a decreased surface area–to–volume ratio, they lyse in less hypotonic solutions than normal-shaped, biconcave RBCs and have increased osmotic fragility. The osmotic fragility is the most useful confirmatory test for HS; however, in about 25% of HS patients, the results of the initial osmotic fragility test are normal when fresh blood is used.[7] Increasing the difference between a normal and an abnormal result is usually possible by incubating the blood at 37° C for 24 hours before performing the test. During this incubation period, HS cells become metabolically deprived and tend to lose membrane surface because of their relative membrane instability. Patients who have increased osmotic fragility only when their blood is incubated tend to be mildly affected and may have less than 1% to 2% spherocytes in the total RBC population; this disease is difficult to diagnose on morphologic grounds. If a patient has normal results on the incubated osmotic fragility test, it is highly unlikely that the patient has HS. In the unincubated osmotic fragility test, a distinct subpopulation of the most fragile cells, those most conditioned by the spleen, is reflected by a "tail" of the osmotic fragility curve (Fig. 23-4).[7,23] After splenectomy is performed, the osmotic fragility improves, and this subpopulation of conditioned cells disappears. Increased osmotic fragility simply indicates the presence of spherocytes and does not differentiate between hereditary spherocytosis and spherocytosis caused by other conditions, such as burns, immune hemolytic anemias, and other acquired conditions.

Autohemolysis. The autohemolysis test is relatively sensitive to HS but is not routinely used in many laboratories

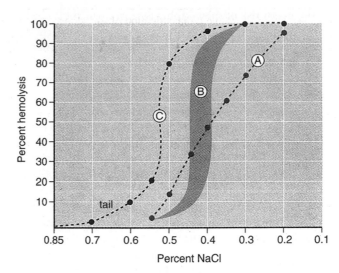

Figure 23-4 Erythrocyte osmotic fragility curve. **A,** Thalassemia showing two cell populations: one with increased fragility *(lower left of curve)* and one with decreased fragility *(upper right of curve)*. **B,** Normal curve. **C,** Increased fragility, as in HS.

because the test is time-consuming, and the results vary.[1,7] When normal RBCs are incubated in their own plasma, hemolysis gradually takes place. In HS, because of the loss of membrane and the inability to maintain the cation gradient, the hemolysis is much greater. Normal samples generally have less than 5.0% hemolysis at the end of the 48-hour incubation, and they have less than 1.0% if a source of glucose is added.[7] The glucose provides energy to drive the cation pumps to help maintain the cells. In HS, the hemolysis is 10% to 50%, which corrects considerably but not to the normal range when glucose is added. An HS patient with numerous conditioned (in vivo by the spleen) microspherocytes may not correct the hemolysis with glucose.

Other Tests. Several other tests have been used to identify patients with HS, including the acidified glycerol lysis test and the hypertonic cryohemolysis test. The acidified glycerol lysis test is based on the rate rather than the extent of hemolysis;[37] there is also an adaptation of the acidified glycerol lysis test, which requires 1-day preincubation.[38] The hypertonic cryohemolysis test is based on the fact that cells from HS are particularly sensitive to cooling at 0° C in hypertonic solutions.[39] It has an advantage over other tests in that it is dependent on primary membrane molecular defects, rather than surface area–to–volume ratio. It is claimed that the test is 100% sensitive for HS, but specificity is only 94% for normal individuals and 86% for patients with autoimmune hemolytic anemia.[39]

Therapy and Outcome. Splenectomy prevents clinically significant hemolysis, and patients with uncomplicated diseases always respond to this treatment.[7] In addition to curing the anemia, splenectomy prevents symptomatic gallbladder disease. This fact is important because of the risks associated with gallbladder surgery, especially in the elderly.

The major risk of splenectomy is sepsis, which may be life-threatening.[7] After splenectomy, infants and young children have increased susceptibility to infection, especially pneumococcal septicemia[40]; the surgery usually is postponed until age 5 to 9, unless the anemia is life-threatening.[7] Even then splenectomy should be avoided before 3 years of age. In older patients, the risk of surgery to prevent persisting hemolysis and pigment gallstones may outweigh the benefits; splenectomy is recommended by some investigators for all HS patients with anemia, significant hemolysis (indicated by repeated reticulocyte counts >5%), or a strong family history of gallbladder disease. Splenectomy can be deferred indefinitely, however, in patients with mild HS and compensated hemolysis.[10,14,26,41] More recently, limited (near-total) splenectomies have been performed with good results.[41]

After splenectomy is performed, spherocytes are still apparent on the blood smear, but conditioned microspherocytes, as evidenced by the change in osmotic fragility, disappear. All of the typical changes in RBC morphology seen after splenectomy also exist, including Howell-Jolly bodies, target cells, siderocytes (Pappenheimer bodies), and acanthocytes (Fig. 23-5). Reticulocyte counts decrease to high-normal levels, and the anemia is usually corrected. Leukocytosis and thrombocytosis are present. Bilirubin levels decrease but may remain in the high-normal range.

Occasionally, an accidental autotransplantation of splenic tissue may occur during splenectomy, and hemolysis may resume years later. The resumption of splenic function can be ascertained from the peripheral blood smear and the increase in pitted RBCs.[7]

Differential Diagnosis. HS must be distinguished from hemolytic anemia with spherocytes that is associated with immune disorders. Family history and evaluation of family members, including parents, siblings, and children of the patient, help differentiate the hereditary origin from the acquired disorder. The immune disorders with spherocytes usually are characterized by a positive result on the direct

antiglobulin test (DAT), whereas the results are negative in HS. The osmotic fragility test is not diagnostic of HS because the cells in acquired hemolytic anemia (AHA) with spherocytes also show increased osmotic fragility.

Spherocytosis also is seen in Heinz body hemolytic anemia during an acute hemolytic crisis and occasionally in a steady state. In Heinz body hemolytic anemia, there are usually bite cells and blister cells on the peripheral smear, and Heinz bodies in RBCs can be detected with methyl violet.[7,14,15,29]

Hereditary Elliptocytosis

History and Mode of Inheritance. HE is characterized by the presence of elliptical or oval erythrocytes on peripheral blood smears. HE was first reported in 1904 by Dresbach,[42] who discovered elliptocytes on a student's blood smear in a histology class at Ohio State University. Clinically, genetically, and biochemically, HE is a very heterogeneous disorder. It reportedly exists in all of its forms in 1 in 2000 to 4000 of the U.S. population.[7] All racial and ethnic groups are represented, but certain types of HE show racial and ethnic preference. Different types of HE have been linked with various blood group antigens, including the Leach phenotype, which lacks the Gerbich antigens and is devoid of glycophorin C and D.[43] Most of the variants are inherited in an autosomal dominant fashion.[1,29]

Pathophysiology. Studies have confirmed the heterogeneity of HE and have indicated several molecular defects in the RBC membrane skeletal proteins that lead to this morphologic abnormality.[7,29] Abnormalities of either α-spectrin or β-spectrin are associated with many cases of HE and HPP. The type of structural change in the membrane protein spectrin seems to be associated with the clinical manifestations. Protein 4.1 deficiencies also have been linked to HE. The defects affect the RBCs' deformability and reflect the failure of RBCs to return to their normal disc shape after being deformed by the shear forces in the microcirculation.[44]

Many patients with common HE have abnormalities of the spectrin heterodimer head region, which cause an inability to associate the dimer form to tetramers and high-order oligomers. These abnormalities commonly involve the N-terminal peptide of the α-chain spectrin, the α^{I} domain, which normally has a molecular mass of 80,000 D ($\alpha^{I/80}$) (Table 23-2). Nine defects that are characterized by the appearance of a new abnormal polypeptide have been identified by using trypsin to cleave the molecule and using isoelectric focusing to identify the abnormal polypeptides. These polypeptides are smaller and are named by their size: $\alpha^{I/78}$, $\alpha^{I/74}$, $\alpha^{I/65-68}$, $\alpha^{I/61}$, $\alpha^{I/50}$, $\alpha^{I/46-50a}$, $\alpha^{I/50b}$, $\alpha^{I/43}$, and $\alpha^{I/33-36}$.[7,45-47] Several specific mutations have been identified that are responsible for some of these α-chain variants. A shortened α-chain also has been discovered, and β-chain abnormalities involving a truncated chain have been reported. In HPP, there exists an α-spectrin mutation that leads to defective spectrin heterodimers and another that leads to partial deficiency of spectrin. Defects in 4.1 protein also are a common cause of elliptocytosis, accounting for 30% to 40% of cases in some Arabic and European populations. It

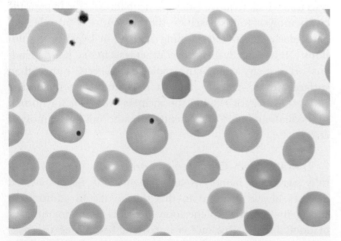

Figure 23-5 RBC morphology of HS after splenectomy, showing Howell-Jolly bodies and spherocytes (PB, ×500).

TABLE 23-2 Hereditary Defects of Red Blood Cell Skeletal Proteins in Elliptocytosis

Protein Deficit	Hereditary Characteristics
Defects in α Chain Spectrin That Impair Spectrin Self-Association	
Spectrin $\alpha^{I/78}$	Silent carrier to moderately severe HE
	Heterogeneous defects seen in North African populations
Spectrin $\alpha^{I/74}$	Generally most severe of common mutations
	Associated with HE, HPP, and HE with infantile poikilocytosis
	Relatively common
	Genetically heterogeneous
Spectrin $\alpha^{I/65-68}$	Silent carrier to mild HE (heterozygous)
	Mild to moderately severe HE (homozygous)
	Common in African Americans of West and Central African ancestry
	Homogeneous defect (extra amino acid [leucine] in α-spectrin)
	Possibly provides protection from malaria
Spectrin $\alpha^{I/46-50a}$	Heterogeneous and variable in severity
Spectrin $\alpha^{I/50b}$	Seen in patients of African ancestry
Spectrin $\alpha^{I/36}$	Shortened α chain
Spectrin α^{LELY} allele	Affects spectrin production or accumulation
	Associated with HPP and hemolytic HE when combined with another spectrin defect
Defects in β Chain Spectrin That Impair Spectrin Self-Association	
Shortened β chain	Heterogeneous mutation that shortens and alters C-terminal sequences and phosphorylation of β chain spectrin
Protein 4.1 defects	Have clinically mild HE; prominent elliptocytosis
Heterozygous protein 4.1 deficiency	
Homozygous protein 4.1 deficiency	Have severe hemolytic anemia
	Prominent elliptocytosis with fragments and poikilocytes

has not been reported in individuals of African ancestry. HE patients all show decreased RBC thermal stability in varying degrees. Patients whose cells show marked thermal sensitivity with fragmentation are classified as having HPP.[45] This fragile self-association of spectrin to spectrin weakens the membrane skeleton of these HE cells and diminishes their resistance to shear stress. Several clinical syndromes are associated with these α-chain defects. Individuals who have only one abnormal allele are silent carriers or have mild common HE or common HE with infantile poikilocytosis.

Clinical and Laboratory Findings.   HE has been subdivided into three types that have different clinical and morphologic syndromes: common HE, spherocytic HE, and Southeast Asian ovalocytosis.[7,23] Southeast Asian ovalocytosis

is an example of an integral protein defect leading to membrane rigidity rather than instability. Most cases of elliptocytosis are caused by membrane instability secondary to skeletal protein defects (Table 23-3). The most common form is common HE, which is composed of several subgroups, including the silent carrier, mild common HE, common HE with chronic hemolysis, and common HE with infantile poikilocytosis.

Common Hereditary Elliptocytosis.   The silent carrier state of HE was identified as the result of studies of asymptomatic members of families with HE or HPP. Individuals with this condition have normal RBC morphology and no evidence of hemolysis, but detailed biochemical studies have revealed subtle defects in the RBC membranes. In mild common HE, many elliptocytes with rod forms are found on the blood smear (Fig. 23-6). The number of these cells always exceeds 30% and may be 100%.[7,23] The patients have no anemia or splenomegaly, however. A mild compensated hemolysis may exist, as evidenced by a slight increase in the reticulocyte count and a decrease in haptoglobin. No budding fragmentation occurs, and no spherocytes are present. Patients with mild HE may develop transient, uncompensated hemolytic anemia secondary to various conditions and infections, including infectious mononucleosis, malaria, cirrhosis, pregnancy, vitamin B_{12} deficiency, disseminated intravascular coagulation, and thrombotic thrombocytopenic purpura. In some families with mild HE, an individual may have more severe hemolysis and anemia; this is common HE with chronic hemolysis. These individuals may have coinherited a spectrin allele that leads to decreased α-spectrin expression, such as the α^{LELY} allele, or one of the more deleterious HE alleles affecting α-spectrin, such as $\alpha^{I/117}$.[46] In other cases, mild HE is accompanied by chronic hemolysis in most family members. These families usually have different molecular defects than those typically found in mild HE; fragmentation and poikilocytosis may be more prevalent. These patients seem to respond to splenectomy.[47,48] *Common HE with infantile poikilocytosis* has budding, fragments, and bizarre poikilocytes and manifests with moderate hemolysis at birth; however, the condition gradually (from 6 months to 2 years of age) converts to a morphologic and clinical picture resembling mild HE.[48] This change corresponds with the change from fetal to adult hemoglobin production; no change in the α-spectrin defect occurs during this time. It has been suggested that because Hb F is elevated in fetal cells and does not bind 2,3-bisphosphoglycerate (2,3-BPG) and that because 2,3-BPG is known to weaken spectrin-actin-protein 4.1 interaction, 2,3-BPG is the crucial agent in this syndrome of common HE.[7,50,51] All of these common HEs have normal osmotic fragility. All HE patients who are significantly anemic and show signs of hemolysis respond well to splenectomy. Common HE RBCs are mildly heat sensitive. They become echinocytic and fragment at 47° C to 48° C, whereas normal RBCs are stable at temperatures of 49° C.

Rarely, parents with mild HE may have offspring who are homozygous for the abnormal gene (homozygous common HE) and present with a moderate to very severe hemolytic state. Some even have transfusion-dependent hemolytic

TABLE 23-3 Clinical and Morphologic Classification of Hereditary Elliptocytosis (HE) and Hereditary Pyroikilocytosis (HPP)

	RBC Morphology	Clinical Manifestations	Heat Sensitivity of RBC	Comments
Common HE				
Heterozygous common HE				
Silent carrier	Normal	Asymptomatic	NA	Family member with HE or HPP
Mild common HE	30% to 100% elliptocytosis	Asymptomatic	Mild	Slightly increased reticulocytes
Common HE with hemolysis	Marked elliptocytosis with fragmentation and poikilocytosis	Chronic hemolytic state	Mild	Increased reticulocytes
Common HE with infantile poikilocytosis	Marked elliptocytosis with budding, fragmentation, and bizarre poikilocytes at birth	Moderate hemolysis at birth	Mild	Converts to mild common HE blood morphology and clinical manifestations from 6 mo to 2 y of age
Homozygous common HE	Elliptocytosis with gross fragmentation, poikilocytosis, and spherocytosis	Moderate to severe hemolytic state	Mild to moderate	Responds to splenectomy
HPP	Elliptocytosis, marked poikilocytes, gross fragmentation, spherocytes, bizarre-shaped RBCs	Severe hemolytic anemia	Marked	Disorder results from an α-spectrin mutation and a partial deficiency of spectrin; responds to splenectomy; most patients are African American
Spherocytic HE	Rounded elliptocytes and spherocytes	Compensated mild hemolysis	Mild	Gallbladder disease common; most patients are of northern European ancestry

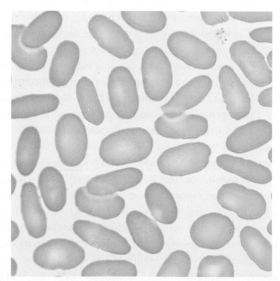

Figure 23-6 Peripheral blood smear of HE (×1000). (From Carr JH, Rodak BF: Clinical Hematology Atlas, 2nd ed. Philadelphia: Saunders, 2004.)

anemia with gross fragmentation, poikilocytosis, and spherocytosis, along with elliptocytosis. These patients also usually respond to splenectomy.[23,52]

Spherocytic Hereditary Elliptocytosis. The second type of HE is a hybrid disorder that combines features of mild HE and mild HS. This disorder is seen in individuals of Northern European origin. Rounded elliptocytes and spherocytes are seen on the blood smear. The RBC morphology varies with different proportions of these abnormal cells, even in the same family. The incidence of this type of HE is unknown but is estimated to be about 5% of HE cases of European ancestry.[7] Most patients have evidence of a mild hemolysis often incompletely compensated.[23,52] Gallbladder disease is common in these patients, and aplastic crises are a risk. Patients show a slightly increased osmotic fragility and an increased glucose-responsive autohemolysis test result. Hemolysis in these patients responds well to splenectomy.

Stomatocytic Hereditary Elliptocytosis. The third major type of HE is stomatocytic HE, or Southeast Asian ovalocytosis, and is common only in the Melanesian and Malaysian populations.[7,23] The elliptocytes are rounded, and some have transverse bars so that they appear like double stomatocytes.[53] The osmotic fragility is usually normal. These cells are resistant to invasion by all forms of malaria.[54] The membrane seems more rigid than a normal RBC membrane, and hemolysis is mild or absent. Many of the blood group antigens are poorly expressed on these cells. The RBCs in this disorder are unusually heat resistant, maintaining their shape at temperatures of 51° C to 52° C (normal 49° C). The cells are strongly resistant to crenation even after several days in storage in plasma or buffered salt solution. All patients with the phenotype of Southeast Asian ovalocytosis are heterozygotes. One band 3 allele is normal, and the other has two mutations. This Southeast Asian ovalocytosis band 3 binds tightly to ankyrin and is unable to transport anions. These cells have a very rigid membrane. No Southeast Asian ovalocytosis homozygotes have been identified; it has been hypothesized that this disorder is incompatible with life.[53]

Hereditary Pyropoikilocytosis

HPP is a rare disorder that manifests in infancy or early childhood as a severe hemolytic anemia with extreme poikilocytosis. It resembles the blood picture of severe burns and homozygous HE. In HPP, there coexist an α-spectrin mutation that leads to defective spectrin heterodimers and another that leads to a partial deficiency of spectrin. HPP traditionally has been described as a separate disease, but many authors believe that it is a subtype of HE.[7,23,52] It seems to be transmitted as a recessive disease but is morphologically similar to homozygous HE. In one third of the reported cases of HPP, one of the parents or siblings has typical mild HE.[7,23,52] In other families, the parents seem normal, but further investigation reveals that at least one of the parents is a silent carrier. Studies of spectrin synthesis and mRNA on a patient who shows no biochemical abnormalities reveal a defect of spectrin synthesis that, when coinherited with the abnormal spectrin, enhances the expression of the mutant spectrin in the cell and leads to a superimposed spectrin deficiency.[55] The HPP phenotype may result from homozygosity for the silent carrier state, homozygosity for one of the mild HE genes, or double heterozygosity for any combination of abnormal genes that cause structural defects of spectrin. In homozygous HE and HPP, osmotic fragility and autohemolysis are markedly increased. The RBCs show marked thermal sensitivity. After 10 to 15 minutes of heating at 45° C to 46° C, RBCs in HPP fragment. Normal cells do not fragment until reaching a temperature of 49° C. RBCs in HPP fragment at 37° C when heated longer than 6 hours.[23,56]

Most patients who have HPP are black. They have a severe hemolytic anemia with facial bone abnormalities (resulting from expanding bone marrow mass), gallbladder disease (resulting from excessive RBC breakdown), and growth retardation. The RBC morphology of these patients shows marked poikilocytosis, including elliptocytes, RBC fragments, budding RBCs, spherocytes, and triangular and other bizarrely shaped cells (Fig. 23-7).[23] The MCV is very low (25-75 fL) because of the RBC fragments. Patients with HPP partially respond to splenectomy, but some hemolysis still remains, probably as a result of the cells fragmenting even at body temperature.[7]

INHERITED DISORDERS OF RED BLOOD CELL CATION PERMEABILITY AND VOLUME

RBC hydration is determined by the intracellular concentration of the monovalent cations Na^+ and K^+. If the total cation content is increased, water enters the cell and forms a hydrocyte, or stomatocyte; if the total cation content is decreased, water leaves the cell and produces a dehydrated RBC, or xerocyte. Many congenital anemias of certain permeability

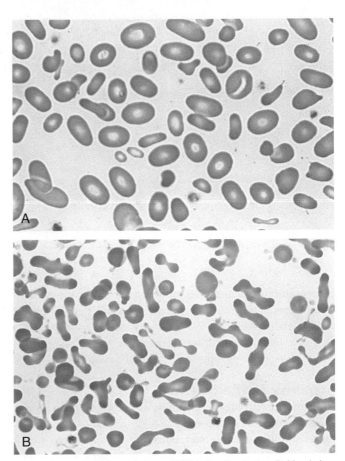

Figure 23-7 A, RBC morphology of HPP before incubation. **B,** Morphology after 1 hour at 45° C (PB, ×500).

have been described in the past 35 years that are clinically, morphologically, genetically, and biochemically diverse.[57]

Hereditary Stomatocytosis (Hydrocytosis)

Hereditary stomatocytosis is a complex mixture of diseases in which hemolysis is mild to severe (Fig. 23-8). It is rare and usually is inherited in an autosomal dominant pattern.[57]

Pathophysiology

Hereditary stomatocytosis is characterized morphologically by stomatocytes and biochemically by the failure of the Na^+ and K^+ pumps and an increase in intracellular water.[7,57] The influx of Na^+ exceeds the loss of K^+, and the cells swell, becoming less dense and more stomatocytic. In most patients, a deficiency of a membrane integral protein called *stomatin* or band 7.2b occurs. The function of stomatin is unknown, but it is hypothesized that it supports or regulates an unidentified ion channel.[56] Studies of Japanese patients with this disorder have shown some with normal stomatin, however.[56,58-61]

Clinical and Laboratory Findings

The disease can cause mild, moderate, or severe hemolysis. The diagnostic features include 5% to 50% stomatocytes on the peripheral blood smear, macrocytes (MCV 110-150 fL), reduced erythrocyte K^+ concentration, elevated erythrocyte Na^+

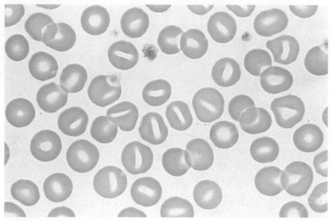

Figure 23-8 RBC morphology of hereditary stomatocytosis (PB, ×500).

concentration, and increased monovalent cation content in the erythrocytes.[7] The RBCs have increased osmotic fragility and are moderately deficient in 2,3-BPG.[7] Patients who have severe hemolysis may benefit from splenectomy, but a high proportion of these patients experience thrombotic complications.[56-62]

Acquired Stomatocytosis

Stomatocytosis occurs frequently as a drying artifact on Wright-stained peripheral blood smears. A clinical laboratory professional should examine many areas on several smears before categorizing the result as stomatocytosis because in true stomatocytosis such cells should be found in all areas of the blood smear. In normal individuals, 3% of RBCs may be stomatocytes.[7] In wet preparations with RBCs diluted in their own plasma and examined under phase microscopy, stomatocytes tend to be bowl shaped or uniconcave, rather than the normal biconcave shape. This technique can eliminate some of the artifactual stomatocytosis, but target cells also may appear bowl shaped in solution. Acute alcoholism and drug therapy have been associated with acquired stomatocytosis.[1,7] Occasionally, the disorder has been seen transiently in marathon runners after a race.[63]

Stomatocytosis in Rh_null Disease

In 1961, a rare condition was discovered in which patients lacked all of the Rh antigens on their RBC membranes,[64,65] thus denoted Rh_null. They also had decreased expression of Ss and U antigens. These patients present clinically with a moderately severe hemolytic anemia, characterized morphologically by stomatocytes and spherocytes.[64] Osmotic fragility is mildly increased. It has been suggested that the Rh antigens are associated with the membrane skeleton and that their loss affects the skeletal stability. Stomatocytosis also occurs in Rh_mod disease, a related anomaly in which the expression of Rh antigens is suppressed but not absent.[7]

Hereditary Xerocytosis

In the rare autosomal dominant hemolytic anemia known as *hereditary xerocytosis,* the RBCs are dehydrated, as evidenced by the elevated MCHC and decreased osmotic fragility.[7,58] These cells lose K⁺ because of an RBC membrane permeability defect; the specific defect has not been discovered. The RBC morphology includes stomatocytes, target cells, spiculated RBCs, and macrocytes. RBCs in which the hemoglobin appears to be puddled in discrete areas on the cell periphery are characteristic. The 2,3-BPG concentration in RBCs is moderately decreased. Removal of the spleen in these patients does not significantly reduce the hemolysis.[58,61] Various other RBC permeability syndromes have been reported that have shared features of hydrocytosis and xerocytosis; these have been termed the *intermediate syndromes.*[58]

Acanthocytosis

Acanthocytes (spur cells) are RBCs with a few irregular projections that vary in width, length, and surface distribution. These are distinct from echinocytes (burr cells), which typically have small, uniform projections evenly spread on the cell circumference.[7] The differentiation is easier to make on scanning electron micrographs and on wet preparation than on dried smears. Echinocytes appear crenated on a stained smear, whereas acanthocytes appear as denser, more contracted, and irregular. Echinocytes have been associated with uremia, defects in glycolytic metabolism, and microangiopathic hemolytic anemias.[7] Echinocytes also are common in neonates, especially premature neonates. Acanthocytes and echinocytes have been associated with severe liver disease, abetalipoproteinemia, infantile pyknocytosis, anorexia nervosa, the McLeod and *In(Lu)* blood groups, and hypothyroidism.

Abetalipoproteinemia is a rare autosomal recessive disorder manifested in the first month of life by steatorrhea. Also associated with the disorder is a progressive neurologic disease, celiac syndrome and retinitis pigmentosa, which often results in blindness. Low-density lipoproteins are absent.[66] Death usually occurs by the teens or 20s. Usually, 50% to 100% of the RBCs are acanthocytes.[66] Affected individuals have a mild hemolytic anemia and normal RBC indices.[7,45,66]

Pathophysiology

Acanthocytes have a normal membrane protein composition, but the membrane lipids are abnormal. An increase in membrane sphingomyelin and a decrease in phosphatidylcholine are present. These changes reflect abnormalities in the distribution of plasma phospholipids that decrease the lipid fluidity of the RBC membrane, resulting in the shape change. The shape defect is not present in developing nucleated RBCs or reticulocytes, but progresses as RBCs age.[66] Patients with other related disorders, such as hypobetalipoproteinemia, normotriglyceridemic abetalipoproteinemia, and chylomicron retention disease, also may have acanthocytosis and neurologic disease, depending on the severity of the lipoprotein defect.[66]

Other Causes of Acanthocytosis

The McLeod blood group phenotype is an X-linked anomaly of the Kell blood group system that causes a lack of Kx, a membrane precursor of the Kell antigens.[67] Men who lack Kx on their RBCs have variable acanthocytosis (8% to 85%) and a mild compensated anemia. Female heterozygote carriers may have an occasional acanthocyte as a result of the X chromosome inactivation. Patients with an *In(Lu)* gene, which is a dominant inhibitor of Lutheran blood group antigens (Lu^a and Lu^b), have abnormally shaped RBCs but no hemolysis. Morphology varies from normal to mild poikilocytosis to marked acanthocytosis. Patients who have malnutrition as a result of conditions such as anorexia nervosa and cystic fibrosis may have acanthocytes on their blood smear that resolve after a normal nutritional state is obtained.[7,45,68]

Patients with vitamin E deficiency may have a variable number of acanthocytes. A syndrome of neonatal jaundice and hemolysis in which a variable number of cells resembling acanthocytes is present has been described in neonates. The abnormal cells peak at 3 to 4 weeks of age and then decline spontaneously. Now that infant formulas contain vitamin E, this syndrome is seldom seen except in fat malabsorption, as in cystic fibrosis and abetalipoproteinemia.

RED BLOOD CELL ENZYMOPATHIES

Glucose-6-Phosphate Dehydrogenase Deficiency

Hemolysis resulting from G6PD deficiency was recognized very early, when Pythagoras, the Greek philosopher and mathematician, warned his followers against the dangers of eating fava beans.[69] Physicians in southern Italy wrote of the clinical picture of this disorder around the turn of the 20th century.[70] The hemolytic effect of the antimalarial drug primaquine was recognized in the early 1950s. Alving et al[71] discovered that primaquine-sensitive individuals had low levels of G6PD activity in their RBCs.

The gene for G6PD is located on the X chromosome and shows a characteristic X-linked pattern. Men can be normal hemizygotes (have the normal allele) or deficient hemizygotes (have a variant allele). Women can be normal homozygotes (both alleles normal), deficient homozygotes (both alleles abnormal), or heterozygotes (one normal allele and one abnormal allele).[72] The heterozygous woman's level of enzyme lies between normal and deficient. This disorder has been considered X-linked recessive, but because heterozygous women have a decreased amount of the enzyme, it is biochemically codominant.[72] Some heterozygous women may have hemolytic attacks, depending on the amount of RBC G6PD activity. Female heterozygotes have two populations of G6PD-producing cells because of the X chromosome inactivation (the Lyon hypothesis). This means that statistically half of the cells are G6PD deficient. In reality, the inactivation is statistically random; in female heterozygotes, the RBCs may be deficient in G6PD, or normal levels of G6PD may be present.[70-78]

The G6PD locus has the greatest apparent extent of variability of any in the human genome. Genetic studies reveal the abnormality is structural (point mutations) rather than resulting from a decrease in the number of normal molecules (deletions).[73,74] These changes in the primary structure (substitution of individual amino acids) cause G6PD deficiency by decreasing its in vivo stability or by affecting its enzymatic functions, or possibly both, depending on the particular variant. (See Luzzatto[73] for a list of human G6PD gene mutations and a map of structural mutations of the variants for which a molecular basis has been elucidated.) The different genetic expressions of G6PD have been divided into classes by the World Health Organization, based on clinical symptoms and amount of enzyme activity.[73,74,79] Class I has severe clinical symptoms (chronic, nonspherocytic hemolytic anemia) and less than 20% G6PD activity. Class II has mild clinical expression with intermittent hemolysis and less than 10% activity. Class III has mild clinical expression with intermittent hemolysis associated with infection or drugs and 10% to 60% activity. Class IV has no clinical expression and 100% activity. Class V has no clinical expression and greater than 100% activity. Within these groups, more than 400 different genetic mutations and enzymes may exist that have many different electrophoretic patterns.[73,80]

Normal G6PD generally has been designated *G6PD-B*. Some G6PD variants are not associated with significant reduced enzyme activity in the RBCs. A common mutant that is clinically normal, has no enzyme deficiency, and is present most often in individuals of African descent is *G6PD-A$^+$*. This common mutant has Asn→Asp at the 126th amino acid position and moves faster on electrophoresis than does G6PD-B.[71] Approximately 20% to 40% of the X chromosomes of Africans have the gene for G6PD-A$^+$. Three clinically deficient mutations are mutations of G6PD-A and are called *G6PD-A$^-$*. These variants have the G6PD mutation plus an additional amino acid substitution. Individuals with a G6PD-A$^-$ mutation are a prototype for class III because of their clinical symptoms and the amount of enzyme activity in their RBCs. In the United States, 10% to 11% of African-American men carry a gene that codes for G6PD-A$^-$.[71] All other variants are designated by geographic names.[79] G6PD Mediterranean (G6PD-Med) is the most common variant enzyme among Caucasians.[71] In this variant, enzyme activity is barely detectable because the G6PD is synthesized in subnormal amounts and is unstable. Patients with this variant are a prototype for class II.[79] The incidence among Kurdish Jews is up to 50%.[79] The Mahidol variant has a high incidence in the populations of Thailand and Vietnam, and the Canton variant is commonly found in the Chinese and in individuals from Southeast Asia.[78]

Pathophysiology

The enzyme G6PD reduces nicotinamide adenine dinucleotide phosphate (NADP) while oxidizing glucose-6-phosphate. It governs the rate of reduction of NADP, which restores reduced glutathione (GSH) through H$^+$ transfer by glutathione reductase in the hexose monophosphate shunt (see Fig. 9-1). G6PD provides the only means of generating the reduced form of nicotinamide adenine dinucleotide phosphate (NADPH), and in its absence the erythrocyte is particularly vulnerable to oxidative damage.[80] Most oxidant drugs enable interaction between molecular oxygen and components of the RBC. RBCs with normal G6PD activity are able to detoxify the oxidative compounds and safeguard the hemoglobin. SH-containing enzymes and membrane thiols (sulfhydryls) allow normal-functioning RBCs to carry enormous quantities of oxygen safely.[80]

In patients with deficient G6PD activity, the exposure of RBCs to oxidative agents causes oxidation of membrane thiols, which produces several consequences, the most conspicuous being the appearance of Heinz bodies (intracellular irreversible precipitates of denatured hemoglobin) along with skeletal abnormalities, causing K^+ and Na^+ leak rates to increase.[81] The mechanism of Heinz body formation is complex and poorly understood but most likely occurs when the NADPH-dependent counteroxidant defenses are overwhelmed and GSH is oxidized to oxidized glutathione (GSSG). Conformational changes occur in the hemoglobin molecule, which also exposes the interior thiols to oxidation. With sustained intracellular production of oxygen free radicals, the three-dimensional structure of hemoglobin is affected sufficiently to lower its solubility, and insoluble hemochromes aggregate as Heinz bodies.[82] A coagulum of hemoglobin separates from the RBC membrane, leaving a clear area similar to a bite being taken out of a cell.[82] These "bite" cells occasionally can be seen on the peripheral blood smear. Other RBCs are less pliable because of the undeformable Heinz body aggregates and are trapped and lysed in the spleen by mechanical hemolysis.[73]

Hemolytic Process

The following clinical syndromes associated with G6PD are recognized: AHA, resulting from drug exposure or infection; favism; neonatal jaundice; and chronic nonspherocytic hemolytic anemia.[74] Hemolysis also has been reported in association with diabetic ketoacidosis and hypoglycemia, but other factors, such as coexistent infection or oxidant drug exposure, cannot always be ruled out as a cause of the hemolysis.

AHA secondary to drug exposure is the classic manifestation of G6PD deficiency. The actual discovery of G6PD deficiency was a direct consequence of investigations into the development of hemolysis after the ingestion of the antimalarial agent primaquine in some individuals (usually African American men). Box 23-2 lists drugs that have a definite association with hemolytic episodes in individuals with G6PD deficiency.[83] Other agents have a less direct association. With some of these drugs, hemolysis occurs in some populations and not in others, and different doses give rise to different degrees of hemolysis, depending on other circumstances, such as a coexisting infection or concomitant use of other drugs.[83] Also, because the oldest RBCs have the lowest amount of enzymes and are the first to lyse, the number of reticulocytes affects the rate of hemolysis, since they are more resistant.

Individuals with G6PD deficiency are clinically and hematologically normal until the offending drug is given. The acute hemolytic episode is caused by a genetic factor (the lack of functional G6PD) and an exogenous factor (the drug).[73,74] Clinical hemolysis and jaundice typically begin 2 to 3 days after the drug is started. Hemoglobinuria is a chief sign and indicates that the hemolysis is intravascular, although some extravascular hemolysis probably also takes place. The anemia worsens until the 7th to 8th day. Heinz bodies can be shown by incubating the blood in a supravital stain. The reticulocyte count generally increases by the 8th to the 10th day, and the hemoglobin level begins to rise.[73,74] With some variants, the hemolytic episode is self-limiting because the newly formed reticulocytes have higher G6PD activity. With other variants that are more severely deficient, however, the hemolytic episode may be longer. The level of the drug dosage also plays a role in the severity and length of the hemolytic episode.[73]

Infection is probably the most common cause of hemolysis in individuals with G6PD deficiency in areas where favism is not prevalent.[71,73,74,84] The clinical picture of hemolysis caused by infection is influenced by several factors, including the concomitant administration of oxidant drugs and the Hb level, the liver function, and the age of the patient. The mechanism of hemolysis induced by acute and subacute infection is poorly understood, but the generation of hydrogen peroxide by phagocytizing leukocytes may play a role.[74,84] Diminished liver function may aggravate further the oxidant stress on the RBCs by allowing the accumulation of metabolites capable of oxidizing RBC-SH groups. Some of the infectious agents associated with hemolysis in G6PD-deficient individuals are salmonellae, coliforms, β-hemolytic streptococci, rickettsiae, influenza virus, and hepatitis virus. In addition to hemolysis, viral hepatitis can cause acute renal failure and hyperbilirubinemia in G6PD-deficient patients.[73,85,86]

Favism results when a small percentage of G6PD-deficient individuals are exposed to the fava bean (*Vicia fava* or broad bean, commonly grown in the Mediterranean area), either by ingesting the bean or inhaling the plant's pollen. Substances capable of oxidizing RBC GSH and capable of causing hemolysis have been isolated from fava beans. Favism clinically manifests with a sudden onset of acute intravascular hemolysis within 24 to 48 hours of exposure.[74] Hemoglobinuria is one of the first signs of the disorder. Only a small percentage of G6PD-deficient individuals are affected, and most of these have the G6PD-Med variant; favism is seen primarily in the Mediterranean area. Rarely, a G6PD-deficient African American patient may be susceptible.[73]

Neonatal jaundice secondary to G6PD deficiency occurs particularly in Greece, Sardinia, Africa, and the United States.[74] Jaundice usually appears by 1 to 4 days after birth, which is slightly earlier than physiologic jaundice but later than in blood group alloimmunization.[74] Genetic factors, which

---

BOX 23-2 Substances That Can Induce Hemolysis in Patients with Glucose-6-Phosphate Dehydrogenase Deficiency

Acetanilid
Doxorubicin
Furazolidone
Methylene blue
Nalidixic acid
Niridazole
Nitrofurantoin
Phenazopyridine
Primaquine
Sulfamethoxazole

include the particular variant of G6PD, and environmental factors (e.g., drugs given to the mother or infant, infection, and gestational age) probably play an important role in this occurrence because a wide variation exists in the frequency and severity in different populations with G6PD deficiency.[87-89]

Most G6PD patients are clinically normal and have only a slightly reduced RBC life span, evidenced only by RBC survival studies, unless they are challenged. A small group of G6PD-deficient patients have chronic, clinically detectable anemia evidenced by chronic hyperbilirubinemia, decreased haptoglobin level, and increased lactate dehydrogenase level. Most of these patients are diagnosed at birth as having neonatal jaundice, and the hemolysis continues into adulthood. They usually do not have hemoglobinuria, suggesting that the chronic hemolysis is extravascular as opposed to the intravascular hemolysis associated with the AHA of G6PD deficiency.[73] There is evidence that normal oxidative stress causes the sulfhydryl groups of the membrane proteins (especially spectrin) to be oxidized and conformational changes to occur so that the RBCs are removed by the spleen, probably by the same mechanism as in hereditary spherocytosis. The RBC morphology is unremarkable and is referred to as "nonspherocytic."[73] These patients also are vulnerable to acute oxidative stress from the same agents as in other G6PD patients and may have acute attacks of hemoglobinuria. The severity associated with chronic, nonspherocytic hemolytic anemia is extremely variable, probably because almost every case that has been evaluated has resulted from a different mutation of the enzyme.[73]

An association between the distribution of G6PD deficiency and the incidence of *Plasmodium falciparum* has been suggested.[74,79] Many epidemiologic studies have supported the hypothesis that malaria selects for G6PD deficiency, which also may explain the genetic heterogeneity of the G6PD alleles and the frequency of the abnormal allele in particular geographic regions. Although earlier studies suggested that this protection was only for G6PD-deficient hemizygous men and not for deficient women, more recent studies have reported that, for G6PD-A⁻ (the most common African deficiency variant), heterozygous women and hemizygous men seem to be protected.[83] The *P. falciparum* parasite invades the G6PD-deficient cell normally, but intracellular development is impaired. This impairment is overcome by repeated schizogonic cycles of the parasite in G6PD-deficient RBCs.[88,90]

Clinical and Laboratory Findings

Most individuals with G6PD deficiency are usually asymptomatic and may never discover their genetic abnormality. Their only clinical manifestation may be acute hemolysis during oxidative stress resulting from drugs or other causes; this hemolysis may go undetected because the bone marrow rapidly compensates for the increased RBC destruction.[71,73,74,79] However, G6PD deficiency can cause clinically recognizable hemolysis (see later).

The anemia occurring during a hemolytic crisis may range from moderate to extremely severe and is usually normocytic, normochromic. The morphology of G6PD-deficient RBCs is normal except during a hemolytic episode. The change in morphology during a hemolytic episode varies depending on the amount of hemolysis. In some patients, such as G6PD-A⁻ individuals, the change is not striking,[71] but in individuals with other variants, marked anisocytosis and poikilocytosis may occur, with distorted RBCs and bite cells in which the cell's margin appears dented.[73] When an offending drug is administered, Heinz bodies (denatured hemoglobin) develop in the RBCs.[83] These cannot be detected with Wright stain, but when exposed to certain basic dyes or supravital stains, such as crystal violet, they assume a purple color and appear at the margin of the RBC. When they are removed by the spleen, bite cells are formed. The reticulocyte count is increased and may reach 30%.[73] Haptoglobin level is severely decreased. In some cases, free hemoglobin may be detected in the plasma. The white blood cell (WBC) count is moderately elevated,[73] and the platelet count varies. The unconjugated (indirect) bilirubin level is elevated. The darkly colored urine tests strongly positive for blood. Few intact RBCs appear in the sediment because the color and blood reaction result from hemoglobinuria and not hematuria.[73]

Quantitative assays of the G6PD enzyme activity in RBCs can be performed to enable the differential diagnosis in G6PD deficiency to be made, but screening tests are usually adequate.[71] The principle of both tests is based on the reduction of an oxidized pyridine nucleotide (NADP-NADPH) during the reaction shown in Figure 23-9. In the quantitative assay, hemolysate of the patient's blood is added to a mixture of reagents that has been constituted in such a way that the amount of enzyme represents the limiting step; the activity is read at 340 ηm with the cuvette thermostat at 37° C. The principle of the screening test is the same except that, rather than measuring the absorption of light by the reduced pyridine nucleotide (NADPH), visual observation of fluorescence of reduced nucleotide, when activated with long-wave ultraviolet light, is used to evaluate visually whether pyridine nucleotide (NADP) has been reduced.[91] This is done by mixing the reagents, placing them on a filter paper, and observing the filter paper under fluorescent light. Because reticulocytes have higher G6PD levels than mature RBCs, assays or screening tests should not be prepared with samples collected after an individual has had a severe hemolytic crisis because the G6PD levels may be falsely elevated. The testing should be performed after mature RBC levels have returned to normal. A normal and

$$\text{Glucose-6-phosphate} + \text{NADP} \xrightarrow{\text{G-6-PD}} \text{6-Phosphogluconate} + \text{NADPH}$$
(no fluorescence) (fluorescence)

Figure 23-9 Principle of G6PD deficiency test. In the screening test, NADPH fluoresces, whereas NADP does not. If glucose-6-phosphate (G6P) is oxidized to 6-phosphogluconate (6PG), the coenzyme NADP is reduced to NADPH with a corresponding increase in fluorescence.

not an increased G6PD assay along with a high reticulocyte count should be a clue that the patient may be G6PD deficient.[74] Other tests that can be used to screen for G6PD deficiency are the methemoglobin reduction test,[92] a sensitive test in which the erythrocytes that are G6PD deficient fail to reduce methemoglobin in the presence of methylene blue, and the ascorbate-cyanide test,[93] which measures peroxidative denaturation of hemoglobin. This last test is not specific for G6PD deficiency and gives positive results with pyruvate kinase (PK) deficiency and with certain unstable hemoglobins.

Therapy and Prognosis

Therapy in patients with G6PD deficiency involves preventing the common manifestations of AHA and neonatal jaundice. Most hemolytic episodes, especially in G6PD-A⁻ individuals, are self-limited. In more severe types, such as G6PD-Med, this is not always the case. Screening is important in populations that have a high incidence of this deficiency.[73] Because neonatal jaundice cannot be prevented, it must be sought in the populations that are high risk and must be treated immediately. Neonatal jaundice is not a major problem in most populations in the United States. The prevention of AHA is more difficult because multiple causes exist; however, some cases of AHA are easily preventable, such as avoiding eating fava beans in families in which this sensitivity exists.

Favism is a relatively dangerous disease, and fatalities were common before transfusion services were available.[71] Prevention of drug-induced AHA is possible by choosing alternate drugs when possible.[78] In cases in which the offending drugs must be used, especially in individuals with G6PD-A⁻, the dosage can be lowered, decreasing the hemolysis to a manageable level.[78] Infection-induced hemolysis is more difficult to prevent but can be detected early in the course of the episode and treated if necessary. Most episodes of AHA resolve without treatment but may be severe enough to warrant a blood transfusion. Hemoglobin levels between 7 and 9 g/dL with evidence of continuing hemolysis have been recommended as criteria for a transfusion. In patients with hemoglobin levels greater than 9 g/dL with persistent hemoglobinuria, close monitoring is important. Infants with neonatal jaundice secondary to G6PD deficiency may require exchange transfusion.

Differential Diagnosis

The drug-induced hemolysis of classes II and III G6PD deficiency must be differentiated from other drug-induced hemolytic anemias. This differentiation can be performed by the screening test or by quantitative assay for G6PD deficiency. Patients with chronic, nonspherocytic hemolytic anemia (class I G6PD deficiency) must be differentiated from patients with HS, hemoglobinopathies, and other enzymopathies.

ENZYMOPATHIES OF THE GLYCOLYTIC PATHWAY

The mature RBC beyond the reticulocyte stage lacks a nucleus, mitochondria, and other organelles and is unable to synthesize proteins and lipids or to perform oxidative phosphorylation.

Its energy requirements are met by the generation of ATP through glycolysis; glycolysis is essential for the function and survival of the RBC (see Fig. 9-1). It is not surprising that enzyme deficiencies or abnormalities in the glycolytic pathway would result in hemolysis or other RBC abnormalities. The most common of these disorders is PK deficiency, but defects of seven other enzymes of the RBC Embden-Meyerhof pathway have been described, including hexokinase, glucose phosphate isomerase, phosphofructokinase, aldolase, triosephosphate isomerase, phosphoglycerate kinase, and enolase deficiencies. In addition, deficiencies of 2,3-BPG mutase and phosphatase and lactate dehydrogenase have been identified, but these do not result in hemolysis.[94] Several good reviews of these enzymopathies of the glycolytic pathway have appeared in the literature.[84,92] All of these deficiencies are autosomal recessive traits except for phosphoglycerate kinase, which is X-linked, and enolase, which is presumably autosomal dominant.[94] Lactate dehydrogenase deficiency is not associated with hemolysis, and deficiencies of 2,3-BPG mutase and 2,3-BPG phosphatase are associated with mild erythrocytosis secondary to the near-absence of 2,3-BPG.[88] Table 23-4 summarizes the features associated with the glycolytic enzymopathies.[49,90,91]

Pyruvate Kinase Deficiency
History and Mode of Inheritance

PK deficiency is the first described defect and the most common one in the glycolytic pathway, accounting for about 90% of the defects of this pathway.[94] Dacie et al[95] first discussed a heterogeneous group of disorders that were referred to as *congenital nonspherocytic hemolytic anemias* in 1953. In 1954, these disorders were classified as types I and II based on the results of their autohemolysis test.[96] Several groups presented evidence that some disorder of glycolysis existed in the erythrocytes in type II cases.[96,97] In 1961 the first deficiency of PK was documented.[97] PK deficiency and class I G6PD deficiency are equally common and together constitute most of the cases of chronic hemolytic anemia that result from erythrocyte enzymopathies.[94] PK deficiency is most common in individuals of Northern European ancestry but has been reported from many areas and seems to have a worldwide distribution.[98] An especially high prevalence of this disorder has been identified in the Mifflin County, Penn., Amish population.[99] PK deficiency is an autosomal recessive disorder with only rare exceptions; both sexes are equally affected.[94] Usually, overt hemolytic disease occurs in homozygotes or compound heterozygotes; simple heterozygotes are not anemic, although their RBCs may show some enzyme alterations.[94]

Pathophysiology

PK is a rate-limiting key enzyme of the glycolytic pathway. It catalyzes the conversion of phosphoenolpyruvate to pyruvate with regeneration of ATP (see Fig. 9-1).[94] The exact mechanisms for hemolysis in PK-deficient cells are poorly understood. The ATP content is often decreased, as are the adenosine diphosphate and adenosine monophosphate contents of the RBC. The 2,3-BPG content is often increased approximately twofold.[94] These alterations in the PK-deficient RBCs result in

TABLE 23-4 Features Associated with Glycolytic Enzymopathies

Enzyme	Incidence	Inheritance	Hemolytic Anemia	Neurologic Abnormalities	Myopathy	Comments
Hexokinase (HK)	<30 cases reported	Autosomal recessive	Yes	—	—	Low 2,3-BPG level; suggestion of poor tolerance of anemia
Glucose phosphate isomerase (GPI)	Second to pyruvate kinase	Autosomal recessive	Yes	Rare	Rare	Propensity for hemolytic crisis during infection
Phosphofructokinase (PFK)	<30 cases reported	Autosomal recessive	Variable	—	Usual	Hemolysis usually fully compensated; may have erythrocytosis; early-onset gout
Aldolase (ALD)	<5 cases reported	Autosomal recessive	Yes	—	—	Only 3 reported cases
Triosephosphate isomerase (TPI)	Rare	Autosomal recessive	Yes	Usual	—	Generalized disorder; most severe of glycolytic deficiencies; neurologic, infectious, and cardiac complications
Phosphoglycerate kinase (PGK)	Rare	X-linked recessive	Yes, usually	Usual	Rare	Mental retardation; neurologic defect most serious manifestation in affected men; multisystem disease
Diphosphoglycerate mutase (DPGM) and diphosphoglycerate phosphatase (DPGP)	Very rare	Autosomal recessive	No	—	—	Both activities reside in the same enzyme protein; near-absence of 2,3-BPG; mild erythrocytosis
Enolase (ENO)	Very rare	Autosomal dominant	Yes	—	—	Partial deficiency with spherocytic phenotype
Pyruvate kinase (PK)	Most common of group	Autosomal recessive	Yes	—	—	First-described and best-studied deficiency; >300 cases reported; prototype for group; increased 2,3-BPG
Lactate dehydrogenase (LDH)	Very rare	Autosomal recessive	No	—	Usual	No hemolysis with lack of H-subunit; myopathy with lack of M-subunit

From Tanaka KR, Zeres CR: Red cell enzymopathies of glycolytic pathway. Semin Hematol 1990;27:165-185.

a rigid cell that is removed by the macrophages of the spleen and the liver.[81,100,101]

Clinical and Laboratory Findings

Individuals with PK deficiency have a wide range of clinical presentations, varying from severe neonatal anemia requiring exchange or multiple transfusions to a fully compensated hemolytic process in apparently healthy adults.[94] PK deficiency generally is more severe than hereditary spherocytosis. Except for patients seriously affected during infancy, most PK-deficient patients have a stable hemoglobin level (range 8-12 g/dL).[94] PK-deficient patients may have a greater tolerance for anemia because of their increased 2,3-BPG levels, which decreases the oxygen affinity of their hemoglobin, delivering more

oxygen to the tissues even though lower amounts of hemoglobin are present.[94] Patients who present with the deficiency in infancy may require transfusions, and splenectomy may be necessary during the first year of life.[98] Viral infections, coexistence of myelodysplastic syndrome,[101] and pregnancy may exacerbate the chronic hemolytic process. Other rare complications include kernicterus, chronic leg ulcers, acute pancreatitis secondary to biliary tract disease, development of iron overload, splenic abscess, spinal cord compression by extramedullary hematopoietic tissue, and migratory phlebitis with arterial thrombosis.[81,88,100]

The RBC morphology is not a prominent factor in the diagnosis of PK deficiency. The RBCs are normochromic with only an occasional spiculated or irregularly contracted cell, except in children with severe anemia.[98] Reticulocytosis leads to a slight to marked macrocytosis. Postsplenectomy features include the usual Howell-Jolly bodies, siderocytes, and target cells. In addition "shrunken echinocytes," crenated RBCs of unusual form, are a characteristic PK deficiency finding.[98] Frequently after splenectomy, a characteristic finding is a high percentage of reticulocytes (range 40% to 70%), which may persist.[98] The WBC and platelet counts are normal or slightly increased. Patients usually display the characteristic hallmarks of chronic hemolytic processes, such as variable degrees of jaundice, slight-to-moderate splenomegaly, and an increased incidence of gallstones. Laboratory indications of hemolysis, including an increased indirect bilirubin level, a decreased haptoglobin level, and an increased fecal urobilinogen level, may be present. The osmotic fragility of fresh cells is usually normal, but the incubated osmotic fragility test may show some abnormality.[98] The results of the incubated Heinz body test show increased numbers of Heinz bodies in the RBCs,[81] and the results of the DAT are negative. The autohemolysis test shows that many PK-deficient cells have increased hemolysis after 48 hours' incubation that is not corrected by glucose. The autohemolysis pattern varies, however, and is not useful in the diagnosis of this disorder.[98]

The diagnosis of PK deficiency depends on the specific demonstration of quantitatively reduced activity or qualitative abnormalities of erythrocyte PK.[99] Most homozygotes or compound heterozygotes have 5% to 25% of enzyme activity, and clinically normal heterozygotes have about half the normal activity.[99] The enzyme can be assayed by a spectrophotometric assay of a hemolysate prepared from RBCs with the WBCs carefully removed. Contaminating WBCs may obscure the correct results because the ratio of WBC to RBC PK activity is about 300:1.[84] The assay uses phosphoenolpyruvate (as substrate), crystalline lactate dehydrogenase, and nicotinamide adenine dinucleotide, reduced form (NADH), constituted in such a way that the oxidation of NADH is followed at 340 ηm, and optical density is decreased according to the amount of NADH oxidized to NAD (Fig. 23-10). PK is an allosteric enzyme, and its activity at low phosphoenolpyruvate concentration strongly depends on the presence of fructose diphosphate.[84] More complex techniques may be necessary when a variant form of PK is suspected.[102] Screening tests for PK deficiency are based on the same principle as that described earlier except that the hemolysate and reagents are absorbed onto filter paper, and the loss of fluorescence, rather than color, is visually evaluated to determine the oxidation of NADH of NAD.[84,88]

Therapy and Prognosis

No specific therapy is available for PK deficiency except supportive treatment and RBC transfusion as necessary. Splenectomy does not correct the hemolysis totally but usually increases the hemoglobin levels from 1 to 3 g/dL, which is enough to reduce or eliminate the need for transfusion.

Differential Diagnosis

Because PK deficiency causes chronic hemolytic anemia, it must be differentiated from hemoglobinopathies, hereditary spherocytosis, and other enzymopathies.[102] The appropriate diagnostic strategy is first to eliminate the hemoglobinopathies (through electrophoresis and morphology) and HS (through morphology, osmotic fragility, and membrane protein studies) and then to proceed to tests for enzyme disorders as have been described.[88,91,94,103,104]

PAROXYSMAL NOCTURNAL HEMOGLOBINURIA

History and Etiology

In the late 1800s, Gull[105] published a case describing a patient with hematuria that was worse in the morning. In 1882, Strubing[106] described a patient with hemoglobinuria after sleep.[106] He suggested that the RBCs were destroyed in the bloodstream. He also found a fine-grained, yellowish-brown sediment in the urine that may have been hemosiderin. In 1911, van Den Berg showed that RBCs from a similar patient were lysed in normal serum and in the patient's serum. Marchiafava and Micheli studied the disorder in detail, and for a time it was designated *Marchiafava-Micheli syndrome*.[107,108]

Paroxysmal nocturnal hemoglobinuria (PNH) is a hemolytic anemia, although it has been further classified as a myeloproliferative disorder. Intravascular hemolysis results from an RBC membrane defect that increases its susceptibility to complement.[109] The membrane defect is also present in platelets and granulocyte membranes and possibly lymphocyte membranes.[110] PNH is the only hemolytic anemia caused by an acquired abnormality (Table 22-1). The lesion arises from a clonal somatic mutation of an X chromosome gene, phosphatidylinositol glycan class A (PIGA), that occurs at the pluripotential stem cell level.[111] Several short insertions and

---

The enzyme pyruvate kinase catalyzes the following reaction:

1. ADP + Phosphoenolpyruvic acid $\xrightarrow{\text{Pyruvate Kinase}}$ ATP + Pyruvic acid

The pyruvic acid formed then takes part in the following reaction:

2. Pyruvic acid + NADH (high fluorescence) $\xrightarrow{\text{Lactate Dehydrogenase}}$ Lactic acid + NAD (no fluorescence)

Figure 23-10 Principle of PK test. In the screening test, an RBC suspension made from blood with the plasma and buffy coat removed is incubated with the reagent that contains adenosine diphosphate (ADP), phosphoenolpyruvic acid, and NADH. Lactate dehydrogenase, which also is required for the reaction, is provided by the RBCs. When PK is present, the NADH is destroyed, which results in a loss of fluorescence when spots made on filter paper are viewed under long-wave ultraviolet light. When pyruvate is deficient in the sample, the NADH remains intact, and no loss of fluorescence occurs.

deletions in the coding area have been identified.[112-115] Investigators observed that the PNH RBC population in G6PD-heterozygous patients possess only one of the enzyme variants G6PD-A or G6PD-B. Both occupy the patient's normal cells; this substantiates the clonal nature of PNH. In most patients, the abnormal clone coexists with normal hematopoiesis, resulting in a dual RBC population.[111] In the most severe cases, 95% of the RBCs are PNH RBCs. The abnormality is well-defined as the absence of glycosyl phosphatidylinositol (GPI)-linked proteins on cell surfaces secondary to the PIGA mutation. Many PNH patients have a history of idiopathic or drug-induced aplastic anemia.[106,109,112]

Pathophysiology

GPI absence and the loss of GPI-linked proteins causes increased susceptibility to complement.[106,109] PNH etiology became clear as two normal complement inhibitory proteins, decay accelerating factor (DAF, CD55) and membrane inhibitor of reactive lysis (MIRL, CD59), were shown to be absent. Consequently, incidental complement and C3 convertase complexes are not cleared from the membrane, leading to formation of the membrane attack complex, membrane pores, and cell lysis. DAF, MIRL, and other proteins require the GPI anchor.[116] GPI is modified phosphatidylinositol on the outer leaflet of the lipid bilayer that is connected to a glycan core of multiple sugars and side chains (Fig. 23-11). DAF and MIRL link through an amide bond to the PIG anchor at their C-terminus. The entire assembly is extracellular, and the surface protein is motile. The additional PIG-anchored proteins are receptors, enzymes, and a number of proteins with unknown functions, and several of these have immunologic significance (Box 23-3). All the normal GPI-linked proteins are absent from PNH cells because of the incomplete bioassembly of the GPI anchors.

PNH erythrocytes have traditionally been classified into subpopulations according to their susceptibility to complement-mediated lysis in laboratory tests. These were PNH-I, nearly normal in their susceptibility to complement; PNH-II, three to five times more sensitive; and PNH-III, 15-25 times more sensitive. Current analysis relies on flow cytometry to identify granulocyte surface expression of GPI-linked proteins CD16, CD48, CD55, and CD59.[117] Based on phenotyping, completely deficient RBCs correspond to PNH type III. Type I cells have normal amounts of PIG-anchored proteins and resist complement.

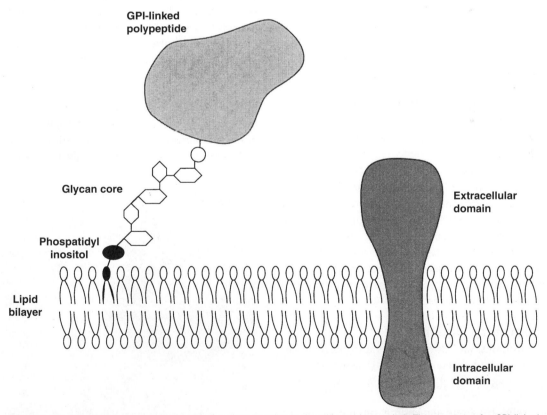

Figure 23-11 GPI anchor for attachment of surface proteins to the cell membrane. *Left,* The structure of a GPI-linked protein. The GPI anchor consists of a phosphatidylinositol molecule in the outer leaflet of the lipid bilayer, which is connected to a glycan core consisting of multiple sugars and side chains. The polypeptide is linked to the anchor at its C-terminus by an amide bond. The result is a surface protein with a fluid and mobile attachment to the cell surface. The entire polypeptide is present in the extracellular milieu. *Right,* In contrast, a transmembrane protein has an extracellular domain, a short transmembrane domain, and an intracellular domain. (From Ware RE, Rosse WF: Autoimmune hemolytic anemia. In Nathan DG, Orkin SH [eds]: Nathan and Oski's Hematology of Infancy and Childhood, 5th ed. Philadelphia: Saunders, 1998:514.)

BOX 23-3 Surface Proteins Absent from Abnormal Hematopoietic Cells in Paroxysmal Nocturnal Hemoglobinuria

Complement Regulatory Proteins
Decay accelerating factor (CD55)
Membrane inhibitor of reactive lysis (CD59)

Immunologically Important Proteins
Lymphocyte function antigen-3 (CD58)
Fc receptor γIII (CD16)
Endotoxin binding protein receptor (CD14)

Receptors
Urokinase receptor
Folate receptor

Enzymes
Alkaline phosphatase
Acetylcholinesterase
5-Ectonucleotidase

Other Proteins with Unknown Functions
CD24
CD48
CD52
CD66
CD67
JMH-bearing protein

Adapted from Rosse WF, Ware RE: The molecular basis of paroxysmal nocturnal hemoglobinuria. Blood 1995;86:3277.

When serum complement is activated, PNH RBCs fix more C3 molecules than normal. The terminal lytic complex C5 through C9 creates membrane lesions; the membrane of a PNH-III cell looks like a sieve. The percentage of PNH-III cells determines the intensity of the clinical symptoms. Fewer than 20% PNH-III yield mild hemolysis. If 20% to 50% PNH-III cells are present, the hemolysis is episodic and sleep induced. If more than 50% of RBCs are PNH-III, perpetual hemoglobinemia and hemoglobinuria exist.[113-115]

Clinical Laboratory Findings

PNH onset is insidious, and 30% of cases arise from severe aplastic anemia for 1 to several years. PNH associates with middle age or young adults of both sexes and can occur at any age.[118]

Anemia is mild to severe depending on the degree of hemolysis. Passage of red urine upon arising from sleep, from which PNH derives its name, is present in only 25% of patients.[109] Nocturnal *hemoglobinemia* is present in most, however. Hemoglobinemia is sleep induced and occurs during daytime or night-time sleep. The cause has been disputed, but many believe that the phenomenon is caused by the lowered blood pH, facilitating complement binding to PNH cells. Other causes of hemoglobinemia are infections, vaccinations, transfusions (which may increase the complement supply), x-ray contrast dye exposure, and possibly even strenuous exercise.

If the free hemoglobin in the plasma is less than 30 to 40 mg/dL, it is catabolized in the proximal tubules, and hemosiderinuria is present. Higher levels cause hemoglobinuria. Even without hemoglobinuria, hemosiderinuria is present and is detected by a Prussian blue iron stain on the urine sediment. The observer sees iron-filled renal tubular epithelial cells with blue granules (Fig. 23-12). Most patients develop iron deficiency anemia because of this heavy loss of iron in the urine. Infections are common because of defects in neutrophil function.

Patients with PNH are predisposed to thrombosis,[119] especially in the hepatic portal circulation or the venous circulation of the brain.[120] Hepatic vein thrombosis or Budd-Chiari syndrome results in severe, colicky abdominal pain, often with a poor prognosis.[118] The thrombosis has been attributed to increased susceptibility of PNH platelets to complement activation.[121] Patients with PNH have self-limited attacks of abdominal pain, presumably caused by intestinal infarction or bleeding. Severe headaches may be caused by thrombi in small vessels of the brain.[121] Severely thrombocytopenic PNH patients may show bleeding tendencies.[109]

PNH may evolve into acute myeloid leukemia with an incidence of 1% to 3%. Leukemia transformation typically occurs within the first 5 years.[118]

Hematologic Findings

PNH is a mild-to-severe pancytopenic normochromic/normocytic anemia. Hemoglobin varies from 6 g/dL to normal. Reticulocyte counts are mildly to moderately elevated,

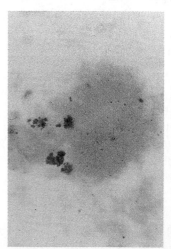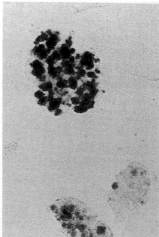

Figure 23-12 Renal tubular cells laden with hemosiderin and ferritin from a patient with PNH. (From Hoffbrand AV, Pettit JE: Clinical Haematology Illustrated: An Integrated Text and Colour Atlas. Edinburgh: Churchill Livingstone, 1987:4.4.)

less than would be expected in other hemolytic anemias of comparable intensity. The MCV may be slightly elevated, reflecting reticulocytosis. Osmotic fragility is normal, and the DAT is negative. If the patient does not receive transfusions, iron deficiency develops, and the RBCs become microcytic and hypochromic. Plasma iron and ferritin are low, and the total iron-binding capacity is elevated. Likewise, folate deficiency often occurs, leading to secondary macrocytosis.[118]

Moderate neutropenia (causing leukopenia) is almost always present, although the neutrophil life span appears normal. The leukocyte alkaline phosphatase level is very low.[122] PNH granulocytes have functional defects that decrease resistance to pyogenic organisms.[123] Infection causes 5% to 10% of fatalities in PNH patients. The platelet count may range from 50-100 × 10^9/L, although the life span seems to be normal.[109,124]

The bone marrow is normocellular with RBC hyperplasia and a reduced M:E ratio. Some patients have aplasia or hypocellularity. Iron is often absent unless the patient has received transfusions, in which case it may be normal or elevated.[109]

Hemosiderinuria is a constant feature of PNH and is of diagnostic importance.[109] A Prussian blue stain of the urine sediment reveals blue-staining hemosiderin granules in sloughed renal tubular epithelial cells (see Fig. 23-12). Hemoglobinuria may be distinguished from hematuria by a positive reagent strip blood result accompanied by absence of RBCs in the urine microscopic examination. Hemoglobinuria may lead to formation and detection of Hb casts. Renal insufficiency resulting from the iron deposition may occur in PNH patients.[109,111,125]

Special Diagnostic Tests

The diagnosis of PNH should be suspected in any patient with idiopathic pancytopenia and acquired nonspherocytic anemia accompanied by reticulocytosis. Screening tests traditionally have been the urine hemosiderin determination and the sugar water test (sucrose hemolysis test). If the sugar water test result was positive, the Ham test (acidified serum lysis test) was used to confirm the diagnosis.[109]

Peripheral blood erythrocytes and granulocytes now can be analyzed by flow cytometry for surface expression of GPI-linked proteins, such as CD16, CD48, CD55, and CD59. The simplest method is to measure the expressed CD59 on the RBCs. Immunophenotype analysis of RBCs in PNH can determine the amount of types I, II, and III cells (Fig. 23-13).[117]

Therapy and Prognosis

The treatment of PNH is mainly supportive, with transfusions, antibiotics, and anticoagulants. Iron therapy is given to help alleviate the iron deficiency caused by the urinary loss of Hb. Steroids given every other day may decrease the hemolysis in some patients. Androgenic steroids seem to be effective in cases with prominent marrow hypoplasia. Anticoagulants are used in the treatment of thrombotic complications, such as Budd-Chiari syndrome. In suitable patients, stem cell transplantation may be an option and can be a curative therapy.[109]

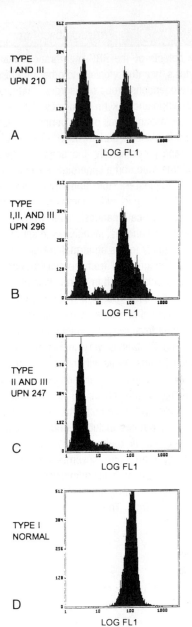

Figure 23-13 Immunophenotype analysis of erythrocytes in PNH by flow cytometry. Examples of surface CD59 expression are shown for three patients and a control. **A,** Data for unique patient number (UPN) 210, who had type I and type III erythrocytes. **B,** Data for UPN 296 with types I, II, and III cells. **C,** Data for UPN 247 with predominantly type III erythrocytes and a few type II cells. **D,** Normal expression from a control. (Data from Ware RE, Rosse WF, Hall SE: Immunophenotypic analysis of reticulocytes in paroxysmal nocturnal hemoglobinuria. Blood 1995;86:1586.)

The clinical course of PNH varies widely. Rarely, a patient dies of the disorder within a few months, but most patients experience a chronic course, with the symptom severity changing from time to time as the amount of normal cells and PNH clone cells change. The disease is very serious, and most patients die from its various complications, such as thrombotic episodes or pancytopenia. Some PNH patients may develop acute leukemia as a terminal event.[126]

CHAPTER at a GLANCE

- Hereditary defects of the RBC membrane include HS, HE, HPP, stomatocytosis, acanthocytosis, and other rare disorders.
- HS is a heterogeneous group of disorders that usually have some degree of spectrin and ankyrin deficiency and are characterized by numerous microspherocytes on the peripheral blood smear.
- The membrane skeletal protein abnormalities cause the RBC to lose membrane progressively and acquire a decreased surface area–to–volume ratio and a spheroidal shape.
- The spleen sequesters the abnormal RBCs, resulting in a decreased RBC life span and a hemolytic process.
- The three key clinical manifestations with which HS patients usually present are anemia, jaundice, and splenomegaly.
- The osmotic fragility test is abnormal in HS.
- HS must be distinguished from hemolytic anemia with spherocytes that is associated with immune disorders.
- HE is a heterogeneous group of disorders characterized by the presence of elliptical or oval erythrocytes on the peripheral blood smear that result from skeletal protein abnormalities.
- The clinical manifestations vary in HE from a silent carrier, to mild common HE that is usually not associated with anemia or splenomegaly, to HE with chronic hemolysis.
- HPP is probably a subtype of HE and presents with a severe hemolytic anemia with marked poikilocytosis on the blood smear.
- The RBC enzymopathies include G6PD deficiency and enzymopathies of the glycolytic pathway.
- G6PD deficiency is an X chromosome–linked genetic abnormality that results in acute hemolytic anemia secondary to drug exposure or infection, favism, or neonatal jaundice or in chronic, nonspherocytic hemolytic anemia. There are more than 400 mutations of G6PD.

- Most individuals with G6PD deficiency are asymptomatic except during oxidative stress resulting from drugs or other causes.
- Quantitative assays of RBC G6PD enzyme activity can be performed to establish the diagnosis.
- PK deficiency is the most common of the glycolytic pathway enzyme deficiencies and can have a wide range of clinical presentations varying from severe neonatal anemia requiring exchange or multiple transfusion to a fully compensated hemolytic process.
- RBC morphology is not a prominent factor in the diagnosis of PK deficiency. Rather, diagnosis depends on the specific demonstration of quantitatively reduced activity or qualitative abnormalities of erythrocyte PK.
- PNH is an acquired blood cell abnormality caused by a myeloproliferative clonal disorder of the bone marrow that results in increased susceptibility of blood cells to complement, causing a hemolytic anemia.
- The genetic defect of PNH is a mutation in the coding area of a gene designated as PIGA on the X chromosome, which causes the absence of proteins that use a glycosyl phosphatidylinositol anchor membrane for membrane attachment.
- Screening tests for PNH include sugar water, acidified serum, and urine hemosiderin tests. Definitive testing relies on the flow cytometric analysis of peripheral blood for CD55 and CD59.

Now that you have completed this chapter, go back and read again the case study at the beginning and respond to the questions presented.

REVIEW QUESTIONS

1. An outstanding abnormality of hereditary spherocytosis noted in the CBC is:
   a. Increased MCV
   b. Increased MCHC
   c. Decreased MCH
   d. Decreased platelet and WBC count

2. The altered shape of the spherocyte in HS is due to:
   a. Abnormal RBC membrane protein
   b. Defective RNA synthesis
   c. An extrinsic factor in the plasma
   d. Abnormality in the globin composition of the Hb molecule

3. Which of the following results are consistent with HS?
   a. Increased osmotic fragility, negative DAT
   b. Decreased osmotic fragility, positive DAT
   c. Increased osmotic fragility, positive DAT
   d. Decreased osmotic fragility, negative DAT

4. RBCs in HE are abnormally shaped and have unstable cell membranes as a result of:
   a. Abnormal shear stresses in the circulation
   b. Fragile self-association of spectrin to spectrin
   c. Ankyrin abnormalities
   d. Lack of all Rh antigens in the RBC membrane

5. The blood picture for patients with mild common HE is characterized by:
   a. Budding and spherocytes along with elliptocytes on the peripheral blood smear and a hemolytic anemia
   b. 100% elliptocytes on the blood smear and a hemolytic anemia
   c. Greater than 30% elliptocytes on the blood smear and no anemia, but patient may have a mild compensated hemolysis
   d. Greater than 50% elliptocytes and greatly increased polychromatophilic RBCs on the peripheral blood smear, but no abnormal hemolysis

6. Laboratory tests for patients with hereditary pyropoikilocytosis include all of the following *except*:
   a. RBCs that show marked thermal sensitivity at 45° C to 46° C
   b. Marked poikilocytosis with elliptocytes, RBC fragments, budding RBCs, spherocytes, and triangular RBCs
   c. Markedly increased osmotic fragility and autohemolysis
   d. Increased MCV and normal RBC distribution width

7. Acanthocytes are found in association with:
   a. Abetalipoproteinemia
   b. G6PD deficiency
   c. Rh_{null} phenotype
   d. Vitamin B_{12} deficiency

8. The classic manifestation of G6PD deficiency is:
   a. Chronic hemolytic anemia owing to cell shape change
   b. Acute hemolytic anemia owing to drug exposure
   c. Mild compensated hemolysis
   d. Chronic hemolytic anemia owing to intravascular RBC lysis

9. A patient experiences an episode of acute intravascular hemolysis after being placed on an antibiotic for the first time. The physician suspects that the patient may have G6PD deficiency and orders an RBC G6PD assay 2 days after the hemolytic episode begins. How should the laboratory professional respond to this test order?

   a. Perform the assay as ordered and report the results.
   b. Refuse to perform the assay at this time, explaining to the physician that it is too late and that the sample should have been drawn during the hemolytic peak.
   c. Refuse to perform the assay at this time, explaining to the physician that the test should be performed 7 to 10 days after the hemolysis begins, coordinating with the increase in reticulocytes.
   d. Refuse to perform the assay at this time explaining to the physician that the test must wait until the patient has recovered from the hemolysis and is again in equilibrium.

10. The most common defect or deficiency in the anaerobic glycolytic pathway is:
    a. PK
    b. Lactate dehydrogenase
    c. G6PD
    d. Methemoglobin reductase

11. Which of the following laboratory tests would be best to confirm PNH?
    a. DAT
    b. Osmotic fragility test
    c. Flow cytometry analysis for CD55 and CD59
    d. Uroporphyrin

ACKNOWLEDGMENT

The author acknowledges Martha S. Payne, who was the principal author of this chapter in the previous edition.

REFERENCES

1. Gallagher PG: Disorders of the red blood cell membrane: hereditary spherocytosis, elliptocytosis and related disorders. In Lichtman MA, Beutler E, Kipps T, et al (eds): Williams Hematology, 7th ed. New York: McGraw-Hill, 2006:571-601.
2. Singer SJ, Nicholson GL: The fluid mosaic model of the structure of cell membranes. Science 1972;175:720-731.
3. Iolascon A, Perrotta S, Stewart GW: Red blood cell membrane defects. Rev Clin Exp Hematol 2003;7:22-56.
4. Vanlair C, Masius JB: De la microcythemie. Bull R Acad Med Belg 1871;5:515.
5. Minkowski O: Ueber eine hereditare, unter dem Bilde eines chronischen lkterus mit Urobilinurie, Splenomegalie und Neirenside-rosis verlaufende Affektion. Verh Dtsch Kongr Med 1900;18:316.
6. Agre P, Orringer EP, Bennett V, et al: Deficient red cell spectrin in severe recessively inherited spherocytosis. N Engl J Med 1982;306:1155-1161.
7. Gallagher PG, Lux SE: Disorders of the erythrocyte membrane. In Nathan DG, Orkin SH, Ginsburg D, et al (eds): Nathan and Oski's Hematology of Infancy and Childhood. Philadelphia: Saunders, 2003:560-684.
8. Savvides P, Shalev O, John KM, et al: Combined spectrin and ankyrin deficiency is common in autosomal dominant hereditary spherocytosis. Blood 1993;82:2953-2960.
9. Inoue T, Kanzaki A, Yawata A, et al: Uniquely higher incidence of isolated or combined deficiency of band 3 and/or band 4.2 as the pathogenesis of autosomal dominantly inherited hereditary spherocytosis in Japanese population. Int J Hematol 1994;60:227-238.
10. Eber SW, Armbrust R, Schroter W: Variable clinical severity of hereditary spherocytosis: relation to erythrocyte spectrin concentration, osmotic fragility and autohemolysis. J Pediatr 1990;117:409-416.
11. Boivin P, Galand C, Devaus I, et al: Spectrin alpha IIa variant in dominant and non-dominant spherocytosis. Hum Genet 1993;92:153-156.
12. Hassoun H, Vassiliadis JN, Murray J, et al: Characterization of the underlying molecular defect in hereditary spherocytosis associated with spectrin deficiency [abstract]. Blood 1995;86(Suppl 1):476a.
13. Heine GH, Sester U, Girndt M, et al: Acanthocytes in the urine: useful tool to differentiate diabetic nephropathy from glomerulonephritis? Diabetes Care 2004;27:190-194.
14. Shah S, Vega R: Hereditary spherocytosis. Pediatr Rev 2004;25:168-172.
15. Jijina F, Ghosh K, Mukherjee M, et al: Hereditary spherocytosis in North India: need for more extensive data. J Assoc Physicians India 2003;51:1025; author reply 1025-1026.
16. Hanspal M, Yoon SH, Yu H, et al: Molecular basis of spectrin and ankyrin deficiencies in severe hereditary spherocytosis: evidence implicating a primary defect of ankyrin. Blood 1991;77:165-173.

17. Eber SW, Gonzalez JM, Lux ML, et al: Ankyrin-1 mutations are a major cause of dominant and recessive hereditary spherocytosis. Nat Genet 1996;13:214-218.

18. Alloisio N, Texier P, Vallier A, et al: Modulation of clinical expression and band 3 deficiency in hereditary spherocytosis. Blood 1997;90:414-420.

19. Jarolim P, Rubin HL, Brabec V, et al: Mutations of conserved arginines in the membrane domain of erythroid band 3 lead to a decrease in membrane-associated band 3 and to the phenotype of hereditary spherocytosis. Blood 1995;85:634-640.

20. Yawata Y: Red cell membrane protein band 4.2: phenotypic genetic and electron microscopic aspects. Biochim Biophys Acta 1994;1204:131-148.

21. Jandl J: Hemolytic anemias caused by primary defects of red cell membranes. In Jandl JH (ed): Blood. Boston: Little, Brown, 1987:237-264.

22. Malorni W, Iosi F, Donelli G, et al: A new, striking morphologic feature for the human erythrocyte in hereditary spherocytosis: the blebbing pattern [letter]. Blood 1993;81:2821-2822.

23. Tse WT, Lux SE: Hereditary spherocytosis and hereditary elliptocytosis. In Scriver CR, Beaudet AL, Sly WS, et al (eds): The Metabolic and Molecular Bases of Inherited Disease, 8th ed. New York: McGraw-Hill, 2001:4665-4727.

24. Pajor A, Lehoczky D, Szakacs Z: Pregnancy and hereditary spherocytosis. Arch Gynecol Obstet 1993;253:37-42.

25. Gallagher PG: Disorders of the red blood cell membrane: hereditary spherocytosis, elliptocytosis and related disorders. In Lichtman MA, Beutler E, Kipps TJ, et al (eds): Williams Hematology, 7th ed. New York: McGraw-Hill, 2006:571-601.

26. Friedman EW, Williams JC, Van Hook L: Hereditary spherocytosis in the elderly. Am J Med 1988;84:513-556.

27. Agre P, Asimos A, Casella JF, et al: Inheritance pattern and clinical response to splenectomy as a reflection of erythrocyte spectrin deficiency in hereditary spherocytosis. N Engl J Med 1986;315:1579-1583.

28. Gehlbach SH, Cooper BA: Haemolytic anaemia in infectious mononucleosis due to inapparent congenital spherocytosis. Scand J Haematol 1970;7:141-144.

29. Mentzer WC, Glader B: Hereditary spherocytosis and other anemias due to abnormalities of the red cell membrane. In Greer JP, Foerster J, Lukens JN, et al (eds): Wintrobe's Clinical Hematology, 11th ed. Philadelphia: Lippincott, Williams & Wilkins, 2004:1089-1114.

30. Kedar PS, Colah RB, Ghosh K, et al: Hereditary spherocytosis in association with severe G6PD deficiency: report of an unusual case. Clin Chim Acta 2004;344:221-224.

31. Davidson RJ, Brown T, Wiseman D: Human parvovirus infection and aplastic crisis in hereditary spherocytosis. J Infect 1984;9:298-300.

32. Dhaliwal G, Cornett PA, Tierney LM Jr: Hemolytic anemia. Am Fam Physician 2004;69:2599-2606.

33. Lawrence P, Aronson I, Saxe N, et al: Leg ulcers in hereditary spherocytosis. Clin Exp Dermatol 1991;16:28-30.

34. Gilsanz F, Richard MP, Millan I: Diagnosis of hereditary spherocytosis with dual-angle differential light scattering. Am J Clin Pathol 1993;100:119-122.

35. Michaels LA, Cohen AR, Zhao H, et al: Screening for hereditary spherocytosis by use of automated erythrocyte indexes. J Pediatr 1997;130:957-960.

36. Emerson CP Jr, Shen SC, Haleham T, et al: Studies of the destruction of red blood cells: IX. Quantitative methods for determining the osmotic and mechanical fragility of red cells in the peripheral blood and splenic pulp: the mechanism of increased hemolysis in hereditary spherocytosis (congenital hemolytic jaundice) as related to the function of the spleen. Arch Intern Med 1956;97:1-38.

37. Marik T, Brabec V: Acidified glycerol lysis test in various haemolytic anaemias. Folia Haematol Int Mag Klin Morphol Blutforsch 1990;117:259-263.

38. Pinto L, Iolascon A, Miraglia del Guidice E, et al: A modification of the "pink test" may improve the diagnosis of hereditary spherocytosis. Acta Haematol 1989;82:53-54.

39. Streichman S, Gesheidt Y, Tatarsky I: Hypertonic cryohemolysis: a diagnostic test for hereditary spherocytosis. Am J Hematol 1990;35:104-109.

40. Eraktis AJ, Kevy SV, Diamond LK, et al: Hazards of overwhelming infection after splenectomy in childhood. N Engl J Med 1967;276:1225-1229.

41. Stoehr GA, Stauffer UG, Eber SW: Near-total splenectomy: a new technique for the management of hereditary spherocytosis. Ann Surg 2005;241:40-47.

42. Dresbach M: Elliptical human red corpuscles. Science 1904;19:469.

43. Telen MJ, Le Van Kim C, Chung A, et al: Molecular basis for elliptocytosis associated with glycophorin C and glycophorin D deficiency in the Leach phenotype. Blood 1991;78:1603-1606.

44. Gallagher PG: Hereditary elliptocytosis: spectrin and protein 4.1R. Semin Hematol 2004;41:142-164.

45. Gallagher PG: Update on the clinical spectrum and genetics of red blood cell membrane disorders. Curr Hematol Rep 2004;3:85-91.

46. Alloisio N, Morle L, Marechal J, et al: Sp $\alpha^{v/41}$: a common spectrin polymorphism at the α^{IV}-α^{V} domain junction: relevance to the expression level of hereditary elliptocytosis due to α-spectrin variants located in trans. J Clin Invest 1991;87:2169-2177.

47. Coetzer T, Sahr K, Prchal J, et al: Four different mutations in codon 28 of α spectrin are associated with structurally and functionally abnormal spectrin $\alpha^{1/74}$ in hereditary elliptocytosis. J Clin Invest 1991;88:743-749.

48. Palek J: Hereditary elliptocytosis and related disorders. Clin Haematol 1985;14:45-87.

49. Zarkowsky HS: Heat-induced erythrocyte fragmentation in neonatal elliptocytosis. Br J Haematol 1979;41:515-518.

50. Mentzer WC Jr, Iarocci T, Mohandas N, et al: Modulation of erythrocyte membrane mechanical fragility by 2,3-diphosphoglycerate in the neonatal poikilocytosis/elliptocytosis syndrome. J Clin Invest 1987;79:943-949.

51. Suzuki Y, Nakajima T, Shiga T, et al: Influence of 2,3 diphosphoglycerate on the deformability of human erythrocytes. Biochim Biophys Acta 1990;1029:85-90.

52. Coetzer T, Lawler J, Prchal JT, et al: Molecular determinants of clinical expression of hereditary elliptocytosis and pyropoikilocytosis. Blood 1987;70:766-772.

53. Liu SC, Zhai S, Palek J, et al: Molecular defect of the band 3 protein in Southeast Asian ovalocytosis. N Engl J Med 1990;323:1530-1538.

54. Cattani JA, Gibson FD, Alpers MP, et al: Hereditary ovalocytosis and reduced susceptibility to malaria in Papua New Guinea. Trans R Soc Trop Med Hyg 1987;81:705-709.

55. Hanspal M, Hanspal JS, Sahr KE, et al: Molecular basis of spectrin deficiency in hereditary pyropoikilocytosis. Blood 1993;82:1652-1660.

56. Kanzaki A, Yawata Y: Hereditary stomatocytosis: phenotypical expression of sodium transport and band 7 peptides in 44 cases. Br J Haematol 1992;82:133-141.

57. Lande WM, Mentzer WC: Haemolytic anemia associated with increased cation permeability. Clin Haematol 1985;14:89-103.

58. Nolan GR: Hereditary xerocytosis: a case history and review of the literature. Pathology 1984;16:151-154.

59. Delaunay J: The hereditary stomatocytoses: genetic disorders of the red cell membrane permeability to monovalent cations. Semin Hematol 2004;41:165-172.

60. Rees DC, Portmann B, Ball C, et al: Dehydrated hereditary stomatocytosis is associated with neonatal hepatitis. Br J Haematol 2004;126:272-276.

61. Jokinen CH, Swaim WR, Nuttall FQ: A case of hereditary xerocytosis diagnosed as a result of suspected hypoglycemia and observed low glycohemoglobin. J Lab Clin Med 2004;144:27-30.

62. Gallagher PG, Chang SH, Rettig MP, et al: Altered erythrocyte endothelial adherence and membrane phospholipid asymmetry in hereditary hydrocytosis. Blood 2003;101:4625-4627.

63. Reinhart WH, Bartsch P, Straub PW: Red blood cell morphology after a 100 km run. Clin Lab Haematol 1989;11:105-110.

64. Ballas SK, Clark MR, Mohandas N, et al: Red cell membrane and cation deficiency in Rh null syndrome. Blood 1984;63:1046-1055.

65. Vos GH, Vos D, Kirk RL, et al: A sample of blood with no detectable Rh antigens. Lancet 1961;1:14-15.

66. Kane JP, Havel RJ: Disorders of the biogenesis and secretion of lipoproteins containing the B apolipoproteins. In Scriver CR, Beaudet AL, Sly WS, et al (eds): Metabolic and Molecular Bases of Inherited Disease. New York: McGraw-Hill, 2001:2717-2752.

67. Redman CM, Marsh WLI, Scarborough A, et al: Biochemical studies on McLeod phenotype red cells and isolation of Kx antigen. Br J Haematol 1988;68:131-136.

68. Udden MM, Umeda M, Hirano Y, et al: New abnormalities in the morphology of cell surface receptors, and electrolyte metabolism of In(Lu) erythrocytes. Blood 1987;69:52-57.

69. Arie THD: Pythagoras and beans. Oxf Med School Gaz 1959;11:75-81.

70. Fermi C, Martinetti P: Studio sul favismo. Ann Ig Sper 1905;15:75.

71. Alving AS, Carson PE, Flanagan CL, et al: Enzymatic deficiency in primaquine sensitive erythrocytes. Science 1956;124:484-485.

72. Beutler E: Disorders of red cells resulting from enzyme deficiencies. In Lichtman MA, Beutler E, Kipps TJ, et al (eds): Williams Hematology, 7th ed. New York: McGraw-Hill, 2006:603-631.

73. Luzzatto L: Glucose-6-phosphate dehydrogenase deficiency and hemolytic anemia. In Nathan DG (ed): Nathan and Oski's Hematology of Infancy and Childhood, 6th ed. Philadelphia: Saunders, 2003:721-742.

74. Luzzatto L, Mehta A, Vulliamy T: Glucose-6-phosphate dehydrogenase. In Scriver CR, Beaudet AL, Sly WS, et al (eds): The Metabolic and Molecular Bases of Inherited Disease. New York: McGraw-Hill, 2001:4517-4554.

75. Iranpour R, Akbar MR, Haghshenas I: Glucose-6-phosphate dehydrogenase deficiency in neonates. Indian J Pediatr 2003;70:855-857.

76. Kaplan M, Hammerman C: Glucose-6-phosphate dehydrogenase deficiency: a hidden risk for kernicterus. Semin Perinatol 2004;28:356-364.

77. Hamilton JW, Jones FG, McMullin MF: Glucose-6-phosphate dehydrogenase Guadalajara—a case of chronic non-spherocytic haemolytic anaemia responding to splenectomy and the role of splenectomy in this disorder. Hematology 2004;9:307-309.

78. Au WY, Ma ES, Lam VM, et al: Glucose 6-phosphate dehydrogenase (G6PD) deficiency in elderly Chinese women heterozygous for G6PD variants. Am J Med Genet 2004;129:208-211.

79. Beutler E: Study of glucose-6-phosphate dehydrogenase: history and molecular biology. Am J Hematol 1993;42:53-58.

80. Beutler E: G6PD deficiency. Blood 1967;84:3613-3636.

81. Borges A, Desforges JF: Studies of Heinz body formation. Acta Haematol 1967;37:1-10.

82. Jacob H: Mechanism of Heinz body formation and attachment to red cell membrane. Semin Hematol 1970;7:341-354.

83. Beutler E: Glucose-6-phosphate dehydrogenase deficiency. N Engl J Med 1991;324:169-174.

84. Glader B: Hereditary hemolytic anemias due to enzyme disorders. In Greer JP, Foerster J, Lukens JN, et al (eds): Wintrobe's Clinical Hematology, 11th ed. Philadelphia: Lippincott, Williams & Wilkins., 2006:1115-1140.

85. Ruwende C, Hill A: Glucose-6-phosphate dehydrogenase deficiency and malaria. J Mol Med 1998;76:581-588.

86. Rother RP, Bell L, Hillmen P, et al: The clinical sequelae of intravascular hemolysis and extracellular plasma hemoglobin: a novel mechanism of human disease. JAMA 2005;293:1653-1662.

87. Beydemir S, Gulcin I, Kufrevioglu OI, et al: Glucose 6-phosphate dehydrogenase: in vitro and in vivo effects of dantrolene sodium. Pol J Pharmacol 2003;55:787-792.

88. Tagarelli A, Piro A, Tagarelli G, et al: G6PD/PK ratio: a reliable parameter to identify glucose-6-phosphate dehydrogenase deficiency associated with microcytic anemia in heterozygous subjects. Clin Biochem 2004;37:863-866.

89. Efferth T, Bachli EB, Schwarzl SM, et al: Glucose-6-phosphate dehydrogenase (G6PD) deficiency-type Zurich: a splice site mutation as an uncommon mechanism producing enzyme deficiency. Blood 2004;104:2608.

90. Usanga EA, Luzzatto L: Adaptation of *Plasmodium falciparum* to glucose-6-phosphate dehydrogenase deficient host red cells by production of parasite-encoded enzyme. Nature 1985;313:793-795.

91. Beutler E: Erythrocyte enzyme assays. In Beutler E, Lichtman MA, Coller BS, et al (eds): Williams Hematology, 5th ed. New York: McGraw-Hill, 1995:L45-L47.

92. Brew GJ, Tarlov AR, Alving AS, et al: The methemoglobin reduction for primaquine-type sensitivity of erythrocytes: a simplified procedure for detecting a specific hypersusceptibility to drug hemolysis. JAMA 1962;180:386-388.

93. Jacob HS, Jandl JA: A simple visual screening test for glucose-6-phosphate dehydrogenase deficiency employing ascorbate and cyanide. N Engl J Med 1966;274:1162-1167.

94. Tanaka KR, Zerez C: Red cell enzymopathies of the glycolytic pathway. Semin Hematol 1990;27:165-186.

95. Dacie JV, Mollison PL, Richardson N, et al: Atypical congential hemolytic anemia. QJM 1953;22:79.

96. Selwyn JG, Dacie JV: Autohemolysis and other changes resulting from the incubation in vitro of red cells from patients with congenital hemolytic anemia. Blood 1954;9:414-438.

97. Robinson MA, Loder PB, DeGruchy GC: Red cell metabolism in non-spherocytic congenital haemolytic anemia. Br J Haematol 1961;7:327-339.

98. Mentzer WC: Pyruvate kinase deficiency and disorders of glycolysis. In Nathan DG, Orkin SH, Ginsburg D, et al (eds): Nathan and Oski's Hematology of Infancy and Childhood, 6th ed. Philadelphia: Saunders, 2003:685-720.

99. Frye RE: Pyruvate kinase deficiency. Available at: http://www.emedicine.com/med/TOPIC1980.htm. Accessed June 3, 2006.

100. Aizawa S, Kohdera U, Hiramoto M, et al: Ineffective erythropoiesis in the spleen of a patient with pyruvate kinase deficiency. Am J Hematol 2003;74:68-72.

101. Ryan C, Percy M, O'Brien D, et al: Myelodysplastic syndrome in a patient with hereditary pyruvate kinase deficiency. Hematol J 2004;5:91-92.

102. Blume KG, Arnold H, Löhr GW, et al: Additional diagnostic procedures for the detection of abnormal red cell pyruvate kinase. Clin Chim Acta 1973;42:443-446.

103. Keitt AS: Diagnostic strategy in a suspected enzymopathy. Clin Haematol 1981;10:3-30.

104. Andersen FD, d'Amore F, Nielsen FC, et al: Unexpectedly high but still asymptomatic iron overload in a patient with pyruvate kinase deficiency. Hematol J 2004;5:543-545.

105. Gull W: A case of intermittent hematuria with remarks. Guys Hosp Rep 1866;12:381.

106. Crosby WH: Paroxysmal nocturnal hemoglobinuria: a classic description by Paul Strubing in 1882, and a bibliography of the disease. Blood 1951;6:270-284.

107. Marchiafava E: Anemia emolitica con emosiderinuria perpituai. Policlinico (sez med) 1931;18:241.

108. Micheli F: Anemia (splenomegalia) emolitica con emoglobinuria-emosiderinuria tipo Marchiafava. Haematologica 1931;12:101.

109. Beutler E: Paroxysmal nocturnal hemoglobinuria. In Lichtman MA, Beutler E, Kipps TJ, et al (eds): Williams Hematology, 7th ed. New York: McGraw-Hill, 2006:469-475.

110. Hillmen P, Bessler M, Crawford DH, et al: Production and characterization of lymphoblastoid cell lines with the paroxysmal nocturnal hemoglobinuria phenotype. Blood 1993;81:193-199.

111. Schwartz RS: Black mornings, yellow sunsets—a day with paroxysmal nocturnal hemoglobinuria. N Engl J Med 2004;350:537-538.

112. Smith LJ: Paroxysmal nocturnal hemoglobinuria. Clin Lab Sci 2004;17:172-177.

113. Schwartz RS: PIG-A: the target gene in paroxysmal nocturnal hemoglobinuria. N Engl J Med 1994;330:249-255.

114. Rosse WF, Ware RE: The molecular basis of paroxysmal nocturnal hemoglobinuria. Blood 1995;86:3277-3286.

115. Ostendorf T, Nischan C, Schubert J, et al: Heterogeneous PIG-A mutations in different cell linages in paroxysmal nocturnal hemoglobinuria. Blood 1995;85:1640-1646.

116. Low MG, Saltiel AR: Structural and functional roles of glycosylphosphatidylinositol in membranes. Science 1988;239:268-275.

117. Hall SE, Rosse WF: The use of monoclonal antibodies and flow cytometry in the diagnosis of paroxysmal nocturnal hemoglobinuria. Blood 1996;87:5332-5340.

118. Ware RE: Autoimmune hemolytic anemias. In Nathan DG, Orkin SH, Ginsburg D, et al (eds): Nathan and Oski's Hematology of Infancy and Childhood, 6th ed. Philadelphia: Saunders, 2003:521-559.

119. Hillmen P, Lewis SM, Bessler M, et al: Natural history of paroxysmal nocturnal hemoglobinuria. N Engl J Med 1995;333:1253-1258.

120. Socié G, Mary JY, de Gramont A, et al: Paroxysmal nocturnal haemoglobinuria: long-term follow-up and prognostic factors. Lancet 1996;348:573-577.

121. Blaas P, Berger B, Weber S, et al: Paroxysmal nocturnal hemoglobinuria: enhanced stimulation of platelets by the terminal complement components is related to the lack of C8bp in the membrane. J Immunol 1988;140:3045-3051.

122. Kawakami Z, Ninomiya H, Tomiyama J, et al: Deficiency of glycosyl-phosphatidylinositol anchored proteins on paroxysmal nocturnal haemoglobinuria neutrophils and monocytes. Br J Haematol 1990;74:508-513.

123. Craddock PR, Fehr J, Jacob HS: Complement-mediated granulocyte dysfunction in paroxysmal nocturnal hemoglobinuria. Blood 1976;47:931-939.

124. Boschetti C, Fermo E, Bianchi P, et al: Clinical and molecular aspects of 23 patients affected by paroxysmal nocturnal hemoglobinuria. Am J Hematol 2004;77:36-44.

125. Clark DA, Butler SA, Braren V, et al: The kidneys in paroxysmal nocturnal hemoglobinuria. Blood 1981;57:83-89.

126. Devine DV, Gluck WL, Rosse WF, et al: Acute myeloblastic leukemia in paroxysmal nocturnal hemoglobinuria clone. J Clin Invest 1987;79:314-317.

Extracorpuscular Defects Leading to Increased Erythrocyte Destruction—Nonimmune Causes

Vishnu V. B. Reddy

24

OBJECTIVES

After completion of this chapter, the reader will be able to:

1. List the five characteristics of thrombotic thrombocytopenic purpura (TTP).
2. Describe red blood cell (RBC) morphology in TTP.
3. State the triad of characteristics of hemolytic-uremic syndrome.
4. Name the most common cause of hemolytic anemia worldwide.
5. Describe the life cycle of the malarial parasite, including the insect vector, and state when in the cycle it is preferable to collect the blood sample to identify the organism.
6. List at least four characteristics that distinguish *Plasmodium vivax*.
7. List three characteristics of *Plasmodium malariae*.
8. List three characteristics of *Plasmodium falciparum*.
9. Distinguish *Babesia microti* from *P. falciparum*.
10. Describe morphologic RBC changes in patients with third-degree burns involving more than 20% of the body.
11. Explain traumatic cardiac hemolytic anemia occurring after corrective cardiac surgery with aortic valve replacement.
12. Recognize laboratory and clinical results consistent with each of the conditions.
13. Describe the preparation of two types of blood smears needed to diagnose malaria and the value of each.
14. Name the normal blood smear finding that can be confused with malarial parasites.

CASE STUDY

After studying the material in this chapter, the reader should be able to respond to the following case study:

A 24-year-old woman from Zaire was brought to the emergency department because of periodic fever, chills, night sweats, and fatigue. Her laboratory data revealed the following:
Hematocrit: 0.35 L/L
Reticulocytes: 275×10^9/L
WBC count: 11×10^9/L
Thin smear: slight variation in diameter of RBCs; inclusions noted in the RBCs (similar to Figs. 24-1 and 24-2); diffusely basophilic RBCs

Thick film (or thick drop preparation): many inclusions observed (similar to Fig. 24-3)
The patient was treated with quinine.

1. Describe the type of inclusions present on the blood smear.
2. Describe the inclusions on the thick film.
3. Justify the diagnosis.

Continued

311

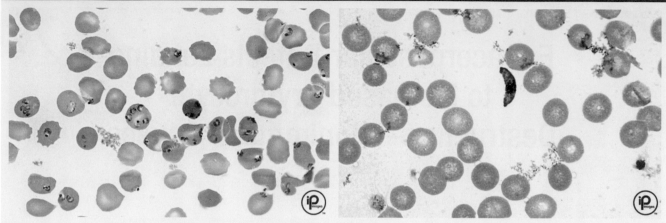

Figure 24-1 Thin blood smear. (From Marler LM, et al: Parasitology Image Atlas CD-Rom. Indiana Pathology Images, 2003, Indianapolis, Ind.)

Figure 24-2 Thin blood smear. (From Marler LM, et al: Parasitology Image Atlas CD-Rom. Indiana Pathology Images, 2003, Indianapolis, Ind.)

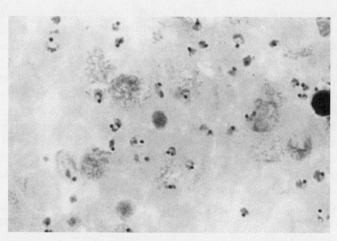

Figure 24-3 Thick film.

MICROANGIOPATHIC HEMOLYTIC ANEMIA

In 1962, Brain et al[1,2] described microangiopathic hemolytic anemias (MAHAs) as a group of clinical disorders characterized by red blood cell (RBC) fragmentation in the circulation, resulting in intravascular hemolysis. The fragmentation occurred as RBCs passed through fibrin deposits inside the lumens of arterioles and capillaries or through damaged epithelium and vessel walls. In vitro studies of RBC fragmentation showed RBCs being forced through a fibrin clot, attaching to fibrin, folding around the strands, and fragmenting by the force of the flowing blood.[1,3,4] Two disorders with severe MAHA are thrombotic thrombocytopenic purpura (TTP) and hemolytic-uremic syndrome (HUS), in which widespread microthrombi occur in arterioles and capillaries. These syndromes include thrombocytopenia, which results from destruction by processes independent of immunologic phenomena.

MAHA may be observed in some patients with sepsis,[5,6] disseminated carcinomatosis,[7,8] and disseminated intravascular coagulation (DIC); after liver or kidney transplantation; and with complications of pregnancy, malignant hypertension,[9,10] and venoms and toxins.[5,11] Several antineoplastic drugs, such as mitomycin and cyclosporine, can cause a disorder similar to HUS.[12]

Thrombotic Thrombocytopenic Purpura

Chapter 43 provides a complete review of TTP and HUS. TTP is a heterogeneous clinical syndrome characterized by the pentad of hemolytic anemia with RBC fragmentation, thrombocytopenia, fluctuating neurologic dysfunction, fever, and progressive renal failure.[13,14] TTP is rare and potentially fatal and is characterized by disseminated thrombotic occlusions of the microcirculation. Deposition of microthrombi that contain platelets and von Willebrand factor is observed in arterioles and capillaries of many organs.[15,16]

The diagnosis can be made readily by observing thrombocytopenia with a marked increase in blood film schistocytes.[1,17,18] Erythrocytes reveal microangiopathic changes: fragmented, small, triangular, and bizarre RBCs, helmet cells, and microspherocytes, all pathognomonic of TTP. Diffusely basophilic RBCs are prominent.

Anemia is always present in TTP and may be severe. Hemoglobin (Hb) is usually less than 10 g/dL.[3] Reticulocytes are increased, and nucleated RBCs and basophilic stippling are present on the peripheral smear (Fig. 24-4).[3]

Severe thrombocytopenia is frequently present, with platelet counts often less than 20×10^9/L. Platelet survival is decreased because of consumption. Megakaryocytes are normal in number but do not often show platelet budding.

The leukocyte count often is increased, and immature granulocytes (left shift) may appear. Erythroid hyperplasia is noted in the bone marrow, and most of the cells are at the polychromatic normoblast stage.

More recently, a severe deficiency of the von Willebrand factor–cleaving protease, now designated as *ADAMTS-13*, has been implicated in pathogenesis of acute TTP.[19-29] It has been reported that patients with TTP in remission may have abnormally large plasma von Willebrand factor molecules, which probably result from endothelial cell damage and the ADAMTS-13 deficiency, and these large molecules may aid in the formation of platelet thrombi.[27]

The febrile nature of TTP is consistent with infection, and there are many cases in the literature of MAHA associated with infection. The disease also has occurred in association with viral infection and immunologic diseases. Pregnancy seems to trigger the onset of TTP. Because TTP has been reported in siblings, hereditary factors may play a role in the cause. Due to the varied causes given for TTP, predisposing factors may not be apparent.

Autopsy findings include prominent microthrombi (hyaline thrombi) in vessels in the brain, heart, kidney, spleen, adrenal glands, pancreas, and lymph nodes. Histopathologic examination shows accumulation of hyaline deposits with a strongly positive periodic acid–Schiff reaction in lumens of arterioles and capillaries and accumulation of fibrin in the lumen of vessels at the site of wall damage. In electron microscopy, the microthrombi contain fibrin-like material, aggregates of platelets, and occasionally white blood cells (WBCs) and RBCs.

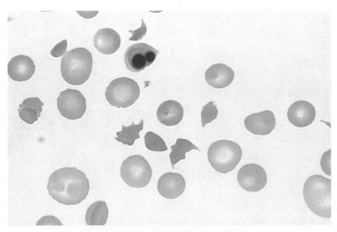

Figure 24-4 TTP with schistocytes.

Most patients may be cured with plasma replacement therapy, and remission may be induced in others.[26,29-32]

Hemolytic-Uremic Syndrome

Chapter 43 contains a complete discussion of HUS. HUS is an acquired disorder that resembles TTP and was described by Gasser et al in 1955.[33] Gasser et al[33] reported on the triad of MAHA, thrombocytopenia, and acute renal failure in young children. HUS is a heterogeneous syndrome with several clinical variants that may be distinguished from TTP by the severity of renal failure and absence of neurologic symptoms.

The typical HUS of childhood resembles enteric infectious disease. A toxin produced by certain serotypes of *Escherichia coli* has been commonly associated with HUS.[34-36] Comparable toxins are produced by other organisms, such as *Shigella dysenteriae*, *Streptococcus pneumoniae*, and *Campylobacter jejuni*.[37-42] The main target seems to be the renal capillary endothelium. The macrophage system is unable to clear fibrin, and deposits are found in glomerular vessels. The deposits persist and produce damage to the glomerulus, renal failure, MAHA, and thrombocytopenia.

Abundant data support the presence of intravascular platelet activation, and possibly the most obvious mechanism is some form of endothelial insult in the kidney. Glomerular lesions of varying severity are observed, as are thrombi in arterioles and capillaries of the glomerulus. Necrosis with proteinaceous material (similar to fibrin) in the glomerular arterioles is common. Fibrosis also may be present.[20,37]

HUS is characterized by the sudden onset of acute renal failure, intravascular hemolysis with MAHA, hemoglobinuria, abdominal pain with vomiting, variable thrombocytopenia, and leukocytosis. HUS rivals TTP in its severity, suddenness, and vascular involvement. Hypertension is present in more than half of patients with HUS.[2,15,42]

Coagulation findings typical of DIC occasionally may be present, and the prothrombin time and partial thromboplastin time occasionally are prolonged. The urine contains protein, RBCs, and often RBC casts.[20,41-43]

Adult HUS is more closely related to TTP in severity and prognosis than to classic HUS. In adult HUS, renal failure is more prominent, and neurologic dysfunction is less severe than in TTP. Most patients with adult HUS are women in whom the condition develops after gram-negative infection, after preeclampsia or eclampsia, in the postpartum period, or after ingestion of oral contraceptives. Enteric infections are seldom seen in adults. More recent reports have shown a link between HUS and malignant disease and HUS and chemotherapeutic agents (e.g., mitomycin).[10,22]

Malignant Hypertension

MAHA may occur in patients with malignant hypertension. The mechanical destruction of RBCs results from fibrin deposition in arterioles and from the forcing of RBCs through damaged endothelium of arterioles. When hypertension is brought under control, RBC fragmentation and hemolytic anemia disappear.[9] It seems that hypertension is the cause of RBC fragmentation and not the reverse.

Disseminated Intravascular Coagulation

RBC fragmentation, which occurs in approximately half of patients with DIC, is the result of fibrin strands in the microvasculature. The hemolysis is not usually severe. Thrombocytopenia of varying degrees is always observed, and platelet function is impaired by fibrin degradation products. DIC accompanies many systemic disorders, such as obstetric complications, disseminated carcinoma, snakebite, heatstroke, and infections (see Chapter 42 for discussion of DIC). DIC is not present in every case of hemolytic anemia and RBC fragmentation associated with infection. When the underlying disease comes under control with appropriate therapy, erythrocyte fragmentation no longer occurs.[4,15,43-45]

Disseminated Carcinoma

MAHA is a complication of disseminated carcinoma, particularly metastatic carcinoma of the stomach. Hemolytic anemia with RBC fragmentation, DIC, hemoglobinemia, increased levels of unconjugated bilirubin, absent or decreased haptoglobin, and increased lactate dehydrogenase, in addition to metastatic infiltration of marrow, may cause a very severe anemia. Fragmentation of RBCs results from shearing of RBCs on fibrin strands that are produced by intravascular coagulation and from contact with tumor cell emboli. The infiltrating tumor releases mucin, which causes fibrin deposition in the microvasculature, resulting in RBC fragmentation.[7,46-48]

Chemotherapy-Induced Microangiopathic Hemolytic Anemia Syndrome

Certain antineoplastic drugs, such as mitomycin combined with other drugs and tamoxifen in combination with cisplatin or other drugs, have led to a syndrome that resembles TTP and sometimes HUS. This syndrome is characterized by MAHA, thrombocytopenia, and renal failure. The pathogenesis of this thrombotic microangiopathy is not definitely established and requires further study. The prognosis of chemotherapy-induced MAHA is poor.[8,21,49,50]

Microangiopathic Hemolytic Anemia Syndrome Associated with Transplantation

A syndrome similar to the chemotherapy-induced MAHA syndrome may occur in patients with organ and marrow allografts. Total-body irradiation and certain drugs are two of many factors that seem to be associated with MAHA syndrome, renal disease, and thrombocytopenia. This disease is difficult to treat with the same measures usually used in patients with TTP.[50]

MACROVASCULAR HEMOLYTIC ANEMIA

Traumatic Cardiac Hemolytic Anemia
History
In the 1950s, when corrective cardiac surgery became possible, it was observed that some patients who had aortic valve replacement developed hemolytic anemia and RBC fragmentation. The anemia was caused by injury and fragmentation of RBCs exposed to high shear stresses on a foreign surface.

The construction of prosthetic valves and surfaces has been improved, and traumatic cardiac hemolytic anemia has diminished.[51]

Pathogenesis
The hemolysis that occurs in patients with valvular disorders is mild and rarely leads to hemolytic anemia except in patients with severe aortic stenosis. Turbulence in blood flowing around or through the artificial valve may occur, the valve may be improperly positioned, or the valve may be spontaneously separated from the natural valve. RBC destruction in flowing blood results not only from turbulence and shear stresses created by artificial prosthetic valves but also from turbulence on an artificial foreign surface, which is no longer covered by a layer of anticoagulating endothelial cells.[51,52]

Clinical and Laboratory Findings
The anemia that occurs in patients with heart valve prosthesis is of variable severity, and usually a mild compensated hemolysis occurs. Rarely, a patient has a severe anemia that requires transfusion. Blood films show helmet cells, triangular crescent cells, often microspherocytes, and other types of fragmented RBCs (Fig. 24-5). The number of fragmented cells in the smear reflects the severity of the hemolytic process. The reticulocyte count is increased despite a normal hematocrit and compensated hemolysis. Platelets may be decreased. Lactate dehydrogenase activity, serum bilirubin, and plasma Hb level are elevated. Haptoglobin concentration is decreased. There may be hemosiderin in the urine and reduced serum ferritin levels owing to loss of iron. Hemoglobinuria may be observed in severe hemolysis.[51,52]

Treatment
If severe anemia is present and lactate dehydrogenase is elevated, the prosthesis should be replaced promptly. If the anemia is mild or compensated, normal erythropoietic activity should be maintained, and administration of ferrous sulfate is recommended to replace urinary iron loss. Folic acid may be beneficial.

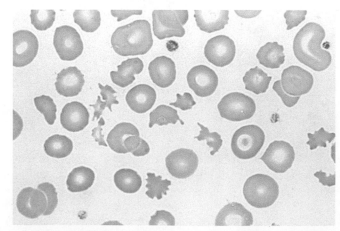

Figure 24-5 Cardiac hemolytic anemia with RBC fragmentation.

March Hemoglobinuria

Definition

March hemoglobinuria refers to hemoglobinuria and hemoglobinemia that result from forceful repeated impact of the feet or other parts of the body on a hard surface or during strenuous exercises.[53-57]

History

In 1881 a soldier in Germany complained of passing dark urine after strenuous marches. His physician found hemoglobin in the urine. Eighty years later, Davidson[58] proposed that RBCs were destroyed in the soles of the feet during long-distance running as a result of the stamping gait of track runners. He recommended that track runners wear soft linings in their shoes, and the hemoglobinuria disappeared. Despite the use of padded insoles, traumatic disruption of RBCs by pressure on soles during running and walking may occur.

Clinical and Laboratory Findings

The physical examination is normal in patients with march hemoglobinuria and sports anemia. Hematocrit and hemoglobin levels are often at the lower limits of normal, but significant anemia is uncommon. RBCs may be slightly macrocytic, but the blood smear does not contain fragmented RBCs. Reticulocyte percentage may be increased after strenuous sports. The urine may be red or dark after exertion and may show hemoglobin casts, hemosiderin, and hemoglobin, but clears after 6 to 12 hours.

Differential Diagnosis

March hemoglobinuria must be distinguished from paroxysmal cold hemoglobinuria that occurs after exposure to cold. Myoglobinuria can be distinguished from hemoglobinuria by solubility of the heme pigments in ammonium sulfate, by electrophoretic comparison with hemoglobin, by high-performance liquid chromatography, and by muscle pain during exercise. Plasma is red or pink during hemoglobinuria but is clear of pigment in myoglobinuria.[58]

Treatment

The physician should reassure the patient that he or she does not have a serious problem. The condition ameliorates when rubberized insoles are added to shoes or when the patient changes his or her gait to a less traumatic running style.

HEMOLYTIC ANEMIA CAUSED BY INFECTION WITH MICROORGANISMS

Intracellular Microorganisms

Malaria

An infection of RBCs by malarial parasites is a common cause of hemolytic anemia worldwide. More than 400 million individuals have the disease. The yearly mortality from malaria exceeds 1 million individuals. Although malaria control measures have been implemented in numerous areas in the world for many years, in the past 40 years a resurgence of the disease has occurred as a result of resistance to many of the antimalarial drugs, particularly chloroquine. The *Anopheles* mosquito also has become resistant to insecticides such as dichlorodiphenyltrichloroethane (DDT), which earlier was highly effective in eradication of the vector.[59-62]

An increase in the disease has occurred in residents of the United States and other countries because of increased air travel to areas in which malaria is endemic and because of increased numbers of immigrants and visitors. Malaria also may be transmitted by blood transfusion, and the diagnosis should be considered in an individual with a febrile illness that occurs several weeks after a transfusion. Malaria may be transmitted by drug abuse and sharing needles.

Life Cycle.   Malaria is an acute, chronic, or recurrent febrile protozoan infection transmitted by the bite of the female *Anopheles* mosquito, which is the insect vector for the organism. Sporozoites in the salivary gland of the mosquito are injected into the human host. Sporozoites of the four species of the genus *Plasmodium* may cause malaria: *P. vivax, P. malariae, P. falciparum,* and *P. ovale.* These microorganisms can parasitize RBCs and a few other body tissues.[63,64]

The sporozoites rapidly leave the circulating blood and invade hepatic parenchymal cells to begin exoerythrocytic schizogony, which occurs 6 to 12 days after exposure. Hepatic cells rupture, releasing merozoites that invade circulating RBCs, and the erythrocytic life cycle schizogony begins. Inside the erythrocyte, the merozoite is nourished by the cell's contents, and it metabolizes the hemoglobin and grows intracellularly. The merozoite becomes a ring form, which grows into a late ring or ameboid trophozoite, then into an early schizont (chromatin dividing), and finally into a schizont that contains merozoites. The merozoites are released from the erythrocyte and invade other cells. The patient experiences chills and fever as the RBCs are ruptured. It has been stated that some of the merozoites in *P. vivax* may reenter the liver to produce an exoerythrocytic cycle again, but this concept is not universally accepted. Other investigators state that some merozoites remain in the hepatocytes and may reappear in the circulation after a considerable length of time.[64]

Some merozoites form male and female gametocytes in the circulating blood. While taking a blood meal, gametocytes (sexual stages) are ingested by an *Anopheles* mosquito. The female gamete is fertilized by the male gamete in the stomach of the mosquito, resulting in a zygote that establishes itself on the outer wall of the mosquito stomach and develops into an ookinete and then an oocyst. The oocyst produces sporozoites. As the abdomen enlarges by the force created by proteolysis of Hb, the sporozoites become free and migrate to the salivary gland of the mosquito. When the mosquito takes a blood meal, the sporozoites inoculate the human host.[15,63,64]

Pathogenesis.   The presence or lack of particular receptors on the surface of the RBC membrane determines the host range of the different plasmodia. RBCs lacking the Duffy determinants (Fy^{a-b-}) are not vulnerable to infection by

P. vivax. The Duffy-negative phenotype has high frequency among West African Americans, and these individuals are resistant to vivax malaria. The number of Duffy-negative individuals is lower and the incidence of *P. vivax* higher as one moves from West to East Africa. The development of the Duffy-negative population helped to prevent the spread of *P. vivax.* The missing or suppressed genes for the Duffy blood group seems to be a highly specific genetic adaptation to vivax malaria.[65-68]

RBCs of patients with hereditary pyropoikilocytosis are not invaded by malaria because the RBC cytoskeleton is altered, and cells lack deformability. The age of the cells determines what species of malaria infects the RBCs. *P. vivax* and *P. ovale* infect young RBCs and reticulocytes. *P. falciparum* infects young and mature RBCs. *P. malariae* infects only mature RBCs.[69]

Having a hemoglobinopathy may in some way guard against malarial infection and lead to an increased incidence of the hemoglobinopathy gene in the population. Hb S,[44,70,71] Hb C, Hb E,[72] and thalassemia[73] have been shown to benefit heterozygotes in combating malaria. The incidence of Hb AS is greatest in areas where *P. falciparum* is prevalent. The specific physiologic benefit that Hb AS provides is unclear. Growth of *P. falciparum* is low in fetal RBCs.[74] Adults with hereditary persistence of fetal Hb have a low rate of parasite growth.

In similar fashion, the growth of *P. falciparum* may be impaired in glucose-6-phosphate dehydrogenase (G6PD)–deficient RBCs. Although there are conflicting studies, one large study provides evidence that G6PD-A, the most common Africa G6PD deficiency variant, is associated with significant reduction in malaria in G6PD-deficient female heterozygotes and male hemizygotes.[59,62,75]

Clinical and Laboratory Findings.   The clinical features of malaria vary with the species. The usual symptoms are fever, chills, rigors, sweating, headache, muscle pain, and prostration. About 25% of patients have hemolytic anemia,[68] which may be accompanied by jaundice, splenomegaly, and hepatomegaly. In patients with chronic malaria or with repeated malarial infection, the spleen may be massively enlarged.

The main cause of anemia is the rupture of infected cells at the end of the asexual cycle; immune complexes also may play a role in the anemia. The amount of hemolysis is related to the number of RBCs parasitized. Hemolysis is greatest in falciparum malaria because this species invades RBCs at all stages of development; hemolysis is less in vivax malaria because the merozoites attach to reticulocytes.[68] Hemolysis is characterized by spherocytosis, reticulocytosis, and shortened RBC survival. The spleen pits out the parasites from the infected RBCs, which are often destroyed. At first, only parasitized RBCs succumb, but after several days, hemolysis becomes worse and nonparasitized cells become spherical and are destroyed, possibly as a result of immunologic factors.[68,76]

A few patients with malaria may have DIC, which occurs with the release of thromboplastin material when RBCs are destroyed or as a result of immune complexes. Thrombocytopenia is found in about 75% of patients with resistance to chloroquine.[59,65]

BOX 24-2 Thick Film Preparation for Malaria

To make a thick film, place three small drops of blood (each drop about the size used to make a thin film) close together near one end of the slide. With one corner of a clean slide, stir the blood to mix the three drops over an area of 2 cm or more in diameter. Stir for about 30 seconds to prevent formation of fibrin strands, which might obscure the parasites. Allow film to dry thoroughly. Stain film in a water-based Giemsa stain for 30 minutes. The erythrocytes are lysed by the water-based Giemsa stain. (Thin blood smears are first fixed in methyl alcohol to preserve the RBCs.) In a thick film, more parasites are seen in each field.

During the infection, the WBC count is normal to slightly increased. Neutropenia may develop during chills and rigors. Monocytes and immature granulocytes may be observed if malaria persists. Malarial infection in patients with symptomatic infection is diagnosed by the presence of parasites in the peripheral blood smear stained with Wright-Giemsa. Smears should be made before the anticipated onset of chills and fever.[68] To concentrate parasites when only a few are present, a thick drop preparation (thick smear) should be made and stained with fresh diluted Giemsa without fixing in methyl alcohol (Box 24-1). RBCs are lysed with water-based Giemsa, and the parasite may be observed more frequently on this thick smear than on the thin smear; however, identification of the species is difficult. To identify the species, a thin smear also must be made. A platelet lying on top of an erythrocyte in a thin smear may be confused with a malarial parasite (Fig. 24-6).

Plasmodium vivax.   *P. vivax* invades young RBCs, or reticulocytes.[64,68] The early trophozoite has a small ring with a red chromatin dot and a blue-staining cytoplasmic circle. The RBC begins to grow larger and becomes pale and misshapen. Schüffner stippling is seen in the late ring stages and all other stages. In the growing trophozoite, the chromatin and cytoplasm increase in amount, and the ring shape is lost. The

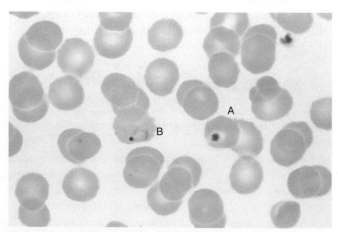

Figure 24-6 Platelet on top of an RBC *(A)* compared with *P. vivax*, ring form *(B)*.

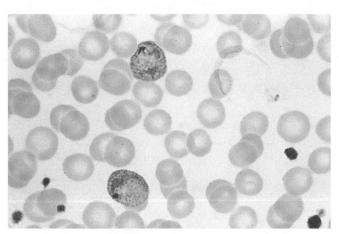

Figure 24-7 *P. vivax:* trophozoite.

ameboid trophozoite almost fills the cell (Fig. 24-7). Yellow-brown pigment from digested Hb appears. In an immature schizont, chromatin begins to divide into two or more masses. The mature schizont usually has 12 to 24 merozoites and yellow-brown hematin and hemosiderin in clumps (Fig. 24-8). The pale or decolorized RBC filled with merozoites soon releases the merozoites and disintegrates. A few merozoites prepare for sexual schizogony and transfer into large gameto-cytes with a bulky nucleus. Gametocytes are rounded with blue cytoplasm and pigment and have a small, eccentrically placed, dispersed chromatin (male microgametocyte) or large, cen-trally located chromatin (female macrogametocyte). The ery-throcytic cell cycle requires 44 to 48 hours.[62,73] *P. vivax* has a worldwide distribution, especially in temperate climates and in the tropics. It is not as common in Africa as are other types.[64] *P. vivax* is difficult to eradicate, and relapses may occur. The schizont of *P. vivax* lies dormant for years in the liver and may become reactivated, causing a recurrence of infection.

Plasmodium ovale.   *P. ovale* parasites invade young RBCs and reticulocytes. The young trophozoite resembles *P. vivax* and *P. malariae.* RBCs become enlarged, oval, and fringed and

have Schüffner stippling. In the schizont stage, the RBCs are oval, and the parasite is round in the center of the cell. Merozoites can number four to eight or more and are found in a rosette around a mass of pigment. Gametocytes cannot be differentiated from *P. vivax.* The length of the asexual cycle is 48 hours[64] (Fig. 24-9).

Plasmodium malariae.   Parasites invade older RBCs, and the infection is usually mild. The ring stage has a single chromatin dot and a blue cytoplasmic ring that is often smaller and heavier than that of *P. vivax,* although the two may be indistinguishable. In growing trophozoites, chromatin is rounded or streaky; cytoplasm forms a narrow band across the cell, and coarse brown pigment is noted. The band form is a characteristic feature of the species (Fig. 24-10). RBCs do not become enlarged, and no stippling occurs in the schizont stage (Fig. 24-11). Eight to 12 merozoites form a rosette around clumped pigment and are expelled from the cell. The asexual cycle is 72 hours, or every third day. Gametocytes are similar to those of *P. vivax* but smaller; pigment may be conspicuous, and few gametocytes are observed.[59,64,77]

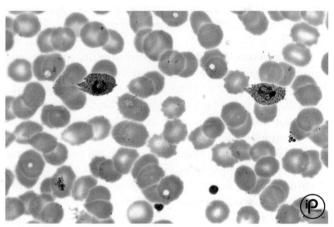

Figure 24-9 *P. ovale:* trophozoite with fimbriated edges. (From Marler LM, et al: Parasitology Image Atlas CD-Rom. Indiana Pathology Images, 2003, Indianapolis, Ind.)

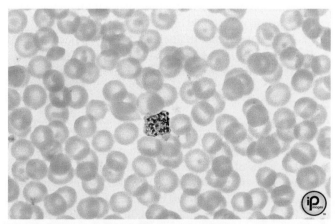

Figure 24-8 *P. vivax:* schizont. (From Marler LM, et al: Parasitology Image Atlas CD-Rom. Indiana Pathology Images, 2003, Indianapolis, Ind.)

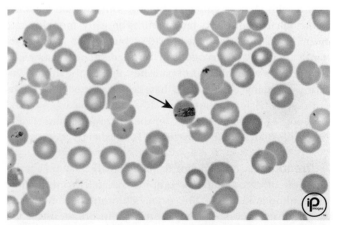

Figure 24-10 *P. malariae:* band form. (From Marler LM, et al: Parasitology Image Atlas CD-Rom. Indiana Pathology Images, 2003, Indianapolis, Ind.)

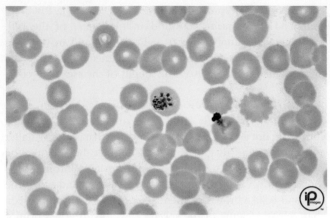

Figure 24-11 *P. malariae:* schizont. (From Marler LM, et al: Parasitology Image Atlas CD-Rom. Indiana Pathology Images, 2003, Indianapolis, Ind.)

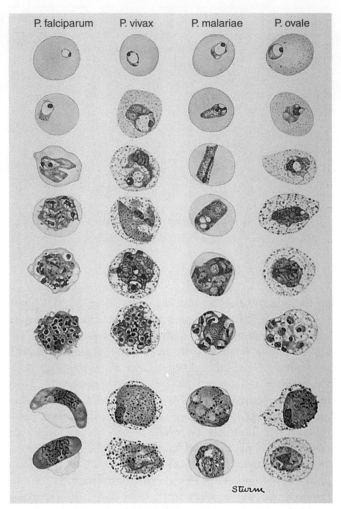

Figure 24-12 Malarial parasites. (From Diggs LW, Sturm D, Bell A: Morphology of Human Blood Cells, 5th ed. Abbott Park, Ill.: Abbott Laboratories, 1985; permission has been granted with approval of Abbott Laboratories, all rights reserved by Abbott Laboratories, Inc.)

P. malariae is found in tropical Africa, India, Burma, Malaysia, and Indonesia.[64] Infection with *P. malariae* is more amenable to chloroquine therapy than is *P. vivax*, but it also may be disabling. Rarely, patients may develop a nephropathy with albuminuria, hematuria, and edema that likely reflects deposition of immune complexes from parasite antigen in the kidney.[72-74]

Plasmodium falciparum.   Parasites invade old and young RBCs, which remain normal in size. Ring forms are numerous (see Fig. 24-1) and may be missed because the ring is small, with a small cytoplasmic circle and one or two little chromatin dots. One or more rings may be at the margin of the cell. The trophozoite grows and is usually the main form seen in circulation. Schizont stages occur in visceral organs and only rarely in peripheral blood, except in severe infections. Crescent-shaped or banana-shaped gametocytes have deep-blue cytoplasm with brownish pigment near the center and are easily recognized on thick preparations (see Figs. 24-2 and 24-3). A cycle is 36 to 48 hours in length.[64]

P. falciparum is the most pathogenic human malaria, and it may run an acute fulminating course, ending in death if prompt treatment is not begun. It is important to make an early and rapid diagnosis. Massive intravascular hemolysis occurs with hemoglobinemia, hemoglobinuria, and jaundice. Acute renal failure also may occur. The early mortality rate from *P. falciparum* approaches 10%, but deaths can be prevented with early recognition and adequate treatment.[69] Erythrocytes with falciparum parasites plug up the microcirculation of many organs. DIC has been reported in patients with severe falciparum infection.[45,61] Cerebral malaria is caused by sludging of damaged RBCs in the microvasculature. Figure 24-12 illustrates the four species of *Plasmodium*.

Treatment.   Therapy for malaria usually includes administration of chloroquine or quinine sulfate. Pyrimethamine and sulfonamides also are given. Chloroquine destroys all stages of malaria in erythrocytes except in drug-resistant falciparum infection; quinine sulfate often is given in combination with pyrimethamine and sulfonamides.[62,65,67,72,74,78]

Primaquine may be used to treat the hepatic stages of vivax malaria. Patients with malaria and G6PD deficiency develop severe hemolysis after treatment with sulfones and primaquine. Because falciparum malaria has the potential for a rapid, fatal course, the infection should be treated as soon as possible after diagnosis. Drug-resistant strains of *P. falciparum* have required various combinations of antimalarial drugs. Eventual cure for malaria lies in the development of a suitable vaccine.[59-61,66,68]

Babesia

Babesia are small, ring-like protozoa (diameter <2 mm) within erythrocytes that resemble the ring stages of falciparum malaria. Babesiosis is an uncommon hemolytic disorder caused by a few of the 71 species of the small protozoan. Most infections result from *Babesia microti,* which is transmitted from wild feral deer mice to humans by the tick *Ixodes dammini*. The disease is thought to be more severe in individuals who have had a splenectomy. Babesiosis has been transmitted by transfusion.[79-81]

Geographic Distribution.   Babesiosis occurs on Nantucket Island, on coastal regions of the northeastern United States, and in California. It has been found in France, Ireland, Scotland, and other European countries.[79-81]

Symptoms.   The incubation period for the infection is 1 to 4 weeks. The infection is characterized by gradual onset of malaise followed by fever, chills, headache, drenching sweats, arthralgias, myalgia, weakness, and fatigue. There is no periodicity to the fever as seen in malaria. There may be a mild to moderately severe hemolytic anemia. Serum bilirubin and transaminase levels are elevated slightly.[64]

Laboratory Diagnosis.   The diagnosis of babesiosis can be made by demonstration of the ring-shaped parasites on Wright-Giemsa–stained smears or by animal inoculation. Thick drop preparations are often preferred to thin smears because the parasites may be scarce. Serologic tests for antibodies to *Babesia* have been described.[80,82,83]

Babesia are tiny rings with a minute chromatin dot and a minimal amount of cytoplasm (Fig. 24-13). They may be round, oval, elongated, or ameboid. One or two chromatin dots, which stain dark purple, may be observed with practically no cytoplasm. More than one ring can be seen in an RBC.[80,82-84] Tetrad forms may be noted and aid in positively identifying *Babesia* (Fig. 24-14).

Treatment.   The antibiotic clindamycin given in combination with quinine has been reported to be a highly effective treatment for babesiosis. A cure should occur about 1 week after the institution of therapy, and consolidation therapy should continue for another week. The failure of chloroquine in human babesiosis has been reported. Exchange transfusion has been used to treat transfusion-transmitted babesiosis.[82,83,85]

Ehrlichia

Ehrlichia, small intracellular bacteria, are transmitted by ticks to humans.[86-89] Transfusion-transmitted tick-borne diseases are definitely a risk; however, transfusion-related cases of

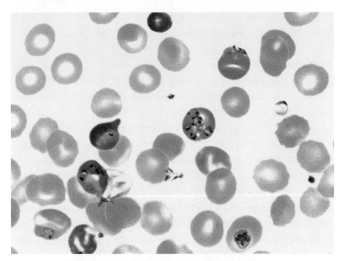

Figure 24-14 *B. microti:* ring and tetrad forms.

ehrlichiosis are rare.[90,91] Ehrlichiosis was first reported in dogs in 1935, and the first human case was documented in the United States in 1986. They grow as a cluster (morula) in neutrophils (*Anaplasma phagocytophilum* and *Ehrlichia ewingii*) (Fig. 24-15A) and in monocytes (*Ehrlichia chaffeensis*) (Fig. 24-15B). The infection may cause necrosis of lymph nodes and liver and is characterized by bone marrow suppression leading to pancytopenia. In the first week of infection, ehrlichiae can be detected by finding intracellular aggregates on the blood and body fluid smears. Immunofluorescent antibody titers and polymerase chain reaction are needed for confirmation. Early diagnosis is essential because antibiotic treatment is very effective.[6]

Extracellular Microorganisms
Clostridial Septicemia

Intravascular hemolysis, which is often fatal, is produced by the gram-positive, spore-forming bacillus *Clostridium perfringens (welchii)*. Clostridial sepsis is a complication of septic abortion, deep wounds, and any condition that leads to destruction of RBCs and to lysis. Leukocytosis with a shift to the left and thrombocytopenia are often present. Swift therapy with transfusions, antibiotics, and other measures is required before the

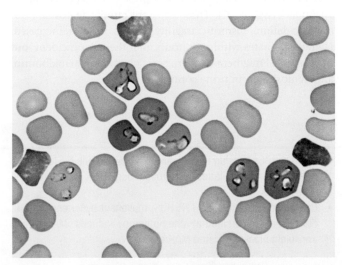

Figure 24-13 *B. microti:* ring forms.

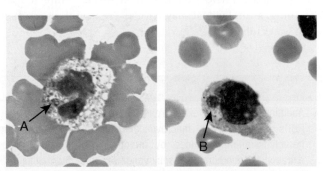

Figure 24-15 A, *A. phagocytophilum* in a neutrophil (×400). **B,** *E. chaffeensis* in monocytic cell (×250). (Courtesy of J. Stephen Dumler, MD, Division of Medical Microbiology, The Johns Hopkins Medical Institutions, Baltimore, Md.)

surgeon removes the infected tissue or organ. The prognosis is grave, and many patients die despite extensive treatment.[92,93]

Bartonellosis

Human bartonellosis (Carrión disease) is transmitted by the sandfly. The RBCs become infected with the organism *Bartonella bacilliformis*, which is thought to adhere to the exterior surface of the RBC. There are two clinical stages: acute hemolytic anemia (Oroya fever) is the early stage; the second stage, verruga peruana, is characterized by eruptions on the face and extremities and by the development of bleeding, warty tumors.

Carrión disease was named for a medical student, Daniel A. Carrión, who in 1885 inoculated himself with blood from a verrucous node on the skin of a patient. He developed a fatal hemolytic anemia similar to the disease Oroya fever, which was first observed in railroad workers near the city of Oroya in the Peruvian Andes.[94] Oroya fever responds to chloramphenicol, penicillin, streptomycin, tetracycline, and the aminoglycosides.[91,94-96]

HEMOLYTIC ANEMIA CAUSED BY CHEMICALS, DRUGS, AND VENOMS

Drugs and Chemicals

There are certain chemical agents that cause the oxidative denaturation of hemoglobin, leading to the formation of methemoglobin, sulfhemoglobin, and Heinz bodies. Examples of such agents are naphthalene (mothballs) and dapsone (for leprosy). Individuals deficient in G6PD or other RBC enzymes are noted to be sensitive to the effects of oxidative agents.

Hemolytic anemia caused by oxidant drugs varies in severity. The signs of hemolysis include anemia, increase in reticulocytes, increase in bilirubin, and hyperplasia of erythroid cells in marrow. In severe hemolytic anemia, Heinz bodies may be observed in RBCs. Heinz bodies result from precipitated hemoglobin clinging to the inner layer of the RBC membrane. This coagulum of Hb separates from the cell membrane, leaving a clear area, similar to a "bite" being taken out of the cell (Chapter 23).

Exposure to high levels of arsenic, copper, and lead can cause intravascular hemolysis, as can the use of water irrigation during surgery. Spherocytes are seen on the blood film. In near-drowning, an individual may have severe hemolysis resulting from water inhalation.[97,98]

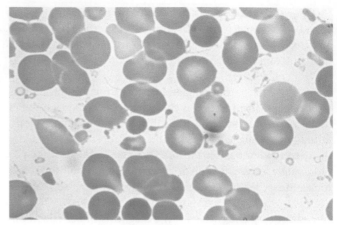

Figure 24-16 Fragmented RBCs from severely burned patient.

Venoms

The brown recluse spider (*Loxosceles reclusa*) injects a venom that leads to a severe hemolytic anemia with local pain, ischemic necrosis, and ulceration at the site of the bite. The venom contains enzymes that act directly on the RBC membrane and produce lysis. Bee and wasp stings have been reported to cause hemolysis in some patients.

The venoms of certain snakes, such as the cobra and the pit viper, contain hemolysins, thrombin-like enzymes, and activators and inactivators of complement. The amount of venom absorbed determines the intensity of the hemolysis.[98] Sometimes the venom causes defibrination but does not affect other coagulation factors.[99-101]

HEMOLYTIC ANEMIA CAUSED BY THERMAL INJURY

Patients with third-degree burns involving more than 20% of the body may have severe, acute hemolytic anemia. Direct thermal damage to RBCs circulating in the involved skin and tissues leads to hemolysis.[58,102,103] Morphologic RBC changes in widespread burns include globular fragmentation, budding, and microspherocytes, which are present for approximately 24 hours (Fig. 24-16). These cells are rapidly removed from the circulation. Osmotic fragility at this time is increased. Hemolysis abates within 48 hours after the burn incident, but tiny spherical fragments, spherocytes, plasma methemalbumin, and hemosiderin in urine continue.

CHAPTER at a GLANCE

- Anemias caused by extracorpuscular abnormalities damaging RBCs include MAHA, macrovascular hemolytic anemia, and hemolytic anemia caused by infection with intracellular or extracellular microorganisms, by venoms, and by thermal injury.
- MAHA is characterized by fragmentation of RBCs in the circulation, resulting in intravascular hemolysis. Fragmentation occurs as a result of RBCs passing through fibrin deposits inside the lumens of arterioles and capillaries or through damaged epithelium and vessel walls.
- Causes of MAHA include TTP, HUS, malignant hypertension, DIC, disseminated carcinoma, chemotherapy-induced MAHA, and transplantation-associated MAHA.

CHAPTER at a GLANCE—cont'd

- TTP is distinguished by the pentad of hemolytic anemia with RBC fragmentation, thrombocytopenia, neurologic dysfunction, fever, and progressive renal failure.
- HUS is an acquired disorder resembling TTP in that it is characterized by MAHA, thrombocytopenia, and renal failure, but it is found primarily in children, and the renal failure is much more severe than in TTP.
- Causes of macrovascular hemolytic anemia include traumatic cardiac hemolytic anemia after prosthetic aortic valve replacement and march hemoglobinuria. With improved construction of prosthetic valves, the incidence of traumatic cardiac hemolytic anemia has diminished.
- March hemoglobinuria is the result of forceful impact of the feet or other parts of the body on hard surfaces without sufficient padding. The anemia is usually minimal and resolves when the patient uses rubberized insoles or changes his or her running style to a less traumatic one.
- Intracellular organisms associated with hemolytic anemia include malaria (four types) and *B. microti*. Infection with malaria is one of the most common causes of hemolytic anemia worldwide.
- The main cause of anemia in malaria is the rupture of infected cells at the end of the asexual cycle, the severity of the anemia being proportional to the number of RBCs parasitized.

- Hemolysis is characterized by spherocytosis, reticulocytosis, and shortened RBC survival. Hemolysis is greatest in *P. falciparum* because all stages of RBC development are invaded by the parasite.
- *Babesia* are small, ring-like protozoa within RBCs that resemble the ring forms of *P. falciparum*. Tetrad forms aid in positively identifying *Babesia*.
- Extracellular organisms that have been implicated in intravascular hemolysis include *C. perfringens* and *B. bacilliformis*.
- Venoms of some spiders, such as the brown recluse, and snakes, such as the pit viper and the cobra, may lead to hemolytic anemia.
- In patients with third-degree burns involving more than 20% of the body, direct thermal damage to circulating RBCs leads to hemolysis. Characteristic morphology includes fragmentation, budding (blistering), and microspherocytes.

Now that you have completed this chapter, go back and read again the case study at the beginning and respond to the questions presented.

REVIEW QUESTIONS

1. A group of disorders characterized by fragmentation of RBCs in the circulation as a result of RBCs being forced through small fibrin clots is known as:
   a. Fibrinolytic hemolytic anemia
   b. MAHA
   c. Myelodysplastic syndromes
   d. Extravascular hemolytic anemia

2. Classic findings in TTP include all of the following *except*:
   a. RBC fragmentation and thrombocytopenia
   b. Neurologic dysfunction
   c. Agglutinated RBCs
   d. Progressive renal failure

3. MAHA, thrombocytopenia, and acute renal failure in children describes the disorder of:
   a. HUS
   b. TTP
   c. DIC
   d. Babesiosis

4. A marathon runner who had just finished a 20K run on hard pavement complained of dark urine. On physical examination, no abnormalities were found, and the next day the dark urine had cleared, and the runner continued with moderate exercise. The most likely cause of this phenomenon was:
   a. DIC
   b. *E. coli* sepsis
   c. Prosthetic heart valve
   d. March hemoglobinuria

5. The insect vector for malaria is the:
   a. Deer tick
   b. *Anopheles* mosquito
   c. Sand fly
   d. Brown recluse spider

6. A patient presents with chills, fluctuating fever, sweating, and muscle pain. The best time to draw blood to search for malaria parasites would be:
   a. When the patient is fasting
   b. During a period of chills and fever
   c. Just before an anticipated episode of chills and fever
   d. As soon as the patient recovers from an episode of fever and chills

7. The malaria species whose gametocyte has been described as "banana shaped" is:
   a. *P. malariae*
   b. *P. vivax*
   c. *P. ovale*
   d. *P. falciparum*

8. Which of the following can be confused with the ring form of malaria?
   a. Platelet on top of an RBC
   b. Stippled RBC
   c. Howell-Jolly body
   d. Reticulocyte

9. A ring-like protozoan with a diameter of less than 2 mm found within RBCs and resembling *P. falciparum* is:
   a. *P. vivax*
   b. *B. bacilliformis*
   c. *Babesia* species
   d. *Toxoplasma gondii*

10. A 32-year-old woman was brought to the emergency department by her husband because she had experienced a seizure. He reported that she had complained of not feeling well for several days. Laboratory studies showed anemia with polychromasia and poikilocytosis including RBC fragments, helmet cells, and microspherocytes. The platelet count was $18 \times 10^9/L$. Chemistry test results included elevated lactate dehydrogenase and total and indirect bilirubin. The urinalysis results were positive for blood, but there were no RBCs in the sediment. Considering the entire clinical and laboratory picture, which of the following is the most likely explanation for her condition?
    a. HUS
    b. Heinz body anemia
    c. Snake bite
    d. TTP

ACKNOWLEDGMENT

The author acknowledges Ann Bell, who was the principal author of this chapter in the previous edition.

REFERENCES

1. Brain MC, Neame PB: Thrombotic thrombocytopenic purpura and hemolytic-uremic syndrome. Semin Thromb Hemost 1982;8:186-187.
2. Brain MC, Dacie JV, Hourhiane DO: Microangiopathic haemolytic anemias: the possible role of vascular lesions in pathogenesis. Br J Haematol 1962;8:358-374.
3. Ridolfi RL, Bell WR: Thrombotic thrombocytopenic purpura: report of 25 cases and review of the literature. Medicine 1981;60:413-428.
4. Burle S, Passi GR, Salgia P, et al: Thrombotic thrombocytopenic purpura. Indian Pediatr 2004;41:277-279.
5. Tarr PI, Gordon CA, Chandler WL: Shiga-toxin–producing *Escherichia coli* and haemolytic uraemic syndrome. Lancet 2005;365:1073-1086.
6. Dumler JS, Walker DH: Tick-borne ehrlichioses: more of them, higher incidences, and greater clinical diversity. Lancet Infect Dis 2001;21-28 (preview edition).
7. Lee JL, Lee JH, Kim MK, et al: A case of bone marrow necrosis with thrombotic thrombocytopenic purpura as a manifestation of occult colon cancer. Jpn J Clin Oncol 2004;34:476-480.
8. Kwaan HC: Miscellaneous secondary thrombotic microangiopathy. Semin Hematol 1987;24:141-149.
9. Capelli JP Wesson LG Jr, Erslev AV: Malignant hypertension and red cell fragmentation syndrome. Ann Intern Med 1966;64:128-136.
10. Nissenson AR, Krumlovsky FA, del Greco F: Postpartum hemolytic-uremic syndrome: late recovery after prolonged maintenance dialysis. JAMA 1979;242:173-175.
11. Hostetler MA, Dribben W, Wilson DB, et al: Sudden unexplained hemolysis occurring in an infant due to presumed *Loxosceles* envenomation. J Emerg Med 2003;25:277-282.
12. Alonso-Santor JE, Gutierrez-Zufiaurre JL, Perez-Castrillon JL: Microangiopathic hemolytic anemia secondary to cyclosporine. Ann Pharmacother 2004;38:903.
13. Moschcowitz C: An acute febrile pleochromic anemia with hyaline thrombosis of terminal arterioles and capillaries: an undescribed disease. Arch Intern Med 1925;36:89-93.
14. Baehr G, Klemperer P, Schifrin A: An acute febrile anemia and thrombocytopenic purpura with diffuse platelet thrombosis of capillaries and arterioles. Trans Assoc Am Physicians 1936;51:43-58.
15. Jandl JH (ed): Blood: Textbook of Hematology, 2nd ed. Philadelphia: Lippincott, Williams & Wilkins, 1996.
16. Rapaport S: Introduction to Hematology. Philadelphia: Lippincott, 1987:500-504.
17. Daram SR, Philipneri M, Puri N, et al: Thrombotic thrombocytopenic purpura without schistocytes on the peripheral blood smear. South Med J 2005;98:392-395.
18. Bull BS, Rubenberg ML, Dacie JV, et al: Microangiopathic haemolytic anemia: mechanisms of red cell fragmentation: in vitro studies. Br J Haematol 1968;14:643-652.
19. Amoura Z, Costedoat-Chalumeau N, Veyradier A, et al: Thrombotic thrombocytopenic purpura with severe ADAMTS-13 deficiency in two patients with primary antiphospholipid syndrome. Arthritis Rheum 2004;50:3260-3264.
20. Kremer Hovinga JA, Studt JD, Lammle B: The von Willebrand factor–cleaving protease (ADAMTS-13) and the diagnosis of thrombotic thrombocytopenic purpura (TTP). Pathophysiol Haemost Thromb 2003;33:417-421.
21. Robson M, Cote I, Abbs I, et al: Thrombotic microangiopathy with sirolimus-based immunosuppression: potentiation of calcineurin-inhibitor-induced endothelial damage? Am J Transplant 2003;3:324-327.
22. Sadler JE, Poncz M: Antibody mediated thrombotic disorders: idiopathic thrombotic thrombocytopenic purpura and heparin-induced thrombocytopenia. In Lichtman MA, Beutler E, Kipps T, et al (eds): Williams Hematology, 7th ed. New York: McGraw-Hill, 2006:2031-2054.
23. Lattuada A, Rossi E, Calzarossa C, et al: Mild to moderate reduction of a von Willebrand factor cleaving protease (ADAMTS-13) in pregnant women with HELLP microangiopathic syndrome. Haematologica 2003;88:1029-1034.
24. Lopez JA, Dong JF: Shear stress and the role of high molecular weight von Willebrand factor multimers in thrombus formation. Blood Coagul Fibrinol 2005;16(Suppl 1):S11-S16.
25. Moake JL, Rudy CK, Troll JH, et al: Unusually large plasma factor VIII: von Willebrand factor multimers in chronic relapsing thrombotic thrombocytopenic purpura. N Engl J Med 1982;307:1432-1435.
26. Ahmad A, Aggarwal A, Sharma D, et al: Rituximab for treatment of refractory/relapsing thrombotic thrombocytopenic purpura (TTP). Am J Hematol 2004;77:171-176.
27. Tsai HM: Molecular mechanisms in thrombotic thrombocytopenic purpura. Semin Thromb Hemost 2004;30:549-557.
28. Khanna A, McCullough PA: Malignant hypertension presenting as hemolysis, thrombocytopenia, and renal failure. Rev Cardiovasc Med 2003;4:255-259.

29. Sadler JE, Moake JL, Miyata T, et al: Recent advances in thrombotic thrombocytopenic purpura. Hematology (Am Soc Hematol Educ Program) 2004;407-423.

30. Stein GY, Zeidman A, Fradin Z, et al: Treatment of resistant thrombotic thrombocytopenic purpura with rituximab and cyclophosphamide. Int J Hematol 2004;80:94-96.

31. Shepard KV, Bukowski RM: The treatment of thrombotic thrombocytopenic purpura with exchange transfusion, plasma infusion and plasma exchange. Semin Hematol 1987;24:178-193.

32. Ziman A, Mitri M, Klapper E, et al: Combination vincristine and plasma exchange as initial therapy in patients with thrombotic thrombocytopenic purpura: one institution's experience and review of the literature. Transfusion 2005; 45:41-49.

33. Gasser C, Gautier E, Steck A, et al: Hamolytisch uramische Syndrom: Bilaterale Nierenrindennekrosen bei akuten erworbenen hamolytischen anamien. Schweiz Med Wochenschr 1955;85:905.

34. Beattie TJ: Recent developments in the pathogenesis of hemolytic uremic syndrome. Ren Fail 1990;12:3-7.

35. Karmali MA, Petric M, Lim C, et al: The association between idiopathic hemolytic uremic syndrome and infection by verotoxin-producing *Escherichia coli*. J Infect Dis 1985; 151:775-782.

36. Delans RD, Binso JD, Saba SR, et al: Hemolytic-uremic syndrome after *Campylobacter*-induced diarrhea in adult. Arch Intern Med 1984;114:1074-1076.

37. Drummond KN: Hemolytic uremic syndrome—then and now. N Engl J Med 1985;312:116-118.

38. Greenough WB 3rd. Hemolytic uremia syndrome after shigellosis [letter]. N Engl J Med 1975;293:305.

39. Moorthy B, Makker SP: Hemolytic-uremic syndrome associated with pneumococcal sepsis. J Pediatr 1979;95:558-559.

40. Raghupathy P, Date A, Shastry JC, et al: Haemolytic-uremic syndrome complicating shigella dysentery in South Indian children. BMJ 1978;1:1518-1521.

41. Blackall DP, Marques MB: Hemolytic uremic syndrome revisited: shiga toxin, factor H, and fibrin generation. Am J Clin Pathol 2004;121(Suppl):S81-S88.

42. Salerno AE, Meyers KE, McGowan KL, et al: Hemolytic uremic syndrome in a child with laboratory-acquired *Escherichia coli* O157:H7. J Pediatr 2004;145:412-414.

43. Liebman HA, Weitz IC: Disseminated intravascular coagulation. In Hoffman R, Benz EJ, Shattil S, et al (eds): Hematology Basic Principles and Practice, 4th ed. Philadelphia: Saunders, 2005:2169-2182.

44. Fleming AF, Storey J, Molineaux L, et al: Abnormal haemoglobinis in the Sudan savanna of Nigeria: I. Prevalence of haemoglobins and relationships between sickle cell trait, malaria and survival. Ann Trop Med Parasitol 1979;73:161-172.

45. Sheehy TW: Disseminated intravascular coagulation and severe falciparum malaria. Lancet 1975;1:516.

46. Carr DJ, Kramer BS, Dragonetti DE: Thrombotic thrombocytopenic purpura associated with metastatic gastric adenocarcinoma: successful management with plasmapheresis. South Med J 1986;79:476-479.

47. Candoni A, Pizzolitto S, Boscutti G, et al: Atypical haemolytic-uraemic syndrome at the onset of acute promyelocytic leukaemia. Br J Haematol 2005;128:274.

48. Ohashi N, Yamamoto T, Kanno D, et al: A case of thrombotic microangiopathy complicated with systemic lupus erythematosus. Am J Med Sci 2003;326:102-104.

49. Lapp H, Shin DI, Kroells W, et al: Cardiogenic shock due to thrombotic thrombocytopenic purpura. Z Kardiol 2004; 93:486-492.

50. Doll DC, Ringenberg QS, Yarbro JW: Vascular toxicity associated with antineoplastic agents. J Clin Oncol 1986; 4:1405-1417.

51. Baker KR, Moake J: Hemolytic anemia resulting from physical injury to red cells. In Lichtman MA, Beutler E, Kipps TJ, et al (eds): Williams Hematology, 7th ed. New York: McGraw-Hill, 2006:709-716.

52. Marsh GW, Lewis SM: Cardiac haemolytic anemia. Semin Hematol 1969;6:133-149.

53. Banfi G, Roi GS, Dolci A, et al: Behaviour of haematological parameters in athletes performing marathons and ultra-marathons in altitude ("skyrunners"). Clin Lab Haematol 2004;26:373-377.

54. Dubnov G, Constantini NW: Prevalence of iron depletion and anemia in top-level basketball players. Int J Sport Nutr Exerc Metab 2004;14:30-37.

55. Fallon KE: Utility of hematological and iron-related screening in elite athletes. Clin J Sport Med 2004;14:145-152.

56. Halm EA, Wang JJ, Boockvar K, et al: The effect of perioperative anemia on clinical and functional outcomes in patients with hip fracture. J Orthop Trauma 2004;18:369-374.

57. Unal M, Ozer Unal D: Gene doping in sports. Sports Med 2004;34:357-362.

58. Davidson RJ: Exertional hemoglobinuria: a report on three cases with studies on the haemolytic mechanism. J Clin Pathol 1964;17:536-540.

59. Peters W: *Plasmodium*: resistance to antimalarial drugs. Ann Parasitol Hum Comp 1990;65(Suppl):103-106.

60. Howard RJ: Malaria: the search for vaccine antigens and new chemotherapeutic strategies. Blood 1989;74:533-536.

61. Gordan DM: Malaria vaccines. Infect Dis Clin North Am 1990;4:299-313.

62. Wyler DJ: Malaria—resurgence, resistance, and research (second of 2 parts). N Engl J Med 1983;308:934-940.

63. Dvorak JA, Miller LH, Whitehorse WC, et al: Invasion of erythrocytes by malaria merozoites. Science 1975;187:748-750.

64. Markell EK, John DT, Krotoski W: Markell and Voge's Medical Parasitology, 8th ed. Philadelphia: Saunders, 1999.

65. White NJ, Warrell DA: Clinical management of chloroquine-resistant *Plasmodium falciparum* malaria in Southeast Asia. Trop Doct 1983;13:153-158.

66. Aleem MA: Epilepsy in malaria. Epilepsia 2005;46:601, author reply 601-602.

67. Ruwende C, Hill A: Glucose-6-phosphate dehydrogenase deficiency and malaria. J Mol Med 1998;76:581-588.

68. Perrin LH, Mackey LJ, Miescher PA: The hematology of malaria in man. Semin Hematol 1982;19:70-82.

69. Jeng MR, Glader B: Acquired nonimmune hemolytic disorders. In Greer JP, Foerster J, Lukens JN, et al (eds): Wintrobe's Clinical Hematology, 11th ed. Philadelphia: Lippincott, Williams & Wilkins, 2004:1223-1246.

70. Allison AC: The distribution of sickle cell trait in East Africa and elsewhere and its apparent relationship to subtertian malaria. Trans R Soc Trop Med Hyg 1954;48:312-318.

71. Allison AC: Protection afforded by sickle cell trait against subtertian malaria infection. BMJ 1954;4857:290-294.

72. Nagel RL, Raventos-Suarez C, Fabry ME, et al: Impairment of the growth of *Plasmodium falciparum* in Hb EE erythrocytes. J Clin Invest 1981;68:303-305.

73. Siniscalco M, Bernini L, Filippi G, et al: Population genetics of haemoglobin variants, thalassemia and glucose-6-phosphate dehydrogenase deficiency, with particular reference to the malarial hypothesis. Bull World Health Organ 1966;34:379-393.

74. Pasvol G, Weatherall DJ, Wilson RJ: The effects of fetal hemoglobin on susceptibility of red cells to *Plasmodium falciparum*. Nature 1977;270:171-173.

75. Elghazali G, Adam I, Hamad A, et al: *Plasmodium falciparum* infection during pregnancy in an unstable transmission area in eastern Sudan. East Mediterr Health J 2003;9:570-580.
76. Vryonia G: Observations on the parasitization of erythrocytes by *Plasmodium vivax*, with special reference to reticulocytes. Am J Hyg 1939;30:41-48.
77. Miller LH, Mason SJ, Clyde DF, et al: The resistance factor to *Plasmodium vivax* in blacks: the Duffy-blind-group phenotype Fy-Fy. N Engl J Med 1976;295:302-304.
78. Susi B, Whitman T, Blazes DL, et al: Rapid diagnostic test for *Plasmodium falciparum* in 32 Marines medically evacuated from Liberia with a febrile illness. Ann Intern Med 2005; 142:476-477.
79. Chisholm ES, Sulzer AJ, Ruebush TK II: Indirect immuno-fluorescence test for human *Babesia microti* infection: antigenic specificity. Am J Trop Med Hyg 1986;35:921-925.
80. Healy GR: Babesia infections in man. Hosp Pract 1979; 14:107-111, 115-116.
81. Ruebush TK II, Cassaday PB, Marsh HJ, et al: Human babesiosis on Nantucket Island. Ann Intern Med 1977;86:6-9.
82. Meer-Scherrer L, Adelson M, Mordechai E, et al: *Babesia microti* infection in Europe. Curr Microbiol 2004;48:435-437.
83. Froberg MK, Dannen D, Bakken JS: Babesiosis and HIV. Lancet 2004;363:704.
84. Healy GR, Ruebush TK II: Morphology of *Babesia microti* in human blood smears. Am J Clin Pathol 1980;73:107-109.
85. Jacoby GA, Hunt JV, Kosinski KS, et al: Treatment of transfusion-transmitted babesiosis by exchange transfusion. N Engl J Med 1980;303:1098-1100.
86. Stone JH, Dierberg K, Aram G, et al: Human monocytic ehrlichiosis. JAMA 2004;292:2263-2270.
87. Garsde M, James R, Cooper N: A diagnosis not to miss. Hosp Med 2004;65:628-629.
88. Wen B, Cao W, Pan H: Ehrlichiae and ehrlichial diseases in China. Ann N Y Acad Sci 2003;990:45.
89. Maender J, Tyring S: Treatment and prevention of rickettsial and ehrrlichial infections. Dermatol Ther 2004;17:499-504.
90. Leiby DA, Gill EJ: Transfusion transmitted tick-borne infections. Trans Med Rev 2004;18:293-306.
91. Smith LA, Wright-Kanuth MS: Transfusion-transmitted parasites. Clin Lab Sci 2003;16:239-245, 251.
92. Beutler E: Hemolytic anemia resulting from infections with microorganisms. In Lichtman MA, Beutler E, Kipps TJ, et al (eds): Williams Hematology. New York: McGraw-Hill, 2006:723-727.
93. Mahn HE, Dantuono LM: Postabortal septicotoxemia due to *Clostridium welchii*. Am J Obstet Gynecol 1955;70:604-610.
94. Ricketts W: *Bartonella bacilliformis* anemia (Oroya fever): a study of 30 cases. Blood 1948;3:1025-1049.
95. Reynafarje C, Ramos J: The hemolytic anemia of human bartonellosis. Blood 1961;17:562-578.
96. Maurin M, Birtles R, Raoult D: Current knowledge of *Bartonella* species. Eur J Clin Microbiol Infect Dis 1997; 16:487-506.
97. Dhaliwal G, Cornett PA, Tierney LM Jr. Hemolytic anemia. Am Fam Physician 2004;69:2599-2606.
98. Beutler E: Hemolytic anemia resulting from chemical and physical agents. In Lichtman MA, Beutler E, Kipps TJ, et al (eds): Williams Hematology. New York: McGraw-Hill, 2006:717-721.
99. Bertazzi DT, de Assis-Pandochi AI, Azzolini AE, et al: Effect of *Tityus serrulatus* scorpion venom and its major toxin, TsTX-I, on the complement system in vivo. Toxicon 2003;41:501-508.
100. Seibert CS, Shinohara EM, Sano-Martins IS: In vitro hemolytic activity of *Lonomia obliqua* caterpillar bristle extract on human and Wistar rat erythrocytes. Toxicon 2003;41:831-839.
101. Tibballs J, Kuruppu S, Hodgson WC, et al: Cardiovascular, haematological and neurological effects of the venom of the Papua New Guinean small-eyed snake (*Micropechis ikaheka*) and their neutralisation with CSL polyvalent and black snake antivenoms. Toxicon 2003;42:647-655.
102. Bergeron MF, Cannon JG, Hall EL, et al: Erythrocyte sickling during exercise and thermal stress. Clin J Sport Med 2004;14:354-356.
103. Lamchiagdhase P, Nitipongwanich R, Rattanapong C, et al: Red blood cell vesicles in thalassemia. J Med Assoc Thai 2004;87:233-238.

Extracorpuscular Defects Leading to Increased Erythrocyte Destruction—Immune Causes

25

Vishnu V. B. Reddy

OBJECTIVES

After completion of this chapter, the reader will be able to:

1. Define immune hemolytic anemia.
2. Explain the mechanism of premature red blood cell (RBC) destruction in autoimmune hemolytic anemia (AHA).
3. Describe how the direct antiglobulin test (DAT) is used as a screening procedure for AHA.
4. List the immunoglobulin type, the maximum temperature reactivity, the role of complement activation, and the type of hemolysis that is usually present in warm-reactive AHA.
5. List the immunoglobulin type and common specificity, the maximum temperature reactivity, the role of complement activation, and the type of hemolysis that is usually present in cold-reactive AHA.
6. List the immunoglobulin type and usual specificity, the maximum temperature reactivity, the role of complement activation, and the type of hemolysis that is usually present in paroxysmal cold hemoglobinuria.
7. Describe the pathogenesis of paroxysmal cold hemoglobinuria.
8. Describe the different mechanisms of drug-induced immune hemolytic anemia with emphasis on the specificity of the antibody.
9. Describe the two types of hemolytic transfusion reactions, the usual immunoglobulin class involved, and the typical type of hemolysis, and list the important laboratory findings.
10. Describe hemolytic disease of the newborn (HDN), including how alloimmunization of the mother occurs, the type of hemolysis affecting the fetus, and commonly involved antigen systems, and describe the laboratory findings for mother and infant.
11. Given results of DAT testing, including tests with drug-treated cells and eluates, distinguish different forms of warm AHA.

CASE STUDY

After studying the material in this chapter, the reader should be able to respond to the following case study:

A 20-year-old woman sought medical attention for an elevated temperature and a possible insect bite. Physical examination revealed a small bite wound on the right lateral area of the chest that was tender and contained a clear fluid with no pus. Necrosis was not evident. A diffuse erythematous rash on most of her body also was observed. The physician prescribed 40 mL of liquid acetaminophen (Tylenol) and 10 days of cephalexin (Keflex). A secretion from the lesion was subjected to culture, but there was no growth after 72 hours. Blood was drawn for cultures, which were reported as negative after 5 days. Four days later, the patient went to the emergency department, complaining of being unable to walk. A complete blood count, urinalysis, urine and sputum cultures, and chemistry profile were ordered.

Laboratory Data	Patient	Reference
WBC ($\times 10^9$/L)	5.9	4.5-11
RBC ($\times 10^{12}$/L)	1.14	4.3-5.9
Hb (g/dL)	3.8	13.9-16.3
Hct (%)	10	39-55

Continued

The platelet count was within normal reference range. The peripheral blood smear revealed normochromic, normocytic RBCs with few spherocytes and an increase in neutrophilic bands, few early WBCs, and 3 nucleated RBCs (Fig. 25-1). Urinalysis yielded 3+ blood. Urine and sputum cultures were negative. Significant values from the chemistry profile included elevated levels of total bilirubin, alkaline phosphatase, lactate dehydrogenase, and aspartate aminotransferase. Subsequently, the patient was typed and crossmatched for 3 units of blood. A positive direct antiglobulin test (DAT) was reported. The indirect antiglobulin test was negative. An eluate prepared from the patient's cells was negative with all panel cells tested.

1. Is this type of anemia caused by intracorpuscular or extracorpuscular defects?
2. What does a positive result of the DAT imply?
3. What mechanisms can lead to the development of drug-related antibodies and drug-induced immune hemolytic anemia?

4. Describe the mechanism that is the most probable cause of this patient's anemia.
5. What is the treatment of choice?

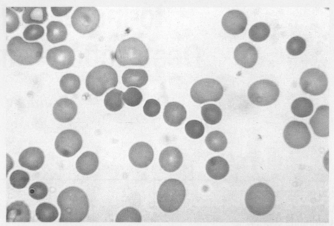

Figure 25-1 Peripheral blood smear of patient in case study.

IMMUNE HEMOLYTIC ANEMIA

The immune hemolytic anemias are extrinsic hemolytic anemias in which auto- or allo-antibodies that bind RBCs and fix complement shorten red blood cell (RBC) life span. Antibody-coated RBCs are removed extravascularly by macrophages equipped with Fc and complement receptors, and in the most severe cases, through intravascular complement lysis. Key laboratory findings are normocytic/normochromic anemia (some may be macrocytic) with spherocytes, schistocytes, and polychromatophilia on blood film examination, reticulocytosis, positive direct antiglobulin test, and increased bone marrow hematopoiesis.

The immune hemolytic anemias are classified as warm-reacting autoimmune hemolytic anemias (AHAs), cold agglutinin disease, drug-induced immune hemolytic anemias, and alloimmune hemolytic anemias.[1-3]

AUTOIMMUNE HEMOLYTIC ANEMIA

Autoimmune hemolytic anemia is characterized by premature RBC destruction caused by autoantibodies that bind the RBC surface (Table 25-1).[3] The disorder is probably secondary to an altered state of immunity with loss of immune tolerance. Normally, autoimmunity is kept in check by T suppressor lymphocytes. In autoimmune hemolytic anemia, this restraint is lost, resulting in the production of autoantibodies against RBC "self-antigens." Association with the following altered states of immunity supports this theory: chronic lymphocytic leukemia, lymphoma, myelodysplastic syndrome,[4] immuno-

globulin deficiency,[5] autoimmune diseases (especially disseminated lupus erythematosus), drug use, and viral infection.[1,3,6-9]

Diagnosis

Diagnosis of autoimmune hemolytic anemia depends on the demonstration of antibody, complement, or both on the RBC surface. Primary AHA has been estimated to occur at an annual incidence of 1 in 80,000 unselected individuals.[1] The direct antiglobulin test (DAT) or direct Coombs' test detects sensitization, antibodies, and complement components coating the surface of RBCs. The DAT defeats the net negative charge of the RBC surface. This charge causes RBCs to repel one another, preventing IgG antibody from bridging the gap between cells to cause agglutination. Polyspecific antihuman globulin provides antibodies against the Fc portion of human IgG and against the C3 complement component. When antihuman globulin is added to RBCs coated with IgG antibody or complement, agglutination is visible. Once agglutination is shown with polyspecific anti-human globulin, monospecific anti-IgG and anti-C3 are used to identify the type of sensitization.[7,10]

Warm-Reactive Antibodies

Warm-reactive autoimmune hemolytic anemia (WAIHA) is responsible for approximately 70% of immune hemolytic anemia cases.[3] Antibodies are primary, in which the cause or underlying defect is not apparent, or secondary. Secondary autoantibodies are associated with systemic autoimmune disease, chronic lymphocytic leukemia, lymphoma, occasional viral infections, and immunodeficiency syndromes.[3,7,8,11]

TABLE 25-1 Characteristics of Autoimmune Hemolytic Anemias

	Warm Reactive	Cold Reactive	Paroxysmal Cold Hemoglobinuria
Immunoglobulin	IgG	IgM	IgG
Maximum temperature reactivity	37° C	4° C	4° C
Complement activation	Variable	Yes	Yes
Hemolysis	Usually extravascular	Intravascular and extravascular	Intravascular
Autoantibody specificity	Rh complex, rarely specific Rh antigen or other	Ii	P
Treatment	Corticosteroids, splenectomy	Avoidance of cold, plasmapheresis	Avoidance of cold, corticosteroids

Patients with human immunodeficiency virus may rarely develop RBC autoantibodies.[12] Evans and associates first noticed the combination of autoimmune anemia with autoimmune thrombocytopenia, now referred to as *Evans syndrome*. A large review of childhood Evans syndrome cases reported that the typical course is chronic and relapsing.[13,14]

The warm-reactive antibody that mediates WAIHA is usually of the IgG isotype and maximum immunogenicity occurs at 37° C. Of IgG1 through IgG4, IgG1 and IgG3 antibodies fix complement.[1] One study comprising several thousand patients found 74% of WAIHA patients had IgG1, 2.1% had IgG3, 20.1% had multiple IgG subclasses including IgG1, and the rest had IgG3 and IgG4.[8] In WAIHA, hemolysis is generally extravascular, with the antibody-coated or antibody and complement–coated cells reacting with Fc and C3 receptors on the membranes of mononuclear phagocytes. Complement-mediated lysis is absent because the antigen against which the antibody is directed is widely spaced, and the lytic sequence cannot be completed. In extravascular hemolysis, a portion of the RBC membrane is removed by the macrophage, and the remaining membrane reanneals, forming a spherocyte. In some cases the entire RBC may be engulfed.[7] Sensitization is particularly common in systemic lupus erythematosus,[15] although not all patients with systemic lupus and a positive DAT develop hemolytic anemia[16,17]

IgG autoantibody is detected using the DAT. About 50% of warm-reactive autoantibodies bind the Rh protein complex. Anti-e is the most common specificity, but anti-c, anti-Sc1, anti-Wr^b, and anti–Gerbich-like autoantibodies have been reported.[3,18] Rare cases of WAIHA have been reported to have IgM autoantibodies. IgM antibodies function best at 20° C to 30° C and are directed against the high-frequency antigenic determinants of glycophorin A. Fatal outcomes of IgM-mediated WAIHA are reported.[18]

Fewer than 10% of WAIHA cases are caused by a combination of isotypes; these are identified as mixed-type WAIHA and usually have simultaneous IgG and IgM autoantibodies. The IgG immunoglobin is most likely responsible for extravascular hemolysis. The IgM is most responsible for comple-

ment activation that may lead to intravascular hemolysis.[3] Patients with mixed-type WAIHA often present with an acute severe anemia that becomes chronic.

The WAIHA patient may present with jaundice or splenomegaly. Sudden onset of severe anemia is possible, and in very severe cases, the patient may have fever, pallor, splenomegaly, hepatomegaly, and tachycardia. An underlying lymphoproliferative disorder is suggested by massive splenomegaly and lymphadenopathy.[18,19]

The blood smear reveals an increase in polychromatophilic RBCs, occasional NRBCs, and spherocytes (see Fig. 25-1). When the diagnosis of hereditary spherocytosis has been ruled out, spherocytes suggest an immune hemolytic process. The reticulocyte count varies between 5% and 10%. The osmotic fragility is increased (Chapter 23), and there is bone marrow erythroid hyperplasia. Indirect bilirubin is increased, as are urinary and fecal urobilinogen levels. Haptoglobin levels are reduced, yet hemoglobinuria is rarely encountered.[7] Mild leukocytosis and neutrophilia are often noted. The DAT is an essential assay in WAIHA. Platelets are normal in number except in Evans syndrome.[13]

Prednisone has improved the management and reduced the mortality in WAIHA. A marked reduction of hemolysis occurs in about two thirds of patients treated. Complete remission occurs in about 20%, but 10% show no response. Prednisone should be administered for several months, and the dosage should be tapered over 1 or 2 months. Relapses of WAIHA may occur, and patients should be observed periodically.[1,3]

Splenectomy may be performed in patients who require long-term, high-dose prednisone therapy to maintain the hemoglobin at a satisfactory level. Splenectomy may not cure AHA, however, and additional immunosuppressive drugs, intravenous immunoglobulin, or antilymphocyte globulin may be used.[1,3]

Cold-Reactive Autoantibodies

Cold agglutinins are usually IgM antibodies whose thermal range is 20° to 30°C.[1,7] Primary cold agglutinin disease is a rare chronic hemolytic anemia in which IgM autoantibody binds complement in vivo while the individual is in a cold environment. Patients are usually 50 or older and suffer anemia, hemoglobinuria, and peripheral vaso-occlusive phenomena (acrocyanosis, Raynaud's phenomenon) when exposed to cold. The skin turns white and then blue with numbness and pain. Hemolysis is predominantly extravascular.

Secondary cold agglutinins appear acutely 2-3 weeks following *Mycoplasma pneumoniae*, infectious mononucleosis, or other viral infections. Chronic lymphocytic leukemia, lymphoma, and other autoimmune disorders are also associated with cold agglutinins.

In both primary and secondary cold agglutinin disease, IgM antibodies arise against the Ii system of RBC antigens. Newborns have the i antigen, which changes to the I antigen in the first few months of life.[7,20]

Full complement activation may cause intravascular hemolysis. Alternatively, complement activation may stop at C3b binding. In this instance, extravascular hemolysis may occur as splenic macrophage receptors bind C3b. Some C3b is transformed to C3d, which is undetected in the spleen.[21]

When a cold agglutinin is present, an anticoagulated blood specimen visibly agglutinates at room temperature or below. When warmed to 37° C, the agglutination often disappears. If not, a new specimen is collected and maintained at 37° C. To avoid blood film RBC agglutination, the slide is first warmed to 37° C.[3] Blood from patients with cold agglutinins must be warmed to 37° C for 15 minutes before it is analyzed. Room temperature agglutination grossly elevates the mean cell volume, reduces the RBC count, and has unpredictable effects on other indices and RBC morphology comments.

The DAT is positive for complement at 15° C to 32° C. A cold agglutinin method is used to titer the antibody, which may reach levels of 1:10,000.[7,21]

The patient avoids exposure to cold and may choose to move to a warm climate.[1,7,21] Plasmapheresis may be used in severe cases but provides only temporary benefit.[21] Anti-CD-20 antibody therapy (Rituximab) elicited at least a partial remission to hemolytic anemia in several studies.[22-26]

Paroxysmal Cold Hemoglobinuria

Paroxysmal cold hemoglobinuria is a rare acute form of cold-generated hemolysis. A complement-binding IgG antibody with specificity for the P antigens reacts at 15° C or below. The reaction is biphasic. Complement binds in cold, but the lytic sequence is completed only after warming. Paroxysmal cold hemoglobinuria is severe and acute but self-limited. It has been associated with congenital, chronic, or tertiary syphilis, acute viral disorders, and idiopathic myelofibrosis.[27,28] The etiology of the autoantibody is unknown.

Donath and Landsteiner first described cold hemoglobinuria in 1904, and it is often called *Donath-Landsteiner hemolytic anemia*. The Donath-Landsteiner antibody dissociates from RBCs at body temperature, so the DAT detects only complement sensitization.[7]

A short time after exposure to cold, the patient develops pain in the back and legs, abdominal cramps, headaches, chills, and fever. Hemoglobinemia and hemoglobinuria

appear as the symptoms develop. Spherocytes and reticulocytosis are noted on the blood film, and monocytes and neutrophils may phagocytize RBCs. At first, leukopenia may be present; later, leukocytosis occurs.[29] The DAT is positive for complement during an attack and the antibody is non-agglutinating. It can be detected by incubating the patient's fresh serum with RBCs at 4° C and warming the mixture to 37° C. Intense hemolysis occurs after warming.[7,29]

DRUG-INDUCED HEMOLYTIC ANEMIA

Drug-induced immune hemolytic anemias are usually self-limiting, but severe, even fatal, cases have been reported. After it is recognized, drug-induced immune hemolysis is easily treated by drug termination, and later episodes are prevented by avoidance of the drug.

Ternary Type Drug-Induced Hemolysis

In ternary drug-induced hemolysis, IgG antibodies bind drug-epitope combination sites, called *neoantigens*. The drug-epitope-antibody complex on the membrane activates complement to trigger acute intravascular hemolysis, often with thrombocytopenia. The drugs most often implicated are quinidine, phenacetin, and stibophen. Hemolysis occurs after short periods of administration or upon readministration. The DAT detects only complement. In the indirect antiglobulin test using reagent RBCs, the serum is reactive in the presence of the drug. The RBC eluate is often nonreactive.[29,33]

Hapten or Drug Adsorption–Induced Hemolysis

In the hapten mechanism the drug is nonspecifically bound or adsorbed to RBCs and remains firmly adherent. The patient develops an antibody directly to the drug. Complement is not usually bound. The drugs implicated are penicillins and, rarely, cephalosporins. Large doses of penicillin (10-20 million U daily) produce a hemolytic reaction 7 to 10 days after administration. The extravascular hemolysis is mild to moderate. The DAT is positive for IgG or, rarely, IgG and complement. In the indirect antiglobulin test the patient's serum or RBC eluate reacts with drug-treated RBCs but not with normal RBCs.[29]

Nonimmunologic Protein Adsorption

High-dose cephalosporins and cisplatin alter the RBC membrane so that numerous proteins, including IgG and complement, are adsorbed. This phenomenon results in a positive DAT, but only rarely has hemolysis been reported. In the indirect antiglobulin test, no serum antibodies are found.[29,34]

Autoantibody-Induced Hemolysis

Methyldopa and procainamide induce gradual-onset, DAT-positive AHA. Only IgG is detected; complement is rarely present. Serum or RBC eluate antibodies agglutinate unaltered homologous or autologous RBCs in the absence of the drug in the indirect antiglobulin test. These antibodies seem to be directed against the RBCs and not a drug-RBC complex.

Hemolysis resolves after withdrawal of the drug, but some patients may retain a positive DAT for 2 years.[29]

Several authors have suggested that all drug-induced immune hemolysis is explained by a single mechanism, the unifying theory. This suggests the drug interacts with the RBC membrane and generates multicomponent immunogenic epitopes that elicit an immune response to the drug alone, the drug-RBC membrane combination, or the RBC alone.

Therapy for Drug-Induced Immune Hemolysis

Several new therapeutic agents, such as the third-generation cephalosporins, ceftriaxone and cefotaxime, have been associated with severe and even fatal AHA. Second-generation cephalosporins (e.g., cefotetan) also have been implicated in AHA but less often. Other drugs involved in AHA are sodium diclofenac, a widely used nonsteroidal anti-inflammatory drug; fludarabine and cladribine, used to treat chronic lymphocytic leukemia; cisplatin; carboplatin; and β-lactamase inhibitors. The list of drugs causing immune hemolysis continues to grow.[6,34,35]

ALLOIMMUNE HEMOLYTIC ANEMIAS

Hemolytic Transfusion Reactions

All transfusions carry the risk of morbidity, and approximately 1 in 500,000 transfusions has a mismatch-related fatal outcome. Most ABO mismatches result from the administration of blood that was given to a misidentified patient.[36] Transfusions may also cause delayed transfusion reactions.

Immediate Hemolytic Transfusion Reaction

Symptoms of severe intravascular hemolysis typical of ABO incompatibility begin within minutes or hours and may include chills, fever, urticaria, tachycardia, nausea and vomiting, chest and back pain, shock, anaphylaxis, pulmonary edema, disseminated intravascular coagulation (DIC), and congestive heart failure. The transfusion is immediately terminated. Treatment is urgent and includes an effort to prevent or correct shock, to maintain renal circulation, and to control DIC.

The laboratory diagnosis provides evidence of hemolysis and of blood group incompatibility. Hemoglobinemia and hemoglobinuria are detectable. The indirect bilirubin level rises, and haptoglobin level drops. The type and crossmatch are repeated to identify the blood group incompatibility. Coagulation tests reveal and assess DIC.

Delayed Hemolytic Transfusion Reaction

A transfusion reaction may occur up to 2 weeks after transfusion as alloantibodies appear. Often, the patient has been alloimmunized by a pregnancy or previous transfusion, but the antibody titer was below the level of serologic detection at the time of administration. The antibody coats the transfused RBCs, leading to hemolysis. Inadequate hemoglobin response, positive DAT, morphologic evidence of hemolysis, and indirect bilirubinemia are the principal signs.[36] Hemolysis also may occur in transmission of malaria and babesiosis, hepatitis, human immunodeficiency virus, and cytomegalovirus.

Rh Blood Group System and Hemolytic Disease of the Newborn

Despite the universal use of Rh immune globulin therapy, the D antigen of the Rh blood group system may occasionally trigger alloimmunization and hemolytic disease of the newborn (HDN). The mother produces an antibody to the fetal antigen she lacks; for example, an Rh (D)-negative woman may develop an alloantibody to a D-positive fetus.

Alloimmune HDN is a disease of the fetus and the newborn characterized by hemolytic anemia, unconjugated bilirubinemia, and extramedullary hematopoiesis. IgG anti-D crosses the placenta and coats the fetal D-positive RBCs. The coated RBCs form rosettes around macrophages, mainly in the spleen. The RBC membrane is phagocytosed by the macrophage causing loss of membrane, sphering, and eventual lysis. The hemolysis causes anemia, splenomegaly, and hepatomegaly, with an outpouring of immature nucleated RBCs in the peripheral blood. Diffusely basophilic cells are also present, reflected in reticulocytosis. Thrombocytopenia may be common in severely affected infants and may lead to hemorrhage. Bilirubin cannot be conjugated by the infant's immature hepatic mechanism. Neuron cell death occurs, and evidence of kernicterus is present at autopsy.[32]

Laboratory Findings

Mothers should be grouped and typed during the first trimester of pregnancy. The unimmunized D-negative mother receives Rh immune globulin at 28 weeks' gestation and again after delivery. To be effective, Rh immune globulin should be given before a suspected Rh immune response. Rh-negative women who experience spontaneous or induced abortion should also receive Rh immune globulin. If a repeat antibody screen is to be done, the specimen should be obtained before the Rh immune globulin is administered; however, the Rh immune globulin may be given before results are returned.[2,38]

If the mother is alloimmunized, the specificity and titer of antibody should be determined by the indirect antiglobulin method. Antibody titers should be repeated at 18 weeks' gestation and every 2 to 4 weeks thereafter until delivery.[38] Titration of the antibody does not predict the severity of HDN; rather, it helps determine when to monitor for HDN by additional methods, such as spectrophotometric analysis of amniotic fluid bilirubin.[38,39] Amniocentesis is accurate at predicting severe fetal anemia, but it is an invasive procedure and carries significant risk.[39]

If severe fetal anemia is suspected, percutaneous umbilical venous fetal blood sampling using ultrasound equipment provides an accurate profile of the severity of hemolytic disease. The DAT, hemoglobin, and bilirubin determinations are performed.[2]

Treatment for the Affected Infant

Treatment for a fetus affected by HDN may include intrauterine transfusion, which can be used to correct fetal anemia and prevent hydrops. After delivery, the neonate may need exchange transfusions and phototherapy.[2]

HDN Caused by Other Blood Group Antigens

ABO HDN is more common than Rh disease and may occur during the first pregnancy. Like Rh disease, ABO disease produces hyperbilirubinemia and anemia. ABO HDN usually occurs in infants with blood groups A or B born to group O mothers who produce IgG anti-A and anti-B. The disease is milder than Rh HDN because most anti-A and anti-B antibodies are IgM isotype and do not cross the placenta. Antigens A and B are found on non-RBC fetal tissue and can absorb the mother's anti-A or anti-B.[2,32]

The DAT result in ABO hemolytic disease is only weakly positive and may be falsely negative. ABO incompatibility results in spherocytes on the peripheral blood smear, whereas Rh incompatibility does not. Table 25-2 presents a comparison of HDN caused by ABO and Rh incompatibility.[2,32]

HDN caused by anti-c and anti-Kell is rare but is similar in severity to anti-D. HDN caused by anti-C or anti-E is usually mild.[45] Jaundice and kernicterus are the adverse clinical outcomes in all forms of HDN.[2,32]

At delivery, cord blood may be collected for ABO and Rh testing for DAT, and for determination of hemoglobin level, unconjugated bilirubin level, enumeration of nucleated RBCs in peripheral blood, and platelet and reticulocyte counts. The cord blood findings and the clinical appearance of the infant determine treatment.[2,32]

TABLE 25-2 Characteristics of Rh and ABO Hemolytic Disease of the Newborn

	Rh	ABO
Blood groups		
Mother	Rh negative	O
Child	Rh positive	A or B
Severity of disease	Severe	Mild
Jaundice	Severe	Mild
Spherocytes on peripheral blood smear	Rare	Usually present
Anemia	Severe	If present, mild
DAT	Positive	Negative or weakly positive

CHAPTER at a GLANCE

- The immune hemolytic anemias are classified into autoimmune, drug-induced, and alloimmune hemolytic anemias.
- AHA is a complex clinical disorder characterized by premature RBC destruction caused by autoantibodies that bind to the antigens on the RBC surface.
- The diagnosis of AHA depends on the demonstration of antibody, complement, or both on the RBC surface.
- AHA antibodies are warm or cold-reactive.
- Warm-reactive AHA is the most common form of AHA and involves IgG antibodies with a maximum reaction at 37° C.
- Warm-reactive AHA varies from mild to severe. Laboratory characteristics are RBCs, spherocytes, possible nucleated RBCs, elevated reticulocyte count, increased osmotic fragility test, erythroid hyperplasia in the bone marrow, increased total bilirubin, and reduced haptoglobin.
- The demonstration of immunoglobulin or complement on the RBCs is necessary to the diagnosis of AHA.
- Cold agglutin disease is caused by IgM anti-RBC autoantibodies with a thermal range of 20°-30° C.

- Cold agglutinin disease is triggered by exposure to cold. Peripheral vaso-occlusion causes intravascular hemolysis with hematuria.
- Paroxysmal cold hemoglobinuria is a rare form of cold-reactive AHA that is characterized by acute episodes of massive hemolysis that occur after exposure to cold.
- Several mechanisms of drug-induced AHA have been described, including ternary, hapten or drug absorption mechanism, non-immunologic protein adsorption, and autoantibodies.
- Before RHIg therapy, alloimmunization by Rh(D) caused the most instances of HDN. ABO incompatibility is now the most prevalent cause.
- HDN is characterized by hemolytic anemia, hyperbilirubinemia, and extramedullary erythropoiesis.
- Other blood group antigens, including ABO, anti-c, and anti-Kell, can cause HDN.

Now that you have completed this chapter, go back and read again the case study at the beginning and respond to the questions presented.

REVIEW QUESTIONS

1. AHA is characterized by:
   a. Membrane abnormalities
   b. Autoantibodies
   c. Abnormal hemoglobin molecule
   d. Alloantibodies

2. The preferred screening test for AHA is:
   a. DAT
   b. Reticulocyte count
   c. Indirect antiglobulin
   d. Direct bilirubin assay

3. The diagnosis of autoimmune hemolytic anemia depends on:
   a. Detecting a low hemoglobin and hematocrit
   b. Observation of spherocytes on the peripheral blood smear
   c. Recognition of a low reticulocyte count
   d. Demonstration of antibody, complement, or both on the RBC surface

4. The antibody that mediates the hemolytic process in warm-reactive AHA is usually of which immunoglobulin class?
   a. A
   b. E
   c. G
   d. M

5. The hemolysis in warm-reactive AHA is usually:
   a. Extravascular
   b. Complement mediated
   c. Intravascular
   d. Not significant

6. Laboratory results in warm-reactive AHA include all of the following *except*:
   a. Spherocytes
   b. Reticulocytosis
   c. Decreased haptoglobin
   d. Elevated direct bilirubin

7. Cold agglutinins are characteristically:
   a. IgA and agglutinate RBCs at 37° C
   b. IgE and agglutinate RBCs at less than 30° C
   c. IgG and agglutinate RBCs at 37° C
   d. IgM and agglutinate RBCs at less than 30° C

8. Cold-reactive hemolytic anemia involves which system?
   a. Rh
   b. Wr^b
   c. Gerbich
   d. Ii

9. Secondary forms of cold-reactive AHA are associated with all of the following *except*:
   a. Antibiotics
   b. *M. pneumoniae* infection
   c. B cell malignancies
   d. Infectious mononucleosis

10. A patient is suspected to have a drug-induced hemolytic reaction. The patient's DAT is positive for complement only, but antibody testing on an eluate of the cells is negative. When the patient's serum is allowed to react with cells pretreated with the suspect drug, the result is positive. This suggests which mechanism of hemolysis for this patient?
    a. Immune complex
    b. Drug absorption
    c. Nonimmunologic drug adsorption
    d. Autoimmune

11. The most important blood group antigen that may cause alloimmunization and HDN is:
    a. c
    b. D
    c. E
    d. e

ACKNOWLEDGMENT

The author acknowledges Martha S. Payne, who was the principal author of this chapter in the previous editions.

REFERENCES

1. Ware RE: Autoimmune hemolytic anemia. In Nathan DG, Orkin SH, Ginsberg G, et al (eds): Nathan and Oski's Hematology of Infancy and Childhood, 6th ed. Philadelphia: Saunders, 2003:521-559.
2. Ramasethu J, Luban NLC: Alloimmune hemolytic disease of the newborn. In Lichtman MA, Beutler E, Kipps TJ, et al (eds): Williams Hematology, 7th ed. New York: McGraw-Hill, 2006:751-766.
3. Smith L: Autoimmune hemolytic anemia: introduction. Clin Lab Sci 1999;12:110-114.
4. Giagounidis AA, Haase S, Germing U, et al: Autoimmune disorders in two patients with myelodysplastic syndrome and 5q deletion. Acta Haematol 2005;113:146-149.
5. Muta T, Yamano Y: Angioimmunoblastic T-cell lymphoma associated with an antibody to human immunodeficiency virus protein. Int J Hematol 2003;78:160-162.
6. O'Brien TA, Eastlund T, Peters C, et al: Autoimmune haemolytic anaemia complicating haematopoietic cell transplantation in paediatric patients: high incidence and significant mortality in unrelated donor transplants for non-malignant diseases. Br J Haematol 2004;127:67-75.
7. Packman CH: Hemolytic anemia resulting from immune injury. In Lichtman MA, Beutler E, Kipps TJ, et al (eds): Williams Hematology, 7th ed. New York: McGraw-Hill, 2006:729-750.
8. Engelfreit CP, Overbeeke MA, von dem Borne AE: Autoimmune hemolytic anemia. Semin Hematol 1992;29:3-13.
9. Stalnikowicz R, Amitai Y, Bentur Y: Aphrodisiac drug-induced hemolysis. J Toxicol Clin Toxicol 2004;42:313-316.
10. Huot AE, Howard PR, Blaney KD: Immunology basics: principles and applications in the blood bank. In Blaney KD, Howard PR (eds): Basic and Applied Concepts of Immunohematology. St Louis: Mosby, 2000:3-35.
11. Ziman A, Hsi R, Goldfinger D: Transfusion medicine illustrated: Donath-Landsteiner antibody-associated hemolytic anemia after *Haemophilus influenzae* infection in a child. Transfusion 2004;44:1127-1128.
12. Telen MJ, Roberts KB, Bartlett JA: HIV-associated autoimmune hemolytic anemia: report of a case and review of the literature. J Acquir Immune Defic Syndr 1990;3:933-937.
13. Pui Ch, Wilimas J, Wang W: Evans syndrome in childhood. J Pediatr 1980;97:754-758.

14. Ramanathan S, Koutts J, Hertzberg MS: Two cases of refractory warm autoimmune hemolytic anemia treated with rituximab. Am J Hematol 2005;78:123-126.
15. Sultan SM, Begum S, Isenberg DA: Prevalence, patterns of disease and outcome in patients with systemic lupus erythematosus who develop severe haematological problems. Rheumatology 2003;42:230-234.
16. Giannouli S, Voulgarelis M, Ziakas PD, et al: Anaemia in systemic lupus erythematosus: from pathophysiology to clinical assessment. Ann Rheum Dis 2006;65:144-148.
17. Budman DR, Steinberg AD: Hematologic aspect of systemic lupus erythrmatosus. Ann Intern Med 1977;86:220-229.
18. Garratty G, Arndt P, Domen R, et al: Severe autoimmune hemolytic anemia associated with autoantibodies directed against determinants on or associated with glycophorin A. Vox Sang 1997;72:124-130.
19. Garratty G: Review: drug-induced immune hemolytic anemia—the last decade. Immunohematology 2004;20:138-146.
20. Sloan SR, Benjamin RJ, Friedman DF, et al: Transfusion medicine. In Nathan DG, Orkin SH, Ginsberg G, et al (eds): Nathan and Oski's Hematology of Infancy and Childhood, 6th ed. Philadelphia: Saunders, 2003:1709-1756.
21. Cunningham MJ, Silberstein LE: Autoimmune hemolytic anemia. In Hoffman R, Benz EJ Jr, Shattil SJ, et al (eds): Hematology Basic Principles and Practice. St Louis: Mosby, 2005:693-707
22. Schollkopf C, Kjeldsen L, Bjerrum OW, et al: Rituximab in chronic cold agglutinin disease: a prospective study of 20 patients. Leuk Lymphoma 2006;47:253-260.
23. Norton A, Roberts I: Management of Evans syndrome. Br J Haematol 2006;132:125-137.
24. Vassou A, Alymara V, Chaidos A, et al: Beneficial effect of rituximab in combination with oral cyclophosphamide in primary chronic cold agglutinin disease. Int J Hematol 2005; 81:421-423.
25. Mantadakis E, Danilatou V, Stiakaki E, et al: Rituximab for refractory Evans syndrome and other immune-mediated hematologic diseases. Am J Hematol 2004;77:303-310.
26. Berentsen S, Ulvestad E, Gjertsen BT, et al: Rituximab for primary chronic cold agglutinin disease: a prospective study of 37 courses of therapy in 27 patients. Blood 2004 15;103:2925-2928.
27. Breccia M, D'Elia GM, Girelli G, et al: Paroxysmal cold haemoglobinuria as a tardive complication of idiopathic myelofibrosis. Eur J Haematol 2004;73:304-306.
28. Mukhopadhyay S, Keating L, Souid AK: Erythrophagocytosis in paroxysmal cold hemoglobinuria. Am J Hematol 2003; 74:196-197.
29. Neff AT: Autoimmune hemolytic anemias. In Greer JP, Foerster J, Lukens JN, et al (eds): Wintrobe's Clinical Hematology, 11th ed. Philadelphia: Lippincott, Williams & Wilkins, 2004:1157-1182.
30. Dlott JS, Danielson CF, Blue-Hnidy DE, et al: Drug-induced thrombotic thrombocytopenic purpura/hemolytic uremic syndrome: a concise review. Ther Apher Dial 2004;8:102-111.
31. Jabr FI, Shamseddine A, Taher A: Hydroxyurea-induced hemolytic anemia in a patient with essential thrombocythemia. Am J Hematol 2004;77:374-376.
32. Liley HG: Immune hemolytic disease. In Nathan DG, Orkin SH, Ginsberg G, et al (eds): Nathan and Oski's Hematology of Infancy and Childhood, 6th ed. Philadelphia: Saunders, 2003:56-85.
33. Rosse WF, Hillmen P, Schreiber AD: Immune-mediated hemolytic anemia. Hematology (Am Soc Hematol Educ Program) 2004;48-62.
34. Shariatmadar S, Storry JR, Sausais L, et al: Cefotetan-induced immune hemolytic anemia following prophylaxis for cesarean delivery. Immunohematology 2004;20:63-66.
35. Koutras AK, Makatsoris T, Paliogianni F, et al: Oxaliplatin-induced acute-onset thrombocytopenia, hemorrhage and hemolysis. Oncology 2004;67:179-182.
36. Beutler E: Preservation and clinical use of erythrocytes and whole blood. In Lichtman MA, Beutler E, Kipps TJ, et al (eds): Williams Hematology, 7th ed. New York: McGraw-Hill, 2006:2159-2173.
37. Franchini M, Gandini G, Aprili G: Non-ABO red blood cell alloantibodies following allogeneic hematopoietic stem cell transplantation. Bone Marrow Transplant 2004;33:1169-1172.
38. Judd WJ, Scientific Section Coordinating Committee of the AABB: Practice guidelines for prenatal and perinatal immunohematology, revisited. Transfusion 2001;41:1445-1452.
39. Sikkel E, Vandenbussche FPHA, Oepkes D, et al: Amniotic fluid ΔOD450 values accurately predict severe fetal anemia in D-alloimmunization. Obstet Gynecol 2002;100:51-57.
40. Harrington K, Fayyad A, Nicolaides KH: Predicting the severity of fetal anemia using time-domain measurement of volume flow in the fetal aorta. Ultrasound Obstet Gynecol 2004; 23:437-441.
41. Hadley AG: Laboratory assays for predicting the severity of haemolytic disease of the fetus and newborn. Transpl Immunol 2002;10:191-198.
42. Rho(D) Immune Globulin (Human)RhoGAM Product insert. Available at: http://www.orthoclinical.com. Accessed July 21, 2006.
43. Pollack W, Gorman JG, Freda VJ, et al: Results of clinical trials of RhoGAM in women. Transfusion 1968;8:151-153.
44. Freda VJ, Gorman JG, Pollack W, et al: Prevention of Rh hemolytic disease—ten years' clinical experience with Rh immune globulin. N Engl J Med 1975;292:1014-1016.
45. Joy SD, Rossi KQ, Krugh D, et al: Management of pregnancies complicated by anti-E alloimmunization. Obstet Gynecol 2005;105:24-28.

Hemoglobinopathies (Structural Defects in Hemoglobin)

26

Tim R. Randolph

OBJECTIVES

After completion of this chapter, the reader will be able to:

1. Compare and contrast structural hemoglobin (Hb) disorders with thalassemias.
2. Briefly describe globin gene structure and the development of normal human hemoglobins throughout prenatal and postnatal life.
3. Characterize the categories of the molecular abnormalities found in the various hemoglobinopathies.
4. Differentiate between homozygous and heterozygous states.
5. Define the pathologic basis of sickle cell disorder.
6. Describe the inheritance pattern of Hb S.
7. State the amino acid substitution found in Hb S.
8. Describe the solubility of Hb S in the deoxygenated state.
9. Discuss the clinical presentation of sickle cell disease, including differentiation among types of sickle cell crises.
10. Locate the geographic region, define the frequency of occurrence, and describe the impact of the incidence of *Plasmodium falciparum* malaria and glucose-6-phosphate dehydrogenase deficiency on Hb variants.
11. Describe the peripheral blood cell profile, chemistries, and other laboratory procedures used in the diagnosis of hemoglobinopathies.
12. Define the treatment goal for Hb S disease, and discuss various treatments and their purposes.
13. Identify the amino acid substitution and electrophoretic mobility of Hb C and Hb C-Harlem.
14. Describe the amino acid substitution in Hb E and the importance of genetic counseling.
15. Explain the importance of and methods for differentiating Hb D and Hb G from Hb S.
16. Describe the laboratory findings in patients who are double heterozygotes for Hb S and Hb D, Hb O-Arab, or Hb Körle Bu.
17. Identify the causes of methemoglobinemia.
18. Describe the inheritance patterns and causes of unstable hemoglobins.
19. Discuss hemoglobins with increased and decreased oxygen affinities, and explain how they differ from unstable hemoglobins.
20. Predict possible inheritance of hemoglobinopathies from the genotype of parents and the inheritance pattern for the gene.
21. Interpret patient hemoglobin electrophoresis patterns on cellulose acetate at pH 8.4 and citrate agar at pH 6.0 to 6.2 when given controls.
22. Correlate hemoglobin electrophoresis and solubility tests to identify hemoglobinopathies.

CASE STUDY

After studying the material in this chapter, the reader should be able to respond to the following case study:

An 18-year-old African American woman was seen in the emergency department for fever and abdominal pain. The following results were obtained on a blood count:

WBC count: 11.9×10^9/L
RBC count: 3.67×10^{12}/L
Hb: 10.9 g/dL
Hct: 32.5% (0.325 L/L)
Platelet count: 410×10^9/L

RDW: 19.5%
Segmented neutrophils: 75%
Lymphocytes: 18%
Monocytes: 3%
Eosinophils: 3%
Basophils: 1%
Reticulocyte count: 3.1%

Continued

Electrophoresis on cellulose acetate at alkaline pH measured 50.9% Hb S and 49.1% Hb C.

1. Select confirmatory tests that should be performed and the expected results.
2. Describe the characteristic RBC morphology on the peripheral blood film (Fig. 26-1).
3. Based on the electrophoresis and RBC morphology results, what diagnosis is suggested?
4. If this patient were to marry a person of genotype Hb AS, what would be the expected frequency of genotypes for each of four children?

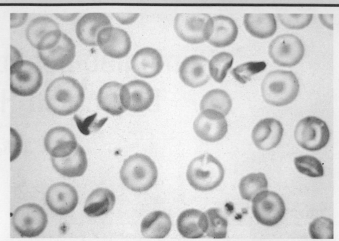

Figure 26-1 Peripheral blood film of patient in case study (×1000). (Courtesy of Ann Bell, Professor emeritus, Department of Clinical Laboratory Sciences, University of Tennessee, Memphis.)

*H*emoglobinopathy refers to a disease state ("opathy") involving the hemoglobin (Hb) molecule. All hemoglobinopathies result from a genetic mutation in one or more genes that affect hemoglobin synthesis. These mutated genes can code for either the proteins that make up the hemoglobin molecule (globin chains) or the proteins involved in synthesizing or regulating synthesis of the globin chains. Regardless of the mutation encountered, all hemoglobinopathies affect hemoglobin synthesis in one of two ways: qualitatively or quantitatively. In qualitative hemoglobinopathies, hemoglobin synthesis occurs at a normal or near-normal rate, but the hemoglobin molecule has an altered amino acid sequence within the globin chains. This change in amino acid sequence alters the structure of the hemoglobin molecule (structural defect) and its function (qualitative). In contrast, quantitative disorders result in a reduced rate of hemoglobin synthesis (quantitative) but do not affect the amino acid sequence of the globin chains. A reduction in the amount of hemoglobin synthesized produces an anemia and stimulates the production of other hemoglobins not affected by the mutation in an attempt to compensate for the anemia. Based on this distinction, hematologists divide hemoglobinopathies into two categories: structural defects (qualitative) and thalassemias (quantitative). To add confusion to the classification scheme, many hematologists also refer to *only* the structural defects as hemoglobinopathies. This chapter describes the structural or qualitative defects that are referred to as hemoglobinopathies; the quantitative defects (thalassemias) are described in Chapter 27.

are referred to as *α-like genes*. The remaining four globin genes, β, γ, δ, and ε, are located on chromosome 11 and are referred to as *β-like genes*. In the human genome, there is one copy of each globin gene per chromatid for a total of two genes per person with the exception of α and γ. There are two copies of the α and γ genes per chromatid for a total of four genes per person. Each globin gene codes for the corresponding globin chain: α globin gene is used as the template to synthesize the α globin chain. The β gene codes for the β chain, and so forth.

HEMOGLOBIN DEVELOPMENT

Each human hemoglobin molecule is composed of four globin chains, a pair of α-like chains and a pair of β-like chains. During the first 3 months of embryonic life, only one α-like gene (ζ) and one β-like gene (ε) are activated, resulting in the production of ζ and ε chains that pair to form a hemoglobin type called *Gower-1*. Shortly thereafter, α and γ chain synthesis begins, resulting in the production of hemoglobins Gower-2 ($α_2/ε_2$) and Portland ($ζ_2/γ_2$). Later in fetal development, ζ and ε synthesis ceases, leaving α and γ chains that pair to produce Hb F ($α_2/γ_2$), also known as *fetal hemoglobin*. During the 6 months after birth, γ chain synthesis gradually decreases and is replaced with β chain synthesis, producing Hb A ($α_2β_2$), also known as *adult hemoglobin*. The remaining globin gene, δ, becomes activated around birth, producing δ chains at low levels that pair with α chains to produce the second adult hemoglobin, called *Hb A_2*. Normal adults produce predominantly Hb A (95%), Hb A_2 (<3.5%), and Hb F (<1% to 2%).

STRUCTURE OF GLOBIN GENES

As discussed in Chapter 10, there are six functional human globin genes located on two different chromosomes. Two of the globin genes, α and ζ, are located on chromosome 16 and

GENETIC MUTATIONS

More than 800 structural hemoglobin variants (hemoglobinopathies) are known to exist throughout the world, and more are being discovered regularly (Table 26-1).[1] Each of

TABLE 26-1 Molecular Abnormalities of Hemoglobin Variants

	NUMBER OF VARIANTS				
	α	β	δ	γ	**Total**
Single amino acid substitution	253	405	34	67	759
Two amino acid substitutions	1	23	0	5	29
Deletions or insertions	14	25	0	0	39
Extended chains	9	9	0	0	18
Fusions	0	9	8	1	18
Totals*	277	471	42	73	863

*The total number of hemoglobin variants (854) is 9 less than the sum of the first four columns because each of the 9 fusion hemoglobins is recorded in multiple columns.
From Lukens JN: The abnormal hemoglobins: general principles. In Greer JP, Foerster J, Lukens J, et al (eds): Wintrobe's Clinical Hematology, 11th ed. Philadelphia: Lippincott, Williams & Wilkins, 2004:1249.

these hemoglobin variants results from one or more genetic mutations that alter the molecular structure of the hemoglobin molecule, ultimately affecting hemoglobin function. The types of genetic mutations that occur in the hemoglobinopathies include point mutations, deletions, insertions, chain extensions, and fusions involving one or more of the adult globin genes—α, β, γ, and δ.[2]

Point mutation is the most common type of genetic mutation occurring in the hemoglobinopathies. Point mutation is the replacement of one original nucleotide in the normal gene with a different nucleotide. Because one nucleotide is replaced by one nucleotide, the codon triplet remains intact, and the reading frame is unaltered. This results in the substitution of one amino acid in the globin chain product at the position corresponding to the location of the original point mutation. As can be seen in Table 26-1, 759 of the 863 known hemoglobin variants result from point mutations that cause a single amino acid substitution. It also is possible to have two point mutations occurring in the same globin gene, resulting in two amino acid substitutions within the same globin chain. Of the 863 variants, 29 occur by this mechanism.

Deletions involve the removal of one or more nucleotides, whereas insertions result in the addition of one or more nucleotides. Usually deletions and insertions are not divisible by three and disrupt the reading frame, resulting in the nullification of synthesis of the corresponding protein. This is the case for the quantitative thalassemias (Chapter 27). In hemoglobinopathies, the reading frame usually remains intact, however, resulting in the addition or deletion of one or more amino acids in the globin chain product affecting the structure and function of the hemoglobin molecule. Of the 863 variants listed in Table 26-1, 29 result from deletions or insertions or both.

Chain extensions occur when the stop codon is mutated, causing translation to continue beyond the typical last codon. Amino acids continue to be added until a stop codon is reached by chance. This process produces globin chains that are longer than normal. Significant globin chain extensions usually result in degradation of the globin chain and a quantitative defect. If the extension of the globin chain is insufficient to produce significant degradation, however, the defect is qualitative in nature and classified as a hemoglobinopathy. Hemoglobin molecules with extended globin chains fold inappropriately, affecting hemoglobin structure and function. Eighteen globin chain extensions have been described (see Table 26-1).

Gene fusions occur when two normal genes break between nucleotides, switch positions, and reanneal with the opposite gene. If the β genes and the δ genes break in similar locations, switch positions, and reanneal, the resultant genes would be β/δ and δ/β fusion genes in which the head of the fusion gene is from one original gene and the tail is from the other. As long as the reading frames are not disrupted and the globin chain lengths are similar, the genes are transcribed and translated into globin chains. The fusion chains fold differently, however, and affect the corresponding hemoglobin function. Eighteen fusion chains have been identified (see Table 26-1).

ZYGOSITY

Zygosity refers to the association between the number of gene mutations and the level of severity of the resultant genetic defect. Generally, there is a level of severity associated with each gene that is normally used to synthesize the protein product. For the globin genes, there are four copies of the α and γ genes and two copies of the β and δ genes. In theory, this could result in four levels of severity for α and γ mutations and two levels of severity for the β and δ mutations. Expressed another way, if all things were equal, it would require twice as many mutations within the α and γ genes to produce the same physiologic effect as within the β and δ genes. Because the γ and δ genes are transcribed and translated at such low levels in adults, however, mutations of both genes would have little impact on overall hemoglobin function.[3] In addition, because the dominant adult hemoglobin, Hb A, is composed of α and β chains, β gene mutations would affect overall hemoglobin function to a greater extent than the same number of α gene mutations. This partially explains the greater number of identified β chain variants compared with α chain variants, in that a single β mutation would be more likely to create a clinical condition, whereas a single α mutation might not.

The inheritance pattern of β chain variants is referred to as *heterozygous* when one β gene is mutated and *homozygous* when both β genes are mutated.[4] The terms *disease* and *trait* also are commonly used to refer to the homozygous (disease) and heterozygous (trait) states.

PATHOPHYSIOLOGY

Pathophysiology refers to the manner in which a disorder translates into clinical symptoms. The impact of these mutations on hemoglobin function depends on the type of amino acid substituted, where it is located in the globin chain, and the number of genes mutated (zygosity). The type of substituted amino acid confers a different charge and size to the protein. A change in charge affects which adjacent amino acids would be attracted to or repelled by the substituted amino acid. In addition, the size of the substituted amino acid confers either a more or a less bulky nature to the protein. The charge and the size of the substituted amino acid determine its impact on hemoglobin structure by altering the tertiary structure of the globin chain and the quaternary structure of the hemoglobin molecule. Changes in hemoglobin structure usually affect function. Location of the substitution within the globin chain also has an impact on the degree of structural alteration and hemoglobin function based on its positioning within the molecule and the interactions with the surrounding amino acids. In the case of the sickle cell mutation, the amino acid substitution results in a change in hemoglobin shape that causes adjacent hemoglobin molecules to polymerize, forming long hemoglobin crystals that stretch the RBC membrane producing the characteristic crescent moon or sickle cell shape.

Zygosity also affects the pathophysiology of the disease. In β-hemoglobinopathies, zygosity predicts two severities of disease. In homozygous β-hemoglobinopathies, in which both β genes are mutated, the variant hemoglobin becomes the dominant hemoglobin type and normal hemoglobin (Hb A) is absent. Examples are sickle cell disease (SCD, Hb SS) and Hb C disease (Hb CC). In heterozygous β-hemoglobinopathies, one β gene is mutated and the other is normal, suggesting a 50/50 distribution. In an attempt to minimize the impact of the abnormal hemoglobin, however, the variant hemoglobin is usually present in lesser amounts than Hb A. In some cases, however, they may be in equal amounts. Examples are Hb S trait (Hb AS) and Hb C trait (Hb AC). Patients with homozygous SCD (Hb SS) inherit a severe form of the disease that occurs less frequently but requires medical intervention early in life, whereas heterozygotes (Hb AS) are much more common but rarely symptomatic.

Fishleder and Hoffman[5] divided the structural hemoglobins into four groups: (1) abnormal hemoglobins that result in hemolytic anemia, such as Hb S and the unstable hemoglobins; (2) methemoglobinemia, such as Hb M; (3) hemoglobins with either increased or decreased oxygen affinity; and (4) abnormal hemoglobins with no clinical or functional effect. Imbalanced chain production also may be associated in rare instances with a structurally abnormal chain, such as Hb

Lepore,[1] because of the reduced production of the abnormal chain. The functional classification of hemoglobin variants is summarized in Box 26-1.

Many of the variants are clinically insignificant because they do not show any physiologic effect. As discussed previously, most clinical abnormalities are associated with the β chain followed by the α chain. Involvement of the γ and δ chains does occur, but because of the small amount of hemoglobin involved, it is rarely detected and is usually of no consequence.[3] Box 26-2 lists clinically significant abnormal hemoglobins. The most frequently occurring of the abnormal hemoglobins and the most severe is Hb S.

NOMENCLATURE

As hemoglobins were reported, they were designated by letters of the alphabet. Normal adult hemoglobin and fetal hemoglobin were called "Hb A" and "Hb F". By the time the middle of the alphabet was reached, it was apparent that the chain would soon be exhausted. Currently, abnormal hemoglobins are assigned a common designation and a scientific designation. The common name is selected by the discoverer and usually represents the geographic area where the hemoglobin was identified. Capital letters are used to indicate a special characteristic of the hemoglobin variants, such as identical electrophoretic mobility but different amino acid substitutions, as in Hb G-Philadelphia, Hb G-Copenhagen, and Hb C-Harlem. The variant description also can involve scientific designations that indicate the variant chain, the sequential and the helical number of the abnormal amino acid, and the nature of the substitution. β_6 (A$_3$) Glu $\rightarrow$ Val for Hb S indicates the substitution of valine for glutamic acid in the A helix in the β chain at the sixth position.[1]

HEMOGLOBIN S

Sickle Cell Anemia
History
Sickle cell anemia was first observed by a Chicago physician, Herrick, in 1910 in a West Indian student with severe anemia. In 1917, Emmel recorded that sickling occurred in nonanemic patients and in patients who were severely anemic. In 1927, Hahn and Gillespie described the pathologic basis of the disorder and its relationship to the hemoglobin molecule. These investigators showed that sickling occurred when a solution of red blood cells (RBCs) was deficient in oxygen and that the shape of the RBCs was reversible when that solution was oxygenated again.[6,7] In 1946, Beet reported that malarial parasites were present less frequently in blood smears from patients with SCD compared with normal individuals.[8] It was determined that sickle cell trait confers a resistance against infection with *Plasmodium falciparum* occurring early in childhood between the time that passively acquired immunity passes and active immunity develops.[9] In 1949, Pauling showed that when Hb SS is electrophoresed, it migrates differently than Hb AA. This difference was shown to be caused by an amino

---

BOX 26-1 Functional Classification of Selected Hemoglobin Variants

I. Homozygous: Hemoglobin polymorphisms: the variants that are most common

Hb S: $\alpha_2\beta_2^{6Val}$—severe hemolytic anemia; sickling

Hb C: $\alpha_2\beta_2^{6Lys}$—mild hemolytic anemia

Hb D-Punjab: $\alpha_2\beta_2^{121Gln}$—no anemia

Hb E: $\alpha_2\beta_2^{261Lys}$—mild microcytic anemia

II. Heterozygous: Hemoglobin variants causing functional aberrations or hemolytic anemia in the heterozygous state

A. Hemoglobins associated with methemoglobinemia and cyanosis

1. Hb M-Boston: $\alpha_2^{58Tyr}\beta_2$
2. Hb M-Iwate: $\alpha_2^{87Tyr}\beta_2$
3. Hb M-Saskatoon: $\alpha_2\beta_2^{63Tyr}$
4. Hb M-Milwaukee: $\alpha_2\beta_2^{67Gu}$
5. Hb M-Hyde Park: $\alpha_2\beta_2^{92Tyr}$
6. Hb FM-Osaka: $\alpha_2\gamma_2^{63Tyr}$

B. Hemoglobins associated with altered oxygen affinity

1. Increased affinity and polycythemia
   a. Hb Chesapeake: $\alpha_2^{92Leu}\beta_2$
   b. Hb J-Capetown: $\alpha_2^{92Gln}\beta_2$
   c. Hb Malmo: $\alpha_2\beta_2^{97Gln}$
   d. Hb Yakima: $\alpha_2\beta_2^{99His}$
   e. Hb Kemp: $\alpha_2\beta_2^{99Asn}$
   f. Hb Ypsi (Ypsilanti): $\alpha_2\beta_2^{99Tyr}$
   g. Hb Hiroshima: $\alpha_2\beta_2^{143Asp}$
   h. Hb Rainier: $\alpha_2\beta_2^{145Cys}$
   i. Hb Bethesda: $\alpha_2\beta_2^{145His}$
2. Decreased affinity—may have mild anemia or cyanosis
   a. Hb Kansas: $\alpha_2^{102Thr}\beta_2$
   b. Hb Titusville: $\alpha_2^{94Asn}\beta_2$
   c. Hb Providence: $\alpha_2\beta_2^{82Asn,Asp}$
   d. Hb Agenogi: $\alpha_2\beta_2^{90Lys}$
   e. Hb Beth Israel: $\alpha_2\beta_2^{102Ser}$
   f. Hb Yoshizuka: $\alpha_2\beta_2^{108Asp}$

C. Unstable Hemoglobins

1. Hemoglobin may precipitate as Heinz bodies after splenectomy ("congenital Heinz body anemia")
   a. Severe hemolysis: no improvement after splenectomy
      Hb Bibba: $\alpha_2^{136Pro}\beta_2$
      Hb Hammersmith: $\alpha_2\beta_2^{42Ser}$
      Hb Bristol: $\alpha_2\beta_2^{67Asp}$
      Hb Olmsted: $\alpha_2\beta_2^{141Arg}$
   b. Severe hemolysis: improvement after splenectomy
      Hb Torino: $\alpha_2^{42Val}\beta_2$
      Hb Ann Arbor: $\alpha_2^{80Arg}\beta_2$
      Hb Geneva: $\alpha_2\beta_2^{28Pro}$
      Hb Shepherd's Bush: $\alpha_2\beta_2^{74Asp}$
      Hb Köln: $\alpha_2\beta_2^{98Met}$
      Hb Wien: $\alpha_2\beta_2^{130Asp}$
   c. Mild hemolysis: intermittent exacerbations
      Hb L Ferrara: $\alpha_2^{47Gly}\beta_2$
      Hb Hasharon: $\alpha_2^{47His}\beta_2$
      Hb Leiden: $\alpha_2\beta_2^{6or7}$ (Glu deleted)
      Hb Freiburg: $\alpha_2\beta_2^{23}$ (Val deleted)
      Hb Seattle: $\alpha_2\beta_2^{76Glu}$
      Hb Louisville: $\alpha_2\beta_2^{42Leu}$
      Hb Zurich: $\alpha_2\beta_2^{63Arg}$
      Hb Gun Hill: $\alpha_2\beta_2^{91-97}$ (5 amino acids deleted)
   d. No disease
      Hb Etobicoke: $\alpha_2^{84Arg}\beta_2$
      Hb Dakar: $\alpha_2^{112Glu}\beta_2$
      Hb Sogn: $\alpha_2\beta_2^{14Arg}$
      Hb Tacoma: $\alpha_2\beta_2^{30Ser}$
2. Tetramers of normal chains; appear in thalassemias
   Hb Bart: γ_4
   Hb H: β_4

From Henry JB: Clinical Diagnosis and Management by Laboratory Methods, 18th ed. Philadelphia: Saunders, 1991:650. Originally modified from Winslow RM, Anderson WF: The hemoglobinopathies. In Stanbury JB, Wyngaarden JB, Fredrickson DS, et al (eds): The Metabolic Basis of Inherited Disease, 5th ed. New York: McGraw-Hill, 1983:Chap. 76.

---

acid substitution in the globin chain. Pauling and coworkers defined the genetics of the disorder and clearly distinguished heterozygous sickle trait (Hb AS) from the homozygous state (Hb SS).[7]

The term *sickle cell diseases* is used to describe a group of symptomatic hemoglobinopathies in which patients express either Hb SS or Hb S in combination with another Hb β chain mutation. SCDs are the most common form of hemoglobinopathy, with the variants Hb SC and Hb S-β-thalassemia (Hb S-β-thal) occurring most frequently.

Genetic Inheritance

As stated earlier, the genes that code for the globin chains are located at specific loci on chromosomes 16 and 11. The α-like genes (α and ζ) are located on chromosome 16, whereas the β-like genes (β, γ, δ, and ε) are located on the short arm of chromosome 11. With the exception of the γ genes, each β-like gene has two loci; β Hemoglobin variants are inherited as autosomal codominants, with one gene inherited from each parent.[1]

Patients with SCD (Hb SS), Hb SC, or Hb S-β-thal have inherited a sickle (S) gene from one parent and an S, C, or

---

BOX 26-2 Clinically Important Hemoglobin Variants

I. Sickle syndromes
  A. Sickle cell trait (AS)
  B. Sickle cell disease
    1. SS
    2. SC
    3. S/D-Los Angeles
    4. S/O-Arab
    5. S/β Thal
    6. S/HPFH
    7. SE
II. Unstable hemoglobins→congenital Heinz body anemia (>200 variants)
III. Hemoglobins with abnormal oxygen affinity
  A. High affinity→familial erythrocytosis (>115 variants)
  B. Low affinity→familial cyanosis (Hbs Kansas, Beth Israel, Yoshizuka, Agenogi, Titusville)
IV. M hemoglobins→familial cyanosis (7 variants)
  Hb M Boston, Hb M Iwate, Hb M Saskatoon, Hb M Hyde Park, Hb M Milwaukee, Hb FM Osaka, Hb FM Fort Ripley
V. Structural variants that result in a thalassemic phenotype
  A. β-Thalassemia phenotype
    1. Lepore hemoglobins (δβ fusion)
    2. Hb E
    3. Hbs Indianapolis, Showa-Yakushiji, Geneva
  B. α-Thalassemia phenotype chain termination mutants (e.g., Hb Constant Spring)

Modified from Lukens JN: Abnormal hemoglobins: general principles (Chap. 39); Wong WC: Sickle cell anemia and other sickling syndromes (Chap. 40); Lukens JN: Unstable hemoglobin disease (Chap. 41). In Greer JP, Foerster J, Lukens JN, et al (eds): Wintrobe's Clinical Hematology, 11th ed. Philadelphia: Lippincott Williams & Wilkins, 2004.

β-thalassemia gene from the other. Individuals with the homozygous state have more severe disease than individuals who are heterozygous for Hb S. Figure 26-2 uses Hb S and Hb C to show inheritance of abnormal hemoglobins involving mutations in the β-like genes.

Incidence

The highest frequency of the sickle cell trait (Hb AS) is in Africa, where the frequency is 20% to 40%.[10] In the United States, approximately 12% of African Americans have a hemoglobin variant. The homozygous state (Hb SS) represents the most severe type of hemoglobinopathy, with an estimated incidence of 1 in 375 live African-American births.[11] The occurrence of heterozygous sickle cell trait is 8% among African Americans, with the serious double heterozygous states of Hb SC and Hb S-β-thal occurring at rates of 1 in 835 (0.12%) and 1 in 1667, (0.16%) respectively.[10] Although in the United States sickle cell anemia is found mostly in individuals of African descent, it also has been found in individuals from the Middle East, India, and the Mediterranean (Fig. 26-3). Sickle cell anemia also can be found in individuals from the

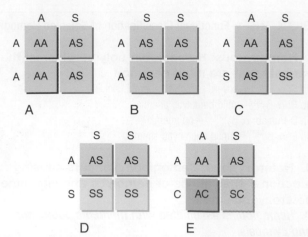

Figure 26-2 Punnett square illustrating the standard method for predicting the inheritance of abnormal hemoglobins. Each parent contributes one gene.

Caribbean and Central and South America.[12] Sickle cell is becoming more prominent in southern India, particularly in certain tribes.[13]

Etiology and Pathophysiology

Hb S is defined by the structural formula $\alpha_2\beta_2^{6Glu \to Val}$, which indicates that on the β chain at the sixth position, glutamic acid is replaced by valine. Glutamic acid has a net charge of (−1), whereas valine has a net change of (+0). This amino acid substitution results in a change in charge of (+1), resulting in a structural change in the hemoglobin molecule. Alterations in Hb S structure and the resultant change in RBC shape relates to the amount of oxygen bound to the hemoglobin molecules. When Hb S is fully oxygenated, it remains soluble in the erythrocyte similar to Hb A, maintaining the normal biconcave disc shape of the RBCs. On deoxygenation, however, Hb S in the RBCs becomes less soluble, forming tactoids or liquid crystals of Hb S polymers that grow in length beyond the diameter of the RBC and causing sickling. In homozygotes, the sickling process begins when oxygen saturation decreases to less than 85%. In heterozygotes, sickling does not occur unless the oxygen saturation of hemoglobin is reduced to less than 40%.[14] The blood becomes more viscous when polymers are formed and sickle cells are created.[14] Increased blood viscosity and sickle cell formation slow blood flow. In addition to a decrease in oxygen tension, the pH is reduced, and there is an increase in 2,3-diphosphoglycerate. Reduced blood flow prolongs the exposure of Hb S-containing erythrocytes to a hypoxic environment, and the lower tissue pH decreases the oxygen affinity, which further promotes sickling. The end result is occlusion of capillaries and arterioles by sickled RBCs and infarction of surrounding tissue.

Sickle cells occur in two forms: reversible sickle cells and irreversible sickle cells.[15] Reversible sickle cells are Hb S–containing erythrocytes that change shape in response to oxygen tension. Reversible sickle cells circulate as normal biconcave discs when fully oxygenated but undergo hemo-

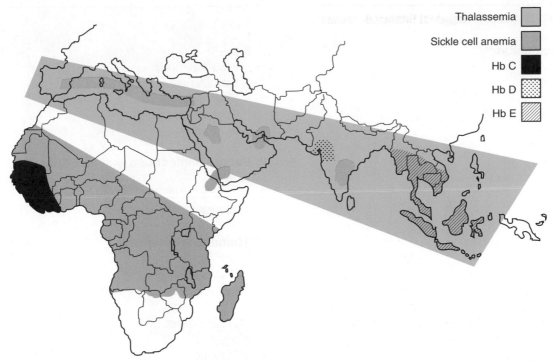

Thalassemia

Sickle cell anemia

Hb C

Hb D

Hb E

Figure 26-3 Geographic distribution of common inherited structural hemoglobin variants and the thalassemias. (From Hoffbrand AV, Pettit JE: Essential Haematology, 3rd ed. Oxford: Blackwell Scientific, 1993.)

globin polymerization, show increased viscosity, and change shape on deoxygenation. The vaso-occlusive complications of SCD are thought to be due to reversible sickle cells that are able to travel into the microvasculature in the biconcave disk conformation due to their normal rheologic properties when oxygenated and then become distorted and viscous as they become deoxygenated, converting to the sickle cell configuration in the vessel.

In contrast, irreversible sickle cells do not change their shape regardless of the change in oxygen tension or degree of hemoglobin polymerization. These cells are seen on the peripheral blood smear as elongated sickle cells with a point at each end. It is thought that irreversible sickle cells are recognized as abnormal by the spleen and removed from circulation, preventing them from entering the microcirculation and causing vaso-occlusion.

In addition to oxygen tension, the level of intracellular hydration exacerbates the sickling process. When RBCs containing Hb S are exposed to a low oxygen tension, hemoglobin polymerization occurs. Polymerized deoxy-Hb S activates a membrane channel called P_{sickle} that is otherwise inactive in normal RBCs. These membrane channels open when the blood Po_2 decreases to less than 50 mm Hg. Open P_{sickle} channels allow the influx of Ca^{2+}, raising the intracellular calcium levels and activating a second membrane channel called the *Gardos channel*. An activated Gardos channel causes the efflux of K^+ that stimulates the efflux of Cl^- through another membrane channel to maintain charge equilibrium across the RBC membrane. The efflux of these ions leads to dehydration, effectively increasing the intracellular concentration of Hb S and inten-

sifying polymerization. Another contributor to K^+ and Cl^- efflux and the resultant dehydration is the K^+/Cl^- cotransporter system. Ironically, this system is activated by dehydration and positively charged hemoglobins such as Hb S and Hb C. The K^+/Cl^- cotransporter pathway also is activated by the low pH encountered in the spleen and kidneys. One potential explanation for the altered function of the membrane channels is oxidative damage triggered by Hb S polymerization. Injury to the RBC membrane induces adherence to endothelial surfaces, causing RBC aggregation, producing ischemia, and exacerbating Hb S polymerization.[9]

Clinical Features

The clinical manifestations of the sickle cell syndrome can vary from asymptomatic to a potentially lethal state as characterized by SCD (Box 26-3). Several hundred hemoglobin variants are known; however, only four are clinically significant (Hb SS, Hb SC, Hb S-β⁰thal, and Hb S-β⁺thal). These four clinically severe forms have high morbidity and mortality rates. The average life expectancy has improved over the past decades as a result of valuable research and improved care. Average life span for Hb SS patients is 45 years; for Hb SC patients, is 65 years.[16] Individuals affected with SCD are characteristically symptom-free until the second half of the first year of life owing to the protective effect of Hb F.[17] During the first 6 months of life, mutated β chains are produced to gradually replace normal γ chains, causing Hb S levels to increase as Hb F levels decrease. Erythrocytes containing Hb S become susceptible to hemolysis, and a progressive hemolytic anemia and splenomegaly may become evident.

BOX 26-3 Clinical Features of Sickle Cell Anemia

I. Vaso-occlusion
A. Causes
    Acidosis
    Hypoxia
    Dehydration
    Infection
    Fever
    Extreme cold
B. Clinical manifestations
  1. Bones
    Pain
    Hand-foot dactylitis
    Infection (osteomyelitis)
  2. Lungs
    Pneumonia
    Acute chest syndrome
  3. Liver
    Hepatomegaly
    Jaundice
  4. Spleen
    Sequestration splenomegaly
    Autosplenectomy
  5. Penis
    Priapism

6. Eyes
    Retinal hemorrhage
7. Central nervous system
8. Urinary tract
    Renal papillary necrosis
9. Leg ulcers

II. Bacterial infections
A. Sepsis
B. Pneumonia
C. Osteomyelitis

III. Hematologic defects
A. Chronic hemolytic anemia
B. Megaloblastic episodes
C. Aplastic episodes

IV. Cardiac defects
A. Enlarged heart
B. Heart murmurs

V. Other clinical features
A. Stunted growth
B. High-risk pregnancy

Many individuals with SCD undergo episodes of recurring pain termed *crises*. Sickle cell crises were described by Diggs[18] as "any new syndrome that develops rapidly in patients with SCD owing to the inherited abnormality." The pathogenesis of the acute painful episode first described by Diggs is not fully understood. Various crises may occur: vaso-occlusive or "painful," aplastic, megaloblastic, sequestration, and chronic hemolytic.

The hallmark feature of SCD is vaso-occlusion, accounting for most hospital and emergency department visits. This acute, painful aspect of SCD occurs with great predictability and severity in many individuals and can be triggered by acidosis, hypoxia, dehydration, infection and fever, and exposure to extreme cold. Painful episodes manifest most often in the bones, lungs, liver, spleen, penis, eyes, central nervous system, and urinary tract.

The pathogenesis of vaso-occlusion in SCD is not fully understood, but Hb S polymerization and sickling of RBCs plays a major role with other factors also affecting this process. The list of possible risk factors includes polymerization, decreased deformability, sickle cell–endothelial cell adherence, endothelial cell activation, white blood cell (WBC) and platelet activation, hemostatic activation, and vascular tone.[18] The interrelationship of these risk factors is shown in Figure 26-4. Vaso-occlusion can be triggered by any of these factors under various circumstances. During inflammation, increased WBCs interacting with endothelium, platelet activation causing elevation of thrombospondin level, or clinical dehydration resulting in increased von Willebrand factor could trigger RBC adherence

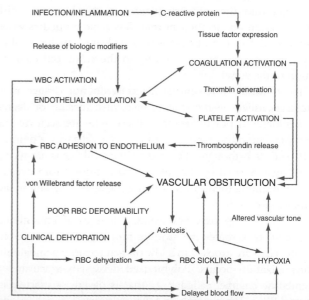

Figure 26-4 Numerous risk factors for vaso-occlusion are highly interrelated physiologically, as shown here. (From Embury SH, Hebbel RP, Mohandas N, et al: Sickle Cell Disease: Basic Principles and Clinical Practice. Philadelphia: Lippincott, Williams & Wilkins, 1994:322.)

to endothelium, precipitating vascular obstruction. Another mechanism of obstruction can be dense cells, which are less deformable and are at greatest risk for intracellular polymerization because of their higher Hb S concentration.[19,20]

The abnormal interaction between sickle cells and vascular endothelium seems to have a great impact on the vaso-occlusive event. Endothelial adherence correlates significantly with the severity of painful episodes. Cells of patients with Hb SC disease produce less sickling and tend to have fewer adherent RBCs.[7,21]

The frequency of painful episodes varies from none to six per year.[7] On average, each episode persists for 4 to 5 days, although protracted episodes may last for weeks. Repeated splenic infarcts produce scarring, resulting in diminished splenic tissue and abnormal function. Gradual loss of splenic function is referred to as *autosplenectomy* and is evidenced by the presence of Howell-Jolly and Pappenheimer bodies on the peripheral smear. In the lungs, pulmonary infarction from sickling in microvasculature causes acute chest syndrome, characterized by fever, chest pain, and presence of pulmonary infiltrates on the chest x-ray. In children, acute chest syndrome generally is precipitated by infection characterized by fever, cough, and tachypnea. In adults, organ failure is the most common cause of death. Vaso-occlusive episodes gradually consume the patient organ by organ, through the destructive and debilitative effects of cumulative infarcts. Approximately 8% to 10% of SCD patients develop cutaneous manifestations in the form of ulcers or sores on the lower leg.[10]

Splenic sequestration is characterized by a sudden trapping of blood in the spleen, resulting in a rapid decline in hemoglobin, often to less than 6 g/dL.[15] This phenomenon occurs most often in infants and young children whose spleens are chronically enlarged. Children experiencing splenic sequestration episodes may have earlier onset of splenomegaly and a lower level of Hb F at 6 months.[7] Crises often are associated with respiratory tract infections.

Bacterial infections pose a major problem for SCD patients. These patients have increased susceptibility to life-threatening infection from *Staphylococcus aureus*, *Streptococcus pneumoniae*, and *Haemophilus influenzae*. Acute infections are common causes of hospitalization and have been the most frequent cause of death, especially in the first 3 years of life.[1] Bacterial infections of the blood (septicemia) are exacerbated by the autosplenectomy effect as the spleen gradually loses its ability to function as a secondary lymphoid tissue to clear organisms effectively from the blood.

Chronic hemolytic anemia is characterized by a shortened RBC survival with a corresponding decrease in hemoglobin and hematocrit, an elevated reticulocyte count, and jaundice. Continuous screening and removal of sickle cells by the spleen perpetuate the chronic hemolytic anemia and autosplenectomy effect. Because other conditions, such as hepatitis and gallstones, may cause jaundice, chronic hemolysis is difficult to diagnose in sickle cell patients.[15]

Megaloblastic episodes result from the sudden arrest of the erythropoiesis due to folate depletion. Folic acid deficiency, as a cause for exaggerated anemia in SCD, is extremely rare in the United States. It is common practice to prescribe prophylactic folic acid to patients with SCD, however.[7]

Aplastic episodes (bone marrow failure) are the most common life-threatening hematologic complications and usually are associated with infection, particularly with parvoviruses.[20] Aplastic episodes present clinical problems similar to those seen in other hemolytic disorders.[22] Sickle cell patients usually can compensate for the decrease in RBC survival by increasing bone marrow output. When the bone marrow is suppressed temporarily by bacterial or viral infections, however, the hematocrit decreases substantially with no reticulocyte compensation. The spontaneous recovery phase is characterized by nucleated RBCs and reticulocytosis. Most aplastic episodes are short-lived and require no therapy. If anemia is severe and the bone marrow remains quiescent, transfusions become necessary. If patients are not transfused in a timely fashion, death can occur.[22]

Patients also experience cardiac defects, including enlarged heart and heart murmurs. In addition, children exhibit a reduced growth rate. When patients enter childbearing age, pregnancy becomes risky.[1]

Incidence with Malaria and Glucose-6-Phosphate Dehydrogenase Deficiency

The sickle gene occurs with greatest frequency in Central Africa, the Near East, the region around the Mediterranean, and parts of India. The frequency of the gene parallels the incidence of *P. falciparum* and seems to offer some protection in young patients with cerebral falciparum malaria. Malarial parasites are living organisms within the RBCs that use the oxygen within the cells. This reduced oxygen tension causes the cells to sickle, resulting in injury to the cells. These injured cells tend to become trapped within the blood vessels of the spleen and other organs, where they are easily phagocytized by scavenger WBCs. Selective destruction of RBCs containing parasites decreases the number of malarial organisms and increases the time for immunity to develop. One explanation for this phenomenon is that the infected cell is uniquely sickled and destroyed, probably in an area of the spleen or liver where phagocytic cells are plentiful, and the oxygen tension is significantly decreased.[23]

Because of the high incidence of glucose-6-phosphate dehydrogenase (G6PD) deficiency in patients with SCD, it was suggested that G6PD deficiency had a protective effect on these patients,[24] although this correlation has not been confirmed through studies. It also has been postulated that hemolytic episodes are more common in these patients, but studies have shown no relationship between clinical severity of sickling and the presence or absence of G6PD deficiency. Because of the presence of young cells rich in G6PD, however, the increased hemolysis is more likely caused by the enzyme abnormality when the population is shifted to the oldest cells during the aplastic crisis.[25]

Laboratory Diagnosis

The anemia of SCD is a chronic hemolytic anemia, classified morphologically as normocytic, normochromic. The characteristic cell presents as a long, curved cell with a point at each end (Figs. 26-5 to 26-7). Because of its appearance, the cell was named a *sickle cell*.[17] The peripheral blood smear shows marked poikilocytosis and anisocytosis with normal,

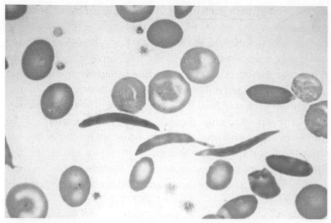

Figure 26-5 SCD with anisocytosis, polychromasia, three sickle cells, target cells, and normal platelets (peripheral blood, ×1000). (Courtesy of Ann Bell, Professor emeritus, Department of Clinical Laboratory Sciences, University of Tennessee, Memphis.)

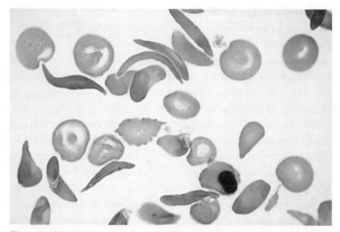

Figure 26-6 SCD with anisocytosis, poikilocytosis, sickle cells, target cells, and one nucleated RBC (peripheral blood, ×1000). Platelets are not present in this field but were adequate in this patient. (Courtesy of Ann Bell, Professor emeritus, Department of Clinical Laboratory Sciences, University of Tennessee, Memphis.)

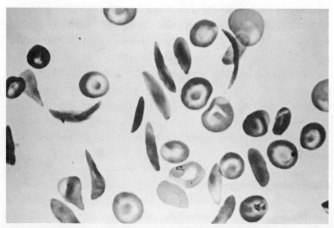

Figure 26-7 SCD with poikilocytosis, several sickle-shaped RBCs, target and oat cells, and Howell-Jolly body (peripheral blood, ×1000). Platelets were adequate in this patient. (Courtesy of Ann Bell, Professor emeritus, Department of Clinical Laboratory Sciences, University of Tennessee, Memphis.)

irreversibly sickled, target, nucleated RBCs; a few spherocytes, basophilic stippling; Pappenheimer bodies; and Howell-Jolly bodies. The presence of sickle cells and target cells is the hallmark of SCD. There is moderate-to-marked polychromasia with reticulocytes between 10% and 25%, corresponding with the hemolytic state and the resultant bone marrow response. The RBC distribution width is increased owing to moderate anisocytosis. The mean cell volume (MCV) is not as elevated, however, as one would expect with the elevated reticulocyte count. An aplastic crisis can be heralded by a decreased reticulocyte count. Moderate leukocytosis is usually present (sometimes $40\text{-}50 \times 10^9/L$) with neutrophilia and a mild shift toward immature granulocytes. Thrombocytosis is usually present. The leukocyte alkaline phosphatase score is not elevated when neutrophilia is due to sickle cell crisis alone and no underlying infection exists. The bone marrow shows erythroid hyperplasia reflecting an attempt to compensate for the anemia and resulting in polychromasia, reticulocytes, and increased nucleated RBCs seen in the peripheral blood. Immunoglobulin levels, particularly IgA, are elevated in all forms of SCD. Serum ferritin levels of young patients are normal but tend to be elevated later in life; however, hemochromatosis is rare. Chronic hemolysis is evidenced by elevated indirect and total bilirubin with the accompanying jaundice.

The diagnosis of SCD is made by showing the insolubility of Hb S in the deoxygenated form using a screening test and confirming its presence on hemoglobin electrophoresis. One screening test shows the insolubility of Hb S by inducing the RBC sickling phenomenon on a glass slide. A drop of blood is placed on a slide, a drop of reducing agent (2% sodium metabisulfite) is added, and the mixture is sealed under a coverslip. RBCs are exposed to this oxygen-poor environment, where they become sickled and can be identified by microscopy.

The decreased solubility of deoxygenated Hb S in solution forms the basis for the hemoglobin solubility test, the most common screening test. Blood is added to a buffered solution of a reducing agent, such as sodium dithionite, and a lysing agent that releases the hemoglobin from the RBCs. Deoxygenated Hb S is insoluble and precipitates in solution, rendering it turbid, whereas solutions containing non-sickling hemoglobins remain clear (Fig. 26-8). False-positive results for Hb S occur with hyperlipidemia; false-negative results occur because of an inadequate number of RBCs or a low hematocrit. Other hemoglobins that give a positive solubility test include Hb C-Georgetown (Harlem), Hb C-Ziguinchor, Hb S-Memphis, Hb S-Travis, Hb S-Antilles, Hb S-Providence, Hb S-Oman, Hb Alexander, and Hb Porte-Alegre.[1,7] All of these hemoglobins have the same amino acid substitution ($\beta^{6Glu \rightarrow Val}$) found in Hb S, in addition to a second substitution. Hb S-Antilles is particularly important because it can cause sickling in the heterozygous state.

Alkaline electrophoresis is the first step in the definitive diagnosis of all hemoglobinopathies including SCD. Because some hemoglobins have the same electrophoretic mobility patterns, hemoglobins that exhibit an abnormal electrophoretic pattern in an alkaline pH may be electrophoresed at an acid

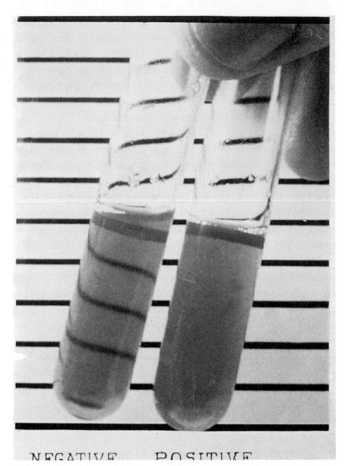

Figure 26-8 Tube solubility screening test for presence of Hb S in sickle cell anemia. (Courtesy of Ann Bell, Professor emeritus, Department of Clinical Laboratory Sciences, University of Tennessee, Memphis.)

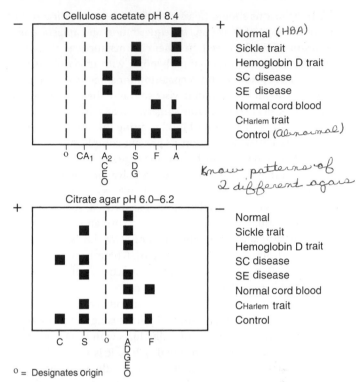

Figure 26-9 Hemoglobin electrophoresis on cellulose acetate and citrate agar, showing relative mobilities of various samples. The relative amounts of hemoglobin are not proportional to the size of the band; for example, in sickle cell trait (AS), the bands may appear equal, but the amount of Hb A always exceeds that of Hb S. (From Schmidt RM, Brosious EF: Basic Laboratory Methods of Hemoglobinopathy Detection, 6th ed [HEW Pub No. (CDC) 77-8266]. Atlanta: Centers for Disease Control and Prevention, 1976.)

pH for definitive separation. Figure 26-9 shows electrophoretic patterns for abnormal hemoglobins. Patients with Hb SS or Hb SC disease lack normal β polypeptide chains, so they have no Hb A. Hb S is usually greater than 80%. Fetal Hb is usually increased (1% to 20%), and when it constitutes more than 20% of hemoglobin, it has a tendency to moderate the severity of the disease. This is especially true in newborns and in hereditary persistence of fetal hemoglobin.[20] Hb A_2 is 2% to 5%, and its quantitation is useful in differentiating sickle cell anemia from sickle $β^0$-thalassemia, in which Hb A_2 is increased (Chapter 27). Hb G, Hb D, and Hb S all migrate in the same position on cellulose acetate electrophoresis, but Hb G and Hb D do not give a positive solubility test.

Treatment

Supportive care has been the mainstay of therapy for SCD. New therapies have evolved, however, that are actually modifying the genetic pathogenesis of the disease. Neonatal screening, childhood prophylactic penicillin, bone marrow transplantation, and treatment with hydroxyurea in adults may extend the life of the SCD patient further.

The main foci of supportive therapy include maintaining adequate hydration, prophylactic vitamin therapy, avoidance of low-oxygen environments, analgesics for pain, and aggres-

sive antibiotic therapy with the first signs of infection. Hydration maintains good blood flow and reduces vaso-occlusive crises. Avoiding strenuous exercise, high altitudes, and unpressurized air travel maintains high oxygen tensions and reduces the sickling phenomenon. Prompt antibiotic treatment reduces the morbidity and mortality associated with infections.[7]

Treatment for painful episodes includes ensuring optimal hydration, rapidly treating associated infection, and effectively relieving pain. Analgesics are the foundation of pain management, with nonsteroidal anti-inflammatory drugs administered to manage mild ischemic attacks. Opioids are recommended when pain becomes chronic in nature.[26] The patient should be examined on a regular basis, and routine testing should be done to establish normal values for the patient during nonsickling periods.

Children younger than 3 years often experience *hand and foot syndrome*, characterized by pain and swelling in the hands and feet.[18] Treatment usually consists of increasing intake of fluids and giving analgesics for pain.

Pneumococcal disease has been a leading cause of morbidity and mortality in children, especially children younger than 6 years. With immunization and prophylactic antibiotics, however, this is now a preventable complication.[6] The risk of bacterial infection probably increases in mature patients with Hb SC disease and homozygous SCD.[15]

Transfusions should be used only for the prevention of the complications of SCD (e.g., in sequestration and aplastic crises to restore the RBC mass). In other circumstances, such as central nervous system infarction, hypoxia with infection, stroke, acute chest episodes, and preparation for surgery, transfusions are used to decrease blood viscosity and the percentage of circulating sickle cells. Before surgery, Hb SS patients are transfused with normal Hb AA blood to bring the volume of Hb S to less than 50% in an effort to prevent complications in surgery.[27] Maintenance transfusions in pregnancy should be done if the mother experiences vaso-occlusive or anemia-related problems or if there are signs of fetal distress or poor growth.[15]

Bone marrow transplantation has proved successful for some individuals. Patients chosen for transplants are generally children with severe complications of SCD (i.e., stroke, acute chest syndrome, and refractory pain). There is evidence that transplantation restores some splenic function, but its effect on established organ damage is unknown.[28]

Hydroxyurea or butyrate therapy has offered some promise in relieving the sickling disorder by increasing the proportion of Hb F in the erythrocytes of individuals with SCD.[29] Because Hb F does not copolymerize with Hb S, it is believed that if the production of Hb F could be sufficiently augmented, the complications of SCD might be avoided. It has been found that the severity of the disease expression and the number of irreversible sickle cells are inversely proportional to the extent to which Hb F synthesis persists. Individuals in whom Hb F stabilizes at 12% to 20% of total hemoglobin may have little or no anemia and few, if any, vaso-occlusive attacks. Levels of 4% to 5% Hb F may moderate the disease, and levels of 5% to 12% may suppress the severity of hemolysis and lessen the frequency of violent episodes.[20]

Course and Prognosis

Proper management of SCD has increased the life expectancy of patients from 14 years in 1973 to the current average life span of 50 years.[30] For men and women heterozygous for Hb SC, the average life span is 60 and 68 years, with a few patients living into their 70s.[17,31] Individuals with Hb SS can pursue a wide range of vocations and professions. They are discouraged, however, from jobs that require strenuous physical exertion, exposure to high altitudes, or extreme environmental temperature variations.

Sickle Cell Trait

The term *sickle cell trait* refers to the heterozygous state (Hb AS) and describes a benign condition that generally does not affect mortality or morbidity. The trait occurs in approximately 8% of African Americans. It also can be found in Central Americans, Asians, and people from the region around the Mediterranean.[1]

Individuals with sickle cell trait are generally asymptomatic and present with no significant clinical or hematologic manifestations. Under extreme hypoxic conditions, however, systemic sickling and vascular occlusion with pooling of sickled cells in the spleen, focal necrosis in the brain, and even death can occur. In conditions such as severe respiratory infection, unpressurized flights at high altitudes, and anesthesia in which

pH and oxygen levels are sufficiently lowered to cause sickling, patients may develop splenic infarcts.[7] Failure to concentrate urine is the only consistent abnormality found in these patients.[32] This abnormality is caused by diminished perfusion of the vasa recta of the kidney, which impairs concentration of urine by the renal tubules. Renal papillary necrosis with hematuria has been described in some patients.[7]

The blood smear of a patient with sickle cell trait has normal RBC morphology, with the exception of a few target cells. No abnormalities in the leukocytes and thrombocytes are seen. The hemoglobin solubility screening test is positive, and sickle cell trait is diagnosed by detecting the presence of Hb S and Hb A on hemoglobin electrophoresis. On electrophoresis, sickle cell trait has approximately 40% of Hb S and 60% or more of Hb A, Hb A_2 is slightly increased, and Hb F is within normal limits. Levels less than 40% of Hb S can be seen in patients who also have α-thalassemia or iron or folate deficiency.[15] No treatment is required for this benign condition, and the patient's life span is not affected by sickle cell trait.

HEMOGLOBIN C

Hb C was the next hemoglobinopathy after Hb S to be described and is found almost exclusively in the African-American population. Spaet and Ranney reported this disease in the homozygous state (Hb CC) in 1953.[6]

Incidence, Etiology, and Pathophysiology

Hb C is found in 17% to 28% of people of West African extraction and in 2% to 3% of African Americans. It is the most common nonsickling variant encountered in the United States and the third most common in the world.[1] Hb C is defined by the structural formula $\alpha_2\beta_2^{6Glu \to Lys}$, in which lysine is substituted for glutamic acid in the sixth position of the β chain. Lysine has a +1 charge resulting in a net change in charge of +2 and a different structural effect on the hemoglobin molecule compared with the Hb S substitution.

Hb C is inherited in the same manner as Hb S but manifests as a milder disease. Similar to Hb S, Hb C polymerizes under low oxygen tension, but the structure of the polymers differs. Hb S polymers are long and thin, whereas the polymers in Hb C form a short, thick crystal within the RBCs. The shorter Hb C crystal does not alter RBC shape to the extent of Hb S resulting in diminished splenic sequestration and hemolysis. In addition, vaso-occlusive crisis does not occur.

Laboratory Diagnosis

A normochromic, normocytic anemia occurs in homozygous Hb C. Occasionally, some microcytosis and mild hypochromia may be present. The MCV and mean cell hemoglobin concentration (MCHC) are normal or increased. There is a marked increase in the number of target cells and reticulocytes. Nucleated RBCs may or may not be present.

Tetragonal crystals of Hb C form within the erythrocyte and may be seen on the blood smear (Figs. 26-10 and 26-11). Many crystals appear free with no evidence of a cell membrane.[33,34] In some cells, the hemoglobin is concentrated within the

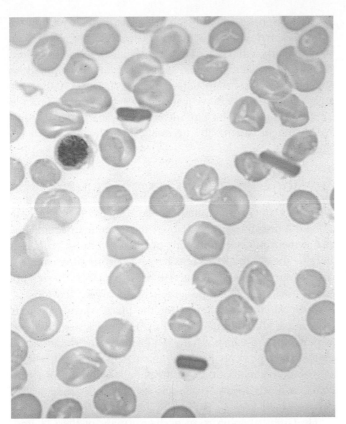

Figure 26-10 Cells from the peripheral blood of a patient with CC disease, showing several bar-shaped crystals in the RBC with visible membrane. (Courtesy of Ann Bell, Professor emeritus, Department of Clinical Laboratory Sciences, University of Tennessee, Memphis.)

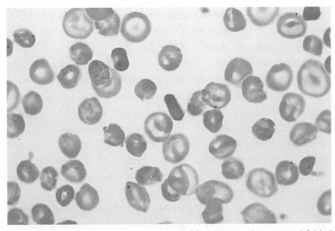

Figure 26-11 Hb C disease with one CC crystal and target and folded cells (peripheral blood, ×1000). (Courtesy of Ann Bell, Professor emeritus, Department of Clinical Laboratory Sciences, University of Tennessee, Memphis.)

boundary of the crystal. The crystals are densely stained and vary in size and appear oblong with pyramid-shaped or pointed ends. These crystals may be seen on wet preparation by washing RBCs and resuspending them in a solution of sodium citrate.[10]

Hb C yields a negative hemoglobin solubility test, and definitive diagnosis is made with electrophoresis. On cellulose acetate electrophoresis, no Hb A is present in Hb CC. In addition, Hb C is present at levels of greater than 90%, with Hb F at less than 7% and Hb A_2 at approximately 2%. In the trait Hb AC, about 60% of Hb A and 30% of Hb C are present. On cellulose acetate agar in an alkaline pH, Hb C migrates in the same position as Hb A_2, Hb E, and Hb O-Arab (see Fig. 26-9). Hb C is separated from these other hemoglobins on citrate agar at an acid pH (see Fig. 26-9). No specific treatment is required. This disorder becomes problematic only if infection occurs or if mild chronic hemolysis leads to gallbladder disease.

HEMOGLOBIN C-HARLEM (HEMOGLOBIN C-GEORGETOWN)

Hb C-Harlem (also known as Hb C-Georgetown) has a double substitution on the β chain.[15,35] The substitution of valine for glutamic acid at the sixth position of the β chain is identical to the Hb S substitution, and the substitution at the 73rd position of aspartic acid for asparagine is the same as that in the Korle Bu mutation. The double mutation is termed *Hb C-Harlem (Hb C-Georgetown)* because the abnormal hemoglobin migrates with Hb C on cellulose acetate electrophoresis at an alkaline pH. Patients with this anomaly are asymptomatic, but patients with double heterozygosity for Hb S and Hb C-Harlem have crises similar to Hb SS disease.

A positive solubility test may occur with Hb C-Harlem and hemoglobin electrophoresis is necessary to confirm the diagnosis. On cellulose acetate at pH 8.4, Hb C-Harlem migrates in the C position (see Fig. 26-9). Citrate agar electrophoresis at pH 6.2 shows migration of Hb C-Harlem in the S position, however (see Fig. 26-9). Because so few cases have been identified, the clinical outcome of individuals affected with this abnormality is uncertain.[35]

HEMOGLOBIN E

Incidence, Etiology, and Pathophysiology

Hb E was first described in 1954.[35,36] The variant occurs with an incidence of 30% in Southeast Asia. As a result of the influx of immigrants from this area, Hb E prevalence has increased in the United States.[37] It occurs infrequently in African Americans and Caucasians. Hb E is a β chain variant in which lysine is substituted for glutamic acid in the 26th position ($\alpha_2\beta_2^{26Glu\rightarrow Lys}$). Similar to Hb C, this substitution results in a net change in charge of +2, but the position of the substitution does not cause polymerization to occur.

Clinical Features

The homozygous state (>90% Hb E) manifests as a mild anemia with microcytes and target cells (Fig. 26-12). The RBC survival time is shortened. The condition is not associated with clinically observable icterus, hemolysis, or splenomegaly. The main concern of identifying homozygous Hb E is differentiating it from iron deficiency, β-thalassemia trait, and Hb E-β-thal (Chapter 27).[38] The disease, Hb EE, resembles thalassemia trait. Because the highest incidence of the Hb E gene is in the

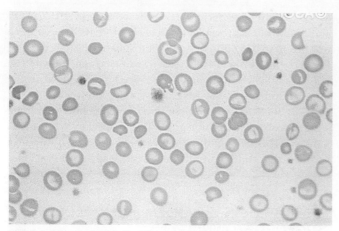

Figure 26-12 Hb E trait with many microcytes and target cells. (From Hematology Tech Sample H-1. Chicago: American Society of Clinical Pathologists, 1991.)

areas of Thailand where malaria is most prevalent, it is thought that *P. falciparum* multiplies more slowly in Hb EE RBCs than in Hb AE or Hb AA RBCs and may give some protection against malaria.[1] Hb E trait is asymptomatic. When Hb E is combined with β-thalassemia, however, the disease becomes more severe than Hb EE and more closely resembles β-thalassemia major, requiring regular blood transfusions.[1]

Laboratory Diagnosis

Hb E does not produce a positive hemoglobin solubility test result. The homozygous state manifests with mostly Hb E on electrophoresis, a very low MCV (55-65 fL), few to many target cells, and a normal reticulocyte count. The heterozygous state is associated with microcytosis (mean MCV 65 fL), slight erythrocytosis, and target cells,[1] and approximately 30% to 40% of the hemoglobin is Hb E on electrophoresis. In alkaline medium (cellulose acetate), Hb E migrates with Hb C, Hb O, and Hb A$_2$ (see Fig. 26-9). On acid agar (citrate), Hb E can be separated from Hb C and Hb O, but it co-migrates with Hb A (see Fig. 26-9).

Treatment and Prognosis

No therapy is required because the patient's health usually is not affected. Some patients may experience splenomegaly and fatigue, however. Genetic counseling is recommended, and the Hb E gene should be discussed in a similar manner as is a mild thalassemia allele.[38]

HEMOGLOBIN O-ARAB

Hb O-Arab is a β chain variant caused by the substitution of lysine for glutamic acid at the 121st amino acid position ($\alpha_2\beta_2^{121\,Glu\rightarrow Lys}$).[7,15,18] It is a rare disorder found in Kenya, Israel, Egypt, and Bulgaria, and it is found in 0.4% of African Americans. No clinical symptoms are exhibited by individuals affected with this variant, except for a mild splenomegaly in homozygotes. When Hb O-Arab is inherited with Hb S, severe clinical conditions similar to those in Hb SS result.

The peripheral smear of homozygous individuals shows a mild hemolytic anemia with many target cells. Because Hb O-Arab migrates with Hb A$_2$, Hb C, and Hb E on cellulose acetate, citrate agar electrophoresis at an acid pH is required to differentiate it from Hb C (see Fig. 26-9). Hb O-Arab is the only hemoglobin to move just slightly away from the point of application toward the cathode on citrate agar at an acid pH. No treatment is generally necessary for individuals with Hb O-Arab.

HEMOGLOBIN D AND HEMOGLOBIN G

Hb D and Hb G are a group of at least 16 β chain variants (Hb D) and 6 α chain variants (Hb G) that migrate in an alkaline pH at the same electrophoretic position as Hb S.[6-8,35] This is because their α and β subunits have one less negative charge at an alkaline pH compared with Hb A, as does Hb S. They do not sickle, however, when exposed to reduced oxygen tension.

Most variants are named for the place where they were discovered. Hb D-Punjab and Hb D-Los Angeles are identical hemoglobins in which glycine is substituted for glutamic acid at the 121st position in the β chain ($\alpha_2\beta_2^{121\,Glu\rightarrow Gln}$). Hb D-Punjab occurs in about 3% of the population in northwestern India, and Hb D-Los Angeles is seen in fewer than 2% of African Americans.

Hb G-Philadelphia is an α chain variant of the G hemoglobins with a substitution of asparagine by lysine at the 68th position. The Hb G-Philadelphia variant is the most common G variant encountered in African Americans and is seen with greater frequency than the Hb D variants. The Hb G variant also is found in Ghana.

Hb D and Hb G do not sickle and yield a negative solubility test result. On alkaline electrophoresis, Hb D and Hb G have the same mobility as Hb S (see Fig. 26-9). Hb D and Hb G can be separated from Hb S on citrate agar at pH 6.0 (see Fig. 26-9). These variants should be suspected whenever a hemoglobin is encountered that migrates in the S position on cellulose and has a negative solubility test. In the homozygous state, Hb D is present at greater than 95% with normal amounts of Hb A$_2$ and Hb F.[20] It can be confused with the doubly heterozygous state for Hb D and β⁰-thalassemia. The two disorders can be differentiated on the basis of RBC indices, levels of Hb A$_2$, and family studies.

Hb D and Hb G are asymptomatic in the heterozygous state. Hb D disease (Hb DD) is marked by mild hemolytic anemia and chronic nonprogressive splenomegaly. No treatment is required.

DOUBLE HETEROZYGOSITY WITH HEMOGLOBIN S AND ANOTHER β-HEMOGLOBIN DISORDER

Double heterozygosity is the inheritance of two different genetic disorders that share a common genetic locus, in this case the β-globin gene.[33,39-41] Because there are two β-globin genes, these double heterozygotes have inherited Hb S from one parent and another β chain hemoglobinopathy or thalassemia from the other parent. Double heterozygosity of Hb S with Hb C, Hb D, Hb O, or β-thalassemia may produce hemolytic anemia of variable severity. Inheritance of Hb S with other hemoglobins, such as Hb E, Hb G-Philadelphia, and Hb Korle Bu, causes disorders of no clinical consequence.

Hemoglobin SC

Hb SC is the most common double heterozygous syndrome that results in a structural defect in the hemoglobin molecule, wherein different amino acid substitutions are found on each of two β-globin chains. At the sixth position, glutamic acid is replaced by valine (Hb S) on one β-globin chain and by lysine (Hb C) on the other β-globin chain. The frequency of Hb SC is 25% in West Africa. The incidence in the United States is approximately 1 in 833 births.[42]

Clinical Features

Hb SC disease resembles a mild SCD. Growth and development are delayed compared with normal children. In contrast to SCD, significant symptoms of Hb SC usually do not occur until teenage years. Hb SC disease may cause all the vaso-occlusive complications of sickle cell anemia, but the episodes are less frequent, and damage is less disabling. Hemolytic anemia is moderate, and many patients exhibit moderate splenomegaly. Proliferative retinopathy is more common and more severe than in sickle cell anemia.[43] Respiratory tract infections with *S. pneumoniae* are common.[7]

Patients with Hb SC disease live longer than patients with Hb SS and have fewer painful episodes, but this disorder is associated with considerable morbidity and mortality, especially after age 30.[44] In the United States, the median life span for men is 60 years; for women, 68 years.[17]

Laboratory Diagnosis

The complete blood count shows a mild normocytic, normochromic anemia with many of the features associated with sickle cell anemia. The hemoglobin level is usually 11 to 13 g/dL, and the reticulocyte count is 3% to 5%. On the peripheral smear, there are a few sickle cells, target cells, and intraerythrocytic crystalline structures. Crystalline aggregates of hemoglobin (SC crystals) form in some cells, where they protrude from the membrane (Figs. 26-13 and 26-14).[41] Hb SC crystals often appear as a hybrid of Hb S and Hb C crystals. They are longer than Hb C crystals but shorter and thicker than Hb S polymers and are often branched.

The solubility screening test is positive because of the presence of Hb S. Electrophoretically, Hb C and Hb S migrate in almost equal amounts (45%) on cellulose acetate, and Hb F is normal. Hb C is confirmed on citrate agar at an acid pH, where it is separated from Hb E and Hb O. Hb A_2 migrates with Hb C, and its quantitation is of no consequence in Hb SC. Determination of Hb A_2 becomes vital, however, if a patient is suspected of having Hb C concurrent with β-thalassemia (Chapter 27).

Treatment and Prognosis

Therapy similar to that in SCD is given to individuals with Hb SC disorder.[35]

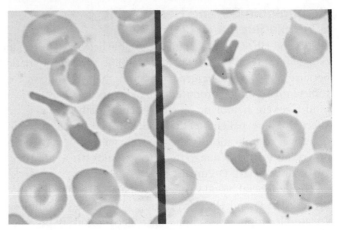

Figure 26-13 Hb SC (peripheral blood, ×1000). Note intraerythrocytic, blunt-ended crystals. (Courtesy of Ann Bell, Professor emeritus, Department of Clinical Laboratory Sciences, University of Tennessee, Memphis.)

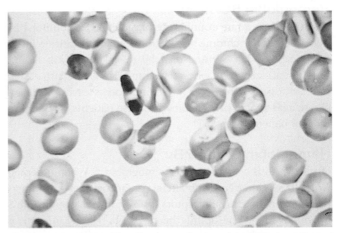

Figure 26-14 Hb SC with two cells containing SC crystals and hypochromic, target, and folded cells (peripheral blood, ×1000). (Courtesy of Ann Bell, Professor emeritus, Department of Clinical Laboratory Sciences, University of Tennessee, Memphis.)

Hemoglobin S/β-Thalassemia

Double heterozygosity for Hb S and β-thalassemia is the most common cause of sickle cell syndrome in patients of Mediterranean descent and is second to Hb SC disease among all double heterozygous sickle disorders. Hb S-β-thal usually causes a clinical syndrome resembling that of mild or moderate sickle cell anemia. The severity of this double heterozygous condition depends on the β chain production of the affected thalassemia β genes. If there is no globin chain production from the β-thalassemia globin gene (S-β⁰-thal), the clinical course is similar to that of homozygous sickle cell anemia. If there is production of β-globin (S-β⁺-thal), patients tend to have a milder condition than patients with Hb SC. These patients can be distinguished from individuals with sickle cell trait because of the presence of greater amounts of Hb S than Hb A, increased levels of Hb A_2 and Hb F, microcytosis from the thalassemia, hemolytic anemia, abnormal peripheral blood morphology, and splenomegaly (Chapter 27).[15]

Hemoglobin SD and Hemoglobin SG-Philadelphia

Hb SD and Hb SG-Philadelphia are double heterozygous sickle cell syndromes.[15,45] Hb SG-Philadelphia is asymptomatic because Hb G is an α gene mutation that still allows for sufficient Hb A to be produced. Hb SD syndrome may cause a mild-to-severe hemolytic anemia because both β chains are affected. Some patients with Hb SD may have severe vaso-occlusive complications. The D Hb syndrome in African Americans is usually due to the interaction of Hb S with Hb D-Los Angeles (Hb D-Punjab).

The peripheral blood smear is comparable to that of Hb SS. Because Hb D and Hb G co-migrate with Hb S on cellulose acetate electrophoresis, citrate agar electrophoresis becomes necessary to separate Hb D from Hb G. The clinical picture is valuable in differentiating Hb SD and Hb SG. The treatment is similar to that in patients with SCD and is administered according to the severity of the clinical condition.

Hemoglobin SO-Arab

Hb SO-Arab is a rare double heterozygous hemoglobinopathy that causes severe chronic hemolytic anemia with vaso-occlusive episodes.[7,15,45] Hb SO-Arab can be mistaken for Hb SC on cellulose acetate electrophoresis because Hb C and Hb O-Arab migrate together; however, differentiation is easily made on citrate agar at acid pH. Therapy for these patients is similar to that for patients with SCD.

Hemoglobin S-Korle Bu

Hb Korle Bu is a rare mutated hemoglobin.[15] When inherited with Hb S, it interferes with lateral contact between Hb S fibers by blocking the crucial receptors for β₆ valine, disrupting Hb S polymerization. The double heterozygote, Hb S-Korle Bu, is asymptomatic.

Hemoglobin SC-Harlem

Hb C-Harlem has two substitutions on the β chain: the sickle mutation and the Korle Bu mutation. Patients heterozygous for only Hb C-Harlem are asymptomatic. The double heterozygous Hb SC-Harlem resembles Hb SS clinically. Hb C-Harlem yields a positive solubility test and migrates to the Hb C position on cellulose acetate electrophoresis at an alkaline pH and to the Hb S position on citrate agar electrophoresis.

Table 26-2 summarizes common clinically significant hemoglobinopathies, including general characteristics and treatment options.

HEMOGLOBIN M

Hb M is caused by a variety of mutations in the α and β genes, all of which result in the production of methemoglobin—hence the Hb M designation.[45,46] These genetic mutations result in a structural abnormality in the globin portion of the molecule. Most M hemoglobins involve a substitution of a tyrosine amino acid for either the proximal (F_8) or the distal (E_7) histidine amino acid in the α or β chains. These substi-

tutions cause heme iron to auto-oxidize, which results in the presence of methemoglobin. Hb M has iron in the ferric state (Fe^{3+}) and is unable to carry oxygen, producing cyanosis. Five hemoglobin variants have been classified as M hemoglobins: Hb M-Hyde Park, Hb M-Boston, Hb M-Iwate, Hb M-Saskatoon, and Hb M-Milwaukee, all named for the locations in which they were discovered.

Hb M variants have altered oxygen affinity and are inherited as autosomal dominant disorders. When Hb M is exposed to certain oxidants, such as sulfonamides or phenacetin, a chocolate-brown color develops. Affected individuals have 30% to 50% methemoglobin and may appear cyanotic because of the chocolate color of circulating hemoglobin causing the blood sample to appear brown. Heinz bodies may be seen sometimes on wet preparations because methemoglobin causes globin chains to precipitate. Diagnosis is made by spectral absorption of hemolysate or by hemoglobin electrophoresis. The absorption spectrum peaks are determined at various wavelengths. The unique absorption range of each Hb M variant is identified when these are compared with the spectrum of normal blood.

Before electrophoresis, all hemoglobin should be converted to methemoglobin by adding potassium cyanide so that any migration differences observed are due to an amino acid substitution instead of due to differences in iron states. On cellulose acetate, Hb M migrates slightly slower than Hb A. The electrophoresis should be performed on agar gel at pH 7.1 for clear separation. Further confirmation with amino acid chain studies must be done. No treatment is necessary. Diagnosis is essential to prevent inappropriate treatment for other ailments, such as cyanotic heart disease.

UNSTABLE HEMOGLOBIN VARIANTS

Unstable hemoglobin variants involve genetic mutations to globin genes creating hemoglobin products that precipitate in vivo, producing Heinz bodies and causing a hemolytic anemia.[45,47] More than 200 variants of unstable hemoglobin exist. Most of these are β chain variants; others are α chain variants. Only a few are γ and δ chain variants. Most unstable hemoglobin variants have no clinical significance, although most have an increased oxygen affinity. About 25% of unstable hemoglobins are responsible for hemolytic anemia, varying from compensated mild anemia to severe hemolytic episodes.

At one time, the anemia was referred to as "congenital non-spherocytic hemolytic anemia" or "congenital Heinz body anemia". This disorder is more properly called *unstable hemoglobin disease*. The syndrome appears at or just after birth depending on the globin chains involved. It is inherited through autosomal dominance. All patients are heterozygous; apparently the homozygous condition is incompatible with life. The instability of the hemoglobin molecule has several causes: (1) substitution in the interior of the molecule of the polar for a nonpolar pocket, (2) substitution around the heme pocket, (3) substitution of the α and β chains at the contact point, (4) replacement of amino acids with proline, and (5) deletion or elongation of the primary structure.

TABLE 26-2 Common Clinically Significant Hemoglobinopathies

Hemoglobin Disorder	Abnormal Hemoglobin	Structural Defect	Individuals Primarily Affected	Hemoglobin Solubility	Hemoglobins Present	Red Blood Cell Morphology	Symptoms/Organ Defects	Treatment
Sickle cell anemia (homozygous)	Hb S	$\alpha_2\beta_2^{6Glu>Val}$	African, African American, Middle Eastern, Indian, Mediterranean	Positive	0% Hb A, >80% Hb S, 1-20% Hb F, 2-5% Hb A$_2$	Sickle cells, target cells, nucleated RBCs, reticulocytes, Howell-Jolly bodies, basophilic stippling spherocytes	Vaso-occlusion, bacterial infections, hemolytic anemia, aplastic episodes, bones, lungs, liver, spleen, penis, eyes, central nervous system, urinary	Transfusions, antibiotics, analgesics, bone marrow transplants, hydroxyurea
Hb C disease (homozygous)	Hb C	$\alpha_2\beta_2^{6Glu>Lys}$	African, African American	Negative	0% Hb A, >90% Hb C, <7% Hb F, 2% Hb A$_2$	Hb C crystals, target cells, reticulocytes, nucleated RBCs, microcytes	Mild splenomegaly, mild hemolysis	Usually none, antibiotics
Hb C-Harlem (Hb C-Georgetown); occurs as double heterozygote with Hb S (Hb S/Hb C-Harlem)	Hb C-Harlem	$\alpha_2\beta_2^{6Glu>Val}$ and $\alpha_2\beta_2^{73Asp>Asn}$ on same gene	Rare, so uncertain; African, African American	Positive	Migrates with Hb C	Target cells	Double heterozygotes have mild symptoms	Usually none
Hb E disease (homozygous)	Hb E	$\alpha_2\beta_2^{26Glu>Lys}$	Southeast Asian, African, African American	Negative	0% Hb A, 95% Hb E, 2-4% Hb A$_2$; migrates with Hb C and Hb 0	Target cells, microcytes	Mild anemia, mild splenomegaly, asymptomatic	Usually none
Hb O-Arab	Hb 0	$\alpha_2\beta_2^{121Glu>Lys}$	Kenya, Israel, Egyptian, Bulgarian, African American	Negative	0% Hb A, 95% Hb O, 2-4% Hb A$_2$; migrates with Hb A$_2$, Hb C, Hb E	Target cells	Mild splenomegaly	Usually none
Hb D disease (rare homozygous)	Hb D, Hb D-Punjab	$\alpha_2\beta_2^{121Glu>Gln}$	Middle Eastern, Indian	Negative	95% Hb D, normal Hb A$_2$ and Hb F; migrates with Hb S	Target cells	Mild hemolytic anemia, mild splenomegaly	Usually none

Asn, asparagine; Asp, aspartate; Gln, glutamine; Glu, glutamate; Lys, lysine; Val, valine.

Continued

TABLE 26-2 Common Clinically Significant Hemoglobinopathies—cont'd

Hemoglobin Disorder	Abnormal Hemoglobin	Structural Defect	Individuals Primarily Affected	Hemoglobin Solubility	Hemoglobins Present	Red Blood Cell Morphology	Symptoms/Organ Defects	Treatment
Hb G disease (rare homozygous)	Hb G, Hb G-Philadelphia	$\alpha_2^{68Asn>Lys}\beta_2$	African American, Ghanan	Negative	95% Hb G, normal Hb A$_2$ and Hb F; migrates with S	Target cells	Mild hemolytic anemia, mild splenomegaly	Usually none
Hb SC disease	Hb S/C	$\alpha_2\beta_2^{6Glu>Val}$ and $\alpha_2\beta_2^{6Glu>Lys}$; separate genes	Same as Hb S	Positive	45% Hb S, 45% Hb C, 2-4% Hb A$_2$, 1% Hb F	Sickle cells, Hb C crystals, Hb SC crystal, target cells	Same as Hb SS except milder	Similar to Hb S
Hb S/β-Thal	Hb S + β mutation	$\alpha_2\beta_2^{6Glu>Val}$ and β^0 or β^+	Same as Hb S	Positive	Hb S variable, some Hb A, increased Hb A$_2$ and Hb F	Sickle cells, target cells, microcytes	Hemolytic anemia, splenomegaly	Some treatment required
Hb SD disease	Hb S/D	$\alpha_2\beta_2^{6Glu>Val}$ and $\alpha_2\beta_2^{121Glu>Gln}$ $\alpha_2\beta_2$	Same as Hb S	Positive	45% Hb S, 45% Hb D, 2-4% Hb A$_2$, 1% Hb F; Hb S/D co-migrate	Sickle cells, target cells	Similar to Hb S but milder	Similar to Hb S but milder
Hb SG	Hb S/G	$\alpha_2\beta_2^{6Glu>Val}$ and $\alpha_2^{68Asn>Lys}\beta_2$	Same as Hb S	Positive	45% Hb S, 45% Hb G, 2-4% Hb A$_2$, 1% Hb F; Hb S/G co-migrate	Sickle cells, target cells	Asymptomatic	Usually none
Hb S/O	Hb S/O	$\alpha_2\beta_2^{6Glu>Val}$ and $\alpha_2\beta_2^{121Glu>Lys}$	Same as Hb S	Positive	45% Hb S, 45% Hb D, 2-4% Hb A$_2$, 1% Hb F	Sickle cells, target cells	Similar to Hb S	Similar to Hb S

Asn, asparagine; Asp, aspartate; Gln, glutamine; Glu, glutamate; Lys, lysine; Val, valine.

Clinical Features

The unstable hemoglobin disorder usually is detected in early childhood in patients with hemolytic anemia concurrent with jaundice and splenomegaly. Elevated fever or ingestion of an oxidant exacerbates the hemolysis. The severity of the anemia depends on the degree of instability of the hemoglobin molecule. The unstable hemoglobin precipitates in vivo and in vitro because of exposure factors that do not affect normal hemoglobins, such as drug ingestion and exposure to heat or cold. The hemoglobin precipitates in the RBC as Heinz bodies. The precipitated hemoglobin attaches to the cell membrane, causing clustering of band 3, attachment of autologous immunoglobulin, and macrophage activation. Additionally, Heinz bodies can be trapped mechanically in the splenic sieve, shortening the RBC survival. The oxygen affinity of these cells is abnormal.

The most prevalent unstable hemoglobin is Hb Köln. Other unstable hemoglobins include Hb Hammersmith, Hb Zurich, Hb Gunn Hill, and Hb Cranston. Because of the large variability in the degree of instability in these hemoglobins, the extent of hemolysis varies greatly. In some of the variants, such as Hb Zurich, an oxidant is required for any significant hemolysis to occur.

Laboratory Diagnosis

The RBC morphology varies. It may be normal or show slight hypochromia and prominent basophilic stippling, which possibly is caused by excessive clumping of ribosomes. Before splenectomy, the hemoglobin level ranges from 7 to 12 g/dL with 4% to 20% reticulocytes. After splenectomy, anemia is corrected, but reticulocytosis persists. Heinz bodies can be shown using a supravital stain. After splenectomy, Heinz bodies are larger and more numerous. Many patients excrete dark urine that contains dipyrrole.

Many unstable hemoglobins migrate in the normal AA pattern and thus are not detected on electrophoresis. Other tests used to detect unstable hemoglobins include the isopropanol precipitation test, which is based on the principle that an isopropanol solution at 37° C weakens the bonding forces of the hemoglobin molecule. If unstable hemoglobins are present, rapid precipitation occurs in 5 minutes, and heavy flocculation occurs after 20 minutes. Normal hemoglobin does not begin to precipitate until approximately 40 minutes. The heat denaturation test also can be used. When incubated at 50° C for 1 hour, heat-sensitive unstable hemoglobins show a flocculent precipitation, whereas normal blood shows little or no precipitation. Significant numbers of Heinz bodies appear after splenectomy, but even in individuals with intact spleens, with longer incubation and the addition of an oxidative substance such as acetylphenylhydrazine, unstable hemoglobins form more Heinz bodies than does the blood from individuals with normal hemoglobins. Newer techniques, such as isoelectric focusing, can resolve many hemoglobin mutations with only a slight alteration in their isoelectric point, and globin chain analysis can be performed by reverse-phase, high-performance liquid chromatography.

Treatment and Prognosis

Patients are treated to prevent hemolytic crises. In severe cases, the spleen must be removed to reduce sequestration and rate of removal of RBCs. Because unstable hemoglobins are rare, prognosis in these affected individuals is unclear. Patients are cautioned against the use of sulfonamides and other oxidant drugs. They also should be informed of the potential for febrile illnesses that may trigger a hemolytic episode.

HEMOGLOBINS WITH INCREASED AND DECREASED OXYGEN AFFINITY

More than 60 hemoglobin variants have been discovered to have abnormal oxygen affinity.[1,45,48,49] Most are high-affinity variants and have been associated with familial erythrocytosis. The remaining mutant hemoglobins are characterized by low oxygen affinity. Many of these are associated with mild-to-moderate anemia.[20]

As described in Chapter 10, normal Hb A undergoes a series of allosteric conformational changes as it converts from fully deoxygenated to fully oxygenated. These conformational changes affect hemoglobin function and its affinity for oxygen. When normal hemoglobin is fully deoxygenated (tense state), it has low affinity for oxygen and other heme ligands and high affinity for allosteric effectors, such as Bohr protons and 2,3-bisphosphoglycerate (diphosphoglycerate). In the oxygenated (relaxed) state, hemoglobin has a high affinity for heme ligands, such as oxygen, and a low affinity for Bohr protons and 2,3-bisphosphoglycerate. The transition from the tense to the relaxed state involves a series of structural changes that have a marked effect on hemoglobin function. If an amino acid substitution lowers the stability of the tense structure, the transition to the relaxed state occurs at an earlier stage in ligand binding, and the hemoglobin has increased oxygen affinity and decreased heme-heme interaction or cooperativity (Chapter 10). One example of a β chain variant is Hb Kempsey. This unstable hemoglobin variant has amino acid substitutions at sites crucial to hemoglobin function.

Hemoglobins with Increased Oxygen Affinity

The high-affinity variants, similar to other structurally abnormal hemoglobins, are inherited through autosomal dominance. Affected individuals have equal volumes of Hb A and the abnormal variant. Exceptions to this are double heterozygotes for Hb Abruzzo and β-thalassemia and for Hb Crete and β-thalassemia, in which abnormal hemoglobin is greater than 85%.

More than 115 variant hemoglobins with high oxygen affinity have been discovered. Such hemoglobins fail to release oxygen on demand, producing hypoxia. The kidneys sense the hypoxia and respond by increasing the release of erythropoietin, causing a compensatory erythrocytosis. These variants differ from unstable hemoglobin, which also may have abnormal oxygen affinity, in that they do not precipitate in vivo to produce hemolysis, and there is no abnormal RBC morphology.

Most individuals are asymptomatic and present with no physical symptoms except a ruddy complexion. Erythrocytosis usually is detected during routine examination because the patient generally has a high RBC count and high hemoglobin and hematocrit results. The WBC count, platelet count, and peripheral blood smear are generally normal. In some cases, hemoglobin electrophoresis may establish a diagnosis. An abnormal band that separates from the A band is present on cellulose acetate in some variants; however, if a band is not found, the diagnosis of increased oxygen affinity cannot be ruled out. Some cases can be separated by using citrate agar (pH 6.0) or by gel electrophoresis. Measurement of oxygen affinity is required for definitive diagnosis.

Patients with high-oxygen-affinity hemoglobins live normal lives and require no treatment. Diagnosis should be made to avoid unnecessary treatment of the erythrocytosis as a myeloproliferative disorder or a secondary erythrocytosis.

Hemoglobins with Decreased Oxygen Affinity

Hemoglobins with decreased oxygen affinity quickly release oxygen to the tissues, resulting in normal to decreased hemoglobin concentration and slight anemia. The best known is Hb Kansas, which has an amino acid substitution of asparagine by threonine at the 102nd position of the β chain. These hemoglobins may be present when cyanosis and a normal arterial oxygen tension coexist, and most may be detected by starch gel electrophoresis.

CHAPTER at a GLANCE

- Hemoglobinopathies are genetic disorders of globin genes that produce structurally abnormal hemoglobins with altered amino acid sequences that affect hemoglobin function and stability.
- Hb S is the most common hemoglobinopathy, resulting from a substitution of valine for glutamic acid at the sixth position of the β globin chain, and primarily affects people of African descent.
- Hb S polymerizes in the RBC because of abnormal interaction with adjacent tetramers when it is in the deoxygenated form, producing sickle-shaped RBCs.
- In SCD (homozygous SS), the polymerization of hemoglobin may result in severe episodic conditions; however, factors other than hemoglobin polymerization may account for vaso-occlusive episodes in sickle cell patients.
- The most clinically significant hemoglobinopathies are Hbs SS, SC, and S-β-thalassemia, with Hb SS being the most severe.
- Individuals with sickle cell trait (Hb AS) are clinically asymptomatic.
- Sickle cell anemia is a normocytic, normochromic anemia, characterized by a single band in the S position on hemoglobin electrophoresis and a positive solubility test.
- The median life expectancy of patients with SCD has been extended to approximately 50 years.
- Hbs C and E are the next most common hemoglobinopathies after Hb S and cause mild hemolysis in the homozygous state. In the heterozygous states, these hemoglobins are asymptomatic.

- Hb C affects primarily people of African descent.
- On peripheral blood smear from patients with Hb CC, tetragonal crystals may be seen with and without apparent RBC membrane surrounding them.
- Hb EE results in a microcytic anemia and affects people primarily of Southeast Asian descent.
- Other variants, such as unstable hemoglobins and hemoglobins with altered oxygen affinity, can be identified, and many cause no clinical abnormality.
- Laboratory procedures employed to determine the presence of an abnormal hemoglobin are complete blood count, peripheral smear evaluation, reticulocyte count, hemoglobin solubility, hemoglobin electrophoresis (acid and alkaline pH), and measurement of Hb A_2 and Hb F.
- Advanced techniques available for hemoglobin identification include high-performance liquid chromatography, globin electrophoresis, and isoelectric focusing.

Now that you have completed this chapter, go back and read again the case study at the beginning and respond to the questions presented.

REVIEW QUESTIONS

1. A qualitative abnormality in hemoglobin may involve all of the following *except*:
   a. Replacement of an amino acid or amino acids in a globin chain
   b. Addition of an amino acid or amino acids in a globin chain
   c. Deletion of an amino acid or amino acids in a globin chain
   d. Decreased production of a globin chain

2. The substitution of valine for glutamic acid at the sixth position of the β chain of hemoglobin results in hemoglobin that:
   a. Is unstable and causes formation of Heinz bodies
   b. Polymerizes to form tactoid crystals
   c. Crystallizes in a tetragonal shape
   d. Contains iron in the ferric (Fe^{3+}) state

3. Patients with SCD usually do not exhibit symptoms until 6 months of age as a result of:
   a. Protective effect of mother's blood
   b. Higher hemoglobin level in infants at birth
   c. Presence of higher levels of Hb F
   d. Immune system not being fully developed

4. Megaloblastic episodes in SCD can be prevented by prophylactic administration of:
   a. Iron
   b. Folate
   c. Steroids
   d. Erythropoietin

5. Which of the following is the most definitive test for Hb S?
   a. Hemoglobin solubility test
   b. Hemoglobin electrophoresis at alkaline pH
   c. Osmotic fragility
   d. Hemoglobin electrophoresis at acid pH

6. A patient presents with mild normochromic, normocytic anemia. On the peripheral smear, there are a few target cells, a rare nucleated RBC, and tetragonal crystals within and lying outside of the RBCs. Which abnormality in the hemoglobin molecule is most likely?
   a. Decreased production of β chains
   b. Substitution of lysine for glutamic acid at the sixth position of the β chain
   c. Substitution of a tyrosine amino acid for the proximal histidine amino acid in the β chain
   d. Double substitution on the β chain

7. A well-mixed specimen for a complete blood count has a brown color. The patient is being treated with a sulfonamide for a bladder infection. Which of the following could explain the brown color?
   a. The patient has Hb M.
   b. Double heterozygosity for Hb S and thalassemia
   c. The incorrect anticoagulant was used.
   d. High levels of Hb F

8. Through routine screening, prospective parents discover that they are both heterozygous for Hb S. What percentage of their children potentially could have SCD?
   a. 0
   b. 25
   c. 50
   d. 100

9. Painful crises in patients with SCD occur as a result of:
   a. Splenic sequestration
   b. Aplasia
   c. Vaso-occlusion
   d. Anemia

10. The screening test for Hb S that uses a reducing agent, such as sodium dithionite, is based on the fact that hemoglobins that sickle:
    a. Are less soluble than normal reduced hemoglobins in a salt solution
    b. Form methemoglobin more readily and cause a color change
    c. Are unstable and precipitate easily, forming Heinz bodies
    d. Oxidize quickly and cause turbidity

REFERENCES

1. Lukens JN: Abnormal hemoglobins: general principles. In Greer JP, Foerster J, Lukens J, et al (eds): Wintrobe's Clinical Hematology, 11th ed, vol 1. Philadelphia: Lippincott, Williams & Wilkins, 2004:1247-1262.
2. Fishleder AJ, Hoffman GC: A practical approach to the detection of hemoglobinopathies. Part I: the introduction and thalassemia syndrome. Lab Med 1987;18:368-372.
3. Bauer JD: Clinical Laboratory Methods, 6th ed. St Louis: Mosby, 1982:72-74.
4. Elghetany MT, Davey FR: Erythrocyte disorders. In Henry JB (ed): Clinical Diagnosis and Management by Laboratory Methods, 20th ed. Philadelphia: Saunders, 2001:542-585.
5. Fishleder AJ, Hoffman GC: A practical approach to the detection of hemoglobinopathies. Part II: the sickle cell disorders. Lab Med 1987;18:441-443.
6. Beutler E: Disorders of hemoglobin structure: sickle cell anemia and related abnormalities. In, Lichtman MA, Beutler E, Kipps TJ, et al (eds): Williams Hematology, 7th ed. New York: McGraw-Hill, 2006:667-700.
7. Wang WC: Sickle cell anemia and other sickling syndromes. In Greer JP, Foerster J, Lukens J, et al (eds): Wintrobe's Clinical Hematology, 11th ed. Philadelphia: Lippincott, Williams & Wilkins, 2004:1263-1311.
8. Serjeant GR: Historical review: the emerging understanding of sickle cell disease. Br J Haematol 2001;112:3-18.
9. Park KW: Sickle cell disease and other hemoglobinopathies. Int Anesth Clin 2004;42:77-93.
10. Sickle Cell Disease Guideline Panel: Sickle Cell Disease: Screening, Diagnosis, Management, and Counseling in Newborns and Infants. Clinical Practice Guideline (AHCPR Pub No. 93-0562). Rockville, Md.: Agency for Health Care Policy and Research, 1993.
11. Weatherall DS: ABC of clinical haematology: the hereditary anaemias. BMJ 1997;314:492-496.
12. Smith JA, Kinney TR (co-chairs), Sickle Cell Disease Guideline Panel: Sickle cell disease: guideline and overview. Am J Hematol 1994;47:152-154.
13. Shah A: Hemoglobinopathies and other congenital hemolytic anemia. Ind J Med Sci 2004;58:490-493.
14. Phillips JA III, Kazazian HH Jr: Hemoglobinopathies and thalassemias. In Spivak JL, Eichner ER (eds): Fundamentals of Clinical Hematology, 3rd ed. Baltimore: The Johns Hopkins University Press, 1993:47-76.
15. Dover GJ, Platt OS: Sickle cell disease. In Nathan DG, Orkin SH (eds): Nathan and Oski's Hematology of Infancy and Childhood, 6th ed. Philadelphia: Saunders, 2003:762-780.
16. Noguchi CT, Rodgers GP, Sergeant G, et al: Level of fetal hemoglobin necessary for treatment of sickle cell disease. N Engl J Med 1988;318:96-99.
17. Platt OS, Brambilla DJ, Rosse WF, et al: Mortality in sickle cell disease: life expectancy and risk factors for early death. N Engl J Med 1994;330:1639-1644.
18. Diggs LW: Sickle cell crises. J Clin Pathol 1965;44:1-19.
19. Embury SH, Hebbel RP, Steinberg MH, et al: Pathogenesis of vasoocclusion. In Embury SH, Hebbel RP, Mohandas N, et al (eds): Sickle Cell Disease: Basic Principles and Clinical Practice. Philadelphia: Lippincott Williams & Wilkins, 1994:311-323.
20. Jandl JH: Blood: Textbook of Hematology, 2nd ed. Philadelphia: Lippincott, Williams & Wilkins, 1996:531-577.
21. Bunn HF: Pathogenesis and treatment of sickle cell disease. N Engl J Med 1997;337:762-769.

22. MacIver JE, Parker-Williams EJ: Aplastic crisis in sickle cell anemia. J Lab Clin Med 1950;35:721.

23. Nagel RL: Innate resistance to malaria: the intraerythrocytic cycle. Blood Cells 1990;16:321-339.

24. Beutler E, Johnson C, Powars D, et al: Prevalence of glucose-6-phosphate dehydrogenase deficiency in sickle cell disease. N Engl J Med 1974;290:826-828.

25. Steinberg MH, West MS, Gallagher D, et al: Effects of glucose-6 phosphate dehydrogenase deficiency upon sickle cell anemia. Blood 1988;71:748-752.

26. Preboth M: Management of pain in sickle cell disease. Am Fam Physician 2000;61:1-7.

27. Bunn HF, Forget BG: Sickle cell disease—clinical and epidemiological aspects. In Bunn HF, Forget BG (eds): Hemoglobin: Molecular, Genetic and Clinical Aspects. Philadelphia: Saunders, 1986:503-510.

28. Martin HS: Review: sickle cell disease: present and future treatment. Am J Med Sci 1996;312:166-174.

29. Reid CD, Charache S, Lubin B, et al: Management and Therapy of Sickle Cell Disease, 3rd ed (Pub No. 95-2117). Bethesda, Md.: National Heart, Lung and Blood Institute, 1995.

30. Claster S, Vichinsky E: Managing sickle cell disease. BMJ 2003;327:1151-1155.

31. Steinberg MH, Ballas SK, Brunson CY, et al: Sickle cell anemia in septuagenarians. Blood 1995;86:3997-3998.

32. Schlitt LE, Keital HG: Renal manifestations of sickle cell disease: a review. Am J Med Sci 1960;239:773-778.

33. Diggs LW, Bell A: Intraerythrocytic hemoglobin crystals in sickle cell hemoglobin C disease. Blood 1965;25:218-223.

34. Bell A: Homozygous C disease. Hematology Tech Sample H-71. Chicago: American Society of Clinical Pathologists, 1974.

35. Rabinovitch A (Chair): Hemoglobinopathy survey, Set HG-B. Northfield, Minn.: CAP, 1992:2-3.

36. Fairbanks VF, Gilchrist GS, Brimhall B, et al: Hemoglobin E trait reexamined: a cause of microcytosis and erythrocytosis. Blood 1979;53:109-115.

37. Anderson HM, Ranney HM: Southeast Asian immigrants: the new thalassemias in America. Semin Hematol 1990;27:239-246.

38. Brewer GJ, Iyengar V, Prasad AS: Clinical aspects of hemoglobinopathies. In Bick RL, Bennett JM, Brynes RK, et al (eds): Hematology: Clinical and Laboratory Practice. St Louis: Mosby, 1993:307-326.

39. Hoffman GC: The sickling disorders. Lab Med 1990;21:797-807.

40. Moewe C: Hemoglobin SC: a brief review. Clin Lab Sci 1993;6:158-159.

41. Nagel RL, Lawrence C: The distinct pathobiology of sickle cell-hemoglobin C disease: therapeutic implications. Hematol Oncol Clin N Am 1991;5:433-451.

42. Lawrence C, Fabry ME, Nagel RL: The unique red cell heterogeneity of SC disease: crystal formation, dense reticulocytes and unusual morphology. Blood 1991;78:2104-2112.

43. Platt OS, Thorington BD, Brambilla DJ, et al: Pain in sickle cell disease: rates and risk factors. N Engl J Med 1991;325:11-16.

44. Steinberg MH: Review: sickle cell disease: present and future treatment. Am J Med Sci 1996;312:166-174.

45. Safko R: Anemia of abnormal globin development—hemoglobinopathies. In Stiene-Martin EA, Lotspeich-Steininger C, Koepke JA (eds): Clinical Hematology: Principles, Procedures, Correlations, 2nd ed. Philadelphia: Lippincott Raven, 1990:192-216.

46. Lukens JN: Hemoglobins associated with cyanosis: methemoglobin and low-affinity hemoglobins. In Greer JP, Foerster J, Lukens J, et al (eds): Wintrobe's Clinical Hematology, 11th ed. Philadelphia: Lippincott, Williams & Wilkins, 2004:1487-1493.

47. Lukens JN: Unstable hemoglobin disease. In Greer JP, Foerster J, Lukens J, et al (eds): Wintrobe's Clinical Hematology, 11th ed. Philadelphia: Lippincott, Williams & Wilkins, 2004:1313-1318.

48. Williamson D: The unstable haemoglobins. Blood Rev 1993;7:146-163.

49. Bunn HF: Hemoglobinopathy due to abnormal oxygen binding. In Bunn HF, Forget BG (eds): Hemoglobin: Molecular, Genetic and Clinical Aspects. Philadelphia: Saunders, 1986:595-616.

Thalassemias

Rakesh Mehta

OUTLINE

Definitions and History
Epidemiology
Genetic Control of Globin
  Synthesis
Categories of
  Thalassemia
Pathophysiology
Genetic Defects Causing
  Thalassemia
β Cluster Thalassemias
α-Thalassemias
Thalassemia Associated
  with Structural
  Hemoglobin Variants
Diagnosis of Thalassemia
Differential Diagnosis of
  Thalassemia and Iron
  Deficiency Anemia

OBJECTIVES

After completion of this chapter, the reader will be able to:

1. Describe the hemoglobin (Hb) defect found in thalassemias.
2. Name the chromosomes that contain the alpha (α) gene and the beta (β) gene clusters and the globin chains produced by each.
3. Discuss the geographic distribution of thalassemia, and explain its association with malaria.
4. Explain the pathophysiology caused by the imbalance of the globin chain synthesis in thalassemia.
5. List the clinically defined thalassemic syndromes associated with genetic defects of the β gene cluster, and describe the clinical expression of each heterozygous and homozygous form.
6. Describe the type of genetic mutations that result in β-thalassemias, including hereditary persistence of fetal hemoglobin (HPFH).
7. Recognize the pattern of laboratory findings in heterozygous and homozygous β-thalassemias, including HPFH.

8. Describe the treatment of homozygous β-thalassemias and the risks involved, and why it is necessary to monitor iron levels.
9. Correlate the clinical syndromes of thalassemia associated with genetic defects of the α genes with the number of α genes present.
10. Justify genetic testing and counseling for individuals of Southeast Asian descent who have α-thalassemia trait.
11. Describe the clinical syndromes of thalassemia associated with structural hemoglobin variants.
12. Specify the erythrocyte indices that are important in screening for thalassemia.
13. Correlate bone marrow evaluation, hemoglobin electrophoresis, and quantitation of Hb F and Hb A_2 with the various thalassemia syndromes.
14. Differentiate thalassemia from iron deficiency anemia.
15. Recognize the laboratory findings associated with various α thalassemia syndromes.
16. Calculate and interpret results of the Mentzer index.

CASE STUDY

After studying the material in this chapter, the reader should be able to respond to the following case study:

A 24-year-old male medical student in the United States was found to have a hemoglobin of 10.2 g/dL in a hematology laboratory class. A hematologist at the university discovered during a family history of this student that his mother had always been anemic, had periodically been given iron shots, and had had several gallbladder "attacks." Both of his parents had been born in Sicily. A cousin on the student's mother's side had two children who had died at the ages of 4 and 5 of thalassemia major and had a third young daughter who also received a diagnosis of thalassemia major and was being treated by frequent blood transfusions. The student's laboratory results were as follows:

Hct: 0.35 L/L (35%)
Hb: 10.2 g/dL
RBC count: 5.74 × 1012/L
MCV: 61.3 fL

MCH: 18 pg
MCHC: 29%

The peripheral RBC morphology exhibited moderate anisocytosis with microcytic RBCs, slight hypochromia, slight poikilocytosis with occasional target cells, and several RBCs with basophilic stippling. Hb A_2 was 4.9% by high-performance liquid chromatography.

1. Why was the family history so important in this case, and what diagnosis did it suggest?
2. What laboratory value helped confirm the diagnosis?
3. From what other disorders should this anemia be differentiated? What laboratory test would be helpful? Why is differentiation important?
4. If this individual were planning to have children, what genetic counseling should be done?

DEFINITIONS AND HISTORY

The thalassemias are a diverse group of inherited disorders caused by genetic alterations that reduce or preclude the synthesis of one or more of the globin chains of the hemoglobin (Hb) tetramer. Since it was first described in 1925 by Cooley and Lee,[1] investigators have worked to define and better understand this fascinating but often confusing condition. Cooley and Lee[1] described four children who had anemia, splenomegaly, and mild hepatomegaly who also had mongoloid facies. These characteristics later would become typical findings in young children with β-thalassemia major and were occasionally referred to as "Cooley's anemia". Seven years later, Whipple and Bradford published a paper outlining the detailed autopsy studies of children who died from this disorder.[2] Because of the high incidence of patients of Mediterranean descent with this disorder, Whipple called this disease *Thalassic* (from Greek for "great sea") anemia, which was shortened to *thalassemia*.[2] Several investigators in the 1940s showed the genetic basis for this anemia and were able to show that homozygotes for this condition (thalassemia major) had a severe course. The heterozygotes were not only carriers, however, but also had a milder anemia (thalassemia minor). In the 1950s, thalassemias resulting from defects in the α chain were described.[2] Together, the thalassemias are the most common single gene disorder in humans. The clinical outcome from the genetic mutation is extremely wide-ranging, however, with certain defects causing no anemia and other defects leading to fetal death. Ultimately, thalassemia results from a reduction in the rate of synthesis of one or more of the globin chains. This decreased globin production leads to imbalanced globin chain synthesis, defective hemoglobin production, and damage to the red blood cells (RBCs) or their precursors by the buildup of the globin chain that is produced in excess.[3] Usually, the synthesis of either the α or the β chains of Hb A ($\alpha_2\beta_2$) is impaired; the thalassemias are named according to the chain with reduced or absent synthesis.

EPIDEMIOLOGY

Although approximately 7% of the world's population have a thalassemic condition, the distribution is concentrated in the "thalassemia belt," which extends from the Mediterranean east through the Middle East and India to Southeast Asia and south through Africa.[4,5] The incidence of β-thalassemia ranges from 1% to 20% depending on the region, with Sardinia, Cyprus, and Greece having the highest numbers in Europe (6% to 19%), and Thailand and Cambodia having the highest numbers in Southeast Asia (1% to 11%).[5] The incidence of α-thalassemia varies considerably. In Europe, Sardinia has the highest carrier frequency (12%), whereas in a tribe in India (Koya Dora) and in Papua New Guinea, the frequency is 80%.[5]

The distribution of thalassemia seems to follow the belt along the tropics where malaria is prevalent (see Fig. 26-3). The high frequency of thalassemia in areas where malaria is endemic is believed to be due to the selective advantage of individuals with heterozygous thalassemia to be resistant to malaria.[6,7]

Several case-control studies evaluated the incidence of thalassemia in subjects with severe malaria compared with the control population and consistently found a lower incidence of thalassemia in the malaria population compared with the normal population. In one study, the risk of death in the hospital was 40% lower in heterozygotes with α-thalassemia and more than 60% lower in homozygotes for α-thalassemia.[7] The mechanism of this resistance is still not fully elucidated; however, two major theories have been developed: defective growth of the parasite in the affected cell and increased phagocytosis of the infected cell.[8,9] Although the exact mechanism is unknown, the distribution and the case-control studies do corroborate the protective quality of the thalassemias in malaria.

GENETIC CONTROL OF GLOBIN SYNTHESIS

The normal hemoglobin molecule is a tetramer (double dimer) of two α-like chains (α or zeta, ζ) with two β-like chains (β, gamma γ, delta δ, or epsilon ε). Combinations of these chains produce six normal Hbs. Three are embryonic Hbs: Hb Gower-1 ($\zeta_2\varepsilon_2$), Hb Gower-2 ($\alpha_2\varepsilon_2$), and Hb Portland ($\zeta_2\gamma_2$). The others are fetal Hb (Hb F, $\alpha_2\gamma_2$) and two adult hemoglobins: Hb A ($\alpha_2\beta_2$) and Hb A$_2$ ($\alpha_2\delta_2$). The α-like chains are located on chromosome 16, whereas the β-like globin chain cluster is on chromosome 11 (Fig. 27-1). The α-like globin cluster contains the functional embryonic globin gene (labeled ζ_2) and two functional adult genes (α_1 and α_2). The β-like globin gene cluster contains five functional genes: ε, $^G\gamma$, $^A\gamma$, δ, and β.[10] These genes are positioned in the order that corresponds with their developmental stage of expression. During weeks 6 to 11 of gestation, the ζ and ε genes are expressed, generating Hb Gower-1 ($\zeta_2\varepsilon_2$). Close to the 11th week, the α genes start to be expressed, and the ζ gene is gradually switched off so that Hb Gower-2 ($\alpha_2\varepsilon_2$) is produced. At the 11th week, the ε is switched off, and γ chain synthesis begins. The γ chains combine with the remaining ζ chains to make Hb Portland ($\zeta_2\gamma_2$) or with the α chains to make Hb F ($\alpha_2\gamma_2$), the predominant Hb of fetal life. After birth, γ chain synthesis decreases, and β and δ chain synthesis begin so that by 6 months, Hb A ($\alpha_2\beta_2$) becomes the predominant Hb (with a low percentage of Hb A$_2$ [$\alpha_2\delta_2$]) (Table 27-1; see Fig. 10-6).[11,12]

Two peptides that differ by a single amino acid (glutamic acid or alanine) are coded for by the γ genes and are designated $^G\gamma$ and $^A\gamma$. Both of these globin chains are expressed in fetal Hb, and there does not seem to be a functional difference. Similarly, the α gene loci are duplicated on each chromosome 16 and are denoted α_1 and α_2. Either of these genes can contribute to the two α-globin molecules in the hemoglobin tetramer, and no functional difference seems to exist between the two. Interspersed between the functional genes on these chromosomes are four functionless gene-like loci or pseudogenes that are designated by the prefixed symbol ψ. The purpose of these pseudogenes is unknown.[11] The organization of these genes on chromosomes 16 and 11 is shown in Figure 27-1.

An individual inherits one cluster of the five functional genes on chromosome 11 from each parent. The genotype for

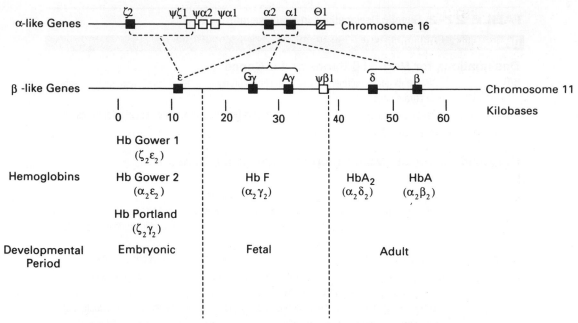

Figure 27-1 Chromosome organization of globin genes and their expression during development. The *solid boxes* indicate functional globin genes; the *open boxes* indicate pseudogenes. The scale of the depicted chromosomal segments is in kilobases (kb) of DNA. The switch from embryonic to fetal Hb occurs between 6 and 10 weeks of gestation, and the switch from fetal to adult Hb occurs at approximately the time of birth. (From Nathan DG, Orkin SH [eds]: Nathan and Oski's Hematology of Infancy and Childhood, 5th ed. Philadelphia: Saunders, 1998:811-886.)

TABLE 27-1 Normal Percentages of Hemoglobins in Adults

Hb A ($\alpha_2\beta_2$)	95-97%
Hb A$_2$ ($\alpha_2\delta_2$)	2-3%
Hb F ($\alpha_2\gamma_2$)	2%

normal β chain synthesis would be designated as β/β. Because the α gene loci are duplicated, two α genes are inherited on each chromosome 16. A normal genotype would be designated $\alpha\alpha/\alpha\alpha$.

CATEGORIES OF THALASSEMIA

The thalassemias are divided into β-thalassemias, which include all the disorders of reduced globin chains arising from the β cluster of genes on chromosome 11, and α-thalassemias, which involve the α_1 and α_2 loci on chromosome 16. Various deletion (absence of a portion of a gene) and non-deletion defects can cause each of these disorders. Even defects that seem the same clinically are often heterogeneous at the genetic level.[3,10] The β-thalassemias affect mainly the β chain production but also may involve the δ, $^G\gamma$, $^A\gamma$, and ε chains. Included in this group is β^0 thalassemia, in which no β chains are produced from the β gene locus on one chromosome 11, and β^+ thalassemia, which is the designation for a partial deficiency in the production of the β chains. The $(\delta\beta)^0$ thalassemias are those where no δ or β chains are produced. In the

homozygous state, these are included in the heterogeneous hereditary persistence of fetal hemoglobin (HPFH) thalassemic disorders. α-Thalassemia, usually caused by a deletion, involves the α_1 or the α_2 gene on chromosome 16 (α^+ thalassemia, designated as $-\alpha$) or the α_1 and the α_2 on chromosome 16 (α^0-thalassemia, designated as $--$).[3,10] These are summarized in Table 27-2.

PATHOPHYSIOLOGY

The clinical sequelae of thalassemia stem from not only a decreased production of a particular globin chain but also, more importantly, from an imbalance of all of globin synthesis.[3,10,13] For α-thalassemia and β-thalassemia, the resultant lack of hemoglobin produces the microcytic, hypochromic RBC (essentially, not enough hemoglobin to fill up the RBC). The mismatched globin chains (from an unequal production of these globin chains) lead to decreased RBC survival, which contributes to a significant component of the anemia. The mechanism and the degree of shortened RBC survival are slightly different, however, for the α-thalassemias and β-thalassemias. In the β-thalassemias, the unpaired α-chains precipitate in the developing cells, which leads to damage to the RBC surface. These damaged RBCs subsequently are destroyed by the macrophages in the bone marrow or in the circulation. The premature death of RBCs in the bone marrow leads to *ineffective erythropoiesis*, a term that indicates that although the bone marrow is attempting to produce cells, it is not able to release viable cells into the circulation. Some of these cells escape the bone marrow only to be destroyed in the spleen, otherwise

TABLE 27-2 Genetic Designations in Thalassemia

Designation	Definition
Designations for Normal β Genes and α Genes	
β/β	Normal β genes, normal amount of β chains produced; one inherited from each parent on chromosome 11
αα/αα	Normal α genes, normal amount of α chains produced; two genes inherited from each parent on chromosome 16
Designations for the Main Group of Thalassemic Genes	
β^0	Abnormal β gene; no β chains produced
β^+	Abnormal β gene; 10-50% of normal chains produced
β^{++} (β^{+s})	Abnormal β gene; small reduction in β chain production; nearly normal α/β chain ratio
$\delta\beta^0$	Abnormal mutation affecting δ and β genes; no β or δ chains produced; only $^A\gamma$ and $^G\gamma$ chains produced from β cluster
$(^A\gamma\delta\beta)^0$	Mutation affecting $^A\gamma\delta\beta$ genes; only $^G\gamma$ chains produced from the β gene cluster
(δβ) Lepore	A non–α globin chain that is a δ-β fusion chain. Lepore Hb is synthesized in small amounts, resulting in thalassemia
HPFH	Hereditary persistence of Hb F: nondeletion thalassemia that results in the production of more Hb F than normal in adulthood
α^0 (α-thal-1)	Deletion of both α genes (– –) from the α gene complex on one chromosome; no α globin is produced
α^+ (α-thal-2)	Deletion of one gene from the α gene complex (–α); decreased production of the α chains from the α gene complex
α^T	Abnormal α gene resulting in decreased production of α chains from the α gene complex (*T* denotes thalassemia)

known as *hemolysis*. In β-thalassemia, the anemia is multifactorial and results from decreased *effective* production and from increased destruction. Typically, individuals with β-thalassemia are asymptomatic during fetal life through 4 to 6 months of age because Hb F ($\alpha_2\gamma_2$) is the predominant circulating hemoglobin. They become symptomatic only after the γ-to-β switch.[12] In α-thalassemia, non-α chain production has different consequences. Because α chains are shared by fetal and adult hemoglobins, defective α chain production results in excess chain production in fetal and adult life. In the fetus, there is excess γ chain production. This excess production occurs even if only one α gene is nonfunctioning. The more nonfunctioning genes, the more excess γ chains are present. These excess γ chains bind one another, resulting in γ_4 tetramers of hemoglobin (called *Hb Bart*). Because these tetramers are soluble, they do not precipitate to any significant degree in the marrow and do not cause severe ineffective erythropoiesis. These tetramers do precipitate as the mature RBCs age in the blood and form inclusion bodies. The spleen removes the cells with inclusions, resulting in hemolysis. The RBCs are microcytic and hypochromic in α-thalassemia owing to the lack of hemoglobin synthesis.[3,10] The anemia is a result not only of decreased effective production, but also shortened RBC survival. Hb Bart (γ_4) has high affinity for oxygen and is an ineffective oxygen carrier. Because of this inability to deliver oxygen adequately, the fetus cannot survive with only Hb Bart (found when all four α genes are absent), resulting in fetal demise in utero, also known as *hydrops fetalis*.[14] Hb H, β chain tetramers in the adult, are discussed in the α-thalassemia section later.

GENETIC DEFECTS CAUSING THALASSEMIA

Molecular cloning, DNA sequencing, and functional analysis of cloned genes have revealed many different types of defects at the molecular level.[3,10,15] Among the types of genetic defects that cause a decrease in or lack of production of a particular globin chain and thalassemia are the following:

- *Single-nucleotide (or point) mutation* that interferes with one of the crucial steps in messenger RNA (mRNA) production, causing the amount of mRNA to be decreased
- *Base substitutions* that alter promoter function, RNA processing, or mRNA translation or modify a codon into a "nonsense codon" that leads to premature termination of translation or to the substitution of an incorrect amino acid
- *Insertion or deletion mutations within the coding region of the mRNA*, creating "frameshifts" that prevent the synthesis of a complete, normal globin polypeptide
- *Large deletion within the α-globin or β-globin clusters* that removes one or more genes or alters the regulation of the remaining genes in the cluster[3,10,15]

All of these heterogeneous genetic defects or mutations cause a decrease in or lack of synthesis of one globin chain, resulting in the thalassemia syndromes.

β CLUSTER THALASSEMIAS

With modern advances in genetic technology, the heterogeneity of the defects in the DNA of the β cluster gene that lead to the clinical syndrome of β-thalassemia has been revealed.[15] More than 200 genetic abnormalities have been discovered in the β cluster gene, including mutations in each of the β, δ, and γ genes or of the combined sections of the β cluster gene.[16] Although there are numerous different mutations, a small subset of only four to six mutations account for more than 90% of the mutant alleles within a single ethnic group or geographic area affected by β-thalassemia.[16] Because there are multiple mutations present in each population, most individuals with severe β-thalassemia are genetic compound heterozygotes for two different thalassemia mutations. The frequency of specific β-thalassemia mutations has been completed for numerous ethnic groups, and this information is particularly relevant to prenatal diagnosis of β-thalassemia.[5]

Clinical Syndromes of β-Thalassemia

Historically, β-thalassemia has been divided into three clinical syndromes: β-thalassemia minor (heterozygous), a mild microcytic, hypochromic hemolytic anemia; β-thalassemia major (homozygous), a severe transfusion-dependent anemia; and β-thalassemia intermedia, with symptoms of severity between the other two.[3,10,13,15] A fourth syndrome is now recognized, which has been designated as *silent carrier status*, for patients with genetic changes in one of the two β genes that results in *no* hematologic abnormalities (Table 27-3).[15] The clinical manifestations of the genetic changes depends on whether one or both of the β genes is affected and the extent to which the gene or genes are expressed. Several mutations result in the absence of production of the β chain, and these mutations are designated as a β^0 gene. Other mutations lead to production of the β chains but at a significantly reduced rate, and these are designated as β^+ genes.[10] The range of production in these β^+ genes varies from 10% to 50% of normal β chain synthesis. The

TABLE 27-3 Clinical Syndromes of β-Thalassemias

Genotype	Hb A	A$_2$	F	Lepore
Normal (Normal Hematologic Parameters)				
ββ	nl	nl	nl	—
Silent Carrier (Usually Normal)				
β^{++s} thalassemia (β^{++s}/β)	nl	nl	nl	—
Thalassemia Minor (Mild Hemolytic Anemia; Microcytic, Hypochromic)				
β^+ thalassemia (β^+/β)	↓	↑	nl to sl ↑	—
β^0 thalassemia (β^0/β)	↓	↑	nl to sl ↑	—
$\delta\beta^0$ thalassemia ($\delta\beta^0/\delta\beta$)	↓	↓	5-20%	—
Hb Lepore thalassemia (Hb Lepore/β)	↓	↓	↑	5-15%
Thalassemia Major (Severe Transfusion-Dependent Hemolytic Anemia; Microcytic, Hypochromic)				
β^+ thalassemia				
β^+/β^+	↓↓	v	↑	—
β^+/β^0	↓↓↓	v	↑	—
β^0 thalassemia ($\beta^0\beta^0$)	—	v	nl to ↑	—
Hb Lepore (Hb Lepore/Hb Lepore)	—	—	75%	25%
Thalassemia Intermedia (Moderate Hemolytic Anemia with Few Transfusion Requirements; Microcytic, Hypochromic)				
Homozygous				
β^{+s} thalassemia (β^{+s}/β^{+s})	↓	↓	↑	—
$\delta\beta^0$ thalassemia ($\delta\beta^0/\delta\beta^0$)	—	—	100%	—

nl, normal; sl, slight; v, variable.

clinical phenotype depends on the severity of the production defect (reduction or absence of globin chain generation) and whether one or both genes are abnormal.

Silent Carrier State of β-Thalassemia

The silent carriers are the various heterogeneous β mutations that produce only a small decrease in production of the β chains and that result in nearly normal α/β chain ratios and no hematologic abnormalities.[17,18] The silent carrier state was recognized through a study of families in which the affected children had a more severe β-thalassemia syndrome than a parent with the typical β-thalassemia trait.[13,17,18] These parents had normal levels of Hb A_2 and a slight microcytosis. Several patients who are homozygous for the silent carrier thalassemia gene have been described. They have a moderate microcytic, hypochromic anemia with a hemoglobin level in the range of 7 to 9 g/dL. The Hb F values range from 2% to 19%, and the Hb A_2 level is elevated to the range normally seen in individuals with thalassemia trait.[19]

β-Thalassemia Minor

β-Thalassemia minor results when one of the two genes that produce the β globin chains is defective (heterozygous state). It usually presents as a mild, asymptomatic anemia.[3,10,15] One β gene is affected by a mutation that decreases or abolishes its function, whereas the other β gene is normal. The peripheral blood count reveals a hemoglobin level in the 10- to 13-g/dL range, and the RBC count is normal or slightly elevated. The anemia is microcytic and hypochromic, with the peripheral smear showing some degree of poikilocytosis, including target cells and elliptocytes. An increased number of stippled RBCs may be seen on the Wright-Giemsa–stained smear (Fig. 27-2). The bone marrow reveals mild-to-moderate erythroid hyperplasia, with slight ineffective erythropoiesis. Hepatomegaly and splenomegaly are seen in a few patients. The most common β-thalassemia syndromes characteristically have a high Hb A_2 level, which can vary from 3.5% to 8%. Hb F levels usually range from 1% to 5%. Less-common variants of β-thalassemia traits exist; one has a Hb A_2 level elevated as just described, but with the Hb F in the 5% to 20% range.[20] Other variants also are found in which the Hb A_2 level is not elevated.[21]

β-Thalassemia Major

β-Thalassemia major is characterized by a severe anemia first detected in early childhood as the γ-to-β switch takes place. At birth, the predominant hemoglobin is Hb F, but over the next 6 months, Hb A levels increase and Hb F levels decrease (see Fig. 10-6).[3,10,12] Patients with severe β-thalassemia usually are diagnosed between 6 months and 2 years of age because the Hb A does not increase as it should. The natural history of this condition (an untreated patient or an inadequately treated patient) results in increasing hepatosplenomegaly, jaundice, and marked bone changes secondary to an expanded marrow cavity caused by extreme erythroid hyperplasia. Radiography shows the typical "hair-on-end" appearance on skull radiographs, whereas the long bones develop a lacy appearance from thinning of the bony cortex due to marrow expansion, which predisposes to pathologic fracture (Fig. 27-3). A typical facies results, with prominence of the forehead (also known as *frontal bossing*), cheekbones, and upper jaw (Fig. 27-4). Physical growth and development are delayed.

The hemoglobin level falls to 3 to 4 g/dL. The RBCs are markedly hypochromic with extreme poikilocytosis, including target cells, teardrop cells, and elliptocytes. RBC fragments and microspherocytes are present as a direct consequence of unbalanced globin chain synthesis. Stippled and many nucleated RBCs are found on the blood smear (Fig. 27-5). The mean cell volume (MCV) is very low. A characteristic RBC finding is enlarged and very thin, often wrinkled and folded cells containing clumps of hemoglobin. A reticulocyte count of 2% to 8% is noted, which is low in relationship to the amount of RBC hyperplasia and hemolysis present. The inappropriate reticulocytosis results from the death of the RBC precursors in the bone marrow (ineffective erythropoiesis). The α chains with no complementary chain form insoluble tetramers that damage the cell membrane, leading to destruction of the cell in the bone marrow.[3]

Electrophoresis shows that most of the hemoglobin is Hb F, with a slightly increased Hb A_2, whereas Hb A is absent or nearly absent, depending on the precise genotype that determines whether none (β^0) or only a small amount of β chains (β^+) are produced. Hb A is present only if a severe β^+ gene is present. The bone marrow shows marked erythroid hyperplasia, with an erythroid-to-myeloid (E:M) ratio of 20:1 (normal E:M ratio is 0.5:1). As a result of the ineffective erythropoiesis and the peripheral hemolysis, the haptoglobin is low, and the lactate dehydrogenase level is elevated.

Transfusions are the major therapeutic option for patients with thalassemia major and typically are initiated in the first year of life.[22,23] Beginning in the mid-1970s, it became the practice to give regular transfusions to prevent not only the anemia, but also the other consequences of the disorder. The hemoglobin usually is maintained between 9.5 and 11.5 g/dL. These transfusion regimens are termed *hypertransfusion* and are used to correct the anemia and to suppress

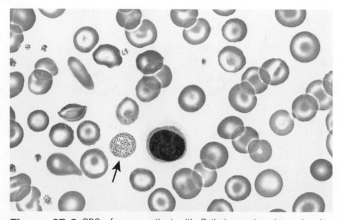

Figure 27-2 RBCs from a patient with β-thalassemia minor, showing microcytic, hypochromic RBCs with target cells, other poikilocytes, and a stippled RBC *(arrow)*.

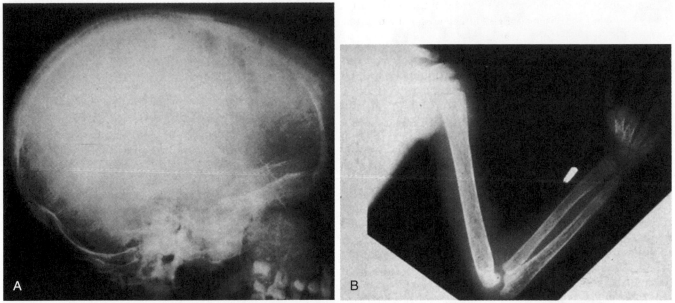

Figure 27-3 Bone changes in severe β-thalassemia major. **A,** Skull radiograph. **B,** Radiograph of forearm and hand. (**A** from Beck WS [ed]: Hematology, 2nd ed. Boston: MIT Press, 1976; **B** from Nathan DG: Thalassemia. N Engl J Med 1972;286:586. Copyright © 1972 Massachusetts Medical Society. All rights reserved; reprinted with permission.)

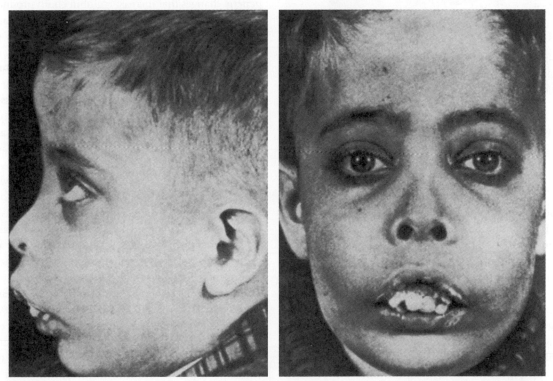

Figure 27-4 Typical facial appearance of a child with untreated homozygous β-thalassemia major. (From Jurkiewicz MJ, Pearson HA, Furlow LT Jr: Reconstruction of the maxilla in thalassemia. Ann N Y Acad Sci 1972;165:437-442.)

the marked erythropoiesis. With erythropoiesis suppressed, the marked marrow expansion does not occur, and the bone changes do not take place. These children have much-improved growth and development. Enlargement of the liver and spleen (hepatosplenomegaly) does not develop.[24] The transfusion regimens lead to an excess iron burden in the patients. Because there is no physiologic pathway for iron excretion in the body, the iron contained within the RBCs in the transfusion accumulates in the body. This iron is stored in organs (e.g., liver, heart, pancreas) outside the bone marrow, which leads to damage of those organs. The accumulation of iron in the liver leads to cirrhosis, and the deposition of iron in the heart leads

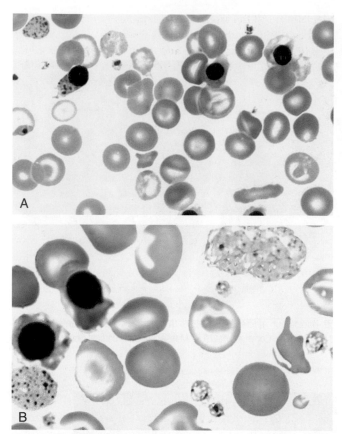

Figure 27-5 RBCs from a patient with β-thalassemia major. **A,** ×500. **B,** ×1000. (Adapted from Carr JH, Rodak BF: Clinical Hematology Atlas, 2nd ed. Philadelphia: Saunders, 2004.)

to cardiac dysfunction and arrhythmias. With transfusion therapy alone, the thalassemic patients died in their teens, typically from cardiac failure. With the beginning of transfusion therapy, these patients now begin iron chelation therapy as well. The medication, desferrioxamine, is able to bind excess iron and is excreted with the iron by the kidney. This agent has been able to prevent iron accumulation and the subsequent complications of iron overload, helping to extend life expectancy into the 30s (Chapter 19).[24]

Bone marrow transplantation has been successful in thalassemia major.[25-27] The average event-free survival is greater than 80% in good-risk children. Patients with good chelation therapy regimens, no hepatomegaly, and no portal fibrosis have the highest success rate. Bone marrow transplantation is not available to all patients, however. In some cases, drugs that cause the γ gene to "switch on" so that the patient's RBCs produce higher levels of Hb F have had some success.[28] Hydroxyurea has been shown to increase the Hb F levels enough to eliminate transfusion requirements for patients with thalassemia major. Not all patients seem to respond to this therapy.[29] Ideally, in the future, gene therapy will be able to correct the genetic defect.[30]

β-Thalassemia Intermedia

Thalassemia intermedia is a term used to describe patients with a more severe anemia than β-thalassemia minor but who do not require regular transfusions to maintain their RBC counts and their quality of life.[3,13] Typically, although these patients maintain an hemoglobin greater than 7 g/dL, the level of hemoglobin is *not* the determinant of this diagnosis, but rather the clinical scenario.[31] Their imbalance in the α and β chain synthesis falls between that observed in β-thalassemia minor and β-thalassemia major, and their general clinical phenotype falls between the extremes of transfusion-dependent thalassemia major and asymptomatic trait. The genotypes of thalassemia intermedia have great heterogeneity. These patients can be homozygotes for mutations that cause a mild decrease in β globin expression. Conversely, they may be doubly heterozygous, with one gene having a mild decrease in β globin production, whereas the other has a marked reduction in β globin production.[13] In some instances, only one of the β genes carries a mutation, but it is severe enough to cause a significant anemia. Many of the thalassemia intermedia phenotypes are generated from the coinheritance of one or two abnormal β globin genes with another hemoglobin defect, such as abnormal α genes or unstable hemoglobins.[31] The coinheritance of α-thalassemia may permit homozygotes for more severe β-thalassemia mutations to remain transfusion independent because the α/β chain ratio is more even.[32] When genetic changes that increase γ globin chain production, which results in increased in Hb F levels, are combined with minimal β globin chain production, a less severe anemia develops, as the Hb F compensates for the reduction in Hb A. Examples of these situations are the deletion forms of δβ-thalassemia. Individuals homozygous for these mutations or compound heterozygotes for δβ-thalassemia and a β-thalassemia mutation have thalassemia intermedia.[13] Coinheritance of a triplicated α globin locus (ααα) (see section on α-thalassemia) is also a cause of thalassemia intermedia in individuals heterozygous for β-thalassemia.[33]

Because of the heterogeneity of this clinical syndrome, the laboratory and clinical features vary. The RBC morphology of thalassemia intermedia is similar to that previously described for thalassemia major. The degree of anemia and jaundice varies depending on the severity of the genetic defect. As a result of the presence of splenomegaly, the platelet count and neutrophil counts may be low. The clinical course varies from minimal symptoms despite moderately severe anemia to severe exercise intolerance and pathologic fractures.[31] Patients with thalassemia intermedia also may have problems of iron overload even though they are not transfused. The markedly accelerated, although ineffective, erythropoiesis, with the resulting increase in plasma iron turnover, provokes an increase in gastrointestinal iron absorption.[34] For this reason, cardiac and endocrine complications present 10 to 20 years later in thalassemia intermedia patients than in patients who are regularly transfused.

Other Thalassemias Caused by Defects in β Cluster Genes

Other thalassemias may be caused by deletion or inactivation of only certain genes of the β cluster, such as δ-thalassemia and γδβ-thalassemia.[35,36]

Thalassemias with Increased Levels of Fetal Hemoglobin

HPFH and δβ-thalassemia are closely related conditions that are characterized by continued synthesis of increased levels of Hb F in adult life. Typically, the increase in Hb F leads to the absence of the usual clinical and hematologic features of thalassemias.[10] These conditions are quite similar and are differentiated by the amount of Hb F produced and the distribution of the Hb F in the RBCs (heterocellular versus pancellular).[10,37] Because these individuals are characteristically asymptomatic, this condition is of little significance except as it interacts with other forms of thalassemia or structural hemoglobin variants, such as Hb S. The additional γ chains produced are able to replace the lacking β chains and help to restore the balance of α and non–α chains (γ or β), raising the hemoglobin level. In sickle cell anemia, the increased Hb F reduces the percentage of Hb S, producing a milder clinical course.

The β gene cluster in HPFH typically contains a deletion in the δγ region that leads to the increased production of Hb F; however, there also are HPFH conditions that have intact β gene clusters (nondeletional changes) that lead to the increased production of Hb F.[3,10,38] The δβ-thalassemias also are characterized by deletions in the δ and β genes. The difference between these two conditions is based on their clinical presentations. HPFH heterozygotes have significant variation but typically have normal-sized RBCs and Hb F levels of 15%

to 30%. The δβ-thalassemia heterozygotes have hypochromic, microcytic RBCs with Hb F levels of 5% to 20%. Homozygotes for HPFH are asymptomatic and have slightly hypochromic, microcytic RBCs with 100% Hb F levels. Homozygous δβ-thalassemia individuals have 100% Hb F and have a mild β-thalassemia intermedia phenotype.[3,10]

Hemoglobins Lepore and Kenya

A rare class of δβ-thalassemias results in structural hemoglobin variants called *Lepore* that have, as the non–α globin chain, a δβ fusion chain that is composed of the first 50 to 80 amino acid residues of the δ chain and the last 60 to 90 residues of the normal C-terminal amino acid sequence of the β chain.[3,10] This fusion event occurs during meiosis, from nonhomologous crossing over between the δ locus on one chromosome and the β locus on the other chromosome (Fig. 27-6). Patients with the Lepore globin chain have reduced production of the fusion globin chain because the transcriptional control is from the δ chain promoter, which is much less active than the β chain promoter (normal Hb A$_2$ levels 2% to 3%). Heterozygotes for Hb Lepore are similar to β-thalassemia minor, whereas homozygotes act more like β-thalassemia major. Conversely, in anti-Lepore, the β gene locus is still intact so that normal production of the β chain occurs (see Fig. 27-6).[3] Unequal crossover events also result in Hb Kenya (see Fig. 27-6). Only heterozygotes have been identified with this gene product and have a normal blood picture with 5% to 20% Hb Kenya.[10]

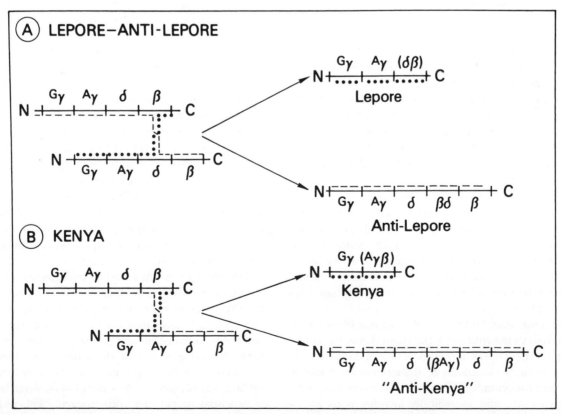

Figure 27-6 Representation of the unequal crossover events that occurred during meiosis and resulted in formation of the Lepore and anti-Lepore **(A)** and Kenya **(B)** genes. (From Nienhuis AW, Benz EJ Jr: Regulation of hemoglobin synthesis during the development of the red cell [part 1]. N Engl J Med 1977;297:1318-1328. Copyright © 1977 Massachusetts Medical Society. All rights reserved; reprinted with permission.)

Screening for Thalassemia

Because of the high frequency of thalassemia in several areas of the world, screening has become an important global health issue.[5] Mass screening programs in Italy and Greece combined with prenatal diagnosis have led to a significant reduction in the number of children born with β-thalassemia major.[3] Identifying potential carriers for these disorders can be accomplished by measuring hemoglobin levels, MCV, Hb A_2 and Hb F concentrations, and osmotic fragility.[3,39] Other causes of microcytic anemias, such as iron deficiency, need to be ruled out. When parents are identified as potential carriers, DNA can be analyzed by polymerase chain reaction and molecular hybridization techniques for the presence of thalassemia mutations. When the parents' defect is known, more focused (and less costly) DNA analyses can be performed in the antenatal period.[39]

α-THALASSEMIAS

In contrast to the β globin cluster, in which point mutations are the most common cause of thalassemia, large deletions in the α globin genes are the predominant cause of α-thalassemia.[3,10] The extent of decreased production of the α chain depends on the specific mutation, the number of α genes affected, and whether an α2 or α1 gene is affected. The α2 gene seems to produce approximately 75% of the α globin in normal RBCs. Notation for the normal α gene complex or haplotype is expressed as αα, signifying the two normal genes (α2 or α1) on one chromosome 16; a normal genotype is αα/αα. The α-thalassemias can be divided into $α^+$ thalassemia (haplotype –α), which have decreased production from the α chain complex (originally named α-thal-2), and $α^0$ thalassemias (originally named α-thal-1), in which no α globin is produced from the α gene complex (haplotype – –).[40]

Point mutations (rather than deletions) that affect the predominant α2 gene (haplotype designated as $α^Tα$) may also produce the α-thalassemia trait ($α^Tα/αα$).[10] These point mutations reduce the expression from the α2 gene ($α^Tα$) and result in $α^+$ thalassemia. In this form of α+ thalassemia there exist unstable α globin chains or fewer α globin chains than in the deletion $α^+$ haplotype (–α). The $α^Tα$ genotype is more severe than the –α genotype. Homozygosity for point mutations in both α2 genes ($α^Tα/α^Tα$) phenotypically produces Hb H disease and not the α-thalassemia trait. Hb H is a tetramer of β chains—$β_4$. There is also a nondeletion $α^+$ haplotype in which the $α^0$ thalassemia (– –/$α^Tα$) produces a more severe Hb H disease than the $α^0$ interaction with the $α^+$ haplotype (– –/–α).[10]

There are more than 20 known deletions that involve both the α genes ($α^0$) or the entire α globin chain cluster (γα globin chain cluster). These result in no production of α chains from that chromosome.[10,41] Genes for $α^0$ thalassemia are found in 4% of the population in Southeast Asia, less frequently in the Mediterranean area, and sporadically in other parts of the world.[5] Further, $α^0$ thalassemia is found infrequently in Africa and in individuals of African ancestry.

Clinical Syndromes of α-Thalassemia

Four clinical syndromes are present in α-thalassemia depending on the gene number, *cis* or *trans* pairing and the amount of α chains produced.[3,10] The four syndromes are silent carrier, α-thalassemia trait (α-thal minor), Hb H disease, and homozygous α-thalassemia (hydrops fetalis) (Table 27-4).

Silent Carrier

The deletion of one α globin gene, leaving three functional α globin genes (–α/αα), causes the silent carrier syndrome. The α/β chain ratio is nearly normal, and no hematologic abnormalities are present.[3,10] Because one α chain is absent, there is a slight decrease in α chain production. There is a slight excess of γ chains at birth, which bind together to generate Hb Bart ($γ_4$) in the range of 1% to 2%. There is no reliable way to diagnose silent carriers other than genetic analysis.

α-Thalassemia Trait

α-thalassemia trait can be caused by the homozygous $α^+$ (–α/–α) or heterozygous $α^0$ (– –/αα) form.[3,10] This syndrome exhibits a mild anemia with marked microcytic, hypochromic RBCs. At birth, Hb Bart is in the range of 2% to 10%. In adults, the production of α and β chains is balanced so that no Hb H ($β_4$) is usually present.

Hemoglobin H Disease

Hb H disease is usually caused by the presence of only one gene producing α chains (– –/–α).[3,10] It also can be caused by the combination of $α^0$ and non-deletion mutations (– –/$α^Tα$) or $α^0$ and Hb Constant Spring (– –/$α^{CS}α$).[41] This genetic abnormality is particularly common in Asians because the $α^0$ gene (haplotype – –) is prevalent and is characterized by the accumulation of excess unpaired β chains, which form tetramers of Hb H. In the newborn, 10% to 40% of the hemoglobin is Hb Bart, with the remainder being Hb F and Hb A. After the γ-to-β switch, Hb H replaces Hb Bart. The hemoglobin percentages are 30% to 50% Hb H, reduced amount of Hb A_2, and traces of Hb Bart, with the remainder being Hb A.[42]

Hb H disease is characterized by a mild-to-moderate, chronic hemolytic anemia with hemoglobin concentrations averaging 7 to 10 g/dL and reticulocytes from 5% to 10%.[3,41,42] The bone marrow exhibits erythroid hyperplasia, and the spleen is usually enlarged. As with most chronic hemolytic states, infection, pregnancy, or exposure to oxidative drugs may cause a hemolytic crisis.

Hemolytic crises often lead to the detection of the disease as individuals with Hb H disease may otherwise lead normal lives. The RBCs are microcytic, hypochromic with marked poikilocytosis, including target cells and bizarre shapes. Hb H is vulnerable to oxidation and gradually precipitates in vivo to form Heinz-like bodies of denatured hemoglobin.[42] These inclusions alter the shape and viscoelastic properties of the RBCs, contributing to the decreased RBC survival. Splenectomy is beneficial in patients with markedly enlarged spleens.[41] When incubated with brilliant cresyl or new methylene blue, RBCs with Hb H display fine, evenly distributed, granular

TABLE 27-4 Clinical Syndromes of α-Thalassemias

Genotype	Hb A	Hb Bart (in Newborn)	Hb H (in Adult)	Constant Spring
Normal (Normal Hematologic Parameters)				
αα/αα	97-98%	0	0	0
Silent Carrier (Normal Hematologic Parameters)				
−α/αα	97-98%	0-2%	0	0
ααCS/αα	96%	0	0	2%
α-Thalassemia Minor (Normal to Mild Hemolytic Anemia; Microcytic, Hypochromic)				
− −/αα	90-95%	5-10%	0	0
−α/−α	90-95%	5-10%	0	0
ααCS/ααCS	85-90%	5-10%	0	6%
HBH Disease (Moderate Hemolytic Anemia with Few Transfusion Requirements; Microcytic, Hypochromic)				
− −/−α	↓	25-40%	2-40%	0
− −/−ααCS	↓	25-40%	2-40%	1.5-2.6%
Hydrops Fetalis (Lethal: Infants Stillborn or Die Within Hours of Birth; Severe Anemia)				
− −/− −	0	80% (with 20% Hb Portland)	0-20%	0

CS, Constant Spring.

inclusions. These inclusions typically are removed as the RBC passes through the spleen. Before splenectomy, only a portion of the cells have this characteristic, but after the spleen is removed, most of the RBCs are full of these inclusions. These cells often are described as golf balls or raspberries (Fig. 27-7).

Thus far, two distinct conditions have been described as being associated with Hb H disease and mental retardation: ATR-16 syndrome and ATR-X syndrome. Chromosomal rearrangements that alter the short arm of chromosome 16 (which includes the γα globin chain cluster) seem to lead to congenital abnormalities, mental retardation, and Hb H disease and have been labeled the ATR-16 syndrome.[41,43] The genes responsible for the mental retardation are not yet known. The X-linked disorder (ATR-X syndrome) is a result of mutations of the ATRX gene located on the X chromosome.[41] This ATR-X syndrome is more common than ATR-16 and is

characterized by pronounced intellectual and physical deficits. The function of the ATRX protein (the product of the ATRX gene) is not well known, but it is believed to play a role in genetic expression of various proteins that may aid in the development of RBCs.[41] An acquired Hb H disease also has been associated with marrow disorders, such as erythroleukemia, acute myelogenous leukemia, and myelodysplasia.[41]

Hydrops Fetalis
Homozygous α-thalassemia (− −/− −) results in the absence of all α chain synthesis and is incompatible with life.[3,14] The infant is born with hydrops fetalis, edema in the fetal subcutaneous tissues, in this case as a result of severe anemia. The predominant hemoglobin is Hb Bart (γ_4), along with 5% to 20% Hb Portland ($\zeta_2\gamma_2$) and traces of Hb H.[14,42] Hb Bart has high oxygen affinity; it cannot transport oxygen to the

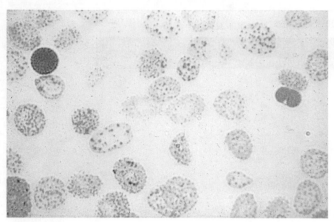

Figure 27-7 RBCs from a patient with Hb H, incubated with brilliant cresyl blue, that have acquired fine, evenly dispersed granular inclusions. (From the American Society for Hematology slide bank.)

tissues. The fetus survives until the third trimester because of Hb Portland, but this Hb cannot support the later stages of fetal growth, and the affected fetus is anoxic. The fetus is delivered prematurely and is stillborn or dies shortly after birth. In addition to anemia, edema, and ascites, the fetus has gross hepatosplenomegaly and cardiomegaly. At delivery, there is a severe microcytic, hypochromic anemia with numerous nucleated RBCs in the peripheral blood. The bone marrow cavity is expanded, and marked erythroid hyperplasia is present, as is extramedullary erythropoiesis.

Hydropic pregnancies are hazardous to the mother, resulting in toxemia and severe postpartum hemorrhage.[14] These changes are detected in mid-gestation by means of ultrasound testing.[44] If both parents carry the α-thalassemia minor gene, prenatal diagnosis of homozygosity can be made by various DNA analyses of tissues obtained from chorionic villus sampling, amniotic fluid, or cordocentesis.[14] Absence of the α globin genes establishes the diagnosis. Early termination of the pregnancy prevents serious maternal complications.

THALASSEMIA ASSOCIATED WITH STRUCTURAL HEMOGLOBIN VARIANTS

Hemoglobin S–Thalassemia

Hb S–thalassemia is a double heterozygous abnormality in which the abnormal genes for Hb S and thalassemia are co-inherited. Hb S–α-thalassemia is fairly common because the gene for Hb S and α[+] thalassemia are common in populations of African ancestry. These individuals have less Hb S than individuals with only sickle cell trait and are usually asymptomatic.[45] The clinical expression of Hb SS–α-thalassemia is milder than sickle cell anemia. There is an increased percentage of Hb F, which reduces the severity of the sickling process. The amount of Hb F is proportional to the number of α genes affected. Patients with α[0]-thalassemia have approximately 16% Hb F, and patients with α[+] have approximately 8%.[45]

Hb S–β-thalassemia results from the inheritance of a β-thalassemia gene from one parent and a Hb S gene from the other. This syndrome has been reported in the populations of Africa, the Mediterranean area, Middle East, and India.[10] The clinical expression of Hb S–β-thalassemia depends on the type of β-thalassemia mutation inherited.[46] The interaction of β[0] or β[+] thalassemia produces only a small amount of β chain, so its association with sickle hemoglobin causes a clinical syndrome similar to sickle cell anemia. Hemoglobin electrophoresis demonstrates mostly Hb S with slightly elevated Hb A₂ and variable amounts of Hb F and Hb A, depending on the specific abnormal β gene inherited. These patients typically can be distinguished from patients with sickle cell anemia by their microcytosis and splenomegaly. One parent has sickle cell trait, and the other has β-thalassemia minor.[46]

The interaction of mild β[+] thalassemia, in which β chains are produced at reduced levels, with Hb S results in a condition that may be slightly more severe than sickle cell trait. Typically there is mild hemolytic anemia with splenomegaly. These patients can be distinguished from patients with sickle cell trait by the presence of microcytosis and splenomegaly. Hemoglobin electrophoresisconfirms this condition when the quantity of Hb S exceeds Hb A. In sickle cell trait, the predominant hemoglobin is A.

The combination of β[0] thalassemia and Hb S produces a phenotype similar to sickle cell anemia with a similar incidence of stroke and life expectancy.[47] Both conditions produce severe pain crises as the predominant symptom. Typically, the microcytosis and an elevated Hb A₂ on electrophoresis distinguish sickle cell anemia from sickle–β[0] thalassemia.

Hemoglobin C–Thalassemia

β-thalassemia is also inherited with Hb C, producing moderately severe hemolysis splenomegaly, hypochromia, and microcytosis with numerous target cells. The hemoglobin electrophoresis pattern varies depending on the type of β-thalassemia gene, with higher Hb C concentrations in patients when there is minimal or no β globin production.[10]

Hemoglobin E–Thalassemia

Hb E–thalassemia is a significant concern in Southeast Asia owing to the high prevalence of both genetic mutations. Because Hb E is synthesized at a reduced rate, it clinically appears as a mild β-thalassemia. When the mutations are co-inherited there may be a marked reduction of β chain production. The clinical picture ranges from thalassemia intermedia to a transfusion-dependent condition indistinguishable from homozygous β-thalassemia.[10]

DIAGNOSIS OF THALASSEMIA

History and Physical Examination

Individual and family histories are paramount in thalassemia diagnosis. The race or ethnic background of the individual should be investigated because of the increased frequency of the various abnormal genes in certain populations. In the clinical examination, pallor indicating anemia, jaundice indicating hemolysis, splenomegaly caused by pooling of the abnormal cells, and skeletal deformities, especially in

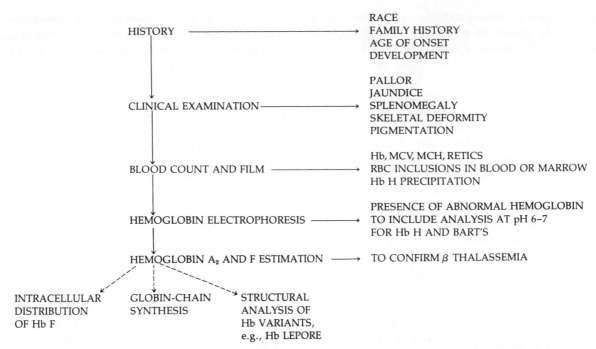

Figure 27-8 Flow chart showing the approach to the diagnosis of the thalassemia syndromes. (From Weatherall DJ: The thalassemias. In Beutler E, Lichtman MA, Coller BS, et al [eds]: Williams Hematology, 6th ed. New York: McGraw-Hill, 2001:533.)

β-thalassemia major as a result of expansion of the bone marrow cavities, are findings that suggest thalassemia (Fig. 27-8).[10]

Laboratory Findings
Complete Blood Count

Most thalassemias are microcytic and hypochromic. The hemoglobin and hematocrit are decreased, but the RBC count is disproportionately high relative to the degree of anemia, generating a very low MCV. The MCHC is slightly decreased. In untreated thalassemia major, the RDW is elevated, reflecting anisocytosis. A normal RDW differentiates thalassemia minor from iron deficiency anemia, which has an elevated RDW, a less-striking MCV and a decreased RBC count.

On a Wright-stained smear, the RBCs are typically microcytic and hypochromic except in the silent carrier phenotype, in which the RBCs appear normal. In heterozygous β-thalassemia and Hb H disease, the cells are microcytic with slight-to-moderate poikilocytosis. In heterozygous α^0 thalassemia, there is mild hypochromia and microcytosis but less poikilocytosis. In homozygous and double heterozygous β-thalassemia, extreme poikilocytosis may be present, including target cells, elliptocytes, polychromasia, basophilic stippling, and nucleated RBCs.

Reticulocyte Count

The reticulocyte count is elevated, indicating that the bone marrow is responding to a hemolytic process. In Hb H disease, the typical reticulocyte count is 5%.[10] In homozygous β-thalassemia, it is 2% to 8%, disproportionately low relative to the degree of anemia. An inadequate reticulocytosis reflects ineffective erythropoiesis.[3]

Bone Marrow

The bone marrow in untreated homozygous β-thalassemia is hypercellular with extreme erythroid hyperplasia. Extramedullary hematopoiesis is prominent. Hb H disease shows less bone marrow erythroid hyperplasia. The heterozygous thalassemias have only slight erythroid hyperplasia.

Osmotic Fragility

The microcytic, hypochromic RBCs of the thalassemias have a decreased osmotic fragility. This trait has been used to screen for the thalassemia carrier state in populations in which thalassemia is common and has been found to have an excellent negative predictive value (>99%).[48] Because iron deficiency also has decreased osmotic fragility, the test does not differentiate between these two conditions. Other tests requiring lysis of RBCs, such as urine chemical strip analysis for hemoglobin, can be affected by the diminished osmotic lysis of the thalassemia.

Supravital Stain

In α-thalassemia trait, Hb H disease, and silent α-thalassemia, the brilliant cresyl or new methylene blue test may be used to induce precipitation of the intrinsically unstable Hb H.[49] Hb H inclusions (denatured β globin chains) typically appear as small, multiple, irregularly shaped, greenish-blue bodies with a pitted pattern similar to that of a golf ball or a raspberry (see Fig. 27-7). They uniformly distribute throughout the RBC. In Hb H disease, almost all RBCs contain these inclusions. In α-thalassemia trait, only a few cells may contain these inclusions, and in silent carrier α-thalassemia, only a rare cell does. These inclusions appear different from Heinz bodies, which are larger and fewer in number and most often appear eccentrically along the membrane of the RBC. This test can be sensitive in detecting Hb H in α-thalassemias.[49]

Electrophoresis

Hemoglobin electrophoresis on cellulose acetate at alkaline pH classically has been the major diagnostic tool used to detect and identify thalassemia. This technique is able to differentiate hemoglobin variants, such as Hb E and Hb Lepore,[51] and is able to distinguish the fast-moving Hb H and Hb Bart.[52] Electrophoresis is used to screen for elevated Hb A$_2$ associated with β-thalassemia trait, although specific tests for Hb A$_2$ quantitation may be more accurate.[51] Increased Hb F can be detected on electrophoresis, which is important in δβ-thalassemia, HPFH, and other β-thalassemia variants (Fig. 27-9). Hb F should be quantitated by other methods. Citrate agar gel electrophoresis performed at an acid pH differentiates between Hb E and Hb C.[50] Emerging technologies such as isoelectric focusing and high-performance liquid chromatography may expand upon or replace hemoglobin electrophoresis.[50]

Hemoglobin A$_2$ and Hemoglobin F Estimation

Quantitation of Hemoglobin A$_2$. Hb A$_2$ is separated by column from other hemoglobins and measured. Several techniques are available to quantitate Hb A$_2$, but automated HPLC is most commonly used.[51] HPLC may be used to simultaneously measure Hb F. This technique is unable to differentiate Hb E from Hb A$_2$, however, so its use is limited when Hb E is present.[51] The accuracy of HPLC is diminished in sickle cell trait, iron deficiency, or α-thalassemia because Hb A$_2$ can be slightly elevated in association with sickle cell trait and decreased in iron deficiency or α-thalassemia.[53] Micro-column chromatography may be more accurate in these cases, but HPLC still can be used effectively if combined with the RBC indices.[51]

Quantitation of Hemoglobin F. Elevated Hb F is present in homozygous β^0 thalassemia, β$^+$ thalassemia, δβ-thalassemia, Hb Lepore, and HPFH. A moderate or slight elevation is seen in β-thalassemia minor.

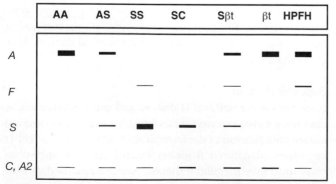

	AA	AS	SS	SC	Sβt	βt	HPFH
A	▬	▬			▬	▬	▬
F			—		—		—
S		—	▬	▬	—		
C, A2	—	—	—	—	—	—	—

Figure 27-9 Relative electrophoretic mobilities on cellulose acetate (pH 8.4) of various hemoglobins that are important in the diagnosis of thalassemia syndromes and hemoglobinopathies. AA, normal Hb; AS, sickle cell trait; SS, sickle cell disease; SC, hemoglobin SC disease; Sβ, sickle/β-thalassemia; βt, β-thalassemia; HPTH, hereditary persistence of fetal hemoglobin. Hb H migrates faster than Hb A.

The classic *alkali denaturation* test is accurate and precise for the quantitation of Hb F in the 0.2% to 50% range.[51] Most hemoglobins are denatured on exposure to strong alkali, but Hb F is not. The Hb F can be separated and its concentration compared with the other hemoglobins. Consistent methodology is required to ensure accurate results.[51] As with Hb A$_2$ quantitation, HPLC is now often used for quantitative measurement of Hb F.

In the acid elution (Kleihauer-Betke) slide test, blood films are immersed in an acid buffer. Adult hemoglobin is eluted from the RBCs, whereas fetal hemoglobin resists acid elution and remains in the cell. When subsequently stained, Hb F RBCs take up the stain, whereas RBCs containing only adult hemoglobin appear as "ghosts."[54] Although this test is fairly accurate, it can be cumbersome to perform. Finally flow cytometry may become the standard test to measure Hb F levels.[55]

Other Special Procedures

Other special procedures, such as mass spectrometry and DNA analysis, can be used to identify specific genotypes for research purposes, to differentiate an α-thalassemia carrier from an αβ-thalassemia carrier, to identify a silent carrier gene, or to examine for family inheritance patterns with multiple genes. This further testing is done in reference or tertiary care laboratories.

Mass Spectrometry. Using whole blood, mass spectrometry assesses the difference in mass of the globin chains, which detects single amino acid substitutions in the globin chain. This technique typically is used in conjunction with electrophoresis to identify variant hemoglobin molecules.[51]

DNA Analysis. Molecular techniques identify globin gene mutations.[39,50] With these detailed analyses, gene frequency and geographic distribution now can be determined. Current methods include polymerase chain reaction, real-time polymerase chain reaction, and signal amplification systems.[39] Many new and rare mutations have been identified. Molecular techniques are used in difficult-to-diagnose cases and, more importantly, for genetic counseling purposes. They also can be used in antenatal diagnosis, especially if the parents' genetic mutations are known.[39]

Indirect Serum Bilirubin. An increased indirect bilirubin level is present in thalassemias, confirming the hemolytic component. Increase is mild in trait but moderate in thalassemia intermedia and Hb H disease. Thalassemia major also shows bilirubinemia; however, the elevation is mild because of the inability to produce hemoglobin.

DIFFERENTIAL DIAGNOSIS OF THALASSEMIA AND IRON DEFICIENCY ANEMIA

Heterozygous thalassemias are microcytic and hypochromic and must be differentiated from iron deficiency and other microcytic, hypochromic anemias. The differential diagnosis for microcytic, hypochromic anemias is relatively limited (see

Table 19-1). Differentiating thalassemia and iron deficiency is important to avoid unnecessary tests or treatments. Assuming iron deficiency may lead to inappropriate iron therapy or to unnecessary diagnostic procedures such as colonoscopy to identify a source of blood loss.

Clinical history is crucial. A family history of thalassemia raises the suspicion for this diagnosis. A history of previously normal hemoglobin and RBC indices, of significant bleeding, or of pica would lead to the diagnosis of iron deficiency.[57] *Pica* means cravings for nonfood items such as clay, dirt, or starch in iron deficiency. The most common pica symptom in the United States is pagophagia, the craving to chew on ice.[56]

A mild erythrocytosis (high RBC count) and marked microcytosis (low MCV) are characteristic of thalassemia trait. The RBC count usually is decreased in patients with iron deficiency. The MCV may be normal or decreased depending on whether the iron deficiency is developing or long-standing but is usually not as decreased as in thalassemia.[58] The RDW is normal in thalassemia minor and elevated in iron deficiency anemia. The Mentzer index may be used; it is determined by dividing the MCV by the RBC.[58] Values greater than 14 indicate iron deficiency, whereas values less than 12 are more indicative of thalassemia trait. Although this index may be useful, its sensitivity is only 80% to 90% and may be even lower in pregnant women, children, or individuals with α-thalassemias and β-thalassemias.[31]

The peripheral blood film demonstrates basophilic stippling and target cells in thalassemia but not in iron deficiency. Iron deficiency is determined using serum iron, total iron-binding capacity, transferrin saturation, serum ferritin, soluble transferrin receptor, and zinc protoporphyrin levels (Chapter 19).[57]

Before evaluating for thalassemia, iron deficiency should be ruled out. Low iron levels in patients with β-thalassemia minor lower the Hb A_2 levels. The iron stores need to be replenished before embarking on the laboratory analysis for thalassemia.

CHAPTER at a GLANCE

- Thalassemias are a group of heterogeneous disorders in which one or more globin chains are reduced or absent.
- Thalassemias result in a hypochromic, microcytic anemia caused by decreased production of hemoglobin.
- The imbalance of globin chain synthesis causes an excess of the normally produced globin chain, which damages the RBCs or their precursors, resulting in hemolysis.
- $β^0$ refers to a thalassemic gene that produces no β chains.
- $β^+$ refers to a thalassemic gene that produces reduced amounts of β chains.
- β-thalassemia is clinically manifested as a silent carrier, thalassemia minor, thalassemia intermedia, or thalassemia major.
- The silent carrier state is caused by a mutated gene that produces a small decrease in β chains. The blood picture is completely normal in the silent carrier heterozygous state.
- Heterozygous β-thalassemia minor, a mild, asymptomatic, microcytic, hypochromic anemia, usually has an elevated Hb A_2 level, which aids in diagnosis.
- Homozygous β-thalassemia major is a severe, transfusion-dependent anemia.
- β-thalassemia intermedia manifests with abnormalities whose level of severity is between those of β-thalassemia major and β-thalassemia minor.
- Hb Lepore, hereditary persistence of fetal hemoglobin, and δβ-thalassemia are other thalassemia syndromes involving the β globin cluster on chromosome 11.
- The α-thalassemias usually are caused by a deletion of one or both of the α genes on chromosome 16, resulting in reduced or absent production of α chains.

- In α-thalassemias, tetramers of γ chains may precipitate as Hb Bart.
- Tetramers of β chains may precipitate as Hb H.
- α-thalassemias are divided clinically into silent carrier, α-thalassemia trait, Hb H disease, and hydrops fetalis.
- α-thalassemia's silent carrier status is the result of the deletion of one of four α genes (–α/αα) it has a normal RBC profile and is totally asymptomatic.
- α-thalassemia trait is the result of the deletion of two α genes—(–α/–α) or (– –/αα)—and is clinically similar to β-thalassemia minor except with no increase in Hb A_2.
- Hb H disease is the result of the deletion of three of the four α genes (– –/–α), which causes excess β chains that precipitate, causing a hemolytic anemia. The blood picture is microcytic, hypochromic, and the disease is clinically similar to β-thalassemia intermedia.
- Hydrops fetalis, in which all four of the α genes are deleted (– –/– –), is incompatible with life.
- The diagnosis of thalassemia is made from the RBC morphology, hemoglobin electrophoresis, supravital stain, and Hb A_2 and Hb F quantitation.
- Thalassemia must be differentiated from other microcytic, hypochromic anemias, especially iron deficiency anemia. Iron studies are important for this differentiation.

Now that you have completed this chapter, go back and read again the case study at the beginning and respond to the questions presented.

REVIEW QUESTIONS

1. The thalassemias are caused by:
   a. Structurally abnormal hemoglobins
   b. Absent or defective synthesis of a polypeptide chain in hemoglobin
   c. Excessive absorption of iron
   d. Abnormal or defective synthesis of porphyrin synthesis

2. Thalassemia is more prevalent in individuals from areas along the tropics because it confers:
   a. Heat resistance to those heterozygous for the thalassemia gene
   b. Selective advantage against tuberculosis
   c. Selective advantage against malaria
   d. Resistance to mosquito bites

3. The hemolytic anemia associated with the thalassemias is due to:
   a. Imbalance of globin chain synthesis
   b. Microcytic, hypochromic cells
   c. Ineffective erythropoiesis owing to immune factors
   d. Abnormal hemoglobin

4. β-thalassemia minor (heterozygous) usually has:
   a. Increased Hb Constant Spring
   b. 50% Hb F
   c. No Hb A
   d. Increased Hb A_2

5. The RBC morphology in β-thalassemia would most likely include:
   a. Microcytic cells, hypochromic cells, target cells, stippled cells
   b. Macrocytic cells, ovalocytes, target cells, stippled cells
   c. Microcytic cells, target cells, sickle cells
   d. Macrocytic cells, hypochromic cells, target cells, stippled cells

6. The major Hb present on electrophoresis in β-thalassemia major is Hb:
   a. A
   b. A_2
   c. F
   d. C

7. Heterozygous hereditary persistence of fetal hemoglobin (HPFH) has:
   a. 15% to 30% of Hb F with normal RBC morphology
   b. 100% Hb F with slightly hypochromic, microcytic cells
   c. A decreased amount of Hb F with normal RBC morphology
   d. 5% to 15% Hb F with hypochromic, macrocytic cells

8. Hb H is composed of:
   a. Two α and two β chains
   b. Two ε and two γ chains
   c. Four β chains
   d. Four γ chains

9. Hb Bart is composed of:
   a. Two α and two β chains
   b. Two ε and two γ chains
   c. Four β chains
   d. Four γ chains

10. When one α gene is missing ($\alpha-/\alpha\alpha$), a patient has:
    a. Normal Hb
    b. Mild anemia (Hb range 9-11 g/dL)
    c. Moderate anemia (Hb range 7-9 g/dL)
    d. Marked anemia requiring regular transfusions

11. In which part of the world is hydrops fetalis ($--/--$) most common?
    a. Northern Africa
    b. Mediterranean
    c. Middle East
    d. Southeast Asia

12. The condition of Hb S–β-thalassemia has a clinical course that resembles:
    a. Sickle cell trait
    b. Sickle cell anemia
    c. β-Thalassemia minor
    d. β-Thalassemia major

13. Hb H inclusions in supravital stain appear as:
    a. A few large, blue, round bodies in the RBCs with aggregated reticulum
    b. Uniformly stained blue cytoplasm in the RBC
    c. Small, multiple, irregularly shaped, greenish-blue bodies that resemble golf balls
    d. Uniform round bodies that adhere to the RBC membrane

14. Which of the following laboratory values is *inconsistent* with thalassemia?
    a. A high RBC count and marked microcytosis (low MCV)
    b. Target cells and basophilic stippling on the peripheral smear
    c. The transferrin saturation and the serum ferritin are normal to increased.
    d. Elevated MCHC consistent with spherocytic RBCs

15. A 5-month-old infant of Asian heritage is seen for a well-baby check. Because of pallor, the physician suspects anemia and orders a complete blood count and iron studies. The results indicate Hb of 100 g/L (10 g/dL) with microcytosis, hypochromia, poikilocytosis, and mild polychromasia. The physician performs a rough Mentzer calculation in her head with a result of 17. These findings lead the physician to suspect:
    a. β-thalassemia major
    b. α-thalassmia silent carrier
    c. Iron deficiency anemia
    d. Homozygous α-thalassmia ($--/--$)

ACKNOWLEDGMENT

The foundation for this chapter is based on the work of Martha Payne. The author expresses his gratitude for the opportunity to amend her fine endeavor.

REFERENCES

1. Cooley TB, Lee P: A series of cases of splenomegaly in children with anemia and peculiar bone changes. Trans Am Pediatr Soc 1925;37:29-30.
2. Lichtman MA, Spivak JL, Boxer LA, et al: Hematology: Landmark Papers of the Twentieth Century. San Diego: Academic Press, 2000.
3. Forget BG, Cohen AR: Thalassemia syndromes. In Hoffman R, Benz EJ Jr, Shattil SJ, et al (eds): Hematology: Basic Principles and Practice, 4th ed. Philadelphia: Churchill Livingstone, 2005:557-589.
4. Angastiniotis M, Modell B: Global epidemiology of hemoglobin disorders, Ann N Y Acad Sci 1998;850:251-269.
5. Weatherall DJ, Clegg JB: Inherited haemoglobin disorders: an increasing global health problem. Bull World Health Organ 2001;79:704-712.
6. Mockenhaupt FP, Ehrhardt S, Gellert S, et al: Alpha(+)-thalassemia protects African children from severe malaria. Blood 2004;104:2003-2006.
7. Williams TN, Wambua S, Uyoga S, et al: Both heterozygous and homozygous α+ thalassemia protect against severe and fatal *Plasmodium falciparum* malaria on the coast of Kenya. Blood 2005; 106:368-371.
8. Pattanapanyasat K, Yongvanitchit K, Tongtawe P, et al: Impairment of *Plasmodium falciparum* growth in thalassemic red blood cells: further evidence by using biotin labeling and flow cytometry. Blood 1999;93:3116-3119.
9. Ayi K, Turrini F, Piga A, et al: Enhanced phagocytosis of ring-parasitized mutant erythrocytes: a common mechanism that may explain protection against falciparum malaria in sickle trait and beta-thalassemia trait. Blood 2004;104:3364-3371.
10. Weatherall DJ: The thalassemias. In Beutler E, Lichtman MA, Coller BS, et al (eds): Williams Hematology, 6th ed. St Louis: McGraw-Hill, 2001:547-580.
11. Steinberg MH, Benz EJ Jr, Adewoye HA, et al: Pathobiology of the human erythrocyte and its hemoglobins. In Hoffman R, Benz EJ Jr, Shattil SJ, et al (eds): Hematology: Basic Principles and Practice, 4th ed. Philadelphia: Churchill Livingstone, 2005:442-454.
12. Harju S, McQuenn KJ, Peterson KR: Chromatin structure and control of beta-like globin gene switching. Exp Biol Med 2002;227:683-700.
13. Galanello R, Cao A: Relationship between genotype and phenotype: thalassemia intermedia. Ann N Y Acad Sci 1998;850:325-333.
14. Chui DHK, Waye JS: Hydrops fetalis caused by α-thalassemia: an emerging health care problem. Blood 1998;91:2213-2222.
15. Thein SL: Genetic insights into the clinical diversity of beta thalassaemia. Br J Haematol 2004;124:264-274.
16. Huisman THJ, Carver MFH, Baysal E: A Syllabus of Thalassemia Mutations. Augusta, Ga.: The Sickle Cell Anemia Foundation, 1997.
17. Thein SL, Kazazian HH Jr, Orkin SH, et al: Molecular characterization of seven beta-thalassemia mutations in Asian Indians. EMBO J 1984;3:593-596.
18. Murru S, Loudianos G, Deiana M, et al: Molecular characterization of beta-thalassemia intermedia in patients of Italian descent and identification of three novel beta-thalassemia mutations. Blood 1991;77:1342-1347.
19. Gasperini D, Perseu L, Melis MA, et al: Heterozygous beta-thalassemia with thalassemia intermedia phenotype. Am J Hematol 1998;57:43-47.
20. Gilman JG, Huisman TH, Abels J: Dutch beta 0-thalassaemia: a 10 kilobase DNA deletion associated with significant gamma-chain production. Br J Haematol 1984;56:339-348.
21. Oggiano L, Pirastu M, Moi P, et al. Molecular characterization of a normal Hb A2 beta-thalassaemia determinant in a Sardinian family. Br J Haematol 1987;67:225-229.
22. Fosburg MT, Nathan DG: Treatment of Cooley's anemia. Blood 1990;76:435-444.
23. Dover GJ, Valle D: Therapy for beta-thalassemia—a paradigm for the treatment of genetic disorders. N Engl J Med 1994;331:609-610.
24. Olivieri NF, Nathan DG, MacMillan JH, et al: Survival in medically treated patients with homozygous beta-thalassemia. N Engl J Med 1994;331:574-578.
25. Lawson SE, Roberts IA, Amrolia P, et al: Bone marrow transplantation for beta-thalassaemia major: the UK experience in two paediatric centres. Br J Haematol 2003;120:289-295.
26. Mentzer WC, Cowan MJ: Bone marrow transplantation for beta-thalassemia: the University of California San Francisco experience. J Pediatr Hematol Oncol 2000;22:598-601.
27. Giardini C, Lucarelli G: Bone marrow transplantation for beta-thalassemia. Hematol Oncol Clin N Am 1999;13:1059-1064.
28. Bradai M, Abad MT, Pissard S, et al: Hydroxyurea can eliminate transfusion requirements in children with severe beta-thalassemia. Blood 2003;102:1529-1530.
29. Choudhry VP, Lal A, Pati HP, et al: Hematological responses to hydroxyurea therapy in multitransfused thalassemic children. Indian J Pediatr 1997;64:395-398.
30. Puthenveetil G, Scholes J, Carbonell D, et al: Successful correction of the human beta-thalassemia major phenotype using a lentiviral vector. Blood 2004;104:3445-3453.
31. Borgna-Pignatti C, Galanello R: Thalassemias and related disorders: quantitative disorders of hemoglobin synthesis. In Greer JP, Foerster J, Lukens JN, et al (eds): Wintrobe's Clinical Hematology, 11th ed. Philadelphia: Lippincott, Williams & Wilkins, 2004:1319-1366.
32. Galanello R, Dessi E, Melis MA, et al: Molecular analysis of beta zero-thalassemia intermedia in Sardinia. Blood 1989;74:823-827.
33. Oron V, Filon D, Oppenheim A, et al: Severe thalassaemia intermedia caused by interaction of homozygosity for alpha-globin gene triplication with heterozygosity for beta zero-thalassaemia. Br J Haematol 1994;86:377-379.
34. Cazzola M, Beguin Y, Bergamaschi G, et al: Soluble transferrin receptor as a potential determinant of iron loading in congenital anaemias due to ineffective erythropoiesis. Br J Haematol 1999;106:752-755.
35. Kan YW, Forget BG, Nathan DG: Gamma-beta thalassemia: a cause of hemolytic disease of the newborn. N Engl J Med 1972;286:129-134.
36. Bollekens JA, Forget BG: Delta beta thalassemia and hereditary persistence of fetal hemoglobin. Hematol Oncol Clin N Am 1991;5:399-422.
37. Craig JE, Barnetson RA, Prior J, et al: Rapid detection of deletions causing delta beta thalassemia and hereditary persistence of fetal hemoglobin by enzymatic amplification. Blood 1994;83:1673-1682.
38. Tuan D, Feingold E, Newman M, et al: Different 3' end points of deletions causing delta beta-thalassemia and hereditary persistence of fetal hemoglobin: implications for the control of gamma-globin gene expression in man. Proc Natl Acad Sci U S A 1983;80:6937-6941.
39. Old JM: Screening and genetic diagnosis of haemoglobin disorders. Blood Rev 2003;17:43-53.
40. Higgs DR, Vickers MA, Wilkie AO, et al: A review of the molecular genetics of the human alpha-globin gene cluster. Blood 1989;73:1081-1104.
41. Chui DH, Fucharoen S, Chan V: Hemoglobin H disease: not necessarily a benign disorder. Blood 2003;101:791-800.
42. Weatherall DJ: The thalassemias. In Stamatoyannopoulos G, Majerus PW, Perlmutter RM, et al (eds): The Molecular Basis of Blood Diseases, 3rd ed. Philadelphia: Saunders, 2001:183-226.

43. Wilkie AO, Zeitlin HC, Lindenbaum RH, et al: Clinical features and molecular analysis of the alpha thalassemia/mental retardation syndromes: II. Cases without detectable abnormality of the alpha globin complex. Am J Hum Genet 1990;46:1127-1140.

44. Ko TM, Tseng LH, Hsu PM, et al: Ultrasonographic scanning of placental thickness and the prenatal diagnosis of homozygous alpha-thalassaemia 1 in the second trimester. Prenat Diagn 1995;15:7-10.

45. Steinberg MH, Rosenstock W, Coleman MB, et al: Effects of thalassemia and microcytosis on the hematologic and vaso-occlusive severity of sickle cell anemia. Blood 1984;63:1353-1360.

46. Saunthararajah Y, Vichinsky E, Embury SH: Sickle cell disease. In Hoffman R, Benz EJ Jr, Shattil SJ, et al (eds): Hematology: Basic Principles and Practice, 4th ed. Philadelphia: Churchill Livingstone, 2005:605-644.

47. Quinn CT, Rogers ZR, Buchanan GR: Survival of children with sickle cell disease. Blood 2004;103:4023-4027.

48. Sirichotiyakul S, Tantipalakorn C, Sanguansermsri T, et al: Erythrocyte osmotic fragility test for screening of alpha-thalassemia-1 and beta-thalassemia trait in pregnancy. Int J Gynaecol Obstet 2004;86:347-350.

49. Pan LL, Eng HL, Kuo CY, et al: Usefulness of brilliant cresyl blue staining as an auxiliary method of screening for alpha-thalassemia. J Lab Clin Med 2005;145:94-97.

50. Chui DHK, Steinberg MH: Laboratory diagnosis of hemoglobinopathies and thalassemias. In Hoffman R, Benz EJ Jr, Shattil SJ, et al (eds): Hematology: Basic Principles and Practice, 4th ed. Philadelphia: Churchill Livingstone, 2005:2687-2695.

51. Wild BJ, Bain BJ: Detection and quantitation of normal and variant haemoglobins: an analytical review. Ann Clin Biochem 2004;41:355-369.

52. Perkins S: Disorders of hemoglobin synthesis. In Kjeldsberg CR (ed): Practical Diagnosis of Hematologic Disorders, 3rd ed. Chicago: ASCP Press, 2000:146-169.

53. Head CE, Conroy M, Jarvis M, et al: Some observations on the measurement of haemoglobin A2 and S percentages by high performance liquid chromatography in the presence and absence of thalassaemia. J Clin Pathol 2004;57:276-280.

54. Pelikan DM, Mesker WE, Scherjon SA, et al: Improvement of the Kleihauer-Betke test by automated detection of fetal erythrocytes in maternal blood. Cytometry B Clin Cytom 2003;54:1-9.

55. Mundee Y, Bigelow NC, Davis BH, et al: Simplified flow cytometric method for fetal hemoglobin containing red blood cells. Cytometry 2000;42:389-393.

56. Brittenham GM: Disorders of iron metabolism: iron deficiency and overload. In Hoffman R, Benz EJ Jr, Shattil SJ, et al (eds): Hematology: Basic Principles and Practice, 4th ed. Philadelphia: Churchill Livingstone, 2005:481-498.

57. Cook JD: Diagnosis and management of iron-deficiency anaemia. Best Pract Res Clin Haematol 2005;18:319-332.

58. Glader B: Anemia: general considerations. In Greer JP, Foerster J, Lukens JN, et al (eds): Wintrobe's Clinical Hematology, 11th ed. Philadelphia: Lippincott, Williams & Wilkins; 2004:947-978.

Morphologic and Distributive Leukocyte Disorders

28

Susan J. Leclair

OUTLINE

Distributive Leukocyte
  Disorders
Morphologic Alterations
  of Leukocytes

OBJECTIVES

After completion of this chapter, the reader will be able to:

1. Define relative and absolute leukocyte counts.
2. Use proper terminology for variations in the number of each type of leukocyte.
3. Compare leukocyte values with reference ranges to recognize deviations from normal numbers.
4. Calculate absolute values of types of leukocytes.
5. Discuss physiologic factors that affect numbers of circulating leukocytes and explain the cause of the change.
6. Differentiate leukemoid and leukoerythroblastic reactions when given test results.
7. Correlate peripheral blood leukocyte numbers and types with possible causes.
8. Compare and contrast nonmalignant changes in granulocytes, using criteria such as mechanism of formation, cellular location, potential cellular dysfunction, and clinical significance.
9. Recognize descriptions of the nonmalignant changes seen in leukocytes.
10. Explain the biochemical or ultrastructural origins (if known) for each of the changes seen in granulocytes.
11. Correlate the presence of nonmalignant granulocytic changes with possible diagnoses or prognoses.
12. List the nonmalignant morphologic changes observed in monocytes and macrophages.
13. Correlate the presence of nonmalignant lymphocytic changes with possible diagnoses or prognoses.
14. Compare and contrast nonmalignant changes in lymphocytes, using criteria such as mechanism of formation, cellular location, potential cellular dysfunction, and clinical significance.
15. Explain the biochemical or ultrastructural origins (if known) for each of the morphologic changes seen in lymphocytes.

CASE STUDIES

After studying the material in this chapter, the reader should be able to respond to the following case studies:

Case 1

A patient with colon cancer had an admitting complete blood count (CBC) that included a white blood cell (WBC) count of 25×10^9/L and a differential of 70% polymorphonuclear cells, 10% bands, 5% metamyelocytes, 10% lymphocytes, and 5% monocytes. Two nucleated red blood cells were seen in the 100-cell differential. Appropriate oncologic therapy was instituted, and 48 hours later, the WBC count decreased to 2.1×10^9/L with 35% polymorphonuclear cells, 55% lymphocytes, and 10% monocytes. Forty-eight hours later, the WBC count had decreased to 0.9×10^9/L with a similar differential. Granulocyte-macrophage colony-stimulating factor (GM-CSF) was administered. On the fifth day after the infusion of GM-CSF, the WBC count increased to 3.4×10^9/L with a differential of 45% polymorphonuclear cells, 5% bands, 42% lymphocytes, and 8% monocytes.

1. What was the interpretation of the first CBC?
2. When the WBC count decreased to less than 1×10^9/L, what possible outcome became a serious concern?
3. Why was GM-CSF used?
4. Which cells were most affected by the chemotherapy and the GM-CSF? Explain.

Continued

DISTRIBUTIVE LEUKOCYTE DISORDERS

The absolute peripheral blood count for each leukocyte (white blood cell, WBC) category has clinical significance. Reference values for WBC counts are established for each population. Although pediatric values have been well established for some time, the need for geriatric reference ranges is growing as life expectancy increases.[1] Absolute WBC counts are more informative than relative percentages when determining whether there is a significant increase or decrease in a cell type. Profiling instruments provide both relative and absolute values (total number per 10^9/L). The absolute value also may be determined manually by multiplying the total WBC count by the relative value, as follows: 10×10^9/L (WBC) $\times$ 0.40 (percentage of neutrophils) = 4×10^9/L. Manual computation does not match instrument accuracy.

Reference Range

The total circulating WBC count is 4.5 to 11.5×10^9/L. Elevations *(leukocytosis)* and decreases *(leukopenia)* provide only part of the hematologic picture. Determining which type of WBC is affected provides more definitive information. Because neutrophils normally constitute the largest adult percentage of WBCs, variations have the greatest impact on the total WBC count. The WBC counts of neonates are higher than in adults but decrease within days after birth (see table on inside cover). Although the high end of the accepted range is higher for children than adults, the range gradually narrows until adolescence, at which time a relatively steady WBC count is maintained. Elderly patients may have lower WBC counts (Chapter 38). Counts in African Americans may be slightly lower than in Caucasians, primarily as a result of lower concentrations of neutrophils, but not all studies have confirmed this.[2]

Granulocyte kinetics are influenced by input from the bone marrow, changes in the proportion of marginating to circulating pools, and changes caused by disease. Transient elevated counts may be seen when granulocytes leave the marginating pool, increasing the circulating pool. Transiently decreased peripheral blood WBC counts may be seen when granulocytes move to the marginating or storage pool. The causes of leukocytosis and leukopenia are many, and in view of the dynamic interactions that are required for WBC number, it is not surprising that many of the causes of leukocytosis are also the causes of leukopenia.

Alterations in Granulocyte Count and Maturity

Neutrophilia is an absolute count of neutrophils greater than 8.6×10^9/L. This is often accompanied by bone marrow myelocytic hyperplasia. Benign neutrophilia occurs in stress, tachycardia, fever, labor, strenuous exercise, and epinephrine and cortisone therapy.

Pathologic causes of neutrophilia include inflammatory states (e.g., acute infection, trauma, diabetes mellitus), intoxications (e.g. uremia), acute hemorrhage, hemolysis, and malignancy.[3] In malignancy, the term *leukoerythroblastic* is often used because of the presence of nucleated RBCs. The most dramatic neutrophilia is a *leukemoid reaction*. This is a WBC count greater than 50×10^9/L and may be considered an exaggerated response to an infection. To differentiate a leukemoid reaction from chronic myelogenous leukemia (CML), the laboratory professional performs the leukocyte alkaline phosphatase stain, which is markedly decreased in CML (Chapter 30). The term *left shift* is sometimes used to describe an increased immature granulocyte count (see Chapter 15).

Neutropenia is an absolute count less than 2.3×10^9/L neutrophils. If input from the bone marrow functional storage pool fails to satisfy tissue demand, fewer neutrophils reach the peripheral blood. These cells may be less mature as depletion of the functional storage pool forces cells from the maturation pool to enter the bloodstream. Transient neutropenia can be seen after exposure to certain medications, such as tranquilizers, sedatives, or antimicrobial agents, and procedures such as hemodialysis.

In *cyclic neutropenia* the peripheral blood neutrophil count oscillates with a 21-day periodicity.[5] This may reflect autosomal dominant mutations in the *ELA2* gene that encodes for neutrophil elastase.[4] The nadir may reach zero, rendering the patient susceptible to infection. Other, more rare cyclic neutropenias include Kostmann neutropenia (severe congenital neutropenia)[6] and Hermansky-Pudlak syndrome.[7]

Neutropenia with fully mature granulocytes arises from vitamin B_{12} or folate deficiency, ingestion of medications, and Job syndrome, all suppressing the mitotic pool.[8] Myelocytic suppression is also seen with antimicrobials and calcium channel blockers. Neutropenia with mature granulocytes is associated with increased morbidity and mortality.[9]

In rare immune neutropenia, neutrophils are destroyed in the spleen or portal circulation as a result of autoantibodies. Autoantibodies can be detected by agglutination assays, immunofluorescence, or enzyme immunoassays.[10] Alloimmunization may occur at birth as a result of the passage of maternal antibodies to the fetus via the placenta. Autoantibodies to neutrophils arise following childhood infection, as a complication of systemic lupus erythematosus, and in Felty syndrome in conjunction with rheumatoid arthritis. More than five antibodies have been detected and identified.[11] Although immune neutropenia is not associated with high rates of mortality, the frequency of infections is a concern.

Autoinfection (infection by an agent present in the body) becomes a possibility when the neutrophil count is less than 1×10^9/L and is almost a certainty with a count less than 0.5×10^9/L. The absolute neutrophil count is monitored closely in patients who are receiving chemotherapy or who have received a stem cell transplant to determine whether it is appropriate to give scheduled chemotherapy, continue with granulocyte-macrophage colony-stimulating factor, or initiate or maintain protective isolation measures. Causes of neutrophilia and neutropenia are summarized in Table 28-1.

In neutrophilia and neutropenia, laboratory professionals enumerate peripheral blood immature forms: bands, metamyelocytes, and myelocytes. Neutrophilia with predominantly mature forms may have a better prognosis than with immature forms. Immaturity implies a diminution of storage pools and maturation pool stress. The *morphology* of neutrophils is also recorded. The discussion of cytoplasmic abnormalities such as Döhle bodies, toxic granulation, degranulated areas, and vacuoles is considered in detail later in this chapter. It is important to list them here, however, because qualitative changes reflect a poorer prognosis.

Alterations in Eosinophil Count

Eosinophilia ($>0.5 \times 10^9$/L) is common in allergic responses and dermatitis, parasitic infections. some autoimmune disorders, and some malignancies.[12] Numbers of eosinophils may be reduced in response to adrenocorticotropic hormone.

Alterations in Basophil Count

Basophilia ($>0.15 \times 10^9$/L) is seen in patients with hypoactive thyroid conditions, ulcerative colitis, some types of nephrosis, and certain malignancies, including chronic myelogenous leukemia.[13] Since the number of basophils is so low, basopenia is hard to assess.

Alterations in Monocyte/Macrophage Count

Monocytosis ($>0.8 \times 10^9$/L) indicates strenuous exercise, active tuberculosis, subacute bacterial endocarditis, syphilis, parasitic and rickettsial infections, certain autoimmune diseases, and trauma.[14] Monocytes also are increased during recovery from acute infections. Monocytopenia may be seen after glucocorticoid administration.[13]

Alterations in Lymphocyte Count

Lymphocyte count reference intervals vary by age (see chart on inside cover).[10] The count is higher in children and ranges up to 70%, or 2 to 7×10^9/L. Lymphocytosis is considered to be present in an adult when the absolute lymphocyte count is greater than 5.5×10^9/L.

Lymphocytosis is seen in patients with exanthems (skin rashes) from certain viral diseases such as measles and mumps, in thyrotoxicosis, and in patients recovering from certain acute infections (Box 28-1). Lymphocytosis is rare in children with bacterial infection. The exception, *Bordetella pertussis* infection, causes a significant elevation in small lymphocytes.[15] More common in viral infections, lymphocytosis is seen with hepatitis A, infectious mononucleosis, and infectious lymphocytosis. It also is seen in cases of congenital and secondary-stage syphilis and brucellosis.

Lymphopenia ($<0.6 \times 10^9$/L) is seen in heart failure, uremia, systemic lupus erythematosus, and malaria.[16] It is associated with a leukoerythroblastic picture and, in the elderly, with bone marrow depletion. It is also seen in infectious hepatitis, certain types of Hodgkin lymphoma and other malignancies, active tuberculosis, and endocrine disorders. Other conditions are post–stem cell transplant, human immunodeficiency virus, and drug exposure.[17]

TABLE 28-1 Causes of Neutrophilia and Neutropenia

Neutrophilia	Neutropenia
Acute infections	Acute infections
Hemorrhage or hemolysis	Hemodialysis
Inflammatory changes	Overwhelming inflammation/infection
Intoxications (drugs, metabolic, poisons)	Medications
Medications	Physical agents (x-rays)
Myeloproliferative disorders	Secondary to autoimmune disorders
Malignancy (leukoerythroblastic picture)	Aplastic/hypoplastic states
Physiologic response to stress	

BOX 28-1 Causes of Lymphocytosis

Beta streptococcus
Cytomegalovirus
Drugs
Epstein-Barr virus (infectious mononucleosis)
T. palidium
Toxoplasma gondii
Vaccination
Viral hepatitis

MORPHOLOGIC ALTERATIONS OF LEUKOCYTES

Some inherited morphologic changes are clinically insignificant and of interest only to morphologists, whereas others indicate a life-threatening disorder. Most acquired changes may be used as indicators of disease states in conjunction with their clinical description. Morphologic changes are seldom unique to a disorder in the way that presence of the Sézary cells, for example, define Sézary syndrome. Each discussion of cellular morphology provides a typical description and the underlying structural or functional aberration.

Morphologic Alterations of Neutrophil Nuclei
Pelger-Huët Anomaly

Autosomal dominant neutrophil nuclear hyposegmentation appears in 1 in 6000 unselected individuals. Known as the *Pelger-Huët anomaly,* it is clinically insignificant because there is no loss of cellular function, although the nuclear matrix proteins are abnormal.[18] The nuclei are round, oval, or bilobed with a characteristic pinched or "pince-nez" appearance; chromatin is clumped and overly mature in contrast to the immature shape of the nucleus; and the population of neutrophils is uniform (Fig. 28-1). The rare homozygote has neutrophils with a round nucleus. Pelger-Huët homozygotes have varying degrees of skeletal and neurologic abnormalities.[19] Inexperienced morphologists may report Pelger-Huët cells incorrectly as myelocytes, metamyelocytes, or bands. An appropriate report would indicate mature cells but remark on the possibility of the Pelger-Huët anomaly. True Pelger-Huët anomaly is usually an incidental finding; however, there is a need to differentiate these cells from pseudo–Pelger-Huet cells. Pseudo–Pelger-Huët cells are acquired phenomena that may be clinically significant. These cells have nuclei that are less dense than those of normal cells or true Pelger-Huët cells, and they may have hypogranular cytoplasm. Pseudo–Pelger-Huët cells are found in burns, drug reactions, infections, myelodysplastic syndromes, chronic myelogenous leukemia, and acute leukemia as well as during chemotherapy.

Hereditary Hypersegmentation, Twinning, and Drumsticks

Autosomal dominant neutrophil hypersegmentation is clinically insignificant but must be distinguished from the hypersegmentation seen in the megaloblastic anemias (Chapter 20; Fig. 28-2) and from twinning deformity.

Twinning describes a nucleus with axial symmetry (mirror-image). Twinning is acquired in malignancies and chemotherapy (Fig. 28-3).

Increased "drumsticks," small chromatin extensions, may be found in trisomy of group E chromosomes, extra X chromosomes, or with other aneuploid states (Fig. 28-4).

Morphologic Alterations of Neutrophil Cytoplasm
Alder-Reilly Anomaly

Alder-Reilly anomaly may be transmitted as a recessive disorder in which decreased mucopolysaccharide degradation results in deposition of mucopolysaccharides (lipids) in the cytoplasm of most, if not all, cells.[20] There also appears to be a structural abnormality of the myeloperoxidase gene. When stained, these deposits, called *Alder-Reilly bodies,* appear as metachromatic (deep purple to lilac) granules and may be difficult to distinguish from toxic granulation (see later). Variable penetrance results in phenotypes ranging from abnormal granulation found only in neutrophils to abnormal granulation in all WBCs. In the extreme manifestation, eosinophils and basophils may possess unusual granulation,

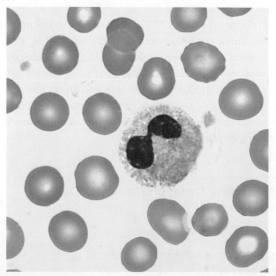

Figure 28-1 Pelger-Huët neutrophil with characteristic bilobed nucleus, dense heterochromatin, and incomplete nuclear segmentation. (From Carr JH, Rodak BF: Clinical Hematology Atlas, 2nd ed. Philadelphia: Saunders, 2004.)

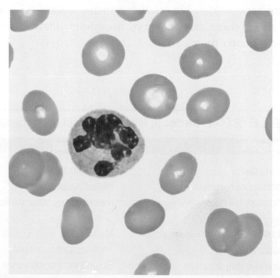

Figure 28-2 Hypersegmented neutrophil (macropolycyte) with six or more twisted and rounded nuclear segments. Present in megaloblastic anemia with macrocytes. (From Carr JH, Rodak BF: Clinical Hematology Atlas, 2nd ed. Philadelphia: Saunders, 2004.)

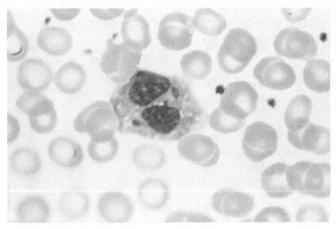

Figure 28-3 Twinning. This type of mirror image is seen in a variety of conditions and may or may not be significant.

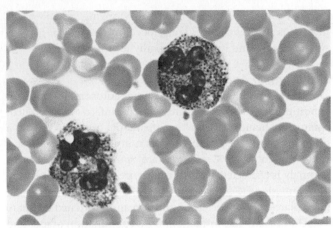

Figure 28-5 Alder-Reilly anomaly. Deep-purple to lilac granules appear in neutrophils (and occasionally eosinophils and basophils). (Courtesy of Dennis P. O'Malley, M.D., US Labs; Irvine, Calif.)

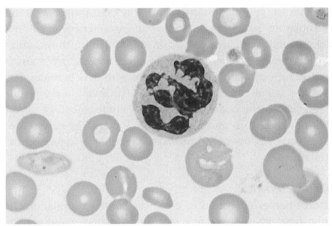

Figure 28-4 Hypersegmented neutrophil with multiple nuclear extrusions. Extrusions may be inactivated X chromosomes (in women). In normal neutrophils extrusions are called Barr bodies and are shaped like drumsticks.

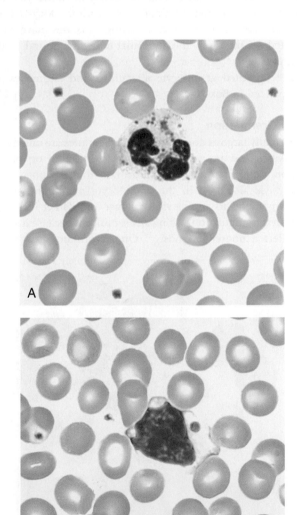

Figure 28-6 Chédiak-Higashi syndrome. **A,** The cytoplasm contains gray-blue granules that are larger in size and fewer in number than normal. **B,** The lymphocyte contains a large red-purple granule. (From Carr JH, Rodak BF: Clinical Hematology Atlas, 2nd ed. Philadelphia: Saunders, 2004.)

which makes it difficult to distinguish between them. These are commonly seen in patients with Hurler and Hunter syndromes[21] (Fig. 28-5).

Chédiak-Steinbrinck-Higashi Syndrome

Chédiak-Steinbrinck-Higashi syndrome, more commonly known as *Chédiak-Higashi syndrome*, is a rare autosomal recessive state in which abnormally large peroxidase-positive lysosomes[22] are seen in most cells of the body. This fusion of granules is seen in many sites, such as melanosomes, the disturbance of which results in albinism. Apparently, uncontrolled activity of the granular membrane creates large primary, secondary, and mixed primary/secondary granules (Fig. 28-6).[23] Increased precursor death in the marrow causes moderate peripheral blood neutropenia that, in addition to slowed bactericidal function, may explain the increased susceptibility to infections.[24] Affected patients also exhibit mucocutaneous hemorrage caused by thrombocytopenia. Platelets have large granules. The bleeding time is prolonged, and platelet aggregometry reveals a reduced response. The syndrome progresses through peripheral neuropathy, pancytopenia, and systemic infections associated with lymphocytic proliferation, hepatosplenomegaly, and lymphadenopathy to death.

May-Hegglin Anomaly

The May-Hegglin anomaly is a rare autosomal dominant condition in which patients are at risk for infections and mucocutaneous hemorrhage. It is apparently associated with a mutation in *MYH9*, which encodes non-muscle myosin heavy chain A. About 20% of cases are sporadic.[25] May-Hegglin anomaly is characterized by the presence of large Döhle body–like formations (Fig. 28-7) in all cells, thrombocytopenia, and giant platelets with decreased function and shortened life span. The Döhle body-like formations are a combination of rods and granules that are ribosomal in origin. Unlike Döhle bodies (see later), May-Hegglin inclusions are larger, more spindle shaped than oval, are permanent, and are found in monocytes and lymphocytes.[26] Although most patients with the May-Hegglin anomaly are asymptomatic, bleeding episodes have been reported secondary to the abnormal structures found in the platelets.

The inherited granulocyte alterations and anomalies are summarized in Box 28-2.

Toxic Granulation

Abnormally large or dominant primary granules are called *toxic granulation* and are a stress response to infection or inflammation. Cellular stimulation, particularly in the younger cells, may cause alteration in the granulocyte membrane, which causes granules to appear visibly larger and darker in Wright stain. Toxic granulation is clinically significant because it seems to reflect a poorer prognosis.[27] One important situation in

BOX 28-2 Inherited Granulocyte Alterations and Anomalies*

Nucleus
Pelger-Huët anomaly
Hereditary hypersegmentation

Cytoplasm
Chédiak-Higashi syndrome
May-Hegglin anomaly
Alder-Reilly granulation

*Inherited morphologic anomalies of granulocytes occur in the nucleus and cytoplasm. Both of the inherited nuclear anomalies are without clinical significance and need only be differentiated from similar manifestations that are acquired and significant. Inherited morphologic cytoplasmic anomalies are always significant.

which toxic granulation does not imply poor prognosis is the granulation pattern seen in granulocyte-monocyte colony-stimulating factor treatment.[28] In this situation, the stimulation is thought to speed up development and shorten marrow transit time, resulting in younger cells with dark granules that are functionally normal (Fig. 28-8). Artifactual heavy granulation caused by poor staining is seen homogeneously spread within each cell and in all granulocytes, whereas toxic granulation is unevenly spread throughout the cytoplasm of certain cells.

Döhle Bodies

Döhle bodies are round to oval neutrophil accumulations of ribosomal RNA. They are 1 to 5 μm in diameter and gray to light blue in Wright stain. Although no clear mechanism for their production is known, they are associated with a wide range of chemical and physical insults, such as burns, infections, surgery, pregnancy, and use of granulocyte-macrophage colony-stimulating factor.[29,30] Döhle bodies appear shortly after the stimulating event, which suggests that they first appear in storage pool cells.

Vacuolization

Vacuoles form by the ingestion and degradation of bacteria or fungi and are unevenly distributed. Vacuoles are clinically significant when associated with toxic granulation, degranulation, or Döhle bodies.[32] Autophagocytosis (phagocytosis of self) is seen with prolonged exposure to drugs such as antimicrobial agents and alcohol or radiation. In autophagocytosis the vacuoles are smaller and more evenly spaced.[31] Jordan's anomaly is a familial disorder in which vacuoles are present in the cytoplasm of granulocytes, lymphocytes, and monocytes.[33] There is no apparent disease correlation, although special staining shows that these vacuoles are filled with lipids.

Necrobiosis

Large numbers of dead granulocytes in the peripheral blood smear indicate a severe strain in the granulocyte development pools. These cells appear to have exploded nuclei and pale or

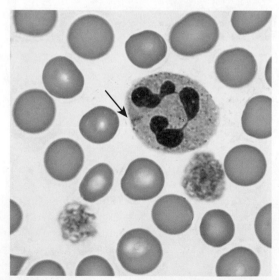

Figure 28-7 May-Hegglin anomaly. Although Döhle bodies (realigned RNA) may be found in occasional cells in patients experiencing bacterial infection or other stress, in May-Hegglin anomaly such inclusions are found in essentially every cell. Electron microscope techniques are usually necessary to visualize this phenomenon, however. Notice the large and bizarre platelets that accompany May-Hegglin anomaly. (From Carr JH, Rodak BF: Clinical Hematology Atlas, 2nd ed. Philadelphia: Saunders, 2004.)

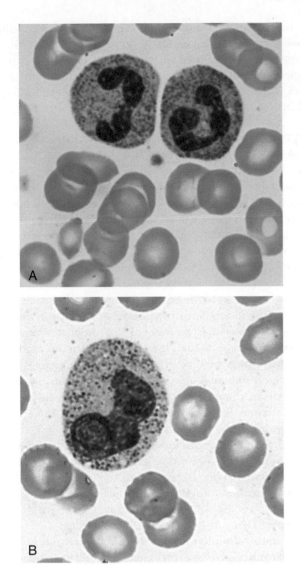

Figure 28-8 Toxic granulation. The number and size of the primary granules give the cell a bluish appearance. (From Carr JH, Rodak BF: Clinical Hematology Atlas, 2nd ed. Philadelphia: Saunders, 2004.)

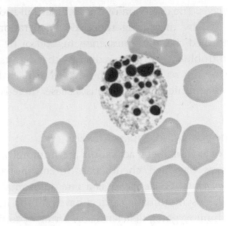

Figure 28-9 Necrobiotic WBC displays nuclear degradation or karyorrhexis. Indicates cell death in chemotherapy or a poorly preserved specimen. (From Carr JH, Rodak BF: Clinical Hematology Atlas, 2nd ed. Philadelphia: Saunders, 2004.)

> **BOX 28-3** Acquired Granulocyte Alterations and Anomalies*
>
> **Nucleus**
> Pseudo–Pelger-Huët anomaly
> Megaloblastic hypersegmentation
> Nuclear distortions (projections/ring forms)
> Pyknotic or necrobiotic forms
> Twinning deformity
>
> **Cytoplasm**
> Toxic granulation
> Döhle bodies
> Degranulation
> Vacuolization
> Pseudopodia

*Most acquired morphologic cytoplasmic anomalies are seen in severe stress situations, such as burns and infections. Acquired morphologic nuclear anomalies other than megaloblastic hypersegmentation are seen in infections and malignancies.

nongranular cytoplasm (Fig. 28-9). The acquired granulocyte alterations and anomalies are summarized in Box 28-3.

Cytoplasmic/Nonmorphologic (Functional) Alterations of Granulocytes

Chronic Granulomatous Disease of Childhood

Chronic granulomatous disease of childhood is a collection of rare genetic disorders in which the intracellular killing mechanism of the granulocyte is defective. Several patterns of inheritance may govern this disease; the two most common are sex-linked and autosomal recessive.[34] The ratio of affected boys to girls is 6:1. Chronic granulomatous disease results in death from bacterial infection, usually at 5 to 7 years of age. The manifestations of this disease are biochemically variable, resulting from combinations of defective/absent respiratory burst, membrane reduced nicotinamide adenine dinucleotide or reduced nicotinamide adenine dinucleotide phosphate oxidase, reduced cytosolic factor, or cytochrome B defects.[35] In

normal systems, hydrogen peroxide is concentrated in neutrophil phagosomes. This peroxide absorbs hydrogen ions, maintaining the neutral pH necessary for the action of bacteriocidal proteases. Because of failure to metabolize oxygen to superoxide anion and hydrogen peroxide, chronic granulomatous disease cells cannot kill catalase-positive or non–hydrogen peroxide–producing microorganisms such as *Staphylococcus*, Enterobacteriaceae, or *Candida*. As a result of the increased susceptibility and subsequent cellular protection for the ingested microorganism, chronic pyogenic infections of all systems, abscess formation, lymphadenopathy, and hepatosplenomegaly are common findings. Anemia of chronic disease is induced. The neutrophil picture includes toxic granulation, degranulation, vacuoles, Döhle bodies, and immature cells. The detection of intracellular kill mechanisms is determined by measuring superoxide generation via the rarely performed chemiluminescence method or by the more common nitroblue tetrazolium reduction that detects peroxide formation by the reduction of the dye to a black formazan deposit.[36] In chronic granulomatous disease, there is no color change.

Miscellaneous Deficiencies

Disorders of complement activation are humoral abnormalities, whereas impaired chemotaxis or enzymopathies are cellular. *Congenital C3 deficiency* is a rare autosomal recessive trait in which asymptomatic carriers have half the normal C3 activity. In homozygotes, deficiencies of serum opsonic activity result in recurrent pyogenic infections.[37]

Job syndrome (hyperimmunoglobulin E) and *lazy leukocyte syndrome* are rare neutrophil directional motility disorders. Their mode of inheritance is unknown, but they are differentiated by motility studies and by their clinical manifestations. In Job syndrome, neutrophils have poor directional motility, and boils are persistent. In patients with lazy leukocyte syndrome, cells have poor directional and random movement, and there are recurrent mucous membrane infections.

Myeloperoxidase deficiency was discovered as a result of the use of peroxidase indicators in automated differential instruments. It is a relatively mild disorder, and compensation occurs through increased frequency of respiratory bursts.[38]

The World Health Organization has clustered a group of disorders characterized by poor leukocyte adherence. Neutrophils and monocytes share a defect in surface glycoproteins CD11/CD18. There are abnormalities in adherence, aggregation, and complement receptor 3 activities, and lymphocytes may have reduced natural killer function.[39]

Individuals with non–insulin-dependent diabetes mellitus have granulocytes that are slower to respond to usual stimuli. Hyperglycemia has been associated with leukocytes that are deficient in chemotaxis, adhesion, and oxidative burst activities. This is a state that waxes and wanes in proportion to diabetic control.

Cytoplasmic/Morphologic Alterations of the Monocyte/Macrophage

Cells of the monocyte/macrophage system are rich in cytoplasmic lysosomes containing hydrolytic enzymes that digest products of cellular metabolism. Monocytes and macrophages store materials that are unsatisfactorily degraded, regardless of whether this partial degradation is due to intrinsic cellular enzyme defects, over-accumulation of substrate, or unsuitability of the material to the cell's enzymatic processes.

Lysosomes fuse to form a phagocytic vacuole containing the ingested material. Hereditary absence or dysfunction of any enzyme in a metabolic pathway causes an increase in substrate concentration and a decrease of the product. Commonly known as *storage diseases,* these are disorders in which one or more tissues become engorged with a substance whose type and distribution have a characteristic pattern. Table 28-2 summarizes common storage disorders, along with the deficient enzyme and subsequent storage product. These abnormalities are discussed briefly in this chapter.

A defect in the degradation of mucopolysaccharides results in enlarged cytoplasm with clear areas that are filled with mucopolysaccharides. Occasionally, granulocytes from affected patients manifest with Alder-Reilly bodies.

Gaucher Disease

Lipid storage disorders parallel mucopolysaccharide disorders in that a missing enzyme results in long-term storage of incom-

TABLE 28-2 Variants of Monocyte/Macrophage Storage Diseases*

Name	Enzyme Deficiency	Substance Stored
Hurler syndrome	α-L-iduronidase	Mucopolysaccharide I
Hunter syndrome	Iduronidate sulfatase	Mucopolysaccharide II
Sanfilippo syndrome	Form A: heparan *N*-sulfatase	Mucopolysaccharide III
	Form B: *N*-acetyl α-glucosaminidase	
Morquio syndrome	Unknown	Mucopolysaccharide IV
Scheie syndrome	α-L-iduronidase	Mucopolysaccharide V
Maroteaux-Lamy syndrome	Arylsulfatase	Mucopolysaccharide VI
Hand-Schüller-Christian disease	—	Cholesterol
Gaucher disease	β-Glucocerebrosidase	Glucocerebroside
Niemann-Pick disease	Sphingomyelinase	Sphingomyelin
Gangliosidosis	β-Galactosidase	GM_1 ganglioside
Tay-Sachs disease	Hexosaminidase A	GM_2 ganglioside
Sandhoff disease	Hexosaminidase A	GM_2 ganglioside
Fabry disease	α-Galactosidase	Ceramide trihexoside
Wolfman disease	Acid esterase	—

*Many dysfunctions result in monocyte/macrophage storage diseases; however, most of them are morphologically similar, and cytochemical testing is necessary for determining the specific product stored.

pletely processed lipids. Figure 28-10 summarizes the pathways and diseases associated with lipid metabolism. The most common lipid storage disorder is Gaucher disease, in which there is an inability to degrade glucocerebroside because of a deficiency of glucocerebrosidase (glucosidase; Enzyme Commission [EC] number 3.2.1.45). This deficiency causes accumulation of glucocerebroside in the monocytes and macrophages of the bone marrow, spleen, and liver. Neurons in the central nervous system also may be affected. Gaucher disease is inherited as an autosomal recessive trait; there are more than 65 mutations in the glucocerebrosidase gene known to cause Gaucher disease. Gaucher disease has three manifestations: type 1, or chronic

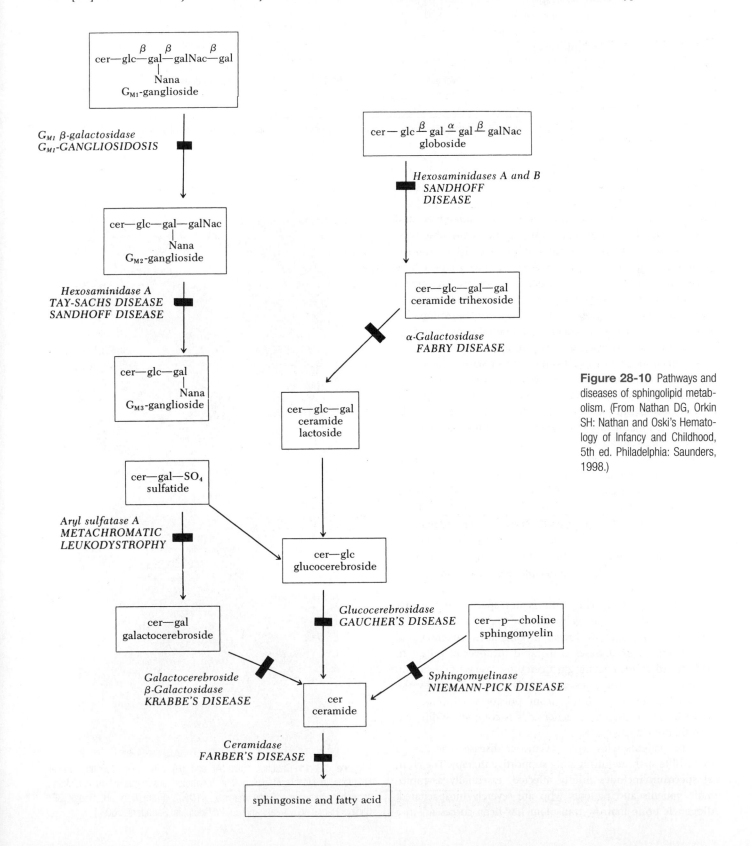

Figure 28-10 Pathways and diseases of sphingolipid metabolism. (From Nathan DG, Orkin SH: Nathan and Oski's Hematology of Infancy and Childhood, 5th ed. Philadelphia: Saunders, 1998.)

TABLE 28-3 Gaucher Disease: Clinical Subtypes

Clinical Features	Type 1: Non-neuronopathic	Type 2: Acute Neuronopathic	Type 3: Subacute Neuronopathic
Clinical onset	Childhood/adulthood	Infancy	Childhood
Hepatosplenomegaly	+	+	+
Hematologic complications secondary to hypersplenism	+	+	+
Skeletal deterioration	+	–	+
Neurodegenerative course	–	+++	++
Death	Variable	By 2 years	2nd-4th decade
Ethnic predilection	Ashkenazi Jewish	Panethnic	Swedish

From Gaucher disease (1882-1982): centennial perspectives on the most prevalent Jewish genetic disease. Mt Sinai J Med 1982;49:443-453.

adult type; type 2, or acute infantile neuronopathic type; and type 3, which is a less-defined subacute neuronopathic type. Characteristics of these types are listed in Table 28-3. Type 1 is found primarily in Ashkenazi Jews. Patients with type 1 have reduced but detectable levels of glucocerebrosidase. This type is often referred to as the *adult* type, but it may develop any time from infancy to old age. Type 1 is called non-neuronopathic because there is no involvement of the central nervous system. Type 2, or *acute neuronopathic,* is a much rarer disorder and shows no ethnic preference. It is much more severe than type 1 because of the central nervous system involvement. Glucocerebrosidase levels are undetectable, and glucocerebroside accumulates in all tissues, including the brain. Type 3, or subacute neuronopathic, has enzyme levels intermediate between those of types 1 and 2.[40]

The characteristic Gaucher cell is large and has an eccentric nucleus and cytoplasm that appears as "crumpled tissue paper" or "chicken scratch"; the latter because it appears as if a chicken walked across it and made scratch marks (Fig. 28-11). Although Gaucher cells are usually seen in the bone marrow, they do not greatly affect erythropoiesis. Hypersplenism probably accounts for anemia, rather than crowding out of normal marrow by Gaucher cells. Hypersplenism also may lead to thrombocytopenia.

The finding of Gaucher cells is not specific to Gaucher disease; pseudo-Gaucher cells may be seen in myeloproliferative disorders, such as chronic myelogenous leukemia, and other hematologic diseases with rapid turnover of cells.[41] In these disorders, the enzyme glucocerebrosidase is not deficient; however, the macrophages are simply overwhelmed by the increased amounts of lipids from phagocytized cells. The ultrastructure of pseudo-Gaucher cells is completely different from that of Gaucher cells.

Many patients with type 1 Gaucher disease may have a normal life span, requiring only supportive therapy. The clinical spectrum includes mildly affected, essentially asymptomatic patients and patients who are severely incapacitated. Allogeneic bone marrow transplant has been successful in a

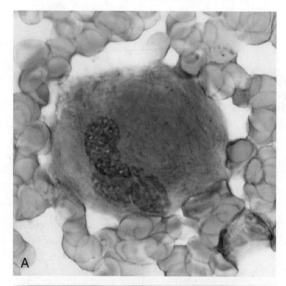

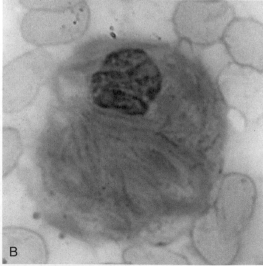

Figure 28-11 Gaucher cells **(A)** and **(B)** with characteristic parallel striations in cytoplasm giving it a "crumpled tissue paper" or "chicken-scratch" appearance (bone marrow, ×1000). (From Carr JH, Rodak BF: Clinical Hematology Atlas, 2nd ed. Philadelphia: Saunders, 2004.)

few patients. Enzyme infusion therapy with glucocerebrosidase is aimed at partially restoring the levels and action of glucocerebrosidase. A recombinant form of the enzyme, imiglucerase (Cerezyme; Genzyme Corp, Boston, Mass.), produced in Chinese hamster ovary cells, has been shown to be as effective as the placental derivative, and the supply is theoretically unlimited.[41] Studies are being performed in mice using retroviral and adenoviral vectors containing normal human glucocerebrosidase to transduce human hematopoietic progenitor cells. It may be possible to introduce autologous hematopoietic stem cells that have been transduced with the glucocerebrosidase gene and are capable of high levels of enzyme expression.

Niemann-Pick Disease

Niemann-Pick disease is caused by a deficiency of sphingomyelinase (EC 3.1.4.12) that allows sphingomyelin to accumulate in the spleen, liver, lungs, bone marrow, and, in some patients, brain. Cholesterol and other lipids accumulate to a lesser degree, along with a subsequent decrease in ceramides.[42] Sphingomyelin is a constituent of cell membranes and cellular organelles, so this deficiency can be quite serious. The disorder may be divided into five types: the neuronopathic types A-D, and an adult non-neuronopathic type E. Although the groups share the same enzyme deficiency, the defect is found on different genes. This classification is based on clinical features, not genetic similarities.[43] Inheritance is autosomal recessive.

Type A, the acute neuronopathic type, manifests in infancy (around 2 to 4 months). It is seen largely in Ashkenazi Jews. Patients have hepatosplenomegaly and serious brain involvement. Type B is the chronic form without central nervous system involvement. Types C and D are the chronic neuronopathic types and differ primarily in the ancestral backgrounds of the individuals affected. Type E, the adult non-neuronopathic type, has normal sphingomyelinase levels, but affected patients store sphingomyelin in cells of the monocyte/macrophage system.[44]

Type C constitutes the largest group of chronic sphingolipidoses and affects the brain, liver, and spleen. Approximately 200 to 300 Americans have Niemann-Pick disease type C. Patients present with symptoms about the time that they begin school. The symptoms may start as subtle changes in performance or declining grades. As damage to the brain increases, more noticeable abnormalities develop, such as difficulty with motor functions, including swallowing, walking, and talking. Progressive dementia becomes evident. Ultimately, the patient becomes nonambulatory and vegetative. Death often occurs by age 5 or 6, although some patients live into the teenage years. In a few patients, symptoms do not appear until teenage or adult years. The initial presentation may be as progressive dementia or psychosis. Type D has essentially the same abnormalities as found in type C, and the genetic defect is in the same region of chromosome 18. The only difference is in the population affected. Type D affects only a small group of Nova Scotian parentage, whereas type C shows no ethnic preference.

The characteristic Niemann-Pick cell (Fig. 28-12) is 20 to 90 μm in diameter and has an eccentric nucleus and a foamy cytoplasm, filled with uniformly sized droplets of accumulated lipid. The Niemann-Pick cell is not specific for Niemann-Pick disease but may be seen in GM_1 gangliosidosis, lactosylceramidosis, and Fabry disease. At this writing, there has been no successful treatment.

Other *inherited* storage cell diseases, such as gangliosidosis, Tay-Sachs disease, and Fabry disease, do not have significant hematologic implications. *Acquired* hyperlipidemias occur when a condition produces an abnormal amount of lipids for monocyte/macrophage cells to process.

Morphologic Alterations of Lymphocytes

Nonmalignant morphologic variants in lymphocytes are neither as frequent nor as dramatic as those seen in neutrophils. Most changes seen in lymphocytes are directly related to antigenic stimulation and can be considered normal activity. Lymphocytes with changes are more correctly referred to as *reactive, stimulated, committed,* or *variant,* rather than the older term "atypical". Mature B cells are capable of expressing surface immunoglobulins of a single specificity. They migrate to lymphoid organs where they may contact antigens and leave (the G_0 or resting stage). When an antigen binds the surface immunoglobulin receptor, B lymphocytes proliferate.

Morphologic changes include enlarged nuclei containing more euchromatin and visible nucleoli, as well as cytoplasmic basophilia. Morphologic changes become apparent and then regress over time. There is a wide range of manifestations based on altered euchromatin-to-heterochromatin ratios and increasing basophilia secondary to increased sophistication of the rough endoplasmic reticulum. Proliferating B cells mature into plasma cells that synthesize and secrete copious quantities of immunoglobulin whose binding specificity matches that present on the initially stimulated cell.

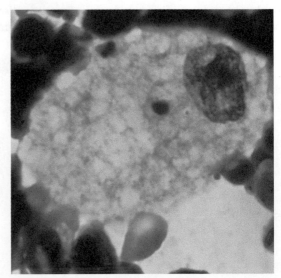

Figure 28-12 Niemann-Pick cell with eccentric nucleus and bubble-like pattern of storage deposit in the cytoplasm (bone marrow, ×1000). (From Carr JH, Rodak BF: Clinical Hematology Atlas, 2nd ed. Philadelphia: Saunders, 2004.)

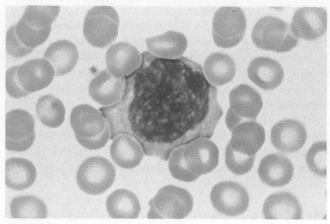

Figure 28-13 Variant (reactive) lymphocyte with expanded open nuclear pattern and peripheral basophilia in scalloped cytoplasm. Cell diameter exceeds normal but cell appearance is non-malignant.

Antigenic stimulation of T cells is more varied because of their range of activity. On stimulation, T cells undergo clonal expansion and pass through a series of stages detectable as gene rearrangements and surface markers. During clonal expansion, the nuclei of the cells contain more euchromatin. This metamorphosis is reflected in cells that are larger in size and that contain azurophilic cytoplasmic granulation (Figs. 28-13 and 28-14).

Nuclear Abnormalities

Clefting of the nucleus is sometimes seen in malignancies, especially lymphomas. Abnormal nuclei with a peculiar cerebriform pattern of heterochromatin are seen in patients with Sézary syndrome (Chapter 37).

Cytoplasmic Abnormalities

Vacuolization of the cytoplasm can be seen in the genetic mucopolysaccharidoses, Gaucher disease, Tay-Sachs disease, Niemann-Pick disease, and Pompe disease. Azurophilic granu-

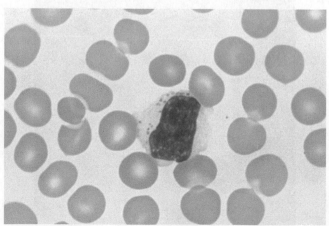

Figure 28-14 Variant (reactive) lymphocyte with expanded nucleus, increased cytoplasmic volume and cytoplasmic granules. Diameter is slightly greater than normal.

lation can be seen in response to antigenic stimulation and in Hunter syndrome, a genetic disease. Increased amounts of non-staining materials, such as Golgi apparatus or polypeptides, are a result of increased activity in response to antigenic stimulation or malignancy. Box 28-4 summarizes morphologic alterations in lymphocytes. Vacuolization also occurs in Burkitt lymphoma (Chapter 37).

Variant Lymphocytes (Infectious Mononucleosis)

Although variant (reactive) lymphocytes may be seen in other disorders, infectious mononucleosis is a frequent cause. This disease was first recognized in the early part of the 20th century and has been irrevocably connected to the presence of reactive lymphocytes by the 1923 work produced by Downey.[45]

Epstein-Barr virus (EBV) type A (EBV-1) and type B (EBV-2) cause infectious mononucleosis. Both strains are common but differ in their abilities to produce memory B cells. EBV infects children and young adults. The childhood form of the disease seems to be less severe than that seen in teenagers. The virus is found in body fluids, especially saliva, which gives rise to one of its nicknames, "the kissing disease," although the sharing of eating utensils has the same effect.

BOX 28-4 Lymphocyte Morphologic Abnormalities*

Abnormalities in the Nucleus
Clefting
Some malignancies, especially lymphomas

Cerebriform Heterochromatin
Sézary syndome

Abnormalities in the Cytoplasm
Vacuolization
Genetic mucopolysaccharidosis
Tay-Sachs disease
Pompe disease
Niemann-Pick disease
Gaucher disease
Chediak-Higashi syndrome

Azurophilic Granulation
Response to antigenic stimulation
Hunter syndrome

Increased Amounts of Nonstaining Materials†
Response to antigenic stimulation
Increased activity of cell as a result of
  Multiple myeloma
  Waldenström macroglobulinemia
  Immune system malignancies

*Unusual morphologic presentations of lymphocytes can be expected as in the case of reactivity, inherited as in the storage diseases, or as a result of malignancy.
†For example, polypeptides in rough endoplasmic reticulum in a plasma cell.

Infectious mononucleosis is diagnosed through the use of current kit modifications of the old Paul Bunnell or heterophile antibody test. Later-stage disease and long-term presence of EBV antigen is confirmed by molecular diagnostic tests.

The incubation period is 3 to 7 weeks, with sudden onset of signs and symptoms. Lassitude, malaise, chills and fever, loss of appetite, sore throat, and nausea are frequently cited. Bilateral lymph node enlargement is also common early in the disease process. By the midpoint of the disease, splenomegaly is common, but hepatomegaly is rare. With the exception of hepatic or splenic concerns, the resolution of the disease is typically uneventful.

The hematologic findings resemble those in many viral diseases. The RBC count may be lowered as a result of a transient hemolysis, caused in part by splenomegaly and in some cases by the presence of cold agglutinins. The RBC morphology is normochromic, normocytic, and the platelet count may be mildly decreased. The WBC count is often elevated to the range of 11 to 20×10^9/L. The differential shows a pleomorphic picture with relative neutropenia, absolute lymphocytosis, possibly a monocytosis, and the continued presence of eosinophils. Lymphocytosis may exceed 60%. Of these, there is significant variation, with non-reactive lymphocytes and large, non-granular, vacuolated lymphocytes. Reactive lymphocytes vary in size but exhibit increased cytoplasm and lobulated or oval nuclei with strands and clumps of chromatin. Reactive (variant) lymphocytes are differentiated T cells.[46]

Although hepatitis and splenomegaly may be significant, most patients recover without incident. There may be a relationship between EBV and Hodgkin lymphoma, chronic fatigue syndrome, and Burkitt lymphoma.

Non-Morphologic Alterations of Lymphocytes

Most non-morphologic alterations are seen in diseases of immunologic function. The alterations result from a deficient cell type or a failure of lymphocyte function. B cell alterations are responsible for hypogammaglobulinemia, agammaglobulinemia, and dysgammaglobulinemia. Quantitative and qualitative defects in T cells are detected by cell marker phenotypes in flow cytometry. (Chapter 33)

T Cell Abnormalities

Patients with Wiskott-Aldrich syndrome, a rare X-linked recessive disorder, have defects in platelet number, size, and function in addition to defects in B cell and T cell function. Caused by an abnormality in CD43, this condition results in diminished humoral and cellular immunity with increased susceptibility to infection.[47] In 1968, DiGeorge first described a condition that included parathyroid, cardiac, and skeletal abnormalities. Patients with DiGeorge syndrome have been shown to have <10% of normal circulating T cells.[48,49] The most well-known acquired disease of T lymphocytes is acquired immunodeficiency syndrome caused by the human immunodeficiency virus (Chapter 33).[50]

B Cell Abnormalities

Sex-linked agammaglobulinemia may present with an absence of B cells, although some pre-B cells may be shown.[51] This condition differs from congenital agammaglobulinemia, in which the defect is either in the pre-B cell or in a qualitative interaction between the mature B cell and its counterpart T cell.

CHAPTER at a GLANCE

- The number, population type, and significance of leukocytes found in the peripheral blood vary with the individual patient.
- The number of circulating (and countable) WBCs depends on the age of the patient, overall granulocyte kinetics, and degree of margination.
- Benign neutrophilia occurs most often in such conditions as stress, tachycardia, fever, strenuous exercise, and ingestion of certain medications, such as epinephrine and cortisone.
- Causes of leukopenia with fully mature granulocytes include diminishing of bone marrow mitotic pool as a result of vitamin B_{12}/folate deficiency, ingestion of medications, and lazy leukocyte syndrome.
- Eosinophilia is seen commonly in a wide spectrum of allergic responses, medication usage, many skin diseases, and malignancy.
- Basophilia is seen in patients with hypoactive thyroid conditions, ulcerative colitis, some types of nephrosis, and certain malignancies.

- Monocytosis is seen whenever there is an increased amount of cell damage, such as recovery from an infection.
- Reference values for peripheral blood lymphocytes vary with age, with values higher in children.
- Relative lymphocytosis sometimes can be seen in patients with exanthems (skin rashes) from certain viral diseases, such as measles and mumps; in patients with thyrotoxicosis; and in patients recovering from certain acute infections.
- Although cytoplasmic alterations of the granulocytes can be inherited (recessive) or acquired through exposure to stress or toxins, most of the morphologic cytoplasmic anomalies of granulocytes are acquired in severe stress situations, such as burns and infections.
- The demonstration of acquired, abnormally large or dominant primary granules is called *toxic granulation* and is a stress response to infection or inflammation or following administration of GM-CSF.

Continued

CHAPTER at a GLANCE—cont'd

- Döhle bodies develop in the cytoplasm of granulocytes of patients with infections or in stress states, are round to oval, are approximately 1 to 5 μm in diameter, and are composed of parallel rows of ribosomal RNA.
- Phagocytic vacuoles may be found in neutrophils as a result of various situations, including exposure to drugs and toxins and ingestion and degradation of bacteria.
- Acquired morphologic nuclear anomalies other than megaloblastic hypersegmentation are seen in infections and malignancies.
- Pelger-Huët anomaly is the most common inherited condition in granulocytes. It is clinically insignificant but can be confused with immaturity in granulocytes, giving rise to incorrect differential reporting.
- Inherited alterations of granulocytes include Chédiak-Higashi syndrome (abnormal granules) and May-Hegglin anomaly (abnormal granules, Döhle bodies, thrombocytopenia, and giant platelets).
- Chronic granulomatous disease of childhood is a collection of genetic disorders in which the intracellular kill mechanism of the granulocyte is defective.
- Lipid storage diseases parallel mucopolysaccharide disorders in that a missing enzyme results in the long-term storage of incompletely processed material. The most common lipid storage disease is Gaucher disease, in which there is an inability to degrade glucocerebroside.

- Nonmalignant morphologic variants in lymphocytes are neither as frequent nor as dramatic as those seen in neutrophils. Most changes seen in lymphocytes are directly related to antigenic stimulation and can be considered as normal activity.
- Vacuolization of the cytoplasm of lymphocytes can be seen in the genetic mucopolysaccharidoses, Gaucher disease, Tay-Sachs disease, Niemann-Pick disease, and Pompe disease.
- Alterations in B cells are responsible for a large list of hypogammaglobulinemias, agammaglobulinemias, and dysgammaglobulinemias; quantitative and qualitative defects in T cells can be described by cell marker phenotypes.
- The hematologic findings in viral disease include a normochromic, normocytic anemia; mild thrombocytopenia and relative neutropenia; absolute lymphocytosis; possibly a monocytosis; and the continued presence of eosinophils.
- Reactive lymphocytosis may exceed 60% of the leukocytes counted in the differential, with significant pleomorphism with some nonreactive cells alongside large, nongranular, possibly vacuolated cells.

Now that you have completed this chapter, go back and read again the case studies at the beginning and respond to the questions presented.

REVIEW QUESTIONS

Refer to the following CBC data to answer questions 1-3. Refer to the reference ranges provided inside the book cover.

WBC (× 10³/μL)	75
RBC (× 10⁶/μL)	3.16
Hb (g/dL)	9.5
Hct (%)	26.3
MCV (fL)	83
MCH (pg)	30
MCHC (%)	36
RDW (%)	13
Platelets (× 10³/μL)	512
Mean platelet volume (fL)	9
Differential	
Segmented neutrophils	43
Bands	10
Lymphocytes	5
Monocytes	0
Eosinophils	3
Basophils	7
Metamyelocytes	0
Myelocytes	30
Promyelocytes	1
Blasts	1
Other	
Morphology	2 nucleated RBCs/100 WBCs

1. Which of the following terms would accurately describe the WBC features for the listed case data?
   a. Leukopenic with a left shift
   b. Leukemoid
   c. Leukoerythroblastic
   d. Lymphocytic

2. A description of the relative differential for the case data would include:
   a. Bandophilia
   b. Monocytosis
   c. Lymphocytosis
   d. Neutrophilia

3. A description for the absolute counts for the case data would include:
   a. Lymphopenia
   b. Basophilia
   c. Eosinopenia
   d. Blastocytosis

4. An absolute lymphocytosis with reactive (variant) lymphocytes suggests which of the following conditions?
   a. Lymphocytic leukemia
   b. Bacterial infection
   c. Parasitic infection
   d. Viral infection

5. This morphologic change is seen in association with nonmalignant conditions. It affects mainly neutrophils, although it also can be seen in monocytes or lymphocytes. It appears as round, clear (i.e., white) areas in the cytoplasm that are well demarcated. Name this morphologic variation.
   a. Döhle bodies
   b. Toxic granules
   c. Vacuolization
   d. May-Hegglin bodies

6. What leukocyte cytoplasmic inclusion is composed of ribosomal RNA?
   a. Toxic granulation
   b. Döhle bodies
   c. Howell-Jolly bodies
   d. Tay-Sachs inclusions

7. In which condition does the nucleus of neutrophils have fewer segments than normal?
   a. Tay-Sachs disease
   b. May-Hegglin anomaly
   c. Pelger-Huët anomaly
   d. Alder-Reilly anomaly

8. The leukocytosis associated with exercise is relative:
   a. Lymphocytosis resulting from increased neutrophil margination
   b. Neutrophilia resulting from increased lymphocyte margination
   c. Lymphocytosis resulting from increased lymphocytes in the circulating pool
   d. Neutrophilia resulting from increased neutrophils in the circulating pool

9. Gaucher cells are:
   a. Monocytes/macrophages that contain large amounts of lipids
   b. Neutrophils with abnormally large primary granules
   c. Lymphocytes with deeply blue cytoplasm and eccentric nucleus
   d. Neutrophils with fragmented, pyknotic nuclei

10. The normal distribution of WBCs in children differs from that of adults because children have:
   a. More eosinophils
   b. More lymphocytes
   c. Fewer basophils
   d. More bands

REFERENCES

1. Horne BD, Anderson JL, John JM, et al: Which white blood cell subtypes predict increased cardiovascular risk? J Am Coll Cardiol 2005;45:1638-1643.
2. Cheng CK, Chan J, Cembrowski GS, et al: Complete blood count reference interval diagrams derived from NHANES III: stratification by age, sex, and race. Lab Hematol 2004;10:42-53.
3. Chung FM, Tsai JC, Chang DM, et al: Peripheral total and differential leukocyte count in diabetic nephropathy: the relationship of plasma leptin to leukocytosis. Diabetes Care 2005;28:1710-1717.
4. Horwitz M, Benson KF, Person RE, et al: Mutations in ELA2, encoding neutrophil elastase, define a 21 biological clock in cyclic haematopoiesis. Nat Genet 1999;23:433-436.
5. Dalee DC, Bolyard AA, Aprikan A: Cyclic neutropenia. Semin Hematol 2002;39:89-94.
6. Tankersley MS: Kostmann disease. May 26, 2004. Available at: http://www.emedicine.com/PED/topic1260.htm. Accessed June 4, 2006.
7. Izquierdo NJ, Townsend W: Hermansky-Pudlak syndrome. March 2, 2006. Available at: http://www.emedicien.com/oph/topic713.htm. Accessed June 4, 2006.
8. Virella G: Diagnostic evaluation of phagocytic function. Immunol Ser 1993;58:311-327.
9. Andres E, Kurtz JE, Maloisel F: Nonchemotherapy drug-induced agranulocytsis: experience of the Strasbourg teaching hospital (1985-2000) and review of the literature. Clin Lab Hematol 2002;24:99-106.
10. Bux J: Molecular nature of antigens implicated in immune neutropenias. Int J Hematol 2002;76(Suppl 1):399-403.
11. Berliner N, Horwitz M, Loughran TP Jr: Congenital and acquired neutropenia. Hematology Am Soc Hematol Educ Program 2004;63-79.
12. Perez Arellano JL, Pardo J, Hernandez Cabrera M, et al: Eosinophilia: a practical approach. An Med Interna 2004;21:244-252.
13. Dinauer MC: The phagocyte system and disorders of granulopoiesis and granulocyte function. In Nathan DG, Orkin SH, Ginsburg D, et al (eds): Nathan and Oski's Hematology of Infancy and Childhood, 6th ed. Philadelphia: Saunders, 2003:923-1010.
14. Mayhew DL, Thyfault JP, Koch AJ: Rest-interval length affects leukocyte levels during heavy resistance exercise. J Strength Cond Res 2005;19:16-22.
15. Heininger U, Klich K, Stehr K, et al: Clinical findings in Bordetella pertussis infections: results of a prospective multicenter surveillance study. Pediatrics 1997;100:E10.
16. Fernandez-Fresnedo G, Ramos MA, Gonzalez-Pardo MC, et al: B lymphopenia in uremia is related to an accelerated in vitro apoptosis and dysregulation of Bcl-2. Nephrol Dial Transplant 2000;15:502-510.
17. Griveas I, Visvardis G, Fleva A, et al: Comparative analysis of immunophenotypic abnormalities in cellular immunity of uremic patients undergoing either hemodialysis or continuous ambulatory peritoneal dialysis. Ren Fail 2005;27:279-282.
18. Sjakste N, Sjakste T: Nuclear matrix proteins and hereditary diseases. Genetika 2005;41:293-298.
19. Hoffmann K, Dreger CK, Olins AL, et al: Mutations in the gene encoding the lamin B receptor produce an altered nuclear morphology in granulocytes (Pelger-Huet anomaly). Nat Genet 2002;31:410-414.
20. Presentey B: Alder anomaly accompanied by a mutation of the myeloperoxidase structural gene. Acta Haematol 1986;75:157-159.
21. Clarke JT, Willard HF, Teshima I, et al: Hunter disease (mucopolysaccharidosis type II) in a karyotypically normal girl. Clin Genet 1990;37:355-362.
22. Higashi O: Congenital gigantism of peroxidase granules: first case ever reported of qualitative abnormality of peroxidase. Tohoku J Exp Med 1954;59:315-332.
23. White JG, Clawson CC: The Chédiak-Higashi syndrome: the nature of the giant neutrophil granules and their interactions with cytoplasm and foreign particulates. Am J Pathol 1980;98:151-196.
24. Lazarchick J, McRae B: Chediak-Higashi syndrome. Blood 2005;105:4162.

25. Kunishima S, Matsushita T, Yoshihara T, et al: First description of somatic mosaicism in MYH9 disorders. Br J Haematol 2005;128:360-365.

26. Cawley JJ, Hayhoe FG: The inclusions of the May-Hegglin anomaly and Döhle bodies of infection: an ultrastructural comparison. Br J Haematol 1972;22:491-496.

27. Lin SJ, Huang JL, Chao HC, et al: A follow-up study of systemic-onset juvenile rheumatoid arthritis in children. Acta Paediatr Taiwan 1999;40:176-181.

28. Schmitz LL, McClure JS, Litz CE, et al: Morphologic and quantitative changes in blood and marrow cells following growth factor therapy. Am J Clin Pathol 1994;101:67-75.

29. Kunishima S, Matsushita T, Kojima T, et al: Identification of six novel MYH9 mutations and genotype-phenotype relationships in autosomal dominant macrothrombocytopenia with leukocyte inclusions. J Hum Genet 2001;46:722-729.

30. Elghetany MT, Hudnall SD, Gardner FH: Peripheral blood picture in primary hypocellular refractory anemia and idiopathic acquired aplastic anemia: an additional tool for differential diagnosis. Haematologica 1997;82:21-24.

31. Rautelin H, Blomberg B, Jarnerot G, et al: Nonopsonic activation of neutrophils and cytotoxin production by Helicobacter pylori: ulcerogenic markers. Scand J Gastroenterol 1994;29:128-132.

32. Solberg CO, Hellum KB: Neutrophil granulocyte function in bacterial infections. Lancet 1972;2:727-730.

33. Rozenszajn L, Klajman A, Jaffe D, et al: Jordan's anomaly in white blood cells. Blood 1966;28:258-265.

34. Holland S, Seger R, Sullivan KE: The chronicles of chronic granulomatous disease. Clin Immunol 2005;116:99-100.

35. El-Benna J, Dang PM, Gougerot-Pocidalo MA, et al: Phagocyte NADPH oxidase: a multicomponent enzyme essential for host defenses. Arch Immunol Ther Exp (Warsz) 2005;53:199-206.

36. Ikinciogullari A, Dogu F, Solaz N, et al: Granulocyte transfusions in children with chronic granulomatous disease and invasive aspergillosis. Ther Apher Dial 2005;9:137-141.

37. Overturf GD: Indications for the immunological evaluation of patients with meningitis. Clin Infect Dis 2003;36:189-194.

38. Emmendorffer A, Nakamura M, Rothe G, et al: Evaluation of flow cytometric methods for diagnosis of chronic granulomatous disease variants under routine laboratory conditions. Cytometry 1994;18:147-155.

39. Anderson DC, Schmalsteig FC, Finegold MJ, et al: The severe and moderate phenotypes of heritable Mac-1, LFA-1 deficiency: their quantitative definition and relation to leukocyte dysfunction and clinical features. J Infect Dis 1985;152:668-689.

40. Germain DP: Gaucher's disease: a paradigm for interventional genetics. Clin Genet 2004;65:77-86.

41. MacKenzie JJ, Amato D, Clarke J: Enzyme replacement therapy for Gaucher's disease: the early Canadian experience. Can Med Assoc J 1998;159:1273-1278.

42. Dardis A, Zampieri S, Filocamo M, et al: Functional in vitro characterization of 14 SMPD1 mutations identified in Italian patients affected by Niemann Pick Type B disease. Hum Mutat 2005;26:164-171.

43. Pavlu-Pereira H, Asfaw B, Poupctova H, et al: Acid sphingomyelinase deficiency: phenotype variability with prevalence of intermediate phenotype in a series of twenty-five Czech and Slovak patients: a multi-approach study. J Inherit Metab Dis 2005;28:203-227.

44. Chikh K, Rodriguez C, Vey S, et al: Niemann-Pick type C disease: subcellular location and functional characterization of NPC2 proteins with naturally occurring missense mutations. Hum Mutat 2005;26:20-28.

45. Downey J: Acute lymphadenosis compared to acute lymphatic leukemia. Arch Intern Med 1923;32:82-112.

46. Kotsiopriftis M, Tanner JE, Alfieri C: Heat shock protein 90 expression in Epstein-Barr virus-infected B cells promotes gammadelta T-cell proliferation in vitro. J Virol 2005;79:7255-7261.

47. Deonarain R, Verma A, Porter AC, et al: Free in PMC: critical roles for IFN-beta in lymphoid development, myelopoiesis, and tumor development: links to tumor necrosis factor alpha. Proc Natl Acad Sci U S A 2003;100:13453-13458.

48. DiGeorge AM: Congenital absence of thymus and its immunologic consequences: concurrence with congenital hypoparathyroidism. Birth Defects 1968;4:116-121.

49. Cancrini C, Romiti ML, Finocchi A, et al: Post-natal ontogenesis of the T-cell receptor CD4 and CD8 Vbeta repertoire and immune function in children with DiGeorge syndrome. J Clin Immunol 2005;25:265-274.

50. Stone S, Price P, French M: Dysregulation of CD28 and CTLA-4 expression by CD4 T cells from previously immunodeficient HIV-infected patients with sustained virological responses to highly active antiretroviral therapy. HIV Med 2005;6:278-283.

51. Bruton OC: Agammaglobulinemia. Pediatrics 1952;9:722-727.

Introduction to Leukocyte Neoplasms

29

Peter D. Emanuel

OBJECTIVES

After completion of this chapter, the reader will be able to:

1. Name two viral etiologic factors causing lymphoid malignancies.
2. Define oncogene and tumor suppressor gene and and explain the difference between them, including the mechanisms by which each produces cancer.
3. Explain why oncogenes are described as acting in a dominant fashion.
4. Give two examples of oncogenes and two examples of tumor suppressor genes.
5. Describe how genetic abnormalities can affect molecular pathways within cells.
6. Identify the two basic subgroups of chemotherapeutic agents.
7. Explain why localized treatments are rarely used for leukocyte neoplasms.
8. Describe examples of supportive care that have been developed from molecular biology techniques, including their functions and purposes.
9. Name two examples of targeted therapeutics for chronic myelogenous leukemia, and explain their methods of action.
10. Describe differences between small molecule inhibitors and monoclonal antibodies.
11. Name three sources of hematopoietic stem cells.
12. Compare and contrast allogeneic and autologous bone marrow transplants.

GENERAL CHARACTERISTICS OF LEUKOCYTE NEOPLASMS

Most malignancies of the hematopoietic system are acquired genetic diseases, meaning that most patients are not born with the illness but acquire it sometime later. Most leukocyte malignancies are not localized but rather are systemic at the initiation of the malignant process. The bone marrow, in which the leukemias arise, and the lymphatic system, in which most lymphomas originate, have passages throughout the body. A single leukemia cell arising in the marrow can obtain passage into the bloodstream and travel to any and all locations of the body. With rare exception, most treatments given for curative intent of leukocyte neoplasms are not localized, such as radiation or surgery, but must by nature be systemic-type treatments.

ETIOLOGY OF LEUKOCYTE NEOPLASMS

For most leukocyte neoplasms, causes directly related to the development of the malignancy are unknown. There are, however, a few exceptions. Environmental toxins can induce

genetic changes, as discussed later in this chapter, leading to a malignancy phenotype. Environmental exposures known to lead to hematopoietic malignancies include radiation, as it affects survivors of atomic explosions, and organic solvents, such as benzene. There are two types of lymphoid malignancies in which viruses may play a pathogenetic role. The Epstein-Barr virus has been implicated as an etiologic factor in the development of Burkitt non-Hodgkin lymphoma. Similarly, the human T cell lymphotropic virus type 1 is the likely cause of adult T cell leukemia/lymphoma. As discussed further in this chapter, there are some known familial cancer predisposition syndromes. Additionally, as more cancer survivors live longer, it is clear that some alkylating agents and other forms of chemotherapy used to treat various forms of cancer can induce DNA damage in hematopoietic cells, leading to hematologic malignancies.

CLASSIFICATION SCHEMAS FOR LEUKOCYTE NEOPLASMS

The French-American-British (FAB) classification for the acute leukemias was devised in the 1970s and 1980s. The FAB

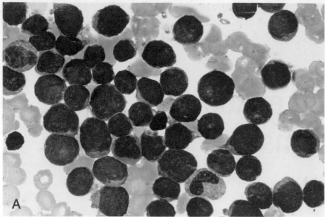

Lymphoblasts:

2-3 times size of lymphocyte diameter
Scant blue cytoplasm
Uniform, coarser than myeloblasts
Inconspicuous nucleoli

Myeloblasts:

3-5 times size of lymphocyte diameter
Moderate gray cytoplasm
Uniform fine chromatin
2 or more prominent nucleoli
Possible Aüer rods

Figure 29-1 A, Lymphoblasts (Wright stain, bone marrow, ×500, and description of morphology). **B,** Myeloblasts (Wright stain, bone marrow, ×500) and description of myeloblasts.

schemas were based largely on morphologic characteristics and relied heavily on examination of routine histologic stains to distinguish lymphoid neoplasms from myeloid neoplasms (Fig. 29-1). Although these types of diagnostic criteria have not been abandoned, there is movement toward more precise classification of some leukocyte neoplasms based on recurring chromosomal and genetic lesions found in many patients. These lesions are related to disruptions of oncogenes, tumor suppressor genes, and other regulatory elements that control proliferation, maturation, apoptosis, and other vital cell functions. In 2001 the World Health Organization (WHO) published new classification schemas for nearly all of the tumors of hematopoietic and lymphoid tissues.[1] The WHO classification scheme for acute myeloid leukemias (AML) includes some remnants of the old FAB classification of AML, while introducing new classifications for leukemias associated with consistently recurring chromosomal translocations.

CHROMOSOMAL ABNORMALITIES IN HEMATOLOGIC NEOPLASMS

In part because of the ease of access to bone marrow compared with other organs of the body, researchers have learned a great deal about the fundamental concepts of cancer biology by studying hematopoietic neoplasms. The study of chromosomal translocations in hematologic malignancies has taught how a single mutation, or series of mutations in stepwise fashion, can lead to malignant transformation by disrupting the molecular machinery of the cell. The first two genetic lesions found in any kind of human cancer were identified as

chromosomal translocations occurring in leukocyte malignancies. The first was the t(9;22) translocation in chronic myelogenous leukemia (CML),[2] and the second was the t(8;14) translocation in Burkitt lymphoma.[3]

ONCOGENES

Oncogenes originally were identified as genes that carried rapidly transforming retroviruses derived from normal cellular homologues, proto-oncogenes. The definition of oncogenes has evolved to refer to genes that cause dominant-acting cancer mutations, regardless of whether they are derived from a retrovirus. Typically, the normal proto-oncogene codes for a protein involved in normal cell cycle regulation. These proteins provide the signal transduction that carries messages about cell division and maturation (differentiation) from outside the cell to the nucleus. Mutations of these genes to form oncogenes result in disruptions of normal cell cycle processes. Most chromosomal translocations in leukemias involve oncogenes. The "dominant" transforming oncogene is able to alter the gene product and transform the cell into a malignant phenotype, even in the presence of a residual normal allele. Even the above-mentioned two examples involve oncogenes in the translocation that are activated when brought into proximity with their new partners on the fusion genes. In the case of CML, the *ABL* proto-oncogene on chromosome 9 is activated when fused to the *BCR* component of chromosome 22. In the case of Burkitt lymphoma, the *MYC* proto-oncogene on chromosome 8 is fused with the immunoglobulin heavy chain locus on chromosome 14. Although oncogenic transformation was first identified by karyotypic analyses, molecular biologic techniques have evolved rapidly over the last 2 decades such that more genetic translocations are being identified that create novel fusion genes invisible at the cytogenetic level.

TUMOR SUPPRESSOR GENES

Tumor suppressor genes are so named because they code for proteins that help cells resist malignant transformation. Rather than acting in a dominant fashion as in the case of oncogenes, these cancer-causing genes transform cells into a malignant phenotype only after both alleles have been lost or otherwise inactivated, the so-called "two-hit" mechanism proposed by Knudson.[4] Although typically much harder to isolate and identify, numerous tumor suppressor genes have now been identified, and many have been found to be associated with autosomal dominant familial cancer predisposition syndromes. Some well-known examples include the *RB1* tumor suppressor gene involved in familial retinoblastoma, the *TP53* gene in the Li-Fraumeni syndrome, the *WT1* gene in Wilms tumor, and the *NF1* gene in familial neurofibromatosis type 1. Perhaps more importantly, many of these tumor suppressor genes and their protein products are altered in many sporadic cancers, including hematologic cancers.

OTHER GENETIC CHANGES

Beyond oncogenes and tumor suppressor genes, researchers have found genes that are involved in DNA repair mechanisms. Mutations in these genes do not lead to cellular transformation by altering signaling pathways, but rather lead to genetic instability and increased mutation rates. Examples of these genes include the DNA mismatch repair genes, *MLH1* and *MSH2*. Another example is the Fanconi anemia gene, *FA*, which is important for maintaining genomic stability in hematopoietic tissues.

MOLECULAR PATHWAYS PERTURBED BY CELLULAR TRANSFORMATION

Regardless of the particular type of chromosomal or genetic abnormality, clinicians recognize the molecular consequences that formation of oncogenes or loss of tumor suppressor genes have on the proliferation and differentiation aspects of hematologic tissues. Several mechanisms are understood, including blocked differentiation, transcriptional repression, disruptions of cell signaling, progression, and apoptosis. The t(15;17) translocation found in acute promyelocytic leukemia (APL), which fuses the *PML* gene to the *RARA* (retinoic acid receptor α) gene, clearly results in a state of *arrested differentiation* because the retinoic acid receptor α–induced differentiation is inhibited. Treating patients with APL with pharmacologically high doses of all-trans retinoic acid can overcome this block and permit APL cells to differentiate to normal neutrophils. In so doing, the APL cells lose their leukemic potential. Other chromosomal abnormalities involve *transcriptional repression* of DNA and condensation abnormalities of chro-

matin, such as those involved in the core-binding factor leukemic subtypes of AML. A similar example on the lymphoid side of hematopoietic neoplasms are the chromosomal translocations involving the *BCL6* gene. Normal *BCL6* encodes for a transcriptional repressor responsible for recruiting the histone deacetylase complex, which regulates germinal center formation in lymph nodes. The mutation of *BCL6* leads to overexpression of this normal protein such that DNA is excessively repressed, in this case preventing lymphocytes from progressing beyond the germinal center stage of development.

Since the initial identification of the *BCR-ABL* fusion gene in CML, there are now many other examples of genetic abnormalities in myeloid malignancies wherein the abnormality leads to disruption of cell signaling, often by way of activation of kinase cascades. *FLT3* is a tyrosine kinase receptor preferentially expressed on hematopoietic stem cells that mediates proliferation and differentiation. A unique mutation resulting in an internal tandem duplication leads to constitutive activation (i.e., always turned on) of this pathway in many forms of AML and other hematopoietic malignancies. Other examples of gene mutations that alter kinase cascades in myeloid or lymphoid cells include *c-KIT*, *NOTCH*, *JAK2*, and *RAS*. Many cyclin-dependent kinases are altered in lymphoid malignancies. The cyclin-dependent kinases serve to regulate tightly *cell cycle progression* through the synthesis, proteolysis, and phosphorylation of cyclins. Finally, another important molecular signaling pathway in cells involves programmed cell death, or apoptosis. This vital process allows organisms to eliminate redundant, damaged, aged, or infected cells. In the hematopoietic environment, apoptosis is essential to contain and control the massive expansion that the hematopoietic system is capable of generating at times of stress, infection, or hemorrhage. Caspases are a family of proteases that participate in the apoptotic cascade within cells that is triggered in response to proapoptotic signals. The culmination of this apoptotic cascade is cellular disassembly. The *BCL* family contains many genes, some of which are proapoptotic and some of which are antiapoptotic. Many of the various forms of non-Hodgkin lymphoma seem to contain disruptions of *BCL2*, *BCL6*, *BCL10*, or other members of the caspase and *BCL* family of genes comprising the apoptotic cascade.

The list of chromosomal and molecular aberrations known to occur in the various leukocyte neoplasms continues to grow on an almost daily basis. Indexing this list is far beyond the scope of this chapter, but some condensed lists are in Chapter 31. More complete indices can be found in other publications such as the WHO reclassification schema[1] or larger hematology textbooks.[5-8,10]

THERAPY FOR LEUKOCYTE NEOPLASMS

The various forms of therapy available today for leukocyte neoplasms can be roughly divided into the following categories: chemotherapy, radiation therapy, supportive therapy, targeted therapy, and stem cell transplantation. In contrast to many solid tumors, numerous hematologic malignancies now carry cure rates that are substantially higher than they were 2 to

3 decades ago. Many new and exciting therapies that are less toxic are now under development or already employed in patient settings. These therapies are bringing more optimism for the care of patients with leukocyte neoplasms than ever before. Choosing the best therapy must start, however, with an accurate diagnosis. Even the most effective therapies do not work if the wrong treatment is applied to the wrong patient. Implementing curative treatment strategies is a realistic goal for most patients with Hodgkin lymphoma, CML, hairy cell leukemia, and some forms of non-Hodgkin lymphoma and children with acute lymphoblastic leukemia. Cure may be attainable in other patients with acute lymphoblastic or myeloblastic leukemia, and long-term remissions may be attainable in adults with multiple myeloma. For other patients with leukocyte neoplasms such as mantle cell lymphoma, chronic lymphocytic leukemia, or a therapy-related leukemia, cure remains elusive, and therapy must be directed more toward attaining remissions or supportive care–type regimens.

Chemotherapy

Chemotherapy can be defined as the treatment of cancer with the use of compounds with antitumor properties, administered orally or parenterally. The methods of action of the chemotherapy drugs vary considerably. Chemotherapy agents can be classified in two ways: by their effects on the cell cycle and by their biochemical mechanism of action. Some chemotherapy drugs can affect only specific phases of the cell cycle (phase specific), whereas other drugs act without regard to the cell cycle (phase nonspecific) and affect any phase of the cell cycle. Agents in this latter category usually have a linear dose-response curve (i.e., the higher the dose, the more cells killed). There are two subgroups:

1. Cycle-specific agents, which kill cells that are moving through the cell cycle, regardless of whether the cells are in G_1, G_2, S, or M phase (e.g., alkylating agents, cisplatin).
2. Cycle-nonspecific agents, which kill nondividing cells or cells in the resting state (e.g., steroids and antitumor antibiotics).

Phase-specific agents are effective only if present during a certain phase in the cell cycle (Chapters 31 and 32). Within a certain dose range, agents of this category show no increase in killing of cells with a further increase in dosage. Examples include L-asparagine amidohydrolase (G_1 phase), antimetabolites such as methotrexate (S phase), and vinca alkaloids (M phase).[1]

Chemotherapeutic agents affect normal and neoplastic cells. The effect is most pronounced with rapidly dividing cells, such as those of the mucosa of the gastrointestinal tract and the bone marrow. This limits the dosage and usually determines the maximum tolerated dose for a patient. Chemotherapy agents are categorized in Table 29-1.

Alkylating Agents

The mechanism of alkylating agents is to ionize within cells, forming highly reactive free radicals that damage DNA. These agents act on any phase of the cell cycle. They include such drugs as nitrogen mustard, cyclophosphamide, chlorambucil, busulfan, and melphalan (Alkeran).

Plant Alkaloids

Plant alkaloids affect microtubules and interrupt the process of mitotic spindle formation during the metaphase stage of mitosis. These agents include vincristine and vinblastine.

Antitumor Antibiotics

Compounds derived from living microorganisms are termed *antibiotics*, and some have antitumor effects. Antibiotics inhibit RNA or DNA synthesis and interfere with the G_2 phase of the cell cycle. Commonly used tumor antibiotics include daunorubicin and doxorubicin (Adriamycin).

Antimetabolites

Antimetabolites interfere with the normal functions of various essential metabolites. Examples include methotrexate, folate antagonists, and the purine analogues such as 6-mercaptopurine and 6-thioguanine, which most often affect cells in S phase.

Glucocorticoids

The synthetic or natural steroids include compounds such as hydrocortisone, prednisone, dexamethasone, and prednisolone. Steroids have a lympholytic effect and affect nonproliferating cells and those in cycle. Protein synthesis and mitosis also may be inhibited.

Radiation Therapy

Shortly after the discovery of x-rays, their usefulness in the treatment of Hodgkin and non-Hodgkin lymphomas was described. Radiation kills cells by producing unstable ions that damage DNA and may cause instant or delayed death of the cell. The toxic effects of radiotherapy can occur during therapy or much later. Complications can be reduced through the use of combined anterior and posterior treatment ports and of maximal shielding techniques to prevent damage to normal tissues. The hematopoietic system, the gastrointestinal tract, and the skin are most often affected during radiotherapy. The toxic effects are usually reversible when radiation is stopped. The epithelium of the entire gastrointestinal tract is a rapidly dividing cellular system that is very sensitive to irradiation. There may be drying-up of saliva and loss of taste. If the stomach is irradiated, anorexia, nausea, and vomiting may occur. Intestinal radiation may result in malabsorption and diarrhea. Irradiated skin becomes erythematous and tender. Permanent loss of body hair and hyperpigmentation also may occur in irradiated areas. Spinal and pelvic irradiation can cause marrow suppression, sometimes lowering blood counts to the life-threatening range.

Supportive Therapy

Numerous substances that are naturally produced in the human body have now been cloned in the laboratory. Several are commercially produced and approved by the Food and

TABLE 29-1 Chemotherapy Agents

Agent	Other Names	Uses	Toxic Effects
Alkylating Agents			
Busulfan	Myleran	CML, pretransplantation	Myelosuppression, infertility
Cyclophosphamide	Cytoxan, Neosar	Lymphoma, MM, ALL, pretransplantation	Marrow suppression, N&V, cystitis
Nitrogen mustard	Mechlorethamine	Hodgkin lymphoma, NHL	Myelosuppression, N&V, infertility
Chlorambucil	Leukeran	CLL, Waldenström macroglobulinemia, NHL, Hodgkin disease	Myelosuppression, hair loss
Melphalan	Alkeran	MM	Myelosuppression
Carmustine	BCNU	Hodgkin disease, NHL, MM	Myelosuppression
Dacarbazine	DTIC	Hodgkin disease	Myelosuppression, N&V
Plant Alkaloids			
Vincristine	Oncovin	ALL, NHL, Hodgkin disease, CLL, MM	Neurotoxicity, hair loss
Vinblastine	Velban	ALL, NHL, Hodgkin disease, CLL, MM	Myelosuppression
Etoposide	VP-16	NHL, pretransplantation	Myelosuppression, hair loss
Antitumor Antibiotics			
Daunorubicin	Daunomycin	AML, ALL	Myelosuppression, cardiotoxicity, N&V, hair loss
Doxorubicin	Adriamycin	ALL, AML, Hodgkin disease, NHL, CLL, MM	Myelosuppression, cardiotoxicity, N&V, hair loss
Bleomycin	Bleo	Hodgkin lymphoma, NHL	Lung toxicity, gastrointestinal toxicity
Idarubicin	Idamycin	AML	Myelosuppression
Antimetabolites			
Methotrexate	Amethopterin, MTX	ALL, NHL	Myelosuppression, gastrointestinal toxicity
Ara-C	Cytosine arabinoside, cytarabine	AML, NHL, Hodgkin disease, hair loss	Myelosuppression, gastrointestinal toxicity
Mercaptopurine	6-MP	ALL, CML	Hepatotoxicity, myelosuppression
Thioguanine	6-TG	AML	Myelosuppression
Pentostatin	2'-Deoxycoformycin	Hairy cell leukemia, CLL, lymphomas	Neurotoxicity, myelosuppression
Fludarabine	—	CLL, lymphomas, Waldenström macroglobulinemia	Neurotoxicity, myelosuppression
2-CDA	CDA, 2-chlorodeoxyadenosine, 2-cladribine	Hairy cell leukemia, CLL, lymphomas, AML, Waldenström macroglobulinemia	Neurotoxicity, myelosuppression
Glucocorticoids			
Prednisone	—	ALL, CLL	Fluid retention, muscle weakness
Methylprednisolone	—	Hodgkin disease, NHL, AMM	Fluid retention, muscle weakness
Hydrocortisone	—	Hodgkin disease, NHL, AMM	Fluid retention, muscle weakness
Decadron	Dexamethasone	MM	Fluid retention, muscle weakness
Others			
Hydroxyurea	Hydrea	CML, PV, AMM	Leukopenia, N&V
Asparaginase	L-asparagine amidohydrolase	ALL, refractory NHL	Nephrotoxicity, N&V
Cisplatin	*Cis*-platinum	Solid tumors, Hodgkin disease, NHL	Nephrotoxicity, ototoxicity
Procarbazine	—	Hodgkin disease, NHL	Myelosuppression

ALL, acute lymphoblastic leukemia; AML, acute myeloid leukemia; AMM, agnogenic myeloid metaplasia; CLL, chronic lymphocytic leukemia; CML, chronic myelogenous leukemia; MM, multiple myeloma; NHL, non-Hodgkin lymphoma; N&V, nausea and vomiting.

Drug Administration and in general use in support of cancer patients, particularly patients with hematologic malignancies. Colony-stimulating factors (CSFs), or cytokines, normally act in the bone marrow microenvironment to stimulate blood cell formation. Erythropoietin is the main stimulatory CSF responsible for red blood cell formation. Normal erythropoietin and a long-acting formulation of this molecule are available to aid in the care of cancer patients with anemia induced by chemotherapy. Similarly, granulocyte colony-stimulating factor (G-CSF) and granulocyte-macrophage colony-stimulating factor (GM-CSF) are used to expand rapidly the number of mature neutrophils capable of fighting infection within the body. Recombinant forms of G-CSF and GM-CSF and a long-acting form of G-CSF are now approved by the FDA and in common practice in the support of cancer patients with neutropenia induced by chemotherapy. All of these CSFs have allowed physicians not only to improve the quality of life of their patients, but also have allowed for more efficient and effective delivery of chemotherapy regimens by preventing delays or dose reductions of chemotherapy courses owing to low blood counts.

Targeted Therapy

As more is learned about the specific genetic lesions that cause cancers, researchers work to develop targeted therapies that specifically "hit" the tumor cell and leave the normal cells untouched. They are in the initial stages of realizing this dream and are slowly moving away from "nonspecific" therapies such as chemotherapy and radiation therapy. The Philadelphia chromosomal abnormality [t(9;22)] associated with CML was first reported in 1960. The Philadelphia chromosome results from the juxtaposition of two genes, *bcr* and *abl*, and the resulting fusion protein has elevated tyrosine kinase activity. It took 40 years to develop an agent that specifically targets the product of the Philadelphia chromosome. Imatinib mesylate (Gleevec) is a tyrosine kinase inhibitor that inhibits the kinase activity of all proteins that contain ABL. Imatinib mesylate is not solely specific for the *bcr/abl* tyrosine kinase; it also inhibits the tyrosine kinase activity of *c-kit* receptor and platelet-derived growth factor. It is through the activity on these other receptors that imatinib has found usefulness in other tumors as a targeted therapeutic. In CML, however, imatinib mesylate has quickly become the new standard treatment for newly diagnosed patients who are not immediate transplant candidates (Chapter 34). Resistance to imatinib has developed in some CML cells, and second-generation, more powerful kinase inhibitors, such as dasatinib and nilotinib (AMN-107), are now being tested. Small molecule inhibitors such as imatinib are typically available in oral form and have relatively few side effects.

Rather than small molecule inhibitors, lymphoid neoplasms have relied more on monoclonal antibodies for targeted therapeutic strategies. Rituximab specifically targets the CD20 antigen present on many non-Hodgkin lymphoma cells. When the antibody binds to the lymphoma cell, complement is activated, and the cell lyses. Other possible scenarios leading to cell death with monoclonal antibodies include antibody-mediated cellular cytotoxicity or stimulation of apoptosis.[10] In contrast to small molecule inhibitors, monoclonal antibodies generally must be delivered by intravenous or subcutaneous route. Monoclonal antibodies such as rituximab have evolved from the original monoclonal antibodies that were derived from mice. Rituximab represents a humanized form of an antibody designed or modified to be "more human" so that the patient's immune system would not raise an antibody against the antibody. Additional modifications are now being developed, such as radioactively labeled monoclonal antibodies that would carry a killing dose of radioactivity directly to the mutated cell.

Stem Cell Transplantation

As more has been learned about hematopoietic stem cells, the therapeutic method of *bone marrow transplantation* has evolved to be more aptly termed *stem cell transplantation* because a variety of different sources in addition to bone marrow can be employed to obtain hematopoietic stem cells. Along with bone marrow, peripheral blood and umbilical cord blood are also rich sources of these cells. Regardless of the source, hematopoietic stem cells are considered *adult stem cells*, even when they come from umbilical cord blood, as opposed to *embryonic stem cells* that are the subject of considerable ethical debate. Stem cell transplantation still remains an expensive and rigorous treatment alternative. When the decision to transplant has been made and a donor has been found, an extensive hospital stay is usually required. The pretransplantation conditioning regimen uses high-dose therapy to kill the patient's cancer cells and bone marrow cells. This regimen reduces the body's immunity to dangerously low levels and necessitates special protective isolation. Granulocyte counts approaching 0 are commonly seen immediately before and after transplantation. After the infusion of donor stem cells, the recipient remains in a severely immunosuppressed condition for 2 weeks or more. Strict isolation of the patient at this point is crucial. Prophylactic antibiotics and intravenous nutrition are also essential in keeping the patient alive until the marrow engrafts. The return of granulocytes, reticulocytes, and platelets to normal levels is monitored closely in the peripheral blood. Hematology laboratory evaluation and management of red blood cell and platelet transfusions are crucial components of stem cell transplantation. After the patient's release from the hospital, the blood counts, along with bone marrow aspirate and core biopsy specimens, continue to be monitored to measure the progress of engraftment of the donor stem cells.

Stem cell transplantations for malignant disease have come from donors of three general types: (1) an identical twin donor (syngeneic transplant), (2) a donor genetically different from the recipient (allogeneic transplant) or (3) the patient's own marrow or peripheral blood stem cells (autologous transplant) (Fig. 29-2). Syngeneic transplants are most desirable because of the perfect match of cells. However, they are rare, for obvious reasons, and are not discussed further in this chapter.

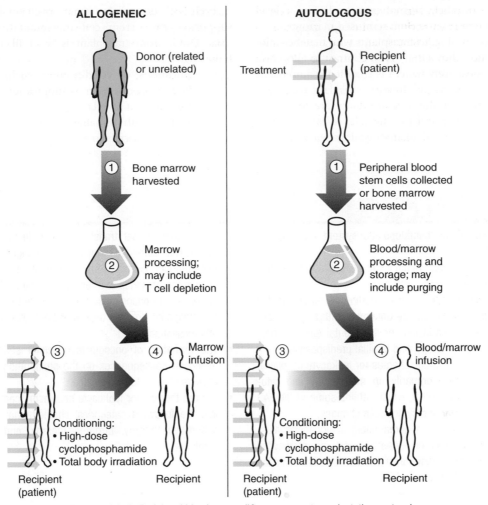

ALLOGENEIC

Donor (related or unrelated)

① Bone marrow harvested

② Marrow processing; may include T cell depletion

③ Conditioning:
• High-dose cyclophosphamide
• Total body irradiation

Recipient (patient)

④ Marrow infusion

Recipient

AUTOLOGOUS

Treatment

Recipient (patient)

① Peripheral blood stem cells collected or bone marrow harvested

② Blood/marrow processing and storage; may include purging

③ Conditioning:
• High-dose cyclophosphamide
• Total body irradiation

Recipient (patient)

④ Blood/marrow infusion

Recipient

Figure 29-2 Peripheral blood stem cell/bone marrow transplantation protocols.

Allogeneic Transplantation

Most stem cell donors are genetically different from the recipient. The intent is to match as many of the human leukocyte antigens (HLAs) as possible. Within any given family, there can be only four HLA haplotypes (two from the mother and two from the father), and there is one chance in four that any sibling of the patient will be HLA identical. In addition to HLA-identical grafts, HLA-mismatched donors within families have been used.

A major complication of an allogeneic marrow graft is the immunologic reaction of donor T cells against the tissues of the recipient, resulting in graft-versus-host disease (GVHD). Two forms of GVHD are recognized: acute and chronic. Acute GVHD develops in the immediate post-transplantation period or shortly thereafter. It is characterized by a skin rash, liver dysfunction, and diarrhea. Chronic GVHD, by definition, develops more than 100 days after transplantation. It is frequently generalized in the form of a multisystem autoimmune disease. Skin lesions, joint contractures, chronic hepatitis, malabsorption, and chronic obstructive pulmonary disease are frequent features of the chronic GVHD syndrome. Clinically significant

GVHD is associated with a risk of fatality that is 25 times higher than that in patients without GVHD.

T cell depletion of donor bone marrow is the most effective means of preventing acute and chronic GVHD, but this benefit has been offset by the substantial increase in the risk of leukemic relapse and infections. There is considerable clinical evidence that allogeneic grafts lower the risk of leukemic relapse. This antileukemia effect is most pronounced in the presence of chronic GVHD.

Autologous Transplantation

In autologous bone marrow transplantation, marrow is harvested from the patients and, after conditioning, transplanted back into them. Harvested remission marrow, presumably contaminated with malignant cells, is purged in vitro through the use of antileukemic monoclonal antibodies or cytotoxic drugs. After conditioning of the patient with cyclophosphamide, total body irradiation, or other techniques to eradicate remaining malignant cells, the purged autologous marrow is reinfused. Requirements for success in autologous transplants are the presence of normal pluripotent stem cells and reduction in the number of malignant cells to a level insufficient to cause recurrence from reinfused marrow.

A comparison of autologous transplants with matched allogeneic transplantation shows that (1) in contrast to allogeneic transplantation, almost every patient is eligible for autologous transplantation; (2) among autologous transplant recipients, post-transplantation morbidity and mortality are lower and hospital stays are shorter; and (3) the relapse rate is higher among autologous recipients than among allogeneic recipients.

Even with the continued improvement in technique and supportive care, stem cell transplantation carries many risks. Death from transplant is most likely caused by the following:

1. Complications of conditioning, such as infections or bleeding from bone marrow suppression
2. Complications of GVHD
3. Relapse (regrowth of malignant cells)
4. Failure of donor cells to engraft

CHAPTER at a GLANCE

- Most malignancies of the hematopoietic system are acquired genetic diseases.
- Most leukocyte malignancies are not localized, but rather systemic at the initiation of the malignant process.
- For most leukocyte neoplasms, causes directly related to the development of the malignancy are unknown, with a few exceptions. Some known causes include environmental toxins, certain viruses, previous chemotherapy, and familial predisposition.
- There are several classification schemas for leukocyte neoplasia, including the FAB, based primarily on morphology and cytochemical staining, and the WHO, which retains some of the FAB but emphasizes molecular and cytogenetic changes.
- Chromosomal translocations in hematologic malignancies illustrate that a single mutation, or series of mutations in stepwise fashion, can lead to malignant transformation by disrupting the molecular machinery of the cell.

- Most chromosomal translocations in leukemias involve oncogenes. The "dominant" transforming oncogene is able to alter the gene product and transform the cell into a malignant phenotype, even in the presence of a residual normal allele.
- In contrast to oncogenes, tumor suppressor genes contribute to the malignant process only after both alleles have been lost or otherwise inactivated.
- The formation of oncogenes or tumor suppressor genes has molecular consequences on the proliferation and differentiation aspects of hematologic tissues.
- Current therapy for leukocyte neoplasms can be roughly divided into the following categories: chemotherapy, radiation therapy, supportive therapy, targeted therapy, and stem cell transplantation.

REVIEW QUESTIONS

1. Which of the following is a virus known to cause lymphoid malignancies in humans?
   a. Human immunodeficiency virus
   b. Epstein-Barr virus
   c. Hepatitis B virus
   d. Parvovirus

2. Tumor suppressor genes cause cancers such as leukemia when mutations result in:
   a. Suppression of cell division
   b. Failure to prevent malignant processes
   c. Induction of cell division
   d. Excessive apoptosis

3. Oncogenes are said to act in a dominant fashion because:
   a. Cancer is a dominating disease that overtakes the individual's health.
   b. The mutation product affects (i.e., dominates) normal cells and the mutated cells.
   c. A mutation in a single allele is sufficient for malignancy to develop.
   d. They are inherited by autosomal dominant transmission.

4. All of the following are among the cellular abnormalities produced by oncogenes *except*:
   a. Apoptotic failure
   b. Suppression of DNA transcription
   c. Acceleration of DNA catabolism
   d. Disruption of cell cycle processes

5. Chemotherapeutic agents are divided into which two major subgroups?
   a. Phase specific and phase nonspecific
   b. Toxic and nontoxic
   c. Oral and intravenous
   d. Traditional and modern

6. G-CSF is provided as supportive treatment during leukemic treatment regimens to:
   a. Suppress GVHD
   b. Overcome anorexia
   c. Prevent anemia
   d. Reduce the risk of infection

7. Imatinib is an example of what type of leukemia treatment?
   a. Supportive care
   b. Chemotherapy
   c. Bone marrow conditioning agent
   d. Targeted therapy

8. Monoclonal antibodies may kill cancer cells by all of the following mechanisms *except*:
   a. Binding to the cancer cells and causing the immune system to destroy them
   b. Stimulating the production of anticancer cell antibodies by the patient's own immune system
   c. Activating complement on the cell surface
   d. Increasing the rate of apoptosis among the cancer cells

9. Hematopoietic stem cells for transplantation are harvested from all of the following tissues *except*:
   a. Bone marrow
   b. Peripheral blood
   c. Spleen
   d. Umbilical cord blood

10. Compared with autologous bone marrow transplantation, allogeneic transplantation has:
    a. Better long-term success (i.e., no relapse)
    b. Reduced occurrence of GVHD
    c. Lower mortality rate
    d. Better-tolerated conditioning phase

REFERENCES

1. Jaffe ES, Harris NL, Stein H, et al (eds): Pathology and genetics of tumours of haematopoietic and lymphoid tissues. In: World Health Organization Classification of Tumours. Lyon, France: IARC, 2001.

2. Rowley JD: A new consistent chromosomal abnormality in chronic myelogenous leukemia identified by quinacrine fluorescence and Giemsa staining [letter]. Nature 1973;243:290-293.

3. Taub R, Kirsch I, Morton C, et al: Translocation of the c-myc gene into the immunoglobulin heavy chain locus in human Burkitt lymphoma and murine plasmacytoma cells. Proc Natl Acad Sci U S A 1982;79:7837-7841.

4. Knudson AG: Hereditary cancer, oncogenes, and antioncogenes. Cancer Res 1985;45:1437-1443.

5. Dewald GW, Ketterling RP: Conventional cytogenetics and molecular cytogenetics in hematologic malignancies. In Hoffman R, Benz EJ, Shattil SJ, et al (eds): Hematology: Basic Principles and Practice, 4th ed. Philadelphia: Saunders, 2005:928-939.

6. Westbrook CA: The molecular basis of neoplasia. In Hoffman R, Benz EJ, Shattil SJ, et al (eds): Hematology: Basic Principles and Practice, 4th ed. Philadelphia: Saunders, 2005:941-954.

7. Huntly B, Gilliland DG: Pathobiology of acute myeloid leukemia. In Hoffman R, Benz EJ, Shattil SJ, et al (eds): Hematology: Basic Principles and Practice, 4th ed. Philadelphia: Saunders, 2005:1057-1069.

8. Gaidano G, Dalla-Favera R: Pathobiology of non-Hodgkin's lymphomas. In Hoffman R, Benz EJ, Shattil SJ, et al (eds): Hematology: Basic Principles and Practice, 4th ed. Philadelphia: Saunders, 2005:1307-1324.

9. Kurzrock R, Kantarjian HM, Druker BJ, et al: Philadelphia chromosome-positive leukemias: from basic mechanisms to molecular therapeutics. Ann Intern Med 2003;138:819-830.

10. Stewart SJ: Immunotherapy. In Greer JP, Foerster J, Lukens JN, et al (eds): Wintrobe's Clinical Hematology, 11th ed. Philadelphia: Lippincott, Williams & Wilkins, 2004:2157-2177.

30

Cytochemistry

Carol A. Bradford

OUTLINE

Basic Principle
Acceptable Specimens
  and Fixatives
Stains and Interpretations
Controls and
  Troubleshooting

OBJECTIVES

After completion of this chapter, the reader will be able to:

1. Discuss the purpose of performing cytochemical stains.
2. Determine appropriate specimen types, handling procedures, and fixatives for cytochemical stains, considering length of stability of specimens if staining is delayed.
3. Discuss the principles and cell staining patterns for the following tests: myeloperoxidase, Sudan black B, esterases, periodic acid-Schiff, leukocyte alkaline phosphatase, and leukocyte acid phosphatase.
4. Name the cell stage that is evaluated using the stains listed in #3.
5. Interpret the results of the stains listed in #3.
6. Discuss the selection of controls in cytochemical staining.
7. Describe routine troubleshooting in cytochemical techniques.

CASE STUDY

After studying the material in this chapter, the reader should be able to respond to the following case study:

A 38-year-old woman presented with a 2-month history of gingival bleeding and gingival hypertrophy. A complete blood count revealed: WBC count, 64×10^9/L; hemoglobin, 7.5 g/dL; and platelet count, 36×10^9/L. The peripheral blood smear and the bone marrow examination revealed greater than 80% abnormal mononuclear cells. The cytochemical characteristics of these cells were as follows:

Myeloperoxidase: Negative
Sudan black B: Negative

α-naphthyl butyrate esterase: Positive
Periodic acid–Schiff: Negative

1. What cell lines stain positive with esterases?
2. What general diagnosis is suggested by the complete blood count values?
3. Based on morphology and cytochemical staining, what is the classification of this disorder?

BASIC PRINCIPLE

Cytochemistry is the study of chemical elements found in cells. These elements may be enzymatic (e.g., peroxidase) or non-enzymatic (e.g., lipids and glycogen). Cellular morphology alone sometimes can be misleading or confusing. Since the early 20th century, cytochemical staining of cells has been a useful tool in differentiating hematopoietic diseases, especially acute and chronic leukemias. With the development of cell surface marker detection by flow cytometry and improved high-resolution techniques for cytogenetics, cytochemistry studies are used mostly in conjunction with these new technologies and not as the sole diagnostic tool. (Leukemias are discussed in Chapters 29, 36, and 37; cytogenetics, in Chapter 31; and flow cytometry, in Chapter 33.)

ACCEPTABLE SPECIMENS AND FIXATIVES

Many specimen types are adequate for cytochemical studies. Smears and imprints made from bone marrow, lymph nodes, spleen, or peripheral blood are preferred. In enzymatic techniques, fresh smears are used whenever possible to ensure optimal enzyme activity. Smears for nonenzymatic stains, such as periodic acid-Schiff (PAS) or Sudan black B (SBB), may remain stable for months if stored at room temperature.

Certain elements may be inhibited during the fixation of smears and imprints; it is important to use the proper fixative for the desired cytochemical stains. Fixatives containing alcohol (methanol or ethanol), acetone, formaldehyde, or a combination of these are commonly used for most cytochemistry studies.

STAINS AND INTERPRETATIONS

Myeloperoxidase

Myeloperoxidase (MPX) (Figs. 30-1 and 30-2) is an enzyme found in the primary granules of neutrophils, eosinophils, and, to a certain extent, monocytes. Lymphocytes do not exhibit MPX activity. This stain is useful for differentiating the blasts of acute myeloid leukemia from acute lymphoblastic leukemia (ALL).

Principle

When hydrogen peroxide is present, MPX oxidizes dye substrates, creating black to red-brown staining (depending on the substrate) at the site of the activity. Benzidine had been the substrate most often used, but because of its carcinogenic properties, other substrates such as 3,3'-diaminobenzidine or *p*-phenylenediamine dihydrochloride and catechol are currently used.[1-3]

Interpretation

MPX is present in the primary granules of myeloid cells, beginning at the promyelocyte stage and continuing throughout maturation. Leukemic myeloblasts also are usually positive. In many cases of the acute myeloid leukemias (without maturation, with maturation, and promyelocytic leukemia), it has been found that more than 80% of the blasts show MPX activity. Aüer rods found in leukemic blasts and promyelocytes are strongly MPX positive. Because of their strong MPX positivity, many Aüer rods that could not be seen with a Wright-Giemsa stain can be seen with the MPX stain.

Monocytes are MPX negative to weakly or diffusely positive. In contrast, lymphoblasts and lymphoid cells are MPX negative; in patients with ALL, less than 3% of the blasts show peroxidase positivity.[4-6]

It is important that the reaction in only the *blast* cells be used as the determining factor for the differentiation of acute leukemias. This is true for MPX and the other cytochemical stains that are mentioned in this chapter. The fact that maturing granulocytes are MPX positive is normal and has little or no diagnostic significance.

Sudan Black B

SBB (Fig. 30-3) is another useful staining technique for the differentiation of acute myeloid leukemia from ALL. The staining pattern is quite similar to that of MPX for the most part; SBB is possibly a little more sensitive for the early myeloid cells.

Principle

SBB stains lipids, such as sterols, neutral fats, and phospholipids, because of the solubility of the dye in lipid particles. These lipids are found in the primary and secondary granules of neutrophils and in the lysosomal granules of monocytes.[2,7]

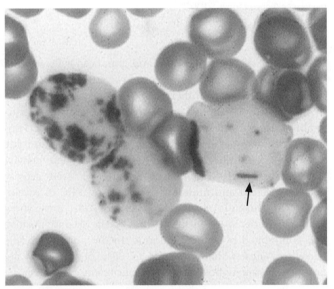

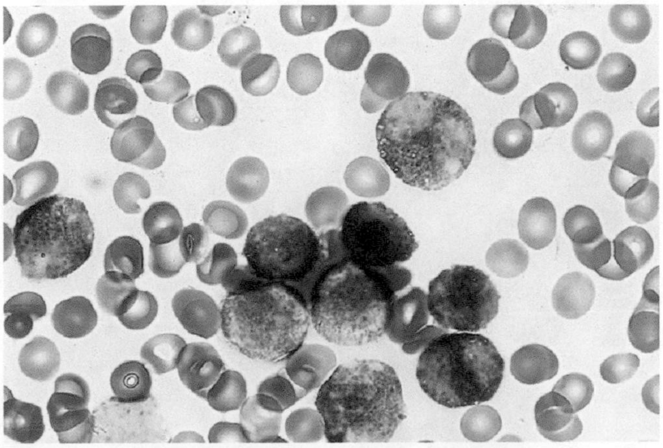

Figure 30-1 MPX stain showing positivity in early myeloid cells. Note Aüer rod at *arrow* (bone marrow, ×1000).

Figure 30-2 MPX stain showing strong positivity in leukemic promyelocytes, from a patient with acute promyelocytic leukemia (bone marrow, ×1000).

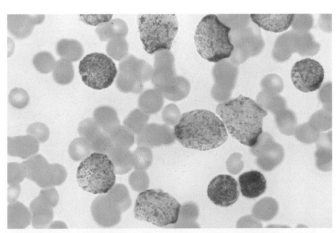

Figure 30-3 SBB reaction. The positivity increases with the maturity of the myeloid cell (bone marrow, ×1000).

Interpretation

Granulocytes (neutrophils) are SBB positive from the myeloblast through the maturation series. The staining becomes more intense as the cell matures, as a result of the increase in the numbers of the primary and secondary granules. Monocytic cells can be negative to weakly positive, showing diffuse activity. Lymphoid cells are generally negative. In ALL, less than 3% of the blast cells show positivity.[4-6]

Esterases

Esterase reactions are used to differentiate myeloblasts and neutrophilic granulocytes from cells of monocytic origin. There are nine isoenzymes of esterases present in leukocytes. Two substrate esters commonly used are α-naphthyl acetate and α-naphthyl butyrate (both nonspecific esterases). Naphthol AS-D chloroacetate esterase (specific) also may be used. The "specificity" refers to staining of only myelocytic cells, whereas nonspecific stains may show positivity in other cells as well.

Principle

Esterases hydrolyze an ester. A naphthol compound is released and combines with a diazonium salt (generally, hexazotized pararosaniline, hexazotized new fuchsin, or fast blue BB), producing a brightly colored compound at the site of the enzyme activity.[1,8]

Interpretation

Esterases can be used to distinguish acute leukemias that are myeloid from leukemias that are mostly cells of monocytic origin. When naphthol AS-D chloroacetate is used as a substrate, the reaction shows positivity in the myeloid cells and negativity to weak activity for the monocytic cells (Fig. 30-4). Chloroacetate esterase is present in the primary granules of neutrophils. Leukemic myeloblasts are generally positive. Aüer rods show positivity as well.

The reaction of α-naphthyl acetate esterase, in contrast to naphthol AS-D chloroacetate, produces strong positive activity in monocytes that can be inhibited with the addition of

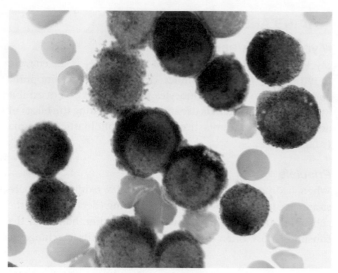

Figure 30-5 α-Naphthyl acetate esterase reaction showing positivity in monocytes (bone marrow, ×1000).

sodium fluoride.[4,9] Granulocytes and lymphoid cells are generally negative for nonspecific esterase (Figs. 30-5 and 30-6).

The reaction of α-naphthyl butyrate esterase is also positive in monocytes. α-Naphthyl butyrate is less sensitive than α-naphthyl acetate, but is more specific. Granulocytes and lymphoid cells are generally negative (Fig. 30-7). Myelomonocytic leukemia should show positive AS-D chloroacetate activity and positive α-naphthyl butyrate or α-naphthyl acetate activity because myeloid and monocytic cells are present. In myelomonocytic leukemia, at least 20% of the cells must show monocytic differentiation that is nonspecific esterase-positive and is inhibited by sodium fluoride. In the pure monocytic leukemias, greater than or equal to 80% of the blasts are nonspecific esterase-positive and specific esterase negative.

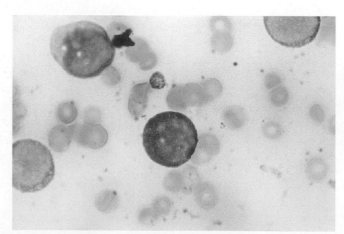

Figure 30-4 AS-D chloroacetate esterase showing positivity in two myeloid cells (bone marrow, ×1000).

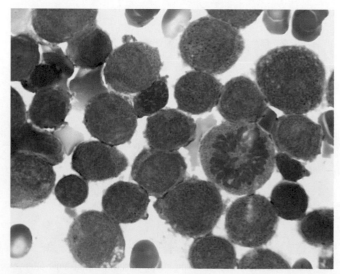

Figure 30-6 Same specimen as Figure 30-5 with sodium fluoride. The esterase reaction in the monocytes is inhibited (bone marrow, ×1000).

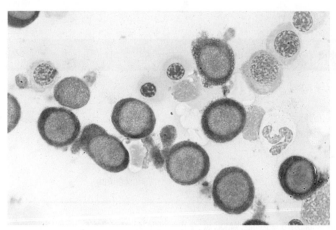

Figure 30-7 α-Naphthyl butyrate esterase positivity in cells of monocytic origin, from a patient with acute monocytic leukemia—poorly differentiated. Note the negative myeloid and erythroid precursors (bone marrow, ×1000).

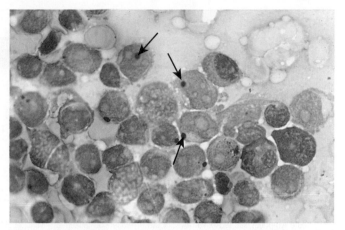

Figure 30-8 PAS reaction showing coarse (block) positivity, from a patient with ALL (bone marrow, ×1000).

Periodic Acid-Schiff

PAS staining may be helpful in the diagnosis of some ALLs and the erythroid type of acute myeloid leukemia.

Principle

Many different cell types contain glycogen. Periodic acid oxidizes glycogen, mucoproteins, and other high-molecular-weight carbohydrates to aldehydes. These aldehydes react with the colorless Schiff reagent, staining them a bright red-pink. The intensity of the staining depends on the number of aldehyde groups liberated by the periodic acid. The PAS stain pattern may be fine and diffuse, coarse and granular (block), or a mixture of both.

Interpretation

Granulocytes are PAS positive; the intensity of staining increases as the cell matures. Megakaryocytes exhibit finely diffuse staining, whereas platelets turn intensely red-pink. Normal erythrocyte precursors do not stain.

In ALL, cells show a varied staining pattern. Lymphoblasts of ALL may show a coarse block pattern of activity, a finely diffuse pattern, or a combination of the two patterns, or they may be negative. Cells from Burkitt lymphoma are generally negative (Fig. 30-8).[10,11]

In the erythroid type of acute myeloid leukemia, PAS-positive erythroblasts may be found. The positivity may be coarse and granular, especially in early normoblasts, or diffusely positive, which is more commonly seen in late normoblasts (Fig. 30-9).[12,13]

Factor VIII Antibodies

Megakaryoblastic leukemia requires immunocytochemical stains for an accurate diagnosis. Monoclonal or polyclonal antibodies against factor VIII–related antigen have given positive results in megakaryoblastic leukemia (Fig. 30-10).[14] A simplified cytochemistry reaction chart intended for quick reference is shown in Table 30-1.

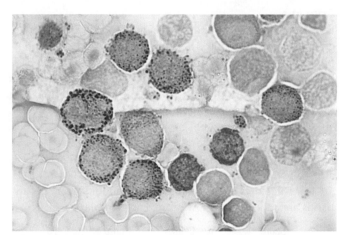

Figure 30-9 PAS reaction showing coarse granular positivity around the nucleus of early erythroid precursors, from a case of acute erythroid leukemia (bone marrow, ×1000).

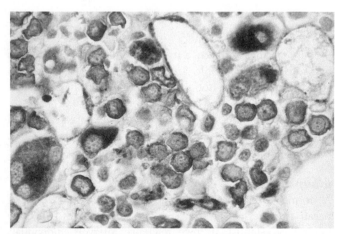

Figure 30-10 Positive factor VIII stain from a patient with acute megakaryocytic leukemia (bone marrow, ×1000).

Leukocyte Alkaline Phosphatase

Leukocyte alkaline phosphatase (LAP) enzyme activity is useful for differentiating chronic myelogenous leukemia from a leukemoid reaction that may be seen in severe infections.

TABLE 30-1 Simplified Acute Leukemia Reaction Chart

Condition	MPX	SBB	NASDA	ANBE	ANAE	PAS	Factor VIII
			CYTOCHEMICAL STAIN				
ALL	–	–	–	–/+ (focal)	–/+ (focal)	Varied	–
AML	+	+	+	–	–	Varied	–
AMML	+	+	+	+ (diffuse)	+ (diffuse)	Varied	–
AMoL	–	±	–	+ (diffuse)	+ (diffuse)	Varied	–
Erythroleukemia	*	*	*	–	–	+; blocky in pronormoblasts	–
Megakaryocytic leukemia	–	–	–	–	+ (localized)	–/+ (localized)	+

*Positive in myeloblasts; negative in normoblasts.

ALL, acute lymphoblastic leukemia; AML, acute myelogenous leukemia; AMML, acute myelomonocytic leukemia; AMoL, acute monocytic leukemia; ANAE, α-naphthyl acetate esterase; ANBE, α-naphthyl butyrate esterase; MPX, myeloperoxidase; NASDA, naphthol AS-D chloroacetate esterase; PAS, periodic acid-Schiff; SBB, Sudan black B.

Principle

LAP is an enzyme found in the membranes of secondary granules of neutrophils. The substrate naphthol AS-BI phosphate is hydrolyzed by the enzyme at an alkaline pH. This hydrolyzed substrate, in combination with a dye such as fast red-violet LB or fast blue BB, produces a colored precipitate at the site of the enzyme activity.

Scoring

LAP activity is scored in the mature polymorphonuclear cells and bands only. The activity scores range from 0 to 4+ (Fig. 30-11). The scores of 100 mature polymorphonuclear cells and bands are added for the LAP score. For example:

Score	No. Cells	Score × No. Cells
0	20	0
1	45	45
2	25	50
3	5	15
4	5	20
Total	100	130 = LAP score

Because scoring is subjective, it is recommended that two slides be scored by two people. These scores should agree within 10%. If the scores do not agree, a third slide from the patient must be scored.

Eosinophils do not show alkaline phosphatase activity and must not be mistaken for mature neutrophils with a score of zero. Eosinophils can be distinguished by their larger granules.

Interpretation

A normal LAP score should be between 20 and 100, but because of the scoring subjectivity, it is important that every laboratory establish its own reference intervals. Individuals with untreated chronic myelogenous leukemia have decreased LAP scores; individuals with leukemoid reactions have scores ranging from high-normal to increased. Other conditions producing higher scores include the third trimester of pregnancy and polycythemia vera. The score is normal in cases of secondary polycythemia. Conditions in which decreased scores are found include paroxysmal nocturnal hemoglobinuria,

sideroblastic anemia, and myelodysplastic disorders. A summary of LAP interpretation is shown in Table 30-2.

Acid Phosphatase (Tartrate Resistant)

Almost all blood cells contain seven nonerythroid isoenzymes of acid phosphatase: 0, 1, 2, 3, 3b, 4, and 5.[15,16] Hairy cells produce isoenzyme 5 in abundance. This makes the acid phosphatase stain a useful diagnostic tool for confirmation of hairy cell leukemia.

Principle

Acid phosphatase hydrolyzes the substrate naphthol AS-BI phosphoric acid. When hydrolyzed, this substrate couples with a dye such as fast garnet GBC and produces a red precipitate at the site of the enzyme activity. When L-(+)-tartaric acid is added, all isoenzymes except isoenzyme 5 are inhibited. Isoenzyme 5 is tartrate resistant. The term *TRAP* (tartrate-resistant acid phosphatase) *stain* is often used to denote this phenomenon.

Interpretation

Most hematopoietic cells show acid phosphatase activity. Granulocytes, lymphocytes, and monocytes all show positivity to some extent until the addition of L-(+)-tartaric acid. The activity is inhibited because isoenzyme 5 is lacking. Hairy cells, which contain isoenzyme 5, remain positive with the addition of L-(+)-tartaric acid. In hairy cell leukemia, at least two or more cells contain 40 or more red granules (Fig. 30-12, Table 30-3).[1]

TABLE 30-2 Results of Leukocyte Alkaline Phosphatase Stain

Finding	Score
Normal	20-100
Chronic myelogenous leukemia	<13
Leukemoid reaction	>100
Polycythemia vera	100-200
Secondary polycythemia	20-100

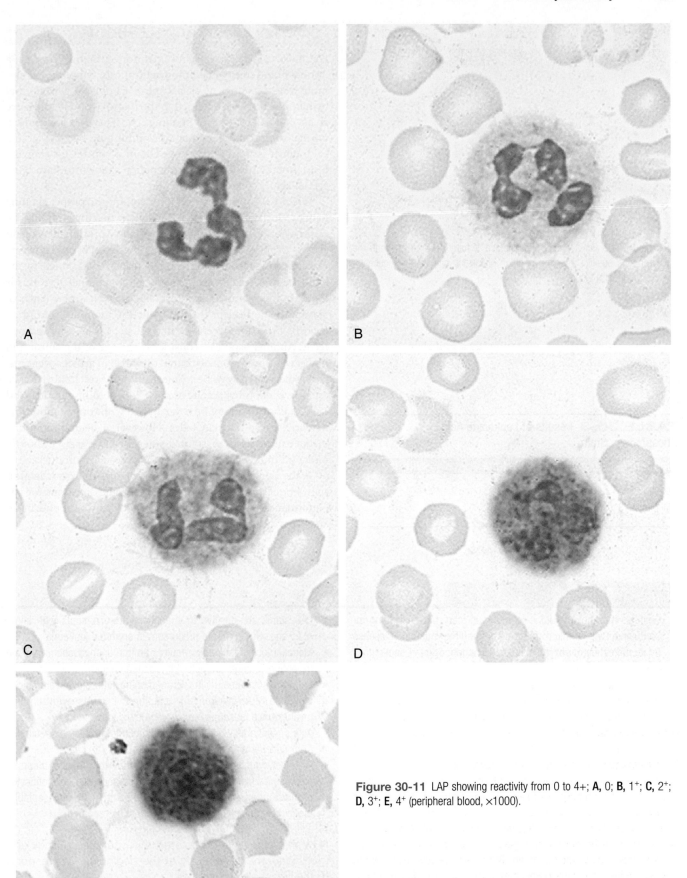

Figure 30-11 LAP showing reactivity from 0 to 4+; **A,** 0; **B,** 1⁺; **C,** 2⁺; **D,** 3⁺; **E,** 4⁺ (peripheral blood, ×1000).

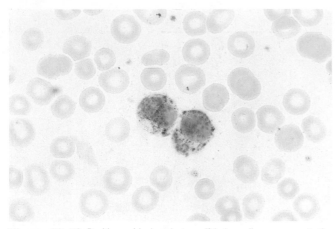

Figure 30-12 Positive acid phosphatase. If hairy cells are present, the stain remains positive after the addition of tartaric acid to the incubation mixture (peripheral blood, ×1000).

TABLE 30-3 Results of Leukocyte Acid Phosphatase Stain

Cell Type	Without Tartrate	With Tartrate
Lymphocytes	+	−
Hairy cells	+	+

CONTROLS AND TROUBLESHOOTING

For most cytochemical stains mentioned in this chapter, a normal blood smear containing neutrophils, lymphocytes, and monocytes is sufficient as a control sample. A few normal hematopoietic cells contained in the marrow aspirate can serve as an internal control for staining. For hairy cell leukemia, a normal smear can be used to show inhibition by L-(+)-tartaric acid, but it is more difficult to obtain a control for showing resistance. Only a smear from a patient known to have hairy cell leukemia could be used.

When the control slides do not exhibit the proper staining pattern, such as showing no activity when they should be positive or exhibiting the wrong color precipitate, certain aspects of the study should be investigated. Possibly a wrong reagent, no reagent, or an expired reagent was added to the test system. A reagent may have been contaminated; if this is the case, the examiner should make or open a new batch of reagent. If the reagent is acceptable, the examiner should go over the procedure to ensure that all steps were followed correctly. Another aspect to consider is the age of the smear and how it was stored. Some enzymes diminish in activity over time. Fresh smears are always best. Smears from the α-naphthyl acetate esterase, α-naphthyl acetate esterase with sodium fluoride, and TRAP stains should not be coverslipped with routine mounting media, because the skin fades. However, a neutral-mounting media can be used, or stained smears can be viewed directly under oil immersion with no effect on reaction products.[17]

If the control results are unacceptable, the cytochemical stain in question must be repeated. Specific directions for test performance are included in test kits or can be found in an atlas of cytochemistry.[1,18]

- Cellular morphology alone sometimes can be misleading or confusing. Cytochemical stains aid in the differentiation of disease by identification of enzymes, lipids, glycogen, or other substances in cells.
- Cytochemistry often is used in conjunction with morphology, immunohistochemistry, flow cytometry, cytogenetics, and molecular biologic techniques in establishing a diagnosis.
- Cytochemical reactions may be enzymatic or non-enzymatic. Fresh smears must be used to detect enzymatic activity, whereas nonenzymatic procedures may be performed on specimens that have been stored at room temperature.
- MPX stains primary granules and is useful in differentiating myeloid from lymphoid cells.
- SBB stains lipids and parallels the results of the MPX stain.
- Esterases help differentiate granulocytes and their precursors from cells of monocytic origin. Butyrate esterase is positive in monocytes but not in myeloid precursors, whereas naphthol AS-D chloroacetate esterase stains myeloid precursors.

- PAS stains are positive in specimens from patients with some ALLs and with erythroid precursors in erythroid leukemia.
- Megakaryocytic leukemia requires an immunohistochemical stain for antibodies against factor VIII–related antigen.
- LAP is most useful in distinguishing chronic myelogenous leukemia from leukemoid reactions. Patients with chronic myelogenous leukemia have a very low score.
- Acid phosphatase with tartrate inhibition is positive in specimens from patients with hairy cell leukemia.
- For most cytochemical stains mentioned in this chapter, a normal blood smear containing neutrophils, lymphocytes, and monocytes is sufficient as a control sample. If the controls are unacceptable, the cytochemical stain in question must be repeated.

Now that you have completed this chapter, go back and read again the case study at the beginning and respond to the questions presented.

REVIEW QUESTIONS

1. Smears for which of the following cytochemical stains may be stable for months if stored at room temperature?
   a. MPX
   b. SBB
   c. LAP
   d. α-Naphthyl butyrate esterase

2. Which cytochemical stain can be used to differentiate acute myeloblastic leukemia from ALL?
   a. TRAP
   b. LAP
   c. MPX
   d. α-Naphthyl acetate

3. SBB stains which of the following component of cells?
   a. Glycogen
   b. Lipids
   c. Structural proteins
   d. Enzymes

4. Hairy cells produce an abundance of which isoenzyme of acid phosphatase?
   a. 1
   b. 3b
   c. 4
   d. 5

5. An LAP score of 250 would be consistent with a diagnosis of:
   a. Normal
   b. Chronic myelogenous leukemia
   c. Hairy cell leukemia
   d. Leukemoid reaction

6. The cytochemical stain α-naphthyl butyrate is a non-specific esterase that stains cells of which lineage?
   a. Erythroid
   b. Monocytic
   c. Myeloid
   d. Lymphoid

7. Which of the following stains is assessed on mature neutrophils and bands?
   a. Leukocyte acid phosphatase
   b. LAP
   c. PAS
   d. SBB

8. Cytochemical staining was performed on the cells from a spleen imprint on a patient with suspected leukemia. The stains were performed promptly, and it was not surprising that the infiltrating cells stained positive for leukocyte acid phosphatase. The acid phosphatase stain was repeated on a second imprint, but the slide was pretreated with tartrate. The slide was still positive for acid phosphatase. This result points to which of the following conditions?
   a. Erythrocytic leukemia
   b. Acute myeloblastic leukemia
   c. Hairy cell leukemia
   d. Acute megakaryoblastic leukemia

9. A normal blood smear provides a suitable positive control for all of the following stains *except*:
   a. MPX
   b. α-Naphthyl acetate esterase
   c. Resistance to tartaric acid effect on acid phosphatase
   d. LAP

10. Which of the following is *not* a suitable fixative for slides that are to be cytochemically stained?
    a. TRIS buffer
    b. Methanol
    c. Acetone
    d. Formaldehyde

REFERENCES

1. Li C-Y, Yam LT, Sun T: Modern Modalities for the Diagnosis of Hematologic Neoplasms: Color Atlas/Text. New York: Igaku-Shoin, 1996.
2. Li C-Y, Yam LT: Cytochemistry and immunochemistry in hematologic diagnoses. Hematol Oncol Clin N Am 1994; 8:665-681.
3. Kaplow IS: Substitute for benzidine in myeloperoxidase stains [letter]. Am J Clin Pathol 1975;63:451.
4. Scott CS, Den Ottolander GJ, Swirsky GA, et al: Recommended procedures for the classification of acute leukemias. Leuk Lymphoma 1993;11:37-49.
5. Cheson BD, Cassileth DR, Schiffer CA, et al: Report of the National Cancer Institute–sponsored workshop on definitions of diagnosis and response in acute myeloid leukemia. J Clin Oncol 1990;8:813-819.
6. Head DR: Revised classification of acute myeloid leukemia. Leukemia 1996;10:1826-1831.
7. Hayhoe FJG: The cytochemical demonstration of lipids in blood and bone marrow cells. J Pathol Bacteriol 1953;65:413-421.
8. Li C-Y, Lam KW, Yam LT: Esterases in human leukocytes. J Histochem Cytochem 1973;21:1-12.
9. Wachstein M, Wolf G: The histochemical demonstration of esterase activity in human blood and bone marrow smears. J Histochem Cytochem 1958;6:457.
10. Lilleyman JS, Hann IM, Stevens RF, et al: Cytomorphology of childhood lymphoblastic leukaemia: a prospective study of 2000 patients. United Kingdom Medical Research Council's Working Party on Childhood Leukaemia. Br J Haematol 1992;81:52-57.
11. Flandrin G, Brouet JC, Daniel MT, et al: Acute leukemia with Burkitt's tumor cells: a study of six cases with special reference to lymphocyte surface markers. Blood 1975;45:183-188.
12. Davey FR, Abraham N, Brunetto VL, et al: Morphologic characteristics of erythroleukemia (acute myeloid leukemia; FAB-M6): a CALGB study. Am J Hematol 1995;49:29-38.
13. Quaglino D, Hayhoe FGJ: Periodic-acid-Schiff positivity in erythroblasts with special reference to Di Guglielmo's disease. Br J Haematol 1960;6:26-33.

14. Bennett JM, Catovsky D, Daniel MT, et al: Criteria for the diagnosis of acute leukemia of megakaryocyte lineage (M7). Ann Intern Med 1985;103:460-462.

15. Hoyer JD, Li C-Y, Yam LT, et al: Immunohistochemical demonstration of acid phosphatase isoenzyme 5 (tartrate-resistant) in paraffin sections of hairy cell leukemia and other hematologic disorders. Am J Clin Pathol 1997;108:308-315.

16. Li C-Y, Yam LT, Lam KW: Acid phosphatase isoenzyme in human leukocytes in normal and pathologic conditions. J Histochem Cytochem 1970;18:473-481.

17. Scott CS, Ottolander GJ, Swirsky D, et al: Recommended procedures for the classification of acute leukaemias. International Council for Standardization in Haematology (ICSH). Leuk Lymphoma, 1993;11:37-50.

18. Sun T, Li C-Y, Yan LT: Atlas of cytochemisty and immuno-cytochemisty of hematologic neoplasms. Chicago: American Society of Clinical Patholgists Press, 1985.

Cytogenetics

31

Gail H. Vance

OBJECTIVES

After completion of this chapter, the reader will be able to:

1. Describe chromosome structure and the methods used in chromosome identification.
2. Explain the basic laboratory techniques for preparing chromosomes for analysis.
3. Differentiate between numeric and structural chromosome abnormalities.
4. Discuss the importance of a karyotype in diagnosis and prognosis in cancer.
5. Explain the basic technique of fluorescence in situ hybridization (FISH).
6. Discuss the advantage of using FISH analysis in conjunction with G-banded analysis of cells.
7. Describe the types of chromosomal abnormalities that are detectable with cytogenetic methods.
8. Given the nomenclature of a chromosome mutation, be able to determine whether the abnormality is numeric or structural, which chromosomes are affected, the type of abnormality, and the portion of the chromosome affected.
9. Given a diagram of a G-banded generic chromosome, name the structures identifiable by light microscopy.

CASE STUDY

After studying the material in this chapter, the reader should be able to respond to the following case study:

A 54-year-old man presented to his physician with a history of fatigue, weight loss, and increased bruising over a 6-month period. A complete blood count was ordered, and the white blood cell count was elevated at $200 \times 10^9/L$. A bone marrow aspirate was sent for cytogenetic analysis. G-banded chromosome analysis of 20 cells from bone marrow cultures showed all cells to be Philadelphia chromosome positive as seen in chronic myelogenous leukemia (Fig. 31-1). Fluorescence in situ hybridization (FISH) studies, with the *BCR* and *ABL* gene probes (Vysis, Downer's Grove, Ill.), produced dual fusion signals, one on the derivative chromosome 9 and one on the derivative chromosome 22, characteristic of the Philadelphia chromosome with the juxtaposition of the *BCR* and *ABL* oncogenes (Fig. 31-2). The patient was treated with imatinib mesylate for the next 2 months. Another cytogenetic study was performed on a second bone marrow aspirate. This analysis showed that 12 of 20 cells analyzed were normal, 46,XY[12]; however, there were still 8 Philadelphia chromosome–positive cells: 46,XY,t(9;22)(q34; q11.2)[8].

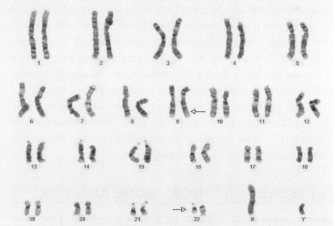

Figure 31-1 Karyotype from the patient in the case study showing a Philadelphia chromosome. (Courtesy of the Cytogenetics Laboratory, Indiana University School of Medicine.)

Continued

After studying the material in this chapter, the reader should be able to respond to the following case study:

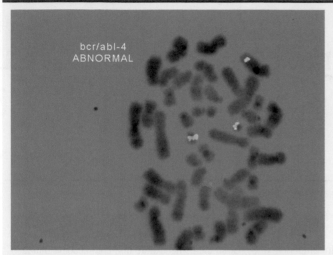

bcr/abl-4
ABNORMAL

Figure 31-2 A bone marrow metaphase from the case study patient hybridized with probes for *BCR* (green) and *ABL* (red) (Vysis). The fusion signals (yellow) represent the translocated chromosomes 9 and 22. (Courtesy of the Cytogenetics Laboratory, Indiana University School of Medicine.)

1. What is a G-banded chromosome analysis?
2. Is the described mutation an example of a numeric or structural abnormality? What type? Which chromosomes are involved? Explain.
3. What is FISH, and how does it complement standard chromosome analysis?

Cytogenetics is the study of chromosomes, their structure, and their inheritance. There are more than 30,000 genes in the human genome, most of which reside on the 46 chromosomes normally found in each somatic cell.

Chromosome disorders are classified as structural or numerical and involve the loss or gain or the rearrangement of a piece of a chromosome or the entire chromosome. Because each chromosome contains thousands of genes, a chromosomal abnormality that is observable by light microscopy causes the disruption of the action and interaction of hundreds of genes. Such disruptions often have a profound clinical effect. Chromosomal abnormalities are observed in approximately 0.6% of all live births.[1] The gain or loss of an entire chromosome other than a sex chromosome is usually incompatible with life and accounts for approximately 50% of first-trimester spontaneous abortions.[2] In leukemia, cytogenetic abnormalities are observed in more than 50% of bone marrow specimens. These recurring abnormalities often define the leukemia and indicate clinical prognosis.

REASONS FOR CHROMOSOME ANALYSIS

Chromosome analysis is an important diagnostic procedure in clinical medicine. Not only are chromosomal anomalies major causes of reproductive loss and birth defects, but also nonrandom chromosome abnormalities are recognized in many forms of cancer.

Physicians who care for patients of all ages may order karyotyping for analysis of mental retardation, infertility, ambiguous genitalia, short stature, fetal loss, risk of genetic or chromosomal disease, and cancer. In the following discussion, basic cytogenetic concepts are presented. This field is in a period of tremendous growth; supplementation of this chapter with the material in Chapter 32 is recommended.

CHROMOSOME STRUCTURE

Chromosome Architecture

A chromosome is formed from a single, long DNA molecule that contains a series of genes. The complementary double-helix structure of DNA was established in 1953 by Watson and Crick.[3] The backbone is a sugar-phosphate-sugar polymer. The sugar is deoxyribose. Attached to the backbone and filling the center of the helix are four nitrogen-containing bases. Two of these, adenine (A) and guanine (G), are purines, and the other two, cytosine (C) and thymine (T), are pyrimidines (Fig. 31-3).

The chromosomal DNA of the cell resides in the cell nucleus. This DNA and its accompanying protein are referred to as *chromatin*. During the cell cycle, at a stage called *mitosis*, the nuclear chromatin condenses approximately 10,000-fold to form chromosomes.[4] Each chromosome results from progressive folding and compaction of the entire nuclear chromatin. This condensation is achieved through multiple levels of helical coiling and supercoiling (Fig. 31-4).

Metaphase Chromosomes

Electron micrographs of metaphase chromosomes have provided models of chromosome structure. In the "beads-on-a-string" model of chromatin folding, the DNA helix is looped around a core of histone proteins.[5] This packaging unit is

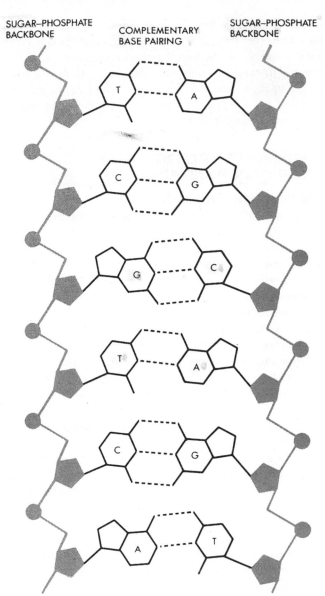

SUGAR–PHOSPHATE BACKBONE   COMPLEMENTARY BASE PAIRING   SUGAR–PHOSPHATE BACKBONE

Figure 31-3 The two DNA chains are held together by the pairing of bases on the interior of the helix. Hydrogen bonds unite a purine base with a pyrimidine base. (From Watson JD, Tooze J, Kurtz DT: Recombinant DNA: A Short Course. New York: WH Freeman, 1983:19. © 1983 James D. Watson, John Tooze, and David T. Kurtz. Used with the permission of WH Freeman and Company.)

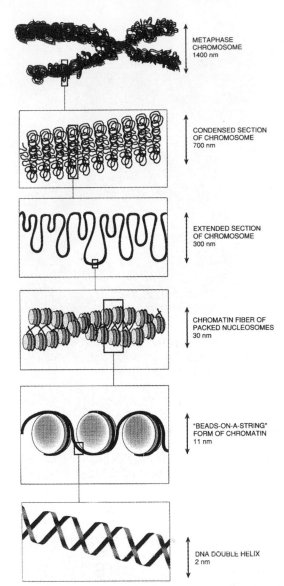

METAPHASE CHROMOSOME 1400 nm

CONDENSED SECTION OF CHROMOSOME 700 nm

EXTENDED SECTION OF CHROMOSOME 300 nm

CHROMATIN FIBER OF PACKED NUCLEOSOMES 30 nm

"BEADS-ON-A-STRING" FORM OF CHROMATIN 11 nm

DNA DOUBLE HELIX 2 nm

Figure 31-4 Chromosome structure. The folding and twisting of the DNA double helix. (From Gelehrter TD, Collins FS, Ginsberg D: Principles of Medical Genetics, 2nd ed. Philadelphia: Lippincott, Williams & Wilkins, 1998.)

known as a *nucleosome* and measures approximately 11 ηm in diameter.[6] Nucleosomes are coiled into regular twisting arrays to form an approximately 30-hm chromatin fiber. This fiber, called a *solenoid,* is condensed further and bent into a loop configuration. These loops extend at an angle from the main chromosome axis (Fig. 31-5).[7]

CHROMOSOME IDENTIFICATION

Cell Cycle

The cell cycle is divided into four stages: G_1, the growth period before DNA synthesis; S phase, DNA synthesis; G_2, the period after DNA synthesis; and M, mitosis or cell division, the

shortest phase of the cell cycle (Fig. 31-6). During mitosis, chromosomes are maximally condensed. While in mitosis, cells can be chemically treated to arrest cell progression through the cycle so that the chromosomes can be isolated and analyzed.

Chromosome Number

In 1956, Tijo and Levan[8] identified the correct number of human chromosomes as 46. This is the *diploid* chromosome number and is determined by counting the chromosomes in dividing somatic cells. The designation for the diploid number is *2n*. Gametes (ovum and sperm) have half the diploid number (23). This is called the *haploid* number of chromosomes and is designated *n*. Different species have different numbers of chromosomes. The reindeer has a relatively high chromosome number for a mammal (2n = 76), whereas the Indian muntjac, or barking deer, has a very low chromosome number (2n = 7 in the male and 2n = 6 in the female).[9]

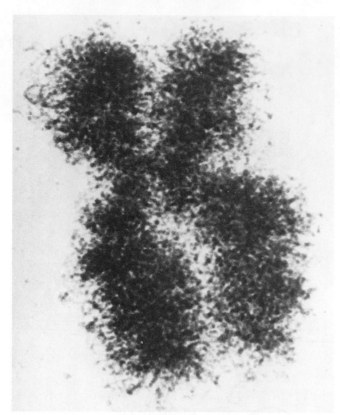

Figure 31-5 Electron microscopy of a human metaphase chromosome showing the looped chromatin attached to a central scaffold. (From Bahr GF: Chromosomes and chromatin structure. In Yunis JJ [ed]: Molecular Structure of Human Chromosomes. New York: Academic Press, 1977:161; reprinted with permission.)

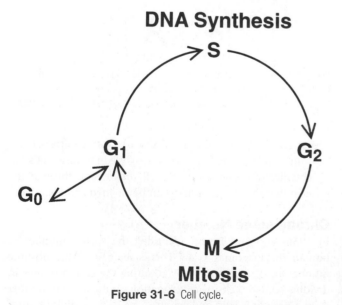

Figure 31-6 Cell cycle.

Chromosome Size and Type

Before banding, chromosomes were categorized by size and the location of the centromere (primary constriction) and assigned to one of seven groups A through G. Group A includes chromosome pairs 1, 2, and 3. These are the largest chromo-somes, and their centromeres are located approximately in the middle (i.e., they are metacentric). Group B chromosomes, pairs 4 and 5, are the next largest chromosomes; their cen-tromeres are off-center, or submetacentric. Group G refers to the smallest chromosomes, pairs 21 and 22, whose cen-tromeres are located at the ends of the chromosomes and are designated as acrocentric (Fig. 31-7).

TECHNIQUES OF CHROMOSOME PREPARATION AND ANALYSIS

Chromosome Preparation

Tissues used for chromosome analysis are composed of cells that exhibit an inherently high mitotic rate (bone marrow cells) or can be stimulated to divide in culture (peripheral blood lymphocytes). Special harvesting procedures are estab-lished for each tissue. Mitogens such as phytohemagglutinin or pokeweed mitogen are added to peripheral blood cultures. Phytohemagglutinin stimulates primarily T cells to divide,[10] whereas pokeweed preferentially stimulates B lymphocytes.[11]

Chromosomes can be obtained from replicating cells by arresting the cell in prometaphase or metaphase. Cells from the peripheral blood or bone marrow are cultured in media for 24 to 72 hours. In standard peripheral blood cultures, a mitogen is added to stimulate cellular division. Neoplastic cells are spontaneously dividing, however, and generally do not require stimulation with a mitogen. After the cell cultures have grown for the appropriate period, Colcemid, an analogue of colchicine, is added to inhibit or disrupt the mitotic spindle fiber attachment to the chromosome. After culture, cells are exposed to a hypotonic (potassium chloride) solution that causes the chromosomes to spread apart. A fixative of methanol and acetic acid is added that "hardens" cells and removes pro-teinaceous material. Cells are dropped onto cold, wet glass slides to achieve optimal dispersal of the chromosomes and aged before banding.

Chromosome Banding

Analysis of each individual chromosome is made possible by staining the chromosome with dye. The name *chromosome* is derived from Greek: *chroma*, meaning "color," and *soma*, mean-ing "body." Hence *chromosome* means "colored body". In 1969, Caspersson et al[12] were the first investigators to stain chromo-somes successfully with a fluorochrome dye. Using quinicrine mustard, which binds to adenine-thymine (AT)–rich areas of the chromosome, they were able to distinguish a banding pattern unique to each individual chromosome. This banding pattern, called *Q-banding*, differentiates the chromosome into bands of differing lengths and relative brightness (Fig. 31-8). The most brightly fluorescent bands of the 46 human chromo-somes are the distal end of the Y chromosome, the centromeric regions of chromosomes 3 and 4, and the acrocentric chromo-somes (13, 14, 15, 21, and 22). Humans are polymorphic (i.e., their chromosomes contain differing amounts of heterochro-matin) for these bright bands, just as they are for the size and fluorescent properties of the satellites located on the short arms of the acrocentric chromosomes.

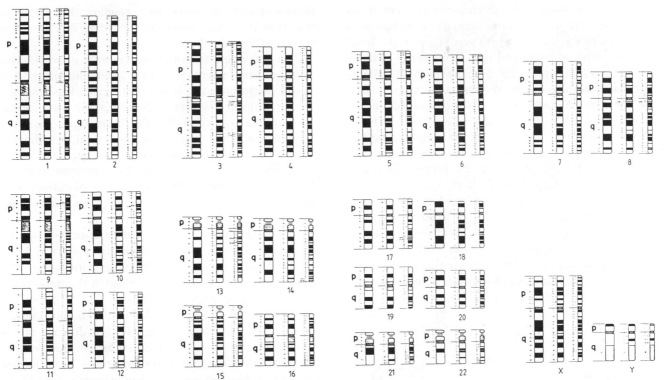

Figure 31-7 International System for Human Cytogenetic Nomenclature. (From Report of the Standing Committee on Human Cytogenetic Nomenclature. Basel, Switzerland: Karger, 1985; reprinted with permission.)

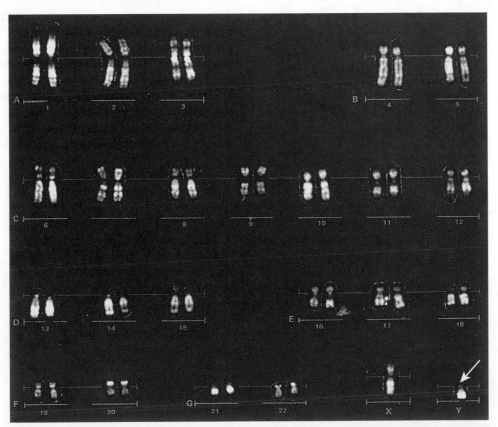

Figure 31-8 Q-banded preparation. Note the intense brilliance of Yq. (Courtesy of the Cytogenetics Laboratory, Indiana University School of Medicine.)

Other stains are used to identify chromosomes, but in contrast to Q-banding, these methods normally necessitate some pretreatment of the slide to be analyzed. Giemsa (G) bands can be obtained by pretreating the chromosomes with the proteolytic enzyme trypsin. GTG banding means "G-banding by Giemsa with the use of trypsin". Giemsa, similar to quinicrine mustard, positively stains AT-rich areas of the chromosome. The dark bands are called *G-positive* (+) bands. Guanine-cytosine (GC)-rich areas of the chromosome have little affinity for the dye and are referred to as *G-negative* (−) bands. G+ bands correspond with the brightly fluorescing bands of Q-banding (Figs. 31-9 and 31-10).

R-banding (reverse Giemsa or G-bands) requires pretreatment of the chromosomes with hot (80° to 90° C) alkali and subsequent staining with Giemsa. As the name implies, this banding pattern is the opposite of Giemsa staining: that is, the G+ bands by Giemsa are light with R-banding, and the G-bands by Giemsa are dark with R-banding. R-banding is often useful for the study of structural changes of the ends of the chromosomes or telomeres. By G-banding, these areas are often light (G−), and thus with R-banding they would be stained positively and be dark.

C-banding stains the centromere (primary constriction) of the chromosome and the surrounding heterochromatin. Constitutive heterochromatin is a special type of late-replicating repetitive DNA that is located primarily at the centromere of the chromosome. In C-banding, the chromosomes are treated first with an acid and then with an alkali (barium hydroxide) before Giemsa staining. C-banding is most intense in human chromosomes 1, 9, and 16 and the Y chromosome. Polymorphisms are also observed in the C-bands from different individuals. These polymorphisms have no clinical significance (Fig. 31-11).

Specific chromosomal regions that are associated with the nucleoli in interphase cells are called *nucleolar organizer regions* (NORs). NORs contain tandemly repeated ribosomal RNA genes. NORs can be differentially stained in chromosomes by a silver stain called *AG-NOR banding*.

Chromosome banding is visible after chromosome condensation, and the banding pattern observed depends on the degree of condensation. By examining human chromosomes early in mitosis, it has been possible to estimate a total haploid genome (23 chromosomes) with approximately 2000 AT-rich (G+) bands.[13] The later the stage of mitosis, the more condensed the chromosome and the fewer total G+ bands.

Metaphase Analysis

After banding, slides are scanned under a light microscope with a low-power objective lens (10×). When a metaphase has been selected for analysis, a 63× or 100× oil immersion objective lens is used. Each metaphase is analyzed first for chromosome number. Then each individual chromosome is analyzed for its banding pattern. A normal somatic cell contains 46 chromosomes, which includes 2 sex chromosomes. Any variation in number and banding pattern is recorded by the technologist. At least 20 metaphase cells are analyzed from leukocyte cultures. If abnormalities are noted, the technologist

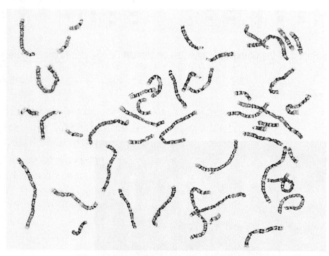

Figure 31-9 Normal male metaphase.

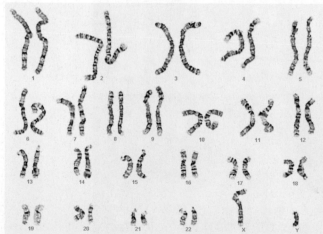

Figure 31-10 Normal male karyotype: GTG-banded preparations. (Courtesy of the Cytogenetics Laboratory, Indiana University School of Medicine.)

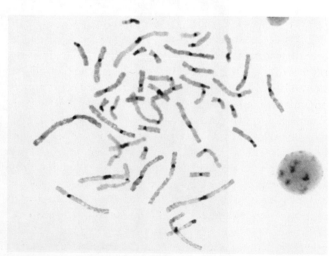

Figure 31-11 C-banded male metaphase. (Courtesy of the Cytogenetics Laboratory, Indiana University School of Medicine.)

General FISH Protocol

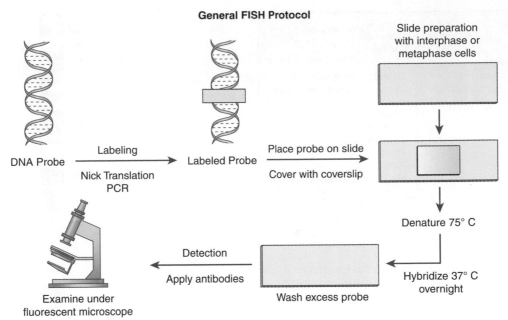

Figure 31-12 General FISH protocol.

may need to analyze additional cells. Computer imaging or photography is used to confirm and record the microscopic analysis. Metaphase cells are selected for imaging on the basis of (1) containing the modal number of chromosomes, (2) having sharply banded chromosomes, (3) containing no artifacts, and (4) having little or no chromosome overlap.[13]

Non-Radioactive In Situ Hybridization

Use of new molecular methods coupled with standard karyotype analysis is improving chromosomal detection capability beyond that of the light microscope. DNA or RNA probes labeled with either fluorescent or enzymatic detection systems are being hybridized directly to metaphase or interphase cells on the glass microscope slide. These probes usually belong to one of three classes: (1) probes for repetitive DNA sequences, primarily generated from centromeric DNA; (2) whole-chromosome probes that include segments of an entire single chromosome; and (3) specific loci or single copy probes.

Fluorescence in situ hybridization (FISH) is a molecular technique commonly used in cytogenetic laboratories. FISH studies are a valuable adjunct to the diagnostic workup and can be used for prognostic stratification, response to treatment, and minimal residual disease. In FISH, the DNA or RNA probe is labeled directly with a fluorophor or indirectly labeled with a hapten, such as biotin, digoxygenin, or dinitrophenyl. Target DNA is treated with heat and formamide to denature the double-stranded DNA, rendering it single-stranded. The target DNA anneals to a similarly denatured, single-stranded, fluorescently labeled DNA or RNA probe with a complementary sequence. After hybridization, the unbound and nonspecifically bound probe is removed by a series of stringent washes, and the cells are counterstained for visualization. If using a hapten label, specific antibodies to the hapten are applied to the cells. These antibodies carry a fluorescent tag. After the

antibodies bind to the DNA or RNA, the cells are washed, and an antifade/counterstain solution is applied. Slides are ready for analysis using a fluorescence microscope to detect and localize the signal (Fig. 31-12).

In situ hybridization with centromere or whole-chromosome painting probes can be used to identify individual chromosomes (Fig. 31-13). Marker chromosomes are found in neoplastic and non-neoplastic specimens and represent chromatin material that has been structurally altered and cannot be identified by a G-band pattern. FISH with a centromere or paint probe, or both, is often helpful in identifying the chromosome of origin (Fig. 31-14).[14]

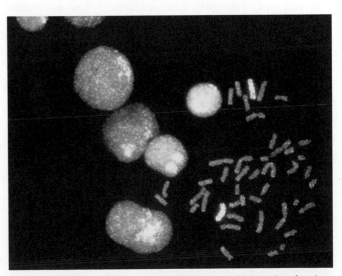

Figure 31-13 A metaphase is "painted" with multiple probes for chromosome 7, producing a fluorescent signal. (Courtesy of the Cytogenetics Laboratory, Indiana University School of Medicine.)

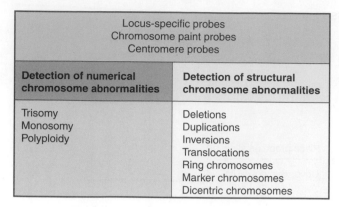

Locus-specific probes Chromosome paint probes Centromere probes	
Detection of numerical chromosome abnormalities	**Detection of structural chromosome abnormalities**
Trisomy Monosomy Polyploidy	Deletions Duplications Inversions Translocations Ring chromosomes Marker chromosomes Dicentric chromosomes

Figure 31-14 FISH in the clinical laboratory.

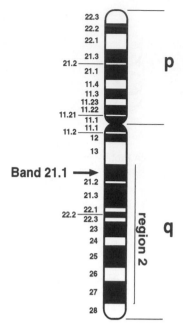

Figure 31-15 Banding pattern of the human X chromosome at the 550-band level.

Specific loci probes can be used to detect structural and numerical abnormalities in cancer (e.g., chronic myelogenous leukemia). FISH also has been extremely helpful in mapping anonymous segments of DNA to chromosomes.

Dividing (metaphase) and nondividing (interphase) cells can be analyzed with FISH. The use of uncultured cells, such as bone marrow smears, allows for a quick FISH result that can be reported in 24 hours. Also, in some cultured bone marrow samples, the number of dividing cells may be limited and insufficient to make a cytogenetic diagnosis by G-banded metaphase analysis. FISH performed on interphase (nondividing) cells with probes for a specific translocation may provide the diagnosis. FISH also can be performed on paraffin-embedded tissue sections, fine needle aspirations, and touch preparations from lymph nodes or solid tumors.

CYTOGENETIC NOMENCLATURE

Banding techniques enabled scientists to identify each chromosome pair by a characteristic banding pattern. In 1971 the Paris conference for nomenclature of human chromosomes was convened to designate a nomenclature system to describe the regions and specific bands of the chromosomes. The chromosome arms were designated *p* (petite) for the short arm and *q* for the long arm. The regions in each arm and the bands contained within each region were numbered consecutively, from the centromere outward to the telomere. To designate a specific region of the chromosome, the chromosome number is written first, followed by location on the short or long arm, then the region of the arm, and finally the specific band. *Xq21* designates the long arm of the X chromosome, region 2, band 1. To designate a sub-band, a decimal point is placed after the original band designation, followed by the number assigned to the sub-band: Xq21.1 (Fig. 31-15).

Cytogenetic nomenclature is a uniform code used by cytogeneticists to communicate chromosome abnormalities. Each nomenclature string begins with the modal number of chromosomes followed by the sex chromosome designation. A normal male karyotype is designated 46,XY, and a normal female karyotype is designated 46,XX. If abnormalities are observed in the cell, the abnormalities are listed in the order of modal chromosome number, sex chromosomes, and autosomes. A cell with trisomy of chromosome 8 (three copies of chromosome 8) in a male is written as 47,XY,+8. The number of cells with this abnormality is indicated in brackets. If 20 cells were examined, trisomy 8 was found in 10 cells, and the remainder were normal, the nomenclature would be written as 47,XY,+8[10]/46,XY[10]. Translocations are designated *t*, with the lowest chromosome number listed first. So a translocation between the short arm of chromosome 12 at band p13 and the long arm of chromosome 21 at band q22 is written as: t(12;21)(p13;q22). A semicolon is used to separate the chromosomes. Deletions are written with the abbreviation *del* preceding the chromosome. A deletion of the long arm of chromosome 5 at band 31 is written as del(5)(q31). There are no spaces entered in nomenclature except between abbreviations.[15]

CHROMOSOME ABNORMALITIES

There are many types of chromosome defects, such as deletions, inversions, ring formations, trisomies, and polyploidy. All these defects can be grouped into two major types: defects involving an abnormality in the *number* of chromosomes and defects involving *structural* changes in one or more chromosomes.

Numeric Abnormalities

Numeric abnormalities often are subclassified into aneuploidy and polyploidy. *Aneuploidy* refers to any number of chromosomes that is not a multiple of the haploid number (23 chromosomes). The common forms of aneuploidy in humans are trisomy (the presence of an extra chromosome) and monosomy (the absence of a single chromosome). Aneuploidy is

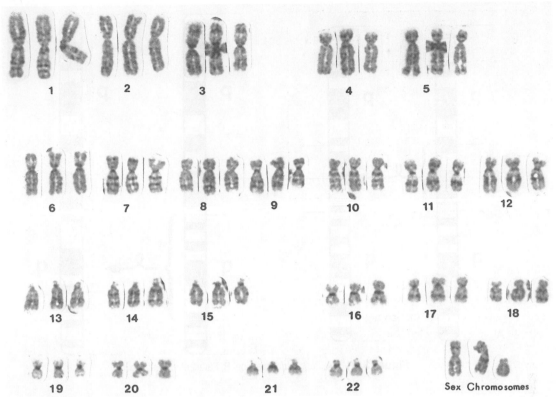

Figure 31-16 A triploid karyotype, 69,XXY. (Courtesy of the Cytogenetics Laboratory, Indiana University School of Medicine.)

the result of nondisjunction, the failure of chromosomes to separate normally during cell division. Nondisjunction can occur during the two types of cell division: meiosis or mitosis. During mitosis, a cell divides once to produce two cells that are identical to the parent cell. Meiosis is a special type of cell division that is used to generate male and female gametes (sperm and ova). In contrast to mitosis, meiosis entails two cell divisions, meiosis I and meiosis II. The end result is a cell with 23 chromosomes, which is the haploid number (n).

In polyploidy, the chromosome number is greater than 46 but is always an exact multiple of the haploid chromosome number of 23. A karyotype with 69 chromosomes is called *triploidy* (Fig. 31-16). A karyotype with 92 chromosomes is called *tetraploidy*.

In cancer, numerical abnormalities in the karyotype may be classified further based on the modal number of chromosomes in a neoplastic clone. *Hypodiploid* refers to a cell with fewer than 46 chromosomes; *near-haploid* cells have from 23 up to approximately 34 chromosomes (Fig. 31-17); *hyperdiploid* cells have greater than 46 chromosomes. *High hyperdiploidy* refers to a chromosome number greater than 50. Finally, the term *pseudodiploid* is used to describe a cell with 46 chromosome and structural abnormalities.

Structural Aberrations

Structural rearrangements result from breakage of a chromosome region with loss or subsequent rejoining in an abnormal combination. Structural rearrangements are defined as *balanced* (no loss or gain of genetic chromatin) or *unbalanced* (addition

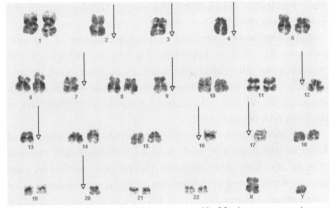

Figure 31-17 A hypodiploid karyotype with 36 chromosomes, (arrows indicate a missing chromosome).

or loss of genetic material). Structural rearrangements of single chromosomes include inversions, deletions, isochromosomes, ring formations, insertions, translocations, and duplications. *Inversions* (Inv) involve one or two breaks in a single chromosome, followed by a 180-degree switch of the segment between the breaks with no loss or gain of material. If the chromosomal material involves the centromere, the inversion is called *pericentric*. If the material that is inverted does not include the centromere, the inversion is called *paracentric* (Fig. 31-18).

Interstitial *deletions* arise after two breaks in the same chromosome and loss of the segment between the breaks. Terminal deletions (loss of chromosomal material from the end of a

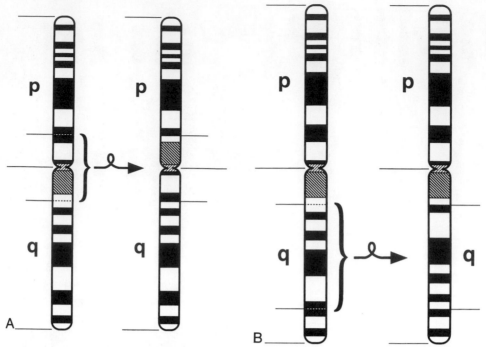

Figure 31-18 A, Pericentric inversion. **B,** Paracentric inversion.

chromosome) and interstitial deletions involve the loss of genetic material. The clinical consequence to the individual with a deletion depends on the extent and location of the deletion (Fig. 31-19).

Isochromosomes arise from abnormal division of the centromeres that divides perpendicular to the long axis of the chromosome rather than parallel to it or from breakage and reunion in chromatin adjacent to the centromere. Each resulting daughter cell has a chromosome in which the short arm or the long arm is duplicated.

Ring chromosomes can result from breakage and reunion of a single chromosome with loss of chromosomal material outside the ring. Alternatively, one or both telomeres may join to form a ring chromosome without significant loss of chromosomal material.

Insertions involve movement of a segment of a chromosome from one area of the chromosome to another area of the same chromosome or movement to another chromosome. The segment is released as a result of two breaks, and the insertion occurs at the site of another break; there are usually three chromosome breaks for an insertion to occur, unless the material inserted is from a terminal segment.

Duplication means partial trisomy for part of a chromosome. This can result from an unbalanced insertion or unequal crossing-over in meiosis or mitosis.

Translocations occur when there is breakage in two chromosomes, and each of the broken pieces reunites with another chromosome. If chromatin is neither lost nor gained, the exchange is called a *balanced reciprocal translocation*. A reciprocal translocation is balanced if all chromatin material is present. A

loss or gain of a rearranged chromosome results in monosomy or trisomy for a segment of the chromosome, however, leading to an imbalance of genetic material.

Another type of translocation involving breakage and reunion near the centromeric regions of two acrocentric chromosomes is known as a *Robertsonian translocation*. Effectively this is a fusion between two whole chromosomes rather than exchange of material as in a reciprocal translocation. These translocations are among the most common balanced structural rearrangements seen in the general population, with a frequency of 0.09% to 0.1%.[16] All five human acrocentric autosomes (13, 14, 15, 21, and 22) are capable of forming a Robertsonian translocation. In this case, the resulting balanced karyotype has only 45 chromosomes, which includes the translocated chromosomes (Fig. 31-20).

CANCER CYTOGENETICS

Cancer cytogenetics is a field that has been built on discovery of nonrandom chromosome abnormalities in many types of cancer. In hematologic neoplasia, specific structural rearrangements are associated with distinct subtypes of leukemia that have characteristic morphologic and clinical features. Cytogenetic analysis of malignant cells can help determine the diagnosis and probable prognosis of a hematologic malignancy, assist the oncologist in the selection of appropriate therapy, and aid in monitoring the effects of therapy. Bone marrow is the tissue most frequently used to study the cytogenetics of a hematologic malignancy. Unstimulated peripheral blood and bone marrow trephine biopsy samples

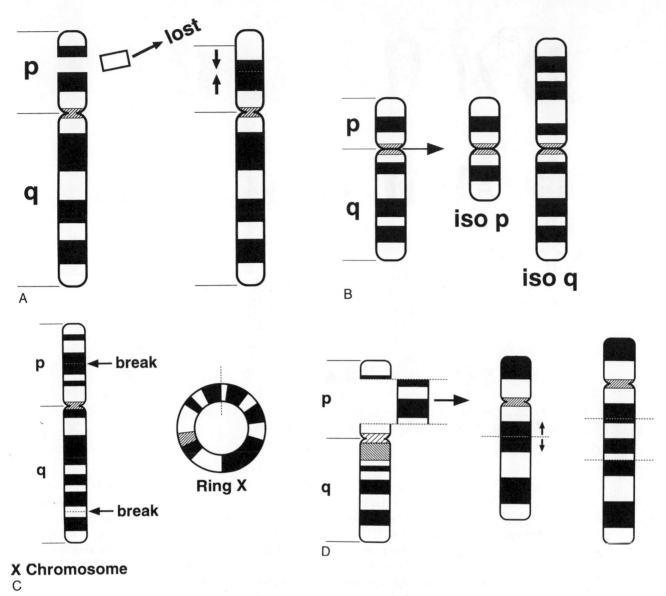

Figure 31-19 **A,** Interstitial deletion. **B,** Isochromosome. **C,** Ring chromosome. **D,** Insertion.

also may be analyzed. Cytogenetic analysis of cancer involving other organ systems can be performed from solid tissue obtained during surgery or by needle biopsy. Chromosomal defects in cancer include a wide range of numeric abnormalities and structural rearrangements (Table 31-1).

Cancer results from multiple and sequential genetic mutations occurring in a somatic cell. At some juncture, a critical mutation occurs, and the cell becomes self-perpetuating or clonal. A *clone* is a cell population derived from a single progenitor.[15] In cytogenetics, a clone exists if two or more cells contain the same structural abnormality or supernumerary marker chromosome or if three or more cells are missing the same chromosome. The primary aberration or stemline of a clone is a cytogenetic abnormality that is frequently observed as the sole abnormality associated with the cancer. The secondary aberration or sideline includes additional abnormal-

ities to the primary aberration.[15] In chronic myelogenous leukemia, the primary aberration is the Philadelphia chromosome resulting from a translocation between chromosomes 9 and 22, t(9;22)(q34;q11.2). A sideline of this clone would include secondary abnormalities, such as trisomy for chromosome 8, written as +8,t(9;22)(q34;q11.2).

Leukemia

Leukemias are clonal proliferations of malignant leukocytes that arise initially in the bone marrow before disseminating to the peripheral blood, lymph nodes, and other organs. They are broadly classified by the type of blood cell giving rise to the clonal proliferation (lymphoid or myeloid) and the clinical course (acute or chronic) of the disease. The four main leukemia categories include acute lymphoblastic leukemia, acute myeloid leukemia, chronic lymphocytic leukemia, and

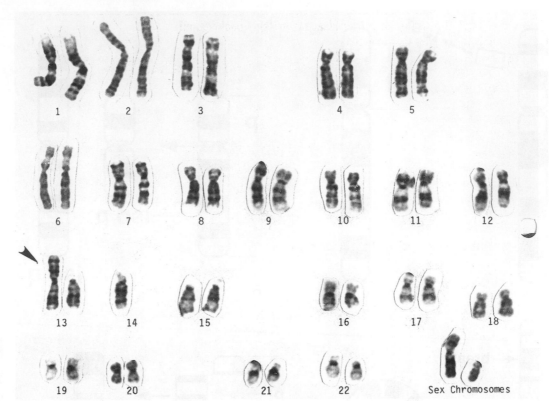

Figure 31-20 A balanced Robertsonian translocation between chromosomes 13 and 14, 45,XY,der(13;14)(q10;q10). (Courtesy of the Cytogenetics Laboratory, Indiana University School of Medicine.)

chronic myelogenous leukemia. The World Health Organization (WHO) classification for myeloid malignancies has classified acute myeloid leukemias (AMLs) into genetic subgroups based on the primary cytogenetic aberration (Box 31-1).[17] There are four subtypes: AML with recurrent cytogenetic abnormalities, AML with multilineage dysplasia, AML and myelodysplasia as a result of therapy, and AML not otherwise classified (Chapter 36). Some of the divisions of the French-American-British (FAB) classification[18] are included in the "not otherwise classified" category. The WHO has classified acute myeloid leukemias into genetic subgroups based on the primary cytogenetic aberration (Box 31-1)[17] and lymphoid leukemias by precursor cell type, B or T (Chapter 36).

BOX 31-1   Acute Myeloid Leukemia with Recurrent Genetic Abnormalities

- Acute myeloid leukemia with t(8;21)(q22;q22); *RUNX/CBFA2T1*
- Acute myeloid leukemia with abnormal bone marrow eosinophils inv(16)(p13.1q22) or t(16;16)(p13.1;q22); *MYH11/CBFβ*
- Acute promyelocytic leukemia, acute myeloid leukemia with t(15;17)(q24;q21); *PML/RARA*
- Acute myeloid leukemia with 11q23 *(MLL)* abnormalities

Modified from Jaffe E, Harris NL, Stein H, et al (eds): WHO Classification of Tumours: Tumours of Haematopoietic and Lymphoid Tissues. Lyon: IARC Press, 2001.

Chronic Myelogenous Leukemia

The first malignancy associated with a specific chromosome defect was chronic myelocytic leukemia, in which approximately 95% of patients were found to have a Philadelphia chromosome, t(9;22)(q34; q11.2).[19,20] The Philadelphia chromosome represents a balanced translocation between the long arms of chromosomes 9 and 22. At the molecular level, the gene for *ABL*, an oncogene, joins a gene on chromosome 22 named *BCR*. The result of the fusion of these two genes is a new fusion protein of about 210 kD with growth-promoting capabilities that over-ride normal cell regulatory mechanisms (Figs. 31-21 and 31-22) (Chapter 34).[21] The fusion protein activates tyrosine kinase signaling to drive proliferation of the cell. This signaling can be blocked by imatinib mesylate (STI-571/Gleevec; Novartis Pharmaceuticals; East Hanover, N.J.).[22] Patient response to imatinib can be monitored by cytogenetics and FISH. At diagnosis, the characteristic karyotype is the presence of the Philadelphia chromosome in all cells analyzed. After treatment for several months with imatinib mesylate, the karyotype typically has a mixture of abnormal cells with the Philadelphia chromosome and normal cells indicating patient response to therapy. *Complete response* is defined as a bone marrow karyotype with only normal cells. Often, a therapeutic response is monitored using peripheral blood instead of a bone marrow aspirate. In contrast to the bone marrow, peripheral blood does not house spontaneously dividing cells. As a result, chromosomal analysis of an unstimulated peripheral blood specimen often is unsuccessful because of the absence

TABLE 31-1 Common Translocations in Hematopoietic and Lymphoid Neoplasia and Sarcoma

Tumor Type	Karyotype	Genes
Myeloid Leukemias		
CML and pre-B-ALL	t(9;22)(q34;q11.2)	BCR/ABL1
AML-M2	t(8;21)(q22;q22)	CBFA2T1/RUNX1
AML-M2	t(7;11)(p15;p15)	HOXA9/NUP98
AML-M3	t(15;17)(q24;q21.1)	PML/RARA
AML-M3, atypical	t(11;17)(q23;q21.1	PZLF/RARA
AML-M3, atypical	t(11;17)(q13;q21.1)	NUMA/RARA
AML-M4 eosinophilia	inv(16)(p13.1q22)	MYH11/CBFB
CMML	t(5;12)(q33;p13)	PDGFRB/ETV6
B Cell Leukemias and Lymphomas		
Pre-pre-B ALL	t(12;21)(p13;q22)	ETV6/RUNX1
	t(1;19)(q23;p13.3)	PBX1/TCF3
B-ALL/AML	t(4;11)(q21;q23)	AF4/MLL
Burkitt lymphoma	t(8;14)(q24;q32.3)	MYC/IGH
	t(2;8)(p12;q24)	IGK/MYC
	t(8;22)(q24;q11.2)	MYC/IGL
Mantle cell lymphoma	t(11;14)(q13;q32.3)	CCND1/IGH
Follicular lymphoma	t(14;18)(q32.3;q21.3)	IGH/BCL2
Diffuse large B cell lymphoma	t(3;14)(q27;q32.3)	BCL6/IGH
Lymphoplasmacytic lymphoma	t(9;14)(p13;q32.3)	PAX5/IGH
MALT lymphoma	t(14;18)(q32.3;q21)	IGH/MALT1
	t(11;18)(q21;q21)	BIRC3/MALT1
	t(1;14)(p22;q32.3)	BCL10/IGH
T Cell Leukemias/Lymphomas		
T-ALL	del(1)(p32p32) or	
	del(1)(p32p36)	SIL/TAL1
T-ALL	t(7;11)(q35;p13)	I MO2/TRB
ALCL	t(2;5)(p23;q35)	ALK/NPM
Sarcomas and Tumors of Bone and Soft Tissue		
Alveolar rhabdomyosarcoma	t(2;13)(q35;q14.1)	PAX3/FOXO1A
	t(1;13)(p36.2;q14.1)	PAX7/FOXO1A
Ewing sarcoma/PNET	t(11;22)(q24;q12)	FLI1/EWSR1
	t(21;22)(q22.3;q12)	ERG/EWSR1
	t(7;22)(p22;q12)	ETV1/EWSR1
Clear cell sarcoma	t(12;22)(q13;q12)	ATF1/EWSR1
Myxoid liposarcoma	t(12;16)(q13;p11.2)	DDIT3/FUS
	t(12;22)(q13;q12)	DDIT3/EWSR1
Synovial sarcoma	t(X;18)(p11.2;q11.2)	SSX1 or 2/SYT
Alveolar soft part sarcoma	t(X;17)(p11.2;q25)	TFE3/ASPSCR1

ALCL, anaplastic large cell leukemia; ALL, acute lymphoblastic leukemia; AML, acute myeloid leukemia; CML, chronic myelogenous leukemia; CMML, chronic myelomonocytic leukemia; MALT, mucosa-associated lymphoid tissue; PNET, primitive neuroectodermal tumor.

of dividing cells. In these cases, FISH with probes for the specific abnormality may be performed on interphase cells of the peripheral blood specimen to search for chromosomally abnormal cells. This is an important advantage of FISH technology.

Acute Leukemia

The Philadelphia chromosome also is observed in acute leukemia. It is seen in about 20% of adults with acute lymphoblastic leukemia, 2% to 5% of children with acute lymphoblastic leukemia, and 1% of patients with acute myeloid

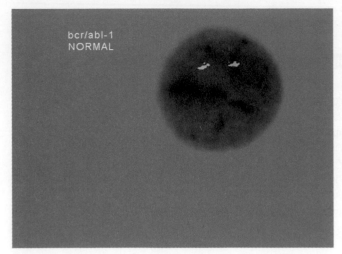

Figure 31-21 Normal bone marrow interphase cell hybridized with the *BCR* (green) and *ABL* (red) genes (Vysis). The two red and two green signals represent the genes on the normal chromosomes 9 and 22. (Courtesy of the Cytogenetics Laboratory, Indiana University School of Medicine.)

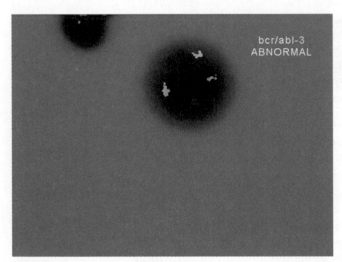

Figure 31-22 Abnormal bone marrow interphase cell with one *BCR* (green) and one *ABL* (red) signal (Vysis) representing the untranslocated chromosomes and two fusion signals from the derivative chromosomes 9 and 22. (Courtesy of the Cytogenetics Laboratory, Indiana University School of Medicine.)

monly found in infants with acute lymphoblastic leukemia. Rearrangements of the *AF4* gene on chromosome 4 and the *MLL* gene on chromosome 11 occur in this translocation.[26] Disruption of the *MLL* gene is seen in both acute lymphoblastic and acute myeloid leukemia (Figs. 31-23 and 31-24)

The acute myeloid leukemias are subdivided into several morphologic classifications ranging from M_0 to M_7 according to the FAB classification[18,27-29] (Chapter 36). Characteristic chromosome translocations are associated with some subgroups and were incorporated into the subsequent WHO classification. Among them is a translocation between the long arm of chromosome 8 and the long arm of chromosome 21,

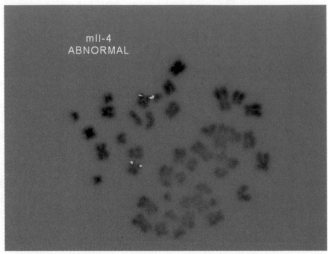

Figure 31-23 Bone marrow metaphase cell with fusion *MLL* signal on the normal chromosome 11 and split red and green signals on the translocated chromosomes, representing a disruption of the *MLL* gene. (Courtesy of the Cytogenetics Laboratory, Indiana University School of Medicine.)

leukemia.[23-25] In childhood acute lymphoblastic leukemia, chromosome number is crucial for predicting the severity of the leukemia. Children whose leukemic cells contain more than 50 chromosomes but with no structural abnormalities have the best prognosis for complete recovery with therapy. Recurring translocations observed in acute lymphoblastic leukemia include t(4;11)(q21;q23), t(12;21)(p13;q22), and t(1;19)(q23;p13.3). Each translocation is associated with a prognostic outcome and assists oncologists in determining patient therapy. The t(4;11) is the translocation most com-

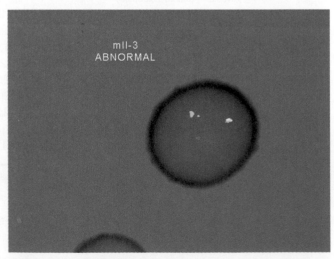

Figure 31-24 Bone marrow interphase cell with a fusion signal and split red and green signals from the *MLL* gene. (Courtesy of the Cytogenetics Laboratory, Indiana University School of Medicine.)

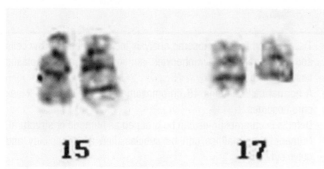

Figure 31-25 Bone marrow metaphase chromosomes 15 and 17 homologues showing a translocation between the long arms of chromosomes 15 and 17, t(15;17)(q22;q21), diagnostic of acute promyelocytic leukemia. The abnormal chromosomes are on the right. (Courtesy of the Cytogenetics Laboratory, Indiana University School of Medicine.)

Solid Tumors

Similar to the recurring structural and numeric chromosome defects observed in the hematologic malignancies, a wide range of abnormalities have been found in solid tumors. Most of these abnormalities confer a proliferative advantage on the malignant cell and serve as useful prognostic indicators. Amplification of the gene, *HER2*, a transmembrane growth factor receptor, is associated with an aggressive form of invasive breast cancer.[31] FISH with probes for the *HER2* gene and an internal control (17 centromere) can determine if there is gene amplification in the tumor (Fig. 31-27).[32] If amplification is present by FISH, the patient is eligible for targeted therapy with a monoclonal antibody, trastuzumab (Fig. 31-28).[33] FISH for *HER2* typically is performed on tissue sections from the paraffin-embedded tumor block.

t(8;21)(q22;q22), which is representative of acute myeloid leukemia with maturation. Acute promyelocytic leukemia is associated with a translocation between the long arms of chromosomes 15 and 17, t(15;17)(q24;q21) (Fig. 31-25). A pericentric inversion of chromosome 16, inv(16)(p13.2q22) is seen in acute myeloid leukemia with increased eosinophils. The inversion juxtaposes the core binding factor β (CBF-β) with the myosin heavy chain gene (*MYH11*) to form a new fusion protein (Fig. 31-26).[30] These recurring translocations have enabled researchers to localize genes crucial to cell growth and regulation. As with acute lymphoblastic leukemia, the particular translocation predicts patient prognosis and response to therapy and is critical for deciding therapeutic strategies. Understanding the molecular consequences of the cytogenetic mutations, like the BCR/ABL translocation, provides the opportunity to develop targeted therapies.

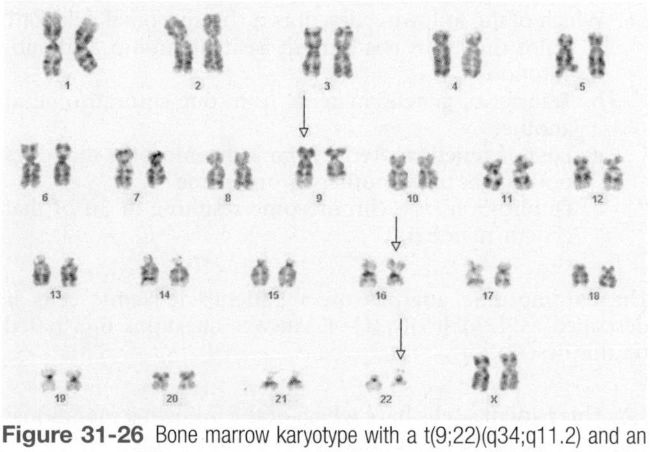

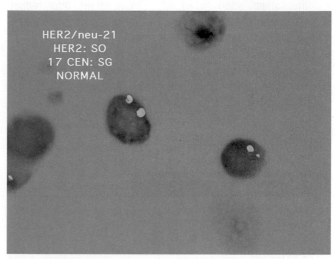

Figure 31-27 Normal interphase nuclei from a paraffin-embedded tissue hybridized with probes for *HER2* (red) and the chromosome 17 centromere (green) (Vysis). Two green and two red signals per cell.

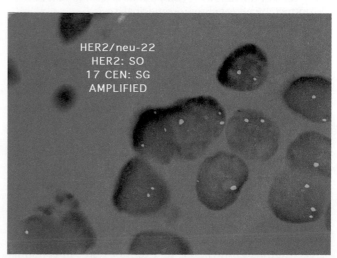

Figure 31-28 Abnormal nuclei from paraffin-embedded tissue section showing amplification of the *HER2* gene (red).

Figure 31-26 Bone marrow karyotype with a t(9;22)(q34;q11.2) and an inverted chromosome 16, inv(16)(p13.1q22), from a patient with acute myeloid leukemia. (Courtesy of the Cytogenetics Laboratory, Indiana University School of Medicine.)

CHAPTER at a GLANCE

- Cytogenetics is the study of chromosome structure and inheritance.
- Chromosome disorders may be structural or numeric, involving the rearrangement or the loss or gain of a piece of a chromosome or the entire chromosome.
- Nonrandom chromosome abnormalities are associated with cancer.
- A chromosome is composed of a complementary double helix of DNA. Attached to the backbone of deoxyribose are adenine (A), guanine (G), cytosine (C), and thymidine (T).
- During mitosis, cells can be chemically treated to arrest cell progression in metaphase so that chromosomes can be analyzed.
- Q-banding differentiates chromosomes into bands of different widths and relative brightness, showing a banding pattern unique to each individual chromosome.
- Other stains used to identify chromosomes may require pretreatment of the slide for analysis. These include G-banding, R-banding, C-banding, and AG-NOR banding.
- FISH, a molecular technique, uses DNA or RNA probes and fluorescence microscopy to identify individual chromosomes. Metaphase and interphase cells can be analyzed by FISH.

- Tissues used for chromosome analysis include bone marrow cells and peripheral blood lymphocytes, amniotic fluid, non-neoplastic tissue, and tumors.
- A normal cell contains 46 chromosomes, which includes 2 sex chromosomes.
- Defects in chromosomes can be grouped as numeric or structural. Numeric abnormalities can be subclassified as aneuploidy and polyploidy.
- Structural rearrangements include inversions, deletions, isochromosomes, ring formations, insertions, translocations, and duplications.
- Specific structural rearrangements are associated with distinct subtypes of leukemias, and analysis may assist in diagnosis, prognosis, and monitoring of therapy. Solid tumors also may be analyzed using cytogenetics.

Now that you have completed this chapter, go back and read again the case study at the beginning and respond to the questions presented.

REVIEW QUESTIONS

1. *G-banding* refers to the technique of staining chromosomes:
   a. To isolate those in G group (i.e. chromosomes 21 and 22).
   b. In the G_0 or resting stage
   c. Using Giemsa stain
   d. To emphasize area high in guanine residues

2. Which of the following compounds is used to halt mitosis in metaphase for chromosome analyses?
   a. Imatinib
   b. Fluoroscein
   c. Trypsin
   d. Colchicine

3. One arm of a chromosome has 30 bands. Which of them would be nearest the centromere?
   a. Band 1
   b. Band 15
   c. Band 30

4. Which of the following is NOT an advantage of the use of FISH?
   a. Can be used on non-dividing cells
   b. Can be used on paraffin-embedded tissue
   c. Can detect mutations that do not result in abnormal banding patterns
   d. Must be performed on dividing cells

5. Which of the following types of mutations would likely NOT be detectable with cytogenetic banding techniques?
   a. Point mutation resulting in a single amino acid substitution
   b. Transfer of genetic material from one chromosome to another
   c. Loss of genetic material from a chromosome that does not appear on any other chromosome
   d. Duplication of a chromosome resulting in 3n of that genetic material

6. Which of the following describes a chromosomal deletion?
   a. Point mutation resulting in a single amino acid substitution
   b. Transfer of genetic material from one chromosome to another
   c. Loss of genetic material from a chromosome that does not appear on any other chromosome
   d. Duplication of a chromosome resulting in 3n of that genetic material

The chromosome analysis on a patient's leukemic cells is described as 47/del(5)(q31)+4. Answer questions 6–8 based on this description.

7. This patient's cells have which of the following mutations?
   a. Loss of the entire number 31 chromosome
   b. Loss of the entire number 5 chromosome
   c. Loss of a portion of the short arm of chromosome 4
   d. Loss of a portion of the long arm of chromosome 5

8. What other mutation is present in this patient's cells?
   a. Polyploidy
   b. Tetraploidy
   c. An extra chromosome 4
   d. Four copies of chromosome 5

9. This patient's leukemic cells demonstrate chromosomal:
   a. Structural defects only
   b. Numeric defects only
   c. Both structural and numeric defects

10. *Aneuploidy* would describe:
   a. A total chromosome number that is a multiple of the haploid number
   b. A total chromosome number that reflects a loss or gain of a single chromosome
   c. A total chromosome number that is diploid but has a balanced deletion and duplication of whole chromosomes
   d. The total chromosome number in gametes; diploid is the number in somatic cells

REFERENCES

1. Buckton KE, O'Riordan ML, Ratcliffe G, et al: A G-band study of chromosomes in liveborn infants. Ann Hum Genet Lond 1980;43:227-239.
2. Boué J, Boué A, Lazar P: Retrospective and prospective epidemiological studies of 1500 karyotyped spontaneous human abortions. Teratology 1975;12:11-26.
3. Watson JD, Crick FHC: Molecular structure of nucleic acids: a structure for deoxyribose nucleic acid. Nature 1953;171:737-738.
4. Earnshaw WC: Mitotic chromosome structure. Bioessays 1988;9:147-150.
5. Olins AL, Olins DE: Spheroid chromatin units. Science 1974;183:330-332.
6. Oudet P, Gross-Bellard M, Chambon P: Electron microscopic and biochemical evidence that chromatin structure is a repeating unit. Cell 1975;4:281-300.
7. Rattner JB: Chromatin hierarchies and metaphase chromatin structure. In Adolph KW (ed): Chromosomes and Chromatin, vol 3. Boca Raton, Fla.: CRC Press, 1988:30.
8. Tijo JH, Levan A: The chromosome number of man. Hereditas 1956;42:1-6.
9. Hsu TC: Human and Mammalian Cytogenetics. New York: Springer-Verlag, 1979:6-7.
10. Nowell PC: Phytohemagglutinin: an initiator of mitosis in culture of normal human leukocytes. Cancer Res 1960;20:462-466.
11. Farnes P, Barker BE, Brownhill LE, et al: Mitogenic activity of *Phytolacca americana* (pokeweed). Lancet 1964;2:1100-1101.
12. Caspersson T, Zech L, Modest EJ, et al: Chemical differentiation with fluorescent alkylating agents in *Vicia faba* metaphase chromosomes. Exp Cell Res 1969;58:128-140.
13. Yunis JJ: Cytogenetics. In Henry JB (ed): Clinical Diagnosis and Management by Laboratory Methods, 16th ed. Philadelphia: Saunders, 1979:825.
14. Plattner R, Heerema NA, Yurov YB, et al: Efficient identification of marker chromosomes in 27 patients by stepwise hybridization with alpha satellite DNA probes. Hum Genet 1993;91:131-140.
15. Mitelman F (ed): ISCN (1995): An International System for Human Cytogenetic Nomenclature. Basel: S. Karger, 1995.
16. Turleau C, Chavin-Colin F, de Grouchy J: Cytogenetic investigation in 413 couples with spontaneous abortions. Eur J Obstet Gynaecol Reprod Biol 1979;9:65.
17. Jaffe ES, Harris NL, Stein H, et al (eds): World Health Organization Classification of Tumours: Pathology and Genetics of Tumours of Haematopoietic and Lymphoid Tissues. Lyon: IARC Press, 2001.
18. Bennett JM, Catovsky D, Daniel MT, et al: Proposals for classification of the acute leukaemias. French-American-British (FAB) Co-operative Group. Br J Haematol 1976;33:451-458.
19. Nowell PC, Hungerford DA: A minute chromosome in human chronic granulocytic leukemia [abstract]. Science 1960;132:1497.
20. Rowley JD: A new consistent chromosomal abnormality in chronic myelogenous leukemia identified by quinacrine fluorescence and Giemsa staining. Nature 1973;243:290-293.
21. Ben-Neriah Y, Daley GQ, Mes-Masson A, et al: The chronic myelogenous leukemia-specific P210 protein is the product of the BCR/ABL hybrid gene. Science 1986;233:212-214.
22. Druker BJ, Tamura S, Buchdunger E, et al: Effects of a selective inhibitor of the Abl tyrosine kinase on the growth of BCR-ABL positive cells. Nat Med 1996;2:561-566.
23. Third International Workshop on Chromosomes in Leukemia: Chromosomal abnormalities in acute lymphoblastic leukemia: structural and numerical changes in 234 cases. Cancer Genet Cytogenet 1981;4:101-110.
24. Ribeiro RC, Abromowitch M, Raimondi SC, et al: Clinical and biologic hallmarks of the childhood ALL. Blood 1987;70:948-953.
25. Crist W, Carroll A, Shuster J, et al: Philadelphia chromosome positive acute lymphoblastic leukemia: clinical and cytogenetic characteristics and treatment outcome. A Pediatric Oncology Group study. Blood 1990;76:489-494.
26. Morrissey J, Tkachuk DC, Milatovich A, et al: A serine/proline-rich protein is fused to HRX in t(4;11) acute leukemias. Blood 1993;81:1124-1131.
27. Bennett JM, Catovsky D, Daniel MT, et al: Proposed revised criteria for the classification of acute myeloid leukemia: a report of the French-American-British Cooperative Group. Ann Intern Med 1985;103:620-625.
28. Bennett JM, Catovsky D, Daniel MT, et al: Criteria for the diagnosis of acute leukemia of megakaryocytic lineage (M7): a report of the French-American-British Cooperative Group. Ann Intern Med 1985;103:460-462.
29. Leblanc T, Berger R: Molecular cytogenetics of childhood acute myelogenous leukemias. Eur J Haematol 1997;59:1-13.
30. Claxton DF, Liu P, Hsu HB, et al: Detection of fusion transcripts generated by the inversion 16 chromosome in acute myelogenous leukemia. Blood 1994;83:1750-1756.
31. Slamon DJ, Godolphin W, Jones LA, et al: Studies of the HER-2 proto-oncogene in human breast and ovarian cancer. Science 1989;244:707-712.
32. Perez EA, Roche PC, Jenkins RB, et al: HER2 testing in patients with breast cancer: poor correlation between weak positivity by immunohistochemistry and gene amplification by fluorescence in situ hybridization. Mayo Clin Proc 2002;77:148-154.
33. Slamon DJ, Leyland-Jones B, Shak S, et al: Use of chemotherapy plus a monoclonal antibody against HER2 for metastatic breast cancer that overexpresses HER2. N Engl J Med 2001;344:783-792.

32

Molecular Diagnostics in the Clinical Laboratory

Mark E. Lasbury

OBJECTIVES

After completion of this chapter, the reader will be able to:

1. Describe the structure of DNA, including the composition of a nucleotide, the helical nature and strand orientation of DNA, and the complementary characteristic of DNA.
2. Predict the nucleotide sequence for a complementary strand of DNA or RNA given the nucleotide sequence of a DNA strand.
3. Explain the relationship between DNA structure and protein production and the relationship between the cell cycle and tumor progression.
4. Discuss the process of DNA replication, including the concepts of replication origin, replication fork, primase, primer, DNA polymerase, Okazaki fragments, leading strand, and lagging strand.
5. When identifying an inherited mutation or somatic disorder, determine the appropriate patient specimen required for DNA isolation.
6. Discuss methods used for isolating DNA.
7. Sequence and explain the purpose of the steps in polymerase chain reaction (PCR), reverse transcription PCR, nucleic acid hybridization, DNA sequencing, and minimal residual disease (MRD) detection.
8. Compare and contrast the following methods for detecting amplified target DNA: (a) gel electrophoresis using ethidium bromide or autoradiography for visualization, (b) restriction fragment length polymorphism, and (c) probe hybridization techniques such as Southern blotting.
9. Interpret an agarose gel result for the factor V Leiden mutation test and a nucleic acid hybridization result for a B and T cell gene rearrangement test.
10. Discuss the use of DNA testing for MRD.
11. Discuss quality control procedures for DNA tests, and interpret the results of quality control samples.

CASE STUDY*

After studying the material in this chapter, the reader should be able to respond to the following case study:

A 42-year-old man presented to the emergency department complaining of pain behind his right knee. He related that he had observed swelling below the knee for the last 2 days. The patient was in no apparent distress and was experiencing no chest pain, shortness of breath, dyspnea, or hemoptysis. The patient reported no history of trauma except for a right leg injury in 1969. He reported that he did not smoke, used alcohol occasionally, was taking no medications, and was in good general health. He was not overweight and had not had any malaise, weight loss, arthralgias, or melena. He reported that he jogged 5 miles daily when possible. Five years previously, he had experienced an episode of deep venous thrombosis (DVT) in his lower leg and was treated with intravenous heparin followed by oral warfarin (Coumadin) for 3 months. Subsequent to treatment, he experienced occasional pain behind both knees, which he treated with aspirin. He noted that his mother had been diagnosed with carpal tunnel syndrome and had developed DVT for which she has been taking oral warfarin for 15 years. There was no family history of collagen diseases. The patient's job requires frequent long airplane flights. He flies first class and walks around occasionally during the long flights. His leg pain had begun 1 week after a flight to Europe.

*This case was provided by George A. Fritsma, MS, MT (ASCP), Associate Professor, Pathology and Clinical Laboratory Science, University of Alabama at Birmingham, Birmingham, Alabama.

CASE STUDY—cont'd

After studying the material in this chapter, the reader should be able to respond to the following case study:

On physical examination, the patient had no evidence of rash or oral ulcers. No petechiae or purpura were noted. He had mild pretibial pitting edema. His right leg measured 36.5 cm at 25 cm distal to the superior aspect of the patella, whereas his left leg measured 33.5 cm in the same location. A complete blood count was unremarkable, and the pro-thrombin time and activated partial thromboplastin time were within the reference ranges. Doppler ultrasound revealed complete occlusion of the distal superficial femoral vein, anterior tibial vein, and popliteal vein. The diagnosis was DVT without pulmonary emboli. The patient was hospitalized and placed on a heparin drip. The hematologist ordered a factor V Leiden analysis. The initial specimen received was drawn in a red-top tube. The laboratory requested a redraw using a lavender-top tube. The patient was still hospitalized, allowing for the collection of a blood specimen in an ethylenediaminetetraacetic acid tube. Figure 32-1 illustrates the results of the factor V test initially done by the molecular

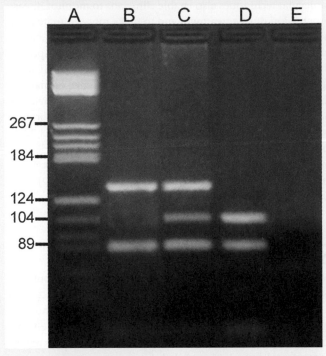

Figure 32-2 The repeated factor V Leiden mutation test done by the molecular technologist in the case study. **A,** Molecular size marker. **B,** Positive control. **C,** Patient's sample. **D,** Negative control. **E,** No DNA control.

technologist. The technologist's supervisor reviewed the gel results and requested the technologist repeat the analysis. Figure 32-2 represents the repeated analysis.

1. What type of specimen is appropriate when analyzing DNA for a hereditary mutation?
2. While examining the first gel result (see Fig. 32-1), determine whether the correct controls are present.
3. After examining the second gel result (see Fig. 32-2) of the patient, what band sizes appear in the patient's sample?
4. What band sizes are expected for an individual who is homozygous, heterozygous, or normal?
5. Why did the laboratory request the blood sample be redrawn?
6. Why was a repeat analysis requested?
7. Does this patient have the factor V Leiden mutation?

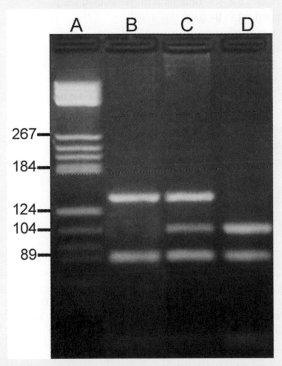

Figure 32-1 Initial factor V Leiden mutation test done by the molecular technologist in the case study. **A,** Molecular size marker. **B,** Positive control. **C,** Patient's sample. **D,** Negative control. The expected banding pattern on an agarose gel for the factor V mutation test is as follows: **B,** homozygous for the factor V mutation (141 bp and 82 bp); **C,** heterozygous for the factor V mutation (141 bp, 104 bp, and 82 bp); **D,** normal individual (104 bp and 82 bp). The band at 37 bp is barely visible. This band is difficult to detect on an agarose gel. This band is not essential for interpreting the results, however.

The application of molecular biology techniques to the clinical laboratory enhances the diagnostic team's ability to identify an increasing number of diseases. Molecular techniques also enable clinicians to monitor disease progression during treatment and to make more accurate prognoses. The short time required to perform and analyze molecular diagnostic tests is often an additional positive aspect of this type of testing, resulting in more efficient patient management. Hematopathology is on the cutting edge of many of these molecular techniques. The three main areas of hematopathology molecular testing include (1) detecting chromosomal translocations in hematologic malignancies (Box 32-1) and inherited hematologic disorders (Box 32-2), (2) identifying hematologically important infectious diseases (Box 32-3), and (3) monitoring minimal residual disease (MRD) after cancer treatment.

STRUCTURE AND FUNCTION OF DNA

DNA to RNA to Protein

Much of the stored information needed to carry out cell processes resides in DNA; proper storage, maintenance, and replication of this information are necessary to ensure homeostasis. Because molecular testing takes advantage of the structure and replication of this stored genetic information, a review of DNA molecular biology is helpful.

The central dogma in molecular biology is that information stored in the DNA is converted to a message (messenger RNA [mRNA]) that is translated into a functional unit (protein) (Fig. 32-3). This DNA to mRNA to protein relationship is essential to carry out cellular functions while preserving a record of the stored information. The copying of the stored sequences of DNA to form messages occurs by a process called *transcription*; DNA is transcribed to mRNA. In eukaryotes, this message is processed to a mature mRNA by processes beyond the scope of this discussion. The mature message is converted

---

BOX 32-1 Hematologic Malignancies Possessing p53 Alterations

Myelodysplastic syndrome
Acute myeloid leukemia
Chronic lymphocytic leukemia
Richter syndrome
Chronic myelogenous leukemia
Hairy cell leukemia
Atypical chronic lymphocytic leukemia
Mantle cell lymphoma
Diffuse large B- cell non-Hodgkin lymphoma
B-cell prolymphoblastic leukemia
B-cell acute lymphoblastic leukemia
T cell acute lymphoblastic leukemia
Splenic lymphoma with villous lymphocytes
Non-Hodgkin lymphoma

Modified from Peller S, Rotter V: TP53 in hematological cancer: low incidence of mutations with significant clinical relevance. Hum Mutat 2003;21:277-284.

BOX 32-2 Detection of Inherited Hematologic Disorders

Hemoglobinopathies
    Sickle cell anemia
    Hemoglobin C disease
    Hemoglobin SC disease
    Hemoglobin E disease
    Hemoglobin D disease
    β-thalassemias
    α-thalassemias
    Hereditary persistence of fetal hemoglobin
Coagulopathies
    Hemophilia A
    Hemophilia B
    Factor V Leiden mutation
Erythrocytic disorders
Lipid storage diseases
Neutrophil disorders

Modified from Crisan MD: Molecular pathology: Part 4. pioneering advances in molecular technology. MLO, 1995;27:52.

BOX 32-3 Detection of Hematologically Important Pathogens

Parasitic pathogens
    Malaria
    Babesiosis
    Leishmania
    Trypanosomiasis
    Filariasis
Fungal pathogens
Bacterial pathogens
Viral pathogens
    Viral pathogens associated with hemolytic anemia
    Parvovirus B19
    Cytomegalovirus
    Epstein-Barr virus
    Human immunodeficiency virus types 1 and 2
    Human T cell lymphoma virus type 1

Modified from Paessler M, Bagg A: Use of molecular techniques in the analysis of hematologic diseases. In Hoffman R, Benz EJ Jr, Shattil SJ, et al (eds): Hematology: Basic Principles and Practice, 4th ed. Philadelphia: Churchill Livingstone, 2005:2713-2726.

---

to a peptide (protein) sequence by translation. This is an enzymatic process wherein the mRNA codons (three member sequence subunits) drive addition of specific protein building blocks (amino acids) to the growing peptide sequence. The mature protein carries out its cellular function, whether it be recognition receptor, structure, enzyme, or regulatory element.

The ability to store information depends on DNA structure. Structural units that carry the message for a single protein are called *genes*. The human β-globin gene is a good example of message storage and retrieval and aberrant sequence maintenance. A normal (or wild-type) β-globin gene contains a

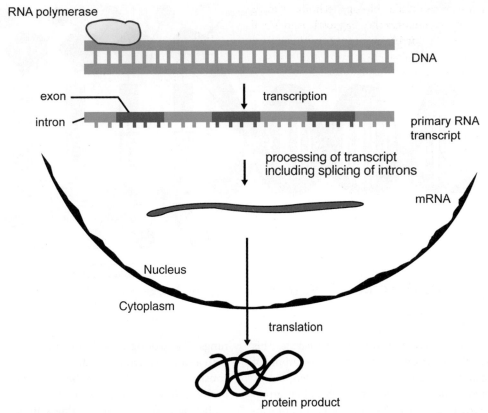

Figure 32-3 RNA polymerase transcribes DNA into a primary RNA transcript. The introns in the primary RNA transcript are spliced out, which is one stage of processing of mRNA. The mRNA enters the cytoplasm of the cell. The ribosomes translate the mRNA into protein.

sequence that codes for a β-globin peptide of 146 amino acids. This protein is part of the hemoglobin A oxygen-carrying complex of the erythrocyte. An inherited mutation results from the change of a single DNA subunit, called a *point mutation*. The mutation occurs in the portion of the DNA sequence that codes for the sixth amino acid of the peptide, resulting in a mutant protein and a disease called *sickle cell anemia*. This change is copied by transcription into the mRNA and translated into the protein, substituting the amino acid valine for the amino acid glutamate in the growing peptide and producing a protein that polymerizes in the presence of low oxygen tension (Chapter 26). The protein modification leads to sickled erythrocytes, circulatory problems, and poor oxygen exchange in the tissues.[1,2]

As described previously, the sequence of the DNA is converted to a functional unit that carries out some activity to benefit the cell, and this process is repeated for every gene of the cell expressed. Human somatic cells contain approximately 20,000 to 25,000 genes[3] along 2 m of DNA[4]; significant packing must occur to reduce the volume of the nucleic acid. DNA packing is reviewed in Chapter 31.

DNA at the Molecular Level

DNA exists as a duplex; two polymer strands of joined subunits called *nucleotides* are hydrogen bonded to each other (Fig. 32-4). Deoxyribonucleotides and ribonucleotides are the basic building blocks of DNA and RNA. Each nucleotide is composed of a sugar, a nitrogenous base, and a phosphate group (Fig. 32-5). The numbers one prime (1′) to five prime (5′) designate the carbons of the sugar. In DNA, the sugar is a ribose in which the hydroxyl group (OH⁻) on the 2′ carbon is replaced by a hydrogen, hence 2′ deoxyribose. In RNA, this ribose has the 2′ hydroxyl group. The hydroxyl group present on the 3′ carbon of the sugar is crucial for polymerization of the nucleotide monomers to form the nucleic acid strand.

The nitrogenous base is linked to the sugar by a glycosidic linkage at the 1′ carbon. There are four different bases in DNA, but the linkage to the sugar is the same for each. The phosphate group is linked to the sugar at the 5′ carbon by a phosphodiester bond. This phosphate group also is crucial for addition of nucleotides to the growing polymer. A sugar, whether ribose or deoxyribose, that is linked to a nitrogenous base but without a phosphate group is called a *nucleoside*. A nucleoside cannot be incorporated into a strand of DNA, and a nucleotide processing of only one phosphate group (deoxynucleotide monophosphate) likewise cannot be incorporated. To be incorporated into a growing strand of DNA, the nucleotide to be added must have three phosphate groups linked to one another, referred to as the α-phosphates, β-phosphates, and γ-phosphates. The α-phosphate is linked to the sugar.

Creating a phosphodiester bond between the 3′ hydroxyl of the existing strand and the 5′ α-phosphate of the nucleotide

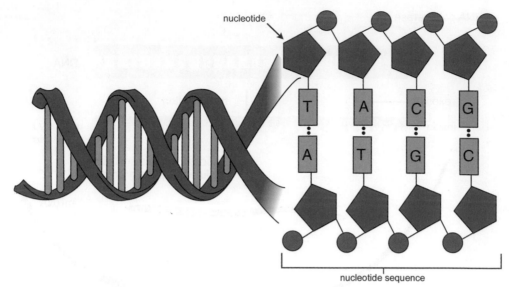

Figure 32-4 DNA is a helical double-stranded macromolecule consisting of nucleotide sequences.

monomer requires the protein enzyme *DNA polymerase*. This enzyme recognizes the hydroxyl group on the 3′ carbon of the sugar and catalyzes bond formation between the 3′ hydroxyl group of one nucleotide with the α-phosphate group of another nucleotide (Fig. 32-6). The polymerization of subsequent nucleotides forms a DNA strand.

DNA consists of two strands that are antiparallel and complementary (Fig. 32-7). One strand begins with a phosphate group attached to the 5′ carbon of the first nucleotide oriented to the left and ends with the hydroxyl group on the 3′ carbon of the last nucleotide oriented to the right. This strand is in the 5′-to-3′ direction. The other strand is in the 3′-to-5′ direction, or antiparallel. The nucleotide sequences comprising these strands are the encoded messages of human genes.

The addition of nucleotides to a growing DNA strand requires a highly regulated process. One mechanism of regulation comes from the complementary characteristic of the nucleotides. A nucleotide's identity depends on the type of base present. There are two categories of nitrogenous bases in nucleic acids, purines and pyrimidines (Fig. 32-8). In DNA, the bases adenine (A) and guanine (G) are double-ringed purines, whereas thymine (T) and cytosine (C) are single-ringed pyrimidines. Adenine forms specific hydrogen bonds at two points with thymine, whereas guanine hydrogen bonds at three points with cytosine. If a 5′-to-3′ DNA strand consists of CTAG nucleotide sequence, the complementary nucleotides on the 3′-to-5′ strand are 3′-GATC-5′. In RNA, the pyrimidine uracil takes the place of thymine and hydrogen bonds to adenine. In DNA, hydrogen bonding between the bases holds the strands together (Fig. 32-9), whereas RNA is most often single stranded.

In addition to conferring identity to the nucleotide, the nitrogenous bases assist in maintaining a constant width between the strands of a DNA molecule. At a molecular level, DNA resembles a ladder with the repeating sugar and phosphate groups as the sides of the ladder and the bases as the rungs. The pairing of a double-ringed purine on one strand with a single-ringed pyrimidine on another strand maintains a consistent distance between the DNA strands. This makes DNA flexible, allowing the DNA molecule to twist and giving DNA its helical character. The twisting stabilizes the molecule and protects the bases from the environment.

Transcription and Translation

DNA contains the permanent set of instructions to synthesize a protein. To make use of these instructions, the DNA code is transcribed into an RNA code through the process of transcription. Although a detailed explanation of transcription and translation is beyond the scope of this chapter, a brief discussion is warranted. An enzyme called *RNA polymerase* recognizes deoxyribonucleotide sequences called *promoters* found in DNA. These sequences lie upstream of coding sequences and promote RNA polymerase binding to the DNA strands as they separate. The RNA polymerase moves along the DNA strand "reading" the deoxyribonucleotide code and polymerizing the complementary ribonucleotides. When the complementary ribonucleotide forms a hydrogen bond with the base of the exposed DNA strand, RNA polymerase creates a phosphodiester bond to extend the single-stranded primary RNA transcript (Fig. 32-10). If the nucleotide sequence of the DNA strand is 3′-CTAG-5′, the primary RNA transcript is 5′-GAUC-3′.

Primary mRNA segments are composed of *introns* and *exons*. Introns are intervening sequences in the coding portions of genes whose functions remain unclear, although recent evidence suggests they play a role in regulation of gene expression.[5] The *exons* provide the nucleotide sequences that encode the protein product. Before mRNA can serve as a template for translation, introns are spliced out of the primary transcript, and the exons are joined. The mature mRNA is formed after other modifications, such as addition of a 5′ cap and a tail of many adenine nucleotides.[6] The mRNA leaves the nucleus and enters the cytoplasm to be translated into protein.

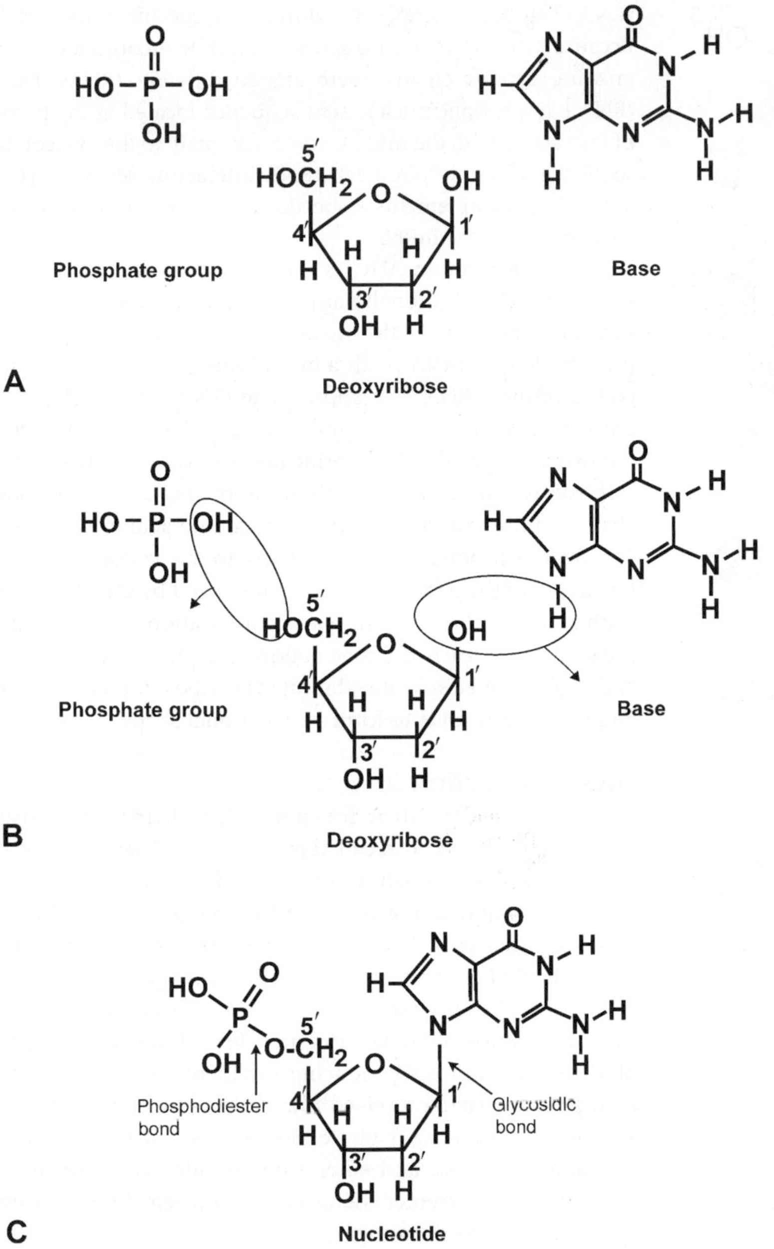

A

Figure 32-5 **A,** The sugar deoxyribose, a phosphate group, and a nitrogenous base comprise a nucleotide of DNA. The carbons of the deoxyribose are numbered 1′ through 5′. **B,** A nucleotide forms by chemical reactions between the nitrogenous base and the hydroxyl group on the 1′ carbon of deoxyribose and the phosphate group and the hydroxyl group on the 5′ carbon of deoxyribose. **C,** A nucleotide showing the glycosidic and phosphodiester linkages.

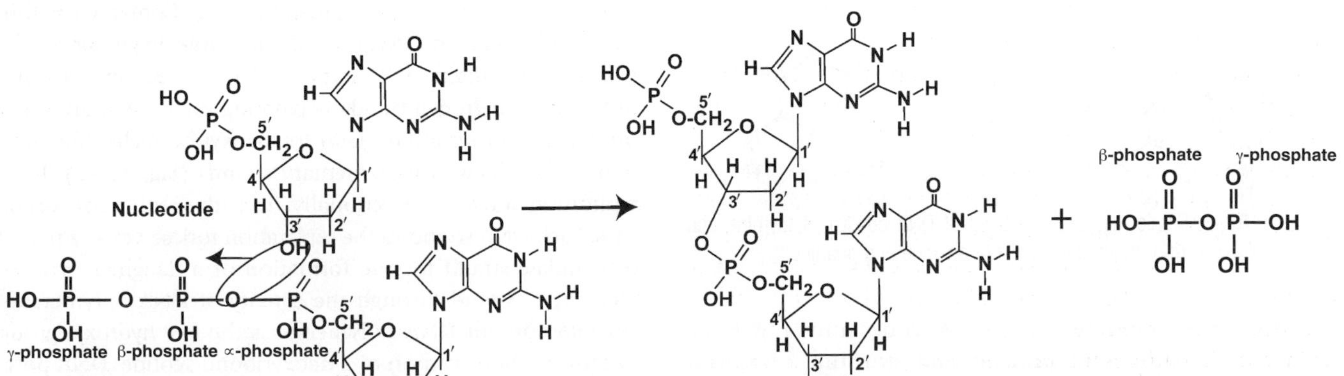

B

C

Figure 32-6 The enzyme DNA polymerase catalyzes the reaction between the hydroxyl group on the 3′ carbon of one nucleotide with the phosphate group bound to the 5′ carbon of the downstream nucleotide. The α-phosphate group is attacked by the 3′-OH, with release of the β-phosphate and γ-phosphate.

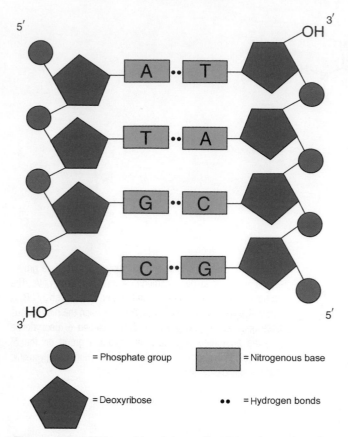

Figure 32-7 DNA consists of two antiparallel and complementary strands. One strand begins with a 5′ phosphate group and ends with a 3′ hydroxyl group. This strand is in the 5′-to-3′ direction. The other strand begins with a 3′ hydroxyl group and ends with a 5′ phosphate group. This strand is in the 3′-to-5′ orientation.

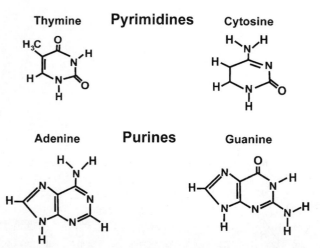

Figure 32-8 Single-ringed pyrimidines of DNA consist of thymine and cytosine. Double-ringed purines consist of adenine and guanine.

Ribosomes translate the mRNA code into a peptide sequence. Complexes of proteins and structural ribosomal RNAs (rRNAs) form the large and small subunits of the ribosome. A mature mRNA in the cytoplasm is bound by a small subunit of the ribosome at the translation start site. At this point, another translation element is introduced, the tRNA. This form of RNA is bound to a specific amino acid. Because there are 20 amino acids that can be incorporated into growing peptide chains, there are 20 different tRNAs. Each tRNA has a specific nucleic acid sequence located at the point of interaction with the mRNA, complementary to the nucleotide sequence of the mRNA. Each tRNA interacting sequence (the anticodon) complements a specific three-nucleotide sequence (the codon) of the mRNA.

The mRNA codon AUG is the most common translation start site and codes for the amino acid methionine. The first step in translation is the hydrogen bonding of the appropriately charged tRNA (with a bound methionine) to the start codon of the mRNA. The appropriate tRNA is bonded to the adjacent codon, and a peptide bond is catalyzed between the two amino acids. The peptide bond is formed between the carboxyl terminus of the methionine or the existing peptide chain and the amino terminus of the amino acid to be added. The hydrogen bonding of the tRNAs to the codons and the formation of the peptide bonds are mediated by the ribosome. With addition of more amino acids, translation proceeds until the stop site is reached. Three codons code for no amino acid and signal the end of translation. The ribosome dissociates, and the peptide folds to form its functional shape.

DNA Replication

After cells carry out their functions, they divide via mitosis or die via apoptosis, also called *programmed cell death*. The cell cycle progresses through a sequence of phases (Fig. 32-11). *Interphase* comprises the G_1, S, and G_2 phases. During the G_1 phase, the cell grows rapidly and performs its cellular functions. The S phase is the synthesis phase, the point in the cell cycle where DNA is replicated. The G_2 phase is the period when the cell produces materials essential for cell division. The M phase refers to mitosis, producing two identical daughter cells, each progeny having received one entire set of the DNA that was replicated during S phase. Some cells exit the cell cycle during the G_1 phase and enter a phase called G_0. Cells in G_0 normally do not reenter the cell cycle and remain alive until apoptosis or necrosis occurs.

DNA replication during S phase requires a complex orchestration of events; this discussion focuses on the events that are exploited for molecular diagnostic testing. Contained within the double-stranded DNA helix are multiple *origins for replication*. At each origin, an enzyme called *helicase* untwists and disrupts the hydrogen bonds, separating the DNA strands and producing two *replication forks* for deoxyribonucleotide addition to form new complementary strands (Fig. 32-12). DNA replication occurs bidirectionally from the replication origin sites. Each DNA strand in the replication fork serves as a parent or template strand for the formation of a daughter or complementary strand through the activity of DNA polymerase.[7] The substrate for DNA polymerase is the free hydroxyl group located on the 3′ carbon of a deoxyribonucleotide. DNA polymerase recognizes this hydroxyl group and catalyzes the joining of the complementary deoxyribonucleotide. DNA is read 3′ to 5′ by DNA polymerase, and the complementary strand is synthesized 5′ to 3′.

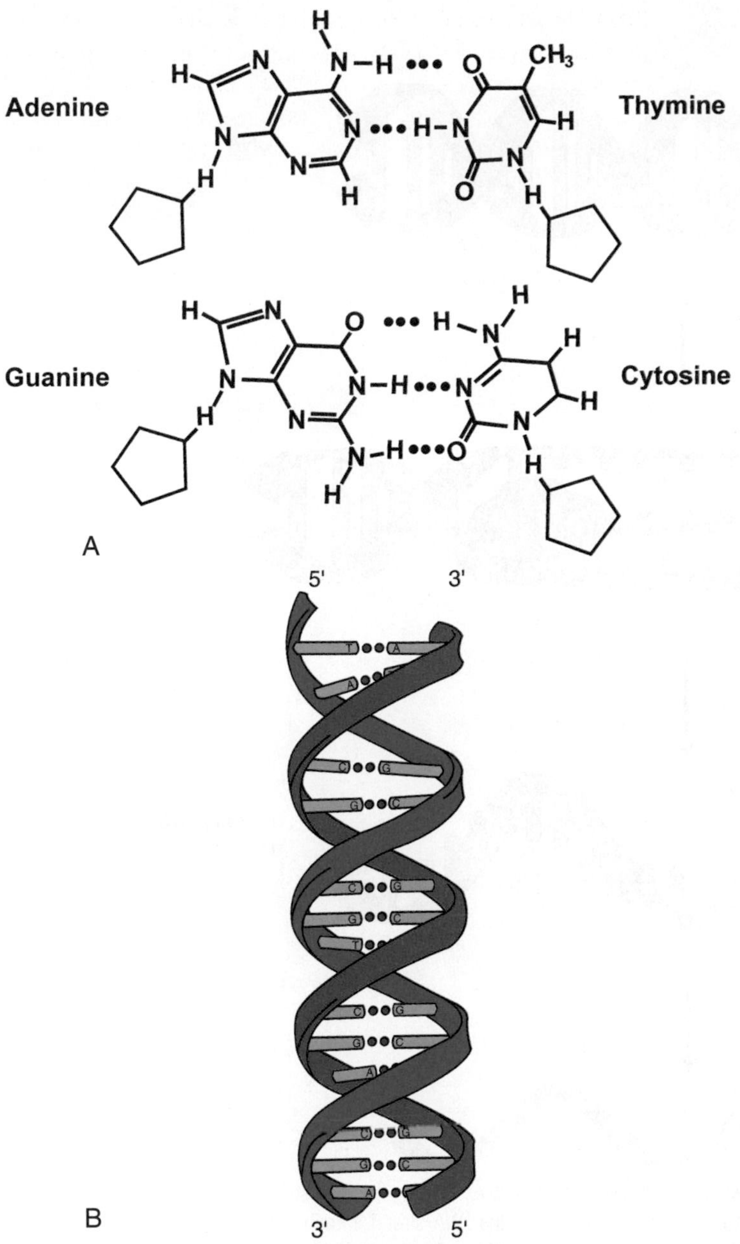

A

B

Figure 32-9 A, The purine adenine hydrogen bonds with the pyrimidine thymine. The purine guanine hydrogen bonds with the pyrimidine cytosine. **B,** The two strands comprising the DNA are equal distances apart, allowing the DNA to twist and forming the helical characteristic of the molecule.

A *primer* provides the free 3′ hydroxyl group required for DNA polymerase activity. Primers are short polymers of nucleotides that are complementary to the template strand. The hybridization of the primer to the template strand requires the enzyme *primase*. At the replication origin, primase joins a primer to the 3′ end of the 5′-to-3′ (top) template strand (Fig. 32-13). DNA polymerase recognizes the free hydroxyl group on the 3′ carbon of the last nucleotide in the primer and catalyzes the formation of the phosphodiester bonds between the correct complementary nucleotide triphosphate and the primer, with the release of the β-phosphate and γ-phosphate groups. DNA polymerase continues adding deoxyribonucleotides along the replication fork, going to the left of the replication origin, producing the complementary strand called the *leading strand*. The other template strand is in the 3′-to-5′

direction. To form this complementary strand, a primer hybridizes to the exposed 3′ end of the replication fork. To proceed in the 5′-to-3′ direction, addition of nucleotides proceeds toward the origin of replication. As the left replication fork extends to open more of the template strands for replication, additional primers are hybridized. DNA polymerase uses the primers to initiate the formation of the complementary strand, continuing until it meets a previously hybridized primer. DNA polymerase not only joins nucleotides but also degrades the RNA primers and fills in the correct complementary deoxyribonucleotides. Because the replication on this *lagging strand* produces many small fragments, it is called *discontinuous replication*, and the small replicated portions are called *Okazaki fragments*. Finally, the enzyme *ligase* is responsible for joining these fragments together. The replication fork to the right (downstream)

Text continued on page 434

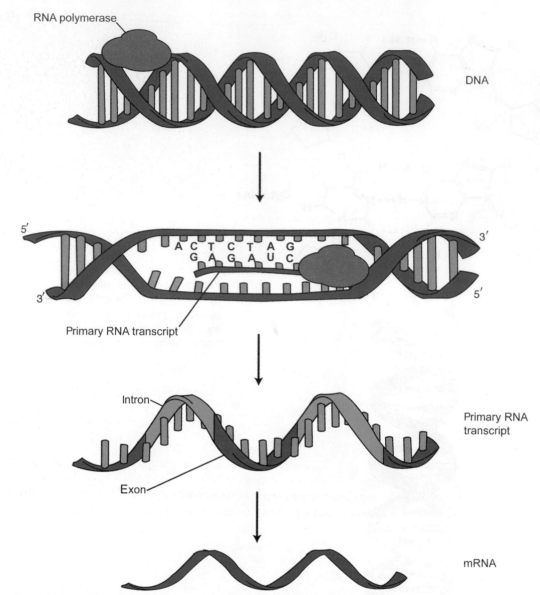

Figure 32-10 RNA polymerase binds to a sequence of DNA called the *promoter,* causing the DNA strands to separate. Using one of the DNA strands as a template, RNA polymerase moves down the DNA strand, forming the primary RNA transcript by reading the DNA strand and joining the complementary ribonucleotides. The primary RNA transcript consists of sequences of ribonucleotides called *exons* that contain coding information and *introns* that contain important information whose functions remain under investigation. The intron sequences are cut out of the primary RNA transcript, forming mRNA.

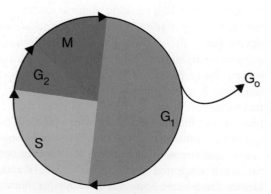

Figure 32-11 The cell cycle consists of interphase and mitosis. Interphase is divided into G_1, S, and G_2 phases. Cell growth occurs during G_1. During the S phase, DNA synthesis occurs. The cell prepares for mitosis during the G_2 phase. Cell division occurs during mitosis, producing two identical cells. Cells also may enter a quiescent phase called G_0.

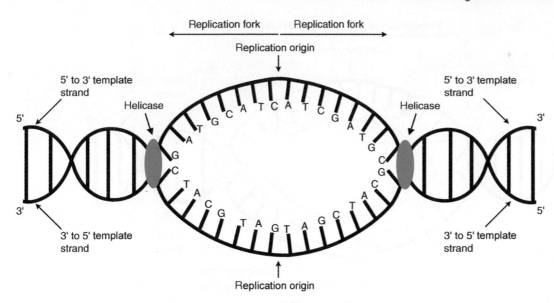

Figure 32-12 DNA replication occurs at replication origin sites throughout the DNA. Helicases separate the DNA strands, producing replication forks to the left and right of the origins.

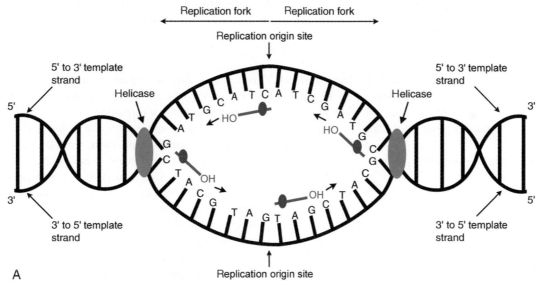

A

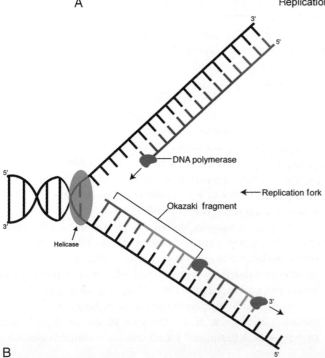

B

Figure 32-13 A, Primases join primers to the single-stranded template strands. The primers must be oriented in such a way that the hydroxyl group on the 3′ end of the primers is available for deoxyribonucleotide addition by DNA polymerase. **B,** DNA polymerase extends the primer located on the 5′-to-3′ template strand, producing the complementary leading strand *(blue).* On the 3′-to-5′ template strand, DNA polymerase extends the primers, producing Okazaki fragments. The primer ribonucleotides *(red)* are replaced with deoxynucleotides by DNA polymerase, producing the complementary lagging strand *(green).*

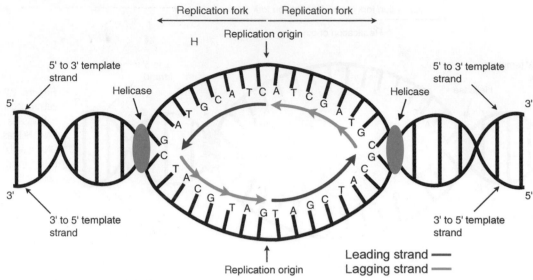

Figure 32-14 Bidirectional DNA replication. The 5'-to-3' parent strand serves as the template for producing the continuous leading strands on a replication fork to the left of an origin. The 3'-to-5' parent strand is the template for the lagging strands, which are produced in a discontinuous manner. The continuous and discontinuous strands are reversed on the replication fork to the right.

is replicated in the same fashion, although the lagging strand is now formed complementary to the top (5'-to-3') strand, and the leading strand is formed from the 3'-to-5' strand, opposite of the situation described for the left replication fork (Fig. 32-14).

The cell cycle is a highly regulated process. At certain critical points within the cell cycle, decisions are made to continue with cell division or begin cell death via apoptosis. This decision may depend on the state of the DNA replicated (Fig. 32-15). Normally, the cell detects errors made during replication and corrects them or begins the process of apoptosis to prevent the production of cells containing errors within genes. If the sensing molecules within a cell fail, cell division may

continue. If debilitating mutations in the genes that mediate cell cycle control are replicated, this may result in the beginning stages of tumor formation.

One protein responsible for sensing damaged DNA is p53, a tumor suppressor protein. Damaged cells with increased p53 protein arrest cell division at G_1, allowing time for DNA repair (Fig. 32-16). Cells with mutant p53 protein are unable to arrest cells in G_1 and continue the process of cell division with damaged DNA.[8-10] If the cell can repair the DNA damage, the cell cycle continues. If the cell damage is too severe, the cell undergoes apoptosis. Hematologic malignancies, such as 21% of chronic myelogenous leukemias,[11-13] 23% of chronic lymphocytic leukemias,[14-16] and 17% of acute lymphoblastic leukemias,[17-19] are associated with p53 mutations or deletions (Box 32-3). DNA synthesis and accurate cell cycle control demand that the integrity of the nucleotide sequence is maintained during DNA replication.

Specimens for DNA Isolation

Most molecular diagnostic tests begin with the isolation of DNA or RNA from the patient specimen. To test for a mutation, the patient's DNA is isolated. To test for microorganism DNA, as in an infection, the patient specimen DNA includes the organism DNA. The preferred nucleic acid used in the clinical setting is DNA because it is inherently more stable than RNA and is less labor intensive to isolate.

Patient specimens for human DNA isolation include peripheral blood, bone marrow, tissue biopsy, needle aspirates, and cheek swabs. A blood specimen is appropriate for identifying an inherited defect. Every nucleated cell (except gametes) contains a full complement of DNA. If an individual has inherited a mutation in the nucleotide sequence of his or her DNA, the mutation is present in the DNA of all the nucleated, nongamete cells. A peripheral blood specimen contains nucleated

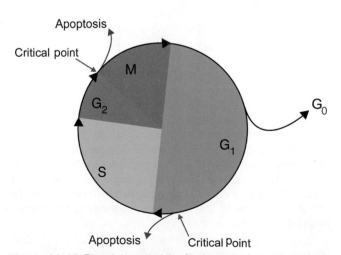

Figure 32-15 Toward the end of the G_1 phase, the first critical point in the cell cycle is reached. At this critical point, the cell either continues into the S phase or goes through apoptosis. The second critical point is located at the end of the G_2 phase. At this point, the cell either continues into mitosis or initiates apoptosis.

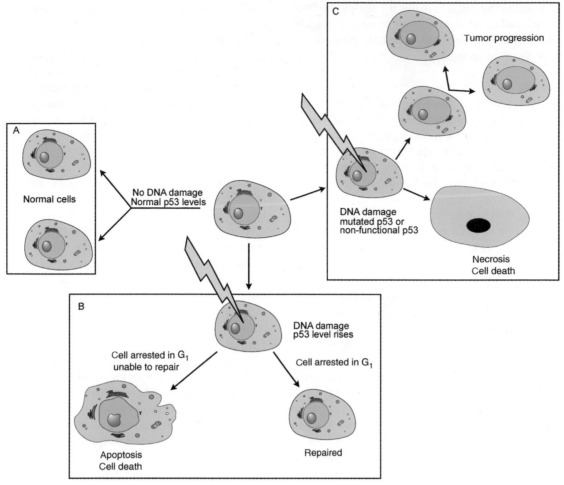

Figure 32-16 A, Cells with no DNA damage and normal levels of p53 divide normally. **B,** Damaged DNA within cells causes an increased level of p53. The physiologic increase in p53 causes the cell to arrest in G_1, allowing for cellular repair. If the cell is too damaged for repair, it goes through apoptosis. **C,** Cells with damaged DNA and mutated or nonfunctioning p53 cannot arrest in G_1 for cell repair. These cells either go through cell death via necrosis or continue cell division, beginning the process of tumor formation.

white blood cells; the DNA can reveal the presence of inherited mutations. In cancers, isolating DNA from the suspect tissue and conducting molecular tests assists in diagnosis of certain *somatic*, or acquired, mutations. For identification of infectious disease organisms by molecular techniques, DNA must be isolated from the affected tissues. Peripheral blood is adequate for viral infections such as human immunodeficiency virus and cytomegalovirus that infect blood cells, whereas diagnosis of meningeal infection requires cerebrospinal fluid.

Whole blood is collected in an ethylenediaminetetraacetic acid (EDTA) tube to prevent clotting and to inhibit enzymes that act on DNA. The white blood cells are separated from the rest of the blood components, and a lysis solution (detergent and proteinase enzyme) ruptures the white blood cells. A concentrated salt solution removes the cellular debris and proteins, leaving the DNA in the aqueous solution. Next, the DNA is precipitated, or taken out of solution. DNA's phosphate backbone is negatively charged, which prevents the DNA strands from coming in close contact with one another, a prerequisite for precipitation. The salt of the protein removal solution neutralizes the charges of the backbone, but the DNA

is still soluble in the aqueous solution. The addition of iso-propanol precipitates the DNA because nucleic acids are insoluble in alcohol. The precipitated DNA appears as long, whitish strands in the solution. After washing with 70% ethanol and resuspending the DNA in an aqueous buffer solution, it is ready for molecular testing. If a delay in the molecular testing occurs, the DNA sample can be stored at −80° C indefinitely. DNA extractions of dispersed cells from bone marrow and needle aspirate specimens follow similar procedures.[20]

DNA from tissue suspected of being cancerous can be isolated from formalin-fixed, paraffin-embedded tissue sections mounted on glass microscope slides. Tissue is obtained from the entire section or from a portion of the section by microdissection, either scraping or by laser. The tissue is degraded by an enzyme called *proteinase K* to break open the cells and release the DNA. The sample is heated to 94° C for several minutes to inactivate the proteinase K and degrade other proteins,[21] and the DNA is purified and precipitated as previously discussed. In addition to paraffin-embedded specimens, fresh or frozen tissue specimens are appropriate for DNA isolation. Quickly thawing and mincing the tissue prepares the sample for DNA isolation. The minced tissue is mixed with an extraction buffer to release the DNA from the cells, which is purified and precipitated as described previously.

RNA Isolation

RNA is trickier to isolate than DNA. Ubiquitous enzymes called *ribonucleases* (RNases) easily degrade RNA. These enzymes are a first line of defense against microorganism pathogens.[22] RNases are found on mammalian epidermal surfaces, making all laboratory surfaces contaminated with RNases. Clinical laboratories isolating RNA must be RNase-free, necessitating many precautions and decontamination steps that increase the cost of conducting RNA testing.[23]

Total RNA isolation includes mRNA, rRNA, tRNA, and small nuclear RNA (snRNA), which are used in protein synthesis. Depending on the cell type, mRNA may represent only 3% to 5% of the total cellular RNA; a larger specimen may be needed to obtain an adequate RNA sample for the analysis. mRNA represents not all the information stored in the cell, only that which is being used by the cell. In this way, assessment of specific mRNA levels provides data on the genes being expressed in a cell and the state of those sequences.

The basic steps of RNA isolation are as follows: (1) releasing the RNA from cells by lysis; (2) inhibiting RNases with strong chemical inhibitors, such as urea or guanidine isothiocyanate; (3) removing any proteins and DNA present; and (4) precipitating the RNA. After lysis of the cells and inhibition of RNases, an extraction using the organic solvent phenol at pH 4, chloroform, and isoamyl alcohol separates the DNA and protein into the organic phase and the RNA into the aqueous phase. RNA is resistant to acidic pH, whereas DNA is readily depurinated in acid solutions; the use of phenol at acidic pH preferentially isolates and maintains the RNA, whereas the genomic DNA is partitioned with contaminating proteins, lipids, and carbohydrates. Similar to DNA isolation, precipitating the RNA from the aqueous phase requires the addition of salt and ethanol.[24,25]

CONCEPTS IN MOLECULAR TESTING

The information stored in the DNA can be used to diagnose and monitor disease processes in tissue and blood. In vitro testing of nucleic acids in molecular diagnostics is based on and uses the enzymes and process of nucleic acid replication. Most molecular testing methods now used in the clinical setting use DNA replication to make millions of copies of a DNA sequence of interest. DNA synthesis reactions allow production of short pieces of DNA in vitro that can be used as probes. The complementary, antiparallel hydrogen bonding of DNA strands mediates hydrogen bonding between the probe and specific target sequences of DNA or RNA within large populations of nucleic acids.

Current applications for molecular testing in hematology are diverse. Mutations associated with malignancies are detected by nucleic acid probes hybridized to amplified patient DNA.

Mutations that lead to hematologic cell dysfunction also are detected by nucleic acid hybridization and DNA sequencing or by a method known as *restriction fragment length polymorphism*. In some cases, copies of a nucleic acid sequence of interest are generated from mRNA rather than from DNA for assessment of the existence of mutations that are not only present, but also are being translated into protein. Assessment of mRNA can show whether a mutation is expressed in a certain cell type or tissue and can be used to determine the level of transcription of a certain gene.

Infectious diseases that affect the hematologic system can be detected using molecular techniques. In these instances, instead of identifying changes in host DNA sequences, tests identify the presence of RNA or DNA sequences that are specific for species of disease-causing organisms. In a similar fashion, kits are available to quantify virus levels in the blood to assess the efficacy of treatments in progress.

It is important to recognize potential negative factors in using molecular tests for hematopathologies and issues that must be kept in mind when analyzing molecular test results. As stated earlier, most molecular-based tests use DNA amplification, generating many copies of the same sequence. Although replication is a similar process for all DNA, amplification for molecular testing is specific to the nucleic acid sequence of interest. The amplification does not differentiate between different sources of the target sequence, however. It is crucial to prevent contamination of the samples or reactions with DNA from previously amplified samples. This problem can be avoided by using meticulous technique, designating an area of the laboratory for each step of the procedure, understanding and using proper controls, and incorporating a procedure to minimize the possible contamination of the samples with previous sample or control nucleic acid. These methods include the use of a ultraviolet (UV) light to induce strand breaks in DNA strands that contaminate surfaces or the air, bleach to rid surfaces of contaminating sequences, or a uracil-N-glycosylase system to destroy previously amplified DNA (amplicons).

The issue of clinical relevance is particularly important when assessing infectious disease occurrence or nucleic acid mutations using molecular techniques. Amplification of DNA sequences from microorganisms and viruses gives millions of copies from a single template sequence. Theoretically, a single organism in the sample would produce a positive test, but a single organism may or may not be clinically relevant. Similarly, when monitoring viral loads, one must remember that these kits are based on amplification of DNA, so standard curves of template number are crucial to interpretation of the data. Also, because DNA can survive the organism, a positive test for the presence of a specific DNA sequence does not guarantee that the organism was viable at the time of sampling, calling into question the clinical relevance of a positive test. In terms of genetically based hematologic disease, mutations may occur without consequence to function. Individuals vary in genetic sequences coding for identical proteins; such single-nucleotide polymorphisms can be detected by molecular methods but may not cause disease. With these caveats in mind, several previously mentioned techniques are discussed as follows and an example from hematopathology is given for each.

MOLECULAR METHODS FOR AMPLIFYING A DNA SEQUENCE

Polymerase Chain Reaction

The principal technique used in the clinical molecular laboratory is the polymerase chain reaction (PCR). PCR is an enzyme-based method for reproducing large numbers of a target sequence of DNA,[26] enabling detection of the sequence of interest from a small amount of starting material. As described previously, sickle cell anemia results from a single-nucleotide substitution (point mutation) in which an adenine replaces a thymine. Detecting this mutation in the 6 billion nucleotides present would be like finding a needle in a haystack if only a few cells were assessed. If millions of β-globin copies are produced, however, the mutation is easily detected by numerous methods. As with DNA replication, amplification of a specific nucleotide sequence by PCR requires the use of primers. When testing for sickle cell mutation, primers flank (i.e., they bind on either side of) the area of the β-globin gene that contains the nucleotide substitution. The total length of the primers and the target sequence can be any number of nucleotides, as determined by the distance between the target sequences bounded by the primers selected, but is often 110 base pairs (bp) for the β-globin test (Fig. 32-17).[27] The other reactants in the PCR reaction are a DNA polymerase called Taq polymerase, isolated from the thermophilic bacterium *Thermus aquaticus,* and deoxyribonucleotides.

The steps of a PCR reaction include denaturing the DNA, allowing hydrogen bonding of the primers to their complementary sequences on the template, and adding nucleotides to the primers through DNA polymerase activity (Fig. 32-18). High temperature (95° C) destroys the hydrogen bonding between the strands of DNA (denaturation). A lower temperature (40° to 60° C) allows hydrogen bonding of the primer to the target (annealing) and must be optimized for each primer

set. Finally, 72° C is the optimum temperature for addition of nucleotides by the DNA polymerase (extension). To facilitate these changes in temperature during the PCR reaction, an instrument called a *thermocycler* is used to modulate and monitor the temperature of the reaction tubes accurately.

When the double-stranded DNA template is denatured, one primer anneals to the 5′-to-3′ strand, and the other primer anneals to the 3′-to-5′ strand. Both these primers possess a free hydroxyl group at their 3′ end. The Taq polymerase recognizes the hydroxyl group, "reads" the template strand, and catalyzes the formation of the phosphodiester bond joining the first complementary deoxyribonucleotide to the primer. Taq DNA polymerase continues down the template strand, elongating the complementary strand, producing a strand of daughter DNA that has the primer sequence at the 5′ end, and continuing to the 3′ end of the template at a rate of nearly 1000 nucleotides per second.[28] This completes one PCR cycle. In the second PCR cycle, the temperature changes are repeated, and the extended product becomes the template for the production of a daughter strand. After the second cycle, the daughter strand is bounded by the primer sequences at the 5′ and 3′ ends, producing a fragment of DNA of the desired length. In subsequent cycles (25-40 total cycles), this DNA of specific length and sequence is reproduced millions of times.[26,29,30]

The annealing of the primers to the template DNA accounts for the specificity of PCR. Primer design is crucial to accurate PCR and for achieving high levels of confidence in data analysis. When testing for a mutation in DNA, the primer set must amplify the target region without annealing to other regions of DNA in the sample. When testing for the presence of DNA from a specific disease-causing microorganism DNA, the primers must anneal specifically to the target region of the organism but not to either the host DNA or the DNA of other organisms. Wherever the primers anneal, whether intended or not, they serve as starting points for extension. Commercial kits contain primer sets that have been tested for specificity of annealing, but care must be taken to use the optimum annealing temperature. Even if the primer is designed to recognize only the target DNA, it can anneal to other regions that are similar to the target if the annealing temperature is too low. When

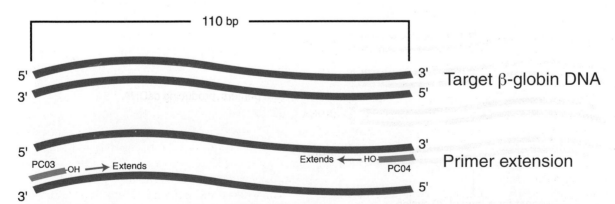

Figure 32-17 Flanking primers are used to amplify the target β-globin DNA. One primer joins with the 3′ end of the 5′-to-3′ DNA strand. The other primer anneals to the 3′ end of the 3′-to-5′ DNA strand. These primers are extended during PCR.

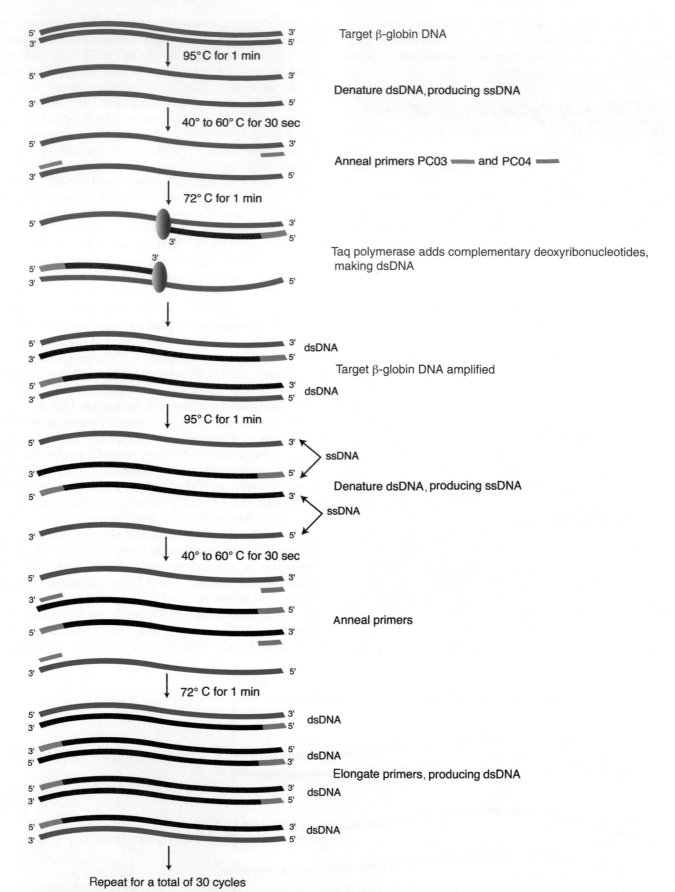

Figure 32-18 PCR of the target β-globin DNA. PCR amplifies the target DNA, making millions of copies of the target DNA after 30 cycles. ds, double stranded; ss, single stranded.

designing primers to amplify a specific target, online algorithms, such as the Basic Local Alignment Sequence Tool (BLAST),[31] are available to assess the specificity of the selected sequences. Finally, complementarities must be avoided between the primers themselves to prevent hybridization of the primers to one another, forming what are known as *primer dimers*.

Proper controls are an essential feature in conducting molecular tests using PCR. The three controls required for PCR are the negative, positive, and "no-DNA" controls, and all three should be included in each PCR run and assessment. The no-DNA control contains all of the reagents used in the PCR, except that water is substituted for the DNA sample. The negative control consists of human DNA known to lack the deoxyribonucleotide sequence of interest. In contrast, the positive control contains the target sequence. Comparing the sample DNA lanes with the negative and positive control lanes on gel electrophoresis determines whether the target DNA sequence is present in the patient's DNA. The no-DNA control shows whether cross-contamination of samples, controls, or reagents occurred during PCR setup. A DNA fragment of any size in the no-DNA control lane indicates that DNA contamination occurred, rendering the entire test result unreliable. Reviewing the techniques used to set up the PCR may reveal where the cross-contamination occurred.[32]

Reverse Transcription Polymerase Chain Reaction

Some molecular hematology testing procedures require mRNA for analysis. Because the translation of mRNA produces proteins, altered ribonucleotide sequences within mRNA may result in an altered protein. Excellent examples of this are leukemias involving the Philadelphia chromosome (Ph; t(9;22) (q[34]1)), present in 95% of chronic myelogenous leukemia cases, 20% of adult acute lymphoblastic leukemia cases, 5% of pediatric acute lymphoblastic leukemia cases,[33] and rare cases of acute myelogenous leukemia.[34] The classic Ph results from a recip-

rocal translocation of the *ABL* gene on chromosome 9 to chromosome 22, producing a *BCR-ABL* hybrid gene (Fig. 32-19).[35-37] Transcription of this target produces a chimeric mRNA comprising portions of the *BCR* and the *ABL* genes. The translation of this chimeric mRNA results in a fusion protein that may alter the normal control of a cell's cycle, eventually resulting in hematologic malignancy.[35,38] A procedure known as *reverse transcription PCR* (RT-PCR) can be performed to detect the presence of the chimeric mRNA and is the preferred template compared with genomic DNA. Although the mutation is present at the DNA level, the position at which the two chromosome sections join varies, whereas the chimeric mRNA always is the same. Also, the genomic sequence includes the intronic sequences, making the chimera too long to perform PCR easily. The splicing of the mRNA yields a much shorter target that is more easily amplified.

In RT-PCR, the reverse transcriptase enzyme produces complementary DNA (cDNA) from mRNA present in a sample of total RNA that has been extracted from a patient's cells (Fig. 32-20). PCR amplifies the number of these cDNA molecules. RT-PCR requires an oligo(dT), random, or specific primer; the enzyme reverse transcriptase; deoxyribonucleotides; primers; the mRNA template; and Taq polymerase. The first step in the procedure involves producing an RNA-cDNA hybrid using the enzyme reverse transcriptase and a *primer*. The primer called *oligo(dT)* consists of many thymine nucleotides. Most mRNAs possess a string of adenine nucleotides on the 3′ end called a *polyA tail*. The oligo(dT) primer anneals to the polyA tail of any mRNA present. Reverse transcriptase recognizes the hydroxyl group on the last nucleotide of the primer and reads the mRNA template strand, then adds the correct complementary deoxyribonucleotide. Reverse transcriptase continues up the mRNA template strand, joining the complementary deoxyribonucleotides to the growing cDNA strand to form the mRNA-cDNA hybrid. Heat denaturation breaks the hydrogen bonds between the mRNA-cDNA hybrid, separating the two strands.

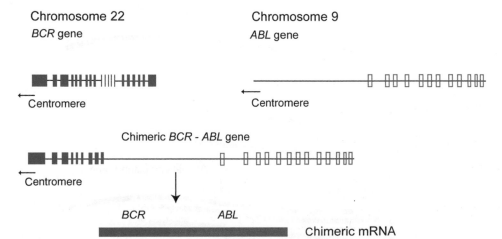

Figure 32-19 The *BCR* gene is present on chromosome 22. The *ABL* gene is found on chromosome 9. The Ph[1] chromosome results from the translocation of the *ABL* gene to chromosome 22, placing the *ABL* gene next to the *BCR* gene and producing a chimeric *BCR-ABL* gene. The transcription of the *BCR-ABL* gene produces a chimeric mRNA consisting of a portion of the BCR gene and a portion of the ABL gene.

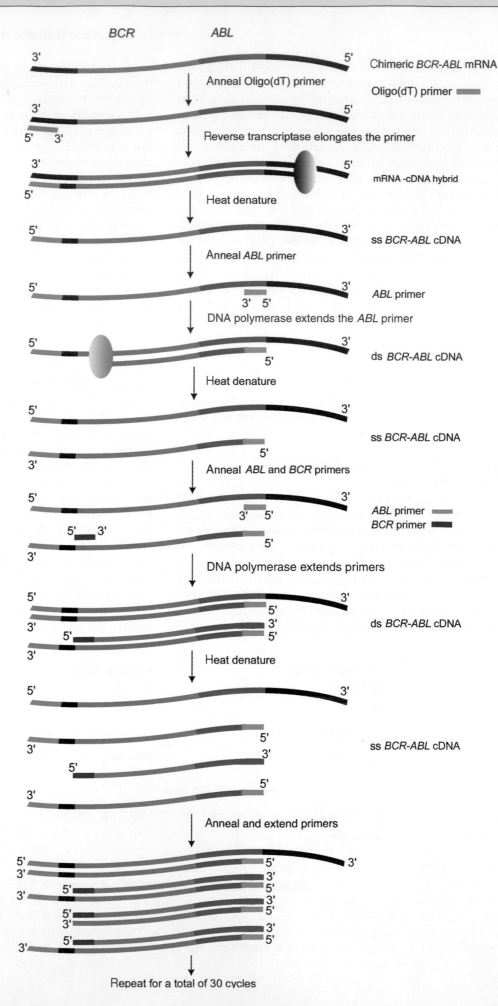

Figure 32-20 RT-PCR produces cDNA from mRNA. This diagram represents the RT-PCR steps used to produce amplified *BCR-ABL* cDNA. Initially an oligo(dT) primer anneals to the 3'-polyA tail of the chimeric *BCR-ABL* mRNA. Reverse transcriptase elongates the primer, producing an mRNA-cDNA hybrid. Heat denaturation breaks the hydrogen bonds holding the hybrid molecule together, releasing the single-stranded (ss) *BCR-ABL* cDNA. Next, a primer specific for the *ABL* gene is annealed to the cDNA. DNA polymerase elongates the primer, producing the double-stranded (ds) *BCR-ABL* cDNA. The cDNA becomes single stranded by heat denaturation. The *ABL* primer and a primer specific for the *BCR* gene anneal to the ss cDNA. DNA polymerase elongates the primers, producing ds *BCR-ABL* cDNA. The cycle is repeated 20 to 40 times, producing millions of copies of the ds *BCR-ABL* cDNA.

The cDNA strand can act as a template for replication. The next step involves amplifying the single-stranded cDNA using primers specific for a target sequence in the *BCR* gene and *ABL* gene. DNA polymerase extends the primers, forming a double-stranded cDNA of the target chimeric gene. The cycling continues, resulting in millions of copies of cDNA representing the sequence of interest.[20,34,39,40]

DETECTING AMPLIFIED DNA

Several methods are available for detecting the amplified target DNA. These methods include (1) gel electrophoresis using ethidium bromide, fluorescence, or autoradiography for visualization; (2) the use of restriction endonuclease enzymes followed by gel electrophoresis; (3) nucleic acid hybridization of a known sequence to the amplified DNA; (4) DNA sequencing; and (5) fluorescent probes and dyes for real-time PCR.

Gel Electrophoresis

Nucleic acids possess an overall negative charge owing to the phosphate groups of the backbone. In addition, the size of the amplified target DNA sequence consists of a specific number of deoxyribonucleotides. DNA lengths are measured in bp or kilobase pairs (kb), which are equal to 1000 bp. Gel electrophoresis provides the means of separating the amplified DNA fragments based on these attributes. To electrophorese DNA or RNA, the nucleic acids are sieved through a polyacrylamide or agarose matrix by passing an electrical current through the gel bathed in a conducting salt solution. During preparation, polyacrylamide or agarose matrices gel by crosslinking, producing pores. The pores of an agarose gel are larger than the pores of a polyacrylamide gel. This difference in pore size determines the gel required for electrophoresis. When separating larger DNA fragments (500 bp to >50 kb), an agarose gel is most effective. For smaller DNA fragments (5-1000 bp), a polyacrylamide gel is used.[3,41]

Whether using an agarose or a polyacrylamide gel, the process of gel electrophoresis is the same. The amplified DNA, the appropriate controls, and a size marker are loaded into the sample wells. An electrical current supplied by the power source moves the negatively charged DNA toward the positive terminal. The fragments migrate through the gel based on their size, three-dimensional shape, and mass-to-charge ratio. Smaller DNA fragments move faster through the gel than the larger fragments. A size marker of DNA fragments of known sizes runs along with the amplified DNA samples with which the sample DNA fragments are compared (Fig. 32-21).

Detecting the controls, size marker, and patient DNA fragments typically involves the use of ethidium bromide, sybr-green, or autoradiography. Ethidium bromide, a hydrophobic molecule about the same size as a DNA or RNA base, *intercalates* between the bases of a DNA double helix or between bases of a segment of secondary structure of a single DNA or RNA strand, labeling the nucleic acid such that it fluoresces when exposed to UV light. Ethidium bromide may be added during the preparation of the gel or after electrophoresis by

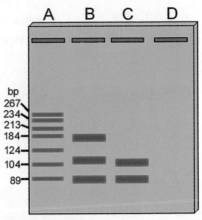

Figure 32-21 Gel electrophoresis of a DNA sample. **A,** Molecular size marker. **B,** Positive control. **C,** Negative control. **D,** No DNA control. By comparing the bands present in the gel with the molecular size markers, the size of each band is determined. In the positive control sample, the sizes of the three bands are 184 bp, 110 bp, and 89 bp. In the clinical laboratory, positive, negative, and no-DNA controls must be used when running a gel. The positive control contains the target DNA sequence, and the negative control lacks this sequence. The no-DNA control sample lacks DNA. There should be no banding present in the no-DNA control. If bands are present, contamination of samples occurred during the testing process.

soaking the gel in an ethidium bromide–containing buffer. Placing the gel under UV light causes the ethidium bromide to fluoresce orange, illuminating the nucleic acid bands. Ethidium bromide is a mutagen, so many laboratories instead use another fluorescing molecule called *sybr-green*. Sybr-green binds to the minor groove of nucleic acid helices and lacks the health risks associated with ethidium bromide.

Another method of visualizing the DNA fragments is autoradiography. During PCR, one of the deoxyribonucleotides, usually the adenine nucleotide, contains a radioactive α-phosphate group ($[\alpha\text{-}^{32}P]dATP$) that is incorporated during the elongation step. After gel electrophoresis, x-ray film is placed over the dried gel. The radioactivity present in the amplified DNA fragments exposes the film, producing a banding pattern that is interpreted by the scientist (Fig. 32-22).[42] The use of gel electrophoresis alone, detecting the bands by any of the described methods, is most appropriate when the presence or absence of the target is the goal of the test. This is often the case in assessing infectious diseases, such as cytomegalovirus infection. Plasma or leukocytes or both are the sample for DNA isolation, and commercially available primers are available for the PCR reaction.

Autoradiography also can be performed after incorporation of an enzyme-conjugated nucleotide into the growing chain or hybridization of a probe containing an enzyme-conjugated nucleotide to the nucleic acid. The enzymes most commonly used are horseradish peroxidase or alkaline phosphatase, which can cleave luminol or other synthetic chemiluminescent substrates with the release of visible light. This light is confined to the bands that contain horseradish peroxidase–conjugated DNAs. This methodology avoids the health hazards associated with radioactivity and now is commonly used in clinical laboratories.

Controls

| Neg | Pos | Sample |

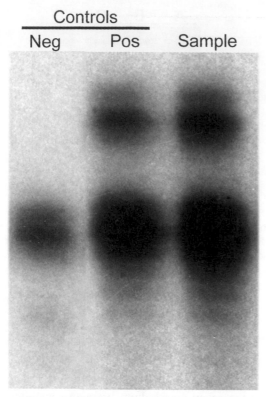

Figure 32-22 Autoradiograph of amplified DNA.

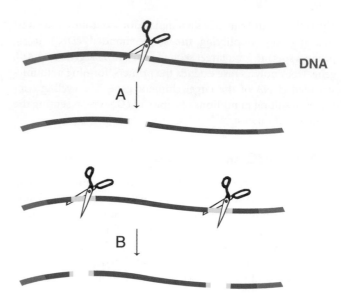

Figure 32-23 Restriction enzymes recognize a specific nucleotide sequence in DNA called the *restriction site* and cut both strands of the DNA. **A,** The scissor represents a restriction enzyme recognizing one restriction site in the amplified DNA, producing two restriction fragments. **B,** Two restriction sites are present in the amplified DNA. After the restriction enzyme cuts the DNA, three restriction fragments are present.

In the clinical laboratory, automation is desired for increasing reproducibility and efficiency, issues that often drive test design of any type. In terms of commercial kits, detection of the amplicon is often not left to human interpretation of the gel, with the storage and reproducibility issues that accompany it. Rather, fluorescently labeled nucleotides often are incorporated into the growing PCR products, and relative fluorescence intensity is monitored to assess the presence or absence of the target band. Likewise, many other molecular-based testing kits use the incorporation of fluorescent molecules for tracking and detecting amplicons, for quantification, for sequence analysis, and for presence or absence of target determinations.

Restriction Endonucleases

One method to determine whether an amplified target DNA contains a mutation of interest uses enzymes called *restriction endonucleases* (also called *restriction enzymes*). These enzymes are present in bacteria and serve to cut (restrict) foreign DNA that may enter the bacterium. Today, they are commonly used in molecular biology procedures. Type II restriction endonucleases recognize specific nucleotide sequences and cut both strands of the target DNA at these specific points i.e., restriction sites, producing DNA fragments called *restriction fragments*. Hundreds of restriction endonucleases are commercially available, allowing restriction of many different DNA sequences. The number of restriction fragments produced depends on the number of restriction sites present in the amplified target DNA.[43,44] One restriction site produces two restriction fragments, two restriction sites produce three restriction fragments,

and so on (Fig. 32-23). If a mutation creates or destroys a sequence pattern recognized by a specific restriction enzyme, that enzyme can be used to detect the mutation in an amplicon population.

The term *restriction fragment length polymorphism* refers to the use of restriction endonucleases to identify mutations within genes by detecting changes in the lengths of the resulting bands after restriction. An excellent example of this is the factor V Leiden mutation. Individuals possessing this mutation have an increased risk of venous thrombosis. The factor V mutation results from the replacement of guanine with adenine within the factor V gene.[45,46] The mutation destroys a restriction site detected by the restriction endonuclease, *Mnl*1. The factor V amplicon is 223 bp, housing two *Mnl*1 sites. One site is destroyed by the mutation. After PCR and incubation with *Mnl*1, the amplicon is reduced to restriction fragments of specific sizes (Fig. 32-24). Polyacrylamide gel electrophoresis separates the fragments, followed by detection using ethidium bromide. Restriction of the wild-type factor V amplicon generates fragments that are 37 bp, 82 bp, and 104 bp long, whereas the mutant gene has restriction fragments with lengths of 82 bp and 141 bp. A normal individual possesses two copies of the wild-type factor V gene. Three bands with the sizes of 37 bp, 82 bp, and 104 bp are present after gel electrophoresis. An individual homozygous for the factor V mutation possess two copies of the mutated factor V gene, resulting in the presence of two bands with sizes of 82 bp and 141 bp. An individual heterozygous for the factor V mutation possesses one normal and one mutated factor V gene. These individuals have four bands present with the sizes of 37 bp, 82 bp, 104 bp, and 141 bp (see Fig. 32-1).

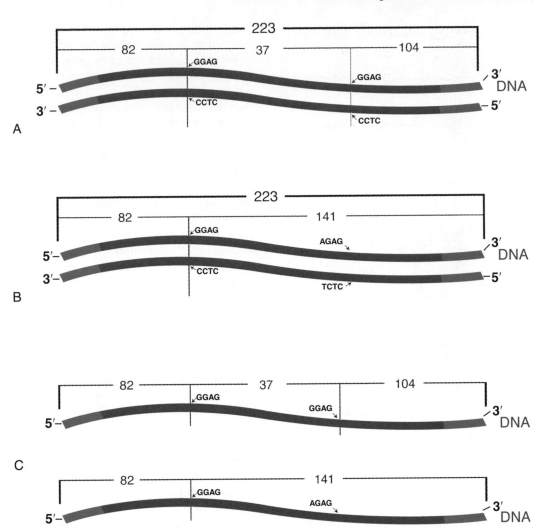

Figure 32-24 The restriction site GGAG is recognized by the restriction enzyme *Mnl*1. The normal coagulation factor V gene contains two restriction sites for *Mnl*1. In the mutated factor V gene, the base substitution of an A for a G destroys one of the restriction sites for *Mnl*1. The mutated factor V gene possesses only one restriction site for *Mnl*1. **A,** The amplified target sequence of a normal individual for the factor V gene contains two restriction sites for *Mnl*1, producing restriction fragments with the sizes of 104 bp, 82 bp, and 37 bp. **B,** An individual who is homozygous for the factor V mutation possesses only one restriction site for *Mnl*1, producing two restriction fragments with the sizes of 141 bp and 82 bp. C, An individual who is heterozygous for the factor V mutation has a normal and a mutated factor V gene. *Mnl*1 produces four restriction fragments with the sizes of 141 bp, 104 bp, 82 bp, and 37 bp.

Nucleic Acid Hybridization

Another method to detect the DNA targets is by hybridization of a nucleic acid probe to the sample or PCR product. This technique makes use of gel electrophoresis and may or may not use restriction endonucleases[47,48] in addition to the hybridization. A Southern blot[47] (named for its developer, Dr. Ed Southern) can use isolated DNA from a patient sample without amplification by PCR but also can be performed on amplified DNA. After the isolation or amplification of the target DNA, a restriction endonuclease called *Eco*RI cuts the DNA (Fig. 32-25). Within human DNA, there are many *Eco*RI restriction sites. Gel electrophoresis separates the fragments, and the DNA is depurinated with acid to nick the DNA fragments. Sodium hydroxide denatures the DNA within the gel, producing single-stranded DNA without changing the

DNA's nucleotide sequence or two-dimensional position. The single-stranded DNA is transferred onto a nitrocellulose filter by electrical current or capillary action so that the nitrocellulose filter exactly represents the gel. Methods used to affix the single-stranded DNA permanently to the nitrocellulose filter include baking and UV cross-linking.[49,50]

In the classic Southern blot, detection of the band containing the DNA sequence of interest involves using a radioactive or enzyme-conjugated (horseradish peroxidase or alkaline phosphatase), single-stranded probe complementary to the target DNA sequence. Hybridization of this single-stranded probe to the target DNA[49,50] is followed by washing off the unhybridized probe. Detecting any bands labeled with the radioactive probe requires apposing the blot to film, called *autoradiography*. Southern blotting may be performed using

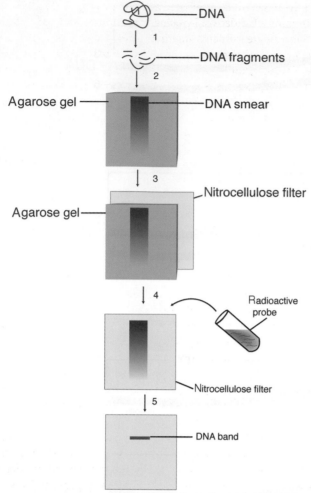

Figure 32-25 Southern blot steps. *1,* DNA is cut with the restriction endonuclease *Eco*RI, producing many restriction fragments. *2,* DNA fragments are separated on an agarose gel. *3,* DNA fragments are transferred to a nitrocellulose filter. *4,* A radioactive probe is hybridized to the filter. *5,* Autoradiography is used to detect the hybridized DNA probe, indicating presence of a complementary sequence to the probe.

hybridization of a fluorescently labeled probe instead of a radioactive one, which eliminates the hazards of working with radioactive labels.[51,52]

An excellent application of the Southern blot technique for hematologic testing is the B cell IgH immunoglobulin gene or T cell receptor gene rearrangement assays. Each B cell or T cell possesses a unique sequence for its IgH or T cell receptor gene as a result of a complex process of rearrangement, joining together distinct segments of the gene from clusters of segments with unique sequences. Each B cell and its progeny produce a specific antibody to an antigen, and each T cell and its progeny possess a specific cell receptor to an antigen.[53-55] Lymphoproliferative disorders arise from a malignant transformation of a B cell or T cell. In other words, a cell containing damaged DNA continues its cell cycle when it should have gone through apoptosis. These damaged cells no longer are under the control of the normal regulators for cell division

and continue to divide uncontrollably, forming a malignant population of cells. Because the cells within the malignant population contain the same gene rearrangement, the cells are monoclonal. Gene rearrangement analysis can determine whether a monoclonal population of cells exists and whether the cell lineage for lymphoproliferative disorders is B or T cell.

The appropriate specimens for gene rearrangement analysis are bone marrow, blood, or tissue from the suspect site. After DNA extraction from the specimen, the restriction enzymes *Eco*RI, *Bam*HI, and *Hin*dIII cut the DNA into fragments. Agarose gel electrophoresis separates the DNA restriction fragments. The DNA is depurinated, denatured, and transferred to a nitrocellulose filter. The hybridization step uses probes specific for nucleotide sequences in either B cell or T cell genes, and autoradiography visualizes the banding pattern. The presence of a distinct band represents a monoclonal population of cells. A polyclonal population consisting of varied cells with unique gene rearrangements appears as a smear with no distinct banding pattern.[56-58] Gene rearrangement analysis provides physicians with an important tool to diagnose and monitor lymphoproliferative disorders in their patients.

Single-stranded DNA probes also can be used to detect sequences of DNA in amplified samples by specific hybridization. The procedures are similar to Southern blotting but use PCR products instead of genomic DNA. These DNAs are blotted onto nitrocellulose by placing the denatured sample directly on the filter or transferred to the filter after gel electrophoresis. Under the proper conditions, the single-stranded probe hybridizes to the single-stranded target DNA (if present in the sample), and the labeled probe is detected according to the label used.

In the clinical setting, radioactivity is not the method of choice for labeling nucleic acid probes for health and safety reasons, but there are many alternative labeling and detection kits and reagents commercially available. Radioactivity is incorporated into the nucleic acid during the synthesis of the probe by using a nucleotide building block that is conjugated to the radioactive molecule. The radioactivity can be detected by apposing to film; thus it is an example of a direct label (Fig. 32-26). *Labels* refer to molecules conjugated to the nucleic acid that can be visualized in some manner and can be direct or indirect. Directly labeling the DNA means that the molecule incorporated into the nucleic acid can be visualized on its own, whereas indirect labels require additional molecules to be visualized. Fluorogenic molecules can be conjugated to nucleotides for incorporation into DNA probes as direct labels. Acridinium ester is a chemiluminescence label for nucleic acids. After it is conjugated to the probe and the probe is hybridized to the target, sodium tetraborate solution containing 1% Triton X-100 degrades the acridinium ester on unhybridized probes, whereas base pairing of the probe to the target protects the ester.[59] The bound ester is detected by a brief emission of light after addition of hydrogen peroxide.

Two commonly used indirect labels for nucleic acids are biotin and digoxygenin. Biotin is conjugated to nucleotides for inclusion in single-stranded probes. The biotin can bind a

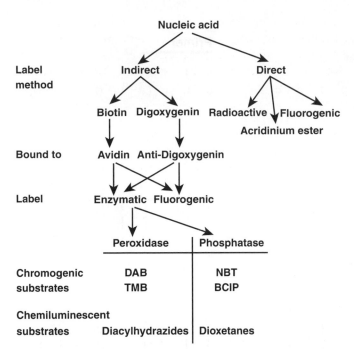

Figure 32-26 Nucleic acids can be labeled directly or indirectly to detect the presence of target sequences in DNA samples. Chromogenic substrates for peroxidase and phosphatase include 3,3'-diaminobenzidine (DAB), 3,3',5,5'-tetramethylbenzidine (TMB), nitroblue tetrazolium (NBT), and 5-bromo-4-chloro-3-indoylphosphate (BCIP).

protein called *avidin,* and the avidin is linked to a fluorescent molecule or to an enzyme for detection (Fig. 32-26). In a similar fashion, digoxygenin is incorporated into probe sequences and bound by an antidigoxygenin antibody conjugated to a fluorescent molecule or enzyme. Alkaline phosphatase and horseradish peroxidase are the enzymes most commonly used in indirect labeling systems. Their enzymatic activities are used to cleave substrates into visible compounds as pigments[60,61] or as chemiluminescence.[62]

DNA Sequencing

The ability to read the sequence of the nucleic acid has been just as important to the development of molecular biology as PCR. A combination of these two important techniques (cycle sequencing) has made DNA sequencing more efficient and its analysis less subjective. DNA sequencing is a procedure whereby the sequence of the nucleotide bases in a strand of DNA is determined, and it is applied in molecular testing to assess amplified sequences for insertions, deletions, or mutations, such as factor V Leiden mutation or the β-globin mutation.

Cycle sequencing is based on dideoxynucleotide terminator sequencing.[63] As discussed previously, the addition of nucleotides to a growing polymer requires a 3' hydroxyl group on the last added nucleotide and a triphosphate group on the 5' end of the next nucleotide to be polymerized. If a nucleotide also lacks the 3' hydroxyl group (a dideoxynucleotide), it can be incorporated into a strand of DNA, but it cannot be added to,

so the fragment is terminated at that base (Fig. 32-27). If small amounts of dideoxyadenosine triphosphate, dideoxycytosine triphosphate, dideoxyguanine triphosphate, and dideoxythymine triphosphate are included in the PCR reaction over numerous strands and numerous cycles, eventually a nested series of fragments is produced with strands that terminate at each successive base. The dideoxynucleotides are fluorescently labeled, a different color for each base. Capillary electrophoresis of the nested series of fragments moves the labels through a detecting laser one at a time based on their length. The sequence of the detected colors would reveal the nucleotide sequence complementary to the template strand. DNA is double stranded, so using two primers for the PCR would produce two series of nested fragments, and the detector would read two bases at each position. The PCR reaction is done with one primer in a reaction called *single-sided PCR.*

Using the sickle cell mutation as an example, DNA sequencing of either strand, but not both strands, shows whether the mutation (adenine to thymine) is present in the DNA. Each cell has two copies (alleles) of somatic genes; sequencing produces a nested series of fragments from each allele. If the patient is homozygotic for this gene, the two nested series of fragments are identical, whether wild-type or mutant. If the patient is heterozygotic for this gene, wild-type and mutant fragments are produced in the single-sided PCR reaction, and two nested series of fragments are produced. In analysis of this sequence, adenine and thymine signals are present at the position of the mutation, but because only half the templates contain each sequence, the signals of the adenine and thymine are half as strong. Sequencing is a reliable method for detection of mutations or single-nucleotide polymorphisms in DNA, but it is expensive and requires significant instrumentation, so it is not often used in the clinical setting.

ASSESSMENT OF MINIMAL RESIDUAL DISEASE

Advances in molecular testing in the diagnosis of hematologic malignancies have led to methods for assessing the effectiveness of treatments and as prognostic indicators for disease remission. Radiologic, chemotherapeutic, or bone marrow transplantation therapies can reduce levels of leukemic cells to below detection levels of traditional morphologic tests, whose limits are approximately 1% to 5%. Significant numbers of malignant cells (10^{10}) may remain, however, in the bloodstream, lymph nodes, or bone marrow. Molecular techniques, such as PCR, real-time quantitative PCR (RQ-PCR), cytogenetics, and flow cytometry, are more sensitive and can identify cells in hematologic specimens. The low level of disease in patients who are in a state of clinical remission is called *minimal residual disease* (MRD). More recent studies have correlated MRD levels to rates of disease relapse.[64-66] With lower levels of MRD detection by molecular methods, even to the point of "molecular remission," the incidence of relapse is recognized earlier. Detection of low levels of disease in patients in clinical remission also can help clinicians with treatment

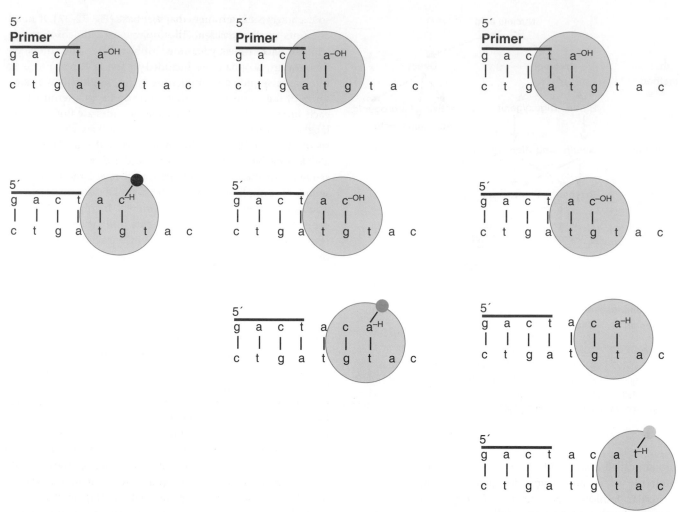

Figure 32-27 Cycle sequencing of a DNA template produces a nested series of fragments that differ by one nucleotide each. The template is amplified by PCR using a single primer sequence (single-sided PCR). The reaction includes small amounts of dideoxynucleotides that are fluorescently labeled, with each of the four bases conjugated to a different fluorophore. When a dideoxynucleotide is incorporated into the growing polymer, extension ceases.

decisions and provide indications of possible drug resistance. For these reasons, sensitive tests designed specifically to assess MRD continue to be developed in many laboratories and by the healthcare industry.

PCR technologies have the ability to detect a single malignant cell in a population of 1 million cells, making it a sensitive method for MRD monitoring. Gene rearrangements and chromosomal deletions, insertions, and translocations can be detected by PCR, whether they are generalized to a cancer type or specific to the individual. The t(9,22) translocation is found in 95% of all chronic myelogenous leukemia cases, making it a good target for PCR detection. The movement of the *c-abl* gene to the *BCR* locus (see Fig. 32-19) produces a nucleic acid sequence unique to the cancer cell. If a forward primer is designed corresponding to a *c-abl* sequence, and a reverse primer is designed to be complementary to the *BCR* sequence, the chimeric sequence can be detected in individuals with this translocation. In contrast, monoclonal antibody-producing rearrangements of immunoglobulin genes may be detected by PCR only if the rearrangement is known. PCR for MRD in these cases requires some knowledge of the rearrangement in the

individual patient, called *allele-specific oligonucleotide PCR*. This technique requires cloning and sequencing of the rearrangement before design of PCR primers. In both cases, gel electrophoresis of the amplification products, followed by ethidium bromide or sybr-green staining, identifies the presence of mutation in the cell population.

Identifying the presence of malignant cells by a sensitive method in a patient in clinical remission often does not provide an adequate level of information for making treatment or prognostic decisions. In many cases, quantifying the copies of the mutation reveals the number of malignant cells present, and this information may facilitate a better outcome. Semi-quantitative PCR can be achieved by comparing the amplification signal from a PCR reaction of the patient sample with PCR reactions using a known number of copies of the target sequence. Although this technique provides some information as to the copy number of the target in the patient sample, a newer technology, RQ-PCR, can determine sensitively the number of copies of the target. Although an in-depth description of RQ-PCR is beyond the scope of this chapter, a brief description of its use is in order. For a detailed description of

RQ-PCR and its use in MRD detection of hematologic cancers, see the review by van der Velden et al.[67] RQ-PCR detects the amplicons of a PCR reaction as they are synthesized. Fluorescent molecules included in the PCR reaction bind the helix in a sequence-specific manner to the amplicon and determine the number of starting copies of this sequence by comparing it with a standard sample of known copy number. This is a fast, sensitive, and reliable method for quantifying the MRD in hematologic malignancies. In the case of chronic myelogenous leukemia, qualitative PCR[68] and RQ-PCR[69,70] methodologies are clinically relevant for prognostic estimations and assessment of therapeutic efficacy.

Although other methods, such as flow cytometric analysis of monoclonal antibody binding to malignant cell markers and cytogenetic or fluorescent in situ hybridization analysis of metaphase chromosomes, also have the ability to identify diseased cells more sensitively than traditional morphologic tests, PCR technologies currently are used more often for MRD detection. Future advances may allow more for sensitive detection of disease states and tailoring of treatments to individual mutations and disease levels.

SUMMARY

When conducted properly and with appropriate controls, molecular testing in the clinical laboratory provides a rapid and accurate means of diagnosing and generating prognoses for many hematologic diseases and infections. Molecular testing in the clinical laboratory is still relatively new and is evolving rapidly. New molecular techniques, such as kinetic (real-time) PCR and amplified fragment length polymorphism, have potential as diagnostic and prognostic tests for hematologic diseases. Patient care will improve as a result of rapid turnaround time for diagnostic tests and more individualized patient treatment resulting from prognostic indicators identified by molecular testing.

CHAPTER at a GLANCE

- Four main areas of hematopathology molecular testing include the detection of:
  Chromosomal translocations in hematologic malignancies
  Inherited hematologic disorders
  Hematologically important pathogens
  Monitoring of cancer therapies
- Most cellular functions are dependent on DNA.
- DNA consists of a five-carbon sugar (deoxyribose), a phosphate group, and a nitrogenous base. The bases are either purines or pyrimidines.
- The purines are adenine (A) and guanine (G); pyrimidines are thymine (T) and cytosine (C).
- DNA is a double-stranded molecule held together by hydrogen bonding between the bases. It is denatured by heating to break the hydrogen bonds, producing single-stranded DNA.
- DNA strands are antiparallel, with bonding of adenine with thymine and guanine with cytosine.
- The tumor suppressor protein p53 detects damaged DNA and halts cell division for DNA repair or begins the process of apoptosis.
- Blood, bone marrow, tissue biopsy, and fine needle aspirates are specimens used for DNA isolation.
- RNA is a single-stranded molecule that contains the sugar ribose instead of deoxyribose found in DNA and the pyrimidine uracil in place of thymine.
- RNA polymerase recognizes a sequence of deoxyribonucleotides called the *promoter* within DNA.
- RNA polymerase separates the DNA strands and begins adding ribonucleotides, forming an initial RNA transcript consisting of introns and exons.

- Transcription of DNA produces mRNA.
- Translation of the mRNA by ribosomes produces protein.
- Proteins function as structural components of the cell, as enzymes involved in metabolism or regulation, as receptors to regulate cellular functions, or as antibodies for the immune system.
- Mutation within a gene ultimately alters the protein, often affecting the function of the protein.
- Molecular methods for amplifying a specific DNA sequence include:
  PCR
  RT-PCR
- Amplified DNA is detected by:
  Gel electrophoresis
  Restriction endonucleases
  Nucleic acid hybridization
  DNA sequencing
- Molecular testing allows more sensitive assessment of therapeutic efficacy and the remaining presence of diseased cells in MRD.
- Molecular testing allows clinicians to make more accurate therapeutic and prognostic decisions in MRD.
- RQ-PCR allows assessment of the level of MRD remaining, not just presence or absence.

Now that you have completed this chapter, go back and read again the case study at the beginning and respond to the questions presented.

REVIEW QUESTIONS

1. If the DNA nucleotide sequence is 5'-ATTAGC-3', the mRNA sequence transcribed from this template is:
   a. 5'-GCUAAU-3'
   b. 5'-AUUAGC-3'
   c. 5'-TAATCG-3'
   d. 5'-UAAUCG-3'

2. Cells with damaged DNA and mutated or nonfunctioning p53:
   a. Arrest the cell in G_1, resulting in DNA repair
   b. Continue to divide, leading to tumor progression
   c. Divide normally, producing identical daughter cells
   d. Go through apoptosis

3. To start DNA replication, DNA polymerase requires an available 3' hydroxyl group found on the:
   a. Leading strand
   b. mRNA
   c. Parent strand
   d. Primer

4. Ligase joins Okazaki fragments of the:
   a. 5'-to-3' template strand
   b. Lagging strand
   c. Leading strand
   d. Primer fragments

5. A 40-year-old patient enters the hospital with a rare form of cancer caused by faulty cell division regulation. This cancer localized in the patient's spleen. An ambitious laboratory developed a molecular test to verify the type of cancer present. This molecular test requires a patient sample taken from which two tissues?
   a. Abnormal growths found on the skin and the bone marrow
   b. Normal splenic tissue and the cancerous tissue
   c. Cancerous tissue in spleen and bone marrow
   d. Peripheral blood and the cancerous tissue in the spleen

6. One main difference between PCR and RT-PCR is that:
   a. PCR requires primers.
   b. PCR uses reverse transcriptase to elongate the primers.
   c. RT-PCR forms billions of cDNA.
   d. RT-PCR requires ligase to amplify the target DNA.

7. Which one of the following statements about gel electrophoresis is *false*?
   a. The gel is oriented in the chamber with the wells at the positive terminal.
   b. A buffer solution is required to maintain the electrical current.
   c. The matrix of a polyacrylamide gel is tighter than that of an agarose gel.
   d. The larger-sized DNA fragments are closest to the wells of the gel.

8. Autoradiography of DNA is the:
   a. Detection of radioactive deoxyribonucleotides
   b. Exposure of the gel to UV light
   c. Transfer of DNA to a nitrocellulose filter
   d. Use of ethidium bromide to visualize the DNA banding pattern

9. The result of a B cell gene rearrangement test showed a smear in the patient's sample. This smear indicates that:
   a. A monoclonal population of B cells exists.
   b. A polyclonal population of B cells exists.
   c. Contamination of the sample occurred.
   d. Too much probe was used during detection.

10. Which of the following statements about MRD is *true*?
    a. Clinical remission of hematologic cancers can be determined by molecular techniques such as PCR and flow cytometry.
    b. RQ-PCR determined copy number of *bcr-abl* rearrangements always is lower in molecular remission compared with clinical remission.
    c. Qualitative PCR that uses a known copy number of a target sequence is useful in determining MRD levels.
    d. MRD assessment can aid physicians in treatment decisions but does not yet offer insights into prognostic estimates.

REFERENCES

1. Kaufman RE: Synthesis of sickle and normal hemoglobins: laboratory and clinical implications. Lab Med 1999;30:129-133.
2. Mayo MM, Samuel SM: Clinical pathology rounds: diagnosing hemoglobin SC. Lab Med 1999;30:98-101.
3. International Human Genome Sequencing Consortium: Finishing the euchromatic sequence of the human genome. Nature 2004;431:931-945.
4. Calladine CR, Drew HR, Luisi BF: Understanding DNA: The Molecule and How It Works, 3rd ed. San Diego: Academic Press, 2004:1-17.
5. Le Hir H, Nott A, Moore MJ: How introns influence and enhance eukaryotic gene expression. Trends Biochem Sci 2003;28:215-220.
6. Lewin B: Messenger RNA. In: Genes VIII, 8th ed. Upper Saddle River, N.J.: Pearson Prentice Hall, 2004:113-133.
7. Lodish H, Berk A, Matsudaira P, et al (eds): Basic molecular genetic mechanisms. In: Molecular Cell Biology, 5th ed. New York: WH Freeman & Co, 2004:101-145.
8. Kastan MB, Onyekwere O, Sidransky D, et al: Participation of p53 protein in the cellular response to DNA damage. Cancer Res 1991;51(23 Pt 1):6304-6311.
9. Fritsche M, Haessler C, Brandner G: Induction of nuclear accumulation of the tumor-suppressor protein p53 by DNA-damaging agents. Oncogene 1993;8:307-318.
10. Lane DP: p53, guardian of the genome. Nature 1992;358:15-16.

11. Kelman Z, Prokocimer M, Peller S, et al: Rearrangements in the p53 gene in Philadelphia chromosome positive chronic myelogenous leukemia. Blood 1989;74:2318-2324.

12. Rovira A, Urbano-Ispizua A, Cervantes F, et al: p53 tumor suppressor gene in chronic myelogenous leukemia: a sequential study. Ann Hematol 1995;70:129-133.

13. Beck Z, Kiss A, Toth FD, et al: Alterations of P53 and RB genes and the evolution of the accelerated phase of chronic myeloid leukemia. Leuk Lymphoma 2000;38:587-597.

14. Cano I, Martinez J, Quevedo E, et al: Trisomy 12 and p53 deletion in chronic lymphocytic leukemia detected by fluorescence in situ hybridization: association with morphology and resistance to conventional chemotherapy. Cancer Genet Cytogenet 1996;90:118-124.

15. Amiel A, Arbov L, Manor Y, et al: Monoallelic p53 deletion in chronic lymphocytic leukemia detected by interphase cytogenetics. Cancer Genet Cytogenet 1997;97:97-100.

16. Lazaridou A, Miraxtsi C, Korantzis J, et al: Simultaneous detection of BCL-2 protein, trisomy 12, retinoblastoma and P53 monoallelic gene deletions in B-cell chronic lymphocytic leukemia by fluorescence in situ hybridization (FISH): relation to disease status. Leuk Lymphoma 2000;36:503-512.

17. Marks DI, Kurz BW, Link MP, et al: Altered expression of p53 and mdm-2 proteins at diagnosis is associated with early treatment failure in childhood acute lymphoblastic leukemia. J Clin Oncol 1997;15:1158-1162.

18. Gustafsson B, Stal O, Gustafsson B: Overexpression of MDM2 in acute childhood lymphoblastic leukemia. Pediatr Hematol Oncol 1998;15:519-526.

19. Zhou M, Gu L, Abshire TC, et al: Incidence and prognostic significance of MDM2 oncoprotein overexpression in relapsed childhood acute lymphoblastic leukemia. Leukemia 2000; 14:61-67.

20. Bartlett JMS, White A: Extraction of DNA from whole blood. In Bartlett JMS, Stirling D (eds): PCR Protocols, 2nd ed. Totowa, N.J.: Humana Press, 2003:29-31.

21. Shimizu H, Burns JC: Extraction nucleic acids: sample preparation from paraffin-embedded tissues. In Innis MA, Gelfand DH, Sninsky JJ (eds): PCR Strategies. San Diego: Academic Press, 1995:32-38.

22. Harder J, Schroder JM: RNase 7, a novel innate immune defense antimicrobial protein of healthy human skin. J Biol Chem 2002;277:46779-46784.

23. Tang YW, Procop GW, Persing DH: Molecular diagnostics of infectious diseases. Clin Chem 1997;11:2021-2038.

24. Miller WH, Kakizuka A, Frankel SR, et al: Reverse transcription polymerase chain reaction for the rearranged retinoic acid receptor α clarifies diagnosis and detects minimal residual disease in acute promyelocytic leukemia. Proc Natl Acad Sci USA 1992;89:2694-2698.

25. Schwartz RC, Sonenshein GE, Bothwell A, et al: Multiple expression of Ig λ-chain encoding RNA species in murine plasmacytoma cells. J Immunol 1981;126:2104-2108.

26. Mullis KB, Faloona FA: Specific synthesis of DNA in vitro via a polymerase-catalyzed chain reaction. Methods Enzymol 1987;155:335-350.

27. Saiki RK, Scharf S, Faloona F, et al: Enzymatic amplification of β-globin genomic sequences and restriction site analysis for diagnosis of sickle cell anemia. Science 1985;230:1350-1354.

28. Studwell PS, O'Donnell M: Processive replication is contingent on the exonuclease subunit of DNA polymerase III holoenzyme. J Biol Chem 1990;265:1171-1178.

29. Saiki RK, Gelfand DH, Stoffel S, et al: Primer-directed enzymatic amplification of DNA with a thermostable DNA polymerase. Science 1988;239:487-491.

30. Wiedbrauk DL: Molecular methods for virus detection. Lab Med 1992;23:737-742.

31. Altschul SF, Gish W, Miller W, et al: Basic local alignment search tool. J Mol Biol 1990;215:403-410.

32. Mifflin TE: Setting up a PCR laboratory. In Dieffenbach CW, Dveksler GS (eds): PCR Primer: A Laboratory Manual, 2nd ed. Cold Spring Harbor: CSHL Press, 2003:5-14.

33. Dewald GW, Ketterling RP: Conventional cytogenetics and molecular cytogenetics in hematologic malignancies. In Hoffman R, Benz EJ Jr, Shattil SJ, et al (eds): Hematology: Basic Principles and Practice, 4th ed. Philadelphia: Churchill Livingstone, 2005:928-939.

34. McClure JS, Litz CE: Chronic myelogenous leukemia: molecular diagnostic considerations. Hum Pathol 1994;25:594-597.

35. Keung YK, Beaty M, Powell BL, et al: Philadelphia chromosome positive myelodysplastic syndrome and acute myeloid leukemia—retrospective study. A review of literature. Leuk Res 2004;28:579-586.

36. Bartram CR, de Klein A, Hagemeijer A, et al: Translocation of the c-abl oncogene correlates with the presence of a Philadelphia chromosome in chronic myelocytic leukemia. Nature 1983;306:277-280.

37. Heisterkamp N, Stephenson JR, Groffen J, et al: Localization of the c-abl oncogene adjacent to a translocation break point in chronic myelocytic leukemia. Nature 1983;306:239-242.

38. Clark SS, McLaughlin J, Crist WM, et al: Unique forms of the abl tyrosine kinase distinguish Ph[1]-positive CML from Ph[1]-positive ALL. Science 1987;235:85-88.

39. Preudhomme C, Revillion F, Merlat A, et al: Detection of BCR-ABL transcripts in chronic myeloid leukemia (CML) using a 'real time' quantitative RT-PCR assay. Leukemia 1999;13:957-964.

40. Hebert J, Cayuela JM, Daniel MT, et al: Detection of minimal residual disease in acute myelomonocytic leukemia with abnormal marrow eosinophils by nested polymerase chain reaction with allele specific amplification. Blood 1994; 84:2291-2296.

41. Sambrook J, Russell DW: Gel electrophoresis of DNA and pulsed-field agarose gel electrophoresis. In Sambrook J, Russell DW (eds): Molecular Cloning: A Laboratory Manual, 3rd ed. Cold Spring Harbor: CSHL Press, 2001:5.4-5.86.

42. Lodish H, Berk A, Zipursky SL, et al (eds): Molecular Cell Biology, 4th ed. New York: WH Freeman & Co, 2000:50-99.

43. Nathans D, Smith HO: Restriction endonucleases in the analysis and restructuring of DNA molecules. Annu Rev Biochem 1975;44:273-293.

44. Ross DW: Restriction enzymes. Arch Pathol Lab Med 1990;114:906.

45. De Stefano V, Finazzi G, Mannucci PM: Inherited thrombophilia: pathogenesis, clinical syndromes, and management. Blood 1996;87:3531-3544.

46. Liu XY, Nelson D, Grant C, et al: Molecular detection of a common mutation in coagulation factor V causing thrombosis via hereditary resistance to activated protein C. Diagn Mol Pathol 1995;4:191-197.

47. Southern EM: Detection of specific sequences among DNA fragments separated by gel electrophoresis. J Mol Biol 1975;98:503-517.

48. Chen CY, Shiesh SC, Wu SJ: Rapid detection of K-ras mutations in bile by peptide nucleic acid-mediated PCR clamping and melting curve analysis: comparison with restriction fragment length polymorphism analysis. Clin Chem 2004;50:481-489.

49. Saiki RK, Walsh PS, Levenson CH, et al: Genetic analysis of amplified DNA with immobilized sequence-specific oligonucleotide probes. Proc Natl Acad Sci U S A 1989;86:6230-6234.

50. Thomas PS: Hybridization of denatured RNA and small DNA fragments transferred to nitrocellulose. Proc Natl Acad Sci USA 1980;77:5201-5205.

51. Yuen E, Brown RD: Southern blotting of IgH rearrangements in B-cell disorders. In Brown RD, Ho P (eds): Multiple Myeloma. Totowa, N.J.: Humana Press, 2005:85-103.

52. Dowton SB, Slaugh RA: Diagnosis of human heritable diseases: laboratory approaches and outcomes. Clin Chem 1995;41:785-794.

53. Cossman J, Uppenkamp M, Sundeen J, et al: Molecular genetics and the diagnosis of lymphoma. Arch Pathol Lab Med 1988;112:117-127.

54. Gill JI, Gulley ML: Immunoglobulin and T-cell receptor gene rearrangement. Diagn Hematol 1994;8:751-770.

55. Griesser H, Tkachuk D, Reis D, et al: Gene rearrangements and translocations in lymphoproliferative diseases. Blood 1989;73:1402-1415.

56. Noorali S, Pervez S, Moatter T, et al: Characterization of T-cell non-Hodgkin's lymphoma and its association with Epstein-Barr virus in Pakistani patients. Leuk Lymphoma 2003;44:807-813.

57. Kurosu K, Yumoto N, Mikata A, et al: Monoclonality of B-cell lineage in primary pulmonary lymphoma demonstrated by immunoglobulin heavy chain gene sequence analysis of histologically non-definitive transbronchial biopsy specimens. J Pathol 1996;178:316-322.

58. Hanson CA: Clinical applications of molecular biology in diagnostic hematopathology. Lab Med 1993;24:562-573.

59. Goto M, Oka S, Okuzumi K, et al: Evaluation of acridinium-ester-labeled DNA probes for identification of *Mycobacterium tuberculosis* and *Mycobacterium avium–Mycobacterium intracellulare* complex in culture. J Clin Microbiol 1991;29:2473-2476.

60. Leary JJ, Brigati DJ, Ward DC: Rapid and sensitive colorimetric method for visualizing biotin-labeled DNA probes hybridized to DNA or RNA immobilized on nitrocellulose: Bio-blots. Proc Natl Acad Sci U S A 1983;80:4045-4049.

61. Morrell JI, Greenberger LM, Pfaff DW: Comparison of horseradish peroxidase visualization methods: quantitative results and further technical specifics. J Histochem Cytochem 1981;29:903-916.

62. Thorpe GH, Kricka LJ: Enhanced chemiluminescent reactions catalyzed by horseradish peroxidase. Methods Enzymol 1986;133:331-353.

63. Sanger F, Nicklen S, Coulson AR: DNA sequencing with chain-terminating inhibitors. Proc Natl Acad Sci USA 1977;74:5463-5467.

64. Osborne D, Frost L, Tobal K, et al: Elevated levels of WT1 transcripts in bone marrow harvest are associated with a high relapse risk in patients autografted for acute myeloid leukemia. Bone Marrow Transplant 2005;36:67-70.

65. Kern W, Voskova D, Schoch C, et al: Determination of relapse risk based on assessment of minimal residual disease during complete remission by multiparameter flow cytometry in unselected patients with acute myeloid leukemia. Blood 2004;104:3078-3085.

66. Fenk R, Ak M, Kobbe G, et al: Levels of minimal residual disease detected by quantitative molecular monitoring herald relapse in patients with multiple myeloma. Haematologica 2004;89:557-566.

67. van der Velden VHJ, Hochhaus A, Cazzaniga G, et al: Detection of minimal residual disease in hematologic malignancies by real-time quantitative PCR: principles, approaches, and laboratory aspects. Leukemia 2003;17:1013-1034.

68. Lion T, Henn T, Gaiger A, et al: Early detection of relapse after bone marrow transplantation in patients with chronic myelogenous leukaemia. Lancet 1993;341:275-276.

69. Stentoft J, Pallisgaard N, Kjeldsen E, et al: Kinetics of BCR-ABL fusion transcript levels in chronic myeloid leukemia patients treated with ST1571 measured by quantitative real-time polymerase chain reaction. Eur J Haematol 2001;67:302-308.

70. Gabert J, Beillard E, van der Velden VH, et al: Standardization and quality control studies of "real-time" quantitative reverse transcriptase polymerase chain reaction of fusion transcripts for residual disease detection in leukemia—a Europe Against Cancer program. Leukemia 2003;17:2318-2357.

Flow Cytometric Analysis in Hematologic Disorders

33

Magdalena Czader

OBJECTIVES

After completion of this chapter, the reader will be able to:

1. Describe the technique of flow cytometry, including specimen selection and preparation, instrumentation, data collection, and antibody panel design.
2. Discuss the pattern recognition approach to analysis of flow cytometric data for diagnosis and follow-up of hematologic malignancies.
3. Identify basic cell populations defined by flow cytometric parameters.
4. Recognize the key immunophenotypic features of normal bone marrow, peripheral blood and lymph node specimens, and specimens with acute leukemia and lymphoma.
5. Discuss novel applications of flow cytometry beyond the immunophenotyping of hematologic malignancies.

CASE STUDIES

After studying the material in this chapter, the reader should be able to respond to the following case studies:

Case 1

A 58-year-old man presented with a 5-month history of extensive right cervical lymphadenopathy and night sweats. His complete blood count was within normal limits. Physical examination showed additional bilateral axillary lymphadenopathy. The cervical lymph node was excised. Histologic examination revealed nodular architecture with predominantly medium-sized lymphoid cells with irregular nuclear outlines. Flow cytometric data are presented in Figure 33-1.

1. What cell subpopulation predominates on the forward scatter (FS)/side scatter (SS) scattergram?
2. List antigens positive in this population.
3. Does the pattern of light chain expression support the diagnosis of lymphoma?

Case 2

A 3-year-old girl presented with fatigue and fevers. The complete blood count revealed a white blood cell count of 3×10^9/L, hemoglobin of 8.3 g/dL, and platelet count of 32×10^9/L. Review of the peripheral blood smear showed rare undifferentiated blasts with occasional cytoplasmic blebs. No granules or Aüer rods were identified. Bone marrow examination showed a marked increase in blasts (79%) and decreased background trilineage hematopoiesis. Flow cytometric analysis was performed. In addition to markers shown in Figure 33-2, the population of interest was positive for CD34, CD33, CD41, and HLA-DR.

1. What abnormal features are observed on the CD45/SS scattergram?
2. What is the most likely diagnosis considering the constellation of markers expressed by the predominant population?

Continued

CASE STUDIES—cont'd

After studying the material in this chapter, the reader should be able to respond to the following case studies:

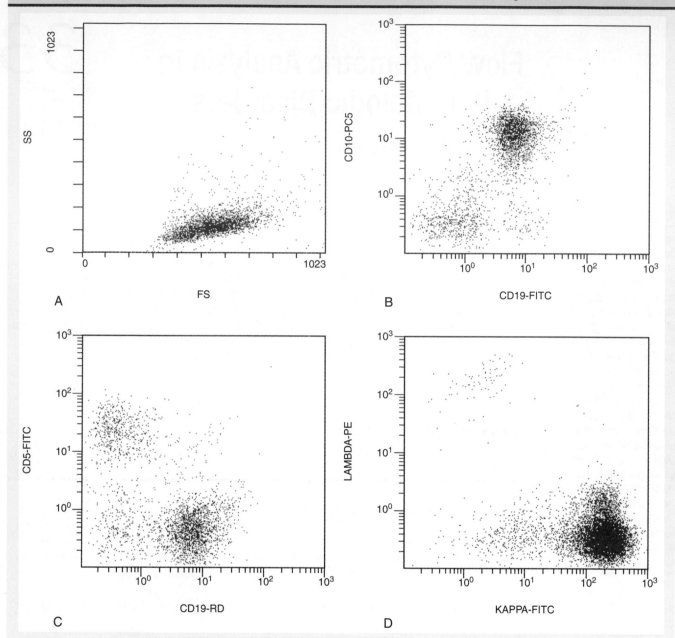

Figure 33-1 Scattergrams showing immunophenotypic features of Case 1.

Flow cytometry originally was designed to measure physical properties of cells based on their ability to deflect light. Over the years, it has evolved to include detection of fluorescent signals emitted by dyes bound directly to specific molecules or attached to proteins through monoclonal antibodies. The development of monoclonal antibodies is the most significant factor that has contributed to today's broad application of flow cytometry. Although the term *flow cytometry* implies the measurement of a cell, this technique is applied successfully to the study of other particles, including chromosomes, microorganisms, and proteins. The main advantage of

flow cytometry over other techniques is the ability to analyze rapidly multiple parameters in a large number of cells. When one adds the capability to identify and quantify rare-event cells in a heterogeneous cell population, the value of flow cytometry to clinical hematology becomes obvious. Currently, this technique not only is applied to the analysis of cell lineage of acute leukemia or the detection of clonality in lymphoid populations but also makes it possible to discern abnormal populations in chronic myeloid disorders, quantitate minimal residual disease, and monitor immunodeficiency states. Immunophenotypes that originally were used to supplement

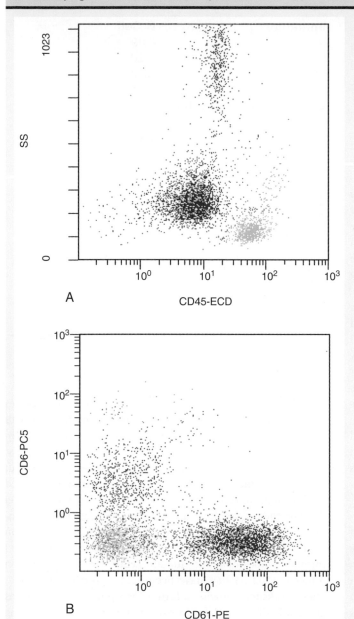

Figure 33-2 Predominant bone marrow population in Case 2.

morphologic classification frequently correlate with specific cytogenetic/molecular abnormalities. According to a classification of hematopoietic neoplasms developed by the World Health Organization,[1] one no longer can rely solely on morphology for diagnosis of hematologic malignancies. The optimal diagnostic algorithm integrates morphology, immunophenotype, and genotype information. This approach solidifies the central role that flow cytometry plays in the hematopathology laboratory.

The review of numerous research applications of flow cytometry is beyond the scope of this chapter. The discussion in this chapter focuses on the use of flow cytometry in the routine hematopathology laboratory. The chapter follows the "life" of the flow cytometric specimen that starts with specimen processing and ends with the final diagnosis. The discussion is divided into preanalytical (specimen processing), analytical (flow cytometric instrumentation and analysis), and postanalytical (immunophenotypic features of hematopoietic disorders) sections.

SPECIMEN PROCESSING

Flow cytometric analysis is particularly useful in diagnosing hematologic malignancies. The specimens most commonly analyzed by this method are bone marrow, peripheral blood, and lymphoid tissues. In addition, immunophenotyping often is performed on body cavity fluids and solid tissues when they are suspected to harbor a hematologic malignancy.[2]

Prolonged transport or transport in inappropriate conditions may render a specimen unsuitable for analysis. Peripheral blood and bone marrow specimens should be processed within 24 to 48 hours from their collection. Certain specimens, such as body cavity fluids or specimens with a high proliferation rate, may require even shorter time intervals between collection and processing.

When cells are suspended in a fluid as in peripheral blood and bone marrow, minimal processing is required. These specimens are collected in an anticoagulant, heparin or ethylenediamine tetraacetic acid (EDTA), and are transported to the flow cytometry laboratory at room temperature. Bone marrow biopsy specimens and solid tissue specimens, including core biopsy samples are submitted in culture media to maintain viability or on saline-moistened gauze. Tissue fragments are mechanically dissociated to yield a cell suspension, usually by mincing with a scalpel.

To purify the specimen, red blood cells are lysed before staining. The analytical process depends on the cellularity and viability of the specimen; both are routinely determined. Cell count can be obtained using automated cell counters or flow cytometry. Trypan blue exclusion, a manual staining method, or flow cytometry of a specimen stained with propidium iodide, a DNA dye, are used to test viability. A cytocentrifuge slide is prepared for the morphologic inspection of the cell suspension.

As soon as these steps are completed, the sample is stained with a cocktail of fluorochrome-conjugated monoclonal antibodies. The analysis of intracytoplasmic markers requires an additional fixation and permeabilization step to allow antibodies to pass through the cell membrane. A predetermined panel of antibodies may be used to detect membrane-bound and intracellular markers. Simultaneous analysis of multiple markers, so-called *multicolor* or *multiparameter flow cytometry*, has numerous advantages. It facilitates visualization of normal antigen expression and maturation pattern, which are often disturbed in hematopoietic malignancies. In addition, regardless of the complexity of the specimen, analysis can be accomplished in a few tubes and with a lower total number of cells, saving on reagents, time, and data storage. There is no consensus on the standardized panel of antibodies to be used in routine flow cytometric evaluation. The U.S.-Canadian Consensus Project in Leukemia/ Lymphoma Immunophenotyping recommends the comprehensive approach with multiple markers for myeloid and lymphoid lineage.[3] Selected markers commonly analyzed by flow cytometry are presented in Table 33-1.

FLOW CYTOMETRY: PRINCIPLE AND INSTRUMENTATION

The most significant discovery that led to the advancement of flow cytometry and its subsequent widespread application to clinical practice was the development of monoclonal anti-

TABLE 33-1 Lineage-Specific Markers Commonly Analyzed in Routine Flow Cytometry

Immature	B Cell
CD34	CD19
CD117	CD20
TdT	CD22
	κ light chain
Granulocytic/Monocytic	λ light chain
CD33	
CD13	**T Cell**
CD15	CD2
CD14	CD3
	CD4
Erythroid	CD5
CD71	CD7
Glycophorin A	CD8
Megakaryocytes	
CD41	
CD42	
CD61	

bodies.[4] In the original *hybridoma* experiments, lymphocytes with predetermined antibody specificity were co-cultured with a myeloma cell line to form immortalized hybrid cells producing specific monoclonal antibodies. For this discovery, which not only fueled the development of flow cytometry but also had innumerable research and, more recently, recognized clinical applications, Köhler and Milstein received a Nobel Prize in 1984. Over the years, numerous antibodies were produced and tested for their lineage specificity. Categorization of these antibodies and associated antigens is accomplished through workshops on Human Leukocyte Differentiation Antigens (HLDA) that have been held regularly since 1982. These workshops provide a forum for reporting new antigens and antibodies and define a cluster of antibodies recognizing the same antigen, called *cluster of differentiation* (CD) (Table 33-2; see also Table 33-1). Consecutive numbers are assigned to each new reported antigen. The VIII HLDA workshop brought the number of characterized antigens to 339.[5]

Monoclonal antibodies have various applications, including immunohistochemistry, immunocytochemistry, immunofluorescence, and Western blotting. These methods study cellular proteins in fixed tissues or in cellular extracts; however, they do not provide the ability to examine antigens in their native state and cannot decipher composite cell populations with complex makeup of antigens. In contrast, flow cytometry can define antigen expression on numerous viable cells. Currently, 17 antigens can be detected simultaneously on an individual cell.[6] This is accomplished by the conjugation of monoclonal antibodies to a variety of fluorochromes that can be detected directly by a flow cytometer. In the flow cytometer,

TABLE 33-2 Hematolymphoid Antigens Commonly Used in Clinical Flow Cytometry

Cluster of Differentiation	Function	Cellular Expression
CD1a	T cell development	Precursor T cells
CD2	T cell activation	Precursor and mature T cells, NK cells
CD3	Antigen recognition	Precursor and mature T cells
CD4	Coreceptor for HLA class II	Precursor T cells, helper T cells, monocytes
CD5	T cell signaling	Precursor and mature T cells, subset of B cells
CD7	T cell activation	Precursor and mature T cells, NK cells
CD8	Coreceptor for HLA class I	Precursor T cells, suppressor/cytotoxic T cells, subset of NK cells
CD10	B cell regulation	Precursor B cells, germinal center B cells, granulocytes
CD11b	Cell adhesion	Granulocytic and monocytic lineage, NK cells
CD13	Unknown	Granulocytic and monocytic lineage
CD14	Monocyte activation	Mature monocytes
CD15	Ligand for selectins	Granulocytic and monocytic lineage
CD16	Low-affinity IgG Fc receptor	Granulocytic and monocytic lineage, NK cells
CD18	Cell adhesion and signaling	Granulocytic and monocytic lineage
CD19	B cell activation	Precursor and mature B cells
CD20	B cell activation	Precursor and mature B cells
CD22	B cell activation and adhesion	Precursor and mature B cells
CD31	Cell adhesion	Megakaryocytes, platelets, leukocytes
CD33	Unknown	Granulocytic and monocytic lineage
CD34	Cell adhesion	Hematopoietic stem cells
CD36	Cell adhesion	Megakaryocytes, platelets, erythroid precursors, monocytes
CD38	Cell activation and proliferation	Hematopoietic cells including activated lymphocytes and plasma cells
CD41	Cell adhesion	Megakaryocytes, platelets
CD42b	Receptor for von Willebrand factor	Megakaryocytes, platelets
CD45	T and B cell receptor activation	Hematopoietic cells
CD56	Cell adhesion	NK cells, subset of T cells
CD61	Cell adhesion	Megakaryocytes, platelets
CD62P	Homing	Platelets
CD63	Unknown	Platelets
CD64	High-affinity IgG Fc receptor	Granulocytic and monocytic lineage
CD71	Iron uptake	High density on erythroid precursors, other proliferating cells
CD79a	B cell receptor signal transduction	Precursor and mature B cells
CD117	Stem cell factor receptor	Hematopoietic stem cells, mast cells

particles are suspended in fluid and pass one by one in front of a light source. As particles are illuminated, they emit fluorescent signals registered by detectors. These results are later converted to digital output and analyzed using flow cytometry software. The flow cytometer consists of fluids, a light source (laser), a detection system, and computer. A brief discussion of these basic components is presented.

To be analyzed as individual events, cells must pass separately, one by one, through the illumination and detection system of the flow cytometer. This passage is accomplished by injecting the cell suspension into a stream of sheath fluid. This technique, called *hydrodynamic focusing*, creates a central core of individually aligned cells surrounded by a sheath fluid (Fig. 33-3). The central alignment is essential for consistent illumination of the cells as they pass before the laser light source.

The laser is composed of a tube filled with gas, most commonly argon or helium-neon, and a power supply. The current that is applied to the gas raises the electrons of gas to the excited state. When electrons return to the ground state, they emit photons of light. Through the amplification system, a strong beam of light with identical direction, polarization

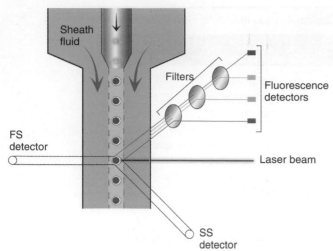

Figure 33-3 Diagram of a flow cytometer. As cells are injected into pressurized sheath fluid, they are positioned in a center of the stream and one by one exposed to the laser light. Forward scatter (FSC or FS) and Side scatter (SSC or SS) are collected by separate detectors.

plane, and spectrum is produced. This narrow coherent beam of light is used to illuminate individual cells, each stained with antibodies conjugated to specific fluorochromes.

After the absorption of laser light, the electrons of fluorochromes are raised from ground to a higher energy state (Fig. 33-4). The return to the original ground level is accompanied

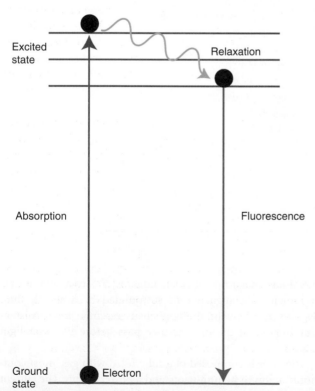

Figure 33-4 Jablonski diagram showing a principle of fluorescence. When electrons absorb energy, they are raised to the excited state. Subsequently, on return to ground state, the absorbed energy is emitted in a form of fluorescence.

by the loss of energy, emitted as light of a specific wavelength. Each flow cytometer is equipped with several photodetectors specific for light of a unique color (wavelength). The fluorescence from an individual cell is partitioned into its different wavelengths through a series of filters (dichroic mirrors) and directed to a corresponding photodetector. Fluorescent signals derived from different fluorochromes attached to particular antibodies are registered separately.

In addition to fluorescence, scatter signals are detected. The detector situated directly in line with the illuminating laser beam measures forward scatter (FSC or FS), which is proportional to particle volume/size. A photodetector located to the side measures side scatter (SSC or SS), reflecting surface complexity and internal structures such as granules and vacuoles. FSC, SSC, and fluorescence are displayed simultaneously on the screen and registered by the computer system.

PATTERN RECOGNITION APPROACH TO ANALYSIS OF FLOW CYTOMETRIC DATA

Concept of Gating

Cell populations with similar physical properties of size, internal and surface complexity, and the presence of a specific antigen form data display *clusters*. A *gate* is an electronic borderline the operator may use to delineate clusters. Gating is a process of selecting, with a cursor or computer mouse, a population of interest as defined by one or more flow cytometric parameters.

Gating can be applied at the time of data acquisition (live gate) or at the time of analysis. For diagnostic purposes, data are collected ungated, meaning all events detected by flow cytometer are recorded. This allows comprehensive testing of the sample and retention of positive and negative internal controls. In addition, unexpected abnormal populations are detected. Gating is most commonly applied after the specimen is run, when the target population is already known. In contrast, live-gating focuses on the acquisition of a specific cell population as defined by flow cytometric parameters. One can collect only CD19⁺ B cells to facilitate detection of a small population of monoclonal B cells.

Analysis of Flow Cytometric Data

Analogous to microscopic examination, proper evaluation of flow cytometric data is based on the inspection of visual patterns. First, the entire display is scanned to detect the presence of abnormal populations. Subsequent analysis focuses on the antigenic properties of abnormal cells.

Analysis begins with inspection of dot-plots presenting cell size, internal complexity, and the expression of pan-hematopoietic antigen CD45, expressed at different levels on all leukocytes. Analogous to low-magnification microscopic examination, at this stage the operator detects specific cell populations based on their physical properties (Fig. 33-5). The identification of particular populations can be confirmed and resolved further on the scattergram of the CD45 antigen and SSC (Fig. 33-6). This display also provides information on the relative proportion of specific cell populations in the flow

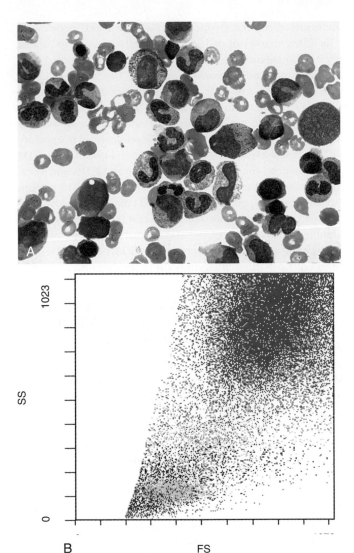

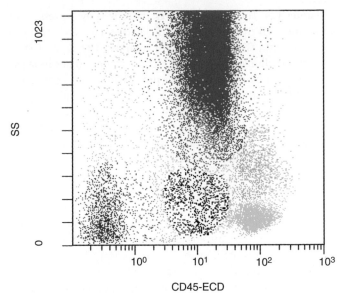

Figure 33-6 Scattergram showing differential densities of pan-hematopoietic marker CD45 on marrow leukocytes. Lymphocytes *(aqua)* and monocytes *(green)* show highest density of CD45 antigen. Intermediate expression of CD45 is seen in granulocytic population *(navy)* and blasts *(black)*. Erythroid precursors *(red)* are CD45⁻.

Figure 33-5 Main cell subpopulations of normal bone marrow. **A,** Bone marrow is composed of a heterogeneous population of cells of different sizes and complexity of cytoplasm (Wright-Giemsa, ×1000). **B,** Dot-plot of FSC (cell size) versus SSC (internal complexity) reflects heterogeneity of bone marrow subpopulations. Lymphocytes are smallest with negligible amount of agranular cytoplasm and are located closest to the origins of the axes *(aqua)*. Monocytes are slightly larger with occasional granules and vacuoles *(green)*. Granulocytic series shows prominent granularity *(navy)*.

CELL POPULATIONS IDENTIFIED BY FLOW CYTOMETRY

The surface and cytoplasmic markers expressed in hematologic malignancies resemble those of normal hematopoietic cell differentiation. Frequently, neoplastic cells arrest at a particular stage of development and display aberrant antigenic patterns. The diagnosis and subclassification of hematologic neoplasms is based on the knowledge of normal hematopoietic maturation pathways.

In the past, the differentiation of hematopoietic cells was defined by morphologic criteria. Over time, it became clear that specific morphologic stages of development are accompanied by distinct changes in immunophenotypes. Approximate morphologic-immunophenotypic correlates exist; hematopoiesis is a continuous process, and transitions between various developmental phases are not discrete.

All hematopoietic progeny are derived from pluripotent stem cells. These cells are morphologically unrecognizable and are defined by their functional and antigenic characteristics. They usually express a combination of CD34, CD117 (c-kit), CD38, and HLA-DR.[9] As hematopoietic cells mature, they lose stem cell markers and acquire lineage-specific antigens. A brief discussion of the maturation sequence of the major hematopoietic cell lineages is presented subsequently.

Myeloid Lineage

The stages of myeloid lineage development, as defined by the expression of specific antigens, correspond closely to the morphologic sequence.[10] The first morphologically recognizable cell committed to the myeloid lineage is a myeloblast

cytometric sample. Lymphocytes show highest-density CD45, with approximately 10% of the cell membrane occupied by this antigen. Granulocytic series show intermediate CD45 density; erythroid precursors and megakaryocytes are negative. The CD45/SSC display is particularly useful for detection of blasts, which overlap with lymphocytes, monocytes, or both on the FSC/SSC.[7,8]

The FSC/SSC and CD45/SSC displays allow the initial identification of the target population. Further analysis focuses on the patterns of antigen expression including qualitative data (antigen present or absent) and fluorescence intensity as a relative measure of surface antigen density.

(Chapter 12). The myeloblast is characterized by expression of immature cell markers CD34, CD38, HLA-DR, and stem cell factor receptor CD117. Pan-myeloid markers, CD13 and CD33, present on all myeloid progeny are first expressed at this stage. As the myeloblast matures to a promyelocyte, it loses CD34 and HLA-DR and acquires the CD15 antigen. Further maturation to the myelocyte stage leads to the expression of CD11b, temporary loss of CD13, and a gradual decrease in the density of CD33. Finally, as myeloid cells near the band stage, CD16 is acquired, and the density of CD13 increases.

Monocytic Lineage

The earliest immunophenotype stage of monocytic development is defined by a gradual increase in the density of CD13, CD33, and CD11b antigens. Subsequent acquisition of CD15 and CD14 marks the transition to a promonocyte and mature monocyte. In contrast to the granulocytic series, bright expression of CD64 and HLA-DR antigens persists throughout monocytic maturation.

Erythroid Lineage

Erythroid precursors are among the few marrow cells that do not express pan-hematopoietic marker CD45. The earliest marker of erythroid differentiation is the transferrin receptor, CD71. The density of this antigen increases starting from the pronormoblast stage and is rapidly down-regulated in reticulocytes.[11] In contrast, glycophorin A, although present on reticulocytes and erythrocytes, first appears at the basophilic normoblast stage.

Megakaryocytic Lineage

The maturation sequence of megakaryocytes is less well defined. CD41 and CD61, referred to as *GP IIb/IIIa complex*, appear as the first markers of megakaryocytic differentiation. These antigens are present on a small subset of CD34+ cells believed to represent early megakaryoblasts.[9] CD31 and CD36, although not entirely specific for megakaryocytic lineage, also are present on megakaryoblasts. Subsequent maturation to megakaryocytes and platelets is characterized by the appearance of additional glycoproteins, CD42, CD62P, and CD63.

Lymphoid Lineage

The B and T lymphocytes are derived from lymphoid progenitors that express CD34, terminal deoxynucleotidyl transferase (TdT), and HLA-DR. The lymphoid differentiation represents a continuum of changes in the surface and cytoplasmic antigen expression. The earliest B cell markers include CD19, cytoplasmic CD22, and cytoplasmic CD79.[12] As B cell precursors mature, they acquire the CD10 antigen. The appearance of the mature B cell marker CD20 coincides with the decrease in CD10 antigen expression. Another specific immature B cell marker is the cytoplasmic μ chain that eventually is transported to the surface and forms the B cell receptor. At this stage, the immunoglobulin chains in so-called *naive B cells* have become rearranged. The normal B cell population now show a mix of κ and λ light chain–expressing cells. The exclusive expression of only κ or λ molecules is a marker of monoclonality, seen frequently in mature B cell neoplasms. The differentiation of mature naive B cells, often recapitulated by B cell malignancies, is discussed in detail in Chapter 37.

Similar to B cell precursors, immature T cells express CD34 and TdT.[13] The first markers associated with T cell lineage include CD2, CD7, and cytoplasmic CD3. These antigens also can be present in natural killer (NK) cells and, along with the CD56 molecule, are used to detect NK cell–derived neoplasms. In T cells, the expression of CD2, CD7, and cytoplasmic CD3 is followed by the appearance of CD1a and CD5 and coexpression of CD4 and CD8 antigens. Finally, the CD3 antigen appears on the cell surface, and CD4 or CD8 is lost. The sequential transition from double-negative (CD4−CD8−) through double-positive (CD4+CD8+) stages generates a population of mature helper (CD4+) and suppressor (CD8+) T cells. The latter stages of T cell differentiation occur in the thymus.

FLOW CYTOMETRIC ANALYSIS OF MYELOID DISORDERS (ACUTE MYELOID LEUKEMIAS AND CHRONIC MYELOID DISORDERS)

In myeloid malignancies, flow cytometry is used for initial diagnosis, follow-up, and prognostication. The specific immunophenotypes are associated with selected cytogenetic abnormalities. Because most myeloid malignancies are stem cell disorders, the evaluation of blast population and maturing myeloid component is considered mandatory. Almost invariably, blasts are characterized by the expression of low-density CD45 antigen. In normal bone marrow, the blast gate includes a relatively low number of cells showing the immature myeloid immunophenotype (see Fig. 33-6). In acute myeloid and lymphoid leukemias, this region becomes densely populated by immature cells reflecting the increase of blasts seen in the bone marrow (Fig. 33-7). The exact location of the immature population on customarily used displays of CD45/SSC depends on the subtype of acute myeloid leukemia (AML). In this chapter, the immunophenotypic features of AMLs and chronic myeloid disorders are discussed in the context of the World Health Organization classification, which introduced categories defined by recurrent cytogenetic abnormalities. These leukemias often show specific immunophenotypes; they are presented separately in the following sections.

Acute Myeloid Leukemias with Recurrent Cytogenetic Abnormalities

In most cases, AML with t(8;21)(q22;q22);(AML1/ETO) shows an immature myeloid immunophenotype with high-density CD34 and coexpression of CD19 (Fig. 33-8).[14] In addition, numerous myeloid antigens, including CD33, CD13, and myeloperoxidase, are expressed. Frequently, there is asynchronous coexpression of CD34 and CD15. TdT is commonly present.

AML with inv(16)(p13q22) or t(16;16)(p13;q22)/(CBFbeta/MYH11) is characterized by the presence of immature cells with expression of CD34, CD117, and TdT and a subpopulation of maturing cells showing monocytic (CD14, CD11b, CD4) and granulocytic (CD15) markers.[15] The coexpression of CD2, more typically seen on T and NK cells, is common.

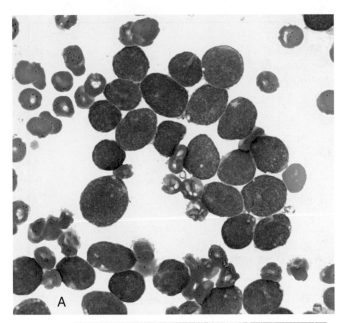

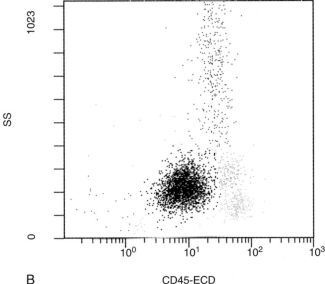

B   CD45-ECD

Figure 33-7 Bone marrow with acute leukemia. Note uniform cytologic and flow cytometric characteristics. **A,** Bone marrow aspirate of ALL (Wright-Giemsa, ×500). **B,** CD45 and SSC show a homogeneous population of blasts with marked decrease in normal hematopoietic elements. Compare with the heterogeneous pattern of normal bone marrow in Figure 33-6.

Acute promyelocytic leukemia (AML with t(15;17)(q22;q12)) shows a highly specific immunophenotype. In contrast to most less-differentiated myeloid leukemias, acute promyelocytic leukemia manifests with high SSC, reflecting the granular cytoplasm of leukemic cells (Fig. 33-9). A constellation of immunophenotypic features used to diagnose acute promyelocytic leukemia include lack of CD34 and HLA-DR antigens, presence of homogeneous CD33 along with myeloperoxidase, and variable CD13 and CD15.[16]

AMLs with 11q23 (*MLL* gene) abnormalities constitute a heterogeneous group most commonly presenting with monocytic differentiation. The immunophenotypic features are nonspecific and can be seen in any acute myelomonocytic or monocytic leukemia (CD34⁻ and positive for CD33, CD13, CD14, CD4, CD11b, and CD64).

Acute Myeloid Leukemias Not Otherwise Categorized

In the least-differentiated AMLs, AML minimally differentiated and AML without maturation, blasts are present in the region of low-density CD45 antigen and display low SSC, reflecting their relatively agranular cytoplasm. Even the least differentiated AMLs usually express myeloid markers. AML, minimally differentiated, and AML without maturation can be positive for CD13, CD33, and CD117. Primitive hematopoietic antigens such as CD34 and HLA-DR are often seen. Myeloperoxidase is negative or expressed only in a few cells. The immunophenotypic profile of AML with maturation is similar, but more mature myeloid markers such as CD15 and myeloperoxidase are often expressed.

Occasionally, there is aberrant coexpression of antigens. Antigens present exclusively in the early or late stages of myeloid differentiation are expressed simultaneously on the leukemic blasts (asynchronous antigen expression). Similarly, markers specific for other lineages such as lymphoid may be seen on myeloid blasts. The most common example is CD7 antigen, usually present in the T/NK cell population (Fig. 33-10).

Acute myelomonocytic leukemia and acute monoblastic leukemia, usually show brighter expression of CD45 similar to normal monocytic precursors. In addition, in acute myelomonocytic leukemia, a population of primitive *myeloid* blasts is often seen (Fig. 33-11). The expression of myeloid markers and antigens associated with monocytic lineage, such as CD14, CD4, CD11b, and CD64, is commonly seen. Although CD14 is present on all mature monocytes, it may be negative in monocytic leukemias.[17] More immature monocytic markers, such as CD64, are more consistently expressed.

Acute erythroid leukemias are categorized into two subtypes: pure erythroid leukemia and erythroid/myeloid leukemia (erythroleukemia). In the latter, similar to acute myelomonocytic leukemia, primitive myeloid blasts and erythroid precursors are present. Erythroid markers, CD71, glycophorin A, and hemoglobin, are seen in leukemic cells. In more immature erythroid leukemias, glycophorin A and hemoglobin may be absent. In these cases, the diagnosis is based on the absence of myeloid markers, presence of bright CD71, and scatter characteristics.

Acute megakaryoblastic leukemia usually shows low SSC and dim to absent CD45. Early megakaryocytic markers, CD41 and CD61, are frequently expressed.[18] Occasionally, the late megakaryocytic marker, CD42, is present. The expression of stem cell markers, CD34 and HLA-DR, on the population of leukemic megakaryoblasts varies.

Myeloproliferative Disorders and Myelodysplastic Syndromes

The knowledge of antigen expression in the normal differentiation of myeloid lineages made it possible to detect the aberrant expression patterns frequently seen in chronic myeloid disorders. The abnormalities detected by flow

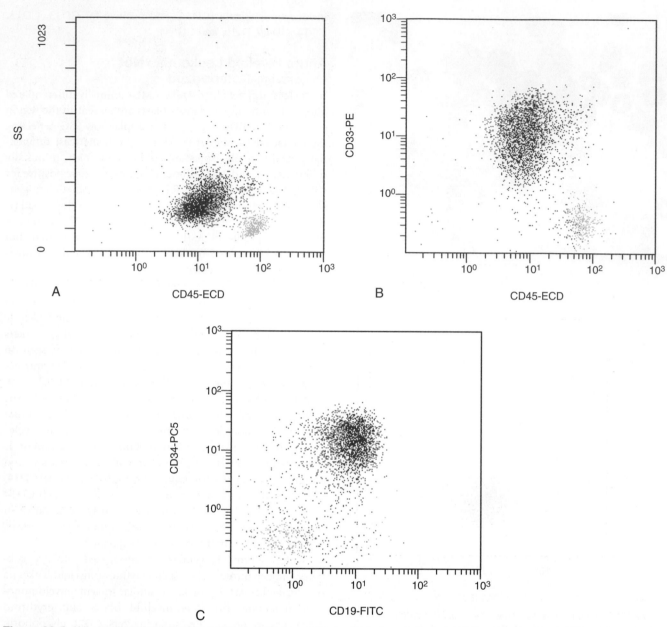

Figure 33-8 AML with t(8;21)(q22;q22);(AML1/ETO). **A,** CD45 versus SSC showing increase in blasts *(red)* with residual lymphocytes *(aqua).* **B** and **C,** Blasts are positive for CD33 and CD34 with characteristic coexpression of CD19 antigen.

cytometry reflect morphologic features of the disorder (e.g., hypogranulation of mature neutrophils in myelodysplastic syndrome detected by low SSC) and changes in the antigen expression. Qualitative (presence or loss of a particular antigen) and quantitative changes (differences in the number of antigen molecules) can be used for diagnostic purposes. The interested reader is referred to review articles discussing the details of immunophenotyping in myelodysplastic syndromes and myeloproliferative disorders.[19,20] A few examples are highlighted to illustrate the role of flow cytometry in diagnosing these diseases.

SSC abnormalities related to hypogranulated neutrophils are seen in approximately 70% of myelodysplastic syndromes (Fig. 33-12). In high-grade myelodysplastic syndrome and

myeloproliferative disorders undergoing transformation, the increase in immature cells is detected easily. Blasts have a variety of aberrant immunophenotypic features, most commonly coexpression of CD7 and CD56 antigens. Blasts and maturing granulocytic precursors may show asynchronous expression of myeloid markers, including retention of CD34 and HLA-DR in late stages of granulocytic lineage or late myeloid markers early in differentiation such as CD15 on myeloblasts. Asynchronous coexpression of markers also can be seen in monocytic and erythroid lineages. Although morphology remains the basis for the diagnosis of myelodysplastic syndrome, aberrant immunophenotypes are seen in 98% of cases. More importantly, in cases with minimal or no myelodysplasia, flow cytometry predicted the future develop-

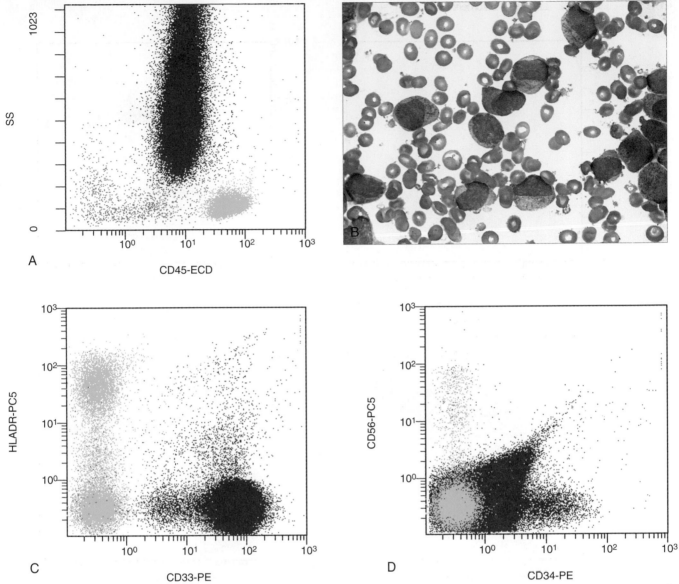

Figure 33-9 Acute promyelocytic leukemia. **A,** Typical SSC pattern of acute promyelocytic leukemia corresponding to prominent granularity of leukemic cells *(red)*. Residual lymphocytes are shown in *aqua*. **B,** Numerous leukemic promyelocytes with distinct granules and occasional Aüer rods (Wright-Giemsa, ×1000). **C,** Acute promyelocytic leukemia shows high-density expression of CD33 antigen and lacks HLA-DR. **D,** Similarly, CD34 antigen is absent or present only in a few leukemic cells.

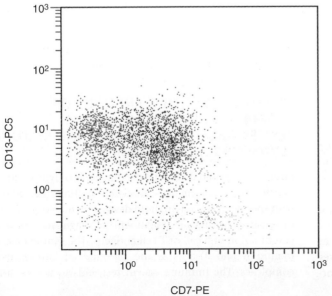

Figure 33-10 Myeloblasts of AML show aberrant coexpression of CD7 antigen.

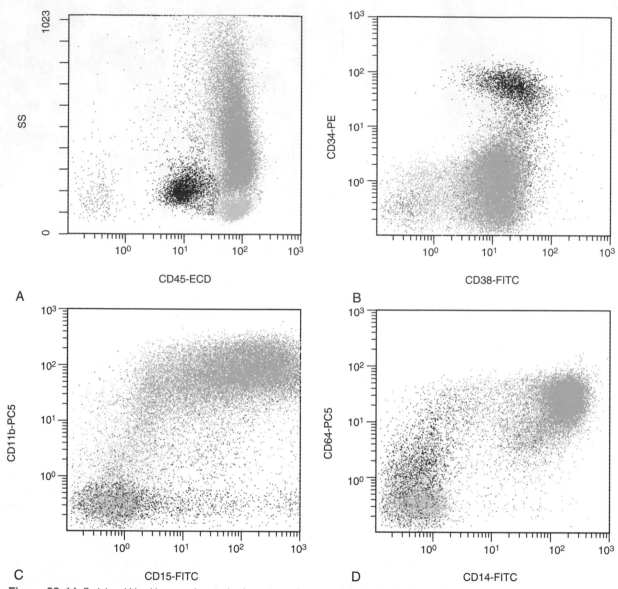

Figure 33-11 Peripheral blood immunophenotyping in acute myelomonocytic leukemia. **A,** CD45/SSC display shows myeloid blasts *(red)* and a monocytic population *(green)*. **B-D,** Primitive leukemic blasts are positive for CD34 and negative for CD14. In contrast, monocytic population does not express CD34 and shows positivity for mature monocyte marker CD14 and characteristic monocytic pattern of CD11b and CD15 expression.

ment of cytogenetic abnormality diagnostic of myelodysplastic syndrome.[19] Other studies underscore the prognostic significance of immunophenotypic abnormalities for the course of the disease and for the outcome after stem cell transplantation.[21,22]

The utility of flow cytometry in myeloproliferative disorders is less well established. Specifically, the application of flow cytometry as a diagnostic tool in chronic myelogenous leukemia is limited to accelerated phase or blast crisis, in which a lineage of an expanding blast population needs to be determined. In the chronic phase, presence of the Philadelphia chromosome as seen on conventional karyotyping or by fluorescent in situ hybridization remains the defining feature. Other myeloproliferative disorders are not well studied. In general, flow cytometric abnormalities are seen in most cases with cytogenetic abnormalities.[20] No consistent set of abnor-

malities was described, however, that can be routinely used in the work-up of myeloproliferative states.

FLOW CYTOMETRIC ANALYSIS OF LYMPHOID NEOPLASMS (ACUTE LYMPHOBLASTIC LEUKEMIA AND MATURE LYMPHOID NEOPLASMS)

Similar to myeloid disorders, the diagnosis of lymphoid malignancies relies on lineage-associated markers corresponding with specific stages of lymphoid development. No single marker can be used for lineage assignment, so diagnosis is based on a combination of B cell or T cell antigens. The sentinel feature of mature B and T cells is the presence of surface receptor complexes. The immune system responds to a wide array of

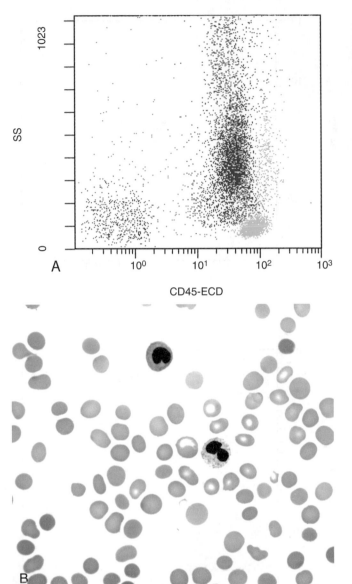

Figure 33-12 A, Low SSC of hypogranular neutrophils seen in most cases of myelodysplastic syndrome (navy blue). **B,** Corresponding photomicrograph of markedly dysplastic, hypogranulated neutrophils in myelodysplastic syndrome (Wright-Giemsa, ×1000).

antigens; in healthy individuals, B and T cells express a great diversity of surface immunoglobulin and T cell receptor complexes (polyclonal populations). A neoplastic lymphoid population is characterized by the monoclonal expression of a single B or T cell receptor. In most cases, clonality confirms the malignant nature of lymphoid proliferation. In contrast, lymphoid precursors are generally negative for surface immunoglobulin and T cell receptors and instead carry immature markers. In lymphoblastic (precursor-derived) neoplasms, the expansion of a population with homogeneous marker expression rather than clonality is diagnostic. The following section presents the key immunophenotypic features of acute lymphoblastic leukemias (ALLs) and lymphomas. Selected examples of the association between the immunophenotype and the genotype are discussed.

Precursor B (Acute) Lymphoblastic Leukemia/Lymphoblastic Lymphoma

Precursor B ALL presents with CD19, cytoplasmic or membranous CD22, CD79a, HLA-DR, and TdT (Fig. 33-13). The expression of CD34 and CD10 is frequently seen. Surface immunoglobulin light chains are not present. Cytoplasmic μ chain or IgM may be detected, however. Because ALL can arise at any stage of B cell differentiation, a combination of markers usually occurs defining an early precursor, intermediate, and pre-B ALL. Frequently, immunophenotypes correlate with specific cytogenetic and clinical features. In routine practice, confirmation of cytogenetic abnormality with conventional karyotyping or molecular techniques is necessary.

Acute Lymphoblastic Leukemia with Rearrangements of 11q23 (MLL Gene)

MLL gene rearrangements occur most frequently in infant ALL. Unlike most ALL, blasts in this leukemia are negative for CD10 antigen.[23] CD19, CD34, TdT, and occasional myeloid markers are positive. The more mature B cell marker, CD20, is negative.

Acute Lymphoblastic Leukemia with BCR/ABL *Translocation*

Philadelphia chromosome (t(9;22); *BCR/ABL*) is a hallmark of chronic myelogenous leukemia but also can occur in pediatric and adult ALL. These cases carry a particularly dismal prognosis, so it is important to identify them promptly. Most *BCR/ABL* cases have a classic intermediate or *common* ALL immunophenotype with the expression of CD19, CD10, CD34, and TdT. The expression of myeloid markers, CD13 and CD33, is common. The density of antigens and their homogeneous or heterogeneous expression within leukemic populations correlates closely with the presence of *BCR/ABL*.[24]

Precursor T (Acute) Lymphoblastic Leukemia/Lymphoblastic Lymphoma

Precursor T ALL and lymphoblastic lymphoma are derived from immature cells committed to T cell lineage. Designation of leukemia or lymphoma depends on the primary site of involvement, bone marrow or lymph node. Both express a combination of markers reflecting the stage of T cell differentiation. CD3 is the most specific T cell marker. Similar to normal T cells, this antigen is seen initially in the cytoplasm before appearing on the cell surface. Other T cell antigens include CD2, CD7, CD5, CD1a, CD4, and CD8. Usually a series of these antigens is detected, recapitulating the T cell differentiation (Fig. 33-14). CD34 and CD10 also may be present. As in other lymphoid neoplasms, the panel of markers determines the lineage of the case. The correlation of the immunophenotype with specific genetic lesions is unclear, and the stage of differentiation of leukemic T cells is not used for prognostication.

Mature Lymphoid Neoplasms

B and T cell lymphomas display immunophenotypes resembling their normal counterparts. The immunophenotypic features of lymphomas are discussed in detail in Chapter 37 and

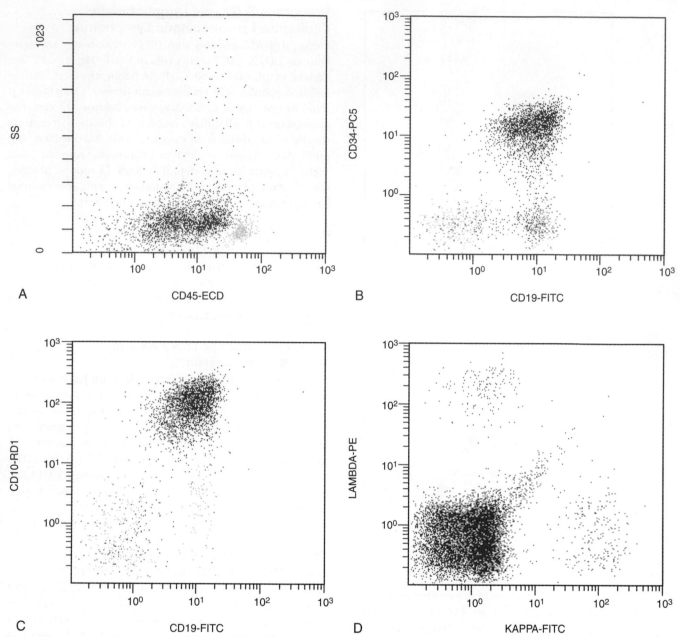

Figure 33-13 Precursor B ALL. **A,** Low-density CD45 antigen characteristic for blast population. **B,** Uniform expression of CD34 and CD19 on leukemic blasts. **C,** High-density CD10 on CD19⁺ blasts. **D,** Lack of surface κ and λ light chains signifies immature B cell population.

summarized in Table 37-2. The flow cytometric work-up of lymphomas assumes that mature lymphoid neoplasms constitute a *clonal* proliferation, implying the malignant lymphoma population is derived from a single cell. All neoplastic cells should show similar genetic and immunophenotypic features. This stands in strong contrast to the variable immunophenotypes of a normal lymphoid population, reflecting a process of antigen-driven selection.

Mature B Cell Neoplasms
Normal precursor B cells randomly rearrange immunoglobulin heavy and light chains. As a result, a mature B cell population expresses a mix of heavy and light chains (Fig. 33-15A). In contrast, a monoclonal surface light chain expression, exclu-

sively κ or λ, is seen in most B cell lymphomas (Fig. 33-15B). Light chain monoclonality along with the expression of pan B cell markers is diagnostic of B cell lymphoma. Rarely, lymphomas may lose the expression of surface light chains, a feature not seen in normal mature B cells.[25] Neoplastic plasma cells lack surface immunoglobulin light chains and express only cytoplasmic κ or λ.

Mature T Cell Neoplasms
Similarly, in T cells, clonality is synonymous with malignancy. Traditionally, the neoplastic nature of T cell population is confirmed only through the molecular analysis of T cell receptor genes. Recently a flow cytometry–based method also has been shown to detect clonality in most T cell lymphomas.[26]

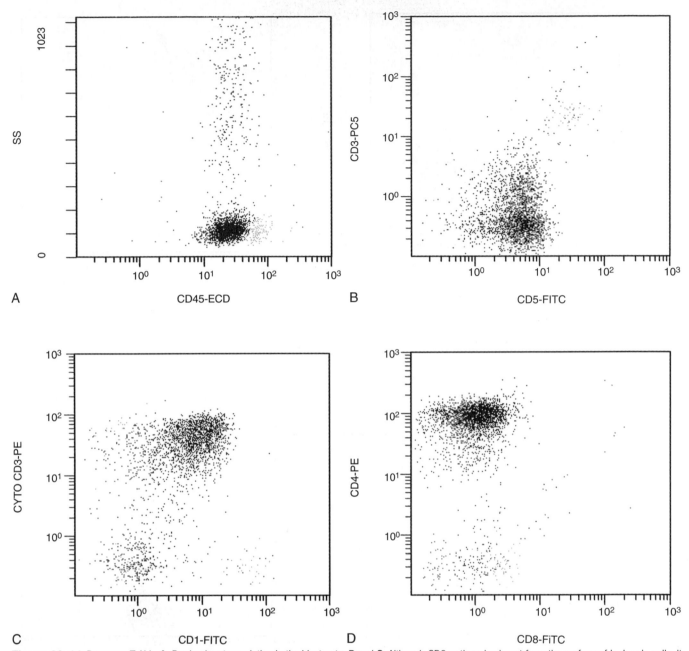

Figure 33-14 Precursor T ALL. **A,** Predominant population in the blast gate. **B** and **C,** Although CD3 antigen is absent from the surface of leukemic cells, it is present in blast cytoplasm, confirming precursor T cell origin of the leukemia (C). Note residual normal T cells *(aqua)* positive for surface CD3 and CD5 antigens. **D,** Simultaneous expression of CD4 and CD8 antigens.

This technique uses a broad array of antibodies against variable regions of T cell receptors. Because this methodology is not yet widely available, often the diagnosis of T cell lymphoma is based on aberrant immunophenotype. In most cases, a loss or atypical expression of a lymphoid marker can be shown using flow cytometry. Mycosis fungoides/Sézary syndrome is characterized by a mature T-cell immunophenotype with expression of CD2, surface CD3, CD5, and CD4 and a loss of the CD7 antigen (Fig. 33-16). The aberrant immunophenotype is a reliable diagnostic feature when the neoplastic population is significant. Because small numbers of T cells with unusual antigen makeup appear in inflammatory conditions,[27] how-

ever, the aberrant immunophenotype alone cannot be considered pathognomonic of the malignancy.

OTHER APPLICATIONS OF FLOW CYTOMETRY BEYOND IMMUNOPHENOTYPING OF HEMATOLOGIC MALIGNANCIES

The immunophenotyping of hematolymphoid neoplasms is one of many applications of flow cytometry. Other common applications include the diagnosis and monitoring of immunodeficiency states, diagnosis of paroxysmal nocturnal

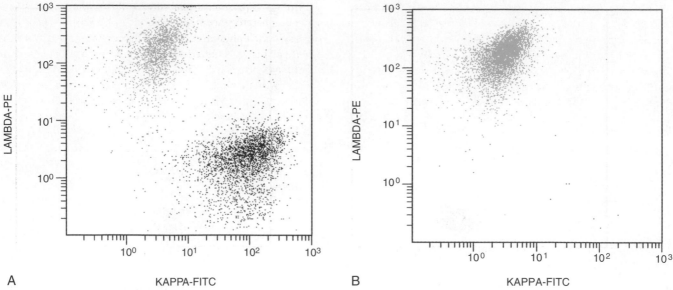

Figure 33-15 Comparison of surface light chain expression in reactive and malignant B cells. **A,** Reactive B cells show heterogeneous expression of κ and λ. **B,** B cell lymphomas are monoclonal with the entire lymphoma population expressing only one type of light chain.

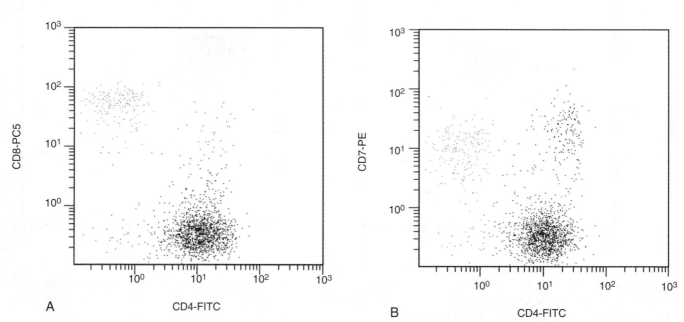

Figure 33-16 Mycosis fungoides. **A,** T cell population is positive for CD4 antigen *(red)*. **B,** Neoplastic T cells show loss of CD7 *(red)*.

hemoglobinuria, stem cell enumeration, cell cycle analysis, detection of fetal hemoglobin, and monitoring of sepsis.

Primary (inherited) and secondary (acquired) immunodeficiency may be diagnosed using flow cytometry. The loss of specific antigens (e. g., CD11/CD18 in leukocyte adhesion deficiency) and functional defects (e.g., oxidative burst evaluation in chronic granulomatous disease) can be assayed.

Human immunodeficiency virus causes a progressive decrease in the number of CD4+ helper T cells. The absolute number of helper T cells in peripheral blood approximately correlates to the stage of the disease and patient prognosis. The

enumeration of T cells and their subsets is easily accomplished by flow cytometry using antibodies against CD4 and CD8 antigens. The absolute numbers are derived from a routine white blood cell count of the concurrent peripheral blood specimen or from special calibrating beads run simultaneously with the patient sample.

The diagnostic approach to paroxysmal nocturnal hemoglobinuria (PNH) is a prime example of how the application of flow cytometry increases understanding of hematologic disorders and directly contributes to clinical decision making (Chapter 23).[28] Before the development of flow cytometric assay, PNH diagnosis was based on detection of increased susceptibility of red blood cells to lysis by the Ham test or sucrose hemolysis test. Intravascular hemolysis, however, decreased the sensitivity of in vitro hemolysis testing. Flow cytometry demonstrates deficiency or absence of involved proteins from red blood cells, granulocytes, monocytes, and lymphoid cells. Absence or decreased expression of CD59 and CD55 antigens is diagnostic for PNH. In addition, the level of CD59 expression correlates with clinical symptoms. (Fig. 33-17).

Another important capability of flow cytometry is cell sorting. A heterogeneous population is physically divided into subsets by their physical or immunophenotypic properties. High-speed sorting is achieved through charging of droplets containing individual cells. As the charged droplet passes through the electrostatic field, it is isolated from the remainder of the sample and collected into a separate container. The primary clinical application of cell sorting is in stem cell transplantation.

For years, flow cytometry remained confined to the hematopathology and research laboratories. Currently, this methodology

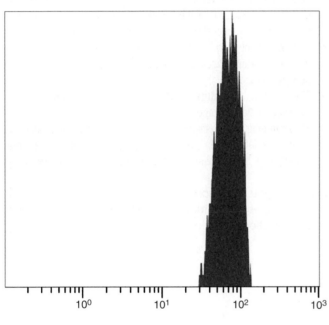

A   CD59-PE

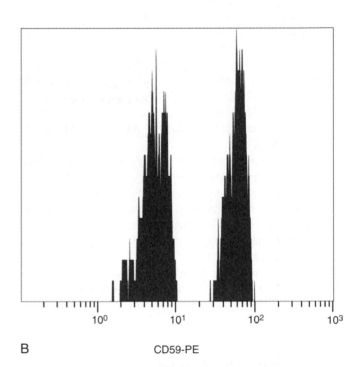

B   CD59-PE

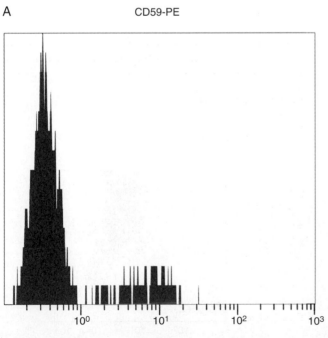

C   CD59-PE

Figure 33-17 The diagnosis of PNH is based on the decreased expression of GPI-linked molecules. Different levels of GPI-anchored proteins are best visualized in red blood cells using an antibody against CD59 antigen. **A,** Red blood cells from a healthy volunteer show a high number of CD59 molecules and correspond with type I cells. **B,** Varying percentage of type I cells (normal level of CD59 antigen) and a population with slight decrease in CD59 expression (type II cells) can be seen in PNH patients. **C,** Granulocytes with a complete loss of CD59 (type III cells) in a patient with PNH. This patient received numerous red blood cell transfusions; the loss of CD59 is best shown on granulocytic and monocytic populations.

is used in bone marrow transplantation, transfusion medicine, coagulation, microbiology, molecular pathology, and drug development. Specific examples of novel applications include tissue typing, molecular testing for neoplasia-associated translocations, and follow-up of drug response exemplified by monitoring of platelet activation after antiplatelet therapy.

Flow cytometry is well suited for the rapid analysis of numerous parameters. The current focus on high-throughput testing for simultaneous analysis of multiple biologic constituents opens new avenues to the mature field of flow cytometry.[28]

CHAPTER at a GLANCE

- Flow cytometry measures physical, antigenic, and functional properties of particles suspended in a fluid.
- Multiparameter flow cytometry is a routine technique for diagnosis and follow-up of hematologic disorders.
- The characterization of complex specimens is achieved through the analysis of individual cells for multiple parameters and the simultaneous display of data for thousands of cells. The cell size, internal complexity, and immunophenotypic features detected by monoclonal antibodies directly conjugated to various fluorochromes are analyzed in clinical specimens.
- A key starting point in flow cytometric analysis is a high-quality fresh specimen.
- A flow cytometer consists of fluids, a light source (laser), multiple detectors, and a computer.
- Analogous to the microscopic examination, proper evaluation of flow cytometric data is based on the inspection of visual patterns. Initially, the entire sample is scanned for the presence of abnormal populations. Subsequently, detailed immunophenotypic features of cell subsets are studied.
- The immunophenotyping of hematologic specimens is based on the knowledge of maturation patterns of hematopoietic cells. In

comparison, myeloid and lymphoid malignancies and cell populations in non-neoplastic hematologic disorders show significant qualitative and quantitative differences in antigen expression.
- Flow cytometric analysis of acute leukemia determines the lineage of leukemic cells. In selected entities, immunophenotype corresponds with the underlying genetic lesion.
- Immunophenotyping of myelodysplastic syndromes and chronic myeloproliferative disorders is an emerging application of clinical flow cytometry.
- The clonality of mature B cell and T cell neoplasms can be detected by flow cytometry.
- Flow cytometric analysis also is used for diagnosis and monitoring of immunodeficiencies, stem cell enumeration, detection of fetal hemoglobin, tissue typing, molecular analysis, and drug testing.

Now that you have completed this chapter, go back and read again the case studies at the beginning and respond to the questions presented.

REVIEW QUESTIONS

1. What is the most common clinical application of flow cytometry?
   a. Diagnosis of platelet disorders
   b. Detection of fetomaternal hemorrhage
   c. Diagnosis of leukemias and lymphomas
   d. Differentiation of anemias

2. Which of the following is *true* of CD45 antigen?
   a. It is present on every cell subpopulation in the bone marrow.
   b. It is expressed on all hematopoietic cells with the exception of megakaryocytes and late erythroid precursors.
   c. It is *not* used routinely in flow cytometry.
   d. It may be present on nonhematopoietic cells.

3. Erythroid precursors are characterized by the expression of CD:
   a. 71
   b. 20
   c. 61
   d. 3

4. In the following figure, the population colored in *aqua* represents:
   a. Monocytes
   b. Nonhematopoietic cells
   c. Granulocytes
   d. Lymphocytes

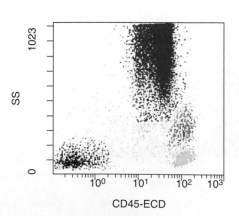

5. Antigens expressed by precursor B ALL include:
   a. CD3, CD4, and CD8
   b. CD19, CD34, and CD10
   c. There are no antigens specific for precursor B ALL.
   d. Myeloperoxidase

6. The following is *true* of flow cytometric "gating":
   a. It is best defined as selection of target population for flow cytometric analysis.
   b. It can be done only at the time of data acquisition.
   c. It can be done only at the time of final analysis and interpretation of flow cytometric data.
   d. It is accomplished by adjusting flow rate.

7. Collection of ungated events:
   a. Facilitates comprehensive analysis of all cells
   b. Does not help in detection of unexpected abnormal populations
   c. Allows the collection of a large number of rare cells
   d. Is used for leukemia diagnosis only.

8. Mycosis fungoides is characterized by:
   a. Loss of certain antigens compared with normal T cell population
   b. Polyclonal T cell receptor
   c. Immunophenotype indistinguishable from that of normal T cells
   d. Expression of CD3 and CD8 antigens

9. Mature granulocytes show the expression of:
   a. CD15, CD33, and CD34
   b. CD15, CD33, and CD41
   c. CD15, CD33, and CD13
   d. CD15, CD33, and CD7

10. During the initial evaluation of flow cytometric data, cell size, cytoplasmic complexity, and expression of CD45 antigen are used to define cell subpopulations. Which of the following parameters defines cytoplasmic complexity/granularity?
    a. SS
    b. FS
    c. CD45
    d. HLA-DR

11. The most important feature of the mature neoplastic B cell population is:
    a. The presence of a specific immunophenotype with expression of CD19 antigen
    b. A clonal light chain expression (i.e., exclusively κ- or λ-positive population)
    c. A clonal TCR expression
    d. Aberrant expression of CD5 antigen on CD19⁺ cells

REFERENCES

1. Jaffe ES, Harris NL, Stein H, et al (eds): World Health Organization Classification of Tumours: Pathology and Genetics: Tumours of Haematopoietic and Lymphoid Tissue. Lyon: IARC Press, 2001.
2. Czader M, Ali SZ: Flow cytometry as an adjunct to cytomorphologic analysis of serous effusions. Diagn Cytopathol 2003;29:74-78.
3. Stewart CC, Behm FG, Carey JL, et al: U.S.-Canadian consensus recommendations on immunophenotypic analysis of hematologic neoplasia by flow cytometry: selection of antibody combinations. Cytometry 1997;30:231-235.
4. Köhler G, Milstein C: Continuous cultures of fused cells secreting antibody of predefined specificity. Nature 1975;256:495-497.
5. Human cell differentiation molecules—collaborative research on cellular markers. Available at: http://www.hlda8.org. Accessed September 7, 2006.
6. Perfetto SP, Chattopadhyay PK, Roederer M: Seventeen-colour flow cytometry: unravelling the immune system. Nat Rev Immunol 2004;4:648-655.
7. Stelzer GT, Shults KE, Loken MR: CD45 gating for routine flow cytometric analysis of human bone marrow specimens. Ann N Y Acad Sci 1993;677:265-281.
8. Borowitz MJ, Guenther KL, Shults KE, et al: Immunophenotyping of acute leukemia by flow cytometric analysis: use of CD45 and right-angle light scattered to gate on leukemic blasts in three-color analysis. Am J Clin Pathol 1993;100:534-540.
9. Macedo A, Orfao A, Ciudad J, et al: Phenotypic analysis of CD34 subpopulations in normal human bone marrow and its application for the detection of minimal residual disease. Leukemia 1995;9:1896-1901.
10. Terstappen LW, Safford M, Loken MR: Flow cytometric analysis

of human bone marrow: III. Neutrophil maturation. Leukemia 1990;4:657-663.
11. Loken MR, Shah VO, Dattilio KL, et al: Flow cytometric analysis of human bone marrow: I. Normal erythroid development. Blood 1987;69:255-263.
12. Ciudad J, Orfao A, Vidriales B, et al: Immunophenotypic analysis of CD19+ precursors in normal human adult bone marrow: implications for minimal residual disease detection. Haematologica 1998;83:1069-1075.
13. Terstappen LW, Huang S, Picker LJ: Flow cytometric assessment of human T-cell differentiation in thymus and bone marrow. Blood 1992;79:666-677.
14. Andrieu V, Radford-Weiss I, Troussard X, et al: Molecular detection of t(8;21)/AML1-ETO in AML M1/M2: correlation with cytogenetics, morphology and immunophenotype. Br J Haematol 1996;92:855-865.
15. Adriaansen H, Boekhorst PAW, Hagemeijer AM, et al: Acute myeloid leukemia M4 with bone marrow eosinophilia (M4Eo) and inv(16)(p13q22) exhibits a specific immunophenotype with CD2 expression. Blood 1993;81:3043-3051.
16. Lo Coco F, Avvisati G, Diverio D, et al: Rearrangements of the RAR-alpha gene in acute promyelocytic leukaemia: correlations with morphology and immunophenotype. Br J Haematol 1991;78:494-499.
17. Krasinskas AM, Wasik MA, Kamoun M, et al: The usefulness of CD64, other monocyte-associated antigens, and CD45 gating in the subclassification of acute myeloid leukemias with monocytic differentiation. Am J Clin Pathol 1998;110:797-805.
18. Helleberg C, Knudsen H, Hansen PB, et al: CD34+ megakaryoblastic leukaemic cells are CD38−, but CD61+ and glycophorin A+: improved criteria for diagnosis of AML-M7?. Leukemia 1997;11:830-834.

19. Stetler-Stevenson M, Arthur DC, Jabbour N, et al: Diagnostic utility of flow cytometric immunophenotyping in myelodysplastic syndrome. Blood 2001;98:979-987.

20. Kussick SJ, Wood BL: Four-color flow cytometry identifies virtually all cytogenetically abnormal bone marrow samples in the workup of non-CML myeloproliferative disorders. Am J Clin Pathol 2003;120:854-865.

21. Ogata K, Nakamura K, Yokose N, et al: Clinical significance of phenotypic features of blasts in patients with myelodysplastic syndrome. Blood 2002;100:3887-3896.

22. Wells DA, Benesch M, Loken MR, et al: Myeloid and monocytic dyspoiesis as determined by flow cytometric scoring in myelodysplastic syndrome correlates with the IPSS and with outcome after hematopoietic stem cell transplantation. Blood 2003;102:394-403.

23. Harbott J, Mancini M, Verellen-Dumoulin C, et al: Hematological malignancies with a deletion of 11q23: cytogenetic and clinical aspects. Leukemia 1998;12:823-827.

24. Tabernero MD, Bortoluci AM, Alaejos I, et al: Adult precursor B-ALL with BCR/ABL gene rearrangements displays a unique immunophenotype based on the pattern of CD10, CD34, CD13 and CD38 expression. Leukemia 2001;15:406-414.

25. Li S, Eshleman JR, Borowitz MJ: Lack of surface immunoglobulin light chain expression by flow cytometric immunophenotyping can help diagnose peripheral B-cell lymphoma. Am J Clin Pathol 2002;118:229-234.

26. Beck RC, Stahl S, O'Keefe CL, et al: Detection of mature T-cell leukemias by flow cytometry using anti T-cell receptor V beta antibodies. Am J Clin Pathol 2003;120:785-794.

27. Alaibac M, Pigozzi B, Belloni-Fortina A, et al: CD7 expression in reactive and malignant human skin T-lymphocytes. Anticancer Res 2003;23:2707-2710.

28. Richards SJ, Rawstron AC, Hillmen P: Application of flow cytometry to the diagnosis of paroxysmal nocturnal hemoglobinuria. Cytometry (Communications in Clinical Cytometry) 2004;2:223-233.

29. Edwards BS, Oprea T, Prossnitz ER, et al: Flow cytometry for high-throughput, high-content screening. Curr Opin Chem Biol 2004;8:392-398.

Myeloproliferative Disorders 34

John Griep

OBJECTIVES

After completion of this chapter, the reader will be able to:

1. Define myeloproliferative disorders (MPDs).
2. List the most common diseases included in the classification of MPDs, and recognize their abbreviations.
3. Define chronic myelogenous (chronic myelocytic) leukemia (CML), with emphasis on the affected cell lines.
4. Discuss the theory of pathogenesis of CML.
5. Describe the peripheral blood and bone marrow in CML.
6. Discuss the cytogenetics of CML.
7. List the clinical phases of CML, and recognize test results expected in each phase.
8. Define polycythemia vera (PV), with emphasis on the affected cell lines.
9. Discuss clinical symptoms commonly observed in patients with PV.
10. Identify major morphologic changes in the bone marrow and peripheral blood in patients with PV.
11. List diagnostic criteria for PV.
12. Discuss the progression of PV.
13. Define essential thrombocythemia (ET), with emphasis on the affected cell lines.
14. List the diagnostic criteria for ET.
15. List the morphologic changes in the peripheral blood in patients with ET.
16. List two complications that may occur in patients with ET.
17. Define chronic idiopathic myelofibrosis (CIMF), with emphasis on the affected cell lines and pathogenesis.
18. Describe the key pathologic features of CIMF in bone marrow, peripheral blood, and tissues.
19. Describe the course of disease of CIMF and current therapy.
20. Given complete blood count results, recognize those consistent with each MPD.
21. Recommend follow-up testing for suspected MPD, and interpret results of testing.

CASE STUDY

After studying the material in this chapter, the reader should be able to respond to the following case study:

A 34-year-old woman presented with a 2-month history of increasing weakness, persistent nonproductive cough, fever and chills accompanied by night sweats, and a 13-lb weight loss over a 6-month period. Chest radiographs and purified protein derivative test (for tuberculosis) were negative. The patient was treated with ciprofloxacin with improvement in her cough, but she continued to grow weaker and was able to consume only small quantities of food. The patient appeared pale and cachectic. There was tenderness and fullness in the left upper quadrant, with the spleen palpable below the umbilicus. No hepatomegaly or peripheral adenopathy was noted. Her laboratory results were as follows:

  White blood cell (WBC) count: 248×10^9/L
  Hemoglobin: 9.5 g/dL
  Hematocrit: 26.3% (0.263 L/L)
  Platelet count: 449×10^9/L
  Segmented neutrophils: 44%
  Band neutrophils: 4%
  Lymphocytes: 10%

Eosinophils: 3%
Basophils: 7%
Myelocytes: 30%
Promyelocyte: 1%
Myeloblast: 1%
Nucleated red blood cells: 2/100 WBCs
Reticulocyte count: 3%
Leukocyte alkaline phosphatase (LAP) score: 20 (reference 40-130)
Lactate dehydrogenase: 692 IU (reference 140-280 IU)
Uric acid: 8.1 mg/dL (reference 4-6 mg/dL)

1. What is the significance of the elevated WBC count and abnormal WBC differential?
2. How does the LAP aid in the diagnosis?
3. Justify the use of cytogenetic studies in a patient with results similar to the results in this case study.
4. What is the usual treatment for this disorder?

The myeloproliferative disorders (MPDs) are clonal hematopoietic stem cell diseases with expansion, excessive production, and overaccumulation of erythrocytes, granulocytes, and platelets. Expansion occurs in varying combinations in the bone marrow, peripheral blood, and tissues.[1-4] The MPDs have pathogenetic similarities and express common clinical and laboratory features.[5]

MPDs are predominately chronic with accelerated, subacute, or acute phases. In certain patients it is difficult to make a clear delineation between subacute and chronic from clinical and morphologic perspectives.

By convention, the MPDs, include chronic myelogenous leukemia (CML), polycythemia vera (PV; also known as polycythemia rubra vera, PRV), essential (primary) thrombocythemia (ET), and agnogenic myelofibrosis with myeloid metaplasia (AMM), also known as chronic idiopathic myelofibrosis (CIMF). CML and PV are defined by their overproduction of granulocytes and erythrocytes, respectively.[2,6,7] CIMF is a combination of overproduction of hematopoietic cells and ineffective hematopoiesis with resultant peripheral blood cytopenias.[8] ET is increased megakaryocytopoiesis and peripheral blood thrombocytosis.[9]

MPDs present as stable chronic disorders that may transform first to a subacute, then to an aggressive cellular growth phase such as acute myeloblastic or lymphoblastic leukemia. They may manifest a depleted cellular phase such as bone marrow hypoplasia, or exhibit clinical symptoms and morphologic patterns resembling first a subacute, then a more aggressive cellular expression

Familial MPDs have been described in families where two or more members are affected.[10] Juvenile MPDs express as chronic myelogenous leukemia and as pediatric myelodysplastic syndrome, both of which exhibit myeloproliferation and are associated with monosomy or deletions of the long arm of chromosome 7.[11]

CHRONIC MYELOGENOUS LEUKEMIA

CML is a MPD arising as a clonal process from a pluripotential hematopoietic stem cell. CML begins with a chronic clinical phase that progresses to an accelerated phase in 3 to 4 years and often terminates as an acute leukemia. The clinical features are frequent infection, anemia, bleeding, and splenomegaly, all secondary to massive pathologic accumulations of myeloid progenitor cells in bone marrow, peripheral blood, and extramedullary tissues. Neutrophilia with all maturational stages, basophilia, eosinophilia, and often thrombocytosis are present in peripheral blood. Verification of the clonal origin of hematopoietic cells in CML is apparent from studies of females heterzygous for glucose-6-phosphate dehydrogenase. Only one isoenzyme is active in affected cells, whereas two isoenzymes are active in nonaffected cells.[12]

Incidence

CML occurs at all ages but predominates at 46 to 53 years. It represents about 20% of all cases of leukemia, is slightly more common in males than females, and manifests a mortality rate of 1.5 per 100,000 per year.

Symptoms associated with clinical onset may be of minimal intensity. Ease of fatigue, decreased tolerance to exertion, anorexia, abdominal discomfort, weight loss, and symptomatic effects from splenic enlargement are commonly encountered.

Cytogenetics

A unique chromosome, the Philadelphia chromosome, is present in proliferating hematopoietic cells. This chromosome is a reciprocal translocation between the long arms of chromosomes 9 and 22 (Chapter 31).[13] This acquired somatic mutation specifically reflects the translocation of an ABL proto-oncogene from band q34 of chromosome 9 to the BCR region of band q11 of chromosome 22, resulting in a unique chimeric gene, BCR/ABL.[14] This new gene produces a 210-kD protein, P210 with enhanced tyrosine kinase activity compared with its natural enzymatic counterpart. P210 catalyzes the transfer of the terminal phosphate of adenosine triphosphate to proteins. This increased tyrosine kinase activity may induce clonal cell proliferation secondary to a reduction of or loss of sensitivity to protein regulators.[15] The mutation affects maturation and differentiation of hematopoietic and lymphopoietic cells whose progeny eventually dominate in the affected individual. Progeny cells that exhibit this chromosome include neutrophils, eosinophils, basophils, monocytes, nucleated erythrocytes, megakaryocytes, and B lymphocytes.[6,16]

Although the cause for Philadelphia chromosome is unknown, it appears more frequently in populations exposed to ionizing radiation.[17,18] In most patients, a cause cannot be identified. Appearance of the Philadelphia chromosome in donor cells after allogeneic bone marrow transplantation implicates a possible transmissible agent.[19]

More than 99% of CML patients have the BCR/ABL fusion gene and produce the fusion protein p210$^{BCR/ABL}$. BCR, the breakpoint cluster region from chromosome 22, and ABL, the Abelson oncogene from chromosome 9, form the fusion gene that is transcribed into a chimeric BCR/ABL mRNA. This is translated into the hybrid protein, p210$^{BCR/ABL}$.[20] The ABL-transcribed portion, when in its normal location on chromosome 9, codes for p125, exhibiting normal tyrosine kinase activity. When activated, p210 causes deregulation of tyrosine kinase, which results in autophosphorylation of other proteins. Increased protein phosphorylation likely alters signal transduction pathways, leading to constitutive tyrosine kinase activity and increased cellular proliferation.

Additionally, the loss of genetic segments in the 5' end of the ABL gene results in an altered protein-binding affinity for F-actin, leading to a reduction in contact binding of hematopoietic CML cells to stromal cells and causing premature release of cells into circulation.[21] One action of interferon-alpha therapy is to reverse the loss of adhesion of CML progenitor cells, reducing premature release of these cells into circulation.[22]

Apoptotic functions are lost because the BCR/ABL fusion protein has a propensity to be sequestered in the cytoplasm, which has antiapoptotic functions. There are slight variations in the structure of the chimeric fusion gene BCR/ABL because the BCR segment has multiple breakage sites. The p210 is necessary for CML transformation of the hematopoietic stem cell.

The *BCR/ABL* fusion is also associated with Philadelphia chromosome–positive acute lymphoblastic leukemia. The chromosome appears in 20% of adults and 2-5% of children with this disease. A minor chimeric *BCL/ABL* gene transforms and translates to a p150 protein that is present in 50% of Philadelphia chromosome–positive acute lymphoblastic leukemia in adults and 75% of Philadelphia chromosome–positive acute lymphoblastic leukemia in children, but it is rarely associated with CML.

Abnormal adhesion between stem cells and stroma may dysregulate hematopoiesis. There is an increase in growth factor–independent cellular proliferation from activation of the *RAS* gene and a decrease in or resistance to apoptosis. New clones of stem cells vulnerable to additional genetic changes lead to accelerated and blast phases. Additionally, the BCR/ABL–produced protein localizes in the cytoplasm, compared with nuclear location for the normal ABL protein.

Peripheral Blood and Bone Marrow

There are dramatic morphologic changes in the peripheral blood and bone marrow that reflect the expansion of the granulocyte pool, particularly in the later maturational stages. In Table 34-1, the common qualitative changes at time of diagnosis in the peripheral blood, bone marrow, and extramedullary tissues are listed. Extramedullary granulopoiesis may involve sinusoids and medullary cords in the spleen and sinusoids, portal tract zones, and solid areas of the liver.

Figure 34-1 illustrates a common pattern in the peripheral blood film of chronic phase CML at the time of diagnosis. Leukocytosis is readily apparent at scanning microscopic powers. Segmented neutrophils, bands, metamyelocytes and myelocytes predominate, and immature and mature eosinophils and basophils are increased. Myeloblasts and promyelocytes are usually present at a rate between 1% and 5%. Lymphocytes and monocytes are present and often increased. Nucleated red blood cells (NRBCs) are rare. Platelets are normal or increased, and some may exhibit abnormal morphology.

Bone marrow changes are illustrated in Figure 34-2. An intense hypercellularity is composed of granulopoiesis that exhibits broad zones of immature granulocytes, usually perivascular or periosteal, differentiating into more centrally placed mature granulocytes. Normoblasts appear reduced in number. Megakaryocytes are normal or increased in number and, when increased, may appear in clusters and exhibit dyspoietic cytologic changes. They often appear small with reduced nuclear size (by approximately 20%) and reduced nuclear lobulations. Reticulin fibers are increased in approximately 20% of patients. Increased megakaryocyte density is associated with an increase in myelofibrosis.[23] The presence of pseudo-Gaucher cells (Chapter 28) usually occurs.

Other Laboratory Findings

Hyperuricemia and uricosuria from increased cell turnover may be associated with secondary gout, urinary uric acid stones, and uric acid nephropathy.[24] Approximately 15% of patients exhibit total white blood cell (WBC) counts greater than $300 \times 10^9/L$.[25] Symptoms in these patients are secondary to vascular stasis and possible intravascular consumption of

TABLE 34-1 Common Morphologic Changes in Chronic Myelogenous Leukemia

Peripheral Blood

Erythrocytes	Normal or decreased
Reticulocytes	Normal
Nucleated RBCs	Present
Total WBCs	Increased
Lymphocytes	Normal or increased
Neutrophils	Increased
Basophils	Increased
Eosinophils	Increased
Myelocytes	Increased
LAP	Decreased
Platelets	Normal or increased
Cytologic anomaly	Present

Bone Marrow

Cellularity	Increased
Granulopoiesis	Increased
Erythropoiesis	Decreased
Megakaryopoiesis	Increased or normal
Reticulin	Increased
Macrophages	
Gaucher-like	
Sea-blue	
Green-gray crystals	Increased
Megakaryocytes	
Small	Increased

Extramedullary Tissue

Splenomegaly	Present
Sinusoidal	
Medullary	
Hepatomegaly	Present
Sinusoidal	
Portal tract	
Local infiltrates	Present

oxygen by the leukocytes. Symptoms are reversible with the lowering of the total WBC count.[26]

Progression

Most patients' disease eventually transforms to acute leukemia.[27] Before blastic transformation, some patients proceed through an intermediate *metamorphosis* or *accelerated* phase. There is an increase in frequency and type of clinical symptoms, adverse changes in laboratory values, and poorer response to therapy than in the chronic phase. Additional chromosome abnormalities may appear, associated with enhanced dyshematopoietic cell maturation patterns and increases in morphologic and functional abnormalities in blood cells. There is often an increasing degree of anemia and, in the peripheral blood, fewer mature leukocytes, increased basophilia, and thrombocytopenia with a greater proportion of abnormal platelets

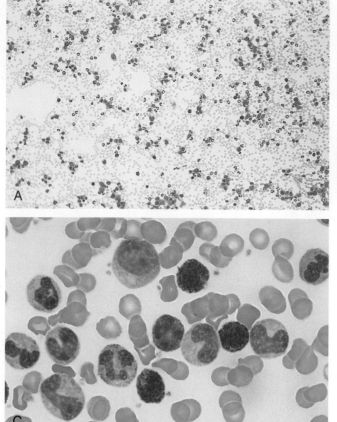

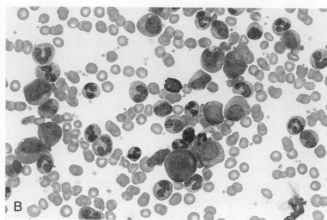

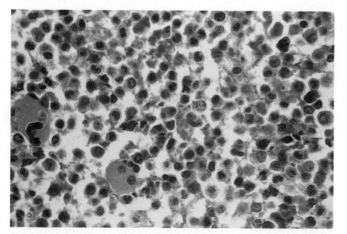

Figure 34-1 Peripheral blood smears in chronic-phase CML. **A,** Leukocytosis is evident at scanning power (×100). **B,** Bimodal population of segmented neutrophils and myelocytes (×500). **C,** Increased basophils and immature neutrophils (×1000).

Figure 34-2 Bone marrow biopsy specimen in chronic-phase CML, showing hypercellularity with increased granulocytes and megakaryocytes (hematoxylin and eosin, ×400).

micromegakaryocytes, and megakaryocytic fragments. The circulating blast count increases to 10%-19%. This total blast percentage, or a combination of 20% blasts and promyelocytes, is proposed as a diagnostic criterion for the accelerated phase.[28]

Blast crisis involves the peripheral blood, bone marrow, and extramedullary tissues. By definition, blasts constitute more than 20% of total bone marrow cellularity; the peripheral blood exhibits increased blasts.[27] Blast crisis leukemia usually is acute myeloid or acute lymphoblastic, but origins from other hematopoietic clonal cells are possible. Extramedullary growth may occur as lymphocytic or myelogenous cell proliferations; the latter are often referred to as *granulocytic sarcoma*. Extramedullary sarcoma is observed at many sites or locations in the body and may precede a marrow blast crisis. The clinical symptoms of blast crisis simulate those of acute leukemia: severe anemia, leukocytopenia, and thrombocytopenia. Chromosome abnormalities accumulate including additional Philadelphia chromosome, isochromosome 17, trisomy 8, loss of Y chromosome, and trisomy 19.[29,30] These occur in approximately 75% of patients.

Related Diseases

Some patients with diseases similar to CML exhibit cells negative for the Philadelphia chromosome and few pseudo-Gaucher cells. Chronic neutrophilic leukemia manifests with peripheral blood, bone marrow, and extramedullary infiltrative patterns similar to those of CML, except that only neutrophilic granulocytes are present and less than 10% of peripheral blood neutrophils are immature.[31] Similarly, chronic monocytic leukemia involves a similar expansion of monocytes, including functional monocytes.[32]

Juvenile myelomonocytic leukemia and adult chronic myelomonocytic leukemia are classified by the World Health Organization as myelodysplastic/myeloproliferative diseases because of the overlap in clinical, laboratory, or morphologic findings. Juvenile myelomonocytic leukemia is observed in children younger than 4 years old and is accompanied by an expansion of monocytes and granulocytes, including immature granulocytes, and manifestations of dyserythropoiesis.[33]

The peripheral blood of adults with chronic myelomonocytic leukemia may have characteristics similar to those in the refractory anemias, such as oval macrocytes and reticulocytopenia. The peripheral WBC concentration may reach $100 \times 10^9/L$. Absolute monocytosis ($>1 \times 10^9/L$) is always present. Clinical features include prominent splenomegaly, symptoms of anemia, fever, bleeding, and infection. Some cases of Philadelphia chromosome–negative CML are likely misdiagnosed chronic myelomonocytic leukemia.[34] Chronic myelomonocytic leukemia is discussed further with myelodysplastic syndromes in Chapter 35.

A puzzling group of patients exhibit Philadelphia chromosome–positive acute leukemia. Studies reveal 2% of acute myeloid leukemia cases exhibit Philadelphia chromosome in a significant proportion of blasts. Further 5% of childhood-onset acute lymphoblastic leukemia and 20% of adult-onset acute lymphoblastic leukemia cases are Philadelphia chromosome positive.[35-38] The proper alignment of these cases within the spectrum of CML is speculative.

Therapy

Initial treatment approaches used measurable parameters for the reduction of tumor burden. More recently, alkylating agents such as nitrogen mustard[39] or busulfan[40] and busulfan in combination with 6-thioguanine were used to achieve this goal. Other drugs eventually used include hydroxyurea and 6 mercaptopurine. Patient survival was improved with the use of these drugs. Introduced in 1983, α-interferon[41] achieved these clinical goals and increased patient survival, induced suppression of the Philadelphia chromosome, reduced the rate of cellular progression to blast cells, and increased the frequency of patient survival.

α-Interferon stimulates a cell-mediated antitumor host response that reduces myeloid cell numbers, induces cytogenetic remissions, and increases survival.[42] It improves the frequency and duration of hematologic remission and reduces the frequency of detection of the Philadelphia chromosome. In some patients, a complete cytogenetic remission is achieved for a time.

Cytarabine given with α-interferon improved the frequency of hematologic remissions but did not eliminate the BCR/ABL gene, which was still detected by molecular and fluorescent methods.[43] Also in some patients, therapy side effects became severe, drug resistance appeared, and relapse rates were not changed compared with other chemotherapies.

Bone marrow and stem cell transplantation, either autologous or allogeneic, have been reported as curative, especially in patients younger than age 55. Relapses occur, but long-term, disease-free survival is possible. Optimal survival occurs when the patient is treated during the chronic phase within 1 year of diagnosis and is younger than age 50. Treatment requires ablative chemotherapy followed by transplant of mobilized normal progenitor cells that exhibit CD34$^+$ surface markers. Allogeneic bone marrow transplants are more successful in patients up to age 55 when donors are matched for HLA antigens A, B, and DR. Donor-matched lymphocyte infusions after allogeneic transplantation from a sibling donor may assist in producing complete remissions.[44]

More recently, therapies focusing on molecular targets that block signal transduction pathways arising from the activity of BCR/ABL fusion protein have emerged. Imatinib mesylate (Gleevec) is a synthetic tyrosine kinase inhibitor intended to inhibit selectively most of the transforming capability stemming from the tyrosine kinase activity of the BCR/ABL fusion protein. Goals of therapy include complete hematologic remission and cytogenetic remission by an apoptotic function.[45] Monitors for effectiveness of imatinib therapy and stem cell transplantation include quantitation of BCR/ABL transcripts and quantitative reverse transcriptase real-time polymerase chain reaction. These monitors of effectiveness are parameters for determining complete cytogenetic remission. More recently, effectiveness is monitored by the log number of reductions of BCR/ABL transcripts, called minimal residual disease (Chapter 32).[46]

A limitation of imatinib therapy is the appearance of resistance with relapse. The use of higher doses benefits some resistant patients, but others continue to have resistance. The problem may reside in the increased rate of mutation occurring in the genome of the cells containing the BCR/ABL gene and in the BCR/ABL gene itself. Currently, studies are under way to evaluate modification of dosage of imatinib used, to identify and develop other tyrosine kinase inhibitors, and to discover new classes of inhibitors that may be more effective than currently known tyrosine kinase inhibitors.

The establishment of a care plan for treating a newly diagnosed patient with CML requires not only the formulation of alternative approaches to achieve complete cellular remission, but also the establishment of parameters to follow that confirm long-term success of therapy. Previous chemotherapies have provided cellular remission but usually do not suppress or defer clinical transitions to accelerated or blast phases. Bone marrow transplantation for patients who qualify is likely the preferred choice, but long-term success (cure) remains at 50% to 70%. Imatinib may be useful to patients with bone marrow transplantation relapse. For patients who are not candidates for bone marrow transplantation, imatinib alone, in conjunction with α-interferon, and as a second-line choice after α-interferon therapy failures are options being evaluated.

POLYCYTHEMIA VERA

PV is a neoplastic clonal MPD that commonly manifests with panmyelosis in the bone marrow and increases in erythrocytes, granulocytes, and platelets in the peripheral blood.[2] Splenomegaly is common. PV arises in a hematopoietic stem cell; the hypothesis of a clonal origin for PV is supported by

X-linked restriction fragment length DNA polymorphism studies that exhibit monoclonal X chromosome inactivation in all blood cells.[47]

In PV, neoplastic clonal stem cells are exquisitely sensitive to erythropoietin for cell growth. Trace levels of erythropoietin in serum stimulate growth of erythroid progenitor cells in in vitro colony-forming growth systems. There is, however, preservation of hypersensitive and normosensitive erythroid colony-forming units, indicating some level of normal hematopoiesis.[48] The adverse clinical progression seems to correlate with the propagation of the erythropoietin-sensitive colony-forming units.[49]

Approximately 80% of patients manifest bone marrow panmyelosis, and 100% of bone marrow volume may exhibit hematopoietic cellularity. Although the bone marrow pattern may simulate other MPDs, the peripheral blood cells appear normal, with normocytic, normochromic erythrocytes; mature granulocytes; and normal-sized, granulated platelets. The other 20% exhibit lesser degrees of cellularity in the bone marrow and peripheral blood. Splenomegaly and hepatomegaly and generalized vascular engorgement and circulatory disturbances increase the risk of hemorrhage, tissue infarction, or thrombosis.

Diagnosis

The diagnosis of PV includes an increased RBC mass of 36 mL/kg or greater in males and 32 mL/kg or greater in females, an arterial oxygen saturation at 92% (normal) or greater, and splenomegaly. Lacking any one of these three parameters, the presence of two of the following parameters is considered diagnostic: thrombocytosis of greater than $400 \times 10^9/L$; leukocytosis of greater than $12 \times 10^9/L$ without fever or infection; or increases in leukocyte alkaline phosphatase (LAP), serum vitamin B_{12}; or unbound vitamin B_{12} binding capacity.[50,51]

It is not always easy to assign an early diagnosis of PV. Individuals with erythrocytosis secondary to hypoxia or erythropoietin-producing neoplasms are the most difficult to diagnose correctly. In these individuals, the bone marrow exhibits erythroid hyperplasia without granulocytic or megakaryocytic hyperplasia. Patients with stress or spurious erythrocytosis exhibit increased hemoglobin and hematocrit without increased erythrocyte mass or splenomegaly.

The World Health Organization criteria for the diagnosis of PV are listed in Table 34-2. The diagnosis of PV is acceptable when A1 and A2 and any other category A are present. Alternatively, the diagnosis can be made when A1 and A2 and any two of the parameters in category B are present.

Peripheral Blood and Bone Marrow

Common peripheral blood, bone marrow, and tissue findings are listed in Table 34-3 for patients with the early or proliferative phase of PV. Figures 34-3 and 34-4 reflect common morphologic patterns of peripheral blood and bone marrow morphologic and cellular changes. In addition to quantitative changes, bone marrow normoblasts may collect in large clusters, megakaryocytes are enlarged and exhibit lobulated nuclei, and bone marrow sinuses are enlarged without fibrosis. Pseudo-Gaucher cells are rare.[23]

TABLE 34-2 World Health Organization Criteria for the Diagnosis of Polycythemia Vera

A1	Elevated RBC mass > 25% above mean normal predicted value or hemoglobin > 18.5 g/dL in men, 16.5 g/dL in women
A2	No cause of secondary erythrocytosis, including
	Absence of familial erythrocytosis
	No elevation of erythropoietin owing to:
	Hypoxia
	High oxygen affinity hemoglobin
	Truncated erythropoietin receptor
	Inappropriate erythropoietin production by tumor
A3	Splenomegaly
A4	Clonal genetic abnormality (other than Ph chromosome or *BCR/ABL* fusion gene) in bone marrow cells
A5	Endogenous erythroid colony formation in vitro
B1	Thrombocytosis > $400 \times 10^9/L$
B2	WBC > $12 \times 10^9/L$
B3	Bone marrow biopsy showing panmyelosis with prominent erythroid and megakaryocytic proliferation
B4	Low serum erythropoietin levels

TABLE 34-3 Common Morphologic Changes in Polycythemia Vera

Peripheral Blood

Hemoglobin	Increased
Hematocrit	Increased
RBC volume	Increased
Erythrocytes	
Normocytic	
Normochromic	
Total WBCs	Increased
Granulocytes	Increased
Platelets	Increased
LAP	Normal or increased

Bone Marrow

Normoblasts	Increased
Granulocytes	Increased
Megakaryocytes	Increased
Reticulin	Increased

Extramedullary Tissue

Splenomegaly	Present
Sinusoidal	
Medullary	
Hepatomegaly	Present
Sinusoidal	

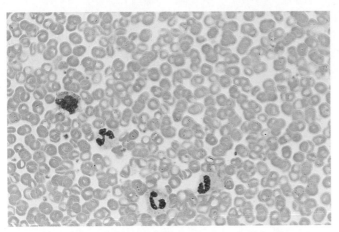

Figure 34-3 Peripheral blood smear in stable phase PV with essentially normocytic normochromic erythrocytes (×500).

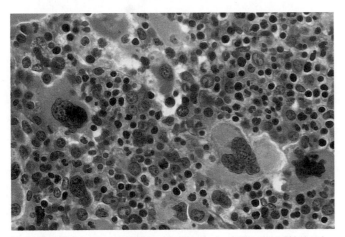

Figure 34-4 Bone marrow biopsy specimen in stable phase PV, showing panmyelosis (hematoxylin and eosin, ×400).

Presentation and Progression

PV initially manifests in a proliferative phase independent of normal regulatory mechanisms. PV is always associated with increased RBC mass. This is the stable phase of PV, which progresses to a spent phase in a few patients. In the spent phase, patients experience progressive splenomegaly (palpable spleen) or hypersplenism (large spleen with bone marrow hyperplasia and peripheral blood cytopenias) and pancytopenia. They may also exhibit the triad of bone marrow fibrosis, splenomegaly, and anemia with teardrop-shaped poikilocytes. The latter pattern is called *postpolycythemic myeloid metaplasia* and its morphologic features are similar to CIMF. Peripheral WBC and RBC counts vary, and nucleated erythrocytes, immature granulocytes, and large platelets are present. Usually, splenomegaly is secondary to extramedullary hematopoiesis.[52] Myelofibrosis occurs within the bone marrow and may come to occupy a significant proportion of bone marrow volume, with subsequent ineffective hematopoiesis.[53]

There is a biologic survival advantage for the PV disease stem cell. PV progenitor cells in vitro grow in the absence of erythropoietin; this may be due to sensitivity to an insulin-like growth factor. They resist erythropoietin-deprivation apoptosis

by upregulation of *BCL-X*, an antiapoptotic protein. PV progenitor cells do not divide more rapidly but accumulate because they do not die normally.

Therapy and Prognosis

The disease progresses to acute leukemia in 15% of patients. Myelosuppressive therapy such as ^{32}P or alkylating agents seems to increase the risk.[51] Only 1% to 2% of cases treated with phlebotomy alone transform. However, there is an increased risk of thrombosis and bleeding in patients treated with phlebotomy alone, so the use of alkylating myelosuppressive agents may be required to control these complications. Some patients may manifest a temporary disease pattern similar to myelodysplasia, and the cell morphology in transformation to acute leukemia may be difficult to classify. Patients with both early and advanced PV may present with clinical, peripheral blood, bone marrow, and extramedullary features that simulate other MPDs.

ESSENTIAL THROMBOCYTHEMIA

ET is a clonal MPD with increased megakaryopoiesis and thrombocytosis greater than $600 \times 10^9/L$, commonly greater than $1000 \times 10^9/L$.[54] Generally appearing after age 60, ET must be differentiated from secondary or reactive thrombocytoses and from other MPDs. Thrombocytosis may be secondary to chronic active blood loss, hemolytic anemia, chronic inflammation or infection, or nonhematogenous neoplasia.

Diagnosis

The diagnostic criteria for ET proposed by the Polycythemia Vera Study Group are intended to distinguish ET from other MPDs and include a platelet count of greater than $600 \times 10^9/L$, hemoglobin less than 13 g/dL or a normal erythrocyte mass, and stainable iron in the bone marrow or a failure of iron therapy. Philadelphia chromosome absence, absent marrow collagen fibrosis (less than one third of a biopsy is fibrous), no splenomegaly, no leukoerythroblastic reaction, and no known cause of reactive thrombocytosis all support the diagnosis.[55] The major peripheral blood, bone marrow, and extramedullary findings are listed in Table 34-4.

Peripheral Blood and Bone Marrow

Figure 34-5 exhibits early-phase thrombocytosis with variation in platelet diameter and shape, including giantism, agranularity, and pseudopods. Commonly, platelets are present in clusters and tend to accumulate near the thin edge of the blood film. Segmented neutrophils may be increased; basophils are not. Erythrocytes are normocytic and normochromic, unless iron deficiency is present secondary to excessive bleeding.

Early-phase bone marrow shows marked megakaryocytic hypercellularity, clustering of megakaryocytes, and increased megakaryocyte diameter with nuclear hyperlobulation and density (Fig. 34-6). Special studies reveal increased smaller and less mature megakaryocytes.[56] Increased granulopoiesis and erythropoiesis may contribute to bone marrow hypercellularity, and in a few patients, reticulin fibers may be increased.

TABLE 34-4 Common Morphologic Patterns in Essential Thrombocythemia

Peripheral Blood

Hemoglobin	Decreased (slight)
Hematocrit	Decreased (slight)
RBC volume	Normal
Total WBCs	Increased (slight)
Neutrophils	Increased (slight)
Platelets	Increased
Platelet function	Decreased

Bone Marrow

Normoblasts	Normal or increased
Granulocytes	Normal or increased (slight)
Megakaryocytes	
Clusters	Present
Large	Present
Hyperlobulated	Present
Dense nuclei	Present
Variability in size	Increased
Reticulin	Normal or increased (slight)

Extramedullary Tissue

Splenomegaly	Present
Sinusoidal	
Medullary	
Megakaryocytic proliferation	Present

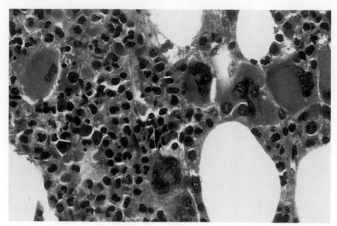

Figure 34-6 Bone marrow biopsy specimen in ET, with marked megakaryocytic hypercellularity (hematoxylin and eosin, ×400).

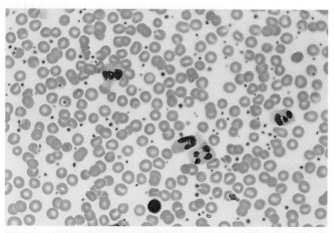

Figure 34-5 Peripheral blood smear in stable phase ET, showing increased numbers of platelets and mature neutrophils (×500).

Presentation, Therapy, and Prognosis

Patients with ET experience relatively long survival rates, provided that they remain free from serious thromboembolic or hemorrhagic complications. Clinical symptoms associated with thromboembolic vaso-occlusive events include the syndrome of erythromelalgia (throbbing and burning pain in the hands and feet, accompanied by mottled redness of areas),

transient ischemic attacks, seizures, and cerebral or myocardial infarction. Other symptoms include headache, dizziness, visual disturbances, and dysesthesias (decreased sensations). Hemorrhagic complications include bleeding from oral and nasal mucous membrane or gastrointestinal mucosa and the appearance of cutaneous ecchymoses (Chapter 43).

Treatment involves prevention or early alleviation of hemorrhagic or vaso-occlusive complications that occur as the platelet count increases. The production of platelets must be reduced by suppressing marrow megakaryocyte production with ^{32}P or one of several alkylating agents. As observed with PV, ET patients so treated may incur an increased risk for disease transformation to acute leukemia or myelofibrosis. Hydroxyurea may achieve a desired reduction of peripheral platelets without the risk of complications experienced with myelosuppressive agents. This may relate to the youth of ET patients in whom the risk of leukemic transformation seems relatively low. More recently, cytoreduction has been achieved with α-interferon.

A median survival of greater than 10 years is common, including instances in which the process arises in younger patients. Adverse prognosis may occur in patients whose cells manifest chromosome abnormalities.[20]

CHRONIC IDIOPATHIC MYELOFIBROSIS

CIMF, previously known as "AMM" and "myelofibrosis with myeloid metaplasia", is a clonal MPD[4] in which there is splenomegaly and ineffective hematopoiesis associated with areas of marrow hypercellularity, fibrosis, and increased megakaryocytes. Megakaryocytes are enlarged with pleomorphic nuclei, coarse segmentation, and areas of hypochromia. The peripheral blood film exhibits immature granulocytes and normoblasts, dacryocytes, and other bizarre RBC shapes.

CIMF clonality was manifest from studies in which cytogenetic abnormalities were detected in normoblasts, neutrophils, macrophages, basophils, and megakaryocytes. Female patients heterozygous for glucose-6-phosphate dehydrogenase isoenzymes demonstrate CIMF cells of a single enzyme isotype whereas tissue cells, including marrow fibroblasts, contained both enzyme isotypes.[4]

Myelofibrosis

The myelofibrosis in this disease comprises three of the five types of collagen; I, III, and IV. Increases in type III are detected by silver impregnation techniques, in type I by staining with trichrome, and in type IV by the presence of osteosclerosis, which may be diagnosed by increased radiographic bone density.[57] In approximately 30% of patients, biopsy specimens may show no fibrosis.[20] Increases in these collagens are not a part of the clonal proliferative process but are considered secondary to an increased release of fibroblastic growth factors, such as platelet-derived growth factor, transforming growth factor-β from megakaryocyte α granules, tumor necrosis factor-α, and interleukin-1α and interleukin-1β. Marrow fibrosis causes expansion of marrow sinuses and vascular volume with an increased rate of blood flow. Bone marrow fibrosis is not the sole criterion for a diagnosis of CIMF because increases in marrow fibrosis may reflect a reparative response to injury from benzene or ionizing radiation, may be a consequence of immunologic-mediated injury, or may represent a reactive response to other hematologic conditions.

Type IV collagen and laminin normally are discontinuous in sinusoidal membranes but appear as stromal sheets in association with neovascularization and endothelial cell proliferation in regions of fibrosis. In addition, deposition of type VII collagen is observed, and this may form a linkage between type I fibers, type III fibers, and types I plus III fibers.[58]

Hematopoiesis and Extramedullary Hematopoiesis

Extramedullary hematopoiesis, clinically recognized as hepatomegaly or splenomegaly, seems to originate from release of clonal stem cells into circulation.[59] The cells accumulate in the spleen, liver, or other organs, including adrenals, kidney, lymph nodes, bowel, breast, lungs, mediastinum, mesentery, skin, synovium, thymus, and lower urinary tract.

The cause of extramedullary hematopoiesis is unknown. In experimental animal models, chemicals, hormones, viruses, radiation, and immunologic factors have been implicated. The disease is associated with an increase in circulating hematopoietic cells, but fibroblasts are a secondary abnormality and not clonal.[60] B and T cells may be involved.[61] There is an increase in circulating unilineage and multilineage hematopoietic progenitor cells,[62] and CD34+ cells may be 300 times normal.[63] The increase of circulating CD34+ cells separates CIMF from other MPDs and predicts risks of degree of splenic involvement and conversion to acute leukemia.

Body cavity effusions containing hematopoietic cells may arise from extramedullary hematopoiesis in the cranium, the intraspinal epidural space, or the serosal surfaces of pleura, pericardium, and peritoneum. Portal hypertension, with its attendant consequences of ascites, esophageal and gastric varices, gastrointestinal hemorrhage, and hepatic encephalopathy, arises from a combination of a massive increase in splenoportal blood flow and a decrease in hepatic vascular compliance secondary to fibrosis around the sinusoids and hematopoietic cells within the sinusoids.[64]

Peripheral Blood and Bone Marrow

CIMF presents with a broad range of changes in laboratory test values, and peripheral blood film and bone marrow biopsy examination provides most of the information for diagnosis. Changes commonly observed in peripheral blood and bone marrow examinations are summarized in Table 34-5.

Abnormalities in erythrocytes noted on peripheral blood films include dacryocytes (teardrop-shaped RBCs), other bizarre shapes, nucleated RBCs, and polychromatophilia.

TABLE 34-5 Common Morphologic Changes in Chronic Idiopathic Myelofibrosis

Peripheral Blood

Hemoglobin	Normal or decreased
Anisocytosis	Present
Poikilocytosis	Present
Teardrop-shaped erythrocytes	Present
Nucleated RBCs	Present
Polychromasia	Normal or increased
Total WBCs	Normal, decreased or increased
Immature granulocytes	Increased
Blasts	Present
Basophils	Present
Leukocyte anomaly	Present
LAP	Increased, normal or decreased
Platelets	Increased, normal or decreased
Abnormal platelets	Present
Megakaryocytes	Present

Bone Marrow

Cellularity	Increased
Granulopoiesis	Increased
Megakaryocytes	Increased
Erythropoiesis	Normal or increased
Myelofibrosis	Increased
Sinuses	Increased
Dysmegakaryopoiesis	Present
Dysgranulopoiesis	Present

Extramedullary Tissue

Splenomegaly	Present
Sinusoidal	
Medullary	
Hepatomegaly	Present
Sinusoidal	
Portal tract	
Local infiltrates	
Other tissues	Present

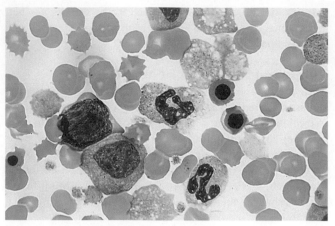

Figure 34-7 Peripheral blood smear in CIMF illustrating nucleated RBCs, giant platelets, and immature myeloid cells (×1000).

Granulocytes are increased, normal, or decreased and may include immature granulocytes, blasts, and cells with nuclear or cytoplasmic anomalies. Platelets may be normal, increased, or decreased with a mixture of normal and abnormal morphology (Fig. 34-7). Micromegakaryocytes may be observed (Fig. 34-8).

Bone marrow biopsy specimens exhibit intense fibrosis, granulocytic and megakaryocytic hypercellularity, dysmegakaryopoiesis, dysgranulopoiesis, and numerous dilated sinuses containing luminal hematopoiesis. Neutrophils may exhibit impairment of physiologic functions, such as phagocytosis, oxygen consumption, and hydrogen peroxide generation, and decreased myeloperoxidase and glutathione reductase activities. Platelets have impaired aggregation in response to epinephrine, decreased adenosine diphosphate concentration in dense granules, and decreased activity of platelet lipoxygenase.

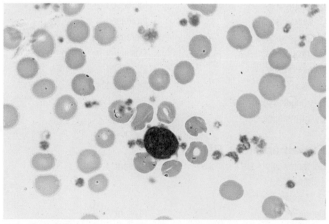

Figure 34-8 Peripheral blood smear in a patient with CIMF exhibiting increased platelets and a micromegakaryocyte (×1000).

Immune Response

Humoral immune responses are altered in approximately 50% of patients and include the appearance of autoantibodies to erythrocyte antigens, nuclear proteins, gamma globulins, phospholipids, and organ-specific antigens.[65] Circulating immune complexes, increased proportions of marrow-reactive lymphocytes, and the development of amyloidosis are evidence for active immune processes. Collagen disorders coexist with CIMF, suggesting that immunologic processes may stimulate marrow fibroblast activity.

Incidence and Presentation

The disease occurs in patients over 60 and may be asymptomatic. CIMF generally presents with fatigue, weakness, shortness of breath, palpitations, weight loss, and discomfort or pain in the left upper quadrant associated with splenomegaly.

Therapy and Prognosis

Average survival from diagnosis is about 5 years, but patients have lived 15 years. During this time, increasing numbers and pleomorphy of megakaryocytes lead to progressive marrow failure. Marrow blasts may increase.[20] Adverse prognostic indicators include the severity of anemia and thrombocytopenia, the magnitude of hepatomegaly, unexplained fever, and hemolysis. Mortality is associated with infection, hemorrhage, postsplenectomy complications, and transformation to acute leukemia.

A diverse spectrum of therapies has been applied to alleviate symptoms or modify clinical problems in these patients. Severe anemia has been treated with androgen therapy and hemolytic anemia with glucocorticosteroids. Reduction of myelofibrosis and of marrow and tissue hypercellularity has been accomplished with busulfan and other alkylating agents, hydroxyurea, and, in a few patients, α-interferon and γ-interferon. Radiotherapy is considered for patients with severe splenic pain, for patients with massive splenomegaly who are not clinical candidates for splenectomy, for patients with ascites secondary to serosal implants (metastatic nodule), and for patients with localized bone pain and other localized extramedullary fibrohematopoietic masses, especially in the epidural space. Splenectomy is performed to end severe pain, excessive transfusion requirements, or severe thrombocytopenia and to correct severe portal hypertension.

Chemotherapy is partially successful in reducing CD34+ cells, immature hematopoietic cells, marrow fibrosis, and splenomegaly.[66] Single-agent chemotherapy is most useful in the early clinical phases of the disease, and agents such as busulfan, 6-thioguanine, and chlorambucil alone or in combination with chemotherapy are useful. Other agents include α-interferon, hydroxyurea, and combinations of the previously-mentioned drugs.[67] The most successful therapy to date for patients under 60 is allogeneic stem cell transplantation. Five-year survival approaches 50%, but 1-year mortality is 27%, and graft-versus-host disease occurs in 33%.[68]

CHAPTER at a GLANCE

- MPDs are clonal hematopoietic stem cell disorders that result in excessive production and overaccumulation of erythrocytes, granulocytes, and platelets in some combination in bone marrow, peripheral blood, and body tissues.
- Within the classification of MPD are CML, PV, ET, and CIMF.
- In CML, there are large numbers of myeloid precursors in the bone marrow, peripheral blood, and extramedullary tissues.
- The peripheral blood exhibits leukocytosis with increased myeloid series, particularly the later maturation stages, often with increases in eosinophils and basophils.
- The LAP score is dramatically decreased in CML.
- Philadelphia chromosome t(9;22) is present in most cases of CML.
- The bone marrow exhibits intense hypercellularity composed of myeloid precursors. Megakaryocytes are normal to increased.
- Patients with CML progress from a chronic stable phase through an accelerated phase into transformation into acute leukemia.
- Bone marrow transplant has been successful in CML, and Gleevec, a tyrosine kinase inhibitor, has shown potential for possible cure.
- PV manifests with panmyelosis in the bone marrow with increases in erythrocytes, granulocytes, and platelets.
- The clinical diagnosis requires an increased RBC mass, normal or increased arterial oxygen saturation, and splenomegaly. If only two of these criteria are present, the diagnosis can be made if two of the following are present: platelet count greater than 400×10^9/L; WBC count greater than 12×10^9/L in the absence of infection; or increases in LAP, serum vitamin B_{12}, or unbound vitamin B_{12} binding capacity.

- ET involves increased megakaryocytes with a platelet count greater than 600×10^9/L.
- Other diagnostic criteria include normal RBC mass, stainable iron in the bone marrow, absence of Philadelphia chromosome, absent marrow collagen fibrosis, absence of splenomegaly or leukoerythroblastic reaction, and no known cause of reactive thrombocytosis.
- In the early phases of ET, peripheral blood shows increased platelets with abnormalities in size and shape. Bone marrow megakaryocytes are increased in number and in size.
- Complications of ET include thromboembolism and hemorrhage.
- CIMF manifests with ineffective hematopoiesis, sparse areas of marrow hypercellularity (especially with increased megakaryocytes), bone marrow fibrosis, splenomegaly, and hepatomegaly.
- The peripheral blood in CIMF exhibits immature granulocytes and nucleated RBCs; teardrop-shaped cells are a common finding.
- Platelets may be normal, increased, or decreased with abnormal morphology. Micromegakaryocytes may be present.
- Immune responses are altered in about 50% of patients.

Now that you have completed this chapter, go back and read again the case study at the beginning and respond to the questions presented.

REVIEW QUESTIONS

1. A peripheral smear with increased neutrophils, basophils, eosinophils, and platelets is highly suggestive of:
   a. AML
   b. CML
   c. Myelodysplastic syndrome
   d. Multiple myeloma

2. Which of the following chromosome abnormalities is associated with most cases of CML?
   a. t(15;17)
   b. t(8;14)
   c. t(9;22)
   d. Monosomy 7

3. A patient presents with a WBC count of 30×10^9/L and the following WBC differential:
   Segmented neutrophils: 38%
   Bands: 17%
   Metamyelocytes: 7%
   Myelocytes: 20%
   Promyelocytes: 10%
   Eosinophils: 3%
   Basophils: 5%
   Which of the following test results would be helpful in determining whether the patient has CML?
   a. Nitroblue tetrazolium increased
   b. Myeloperoxidase increased
   c. Periodic acid-Schiff decreased
   d. LAP decreased

4. A patient with the previous diagnosis of CML presents with circulating blasts and promyelocytes that total 30%. The disease is considered to be in what phase?
   a. Chronic stable
   b. Accelerated
   c. Transformation to acute leukemia
   d. Temporary remission

5. Patients with primary PV usually have blood P_{O_2} that is:
   a. Decreased
   b. Normal
   c. Extremely elevated

6. The peripheral blood in PV typically manifests:
   a. Erythrocytosis only
   b. Erythrocytosis and thrombocytosis
   c. Erythrocytosis, thrombocytosis, and granulocytosis
   d. Anemia and thrombocytopenia

7. A patient presents with a platelet count of 700×10^9/L with abnormalities in size, shape, and granularity of platelets; WBC count of 12×10^9/L; hemoglobin of 11 g/dL; and the absence of the Philadelphia chromosome. The most likely diagnosis would be:
   a. PV
   b. ET
   c. Chronic myeloid leukemia
   d. Leukemoid reaction

8. Complications of ET include all of the following *except:*
   a. Thrombosis
   b. Hemorrhage
   c. Seizures
   d. Infections

9. Which of the following patterns is characteristic of the peripheral blood in patients with CIMF?
   a. Teardrop-shaped erythrocytes, nucleated RBCs, immature granulocytes
   b. Abnormal platelets only
   c. Hypochromic erythrocytes, immature granulocytes, and normal platelets
   d. Spherocytes, immature granulocytes, and increased platelets

10. The myelofibrosis associated with CIMF is a result of:
    a. Apoptosis resistance in the fibroblasts of the bone marrow
    b. Impaired production of normal collagenase from the mutated cells
    c. Enhanced activity of fibroblasts owing to increased stimulatory cytokines
    d. Increased numbers of fibroblasts owing to cytokine stimulation of the pluripotential stem cells

REFERENCES

1. Fialkow PJ, Jacobson RJ, Papayannopoulou T: Chronic myelocytic leukemia: clonal origin in a stem cell common to the granulocytic, erythrocytic, platelet and monocyte/macrophage. Am J Med 1977;63:125-130.
2. Adamson JW, Fialkow PJ, Murphy S, et al: Polycythemia vera: stem-cell and probable clonal origin of the disease. N Engl J Med 1976;295:913-916.
3. Fialkow PJ, Faguet GB, Jacobson RJ, et al: Evidence that essential thrombocythemia is a clonal disorder with origin in a multipotent stem cell. Blood 1981;58:916-919.
4. Jacobson RJ, Salo A, Fialkow PJ: Agnogenic myeloid metaplasia: a clonal proliferation of hematopoietic stem cells with secondary myelofibrosis. Blood 1978;51:189-194.
5. Dameshek W: Some speculations on the myeloproliferative syndromes [editorial]. Blood 1951;6:372.
6. Whang J, Frei E III, Tijo JH, et al: The distribution of the Philadelphia chromosome in patients with chronic myelogenous leukemia. Blood 1963;22:664-673.
7. Spiers AS, Bain BJ, Turner JE: The peripheral blood in chronic granulocytic leukemia: study of 50 untreated Philadelphia-positive cases. Scand J Hematol 1977;18:25-28.
8. Ward HP, Block MH: The natural history of agnogenic myeloid metaplasia (AMM) and a critical evaluation of its relationship with the myeloproliferative syndrome. Medicine (Baltimore) 1971;150:357-420.
9. Mitus AJ, Schafer AI: Thrombocytosis and thrombocythemia. Hematol Oncol Clin N Am 1990;4:157-178.
10. Gilbert HS: Familial myeloproliferative disease. Ballieres Clin Haematol 1998;11:849-858.
11. Cotter FE: Childhood myeloproliferatve disorders. Ballieres Clin Haematol 1998;11:875-898.
12. Barr RD, Fialkow PJ: Clonal origin of chronic myelocytic leukemia. N Engl J Med 1973;289:307-309.
13. Rowley JD: A new consistent chromosome abnormality in chronic myelogenous leukemia identified by quinacrine fluorescence and Giemsa banding. Nature 1973;243:290-293.
14. Stam K, Heisterkamp N, Grosveld G, et al: Evidence of a new chimeric bcr/c-abl mRNA in patients with chronic myelocytic leukemia and the Philadelphia chromosome. N Engl J Med 1985;313:1429-1433.
15. Epner DE, Koeffler HP: Molecular genetic advances in chronic myelogenous leukemia. Ann Intern Med 1990;113:3-6.
16. Douer D, Levine AM, Sparkes RS, et al: Chronic myelocytic leukemia: a pluripotent haemopoietic cell is involved in the malignant clone. Br J Haematol 1981;49:615-619.
17. Bizzozzero OJ, Johnson KG, Ciocco A: Radiation-related leukemia in Hiroshima and Nagasaki, 1946-1964: I. Distribution, incidence, and appearance time. N Engl J Med 1966;274:1095-1101.
18. Brown WM, Doll R: Mortality from cancer and other causes after radiotherapy for ankylosing spondylitis. BMJ 1965;5474:1327-1332.
19. Marmont A, Frassoni F, Bacigalupo A, et al: Recurrence of Ph^1-positive leukemia in donor cells after marrow transplantation for chronic granulocytic leukemia. N Engl J Med 1984;310:903-906.
20. Kurzrock R, Gutterman JU, Talpez M: The molecular genetics of Philadelphia chromosome-positive leukemia. N Engl J Med 1988;319:990-998.
21. Faderl S, Talpaz T, Estrov Z, et al: Mechanisms of disease: the biology of chronic myeloid leukemia. N Engl J Med 1999;341:164-172.
22. Bhatia R, Verfaillie CM: The effects of interferon-alpha on beta-1 integrin mediated adhesion and growth regulation in chronic myelogenous leukemia. Leuk Lymphoma 1998;28:241-254.
23. Georgii A, Buesche G, Krept A: The histopathology of chronic myeloproliferative disorders: review. Ballieres Clin Haematol 1998;11:721-749.
24. Klineberg JR, Bluestone R, Schlosstein L, et al: Urate deposition disease: how it is regulated and how can it be modified? Ann Intern Med 1973;78:99-111.
25. Lichtman MA, Rowe JM: Hyperleukocytic leukemias: rheological, clinical and therapeutic considerations. Blood 1982;60:279-283.
26. Lichtman MA, Heal J, Rowe JM: Hyperleukocytic leukemia. Ballieres Clin Haematol 1987;1:725-746.
27. Muehleck SD, McKenna RD, Arthur DC, et al: Transformation of chronic myelogenous leukemia: clinical, morphologic and cytogenetic features. Am J Clin Pathol 1984;82:1-14.
28. Vardiman JW, Pierre R, Thiele J: Chronic myelogenous leukemia. In Jaffe ES, Harris NL, Stein H, et al (eds): World Health Organization Classification of Tumours: Pathology and Genetics of Tumours of Haematopoietic and Lymphoid tissues. Lyon: IARC Press, 2001:20-26.
29. Bernstein R: Cytogenetics of chronic myelogenous leukemia. Semin Hematol 1988;25:20-34.
30. Sandberg AA: Chromosomes in the chronic phase of CML. Virchows Arch [B] 1978;29:51-55.
31. Bareford D, Jacobs P: Chronic neutrophilic leukemia. Am J Clin Pathol 1980;73:837.
32. Bearman RM, Kjeldsburg CR, Pangalis GA, et al: Chronic monocytic leukemia in adults. Cancer 1981;48:2239-2255.
33. Thomas WJ, North RB, Poplack DG, et al: Chronic myelo-

monocytic leukemia in childhood. Am J Hematol 1981; 10:181-194.

34. Mijovic A, Mufti GJ: The myelodysplastic syndromes: towards a functional classification. Blood Rev 1998;12:73-83.

35. Kurzrock R, Gutterman JU, Talpaz M: The molecular genetics of Philadelphia chromosome positive leukemias. N Engl J Med 1988;319:990-998.

36. Specchia G, Mininni D, Guerrasio A, et al: Ph positive acute lymphoblastic leukemia in adults: molecular and clinical studies. Leuk Lymphoma 1995;18(Suppl):37-42.

37. Faderl S, Talpaz M, Estrov A, et al: Chronic myelogenous leukemia: biology and therapy. Ann Intern Med 1999;131:207-219.

38. Catovsky D: Ph^1-positive acute leukemia and chronic granulocytic leukemia: one or two diseases? Br J Haematol 1979;42:493-498.

39. Wintrobe MM, Huguley CM, McLennan MT, et al: Nitrogen mustard as a therapeutic agent for Hodgkin's disease, lymphosarcoma and leukemia. Ann Intern Med 1947;27:529-539.

40. Galton DA: The use of myleran in chronic myeloid leukemia: results of treatment. Lancet 1953;264:208-213.

41. Lion T, Gaiger A, Henn T, et al: Use of quantitative polymerase chain reaction to monitor residual disease in chronic myelogenous leukemia during treatment with interferon. Leukemia 1995;9:1353-1360.

42. Sawyers CL: Chronic myeloid leukemia. N Engl J Med 1999; 340:1330-1340.

43. Guilhot F, Chastang C, Michallet M, et al: Interferon alpha 2b combined with cytarabine versus interferon alone in chronic myelogenous leukemia. N Engl J Med 1997;337:223-229.

44. O'Brien SG: Autografting for chronic myeloid leukemia. Baillieres Clin Haematol 1997;10:369-388.

45. Druker BJ, Talpaz M, Resta DJ, et al: Efficacy and safety of a specific inhibitor of the BCR-ABL tyrosine kinase in chronic myeloid leukemia. N Engl J Med 2001;344:1031-1037.

46. Lin F, Drummond M, O'Brien S, et al: Molecular monitoring in chronic myeloid leukemia patients who achieve complete remission on imatinib [letter]. Blood 2003;102:1143.

47. Gilliland DG, Blanchard KL, Levy J, et al: Determination of clonality in myeloproliferative disorders: analysis by means of the polymerase chain reaction. Proc Natl Acad Sci U S A 1991;88:6848-6852.

48. Prechal JF, Adamson JW, Murphy S, et al: Polycythemia vera: the in vitro response of normal and abnormal stem cell lines to erythropoietin. J Clin Invest 1978;61:1044-1047.

49. Adamson JW, Singer JW, Catalano P, et al: Polycythemia vera: further in vitro studies of hematopoietic regulation. J Clin Invest 1980;66:1363-1368.

50. Berlin N: Diagnosis and classification of the polycythemias. Semin Hematol 1975;12:339-351.

51. Berk PD, Goldberg JN, Donovan PB, et al: Therapeutic recommendations in polycythemia vera based on Polycythemia Vera Study Group protocols. Semin Hematol 1986;23:132-143.

52. Wolf BC, Bank PM, Mann RB, et al: Splenic hematopoiesis in polycythemia vera: a morphologic and immunohistologic study. Am J Clin Pathol 1988;89:69-75.

53. Ellis JT, Peterson P, Geller SA, et al: Studies of the bone marrow in polycythemia vera and the evolution of myelofibrosis and second hematologic malignancies. Semin Hematol 1986; 23:144-155.

54. Mitus AJ, Schafer A: Thrombocytosis and thrombocythemia. Hematol Oncol Clin N Am 1990;4:157-178.

55. Murphy S, Iland H, Rosenthal D, et al: Essential thrombocythemia: an interim report from the Polycythemia Vera Study Group. Semin Haematol 1986;23:177-182.

56. Kuecht H, Streuli RA: Megakaryopoiesis in different forms of thrombocytosis and thrombocytopenia: identification of megakaryocyte precursors by immunostaining of intracytoplasmic factor VIII-related antigen. Acta Haematol 1985; 74:208-212.

57. McCarthy DM: Fibrosis of the bone marrow, content and causes [annotation]. Br J Haematol 1985;59:1-7.

58. Reilly IF: Pathogenesis of idiopathic myelofibrosis: present status and future directions. Br J Haematol 1994;88:1-8.

59. Wang JC, Cheung CP, Fakhiuddin A, et al: Circulating granulocyte and macrophage progenitor cells in primary and secondary myelofibrosis. Br J Haematol 1983;54:301-307.

60. Jacobson RJ, Salo A, Fialkow PJ. Agnogenic myeloid metaplasia: a clonal proliferation of hematopoietic stem cells with secondary myelofibrosis. Blood 1978;51:189-194.

61. Buschle M, Janssen JY, Drexler H, et al: Evidence for pluripotent stem cell origin of idiopathic myelofibrosis: clonal analysis of a case characterized by a N-ras gene mutation. Leukemia 1988;2:658-660.

62. Juvonen E: Megakaryocyte colony formation in chronic myeloid leukemia and myelofibrosis. Leuk Res 1988;12:751-756.

63. Barosi G, Viarengo G, Pecci A, et al: Diagnostic and clinical relevance of the number of circulating CD34(+) cells in myelofibrosis with myeloid metaplasia. Blood 2001;98:3249-3255.

64. Jacobs P, Maze S, Tayob F, et al: Myelofibrosis, splenomegaly, and portal hypertension. Acta Haematol 1985;74:45-48.

65. Vellenga E, Mulder N, The T, et al: A study of the cellular and humoral immune response in patients with myelofibrosis. Clin Lab Haematol 1982;4:239-246.

66. Pegrum GD, Foadi M, Boots M, et al: How should we manage myelofibrosis? J R Coll Physician Lond 1981;15:17-18.

67. Tefferi A, Silverstein MN: Current perspective in agnogenic myeloid metaplasia. Leuk Lymphoma 1996;22(suppl 1):169-171.

68. Guardiola P, Anderson JE, Bandini G, et al: Allogeneic stem cell transplantation for agnogenic myeloid metaplasia: a European Group for Blood and Marrow Transplantation, Societe Francaise de Greffe de Moelle, Gruppo Italiano per il Trapianto del Midollo Osseo, and Fred Hutchinson Cancer Research Center Collaborative Study. Blood 1999;93:2831-2838.

35

Myelodysplastic Syndromes

Bernadette F. Rodak

OBJECTIVES

After completion of this chapter, the reader will be able to:

1. Define myelodysplastic syndromes (MDS).
2. Explain the sequence of events thought to lead to MDS.
3. Recognize morphologic features of dyspoiesis in bone marrow and peripheral blood.
4. Discuss abnormal functions of granulocytes, erythrocytes, and thrombocytes in MDS.
5. Correlate peripheral blood, bone marrow, and cytogenetic findings in MDS with classification systems.
6. Compare and contrast the French-American-British (FAB) and the World Health Organization (WHO) classifications.
7. Discuss prognostic indicators in MDS.
8. List common causes of death in MDS.
9. Discuss modes of management for MDS.
10. Discuss the epidemiology of MDS, and apply it as a contributor in differential diagnosis.
11. Suggest laboratory tests and their results that would rule out MDS in the differential diagnosis.

CASE STUDY

After studying the material in this chapter, the reader should be able to respond to the following case study:

A 43-year-old man presented with fatigue and malaise. He had pancytopenia (white blood cell count 2.2×10^9/L, hemoglobin 6.1 g/dL, platelet count 51×10^9/L). The white blood cell differential was essentially normal. Mean cell volume was 132 fL (reference range 80-100 fL) in the presence of normal vitamin B_{12} and folate levels. The bone marrow was normocellular with a myeloid-to-erythroid ratio of 1:1 and adequate megakaryocytes. The erythroid component was dysplastic with megaloblastic features. No abnormal localization of immature precursors was noted. Chromosome analysis indicated direct duplication of chromosome 1q. The patient was maintained with transfusions over the next 6 years. At that time, his bone marrow revealed increased erythropoiesis, decreased granulopoiesis, and megakaryopoiesis, all with dysplastic changes. There were 50% to 60% ringed sideroblasts.

1. What should be included in the differential diagnosis of patients with pancytopenia and elevated mean cell volume?
2. Given the normal vitamin B_{12} and folate levels, what is the patient's probable diagnosis?
3. In which classification does this disorder belong?

For decades, laboratory professionals have observed a group of morphologic abnormalities in peripheral blood and bone marrow smears of elderly patients. The findings were heterogeneous in nature, affected all cell lines, and either remained stable for years or progressed rapidly to death.

Historically, this pattern of abnormalities was referred to as *refractory anemia, smoldering leukemia, oligoblastic leukemia,* or *preleukemia.*[1-3] In 1982, the French-American-British (FAB) Cooperative Leukemia Study Group proposed terminology and a specific set of morphologic criteria to describe what are now known as *myelodysplastic syndromes* (MDS).[4] In 1997, a group from the World Health Organization (WHO) proposed a new classification that included molecular, cytogenetic, and immunologic criteria in addition to morphology.[5,6] Both classifications are discussed in this chapter.

MDS are a group of acquired clonal hematologic disorders characterized by progressive cytopenias in the peripheral blood, reflecting defects in erythroid, myeloid, or megakaryocytic maturation.[7,8] The median age at diagnosis is 70. MDS rarely affect individuals younger than age 50, unless preceded by chemotherapy or radiation for another malignancy.[1,9,10] Cases in young adults and children have been reported, however.[11,12] The incidence of these disorders seems to be increasing, but this apparent increase may be attributable in part to improved techniques for identifying these diseases and to improved classification.[13] At this time, the fastest-growing segment of the population is older than 60 years of age; MDS are becoming a more common finding in the hematology laboratory and an essential part of the body of knowledge of all clinical laboratory professionals.

ETIOLOGY

MDS may arise de novo (primary) or as a result of therapy (therapy-related MDS). Some authors also have suggested a familial association.[14] Although MDS seem to be a group of heterogeneous diseases, all are the result of proliferation of abnormal stem cells.[7,8,16,17] The initiating defect in most cases is at the level of the myeloid stem cell because primarily the erythroid, myeloid, and megakaryocytic cells are affected. It may be that the affected hematopoietic stem cell has lost its lymphopoietic potential because only rarely does MDS transform to acute lymphoid leukemia.[18,19] The abnormal stem cell may be the result of the cumulative effects of environmental exposure in susceptible individuals.[20] Mutations may be caused by chemical insult, radiation, or viral infection.[21] There also may be an association with smoking.[20,22] The mutated stem cell produces a pathologic clone of cells that expands in size at the expense of normal cell production.[20,23] Because each mutation produces a unique clone with a specific cellular defect, MDS have a multitude of expressions. Two morphologic findings are common to all types of MDS, however: the presence of progressive cytopenias despite cellular bone marrows and dyspoiesis in one or more cell lines.

Disruption of apoptosis may be responsible for the ineffective hematopoiesis in MDS.[24-29] Apoptosis (programmed cell death) regulates cell population by decreasing cell survival. In MDS, apoptosis seems to be increased in early disease, when peripheral blood cytopenias are evident. Later in MDS, when progression toward leukemia is apparent, apoptosis has been shown to be decreased, allowing increased neoplastic cell survival and expansion of the abnormal clone.[30-33] Other factors include antiangiogenic cytokines, tumor necrosis factor, cellular components of the immune system, and interaction between MDS clonal cells and the hematopoietic inductive microenvironment. Evidence has shown that patients with MDS show increased levels of angiogenic growth factors, including vascular endothelial growth factor.[34,35]

Therapy-related MDS occur in patients who have been treated previously with chemotherapy or radiotherapy or both. Median onset of therapy-related MDS varies with agents used and is usually 2.5 to 5 years after therapy was initiated,[36,37] although cases 7 years after initial exposure to chemotherapy or radiation have been reported.[38] Therapy-related MDS often are more aggressive and may evolve quickly into acute myeloblastic leukemia (AML).[37-39] The primary differences between therapy-related MDS and de novo MDS include

presentation at a younger age, higher incidence of AML, more pronounced bone marrow dysplasia, more severe cytopenias, more pronounced hypocellularity in the bone marrow with greater fibrosis, and a higher incidence of clonal chromosomal aberrations.[36,38] Abnormalities of chromosomes 5 or 7 or both are frequent.[36,37]

MORPHOLOGIC ABNORMALITIES IN PERIPHERAL BLOOD AND BONE MARROW

Each of the three major myeloid cell lines has dyspoietic morphologic features. The following sections provide descriptions of common abnormal morphologic findings.[4,40,41] These descriptions are not all-inclusive because of the large number of possible cellular mutations and combinations of mutations.

Dyserythropoiesis

In the peripheral blood, the most common morphologic finding in dyserythropoiesis is the presence of oval macrocytes (Fig. 35-1). When these cells are seen in the presence of normal vitamin B_{12} and folate values, MDS should be included in the differential diagnosis. Hypochromic microcytes with adequate iron stores also are seen in MDS. A dimorphic red blood cell (RBC) population (Fig. 35-2) is another indication of the clonality of this disease. Poikilocytosis, basophilic stippling, Howell-Jolly bodies, and siderocytes also are indications that the erythrocyte has undergone abnormal development.[23,42]

Dyserythropoiesis in the bone marrow is evidenced by RBC precursors with more than one nucleus or abnormal nuclear shapes. The normally round nucleus may have lobes or buds. Nuclear fragments may be present in the cytoplasm (Fig. 35-3). Internuclear bridging is occasionally present (Fig. 35-4).[41,43] Abnormal cytoplasmic features may include basophilic stippling or heterogeneous staining (Fig. 35-5). Ringed sideroblasts are a common finding. Megaloblastoid cellular development in the presence of normal vitamin B_{12} and folate values is another indication of MDS. These bone marrows may have erythrocytic hyperplasia or hypoplasia (Box 35-1).

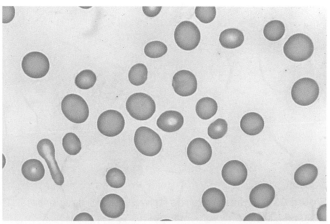

Figure 35-1 Oval macrocytes in peripheral blood (×1000).

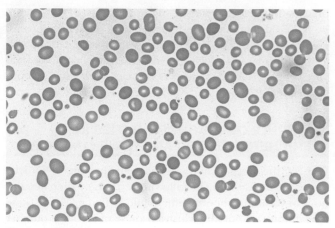

Figure 35-2 Dimorphic erythrocyte population in peripheral blood, showing macrocytic and microcytic cells (×500).

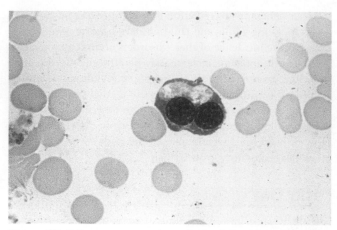

Figure 35-5 Bone marrow specimen showing heterogeneous staining in a bilobed erythroid precursor (×1000).

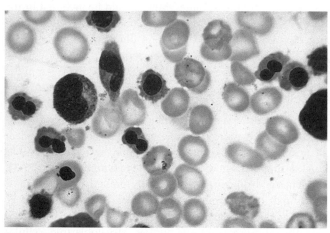

Figure 35-3 Bone marrow specimen showing erythroid hyperplasia and nuclear budding in erythroid precursors (×1000).

BOX 35-1 Morphologic Evidence of Dyserythropoiesis

Oval macrocytes
Hypochromic microcytes
Dimorphic RBC population
RBC precursors with more than one nucleus
RBC precursors with abnormal nuclear shapes
RBC precursors with uneven cytoplasmic staining
Ringed sideroblasts

Dysmyelopoiesis

Dysmyelopoiesis in the peripheral blood is suspected when there is a persistence of basophilia in the cytoplasm of otherwise mature white blood cells (WBCs), indicating nuclear-cytoplasmic asynchrony (Fig. 35-6). Abnormal granulation of the cytoplasm of neutrophils is a common finding, in the form of granules larger than normal, hypogranulation, or the

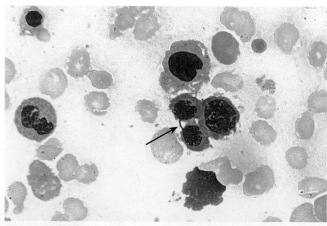

Figure 35-4 Erythroid precursors showing nuclear bridging *(arrow)* (bone marrow, ×1000).

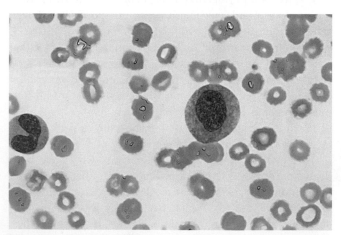

Figure 35-6 This myelocyte *(right)* in peripheral blood has a nucleus with clumped chromatin and a basophilic immature cytoplasm showing asynchrony. Note also the agranular myeloid cell *(left)*. (×1000).

absence of granules. Agranular bands can be easily misclassified as monocytes (Fig. 35-7). Abnormal nuclear features may include hyposegmentation, hypersegmentation, or nuclear rings (Fig. 35-8).[44]

In the bone marrow, dysmyelopoiesis may be represented by nuclear-cytoplasmic asynchrony. Cytoplasmic changes include uneven staining, such as a dense ring of basophilia around the periphery with a clear unstained area around the nucleus or whole sections of cytoplasm unstained with the remainder of the cytoplasm stained normally (Fig. 35-9). There may be abnormal granulation of the cytoplasm in which promyelocytes or myelocytes or both are devoid of primary granules (Fig. 35-10), primary granules may be larger than normal, or secondary granules may be reduced in number or absent, and there may be an occasional Aüer rod.[45,46] Agranular promyelocytes may be mistaken for blasts; this could lead to misclassification of the disease in the AML scheme. Abnormal nuclear findings may include hypersegmentation or hyposegmentation and possibly ring-shaped nuclei (Box 35-2).

The bone marrow may exhibit granulocytic hypoplasia or hyperplasia. Monocytic hyperplasia is a common finding in dysplastic marrows.

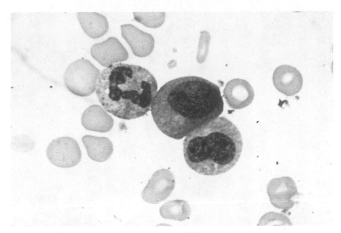

Figure 35-9 Uneven staining of WBC cytoplasm in bone marrow specimen (×1000).

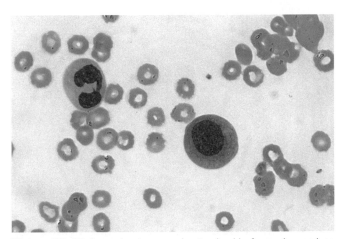

Figure 35-10 Promyelocyte or myelocyte, devoid of granules, and an agranular neutrophil in bone marrow (×1000).

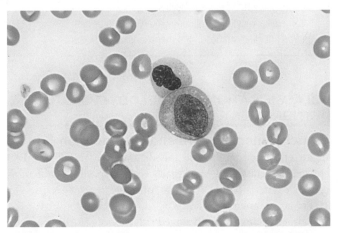

Figure 35-7 Agranular myeloid cells in peripheral blood (×1000).

BOX 35-2 **Morphologic Evidence of Dysmyelopoiesis**

Persistent basophilic cytoplasm
Abnormal granulation
Abnormal nuclear shapes
Uneven cytoplasmic staining

Abnormal localization of immature precursors is a characteristic finding in bone marrow biopsy specimens from patients with MDS.[47] Normally, myeloblasts and promyelocytes reside along the endosteal surface of the bone marrow. In some cases of MDS, these cells tend to cluster centrally in marrow sections.

Dysmegakaryopoiesis

Platelets also exhibit dyspoietic morphology in the peripheral blood. Common changes include giant platelets and abnormal platelet granulation, either hypogranulation or agranulation (Fig. 35-11). Some platelets may possess large fused granules.

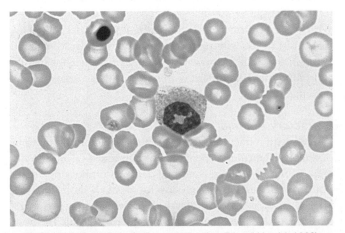

Figure 35-8 Nuclear ring in myeloid cell peripheral blood (×1000).

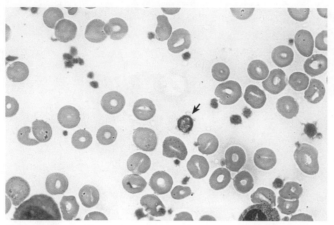

Figure 35-11 Abnormal platelet granulation in peripheral blood *(arrow)* (×1000).

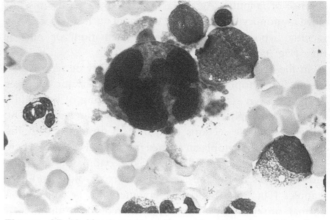

Figure 35-13 Megakaryocyte with small separated nuclei in bone marrow (×1000).

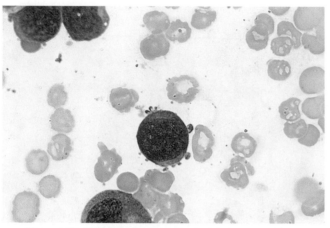

Figure 35-12 Micromegakaryocyte (peripheral blood, ×1000).

Circulating micromegakaryocytes have been described in peripheral blood from patients with MDS (Fig. 35-12).[23]

The megakaryocytic component of the bone marrow may exhibit abnormal morphology: large mononuclear megakaryocytes, micromegakaryocytes, or micromegakaryoblasts. The nuclei in these cells may be bilobed or have multiple small, separated nuclei (Fig. 35-13; Box 35-3).[41]

ABNORMAL CELLULAR FUNCTION

The cells produced by abnormal maturation not only have an abnormal appearance but also have abnormal function.[9,48] The granulocytes may have decreased adhesion,[49,50] deficient phagocytosis,[50] decreased chemotaxis,[49,50] or impaired microbicidal capacity.[51] Decreased levels of myeloperoxidase and alkaline phosphatase may be found.[52] The RBCs may exhibit shortened survival,[53] and erythroid precursors have a decreased response to erythropoietin that may contribute to anemia.[54] Patients may experience increased bleeding despite adequate platelet numbers.[55-57] The type and degree of dysfunction depend on the somatic mutation present in the hematopoietic stem cell.

BOX 35-3 Morphologic Evidence of Dysmegakaryopoiesis

Giant platelets
Platelets with abnormal granulation
Circulating micromegakaryocytes
Large mononuclear megakaryocytes
Micromegakaryocytes or micromegakaryoblasts or both
Abnormal nuclear shapes in the megakaryocytes/blasts

CLASSIFICATION OF MYELODYSPLASTIC SYNDROMES

French-American-British Classification

In an effort to standardize the diagnosis of MDS, the FAB created five classes of MDS, each with a specific set of morphologic criteria (Table 35-1), as follows:

1. Refractory anemia
2. Refractory anemia with ringed sideroblasts (RARS)
3. Refractory anemia with excess blasts (RAEB)
4. Chronic myelomonocytic leukemia (CMML)
5. Refractory anemia with excess blasts in transformation (RAEB-t)

With the exception of the classes of RARS and CMML, the major distinction among the subgroups is the percentage of blasts in the bone marrow. The diagnostic criteria for peripheral blood and bone marrow for each of these categories are presented.[41,58]

Refractory Anemia

Patients with refractory anemia usually have typical symptoms of anemia. Reticulocytopenia is present, and oval macrocytes are a common finding. Neutropenia or thrombocytopenia or both may be present, but dysmyelopoiesis or dysmegakaryopoiesis rarely is present. Blasts, if present in the peripheral blood, constitute less than 1% of the nucleated cells. The bone marrow is normocellular to hypercellular with erythroid hyperplasia or dyserythropoiesis or both. Iron stores are increased.

TABLE 35-1 Features of Peripheral Blood and Bone Marrow in Myelodysplastic Syndrome According to French-American-British Classification

	Refractory Anemia	Refractory Anemia with RS*	Refractory Anemia with Excess Blasts	Refractory Anemia with Excess Blasts in Transformation	Chronic Myelomonocytic Leukemia	Acute Myeloid Leukemia
% Peripheral blood blasts	<1	<1	<5	≥5	<5	NA**
% Bone marrow blasts	<5	<5	5-20	>20, <30	5-20	≥30
Other significant findings	<15% RS; oval macrocytes; cytopenias	>15% RS; dimorphic RBC population; oval macrocytes; cytopenias	Cell dysfunction evident; oval macrocytes; cytopenias	Absolute monocytosis (>1 × 10^9/L); oval macrocytes	Absolute monocytosis (>1 × 10^9/L); oval macrocytes	—

*RS, ringed sideroblasts.
**Diagnosed on bone marrow only.

The granulocytes and megakaryocytes are usually morphologically normal. Less than 5% of the nucleated cells are blasts.

Refractory Anemia with Ringed Sideroblasts

Patients with RARS have all of the signs and symptoms of refractory anemia; in addition, more than 15% of nucleated bone marrow cells are ringed sideroblasts. These cells often appear in clusters. To be considered a ringed sideroblast, an erythroid precursor must contain more than five iron granules/cell, and these iron-containing mitochondria must circle at least one third of the nucleus (Fig. 35-14).[59,60] Acquired sideroblastic anemia, not considered MDS, is discussed in Chapter 19.

Refractory Anemia with Excess Blasts

In many patients with RAEB, oval macrocytes are present in the peripheral blood. Trilineage cytopenias are commonly present, as are significant dysmyelopoiesis or dysmegakaryopoiesis or both. The morphologic abnormalities of WBCs may include hypogranular neutrophils or pseudo–Pelger-Huët cells. The platelets may have abnormal numbers of granules, which may

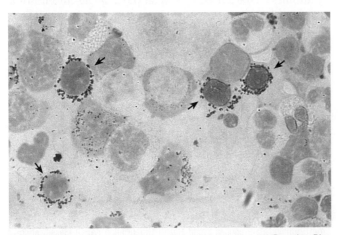

Figure 35-14 Ringed sideroblast *(arrows)* (bone marrow, Prussian Blue stain, ×1000).

exhibit abnormalities in size. There are less than 5% circulating blasts.

The bone marrow is normocellular to hypercellular with granulocytic or erythroid hyperplasia or both. Trilineage dyspoiesis is present, and 5% to 20% of the nucleated bone marrow cells are blasts. These patients present with a wide variety of complaints. The symptoms may include anemia, fever, bleeding, and infection.

Chronic Myelomonocytic Leukemia

The peripheral blood in patients with CMML may have characteristics similar to those of the refractory anemias, such as oval macrocytes and reticulocytopenia. The presence of dyserythropoiesis and dysmegakaryopoiesis varies. Thrombocytopenia may be present. In contrast to other classes of MDS, CMML usually manifests with leukocytosis. The peripheral WBC concentration may be 100 × 10^9/L. Absolute monocytosis (>1.0 × 10^9/L) is always present. Blasts constitute less than 5% of peripheral WBCs. The bone marrow shows granulocytic hyperplasia with dysmyelopoiesis. Monocytosis and dysmegakaryopoiesis are present, and 5% to 20% of nucleated bone marrow cells are blasts. Clinical features include prominent splenomegaly, symptoms of anemia, fever, bleeding, and infection.[14] The inclusion of CMML in the MDS is problematic because it actually fits criteria for the myeloproliferative disorders.[14,43,61] The WHO addressed this in its classification.

Refractory Anemia with Excess Blasts in Transformation

The peripheral blood morphology is the same in RAEB-t as in RAEB, except that there are more than 5% circulating blasts, and Aüer rods may be present. The bone marrow has the same characteristics as RAEB except that in the original FAB classification, RAEB-t included patients with 20% to 29% blasts in the bone marrow, with 30% or greater constituting AML. In the WHO proposed classification, 20% or greater would indicate AML.[51,61]

World Health Organization Classification

The FAB classification provided a framework for discussion of a seemingly heterogeneous group of disorders; however, its reliance on morphology alone limited its usefulness as a prognostic indicator. Additionally, the FAB classification did not view MDS in their totality because it did not address therapy-related or hereditary forms. Advances in medical knowledge, including molecular analysis, have allowed integration of clinical, immunologic, genetic, and molecular data with morphology.[60-63] The WHO classification retains many of the FAB features while recognizing molecular, cytogenetic, and immunologic characteristics of these disorders.[4,36]

The major modifications from the FAB classification of MDS include the reduction of the percentage of blasts required for diagnosis of AML from 30% to 20% and recognition of two new classifications: refractory cytopenia with multilineage dysplasia (RCMD) and the 5q− syndrome. The reduction in the number of blasts eliminates one criterion for RAEB-t.[4,36] That category may completely disappear, although some argue for its continued existence.[64,65] The WHO classification is outlined in Box 35-4.

Refractory Cytopenia with Multilineage Dysplasia

RCMD is categorized by cytopenia and dysplasia in two or more myeloid cell lines and less than 5% blasts in peripheral blood and bone marrow. Occasionally, RCMD has greater than 15% sideroblasts, but its effect on more than one cell line distinguishes it from RARS. This distinction is important because RCMD has a more aggressive course than RARS.[36,41]

Refractory Anemia with Excess Blasts

In the WHO classification, the peripheral blood may contain 19% blasts. In the bone marrow, blasts number 5% to 20%. RAEB is distinguished from RCMD by myeloblast percentage. The proposed WHO classification divides RAEB into two types according to percentage of blasts in blood and bone marrow:
Type 1—5% to 9% blasts
Type 2—10% to 19% blasts

Patients with greater than 10% myeloblasts have a more aggressive course, with a greater percentage transforming to AML.[36,41]

Myeloproliferative Disorders/Myelodysplastic Syndromes

The WHO suggested the removal of CMML from MDS and the creation of a new classification for disorders that overlap characteristics of myeloproliferative disorders and MDS.[4,36] Included in this classification are CMML, juvenile myelomonocytic leukemia, and atypical chronic myelogenous leukemia (Box 35-5).[4]

CYTOGENETICS AND MOLECULAR GENETICS

Cytogenetics

Chromosome abnormalities are found in 40% to 70% of cases of de novo MDS.[66] Of patients with therapy-related MDS, 90% are found to have abnormalities.[12,36,66,67] Translocations, which are common among patients with AML, are rarely found in patients with MDS. The most common abnormalities involve chromosomes 5, 7, 8, and 20.[66,68,69] The most common *single* abnormalities are 5q− and monosomy 7. Less common abnormalities in MDS are 12p−, iso 17, −22, and loss of the Y chromosome.[60,70-73] Newer techniques, such as fluorescence in situ hybridization (Chapters 31 and 32), have increased sensitivity for detecting well-established cytogenetic abnormalities, for example, 5q−, monosomy 7, and trisomy 8.[61]

5q− Syndrome

In patients who have only the deletion of 5q (5q−), the disease represents a fairly well-defined syndrome, affecting predominantly women over age 50. These patients typically have refractory macrocytic anemia, thrombocytosis, hypolobulated megakaryocytes, and erythroid hypoplasia.[16,60,70] Patients with the 5q− syndrome have long-term stable disease (median survival 28 months), and often only supportive therapy is needed.[16,67,70,74]

Other Single-Chromosome Entities

Syndromes characterized by several other single-chromosome abnormalities (including monosomy 7 and iso 17) have been suggested to be distinct MDS subclassifications because of the characteristic clinical and hematologic features they have in common.[60,40,75] None has been as widely studied or accepted, however, as the 5q− syndrome.

BOX 35-4 World Health Organization Classification of Myelodysplastic Syndromes

I. De novo MDS
   Refractory anemia
   RARS
   RARS with unilineage dysplasia
   RARS with multilineage dysplasia
   RCMD
   RAEB
II. Therapy-related MDS
   May classify as de novo, add qualifying term, *therapy-related*
   If case cannot be classified, diagnose as therapy-related MDS, unclassified

From Brunning R: Proposed World Health Organization (WHO) classification of acute leukemia and myelodysplastic syndromes. Abstract presented at Society of Hematopathology meeting: The Myelodysplastic Syndromes (MDS) and Related Disorders: 1999. Mod Pathol 1999;12:101-106.

BOX 35-5 Classification of Myelodysplastic Syndromes/Myeloproliferative Disorders

I. CMML
II. Juvenile myelomonocytic leukemia
III. Atypical chronic myelogenous leukemia

From Brunning R: Proposed World Health Organization (WHO) classification of acute leukemia and myelodysplastic syndromes. Abstract presented at Society of Hematopathology meeting: The Myelodysplastic Syndromes (MDS) and Related Disorders: 1999. Mod Pathol 1999;12:101-106.

Molecular Genetics

Use of Southern blot, restriction-length fragment polymorphism analysis, polymerase chain reaction, and real-time polymerase chain reaction techniques has determined specific oncogenes responsible for mutations in many cases of MDS. Most commonly implicated are the *ras* family and p53 (9% to 40% of cases).[8,12,15,19,43] Among other mutations are *c-fms*,[8] interferon regulatory factor-1,[19,43] and *bcl-2*.[57]

PROGNOSIS

The life expectancy of patients with primary MDS varies from less than 1 year to more than 6 years, with the mean survival varying considerably among series. Patients with therapy-related MDS have a median survival of only 10 months, and progression to AML occurs in 50% to 80% of patients.[15] Some patients require only supportive therapy, such as blood transfusions, whereas in others the disease is much more aggressive and death occurs within 1 year of diagnosis. Acute leukemia is the most common sequela of MDS; however, death is not always caused by a transformation into acute leukemia. Often it results from severe cytopenias, bleeding, bone marrow failure, or organ failure.[19,58] Patients with a favorable prognosis must be identified because certain therapies, even in low dosages, may exacerbate existing cytopenia and increase the risk of morbidity and mortality.[13,45,59]

Prognosis According to French-American-British Classification

The FAB classification divided the MDS into two prognostic groups: those who did fairly well (refractory anemia and RARS) and those who did poorly (RAEB and RAEB-t). Patients with CMML migrated to one of those two groups, primarily on the basis of percentage of bone marrow blasts.[19,58,60] The best prognosis is for patients with refractory anemia or RARS who have a normal karyotype, no neutropenia, and no thrombocytopenia. In this group, median length of survival is 70 months, and there is only a 5% to 10% risk that the disease will transform into acute leukemia. An unrelated problem, such as cerebrovascular accident or heart disease, is often the cause of death in these patients.[13,19] At the other end of the spectrum are patients with RAEB-t: They have the worst prognosis, and in 55%, the disease transforms into acute leukemia.[58]

Prognostic limitations of the FAB classification include the wide range of blasts for RAEB and CMML, absence of indicators such as cytogenetics, and number and severity of cytopenias.[45] Other risk analysis scoring systems have been developed to evaluate clinical outcomes of patients with MDS.[58-63] Essentially all of these systems separate MDS patients into three prognostic groups: *good* (median survival 3-5 years), *intermediate* (median survival 1-2 years), and *poor* (median survival 4-8 months). Each system has drawbacks that limit its universal utility.[45,59]

Prognosis According to International Prognostic Scoring System

In an attempt to develop a consensus of previous systems, an International MDS Risk Analysis workshop combined morphologic, cytogenetic, and clinical data from seven large, previously reported risk-based analyses of patients with primary MDS.[19,45,64] A prognostic model was developed, now known as the *International Prognostic Scoring System* (IPSS). Major variables for evolution to acute leukemia were cytogenetic abnormalities, percentage of blasts, and number of cytopenias. Prediction for survival included the aforementioned parameters plus age and gender.[20,45,59,64]

Cytopenias were defined as hemoglobin less than 10 g/dL, platelet count less than 100,000/μL, and absolute neutrophil count less than 1800/μL.[64] Bone marrow morphology was evaluated according to the FAB classification system.[4] Patients with proliferative CMML (WBC >12,000/μL) were excluded because it was believed that these patients more aptly represented myeloproliferative disorders.

Cytogenetic patterns associated with good outcomes included normal cytogenetics and single deletions of 5q, 20q, or the Y chromosome. Poor outcomes were seen with complex karyotypes (three or more abnormalities) or chromosome 7 defects. Other cytogenetic abnormalities conferred an intermediate prognosis. Combining these three criteria (percent bone marrow blasts, cytopenias, and cytogenetics) produced the IPSS (Table 35-2). Median survival predicted by the IPSS was as follows:

Low: 5.7 years

Intermediate-1: 3.5 years

Intermediate-2: 1.2 years

High: 0.4 years

Adding age-related categories affected survival statistics but not AML evolution.[64]

Other Negative Prognostic Factors

In addition to the factors mentioned previously in this chapter, several other negative prognostic factors have been identified, including incidence of defective granulocyte-monocyte/macrophage colony-stimulating factor (GM-CSF) in bone marrow culture,[19] history of previous alkylating agent chemotherapy or ionizing radiation or both (secondary MDS), presence of abnormal localization of immature precursors in the bone marrow,[19,32] increased incidence of certain antigenic markers (e.g., CD34),[8,45] and fibrosis.[59]

A normal karyotype or the presence of specific single chromosomal abnormalities, such as 5q– and 20q–, suggests a relatively good prognosis. The presence of other single-chromosome aberrations, such as monosomy 7, 7q–, trisomy 8, 12p–, and iso 17, confers a poor prognosis, as do complex abnormalities (abnormalities in three or more chromosomes).[19,53,54,56,64-68]

MANAGEMENT

Although the only "cure" for MDS is bone marrow transplantation, several other therapies are useful, depending on prognostic indicators. Among these are supportive therapy only, vitamins and hormones, chemotherapy (low-dose and aggressive), inducers of differentiation or biologic response modifiers,[15] growth factors,[15] and drugs with antiapoptotic activity.[25,69,70]

TABLE 35-2 International Prognostic Scoring System for Myelodysplastic Syndromes

Prognostic Variable	SCORE VALUE*				
	0	0.5	1	1.5	2
Bone marrow blasts (%)	<5	5-10	—	11-20	21-30
Karyotype[†]	Good	Intermediate	Poor	—	—
Cytopenias	0-1	2-3	—	—	—

*Scores for risk groups are as follows:
  low = 0
  intermediate-1 = 0.5-1
  intermediate-2 = 1.5-2
  high = >2.5
[†]Karyotype: *Good,* normal, −Y, 5q−, 20q− (as single abnormalities); *Poor,* complex (≥3 abnormalities) or chromosome 7
  abnormalities; *Intermediate,* other abnormalities.
Adapted from Greenberg P, Cox E, LeBeau M, et al: International scoring system for evaluating prognosis in myelodysplastic
  syndromes. Blood 1997;89:2079-2088.

Supportive therapy is often all that is needed by patients who do not have an excess of bone marrow blasts, bleeding problems, or infections. They are monitored carefully with periodic blood cell counts, bone marrow examinations, and physical examinations. Antibiotics may be needed to control infections. If severe anemia develops with cardiopulmonary problems or severe bleeding, blood products (RBCs or platelets or both) should be given. The physician must be careful to avoid hemochromatosis as a result of iron overload. Younger patients with refractory anemia and RARS may be given iron chelation therapy to avoid organ failure resulting from hemochromatosis.[15,19,71]

Vitamins and hormones have been tried in patients with MDS, usually with unsatisfactory results. In a small percentage of patients, however, these measures do seem to have some success. Among the agents used are folic acid, vitamin B_{12}, pyridoxine, heme arginate, androgens, and danazol.[3,13,19]

Corticosteroids in general have not been successful because of the potential toxicity of the drugs when given in doses large enough to elicit a response. There is also an association with an unacceptable risk of infection.[3,13,19,71]

Chemotherapy has been used in low-dosage and aggressive protocols. Low-dosage cytosine arabinoside has not prolonged survival and has produced myelotoxicity.[19,71] Aggressive chemotherapy has been successful in treating AML; however, patients with MDS do not respond as well as patients with de novo AML. Remissions are often brief, and mortality is high, especially among elderly patients, who die of severe infections, often from opportunistic organisms. A combination of fludarabine and cytosine arabinoside, preceded by granulocyte colony-stimulating factor (G-CSF) (FLAG protocol), with or without idarubicin, may provide a short-duration remission and allow an opportunity to collect peripheral blood stem cells for transplant.[15]

Biologic response modifiers are theoretically the most desirable management for MDS and other malignancies (Chapter 29). "Traditional" chemotherapy destroys normal cells along with the leukemic ones ("crusader" approach), whereas biologic response modifiers convert the abnormal clone to normal behavior ("missionary" approach).[71] Biologic response modifiers that have been tried in MDS include the following[15]:
CSF (erythropoietin, granulocyte-monocyte/macrophage CSF,
  G-CSF—alone or in combination)

Interleukins, especially interleukin-3 and interleukin-6
13-*cis*-retinoic acid
Vitamins A and D and their analogues
Interferons
Antithymocyte globulin

Most of these agents have met with disappointing or limited success. More recent trials using the following agents have shown response in some patients:
Azacitidine[8,72]
Amifostine[69] (organic thiophosphonate)
Topotecan (topoisomerase I inhibitor) with or without
  cytosine arabinoside[73]

Bone marrow transplantation is, at present, the only real cure for MDS.[8] Although autologous peripheral blood and bone marrow stem cell transplants are possible, they are not effective.[15] Best results from allogeneic bone marrow transplantation occur in patients younger than 40 years old with short disease duration, less than 5% bone marrow blasts, and an HLA-compatible sibling donor. In this group, there is about a 50% disease-free survival at 5 years. This 5-year disease-free survival decreases to 30% if the bone marrow transplantation is performed when there are greater than 20% blasts. Transplants from unrelated donors have a less favorable outcome.[49] Bone marrow transplantation is discussed in detail in Chapter 29.

Newer therapies include the following:
Immunotherapy (cyclosporine and antithymocyte globulin)
  and high-dose glucocorticoids
Azacitidine, decitabine, and other DNA methyltransferase
  inhibitors (demethylation associated with clinical response)
Antiangiogenesis agents (thalidomide)
Anticytokines
Amifostine
Anti–tumor necrosis factor
Cell signaling inhibitors (imatinib, farnesyl transferase)

Lenalidomide (*Revlimid,* Celgene, Summit NJ), a thalidomide analogue less toxic than thalidomide, was FDA approved in 2005 for use in patients with low or intermediate risk MDS.[76-79] It has shown remarkable promise, especially with patients with the 5q-chromosome deletion. Transfusion independence was achieved in 64% of patients with a median increase of 3.9 g/dL of hemoglobin. Complete cytogenetic remissions were seen in 55% of MDS patients taking Lenalidomide as compared in MDS patients taking erythropoietin in which cytogenetic remission is rare. At the time of this writing, median response duration has not yet been reached.[76,77]

The exact mechanism of action of Lenalidomide is unclear, but it is known that it affects angiogenesis, inflammation, cell adhesion, and immune response. The apparent efficacy of Lenalidomide must be balanced against the ability to cause significant myelosuppression.[76]

Future Directions

As research surrounding the role of apoptosis in MDS continues, future therapies may be aimed at controlling apoptosis, with or without the use of chemotherapeutic agents.[25] Because effective treatment for MDS remains limited, it has been suggested that patients be provided with information on their prognosis, available therapies, and success rates and take part in decision making for their treatment.[74] As more is learned about the molecular biology of MDS, it may be possible to develop customized treatment plans for individual patients.[15,69]

CHAPTER at a GLANCE

- MDS are a group of clonal disorders characterized by progressive cytopenias and dyspoiesis of the myeloid, erythroid, and megakaryocytic cell lines.
- The dyspoiesis is evidenced by abnormal morphologic appearance and abnormal function of the cell lines affected.
- Currently, the classification of these syndromes is determined by a strict set of morphologic guidelines (FAB), although a new classification has been proposed that includes molecular, cytogenetic, and immunologic characteristics (WHO).
- As the knowledge of molecular biology expands, cell surface markers and gene rearrangement information presumably will become an integral part of the diagnosis of MDS.
- Prognosis in MDS depends on several indicators, including classification, percentage of bone marrow blasts, cytopenias, and karyotypic abnormalities. Other factors, although less prognostic, are useful in predicting outcome.
- Treatment for MDS depends on the prognosis. Patients with a favorable prognosis may receive only supportive therapy.
- Other treatments that have met with limited success include chemotherapy and biologic response modifiers.
- Currently, the only cure for MDS is bone marrow transplantation.
- Future treatment possibilities include the use of apoptosis-controlling drugs.

Now that you have completed this chapter, go back and read again the case study at the beginning and respond to the questions presented.

REVIEW QUESTIONS

1. MDS are most common in which age group (years)?
   a. 2-10
   b. 15-20
   c. 25-40
   d. >50

2. What is a major indication of MDS in the peripheral blood and bone marrow?
   a. Dyspoiesis
   b. Leukocytosis with left shift
   c. Normal bone marrow with abnormal peripheral blood picture
   d. Thrombocytosis

3. An alert hematologist should recognize all of the following peripheral blood abnormalities as diagnostic clues in MDS *except*:
   a. Oval macrocytes
   b. Target cells
   c. Agranular neutrophils
   d. Circulating micromegakaryocytes

4. For an erythroid precursor to be considered a ringed sideroblast, the iron-laden mitochondria must encircle how much of the nucleus?
   a. One quarter
   b. One third
   c. Two thirds
   d. Entire

5. According to the WHO classification of MDS, what percentage of blasts would constitute transformation to an acute leukemia?
   a. 5
   b. 10
   c. 20
   d. 30

6. A patient presents with anemia, oval macrocytes, and hypersegmented neutrophils. Which of the following tests would be most efficient in differentiating this disorder?
   a. Serum iron and ferritin
   b. Erythropoietin level
   c. Vitamin B_{12} and folate
   d. Chromosome analysis

7. A 60-year-old woman presents with fatigue and malaise. Her hemoglobin is 8 g/dL, hematocrit is 25%, RBC is 2.00×10^{12}/L, platelet count is 550×10^9/L, and WBC is 3.8×10^9/L. Her WBC differential is unremarkable. Bone marrow showed erythroid hypoplasia and hypolobulated megakaryocytes; granulopoiesis appeared normal. Ringed sideroblasts were rare. Chromosome analysis revealed the deletion of 5q only. Based on the classification of this disorder, what therapy would be most appropriate?
   a. Supportive therapy only
   b. Aggressive chemotherapy
   c. Bone marrow transplant
   d. Low-dose cytosine arabinoside, accompanied by *cis*-retinoic acid

8. The following results were noted on a patient who had been treated for breast cancer 5 years earlier:
   WBC—2.3×10^9/L
   Hemoglobin—7.5 g/dL
   Mean cell volume—115 fL
   Differential included 75% polymorphonuclear neutrophils, 8% bands, 3% lymphocytes, 8% monocytes, 3% metamyelocytes, and 3% eosinophils. An occasional nucleated RBC was seen. Chromosome analysis showed −7, +8, and iso 17. This patient's MDS would be considered:
   a. De novo
   b. Therapy related
   c. Familial
   d. Congenital

9. Which of the following is *least* likely to contribute to death for patients with MDS?
   a. Neutropenia
   b. Thrombocytopenia
   c. Organ failure
   d. Neuropathy

10. Into what other hematologic disease does MDS often convert?
   a. Megaloblastic anemia
   b. Aplastic anemia
   c. Acute myelogenous leukemia
   d. Myeloproliferative disease

REFERENCES

1. Layton DM, Mufti GJ: Myelodysplastic syndromes: their history, evolution and relation to acute myeloid leukemia. Blood 1986;53:423-436.
2. Mufti GJ, Galton DAG: Myelodysplastic syndromes: natural history and features of prognostic significance. Clin Haematol 1986;15:953-971.
3. Cheson BD, Bennett JM, Kantarjian H, et al: Report of an international working group to standardize response criteria for myelodysplastic syndromes. Blood 2000;96:3671-3674.
4. Bennett JM, Catovsky D, Daniel MT, et al: Proposals for the classification of the myelodysplastic syndromes. Br J Haematol 1982;51:189-199.
5. Harris NL, Jaffe ES, Diebold J, et al: The World Health Organization classification of hematological malignancies report of the Clinical Advisory Committee Meeting, Airlie House, Virginia, November 1997. Mod Pathol 2000;13:193-207.
6. Vardiman JW, Harris NL, Brunning RD: The World Health Organization (WHO) classification of the myeloid neoplasms. Blood 2002;100:2292-2302.
7. Janssen JWG, Buschle M, Layton M, et al: Clonal analysis of myelodysplastic syndromes: evidence of multipotential stem cell origin. Blood 1989;73:248-254.
8. Greenberg PL: Biologic nature of the myelodysplastic syndromes. Acta Haematol 1987;78(Suppl 1):94-99.
9. List AF, Sandberg AA, Doll DC: Myelodysplastic syndromes. In Greer P, Foerster J, Lukens J, et al (eds): Wintrobe's Clinical Hematology, 11th ed. Philadelphia: Lippincott, Williams & Wilkins, 2004:2207.
10. DeAngelo DJ, Stone RM: Myelodysplastic syndromes: biology and treatment. In Hoffman R, Benz EJ, Shattil SJ, et al (eds): Hematology Basic Principles and Practice, 4th ed. Philadelphia: Saunders, 2005:1195-1208.
11. Jackson GH, Carey PJ, Cant AJ, et al: Myelodysplastic syndromes in children [letter]. Br J Haematol 1993;84:185-186.
12. van Wering ER, Kamps WA, Vossen JM, et al: Myelodysplastic syndromes in childhood: three case reports. Br J Haematol 1985;60:137-142.
13. Hoelzer D: Cytobiology and clinical findings of myelodysplastic syndromes. Recent Results Cancer Res 1988;106:172-179.
14. Mijovic A, Mufti GJ: The myelodysplastic syndromes: towards a functional classification. Blood Rev 1998;12:73-83.
15. Song WJ, Sullivan MG, Legare RD, et al: Haploinsufficiency of CBFA2 causes familial thrombocytopenia with propensity to develop acute myelogenous leukemia. Nat Genet 1999;23:166-175.
16. Beris P: Primary clonal myelodysplastic syndromes. Semin Hematol 1989;26:216-233.
17. Tsukamoto N, Morita K, Maehara T, et al: Clonality in myelodysplastic syndromes: demonstration of pluripotent stem cell origin using X-linked restriction fragment length polymorphisms. Br J Haematol 1993;83:589-594.
18. Kroef MJPL, Fibbe WE, Mout R, et al: Myeloid, but not lymphoid cells carry the 5q deletion: polymerase chain reaction analysis of loss of heterozygosity using mini-repeat sequences on highly purified cell fractions. Blood 1993;81:1849-1854.
19. van Kamp H, Fibbe WE, Jansen RPM, et al: Clonal involvement of granulocytes and monocytes, but not of T and B lymphocytes and natural killer cells in patients with myelodysplasia: analysis by X-linked restriction fragment length polymorphism and polymerase chain reaction of phosphoglycerate kinase gene. Blood 1992;80:1774-1980.
20. Willman CL: The biologic basis of myelodysplasia and related leukemias: cellular and molecular mechanisms. Abstract presented at Society of Hematopathology meeting: The Myelodysplastic Syndromes (MDS) and Related Disorders: 1999. Mod Pathol 1999;12:101-106.
21. Jacobs A, Clark RE: Pathogenesis and clinical variations in the myelodysplastic syndromes. Clin Haematol 1986;15:925-951.
22. Bjork J, Albin M, Mauritzson N, et al: Smoking and myelodysplastic syndromes. Epidemiology 2000;11:285-291.
23. Lichtman MA, Liesveld JL: Myelodysplastic syndromes (clonal cytopenias and oligoblastic leukemia). In Lichtman MA, Beutler E, Kipps TJ, et al (eds): Williams Hematology, 7th ed. New York: McGraw-Hill, 2006:1157-1181.
24. Yoshida Y, Mufti GJ: Apoptosis and its significance in MDS: controversies revisited. Leuk Res 1999;23:777-785.
25. Yoshida Y: Hypothesis: apoptosis may be the mechanism responsible for the premature intramedullary cell death in the myelodysplastic syndrome. Leukemia 1993;7:144.
26. Yoshida Y, Stephenson J, Mufti GJ: Myelodysplastic syndromes: from morphology to molecular biology: Part I. Classification, natural history and cell biology of myelodysplasia. Int J Hematol 1993;57:87.
27. Yoshida Y, Anzai N, Kawabata H: Apoptosis in myelodysplasia: a paradox or paradigm. Leuk Res 1995;19:887.
28. DiGiuseppe JA, Kastan MB: Apoptosis in haematological malignancies. J Clin Pathol 1997;50:361-364.
29. Lepelley P, Campergue L, Grardel N, et al: Is apoptosis a massive process in myelodysplastic syndromes? Br J Haematol 1996;95:368-371.
30. Greenberg PL: Apoptosis and its role in the myelodysplastic syndromes: implication for disease natural history and treatment. Leuk Res 1998;22:1123-1126.
31. Raza A, Gezer S, Mundle S, et al: Apoptosis in bone marrow biopsy samples involving stromal and hematopoietic cells in 50 patients with myelodysplastic syndromes. Blood 1995;86:268-276.
32. Rajapaksa R, Ginzton N, Rott LS, et al: Altered oncoprotein

expression and apoptosis in myelodysplastic syndrome marrow cells. Blood 1996;88:4275-4287.

33. Parker JE, Mufti GJ: The role of apoptosis in the pathogenesis of the myelodysplastic syndromes. Int J Hematol 2001;73:416-428.

34. Wimazal F, Krauth M-T, Vales A, et al: Immunohistochemical detection of vascular endothelial growth factor (VEGF) in the bone marrow in patients with myelodysplastic syndromes: correlation between VEGF expression and the FAB category. Leuk Lymphoma 2006;47:451-460.

35. Brunner B, Gunsilius E, Schumacher P, et al: Blood levels of angiogenin and vascular endothelial growth factor are elevated in myelodysplastic syndromes and in some acute myeloid leukemia. J Haematother Stem Cell Res 2002;11:119-125.

36. Kjeldsberg CR (ed): Practical Diagnosis of Hematologic Disorders, 3rd ed. Chicago: ASCP Press, 2000:369-397.

37. Tsurusawa M, Manabe A, Hayashi Y, et al: Therapy-related myelodysplastic syndrome in childhood: a retrospective study of 36 patients in Japan. Leuk Res 2005;29:625-632.

38. Mufti GJ: Pathobiology, classification, and diagnosis of myelodysplastic syndrome. Best Prac Res Clin Haematol 2004;17:543-557.

39. Giles FJ, Koeffler HP: Secondary myelodysplastic syndromes and leukemias. Curr Opin Hematol 1994;1:256-260.

40. Bick RL, Laughlin WR: Myelodysplastic syndromes. Lab Med 1993;24:712-716.

41. Brunning RD, Bennett JM, Flandrin G, et al: Myelodysplastic syndromes. In Jaffe ES, Harris NL, Stein H, et al (eds): World Health Organization Classification of Tumours: Pathology and Genetics of Tumours of Haematopoietic and Lymphoid Tissues. Lyon: LARC Press, 2001:62-73.

42. Rodak BF, Leclair SJ: The new WHO nomenclature: introduction and myeloid neoplasms. Clin Lab Sci 2002;15:44-54.

43. Head DR, Kopecky K, Bennett JM, et al: Pathologic implications of internuclear bridging in myelodysplastic syndrome. An Eastern Cooperative Oncology Group/Southwest Oncology Group Cooperative Study. Cancer 1989;64:2199-2202.

44. Langenhuijsen MM: Neutrophils with ring-shaped nuclei in myeloproliferative disease. Br J Haematol 1984;58:227-230.

45. Doll DC, List AF: Myelodysplastic syndromes. West J Med 1989;151:161-167.

46. Seymour JF, Estey EH: The prognostic significance of Auer rods in myelodysplasia. Br J Haematol 1993;85:67-76.

47. Tricot G, De Wolf-Peeters R, Vlietinck R, et al: Bone marrow histology in myelodysplastic syndromes. Br J Haematol 1984;58:217-225.

48. Barbui T, Cortelazzo S, Viero P, et al: Infection and hemorrhage in elderly acute myeloblastic leukemia and primary myelodysplasia. Hematol Oncol 1993;11(Suppl 1):15-18.

49. Mazzone A, Ricevuti G, Pasotti D, et al: The CD11/CD18 granulocyte adhesion molecules in myelodysplastic syndromes. Br J Haematol 1993;83:245-252.

50. Mittelman M, Karcher D, Kammerman L, et al: High Ia (HLA-DR) and low CD11b (Mo1) expression may predict early conversion to leukemia in myelodysplastic syndromes. Am J Hematol 1993;43:165-171.

51. Pomeroy C, Oken MM, Rydell RE, et al: Infection in the myelodysplastic syndromes. Am J Med 1991;90:338-344.

52. Boogaerts MA, Nelissen V, Roelant C, et al: Blood neutrophil function in primary myelodysplastic syndromes. Br J Haematol 1983;55:217-227.

53. Verhoef GE, Zachee P, Ferrant A, et al: Recombinant human erythropoietin for the treatment of anemia in the myelodysplastic syndromes: a clinical and erythrokinetic assessment. Ann Hematol 1992;64:16-21.

54. Merchav S, Nielsen OJ, Rosenbaum H, et al: In vitro studies of erythropoietin-dependent regulation of erythropoiesis in myelodysplastic syndromes. Leukemia 1990;4:771-774.

55. Lintula R, Rasi V, Ikkala E, et al: Platelet function in preleukemia. Scand J Haematol 1981;26:65-71.

56. Raman BK, Van Slyck EJ, Riddle J, et al: Platelet function and structure in myeloproliferative disease, myelodysplastic syndrome and secondary thrombocytosis. Am J Clin Pathol 1989;91:647-655.

57. Rasi V, Lintula R: Platelet function in the myelodysplastic syndromes. Scand J Haematol 1986;36(Suppl 45):71-73.

58. Bennett JM, Catovsky D, Daniel MT, et al: Proposed revised criteria for the classification of acute myeloid leukemia. Ann Intern Med 1985;103:626-629.

59. Hast R: Sideroblasts in myelodysplasia: their nature and clinical significance [abstract]. Scand J Haematol 1986;36 (Suppl 45):53-55.

60. Oscier DG: The myelodysplastic syndromes. In Hoffbrand AV, Lewis SM, Tuddenham EGD (eds): Postgraduate Hematology, 4th ed. Oxford: Butterworth-Heinemann, 1999:445-461.

61. Heaney ML, Golde DW: Medical progress: myelodysplasia. N Engl J Med 1999;340:1649-1660.

62. Gallagher A, Darley RL, Padua R: The molecular basis of myelodysplastic syndromes. Haematologica 1997;82:191-204.

63. Greenberg PL, Sanz GF, Sanz MA: Prognostic scoring system for risk assessment in myelodysplastic syndromes. Forum (Geneva) 1999;9:17-31.

64. Albitar M, Beran M, O'Brien S, et al: Differences between refractory anemia with excess blasts in transformation and acute myeloid leukemia (letter to the editor). Blood 2000; 96:372-373.

65. Greenberg P, Anderson J, de Witte T, et al. Problematic WHO reclassification of myelodysplastic syndromes. J Clin Oncol 2000;18:3447-3452.

66. West RR, Stafford DA, White AD, et al: Cytogenetic abnormalities in the myelodysplastic syndromes and occupational or environmental exposure. Blood 2000;95:2093-2097.

67. Secker-Walker LM: Cytogenetics. In Hoffbrand AV, Lewis SM, Tuddenham EGD (eds): Postgraduate Hematology, 4th ed. Oxford: Butterworth-Heinemann, 1999:336-353.

68. White AD, Hoy TG, Jacobs A: Extended cytogenetic follow-up and clinical progress in patients with myelodysplastic syndromes (MDS). Leuk Lymphoma 1994;12:401.

69. Pedersen-Bjergaard J, Rowley JD: The balanced and the unbalanced chromosome aberrations of acute myeloid leukemia may develop in different ways and may contribute differently to malignant transformation. Blood 1994;83:2780-2786.

70. Geddes AD, Bowen DT, Jacobs A: Clonal karyotype abnormalities and clinical progress in the myelodysplastic syndrome. Br J Haematol 1990;76:194-202.

71. Jotterand-Bellomo M, Parlier V, Schmidt PM, Beris P: Cytogenetic analysis of 54 cases of myelodysplastic syndromes. Cancer Genet Cytogenet 1990;46:157-172.

72. Musilova J, Michalova K: Chromosome study of 85 patients with myelodysplastic syndrome. Cancer Genet Cytogenet 1988;33:39-50.

73. Tricot GJ: Prognostic factors in the myelodysplastic syndromes. Leuk Res 1992;16:109-115.

74. Nimer SD, Golde DW: The 5q- abnormality. Blood 1987; 70:1705-1712.

75. Solé F, Torrabadella M, Granada I, et al: Isochromosome 17q as a sole anomaly: a distinct myelodysplastic syndrome entity? Leuk Res 1993;17:717-720.

76. List A, Kurtin S, Roe D, et al. Efficacy of lenalidomide in myelodysplastic syndromes. N Engl J Med 2005;352:549-557.

77. Moyer P. Lenalidomide reduces need for transfusions in patients with MDS. Available at http://www.medscape.com/viewarticle/505142. Accessed October 24, 2006.

78. Witter D. Gaining momentum in MDS. Available at http://www2.mdanderson.org/depts/oncolog/articles/06/7-8-julaug/7-8-06-1.html. Accessed October 24, 2006.

36

Acute Leukemias

Susan J. Leclair

OBJECTIVES

After completion of this chapter, the reader will be able to:

1. Clinically distinguish between acute lymphoblastic and acute myeloid leukemias.
2. Characterize the diagnostic criteria used with these leukemias.
3. Compare and contrast acute lymphoblastic and myeloid leukemias by morphology, presenting signs and symptoms, laboratory analysis, and prognosis.
4. Interpret the results of diagnostic tests for acute leukemias.

CASE STUDY

After studying the material in this chapter, the reader should be able to respond to the following case study:

A 5-year-old child was seen by her family physician because of weakness and headaches. She had been in good health except for the usual communicable diseases of childhood. Physical examination revealed a pale, listless child with multiple bruises. The white blood cell count was 15×10^9/L, the hemoglobin was 8 g/dL, and the platelet count was 90×10^9/L. She had "abnormal cells" in her peripheral blood (Fig. 36-1).

1. What is the most likely diagnosis?
2. What characteristics of this disease indicate a positive prognosis?
3. Which would be considered a "good" phenotype for these cells: CD10 and TdT positivity, surface immunoglobulin positivity, the presence of T cell phenotype, or cytoplasmic immunoglobulin?

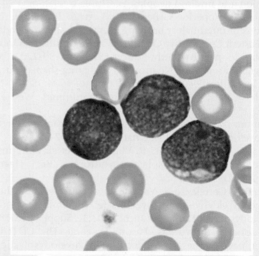

Figure 36-1 Peripheral blood smear of patient in case study (×1000). (From Carr JH, Rodak BF: Clinical Hematology Atlas, ed 2. Philadelphia: Saunders, 2004.)

Our understanding of the acute leukemias has undergone a profound change. The paradigm shift from phenotype assays (morphology and cytochemistry) to genotype assay (karyotyping) to polymerase chain reaction and single-nucleotide polymorphisms is clarifying their cause and prognosis to an extent never before possible. Although cell morphology will remain essential to the investigation of a leukemic process, molecular testing has begun to dominate.

ACUTE LYMPHOBLASTIC LEUKEMIA

Acute lymphoblastic leukemia (ALL) is primarily a disease of childhood; most cases occur between the ages of 2 and 10 years. Although ALL is rare in adults, a second peak in incidence occurs around age 40.[1] Treatment of childhood ALL is a triumph of modern hematology. A uniformly fatal disease before 1970, "good-prognosis" ALL has a 90% complete remission rate and 60% of patients are cured.[2] Adults have a poorer outlook: a 68% to 91% rate of complete remission and a 25% to 41% cure rate.[3] Only half of patients with ALL have leukocytosis, and many may not have circulating lymphoblasts.[4] Neutropenia, thrombocytopenia, and anemia are usually present, leading to fatigue (caused by anemia), fever (caused by neutropenia and infection), and mucocutaneous bleeding (caused by thrombocytopenia). Lymphadenopathy, lymph node enlargement, is often a symptom, and a mediastinal mass is present in 5% to 10% of patients.[5] Enlargement of the spleen (splenomegaly) and of the liver (hepatomegaly) may be seen. Bone pain often results from infiltration of leukemic cells into the bone covering (periosteum). Eventual infiltration of malignant cells into the meninges, testes, or ovaries occurs in 50% of patients, and lymphoblasts are found in the cerebrospinal fluid.[6]

Prognosis

The prognosis for ALL depends on age at the time of diagnosis, lymphoblast "load" (tumor burden), and immunophenotype. Chromosomal translocations are the strongest predictor of adverse treatment outcomes for children and adults.[7] The presence of the Philadelphia chromosome, t(9;22), is an indicator of significant adverse effects. The t(12;21) marker is found in many childhood ALL patients.[8]

Prognosis varies with age; children rather than infants or teens do the best. Peripheral blood lymphoblast counts greater than 20 to 30 × 10⁹/L, hepatosplenomegaly, and lymphadenopathy all adversely affect outcome. T cell and mature B cell immunophenotypes are associated with a poor outcome in children and adults, in contrast to the immature B cell phenotypes.[9] In addition, the presence of an aberrant myeloid surface marker found in ALL (such as CD66c) is associated with a poor outcome in adults.[10] Other variables possibly associated with poorer prognosis are race (Native Americans have a worse prognosis than Caucasians), the presence of karyotypic abnormalities, and male sex.[11,12]

Morphology

Two major groups of ALLs have been recognized by the World Health Organization: precursor B cell and precursor T cell.[13] Lymphoblasts vary in size but fall into two morphologic types. The most common type seen is a small lymphoblast (1-2.5 times the size of a normal lymphocyte) with scant, blue cytoplasm and indistinct nucleoli (see Fig. 36-1); the second type of lymphoblast is larger (2-3 times the size of a lymphocyte) with prominent nucleoli and nuclear membrane irregularities (Fig. 36-2). These cells may be confused with the blasts of acute myeloid leukemia (AML).

Immunophenotyping

Although morphology is the first tool in distinguishing ALL from AML, immunophenotyping and genetic analysis are often the only reliable indicator of a cell's origin. In general, four types of ALL are identified immunologically: CALLa (CD10)-expressing immature B cell ALL, pre-B cell ALL without CALLa (CD10), T cell ALL, and B cell ALL.

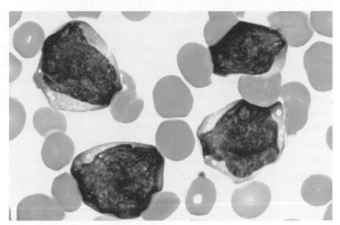

Figure 36-2 ALL. Large lymphoblast with prominent nucleoli and membrane irregularities (peripheral blood, ×1000). (From Carr JH, Rodak BF: Clinical Hematology Atlas, ed 2. Philadelphia: Saunders, 2004.)

In the most common type of immature B cell ALL, the marker CD10 or CALLa (common ALL antigen) is expressed on the cell surface. Other immature B cell markers are expressed such as CD19, CD20, CD22, CD79a, cytoplasmic CD22, and CD9a,[14] but not cytoplasmic immunoglobulin (CIg) or surface immunoglobulin (SIg). Cells typically also are positive for HLA-Dr and terminal deoxyribonucleotidyl transferase (TdT).[15] Advances in molecular diagnostic testing show a wide divergence of mutations for all of these presentations.[16-18]

Pre-B cell ALL is the second most common ALL and differs from immature B cell ALL by the absence of CD10 and the presence of CIg but not SIg.[19] Immature B cell ALL has become associated with the best prognosis subsequent to the introduction of anti-CD20 (rituximab) as a treatment modality.[20]

B cell ALL is the least common ALL, and SIg with κ or λ light chain restriction are expressed. Morphologically, these cells are large and deeply basophilic with an exceptionally high mitotic rate.[21] This condition historically carried a very poor prognosis; however, more recent advances in therapy have improved survival.[22]

In T cell ALL, a variety of T cell surface antigens are expressed.[23] The cells may be TdT positive. T cell ALL is seen most often in teenage males with a mediastinal mass, elevated peripheral blast counts, meningeal involvement, and infiltration of extra marrow sites.[24] Common markers are CD2, CD4, CD5, and CD8. Although this immunophenotype classically has been associated with a poor outcome, aggressive chemotherapy has resulted in improved prognosis with an outcome intermediate between those of B cell ALL and pre-B cell ALL.[25]

Types of Treatment

ALL treatment success varies by age. Most adult cases have a poorer prognosis than in childhood ALL. Patients with childhood ALL may experience some paralysis or ability regression as a result of intrathecal therapy, chemotherapy administered directly into the central nervous system via the cerebrospinal fluid.[26] Methotrexate, commonly used for ALL, is a folate antagonist, causing a megaloblastoid blood or bone marrow film (Chapter 20) with rapid severe leukocytopenia. Drugs used for adult ALL include daunorubicin, vincristine, and prednisone. Daunorubicin frequently causes cardiac complications, so periodic cardiac enzyme assays are required. Vincristine attacks microtubule formation, is toxic to the nervous system, and interferes with platelet activity. Newer agents that employ monoclonal antibodies, such as anti-CD20, are assuming the role of lead therapy, alone or in combination with more traditional chemotherapeutic agents.[27] Transplantation of bone marrow or peripheral stem cells is the last line of treatment for unresponsive or relapsed ALL. (See Chapter 29 for more information on treatment of white blood cell [WBC] neoplasia.)

ACUTE MYELOID LEUKEMIA

AML is the most common family of leukemias in children younger than 1 year of age. It is rare in older children and adolescents, but a second incidence peak occurs at 40 years of age. There has been a dramatic modification in AML classification, relying heavily on cytogenetics and molecular characterization.[28]

Clinical Presentation

The clinical presentation of AML is nonspecific but reflects decreased production of normal bone marrow elements. Most patients with AML present with a total WBC count between $5 \times 10^9/L$ and $30 \times 10^9/L$ although the WBC count may range from $1 \times 10^9/L$ to $200 \times 10^9/L$. Myeloblasts are present in the peripheral blood in 90% of patients. Anemia, thrombocytopenia, and neutropenia give rise to the clinical findings of pallor, fatigue, bruising and bleeding, and fever with infections. In addition, disseminated intravascular coagulation and other bleeding abnormalities are noted.[29] Infiltration of malignant cells into the gums and other mucosal sites and skin also can be seen.[30]

Bone and joint pain are the first symptoms in 25% of patients. Splenomegaly is seen in half of AML patients, but lymph node enlargement is rare. Cerebrospinal fluid involvement in AML is rare and does not seem to be as ominous as in ALL. Patients with AML tend to have few symptoms related to the central nervous system, even when it is infiltrated by blasts.

Other common laboratory abnormalities are elevated serum lysozyme (especially in monocytic subtypes), hyperuricemia (caused by increased cellular turnover), hyperkalemia (caused by cell breakdown), hyperphosphatemia, and hypocalcemia. When cell counts are elevated and these findings are pronounced, this condition is called the *tumor lysis syndrome*,[31] and renal failure, tetany, and lethal heart arrhythmias may develop.

Subtypes of Acute Myeloid Leukemia

Prior to the World Health Organization (WHO) classification, myeloid leukemias were classified according to the system developed by the French-American-British (FAB) cooperative group. The subtypes were based on bone marrow morphology and cytochemical reactions. To the morphologic findings, the WHO system added cytogenetics and molecular characterization. In the WHO classification some of the features of the FAB

classification have been retained in the subgroup of AML not otherwise categorized.[32]

In the WHO classification, there are four categories of AML: AML with recurrent cytogenetic abnormalities, AML with multilineage dysplasia, AML and myelodysplasia as a result of therapy, and AML not otherwise classified.[32] Laboratory diagnosis begins with peripheral blood and bone marrow examinations. The myeloid-to-erythroid ratio should be greater than 1, and 20% or more of the nucleated cells in both peripheral blood and bone marrow are blasts.[33] Each category is discussed, and a summary of the classification is presented in Table 36-1.

Acute Myeloid Leukemia with Recurrent Genetic Abnormalities

Four subtypes of AML with recurrent genetic abnormalities have been identified.

Acute Myeloid Leukemia with t(8;21)(q33:q22). Seen in children and young adults, AML with t(8;21)(q33:q22) has myeloblasts with granular cytoplasm, Aüer rods and some

---

TABLE 36-1 Classification of Acute Myeloid Leukemias (AML)*

AML with Recurrent Abnormal Karyotypes
AML with t(8;21)(q22;q22)
AML with inv(16)9p13q22) or t(16;16)(p13;q22)
AML with t(15;17)(q22;q12) (APL)
AML with 11q23

AML with Dysplasia
AML occurring after a diagnosis of a myeloproliferative or myelodysplastic disease

AML as a Result of Previous Therapy-Related Myelodysplasias
AML with history of alkylating agent exposure
AML with topoisomerase exposure
AML with other exposures such as radiation

AML Not Otherwise Categorized
AML minimally differentiated
AML without maturation
AML with maturation
Acute myelomonocytic leukemia
Acute monoblastic/monocytic leukemia
Acute erythroid leukemia
Acute megakaryocytic leukemia
Acute basophilic leukemia

Acute Leukemia of Ambiguous Lineage
Acute bilineage leukemia
Acute biphenotypic leukemia

*World Health Organization

maturation. Various dysplastic anomalies, such as pseudo–Pelger-Huët cells, hypogranulation or abnormal granulations, and eosinophilia are possible (Fig. 36-3).[34]

Acute Myeloid Leukemia with inv(16)(p13q22) or t(16;16)(p13;q22).   Accounting for approximately 10% of all AML cases, AML with inv(16)(p13q22) or t(16;16)(p13;q22) has an increase in myeloid and monocytic cell lines with occasional eosinophilia (Fig. 36-4).[35]

Acute Myeloid Leukemia with t(15;17)(q22;q12) (Acute Promyelocytic Leukemia).   Acute promyelocytic leukemia occurs in all age groups but is seen most in young adults. Characteristic of this presentation are the abnormal

hypergranular promyelocytes, some with Aüer rods. When Aüer rod bundles are found, the cell is called a "faggot cell" (Fig. 36-5). When promyelocytes release primary granule contents, their procoagulant activity initiates disseminated intravascular coagulation.[36] In one variant of acute promyelocytic leukemia, the granules are so small that the limits of light microscopy give the appearance of no granules. This microgranular variant may be confused with other presentations of AML, but the presence of occasional Aüer rods, the "butterfly" or "bowtie" nucleus and the clinical presentation are clues.[37] Treatment must include a resolution of the disseminated intravascular coagulation. The genetic abnormality seen in this condition results in the ability of the cell to ingest vitamin A, and a successful treatment is to initiate maturation with a vitamin A modification, all-*trans*-retinoic acid.[38]

Acute Myeloid Leukemia with 11q23.   AML with 11q23 is a rare leukemia that presents with an increase in monoblasts and immature monocytes. The blasts are large with abundant cytoplasm and fine nuclear chromatin. The

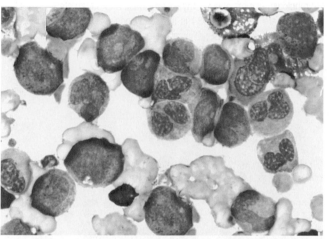

Figure 36-3 AML with t(8;21). Myeloblasts with granular cytoplasm and some maturation (bone marrow, ×500). (From Carr JH, Rodak BF: Clinical Hematology Atlas, ed 2. Philadelphia: Saunders, 2004.)

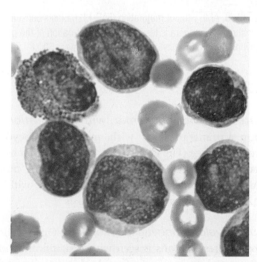

Figure 36-4 AML with inv 16. There is an increase in myeloid and monocytic lines. There may also be eosinophilia (peripheral blood, ×1000). (From Carr JH, Rodak BF: Clinical Hematology Atlas, ed 2. Philadelphia: Saunders, 2004.)

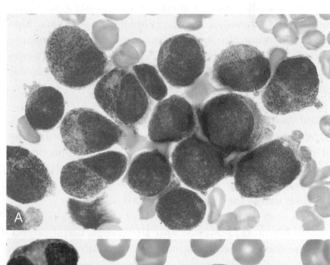

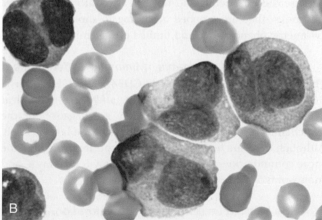

Figure 36-5 AML with t(15;17). Promyelocytic leukemia. **A,** Low-power view of the more common hypergranular variant (peripheral blood, ×500). **B,** Oil immersion view of the microgranular variant showing bilobed nuclear features (peripheral blood, ×1000). (**B** from Carr JH, Rodak BF: Clinical Hematology Atlas, ed 2. Philadelphia: Saunders, 2004.)

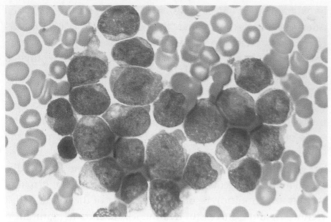

Figure 36-6 AML with 11q23. Increase in both monoblasts and immature monocytes (bone marrow, ×500).

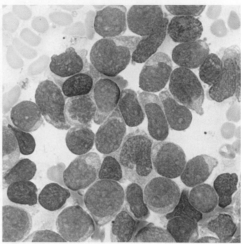

Figure 36-7 AML, minimally differentiated (FAB-M0). Blasts lack myeloid morphologic features and are myeloperoxidase and Sudan black B negative. Aüer rods are not seen. CD34 is frequently positive (bone marrow, ×500). (From Carr JH, Rodak BF: Clinical Hematology Atlas, ed 1. Philadelphia: Saunders, 1998.)

cells may have motility with frequent pseudopodia. Granules and vacuoles can be seen in the blasts (Fig. 36-6).

Acute Myeloid Leukemia with Myelodysplasia

AML with myelodysplasia affects adults and has a poor prognosis.[39] Significant dysplastic morphology includes pancytopenia with neutrophil hypogranulation or hypergranulation, pseudo–Pelger-Huët cells, and unusually segmented nuclei. Erythrocyte precursors have vacuoles, karyorrhexis, megaloblastoid features, and ringed sideroblasts.[40,41]

Treatment-Related Acute Myeloid Leukemia

Treatment with alkylating agents, radiation, or topoisomerase II inhibitors has been associated with the development of a secondary leukemia.[42,43] Similar in morphology to AML with myelodysplasia or monoblastic leukemia, the prognosis parallels that of the corresponding AML.

Acute Myeloid Leukemia Not Otherwise Categorized

Because these leukemias do not fit easily into the first three categories, they are grouped according to morphology, flow cytometric phenotyping, and limited cytochemical reactions.

Acute Myeloid Leukemia, Minimally Differentiated. These blasts are CD13+, CD33+, CD34+, and CD117+ (Fig. 36-7). Aüer rods typically are absent, and there is no clear evidence of cellular maturation. They are negative for the cytochemical stains myeloperoxidase and Sudan black B. Although there are no unique chromosome abnormalities, the more common ones are trisomy 13, trisomy 8, trisomy 4, and monosomy 7.[44]

Acute Myeloid Leukemia without Maturation. Closely aligned with AML, minimally differentiated, these blasts are also CD13+, CD33+, CD34+, and CD117+ (Fig. 36-8). They have Auer rods and are usually positive for myeloperoxidase or Sudan black B dye. There are no specific recurrent chromosome abnormalities.[44]

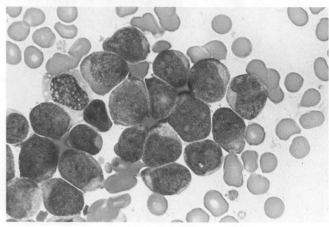

Figure 36-8 AML without maturation (FAB-M1). Blasts constitute 90% of the nonerythroid cells; there is less than 10% maturation of the granulocytic series beyond the promyelocyte stage (bone marrow, ×500.)

Acute Myeloid Leukemia with Maturation. This common variant presents with maturation beyond the promyelocyte stage (Fig. 36-9). Aüer rods and other aspects of dysplasia are present. There is an increase in the monocytic line. Although similar in morphology to AML with t(8;21) (q22;q22), it has a less favorable prognosis.[44]

Acute Myelomonocytic Leukemia. One of the more flamboyant presentations is seen with a significantly elevated WBC count and the presence of myeloid and monocytoid cells in the peripheral blood and bone marrow (Fig. 36-10). Monocytic cells constitute at least 20% of all marrow cells. The monoblasts are large with abundant cytoplasm containing

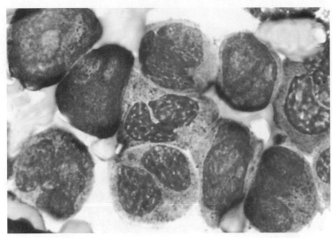

Figure 36-9 AML with maturation. Blasts constitute 20% or more of the nucleated cells of the bone marrow, and there is maturation beyond the promyelocyte stage in more than 10% of the nonerythroid cells (bone marrow, ×1000).

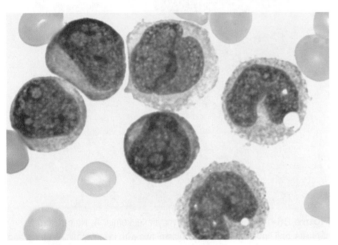

Figure 36-10 Acute myelomonocytic leukemia. Both myeloid and monocytic cells are present. Monocytic cells comprise at least 20% of all marrow cells with monoblasts and promonocytes present (peripheral blood, ×1000). (From Carr JH, Rodak BF: Clinical Hematology Atlas, ed 2. Philadelphia: Saunders, 2004.)

small granules and pseudopodia. The nucleus is large and immature and may contain multiple nucleoli. Promonocytes also are present and may have contorted nuclei. The cells are positive for the myeloid antigens CD13 and CD33 and the monocytic antigens CD14, CD4, CD11c, CD64 and CD36.[44] Nonspecific cytogenetic changes are found in most cases.[44]

Acute Monoblastic Leukemias. Sometimes divided into monoblastic and monocytic leukemias based on the degree of maturity of the monocytic cells present in the marrow and peripheral blood, this leukemia is characterized by having more than 80% of the marrow cells of monocytic origin. These cells are CD14+, CD4+, CD11b+, CD36+, CD64+,

and CD68+ (Fig. 36-11). Monoblastic leukemias displaying specific chromosomal aberrations of chromosome 11 band q23 are included in AML with recurrent cytogenetic abnormalities.

Acute Erythroid Leukemia. According to the WHO classification, there are two subtypes of acute erythroid leukemia, based on the presence of a significant component of myeloblasts. The first is *acute erythroleukemia* (erythroid/ myeloid); 50% or more of nucleated bone marrow cells are normoblasts, and greater than 20% are myeloblasts. In the FAB classification, this type was known as *M6*.

The second type is *pure erythroid leukemia*. It has 50% or more pronormoblasts and 30% or more basophilic normoblasts. Together these two erythroid components involve more than 80% of bone marrow. The myeloblast component is not significant. Distinguishing myeloblasts from primitive normoblasts is difficult.[44,45]

The red blood cell (RBC) precursors have significant dysplastic features, such as multinucleation, megaloblastoid asynchrony, and vacuolization. Abnormal megakaryocytes may be seen. The number of nucleated RBCs in the peripheral blood may account for more than 50% of the total number of nucleated cells. Ringed sideroblasts, Howell-Jolly bodies, and other inclusions are possible (Fig. 36-12).

Leukemic cells express the erythroid markers glycophorin A (CD 71) and transferrin receptor (CD45) and the myeloid markers CD11b, CD13, CD15, and CD33. HLA-DR and CD34 are decreased or absent. The erythroid markers may be increased, but the less mature normoblasts may express glycophorin A only weakly. The absence of erythroid antigens does not exclude erythroleukemia.

Three cytogenetic categories include: normal, fewer than three, and three or more chromosomal abnormalities. There is no specific abnormality, but chromosomes 5 and 7 are frequently affected.[44]

Acute Megakaryocytic Leukemia. Acute megakaryocytic leukemia is the rarest AML, with ≤1% of cases. Incidence

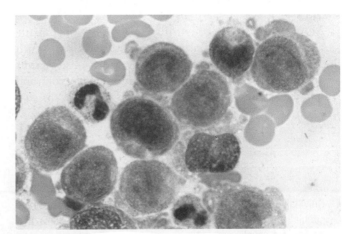

Figure 36-11 Acute monoblastic leukemia. More than 80% of the bone marrow cells are of monocytic origin (bone marrow, ×500).

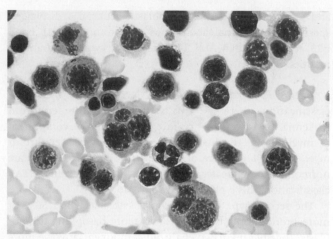

Figure 36-12 Acute erythroid leukemia. Erythroid precursors showing dysplastic features, including multinucleation and megaloblastic asynchrony (bone marrow, ×500). (From Carr JH, Rodak BF: Clinical Hematology Atlas, ed 2. Philadelphia: Saunders, 2004.)

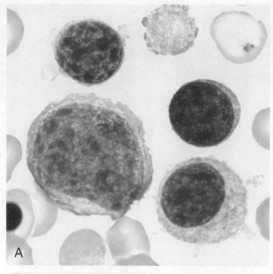

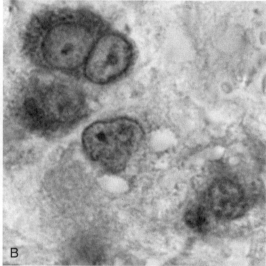

Figure 36-13 A. Acute megakaryocytic leukemia. **A,** Note heterogeneity of blasts, one small with scant cytoplasm, two with cytoplasmic blebbing, and one quite large (peripheral blood ×1000). **B,** Immunoperoxidase reaction showing positivity for Factor VIII (bone marrow, ×1000). (From Carr JH, Rodak BF: Clinical Hematology Atlas, ed 2. Philadelphia: Saunders, 2004.)

may be underestimated because of the difficulty in identifying the megakaryoblast cytochemically. Diagnosis depends on the presence of at least 20% megakaryoblasts.

Megakaryoblasts are heterogeneous in size; some are the size of small lymphoblasts with scant cytoplasm, whereas others are three times that size. Chromatin is delicate, with prominent nucleoli. Immature megakaryocytes may be seen, and cells may have light blue cytoplasmic blebbing (Fig. 36-13A). Megakaryoblasts are identified by positive staining with antibodies to platelet glycoprotein Ib, glycoprotein IIb/IIIa, von Willebrand factor, or detection of platelet antigens CD41, CD42, or CD61 (Fig. 36-13B). Electron microscopy with platelet peroxidase stain has been used in the past.

In adults, acute megakaryocytic leukemia has a varied clinical manifestation. Many patients have a preceding myeloproliferative disorder with pancytopenia or myelofibrosis.[46] Among children, the disorder is seen most often before 3 years of age and in Down syndrome.[47] Response to therapy is poor. No unique chromosomal aberrations are found with megakaryocytic leukemia.

Acute Leukemia of Ambiguous Lineage. Acute leukemia of ambiguous lineage includes leukemia in which the morphology, immunophenotype, or cytochemistry results are not helpful or suggest a combination of myeloid and lymphoid cell lines. Bilineage leukemias contain cells that express either the myeloid or the lymphoid antigens, whereas biphenotypic leukemias contain cells that express the myeloid and the lymphoid antigens on the same cells.[48] Many cases of leukemia of ambiguous lineage show cytogenetic abnormalities, but there is no unique specific aberration.[44]

- Only half of patients with ALL have leukocytosis and may not have circulating lymphoblasts, but neutropenia, thrombocytopenia, and anemia are usually present.

- Childhood ALL is a disease in which the "good prognosis" ALL has a 90% rate of complete remission, whereas adults with ALL have a poorer outlook.

CHAPTER at a GLANCE—cont'd

- Infiltration of malignant cells into the meninges can occur with lymphoblasts found in the cerebrospinal fluid, testes, and ovaries.
- Prognosis in ALL depends primarily on age at the time of diagnosis, lymphoblast "load" (tumor burden), and immunophenotype. Chromosomal translocations seem to be the strongest predictor of adverse treatment outcomes for children and adults.
- The t(12;21) marker is found in a significant number of patients with childhood ALL.
- The presence of the Philadelphia chromosome, t(9;22), in ALL is an indicator of significant adverse effects.
- There are two subtypes of ALL according to the WHO classification system.
- Although morphology is the first tool in distinguishing ALL from AML, immunophenotyping is often the only reliable indicator of a cell's origin.
- AML is the most common leukemia in children younger than 1 year of age. It is rare in older children and adolescents, and a second peak of incidence occurs among adults 40 years of age.

- The clinical presentation of a patient with AML is nonspecific and reflects the decreased production of normal bone marrow elements, an elevated WBC count, and the presence of myeloblasts. Anemia, thrombocytopenia, and neutropenia give rise to the clinical findings of pallor, fatigue, bruising and bleeding, and fever with infections.
- The classification of AML is complicated by the presence or absence of multiple cell lines defined as "myeloid" in origin, specific cells within these cell lines, and specific karyotype abnormalities.
- Leukemias with ambiguous lineage include leukemias with lymphoid and myeloid characteristics.

Now that you have completed this chapter, go back and read again the case study at the beginning and respond to the questions presented.

REVIEW QUESTIONS

1. A 22-year-old patient has an elevated WBC count with 70% blasts, 4% neutrophils, 5% lymphocytes, and 21% monocytes in the peripheral blood. Which of the following karyotypes would be most likely to be expected?
   a. AML with t(8;21)(q33:q22)
   b. AML with t(16;16)(p13;q22)
   c. AML with t(15;17)(q22;q12)
   d. AML with 11q23

2. The flow cytometry report from a patient with suspected ALL shows positivity for CD2, CD5, and CD10. Which of the following subsets of ALL does this patient have?
   a. T cell
   b. B cell
   c. Null cell
   d. Natural killer cell

3. Enlargement of visceral organs observed in patients with acute leukemia is associated with:
   a. Vascular expansion
   b. Hemorrhage
   c. Thrombosis
   d. Leukemic cell infiltration

4. The phenotype antigen that indicates a favorable prognosis in ALL is:
   a. Cellular immunoglobulin
   b. DR(1A) antigen
   c. CALLa (CD10)
   d. Surface immunoglobulin

5. Which acute leukemia commonly has meningeal infiltration requiring intrathecal medication?
   a. Lymphoblastic
   b. Promyelocytic
   c. Monocytic
   d. Megakaryocytic

6. Laboratory abnormalities associated with AML include all of the following *except*:
   a. Hyperuricemia
   b. Hyperkalemia
   c. Hypocalcemia
   d. Hyperproteinemia

7. In which of the acute leukemia subtypes do most cells fail to differentiate beyond the promyelocyte stage and show a translocation between chromosome 15 and 17, t(15;17)?
   a. ALL of childhood
   b. Acute promyelocytic leukemia
   c. Acute erythroid leukemia
   d. AML with eosinophilia

8. A 70-year-old patient presents with fatigue, pallor, easy bruising, and swollen gums. Bone marrow reveals 82% cells with delicate chromatin and prominent nucleoli that show CD14+, CD4+, CD11b+, and CD36+. Which of the following acute leukemias is likely?
   a. Undifferentiated leukemia
   b. Leukemia of ambiguous lineage
   c. Acute monoblastic leukemia
   d. Acute megakaryocytic leukemia

9. Pure erythroid leukemia is a disorder involving:
   a. Pronormoblasts only
   b. Pronormoblasts and basophilic normoblasts
   c. All forms of developing RBC precursors
   d. Equal numbers of pronormoblasts and myeloblasts

10. A leukemia that displays a myeloid-to-erythroid ratio of 5:1 with minimal cellular differentiation, occasional Auer rods, and a normal karyotype would most likely be classified as:
    a. ALL
    b. Acute myeloblastic leukemia without differentiation
    c. Acute monoblastic leukemia
    d. Acute megakaryocytic leukemia

REFERENCES

1. Gurney JG, Davis S, Severson RK, et al: Trends in cancer incidence among children in the U.S. Cancer 1996;78:532-541.
2. Morimoto A, Kuriyama K, Hibi S, et al: Prognostic value of early response to treatment combined with conventional risk factors in pediatric acute lymphoblastic leukemia. Int J Hematol 2005;81:228-234.
3. Castagnola C, Lunghi M, Caberlon S, et al: Long-term outcome of pH-negative acute lymphoblastic leukaemia in adults: a single centre experience. Acta Haematol 2005;113:234-240.
4. Poplack DG, Reaman G: Acute lymphoblastic leukemia in childhood. Pediatr Clin North Am 1988;35:903-932.
5. Onishi Y, Matsuno Y, Tateishi U, et al: Two entities of precursor T-cell lymphoblastic leukemia/lymphoma based on radiologic and immunophenotypic findings. Int J Hematol 2004;80:43-51.
6. Alexander BM, Wechsler D, Braun TM, et al: Utility of cranial boost in addition to total body irradiation in the treatment of high risk acute lymphoblastic leukemia. Int J Radiat Oncol Biol Phys 2005;63:1191-1196.
7. Guillaume N, Alleaume C, Munfus D, et al: ZAP-70 tyrosine kinase is constitutively expressed and phosphorylated in B-lineage acute lymphoblastic leukemia cells. Haematologica 2005;90:899-905.
8. Andersson A, Eden P, Lindgren D, et al: Gene expression profiling of leukemic cell lines reveals conserved molecular signatures among subtypes with specific genetic aberrations. Leukemia 2005;19:1042-1050.
9. Harrison CJ, Foroni L: Cytogenetics and molecular genetics of acute lymphoblastic leukemia. Rev Clin Exp Hematol 2002;6:91-113.
10. Kalina T, Vaskova M, Mejstrikova E, et al: Myeloid antigens in childhood lymphoblastic leukemia: clinical data point to regulation of CD66c distinct from other myeloid antigens. BMC Cancer 2005;5:38.
11. Castagnola C, Lunghi M, Caberlon S, et al: Long-term outcome of pH-negative acute lymphoblastic leukaemia in adults: a single centre experience. Acta Haematol 2005;113:234-240.
12. Garand R, Vannier JP, Bene MC, et al: Correlations between acute lymphoid leukemia (ALL) immunophenotype and clinical and laboratory data at presentation: a study of 350 patients. Cancer 1989;64:1437-1446.
13. Harris NL, Jaffe ES, Stein H, et al: A revised European American classification of lymphoid neoplasms: a proposal from the International Lymphoma Study group. Blood 1994; 84:1361-1392.
14. Harris NL, Jaffe ES, Diebild J, et al: World Health Organization classification of neoplastic diseases of the hematopoietic and lymphoid tissues: report of the Clinical Advisory Committee meeting—Airlie House, Virginia, November 1997. J Clin Oncol 1999;17:3835-3849.
15. Voskova D, Valekova L, Fedorova J, et al: Leukemic cells and aberrant phenotypes in acute leukemia patients: a flow cytometry analysis. Neoplasma 2003;50:422-427.
16. Foubister V: Genes predict childhood leukemia outcome. Drug Discov Today 2005;10:812.
17. Schnakenberg E, Mehles A, Cario G, et al: Polymorphisms of methylenetetrahydrofolate reductase (MTHFR) and susceptibility to pediatric acute lymphoblastic leukemia in a German study population. BMC Med Genet 2005;6:23.
18. Harrison CJ, Moorman AV, Barber KE, et al: Interphase molecular cytogenetic screening for chromosomal abnormalities of prognostic significance in childhood acute lymphoblastic leukaemia: a UK Cancer Cytogenetics Group Study. Br J Haematol 2005;129:520-530.
19. Lenormand B, Bene MC, Lesesve JF, et al: PreB1 (CD10-) acute lymphoblastic leukemia: immunophenotypic and genomic characteristics, clinical features and outcome in 38 adults and 26 children. The Groupe d'Etude Immunologique des Leucemies. Leuk Lymphoma 1998;28:329-342.
20. Corbacioglu S, Eber S, Gungor T, et al: Induction of long-term remission of a relapsed childhood B-acute lymphoblastic leukemia with rituximab chimeric anti-CD20 monoclonal antibody and autologous stem cell transplantation. J Pediatr Hematol Oncol 2003;25:327-329.
21. Chan NP, Ma ES, Wan TS, et al: The spectrum of acute lymphoblastic leukemia with mature B-cell phenotype. Leuk Res 2003;27:231-234.
22. Karimi M, Yarmohammadi H, Sabri MR: An analysis of prognostic factors and the five-year survival rate in childhood acute lymphoblastic leukemia. Med Sci Monit 2002;8:CR792-CR796.
23. Matsubara Y, Hori T, Morita R, et al: Phenotypic and functional relationship between adult T-cell leukemia cells and regulatory T cells. Leukemia 2005;19:482-483.
24. Jaffe ES, Krenacs L, Raffeld M: Classification of T-cell and NK-cell neoplasms based on the REAL classification. Ann Oncol 1997;8(Suppl 2):17-24.
25. Berg SL, Blaney SM, Devidas M, et al: Phase II study of nelarabine (compound 506U78) in children and young adults with refractory T-cell malignancies: a report from the Children's Oncology Group. J Clin Oncol 2005;23:3376-3382.
26. Riva D, Giorgi C, Nichelli F, et al: Intrathecal methotrexate affects cognitive function in children with medulloblastoma. Neurology 2002;59:48-53.
27. Gokbuget N, Hoelzer D: Treatment with monoclonal antibodies in acute lymphoblastic leukemia: current knowledge and future prospects. Ann Hematol 2004;83:201-205.
28. Mano H: Stratification of acute myeloid leukemia based on gene expression profiles. Int J Hematol 2004;80:389-394.
29. Rogers LR: Cerebrovascular complications in cancer patients. Neurol Clin 2003;21:167-192.
30. Wilkins R, Janes S: Aleukaemic leukaemia cutis: case report and review of the literature. Clin Lab Haematol 2004;26:73-75.
31. Seftel MD, Bruyere H, Copland M, et al: Fulminant tumour lysis syndrome in acute myelogenous leukaemia with inv(16)(p13;q22). Eur J Haematol 2002;69:193-199.
32. Harris NL, Jaffe ES, Diebold J, et al: The World Health Organization classification of neoplasms of the hematopoietic and lymphoid tissues: report of the Clinical Advisory Committee meeting—Airlie House, Virginia, November 1997. Hematol J 2000;1:53-66.
33. Harris NL, Jaffe ES, Diebold J, et al: The World Health Organization classification of neoplastic diseases of the hematopoietic and lymphoid tissues: report of the Clinical Advisory Committee meeting—Airlie House, Virginia, November 1997. Ann Oncol 1999;10:1419-1432.
34. Peterson LF, Zhang DE: The 8;21 translocation in leukemogenesis. Oncogene 2004;23:4255-4262.
35. Al Bahar S, Pandita R, Bavishi K, et al: Chromosome aberrations in de novo acute myeloid leukemia patients in Kuwait. Neoplasma 2004;51:223-227.
36. Falanga A, Rickles FR: Pathogenesis and management of the bleeding diathesis in acute promyelocytic leukaemia. Best Pract Res Clin Haematol 2003;16:463-482.
37. Krause JR, Stolc V, Kaplan SS, et al: Microgranular promyelocytic leukemia: a multiparameter examination. Am J Hematol 1989;30:158-163.
38. Zelent A: APL and differentiation therapy—Joint International Congress. Drugs 2001;4:1257-1262.

39. Head DR: Revised classification of acute myeloid leukemia. Leukemia 1996;10:1826-1831.

40. Leith CP, Kopecky KJ, Godwin J, et al: Acute myeloid leukemia in the elderly: assessment of multidrug resistance (MDR1) and cytogenetics distinguishes biologic subgroups with remarkably distinct responses to standard chemotherapy. A Southwest Oncology Group study. Blood 1997;89:3323-3329.

41. Rund D, Ben-Yehuda D: Therapy-related leukemia and myelodysplasia: evolving concepts of pathogenesis and treatment. Hematology 2004;9:179-187.

42. Langer T, Metzler M, Reinhardt D, et al: Analysis of t(9;11) chromosomal breakpoint sequences in childhood acute leukemia: almost identical MLL breakpoints in therapy-related AML after treatment without etoposides. Genes Chromosomes Cancer 2003;36:393-401.

43. Barnard D, Woods W: Treatment-related myelodysplastic syndrome/acute myeloid leukemia in survivors of childhood cancer: an update. Leuk Lymphoma 2005;46:651-663.

44. Brunning RD, Matutes E, Harris NL, et al: Acute myeloid leukemias. In Jaffe ES, Harris NL, Stein H, et al (eds): WHO Classification of Tumours: Tumours of Haematopoietic and Lymphoid Tissues. Lyon: IARC Press, 2001:75-107.

45. Vardiman JW, Harris NL, Brunning RD: The World Health Organization (WHO) classification of the myeloid neoplasms. Blood 2002;100:2292-2302.

46. Imbert M, Nguyen D, Sultan C: Myelodysplastic syndromes (MDS) and acute myeloid leukemias (AML) with myelofibrosis. Leuk Res 1992;16:51-54.

47. Kobayashi K, Usami I, Kubota M, et al: Chromosome 7 abnormalities in acute megakaryoblastic leukemia associated with Down syndrome. Cancer Genet Cytogenet 2005;158:184-187.

48. Brunning RD: Classification of acute leukemias. Semin Diagn Pathol 2003;20:142-153.

37 Mature Lymphoid Neoplasms

Magdalena Czader

OUTLINE

Morphologic and
Immunophenotypic
Features of Normal
Lymph Nodes
Lymph Node Processing
Reactive
Lymphadenopathies
Lymphomas

OBJECTIVES

After completion of this chapter, the reader will be able to:

1. Describe normal lymph node morphology and describe the function of various compartments and constituent cells.
2. Outline the most common histologic patterns of reactive lymphadenopathies.
3. Describe the peripheral blood findings in chronic lymphocytic leukemia and hairy cell leukemia.
4. Describe the approach for the diagnosis of lymphomas as outlined by the World Health Organization classification.
5. Discuss the most commonly occurring mature B and T cell neoplasms including epidemiology, clinical presentation, pathophysiology, lymph node histology, any peripheral blood or bone marrow findings, and diagnostic test results.
6. Given diagnostic test results including immunophenotyping, interpret them to identify lymphoproliferative disorders.

CASE STUDY

After studying the material in this chapter, the reader should be able to respond to the following case study:

A 46-year-old, previously healthy man presented with an enlarged left cervical lymph node. The patient discovered this isolated lymphadenopathy 2 weeks previously and did not complain of any other symptoms. The lymph node measured approximately 2 cm. His physical examination was otherwise unremarkable. Excision of the lymph node was performed, and microscopic examination showed the histologic features presented in Figure 37-1A. Immunohistochemical stains show CD20 (Fig. 37-1B), CD10, BCL-6 positivity, and focal CD30 antigen expression.

1. What is your diagnosis based on the histologic and immunophenotypic features?
2. What additional immunophenotypic features that confirm the diagnosis can be seen using flow cytometry?
3. Is it likely that this patient would show disseminated disease including bone marrow involvement?

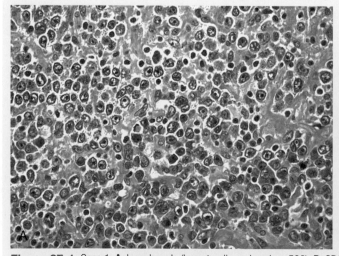
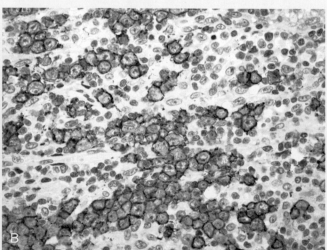

Figure 37-1 Case 1 **A,** Lymph node (hematoxylin and eosin, ×500). **B,** CD20 antigen expression in the lymphoid population (immunoperoxidase, ×500).

Lymphomas are neoplastic lesions of the lymphoid system. Originally microscopic observations and more recently immunophenotypic and molecular studies confirmed that these lesions recapitulate specific stages of differentiation of normal lymphoid cells. The biologic features along with clinical characteristics are the basis for the modern classification of lymphoid neoplasms.[1] It is mandatory that the appropriate steps are taken during initial sample processing to ensure tissue preservation and availability for microscopic examination and immunophenotypic/molecular studies.

Knowledge of normal lymphoid differentiation is a prerequisite for understanding the lymphoid neoplasms. This chapter presents morphologic and immunophenotypic features of normal lymph nodes and selected common lymphomas and lymphoproliferative disorders. Reactive lymphoid hyperplasias, which can resemble neoplastic lesions, also are discussed.

MORPHOLOGIC AND IMMUNOPHENOTYPIC FEATURES OF NORMAL LYMPH NODES

Lymphoid organs serve as sites of antigen recognition, antigen processing, and lymphopoiesis. Most of the lymphoid tissue is concentrated in lymph nodes, which are round-to-oval encapsulated organs serving as primary sites of immunologic response. They are particularly prominent at sites with environmental interface. Large groups of lymph nodes are found draining specific peripheral areas (e.g., cervical, axillary, or inguinal). Similarly, internal organs are served by regional lymph nodes (e.g., mediastinal, hilar, and mesenteric). Respiratory and digestive tracts have additional aggregates of lymphoid tissue located directly in the mucosa called *mucosa-associated lymphoid tissue* (MALT), which is the primary site of antigenic contact at these locations; these aggregates drain directly into regional lymph nodes.

Histologic components of the lymph node include cortex, paracortex, medullary cords, and sinuses (Fig. 37-2). These are not only structural, but also functional compartments serving as sites of immunologic reactions for specific antigenic stimuli.

Cortex

The lymph node is surrounded by a capsule of fibrous tissue. Just within, the cortex is the most superficial portion of the lymph node and consists of primary and secondary follicles. Primary follicles are microscopic aggregates of small round naive B lymphocytes. These lymphocytes express pan-B cell markers, including CD19 and CD20, and are frequently CD5$^+$ (Fig. 37-3). The formation of secondary follicles, including germinal centers, starts with antigen presentation by follicular dendritic cells.[2,3] On antigen encounter, naive B lymphocytes undergo transformation, proliferation, and differentiation into precursors of antibody-producing plasma cells and memory B cells (Fig. 37-3). The remaining naive B cells are displaced into the periphery of the germinal center and form the mantle zone.

Germinal center B cells have a specific immunophenotype. In addition to pan-B cell markers, they express germinal center

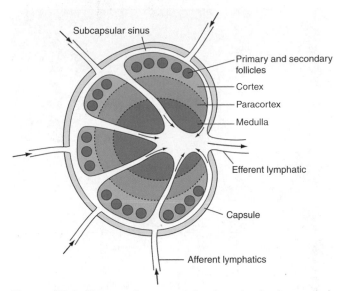

Figure 37-2 Diagram of a normal lymph node showing cortical, paracortical, and medullary compartments.

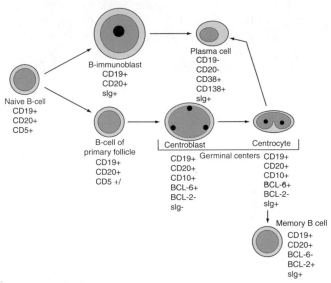

Figure 37-3 Differentiation stages of mature B cells. Note changes in immunophenotype at specific stages of differentiation. CD, cluster of differentiation; sIg, surface immunoglobin; BCL, B cell lymphoma.

cell antigens CD10 and BCL-6, and, in contrast to circulating B cells, lack antiapoptotic BCL-2 protein. The functional compartments of the germinal center include the dark zone occupied by centroblasts, large B cells with round vesicular nuclei, small nucleoli adjacent to nuclear membrane, and basophilic cytoplasm (Fig. 37-4). The dark zone is a site of intense cell proliferation and somatic mutations of B cell immunoglobulin variable regions. The latter process allows for the production of immunoglobulins with the best affinity for a particular antigen.

After completing somatic mutations, centroblasts differentiate into centrocytes, smaller cells with dense chromatin and irregular nuclear outlines, which form the light zone (see

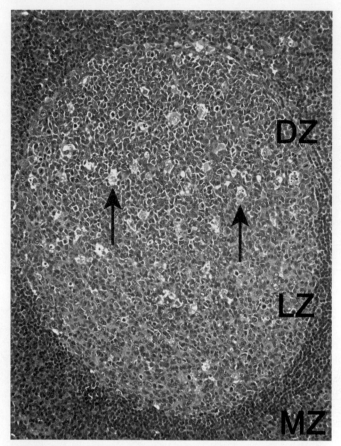

Figure 37-4 Secondary follicle with well-developed polarization in germinal center showing dark zone (DZ) and light zone (LZ). Note the presence of numerous tingible body macrophages *(arrows)*. A distinct mantle zone (MZ) also is present at the periphery of germinal center (hematoxylin and eosin, ×100).

Fig. 37-4). Subsequently, centrocytes with low-affinity ("unfit") surface immunoglobulins undergo apoptosis and are phagocytized by germinal center macrophages (so-called *tingible body macrophages*). Numerous macrophages with apoptotic debris contribute to the characteristic "starry sky" pattern of the germinal center. Centrocytes, with immunoglobulin of high affinity to the particular antigen, lose their germinal center antigens (CD10 and BCL-6) and differentiate into memory B cells that form a marginal zone at the periphery of mantle zone. Marginal zone lymphocytes are medium sized with abundant clear cytoplasm and indented nuclei.

The final step of B cell differentiation is plasma cells that are present in the medullary cords of the lymph nodes and migrate to the bone marrow. Plasma cells are negative for pan-B cell antigens and surface immunoglobulins; however, they express CD138, CD38, and cytoplasmic immunoglobulins.

Paracortex

Paracortex occupies the area separating the follicles and extends toward the medullary cords. This compartment generates immunocompetent T cells and is occupied predominantly by T cells, interdigitating dendritic cells (antigen presenting cells), and high endothelial venules. The latter are specialized vessels serving as a gate of entry of lymphocytes from peripheral blood into the lymph node. T cells express pan-T cell antigens CD3, CD5, CD2, and CD7. CD4+ and CD8+ T lymphocytes are seen in the paracortex. Similar to B cells, T cells transform in response to antigen stimulation. In this process, small lymphocytes become immunoblasts; large lymphoid cells with vesicular nuclei; prominent, often single nucleolus; and abundant basophilic cytoplasm. The paracortex also contains numerous B immunoblasts.

Medulla

The medulla represents the innermost portion of the lymph node surrounding the hilum. This area is composed of medullary cords with plasma cells and medullary sinuses.

Sinuses

The filtration of lymphatic fluid through the lymph node is accomplished through afferent lymphatics communicating with the subcapsular sinus, which is situated immediately beneath the capsule (see Fig. 37-2). The subcapsular sinus drains to cortical sinuses, which run through the cortex and empty to medullary sinuses. The latter converge into the efferent lymphatic vessel at the hilum. The sinuses are filled with macrophages or sinus histiocytes. These cells play an important role in antigen capture and processing.

LYMPH NODE PROCESSING

The current approach to the diagnosis of lymphomas incorporates routine light microscopic examination and ancillary techniques. During sample processing, appropriate steps should be taken to ensure adequate preservation of the tissue and its availability for all necessary studies. The appropriate transport conditions need to be maintained to preserve tissue integrity and prevent drying. Immediately after excision, the lymph node should be transported to the pathology laboratory in a sealed jar on gauze pads moistened with sterile saline. The fresh lymph node is cut into 3-mm-thick sections for the evaluation of nodal architecture. If areas of granulomas or suppuration are present, a portion of the tissue should be sent for cultures.

Touch imprints can be prepared to ensure the adequacy of the specimen and for special studies. To obtain an adequate imprint, a freshly cut tissue surface is gently touched to the glass slide and pulled away. Touch imprints can be fixed in formalin or alcohol solution or air-dried for subsequent Wright-Giemsa staining.

Storing of fixed touch imprints for immunocytochemical studies is optional because currently immunophenotyping is most commonly performed on paraffin-embedded tissue or using flow cytometry, which is particularly helpful in confirming monoclonal light chain expression. Several thin sections of a lymph node are placed in 10% buffered formalin for paraffin embedding. Some pathology laboratories fix additional tissue samples in a variety of fixatives with protein precipitating properties (B5 fixative, zinc chloride formalin) for better preservation of cytologic detail.[4] Regardless of the fixative used, thin sectioning of the fresh lymph node is crucial for the proper permeation of the tissue. A portion of the lymph node is placed in culture medium (Roswell Park Memorial Institute medium) and transported to the flow cytometry laboratory for immunophenotyping. The remaining fresh tissue can be stored at −70° C for further studies.

REACTIVE LYMPHADENOPATHIES

Lymphadenopathy can occur in benign and malignant conditions. Any antigenic stimulation can result in lymph node enlargement. Reactive lymphadenopathies can affect any compartment of the lymph node and present as selective expansion of normal nodal structures. Reactive hyperplasias are classified into several patterns, as follows:

1. Follicular
2. Paracortical
3. Sinusoidal
4. Mixed

Follicular Pattern

Follicular hyperplasia is the most common of the reactive lymphadenopathies. It is seen frequently in lymph nodes and tonsils of children and adolescents as a reaction to infections. In adults, it is present in lymphadenopathy associated with autoimmune disorders (rheumatoid arthritis, systemic lupus erythematosus), syphilis, and early human immunodeficiency virus (HIV) infection. Microscopically, the expansion of reactive follicles can be prominent and extend beyond the cortex into the medulla (Fig. 37-5). The follicles retain all the hallmarks of reactive germinal centers, including cellular pleomorphism with distinct polarization, presence of tingible body macrophages, abundant mitotic figures, and a preserved mantle zone (see Fig. 37-4).

Paracortical Pattern

The paracortical expansion is associated with viral infections (e.g., infectious mononucleosis) and drug reactions and is seen in patients with chronic skin diseases (dermatopathic lymphadenopathy). In addition to small lymphocytes, the paracortex shows numerous immunoblasts, increased mitotic activity, and vascular proliferation (Fig. 37-6). Focal areas of necrosis also may be seen. In dermatopathic lymphadenopathy, the paracortex has a characteristic mottled appearance as a result of an increased number of large cells with abundant clear cytoplasm scattered among small lymphoid cells (Fig. 37-7). These cells include histiocytes, often carrying melanin pigment, and Langerhans cells (Fig. 37-8). Scattered immunoblasts, plasma cells, eosinophils, and vascular proliferation also may be seen.

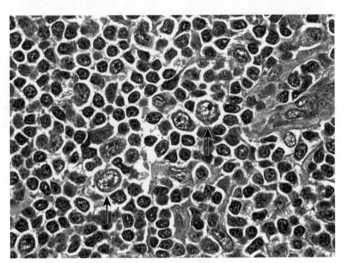

Figure 37-6 Immunoblasts *(arrows)* scattered in the paracortex (hematoxylin and eosin, ×1000).

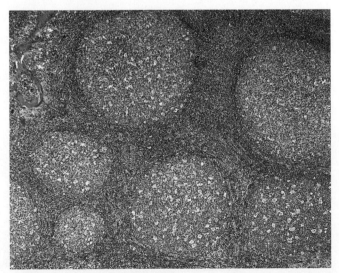

Figure 37-5 Reactive follicular hyperplasia with numerous secondary follicles scattered throughout the lymph node (hematoxylin and eosin, ×40).

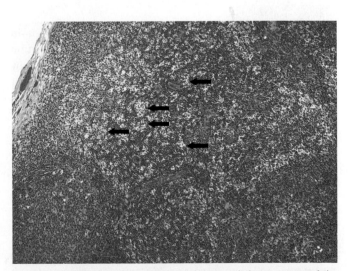

Figure 37-7 Paracortical hyperplasia. Note mottled appearance of the paracortex resulting from multiple scattered histiocytes with abundant cytoplasm *(arrows)* (hematoxylin and eosin, ×40).

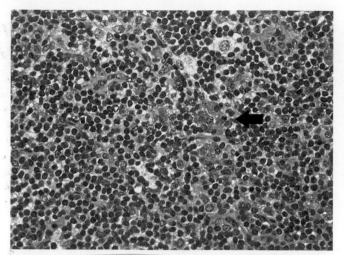

Figure 37-8 Dermatopathic lymphadenopathy in a patient with chronic skin rash. Scattered pigment-laden macrophages *(arrow)* are present in the paracortical area (hematoxylin and eosin, ×400).

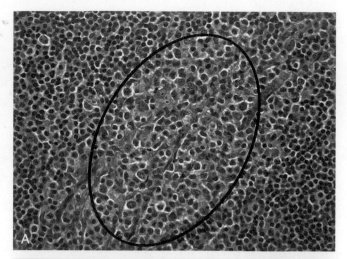

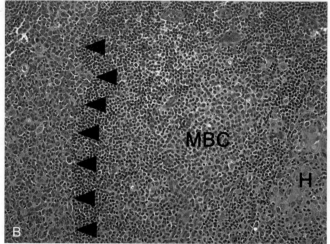

Figure 37-9 *Toxoplasma* lymphadenitis. **A,** Monocytoid B cells are medium sized with irregular nuclear outlines and abundant cytoplasm (shown in *center circle*) (hematoxylin and eosin, ×400). **B,** Classic triad of reactive changes seen in *Toxoplasma* lymphadenitis includes follicular hyperplasia with focal aggregates of histiocytes (H) and monocytoid B cells (MBC). An irregular outline of a secondary follicle is seen on the left *(arrowheads)* (hematoxylin and eosin, ×100).

Sinusoidal Pattern

Expanded subcapsular, cortical, and medullary sinuses are often seen in lymph nodes draining limbs, abdominal organs, various inflammatory lesions, and malignancies. In advanced cases, the prominent sinuses compress the nodal parenchyma. They may be completely filled with histiocytes showing abundant cytoplasm, small oval nucleus with inconspicuous nucleolus, and delicate chromatin. Monocytoid B cells with abundant cytoplasm and oval indented nuclei that may mimic histiocytes are seen in nodal sinuses in HIV-associated lymphadenopathy and *Toxoplasma* lymphadenitis (Fig. 37-9A). Numerous malignant lesions show a predilection to sinuses, such as Langerhans cell histiocytosis, B cell and T cell lymphomas, and carcinomas; a high-power microscopic evaluation of expanded sinuses is always necessary.

Mixed Pattern

A classic example of mixed-pattern hyperplasia is seen in *Toxoplasma gondii* infection, a common protozoal infection typically seen after ingestion of raw meat or contamination by cat feces. Histologically, the expansion of all lymph node compartments is seen (see Fig. 37-9). Florid follicular hyperplasia is accompanied by paracortical expansion, aggregates of histiocytes encroaching on germinal centers, and expanded sinuses. Sinuses are focally filled with a specific subset of B cells, so-called *monocytoid B cells*.

LYMPHOMAS

Approximately 86,000 new cases of lymphoma are diagnosed annually in the United States.[5] Most lymphomas develop in previously healthy individuals. The strongest risk factor for development of lymphoproliferative disorder is altered immune function as seen in immunocompromised patients or individuals with autoimmune disease.[6,7] Similarly, certain viral and bacterial infections are associated with a higher risk for the development of lymphoma.[8] Accumulating evidence indicates that exposure to chemicals and herbicides may predispose to lymphoid neoplasms. Most cases present as a nodal disease. Certain types of lymphoma show a predilection for extranodal sites, however. The frequency of bone marrow and peripheral blood (leukemic phase) involvement varies depending on the lymphoma subtype.

Over the years, numerous classifications have been proposed based mainly on the morphology and clinical characteristics (e.g., Rappaport classification, Kiel system, working formulation). With increased understanding of the development and function of the immune system, however, it became clear that lymphomas, similar to myeloid neoplasms, recapitulate normal stages of lymphoid differentiation. In addition, the elucidation of specific molecular events occurring in lymphomagenesis helps in clinically relevant subclassification, especially in morphologically heterogeneous entities. Currently, numerous subtypes of lymphoma are distinguished based on morphology, immunophenotype, molecular characteristics, and clinical characteristics. The integration of these features is mandatory for comprehensive lymphoma diagnosis. On the basis of cellular origin, lymphomas can be categorized into precursor lesions and neoplasms of mature lymphoid cells (Table 37-1). In this chapter, only mature B cell and T cell neoplasms are discussed; the precursor malignancies are covered in Chapter 36.

Mature B Cell Lymphomas

Mature B cell lymphomas are neoplasms derived from various stages of B cell differentiation. Although they show significant morphologic and immunophenotypic heterogeneity, all B cell lymphomas produce monoclonal light chain immunoglobulins, clonal immunoglobulin gene rearrangements, or both. Follicular lymphoma and diffuse large B cell lymphomas (DLBCLs) are the most common subtypes of B cell lymphoma. Most cases are lymph node–based and occur in elderly individuals. The most common mature B cell neoplasms are discussed subsequently and summarized in Table 37-2.

Chronic Lymphocytic Leukemia/Small Lymphocytic Lymphoma

Definition. Chronic lymphocytic leukemia (CLL) and small lymphocytic lymphoma (SLL) are characterized by the accumulation of small lymphoid cells in the peripheral blood, bone marrow, and lymphoid organs. They are derived from recirculating CD5+, IgM+, IgD+ B cells normally present in the peripheral blood; the World Health Organization (WHO) classification considers CLL and SLL as one entity with different clinical presentations. The diagnosis is based on the predominant site of involvement. CLL, by definition, has peripheral blood (lymphocytosis >10 × 10^9/L) and bone marrow involvement. SLL primarily involves lymph nodes and other lymphoid organs.

Morphology and Immunophenotype. Bone marrow and peripheral blood smears display small lymphoid cells with a coarse chromatin pattern, inconspicuous nucleoli, and scant cytoplasm (Fig. 37-10).[10] Smudge cells, representing disintegrated lymphoid cells, also are present. These cells are of diagnostic significance because they are not seen often in other subtypes of malignant lymphoma. The bone marrow biopsy shows nodular, diffuse, or interstitial infiltrates of small lymphoid cells (Fig. 37-11).

TABLE 37-1 World Health Organization Classification of Mature Lymphoid Neoplasms

Mature B-Cell Lymphomas	Mature T-Cell Lymphomas
Chronic lymphocytic leukemia/small lymphocyte lymphoma (CLL/SLL)	**Leukemic/Disseminated**
B-cell prolymphocytic leukemia	T-cell prolymphocytic leukemia
Lymphoplasmacytic lymphoma	T-cell large granular lymphocytic leukemia
Splenic marginal zone lymphoma	Aggressive natural killer cell leukemia
Hairy cell leukemia	Adult T-cell leukemia/lymphoma
Plasma cell myeloma	**Cutaneous**
Monoclonal gammopathy of undetermined significance (MGUS)	Mycosis fungoides
	Sézary syndrome
Solitary plasmacytoma of bone	Primary cutaneous anaplastic large cell lymphoma
Extraosseous plasmacytoma	Lymphomatoid papulosis
Primary amyloidosis	**Other Extranodal**
Heavy chain disease	Extranodal natural killer/T-cell lymphoma, nasal type
Extranodal marginal zone B-cell lymphoma of mucosa-associated lymphoid tissue (MALT lymphoma)	Enteropathy-type T-cell lymphoma
	Hepatosplenic T-cell lymphoma
	Subcutaneous panniculitis-like T-cell lymphoma
Nodal marginal zone B-cell lymphoma	**Nodal**
Follicular lymphoma	Angioimmunoblastic T-cell lymphoma
Mantle cell lymphoma	Peripheral T-cell lymphoma, unspecified
Diffuse large B-cell lymphomas (DLBCL)	Anaplastic large cell lymphoma
Mediastinal (thymic) large B-cell lymphoma	**Neoplasm of Uncertain Lineage and State of Differentiation**
Intravascular large B-cell lymphoma	Blastic natural killer cell lymphoma
Primary effusion lymphoma	
Burkitt lymphoma/leukemia	

TABLE 37-2 Morphologic and Immunophenotypic Features of Mature B Cell Lymphomas

Subtype	Architectural Features	Cytologic Characteristics	Immunophenotype Cytogenetics	Cell of Origin
CLL/SLL	Diffuse lymphocytic proliferation with growth centers	Small lymphoid cells	CD20+, CD19+, CD5+, CD23+	Naïve or memory B cell
Mantle cell lymphoma	Diffuse, nodular, or mantle zone pattern	Medium-sized lymphocytes with irregular nuclei	CD20+, CD19+, CD5+, FMC7+, cyclin D1+; t(11;14)	Mantle zone cell
Follicular lymphoma	Follicular pattern	Medium-sized lymphocytes with indented nuclei and variable admixture of large lymphoid cells	CD20+, CD19+, CD10+, BCL-6+, BCL-2+; t(14;18)	Germinal center cell
MALT lymphoma	Diffuse lymphoid proliferation, occasionally marginal zone pattern	Medium-sized lymphocytes with clear cytoplasm, indented nuclei, and scattered large lymphoid cells	CD20+, CD19+, CD43+/−	Marginal zone cell
Plasma cell myeloma plasmacytoma	Sheets or large aggregates of plasma cells	Plasma cells, frequently with cytologic atypia	CD20−, CD19−, CD38+, CD138+, cytoplasmic light chain+	Plasma cell
DLBCL	Diffuse proliferation	Large lymphoid cells	CD20+, CD19+, CD10+/−, BCL-6+/−, BCL-2+/−, CD5+/−	Different stages of mature B cell
Burkitt lymphoma	Diffuse lymphoid proliferation with "starry sky" pattern	Medium-sized lymphocytes with evenly distributed chromatin, inconspicuous nucleoli	CD20+, CD19+, CD10+, BCL-6+, BCL-2−; t(8;14)	Germinal center cell

CLL/SLL, chronic lymphocytic leukemia/small lymphocytic lymphoma; MALT, mucosa-associated lymphoid tissue; DLBCL, diffuse large B-cell lymphoma.

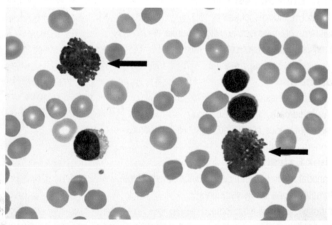

Figure 37-10 CLL/SLL. Peripheral blood smear showing small lymphocytes and smudge cells *(arrows)* (Wright-Giemsa, ×1000).

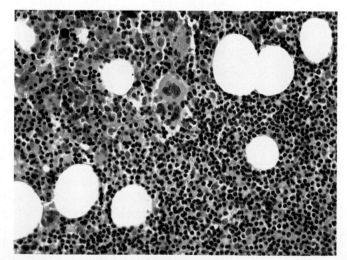

Figure 37-11 CLL/SLL. Bone marrow biopsy specimen with nodular *(right)* and interstitial small lymphocytic infiltrate (hematoxylin and eosin, ×400).

Lymph nodes involved by SLL display a loss of normal nodal architecture (Fig. 37-12A) replaced by a diffuse proliferation of small, round lymphoid cells with coarse chromatin, indistinct nucleoli, and scant cytoplasm. In addition, scattered nodules (so-called *pseudofollicles, growth centers,* or *proliferation centers*) composed of medium-sized and large lymphoid cells with dispersed chromatin and distinct nucleoli are observed

(Fig. 37-12B). The diffuse proliferation of small lymphoid cells with pseudofollicles is pathognomonic for SLL.

CLL/SLL is derived from circulating CD5+, IgM+, IgD+ B cells. Currently, two groups of CLL/SLL are recognized. The first corresponds with the pre–germinal center phenotype with

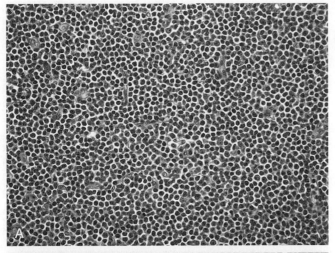

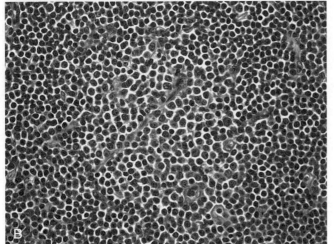

Figure 37-12 CLL/SLL in lymph node. **A,** Diffuse proliferation of small lymphoid cells (hematoxylin and eosin, ×100). **B,** Proliferation center with large and medium-sized lymphoid cells in the background of small lymphocytes (hematoxylin and eosin, ×400).

naïve B cells showing no mutations in the variable region of the immunoglobulin heavy chain (V_H) gene. The second form is derived from memory B cells (the post–germinal center stage), with mutated V_H genes. Both show similar immunophenotype and are positive for pan-B cell antigens, including CD19 and weakly expressed CD20. In addition, the expression of CD5, CD23, and weak surface monoclonal κ *or* λ light chains are seen. The presence of CD23 and absence of FMC7 and cyclin D1 distinguish CLL/SLL from mantle cell lymphoma.

Clinical Features and Prognosis. Overall, CLL/SLL is regarded as an indolent lymphoproliferative disorder of the elderly (median age at diagnosis 65). Although this disease is incurable by current therapeutic approaches, the median survival is 10 years.[12] A variety of features are used to predict patient outcome. Commonly used clinical staging systems are based on the extent of lymphoid organ involvement and degree of cytopenias. In addition, distinct cytogenetic abnormalities that roughly correspond with naïve and memory phenotypes (unmutated and mutated V_H gene) are of prognostic signifi-

cance in CLL/SLL patients.[11] Trisomy of chromosome 12 is seen predominantly in cases of pre–germinal center origin and correlates with a rapidly progressive clinical course. These patients may require aggressive treatment early in the course of the disease. In contrast, the deletion of 13q14 is associated with post–germinal center (memory) phenotype and predicts a more indolent clinical course. Independent of the course of original disease, approximately 5% of patients with CLL/SLL develop a DLBCL (so-called *Richter transformation*).

Hairy Cell Leukemia

Definition. Hairy cell leukemia is composed of small B-lymphocytes with abundant cytoplasm and fine ("hairy") cytoplasmic projections. The postulated cell of origin is peripheral B-cell of post–germinal center stage (memory B-cell).

Morphology and Immunophenotype. Hairy cell leukemia is found predominantly in bone marrow and red pulp of the spleen. A low number of neoplastic B-cells is seen in peripheral blood. Lymph node involvement is rare. The bone marrow infiltrates are interstitial and are composed of small to medium-sized lymphoid cells with abundant cytoplasm (Fig 37-13A). The bone marrow involvement may be subtle with preservation of normal hematopoiesis. As a result of the production of fibrogenic cytokines by the leukemic cells, a bone marrow biopsy shows an increase in reticulin fibers. The characteristic cytology of neoplastic cells is best appreciated in bone marrow aspirate and peripheral blood smears. Neoplastic cells display an indented nucleus, abundant cytoplasm, and fine, hair-like cytoplasmic projections (Fig 37-13B).

Classic cases of hairy cell leukemia show strong positivity for B-cell markers (CD19, CD20, CD22) coupled with bright expression of CD11c, CD25, and CD103. As in other lymphoproliferative disorders, a confident diagnosis can be made using a combination of these markers and characteristic cytologic/histologic features. Tartrate-resistant acid phosphatase (TRAP) cytochemical stain (Chapter 30) and DBA-44 immunostain can be used when only preserved tissues are available (bone marrow/peripheral blood smears, bone marrow biopsy material).

Clinical Features and Prognosis. Hairy cell leukemia is a rare lymphoproliferative disorder occurring in middle-aged individuals (median age 55 years). Patients present with splenomegaly and pancytopenia. Durable remissions can be achieved using interferon-α or purine analogs. Conventional lymphoma therapy is not effective.

Mantle Cell Lymphoma

Definition. Mantle cell lymphoma is a lymphoproliferative disorder composed of medium-sized lymphoid cells with irregular nuclear outlines derived from the follicular mantle zone.[13]

Morphology and Immunophenotype. The main sites of involvement are lymph nodes. Bone marrow, spleen, and gastrointestinal tract also are frequently involved. Most

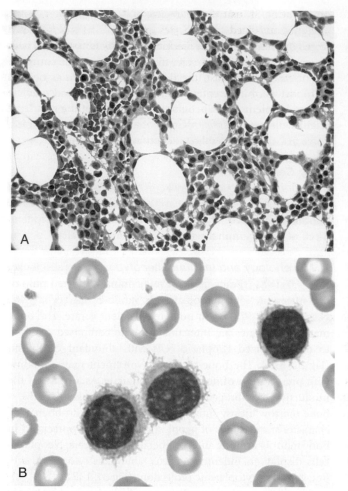

Figure 37-13 Hairy cell leukemia. **A,** Interstitial bone marrow infiltrate composed of widely spaced lymphoid cells with abundant cytoplasm and irregular nuclei (hematoxylin and eosin, ×1000). **B,** Lymphoid cells of hairy cell leukemia show characteristic cytoplasmic projections, which are supported by the peripheral cytoplasmic network of polymerized actin (peripheral blood, Wright-Giemsa, ×1000).

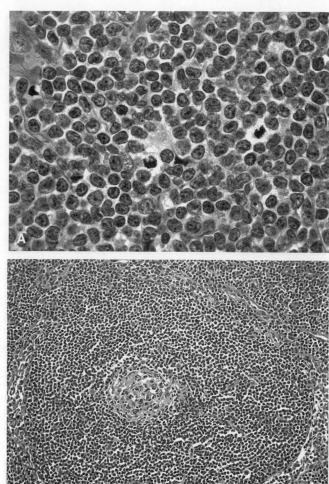

Figure 37-14 Mantle cell lymphoma. **A,** Diffuse proliferation of medium-sized lymphoid cells with irregular nuclei (hematoxylin and eosin, ×1000). **B,** Mantle zone pattern. Regressed germinal center is seen in the center (hematoxylin and eosin, ×100).

commonly, lymph nodes show a loss of normal nodal architecture with a diffuse proliferation of monotonous, medium-sized lymphoid cells with irregular nuclear outlines (Fig. 37-14A). Occasionally, lymph nodes can show a vaguely nodular pattern or partial preservation of nodal architecture with a prominent thickening of mantle zones (Fig. 37-14B).

Similar to other B cell lymphoproliferative disorders, mantle cell lymphoma shows expression of pan-B cell markers (CD19, CD20) and high-density clonal surface light chains. There is coexpression of CD5 antigen; however, CD23 is negative. In contrast to CLL/SLL, the expression of CD20 and light chains is bright, and there is immunoreactivity for cyclin D1. Cyclin D1 (*bcl-1*) is a proto-oncogene involved in the regulation of G_1 to S phase progression. In mantle cell lymphoma, this gene is constitutively expressed through its translocation to the immunoglobulin heavy chain gene, t(11;14). This cytogenetic abnormality is a defining feature of mantle cell lymphoma.

Clinical Features and Prognosis. Mantle cell lymphoma is an aggressive lymphoproliferative disorder with a median survival of 3 to 5 years. Most patients present with disseminated disease, including bone marrow involvement. This lymphoma is incurable with current protocols.

Follicular Lymphoma

Definition. Follicular lymphoma originates from germinal centers and in most cases recapitulates follicular architecture.

Morphology and Immunophenotype. Numerous closely spaced follicles replace the normal nodal architecture (Fig. 37-15). The neoplastic proliferation may extend into the perinodal adipose tissue. In contrast to the reactive secondary follicles, the mantle zone and the polarization are not preserved. The neoplastic follicles are composed of medium-sized lymphoid cells with angular or indented nuclei cytologically

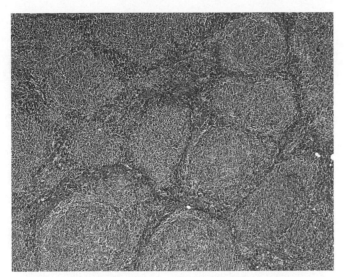

Figure 37-15 Follicular lymphoma. Nodular proliferation replacing normal elements of lymph node architecture (hematoxylin and eosin, ×40).

similar to centrocytes, with a variable admixture of large lymphoid cells. The latter resemble centroblasts and show oval nuclei with vesicular chromatin and multiple, marginally located nucleoli. The relative proportion of medium-sized and large lymphoid cells is of prognostic significance because cases with high numbers of large cells show a significantly more aggressive course, similar to DLBCL. Follicular lymphomas are graded by counting the average number of large cells per high-power field.[1] Three grades are recognized, ranging from grade 1, showing only scattered large lymphocytes, to grade 3, in which numerous centroblasts are seen.

The immunophenotype reflects the follicle center cell origin of this disease. Pan-B cell markers (CD19, CD20) are present along with the coexpression of CD10, BCL-6, and clonal surface immunoglobulin. In contrast to reactive follicles, neoplastic cells express BCL-2 protein. This protein is responsible for the decreased sensitivity to apoptosis observed in follicular lymphomas and allows for the accumulation of neoplastic lymphocytes. The expression of BCL-2 by follicular lymphoma cells is due to the t(14;18)(q32;q21), which places the *bcl-2* gene under a promoter of the immunoglobulin heavy chain gene. This cytogenetic abnormality is present in 95% of cases.[14]

Clinical Features and Prognosis. The median age at diagnosis is 59 years. Most patients present with advanced disease. Bone marrow involvement is seen in approximately 50% of cases. The course of the disease is indolent in grade 1 and 2 lymphoma, whereas grade 3 cases are more aggressive and are treated similar to DLBCL with doxorubicin (Adriamycin)-based regimens.

Extranodal Marginal Zone B Cell Lymphoma of Mucosa-Associated Lymphoid Tissue

Definition. Three subtypes of marginal zone lymphomas are recognized: nodal, extranodal (MALT lymphoma), and splenic. We focus on the extranodal variant derived from marginal zone cells of MALT. In this lymphoma, the neoplastic

proliferation is usually heterogeneous, encompassing small and medium-sized lymphocytes, plasma cells, and scattered large lymphoid cells. This disease frequently is associated with autoimmune conditions (e.g., Sjögren syndrome, Hashimoto thyroiditis) or previous infections (*Helicobacter pylori* gastritis or hepatitis C).[15] Persistent immune stimulation leads to the accumulation of reactive lymphoid tissue and subsequently to the development of marginal zone lymphoma. The importance of continuous antigenic stimulation in the pathogenesis of this lymphoma is shown by a remission of the disease in its early stage when the microorganism is eradicated.[16]

Morphology and Immunophenotype. In most cases, the neoplastic population is composed of a mixture of medium-sized lymphocytes, plasma cells, and occasional large lymphoid cells. Medium-sized marginal zone cells with irregular nuclei and relatively abundant cytoplasm predominate (Fig. 37-16A). Residual reactive germinal centers may be present, which are colonized to variable degrees by the

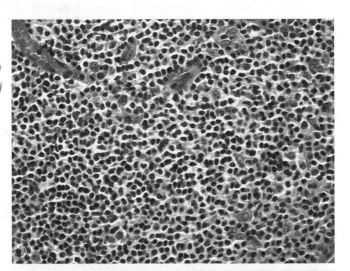

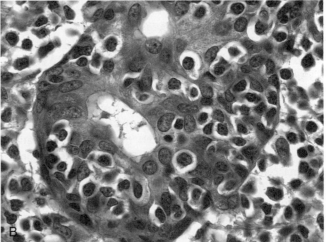

Figure 37-16 MALT lymphoma. **A,** Heterogeneous population of medium-sized lymphoid cells with abundant clear cytoplasm and occasional large cells (hematoxylin and eosin, ×500). **B,** Lymphoepithelial lesion. Malignant lymphocytes invading glandular epithelium (hematoxylin and eosin, ×1000).

neoplastic cells. A characteristic feature of MALT lymphoma is the presence of so-called *lymphoepithelial lesions,* representing the invasion of the neoplastic lymphocytes into the glandular epithelium (Fig. 37-16B). This feature is usually absent from reactive lymphoid proliferations associated with autoimmune processes or infections.

The neoplastic cells of marginal zone lymphoma express CD20, CD19, and monoclonal immunoglobulin chains. CD5 and CD10 are absent. CD43 antigen is coexpressed in 30% of cases and can be a helpful feature in diagnosing marginal zone lymphoma when there is a significant residual reactive component. In selected cases, the demonstration of clonality by flow cytometry or molecular analysis may be necessary to confirm the diagnosis.

Antigenic stimulation and interference with the apoptotic pathway play an important role in the pathogenesis of MALT lymphoma. Fifty percent of cases show a translocation involving apoptosis-inhibitor gene *API2* and *MLT* gene (t[11;18][q21;q21]).[17]

Clinical Features and Prognosis. The gastrointestinal tract is the most common site for extranodal marginal zone lymphoma. The lung, thyroid, ocular adnexae, and breast are other common sites of involvement. In most cases, the disease is limited to the primary site with occasional involvement of regional lymph nodes. Bone marrow is less frequently involved than in other types of indolent lymphoma.[18] In cases of gastric MALT lymphoma positive for *H. pylori,* the antibiotic treatment of the infection may induce a remission of associated lymphoma. Other cases may benefit from local therapy.

Plasma Cell Neoplasms

Definition. Plasma cell neoplasms are characterized by a monoclonal proliferation of terminally differentiated B cells (i.e., plasma cells). These disorders can present as a localized or disseminated process most commonly involving bone marrow and bone. The clinical features and the primary site of involvement define distinct clinicopathologic entities (Table 37-3). *Plasma cell myeloma* is a multifocal accumulation of malignant plasma cells in the bone marrow presenting as lytic bone lesions. In most cases, monoclonal immunoglobulin produced by neoplastic plasma cells is detected in the serum, urine, or both (monoclonal gammopathy). The overt disease may be preceded by an asymptomatic period of monoclonal gammopathy with only mild bone marrow plasmacytosis (<10% plasma cells). Approximately 25% of asymptomatic patients with clonal serum immunoglobulin progress to symptomatic plasma cell myeloma.[19] The term *monoclonal gammopathy of undetermined significance* (MGUS) is used to encompass the entire patient population with clonal serum immunoglobulin and only mild marrow plasmacytosis. *Plasmacytoma,* a localized form of plasma cell neoplasm, may present as a solitary bone lesion or involve an extraosseous/extramedullary site, most commonly the nasopharynx, oropharynx, or sinuses.

Morphology and Immunophenotype. Plasma cell myeloma is characterized by marked bone marrow plasma-

TABLE 37-3 Clinicopathologic Features of Selected Plasma Cell Neoplasms

Plasma Cell Disorder	Defining Features
Plasma cell myeloma	Bone marrow plasmacytosis: >10% plasma cells
	Monoclonal gammopathy
	Serum: IgG >3.5 g/dL, IgA >2 g/dL
	Urine: >1 g/24 h of Bence-Jones protein
	Lytic bone lesions
	Reduced normal immunoglobulins (<50%)
Plasma cell leukemia	Bone marrow plasmacytosis
	Peripheral blood: >2 × 10^9/L or >20% circulating plasma cells
	Lymphadenopathy, organomegaly
	Osteolytic lesions (less frequent than in plasma cell myeloma)
Monoclonal gammopathy of undetermined significance	Bone marrow plasmacytosis (<10%)
	Monoclonal gammopathy (lower level than in plasma cell myeloma)
	No lytic bone lesions or symptoms of plasma cell myeloma
Solitary plasmacytoma of bone	Localized bone mass composed of plasma cells
Extramedullary plasmacytoma	Localized extraosseous mass composed of plasma cells

cytosis. Large aggregates and sheets of plasma cells, frequently with cytologic atypia, are present and often constitute more than 30% of marrow cellularity (Fig. 37-17A). Cytologic atypia seen in plasma cell myeloma includes a high nuclear-to-cytoplasmic ratio, dispersed chromatin pattern, and distinct nucleoli (Fig. 37-17B). These changes are rarely seen in reactive conditions and MGUS. Similarly, in reactive plasmacytosis associated with infections and autoimmune disorders, plasma cells appear scattered throughout the marrow cavity and form small clusters around the vessels. Large aggregates and sheets of plasma cells, which are commonly seen in plasma cell myeloma, are absent from reactive conditions.

Rarely, patients with plasma cell myeloma show a marked increase in circulating plasma cells. The term *plasma cell leukemia* is reserved to cases with more than 20% of circulating plasma cells or plasma cell count exceed 2 × 10^9 cells/L.

Plasmacytoma represents a localized, mass-forming, monoclonal plasma cell proliferation. Neoplastic plasma cells show an immunophenotype similar to that of their normal counterparts. At this terminal stage of differentiation, pan-B cell markers, CD19 and CD20, and surface immunoglobulin chains are usually absent. Plasma cells are positive for CD138 (syndecan-1) and show high-density CD38 antigen and monoclonal cytoplasmic immunoglobulins. These monoclonal proteins, in the form of complete immunoglobulin

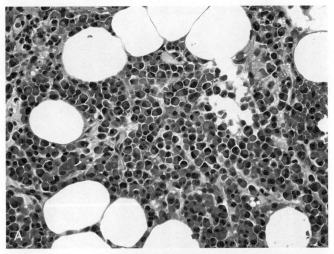

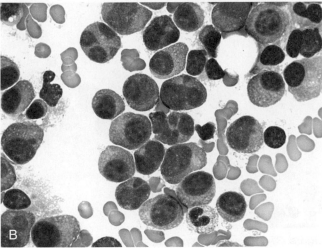

Figure 37-17 Plasma cell myeloma. **A,** Bone marrow biopsy specimen showing large aggregates of plasma cells (hematoxylin and eosin, ×400). **B,** Neoplastic plasma cells with cytologic atypia (bone marrow, Wright-Giemsa, ×1000).

most commonly IgG or IgA, or isolated clonal light chains, are secreted by the neoplastic plasma cells and are seen in serum and urine as monoclonal spikes. In addition, neoplastic plasma cells can show an aberrant expression of other antigens, typically not expressed by normal plasma cells, such as CD56 antigen and myeloid markers.

Clinical Features and Prognosis. Plasma cell myeloma is a disease of older individuals (median age approximately 70 years).[20] Bone pain and pathologic fractures are directly related to proliferation of neoplastic plasma cells. These cells produce factors that cause localized bone destruction (so-called *lytic lesions* on radiographic examination) and hypercalcemia. Renal insufficiency is triggered by the obstruction or direct damage of renal tubules by monoclonal protein. Cytopenias are related to the replacement of normal trilineage hematopoiesis by massive plasma cell infiltrates. Depressed normal immunoglobulin levels confer susceptibility to infections, commonly occurring in patients with plasma cell myeloma. High levels of serum immunoglobulins also may

interfere with the coagulation cascade and impair circulation through an increase in serum viscosity. Tissue deposits of clonal immunoglobulins, called amyloidosis, may compromise kidney, heart, and liver function and cause peripheral neuropathies.

Most of the cases show a rapidly progressive course with a median survival of 3 years. The prognosis is closely related to the number of plasma cells in the bone marrow and to clinical features reflecting overall tumor burden. Patients with more than 50% bone marrow plasma cells, associated renal failure, and severe anemia have a shorter survival than patients with fewer than 20% of plasma cells and preserved renal function.

Typically, patients with bone and extraosseous plasmacytomas are younger and respond favorably to local radiation therapy. Approximately 15% progress to plasma cell myeloma.

Asymptomatic monoclonal gammopathy (MGUS) occurs in less than 5% of individuals older than 70 years.[19] As discussed earlier, 25% may develop overt myeloma. Patients with MGUS should be monitored closely with repeat serum immunoglobulin levels and bone marrow examination.

Diffuse Large B Cell Lymphoma

Definition. The defining feature of DLBCL is its large cell size. In contrast to the lymphoproliferative disorders discussed so far, DLBCL cells are significantly larger than normal lymphocytes. Most show a diffuse histologic growth pattern but differ significantly in cytologic appearance, immunophenotype or both. This is one of the most common lymphomas, accounting for 30% to 40% of all non-Hodgkin lymphoma cases.[9]

Morphology and Immunophenotype. The most common forms show a diffuse proliferation of large lymphoid cells replacing the normal lymph node architecture. Cells are at least twice the size of normal small lymphocytes and show single-to-multiple nucleoli and ample cytoplasm (Fig. 37-18). In rare cases, there is a considerable admixture of background histiocytes and small lymphocytes in addition to the neoplastic large cells.

As in other B cell lymphomas, pan-B cell antigens are expressed. DLBCL can derive from a variety of stages in B cell development; hence the coexpression of other markers is heterogeneous. CD5, CD10, BCL-6, CD30, and CD138 can be present (see Table 37-2).

Clinical Features and Prognosis. Although, as with most lymphomas, the median age of diagnosis is in the 60s, DLBCL also is seen in children and young adults. It presents as a localized disease involving a group of lymph nodes. The bone marrow involvement is rare at presentation but can occur later in the course of the disease. DLBCL also is seen frequently in the extranodal sites, including gastrointestinal tract, central nervous system, and bone. DLBCL is aggressive with a proliferation rate frequently exceeding 40%, which makes it more sensitive to multi-agent chemotherapy. The prognosis depends on a variety of clinical parameters, such as

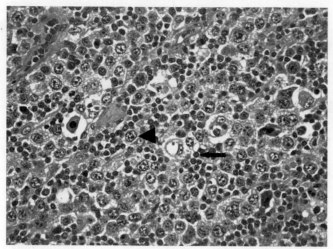

Figure 37-18 DLBCL showing proliferation of large lymphoid cells. Note the size difference between small lymphocytes *(arrow)* and neoplastic B cells *(arrowhead)* (hematoxylin and eosin, ×500).

age, the extent of the disease, and site of involvement. Attempts are being made to include biologic parameters in the prognostication of DLBCL. Initial studies based on morphologic subclassification of DLBCL were flawed with poor intra-observer and interobserver reproducibility.[21] Recent results of gene microarray studies showed, however, that patients with DLBCL of follicle center genotype had better survival than patients with other subtypes.[22]

Burkitt Lymphoma

Definition. Burkitt lymphoma is composed of medium-sized, highly proliferating lymphoid cells with basophilic vacuolated cytoplasm. The WHO classification distinguished three variants of this lymphoma—endemic (occurring predominantly in Africa), sporadic, and immunodeficiency associated.

Morphology and Immunophenotype. The proliferation is diffuse, and low-power microscopy shows a prominent "starry sky" pattern imparted by numerous tingible body macrophages (Fig. 37-19A). The macrophages are responsible for phagocytosing apoptotic debris, a byproduct of the extremely high proliferation rate. Lymphoma cells are medium sized with round nuclei, evenly distributed chromatin, and inconspicuous nucleoli. The cytoplasm is deeply basophilic and highly vacuolated, a feature best displayed on touch imprints or other cytologic preparations (Fig. 37-19B).

The immunophenotype of Burkitt lymphoma reflects germinal center origin. CD19, CD20, CD10, and BCL-6 antigens are positive. There is surface expression of monoclonal immunoglobulin light chains. BCL-2 is negative. The hallmark of Burkitt lymphoma, contributing to its aggressive clinical course, is a high proliferation rate. Nearly 100% of Burkitt lymphoma cells are in active phases of the cell cycle. This feature is linked to the constitutive expression of *MYC* gene (cell cycle gatekeeping gene) secondary to its translocation

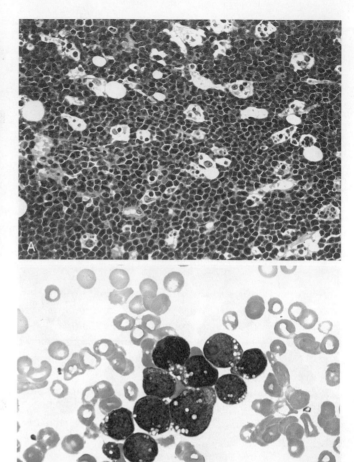

Figure 37-19 Burkitt lymphoma. **A,** "Starry sky" pattern imparted by numerous macrophages with apoptotic debris (hematoxylin and eosin, ×400). **B,** Touch preparation showing characteristic cells of Burkitt lymphoma. Note the deeply basophilic cytoplasm with numerous vacuoles (Wright-Giemsa stain, ×1000).

under the promoter of immunoglobulin heavy or light chain genes (t[8;14], t[2;8], t[8;22]). This translocation is pathognomonic for Burkitt lymphoma, and the diagnosis can be made only in cases showing this cytogenetic abnormality.

Clinical Features and Prognosis. The presentation of Burkitt lymphoma depends on its variant. The endemic form presents in young children (4 to 7 years old), most commonly as a jaw bone mass. The sporadic variant, seen in the United States and Europe, occurs in children and young adults as an abdominal mass. Gastrointestinal tract and abdominal lymph nodes are often involved; however, other extranodal sites, such as gonads and breasts, also can be a site of primary disease. Immunodeficiency-associated Burkitt lymphoma presents most often as nodal disease. Independent of the variant, Burkitt lymphoma commonly involves the central nervous system and can present as Burkitt leukemia with malignant cells in peripheral blood and bone marrow. Epstein-Barr virus (EBV) is present in some patients.

The diagnosis of Burkitt lymphoma is a medical emergency. Because of its high proliferation rate, the doubling time is extremely short. The chemotherapy is significantly different than that used for other types of high-grade lymphoma. These highly aggressive treatment regimens take into account the high proliferation rate and contribute to high cure rates for childhood and adult Burkitt lymphoma—60% to 90% depending on the stage of the disease.[23,24] Immunodeficiency-associated Burkitt lymphoma occurs predominantly in HIV-positive patients; the prognosis is not as favorable as in other variants.

Mature T Cell and Natural Killer Cell Lymphomas

Lymphomas derived from mature T cells and natural killer cells are much less common than the previously discussed mature B cell neoplasms and account for approximately 10% of all lymphomas. The incidence of the specific subtypes of T cell lymphoma shows geographic and ethnic variability, however. In certain regions, T cell malignancies may be more prevalent than in the United States. Compared with B cell lymphoproliferative disorders, T cell neoplasms occur more frequently in extranodal sites. The most common skin lymphoma, mycosis fungoides, is of T cell phenotype.

Although morphology is an important criterion in the diagnosis of T cell lymphomas, a significant morphologic and cytologic variability is seen within specific subtypes. Similarly, the immunophenotypic features are not as specific as those seen in B cell malignancies. Considering these factors, an integration of morphologic, immunophenotypic, cytogenetic, molecular, and clinical information, as stressed by WHO classification, is crucial in diagnosing T cell and natural killer cell malignancies. Until recently, the demonstration of clonality in T cell proliferations was limited to molecular methods detecting T cell receptor gene rearrangements. The development of multiple antibodies directed against the variable region of the T cell receptor allows for the determination of T cell clonality by flow cytometry.[25]

Mycosis Fungoides and Sézary Syndrome

Definition.   Mycosis fungoides is the most common cutaneous lymphoma. It is composed of small to medium-sized lymphoid cells with irregular nuclear outlines. These cells show a predilection for the epidermis (epidermotropism) and dermis and may spread to regional lymph nodes. Sézary syndrome, a variant of mycosis fungoides, presents as a disseminated disease with widespread skin involvement, lymphadenopathy, and circulating lymphoma cells.

Morphology and Immunophenotype.   The degree of cutaneous infiltrate is related to the stage of the disease. Early lesions show patchy or lichenoid infiltrate of the dermis by small to medium-sized lymphoid cells with irregular nuclear outlines (Fig. 37-20A). The colonization of epidermis by neoplastic lymphocytes is seen (Fig. 37-20B), with small aggregates of lymphoma cells forming so-called *Pautrier microabscesses*. Later in the course of the disease, cutaneous infiltrates may become more dense and form tumor-like

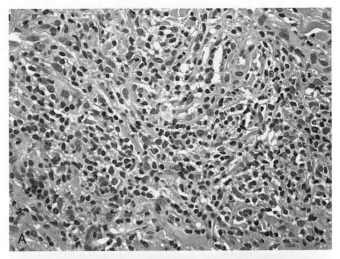

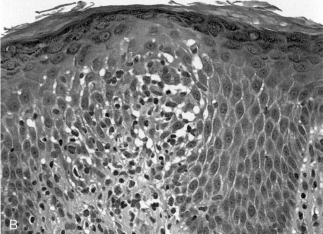

Figure 37-20 Mycosis fungoides. **A,** Dermal infiltrate of medium-sized lymphoid cells with angulated nuclei (hematoxylin and eosin, ×400). **B,** Neoplastic lymphocytes invading the epidermis (hematoxylin and eosin, ×400).

foci. The involvement of regional lymph nodes also may be present.

The immunophenotype is similar to that of T lymphocytes normally present in the skin. The expression of pan-T cell markers CD3, CD5, and CD2 is seen along with CD4 antigen. An important feature, rarely seen in benign lymphoid infiltrates, is the absence of CD7 antigen. The T cell receptor gene is clonally rearranged.

The morphologic, cytologic, and immunophenotypic features of Sézary syndrome are similar. In Sézary syndrome, lymphoma cells can be detected in the peripheral blood.

Clinical Features and Prognosis.   The average age at presentation is 55 to 60 years. The incidence of mycosis fungoides, however, increases with age. The survival of patients with early stage disease is excellent because the progression and development of disseminated lymphoma is very slow.[26] In this patient group, 10-year disease-specific survival was 97% to 98%. In most cases, only local treatment is necessary. In contrast, Sézary syndrome is an aggressive lymphoma with a low (33%) 5-year survival rate.

Peripheral T Cell Lymphoma, Unspecified

Definition. Peripheral T cell lymphoma, unspecified, comprises a morphologically heterogeneous group of lymphomas with mature T cell phenotype.

Morphology and Immunophenotype. Lymph node involvement is usually diffuse. In many cases, a prominent vascular proliferation is seen. The cytologic features range from medium-sized to large cells with atypical and occasionally pleomorphic nuclei (Fig. 37-21). Certain variants show a considerable admixture of reactive small lymphocytes, immunoblasts, histiocytes, and eosinophils. Most cases are derived from CD4$^+$ T cells and retain this immunophenotype. Variable loss of pan-T cell antigens, including CD7, is seen.

Clinical Features and Prognosis. Peripheral T cell lymphoma is an aggressive disease occurring predominantly in older adults (average age 60 years). Generalized lymphadenopathy and a variety of constitutional symptoms, such as fever, night sweats, weight loss, and pancytopenia, are present at diagnosis. The 3-year survival is reported to be approximately 40%.[27] Biologic features and advanced stage at presentation contribute to the dismal prognosis. Additionally, few treatment regimens have been developed specifically for T cell lymphomas; aggressive B cell lymphoma protocols are commonly used to treat these disorders.

Anaplastic Large Cell Lymphoma

Definition. Although a considerable morphologic variability can be seen in this entity, the typical case of anaplastic large cell lymphoma comprises large atypical cells with pleomorphic nuclei and abundant cytoplasm. The expression of CD30 antigen and ALK protein is seen in most cases.

Morphology and Immunophenotype. Numerous morphologic variants have been described. The lymph node architecture is most often diffusely effaced by malignant lymphoid cells (Fig. 37-22). Occasionally, lymph node involvement may be partial with characteristic infiltrates of nodal sinuses. Regardless of the histologic variant, in almost every case, at least a proportion of cells are large with abundant cytoplasm and pleomorphic, frequently multilobulated nuclei.

CD30 antigen and, in most cases, ALK protein are defining immunophenotypic features of this lymphoma. The overexpression of ALK is most often due to t(2;5)(p23;35), between the *ALK* and nucleophosmin genes. Alternative partner genes for *ALK* translocation also have been identified. Although the cytotoxic T cell origin of this lymphoma is indisputable, pan-T cell markers (CD3, CD7, CD5) are often negative. The most commonly expressed T cell lineage-specific antigens are CD4 and CD2 and cytotoxic antigens TIA-1, granzyme, and perforin.[28] Pan-hematopoietic antigen CD45 is expressed only in a proportion of cases (Table 37-4). In cases negative for the T cell–specific antigens and ALK protein, the demonstration of clonal T cell receptor gene rearrangement is pivotal in making the diagnosis.

Clinical Features and Prognosis. Although, similar to other T cell lymphomas, this disease is infrequent in adults, it is one of the most common lymphomas in the pediatric population, representing 10% to 15% of childhood lymphomas. Anaplastic large cell lymphoma presents as disseminated nodal disease with constitutional symptoms. Extranodal sites including skin also can be involved, however. The most important prognostic feature is the expression of ALK protein. ALK$^+$ cases show favorable prognosis, whereas ALK$^-$ disease shows survival rates comparable to peripheral T cell lymphoma, unspecified.

Hodgkin Lymphoma

Hodgkin lymphoma can be divided into two broad categories—nodular lymphocyte-predominant Hodgkin lymphoma and classical Hodgkin lymphoma.[1] Although both disorders

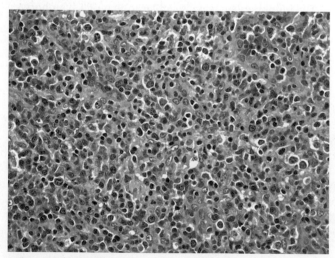

Figure 37-21 Peripheral T cell lymphoma showing heterogeneous population of small, medium-sized, and large lymphoid cells (hematoxylin and eosin, ×500).

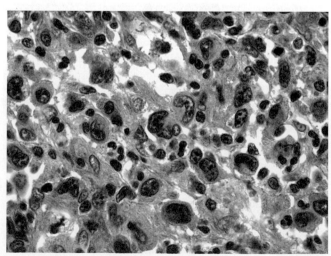

Figure 37-22 Anaplastic large cell lymphoma with large pleomorphic cells (hematoxylin and eosin, ×1000).

TABLE 37-4 Immunophenotypic Features of Lymphomas Composed of Large Lymphoid Cells

Antigen	NLPHL	Classical HL	DLBCL	ALCL
CD30	–	+	+/–	+
CD15	–	+	–	–
CD45	+	–	+	+/–
CD20	+	+/–*	+	–
CD3	–	–	–	–/+†

*If positive, the immunoreactivity is weak and present only in a proportion of neoplastic cells.
†Other T cell markers, such as CD2 and CD4, are more often present.
ALCL, anaplastic large cell lymphoma; DLBCL, diffuse large B cell lymphoma; HL, Hodgkin lymphoma; NLPHL, nodular lymphocyte-predominant Hodgkin lymphoma.

occur preferentially in young individuals and share certain morphologic characteristics, more recent studies have shown that they are biologically distinct entities, and they are discussed separately.

Nodular Lymphocyte-Predominant Hodgkin Lymphoma

Definition. Nodular lymphocyte-predominant Hodgkin lymphoma is a B cell neoplasm composed of relatively rare neoplastic cells (lymphocytic/histiocytic or "popcorn" cells) scattered within nodules of reactive lymphocytes.

Morphology and Immunophenotype. Normal architecture of a lymph node is replaced by a nodular proliferation of small lymphocytes and scattered lymphocytic/histiocytic or popcorn cells (Fig. 37-23). The latter represent the neoplastic cell of nodular lymphocyte-predominant Hodgkin lymphoma. These are large lymphoid cells with abundant cytoplasm and vesicular multilobated nuclei ("popcorn" nuclei). The nucleoli are inconspicuous.

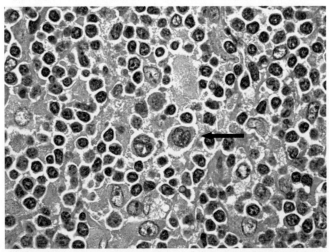

Figure 37-23 Characteristic popcorn (lymphocytic/histiocytic) cells of nodular lymphocyte-predominant Hodgkin lymphoma *(arrow)* (hematoxylin and eosin, ×1000).

The lymphocytic/histiocytic cells are positive for B cell markers, including CD20 antigen (see Table 37-4). These cells are of germinal center cell origin[29]; they express BCL-6 and immunoglobulin chains. The neoplastic cells do not show evidence of EBV infection. The surrounding nodular background is composed of CD20⁺ small B cells and scattered T lymphocytes.

Clinical Features and Prognosis. Most patients are males in their 30s and present with localized disease. Mostly peripheral lymph nodes are involved, and mediastinal lymphadenopathy is rare. As in classical Hodgkin lymphoma, the prognosis is excellent, with survival rates of 80% to 90% in the early stages of the disease.[30]

Classical Hodgkin Lymphoma

Definition. Classical Hodgkin lymphoma comprises a group of heterogeneous germinal center cell disorders.[31] Classical Hodgkin is characterized by the presence of relatively few diagnostic neoplastic cells, Reed-Sternberg cells, in a rich reactive background. The incidence of this disease varies in different geographic regions; in the United States and Europe, it is a common form of lymphoma occurring in young adults. In the United States, approximately 7400 new cases are diagnosed annually.[5] A bimodal age distribution is observed with incidence peaks between 15 and 34 years and older than 54 years.

Morphology and Immunophenotype. On the basis of architectural features, the composition of the reactive background, and relative proportion of neoplastic cells, classical Hodgkin lymphoma can be divided into four subtypes (Table 37-5), as follows:

1. Nodular sclerosis
2. Mixed cellularity
3. Lymphocyte rich
4. Lymphocyte depleted

Despite distinct morphologic characteristics and clinical features, all subtypes share Reed-Sternberg cells with an identical phenotype arising from the germinal center. The classic Reed-Sternberg cell is a large lymphoid cell with a bilobed nucleus or two nuclei with prominent eosinophilic nucleoli and abundant cytoplasm (Fig. 37-24A). When encountered in an appropriate background, Reed-Sternberg cells are pathognomonic for the diagnosis. However, neoplastic cells in classical Hodgkin lymphoma show a striking cytologic variability, and several variants of Reed-Sternberg cells are often encountered in a single lymph node. The most important are Hodgkin cells, mummified cells, and lacunar cells.

Hodgkin cells are mononuclear cells with cytologic features similar to those of Reed-Sternberg cells; large lymphoid cells with oval nucleus, thick nuclear membrane, distinct eosinophilic nucleolus, and abundant cytoplasm. Mummified cells are degenerated or apoptotic cells with pyknotic nucleus and condensed cytoplasm. Lacunar cells occur predominantly in the nodular sclerosis variant of classical Hodgkin lymphoma and are characterized by a lobated nucleus and artifactual

TABLE 37-5 Morphologic Subtypes of Classical Hodgkin Lymphoma

Subtype	Neoplastic Cells	Additional Morphologic Features
Nodular sclerosis	RS cells; Hodgkin cells; lacunar cells	Fibrotic bands; background of small lymphocytes, histiocytes, and eosinophils
Mixed cellularity	RS cells; Hodgkin cells	Background of small lymphocytes, eosinophils, neutrophils, histiocytes, plasma cells; no fibrotic bands
Lymphocyte rich	RS cells; Hodgkin cells	Diffuse nodular background of small lymphocytes; no or few eosinophils and neutrophils
Lymphocyte depleted	RS cells; Hodgkin cells	Numerous RS cells and Hodgkin lymphoma cells; few background lymphocytes

RS, Reed-Sternberg.

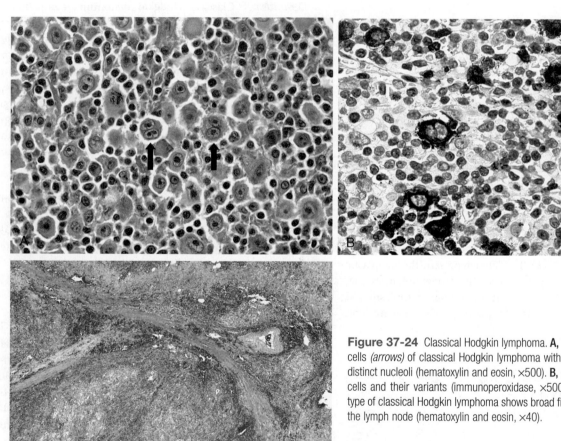

Figure 37-24 Classical Hodgkin lymphoma. **A,** Typical Reed-Sternberg cells *(arrows)* of classical Hodgkin lymphoma with two nuclear lobes and distinct nucleoli (hematoxylin and eosin, ×500). **B,** CD30⁺ Reed-Sternberg cells and their variants (immunoperoxidase, ×500). **C,** Nodular sclerosis type of classical Hodgkin lymphoma shows broad fibrotic bands dissecting the lymph node (hematoxylin and eosin, ×40).

retraction of the cytoplasm secondary to formalin fixation. Because of this artifact, the cells appear to be situated in a clear space (i.e., lacuna).

In all subtypes of classical Hodgkin lymphoma, Reed-Sternberg cells and their variants have a similar immunophenotype (see Table 37-4). They are CD30⁺ in all cases (Fig. 37-24B) and CD15⁺ in approximately 80% of cases. Even in positive cases, however, CD15 immunoreactivity may be weak and seen only in a few malignant cells. The expression of B cell markers including CD20 is weak to absent. Similarly, CD45 antigen is negative. The frequency of EBV infection depends on the subtype of classical Hodgkin lymphoma. The background small lymphocytes are predominantly CD4⁺ T cells.

Nodular Sclerosis Classical Hodgkin Lymphoma. The defining feature of nodular sclerosis subtype is the presence of broad collagen bands with thickening of the nodal capsule

(Fig. 37-24C) and lacunar cells. The background cellularity includes small lymphocytes, eosinophils, and histiocytes. This is the most common of all the subtypes of classical Hodgkin lymphoma, accounting for 70% of the cases. The frequency of immunohistochemically demonstrable EBV infection is lowest in this variant.

Mixed Cellularity Classical Hodgkin Lymphoma. In this subtype, Reed-Sternberg cells and their variants are scattered among the diffuse background proliferation of small lymphocytes, histiocytes, eosinophils, neutrophils, and plasma cells. Typical Reed-Sternberg cells, mononuclear Hodgkin cells, and mummified cells are seen; however, lacunar cells are absent. Similarly, fibrotic bands and capsular thickening are not seen. Approximately 20% of classical Hodgkin lymphomas show this morphology. The association with EBV infection is seen in 75% of cases.

Lymphocyte-Rich Classical Hodgkin Lymphoma. Most commonly, scattered mononuclear Hodgkin and Reed-Sternberg cells are seen along with a vaguely nodular architecture composed of small lymphocytes. Compared with other subtypes of classical Hodgkin lymphoma, the background cellularity is less heterogeneous.

Lymphocyte-Depleted Classical Hodgkin Lymphoma. This is an uncommon variant of classical Hodgkin lymphoma occurring predominantly in immunodeficient patients. There is a paucity of cells of reactive background, and neoplastic Reed-Sternberg cells and their variants are much more common. In most cases, neoplastic cells show evidence of EBV infection.

Clinical Features and Prognosis. With the exception of the lymphocyte rich variant, which occurs in a slightly older population, classical Hodgkin lymphoma is a disease of young adults with peak incidence at 15-35 years. Mostly peripheral lymph nodes are involved with the exception of the nodular sclerosis variant, which often shows mediastinal lymphadenopathy. Contemporary treatment protocols combine chemotherapy and radiotherapy to reach survival and cure rates of 80% to 90% depending on the stage of the disease, patient age, and clinical symptoms. The best prognosis is seen in the nodular sclerosis subtype. Lymphocyte depleted Hodgkin lymphoma is the most aggressive variant of classical Hodgkin lymphoma, especially in HIV-positive patients. In this patient group, Hodgkin lymphoma also may manifest in unusual extranodal sites, including bone marrow. Patients with classical Hodgkin lymphoma treated with a combination of chemotherapy and radiotherapy are at high risk of developing secondary malignancies, including lung and breast carcinomas and acute leukemia.

CHAPTER at a GLANCE

- Histologic components of normal lymph nodes include the cortex, paracortex, medullary cords, and sinuses. These are structural and functional compartments from which reactive hyperplasias and malignant disorders originate.
- Lymphomas are neoplastic lesions of the lymphoid system arising at specific stages of differentiation of normal lymphoid cells.
- Modern lymphoma classification incorporates morphologic, immunophenotypic, molecular, and clinical characteristics.
- Lymphomas are broadly divided into precursor and mature lesions and B cell and T cell neoplasms.
- The most common mature B cell lymphomas are follicular and diffuse large B cell subtypes.
- T cell neoplasms most common in the United States and Europe are peripheral T cell lymphoma, unspecified, and anaplastic large cell lymphoma.
- In CLL, the peripheral blood and bone marrow display smudge cells and small lymphoid cells with coarse chromatin, inconspicuous nucleoli and scant cytoplasm.
- In HCL, small B-lymphocytes have abundant cytoplasm and fine cytoplasmic projections.

- Hodgkin lymphoma has been shown to be of B cell origin.
- Hodgkin lymphoma is subclassified based on morphologic and immunophenotypic features.
- B cell and T cell lymphomas and Hodgkin lymphoma involve mainly lymph nodes; however, extranodal sites and bone marrow/peripheral blood involvement also occur with varying frequency.
- In general, lymphomas occur in elderly individuals; however, specific subtypes such as Hodgkin lymphoma show a predilection for younger age groups.
- The prognosis depends on lymphoma subtype. Indolent lymphomas show a protracted course but are largely incurable with current chemotherapeutic regimens. In contrast, although aggressive lymphomas have a more progressive course, the cure rates are higher.

Now that you have completed this chapter, go back and read again the case study at the beginning and respond to the questions presented.

REVIEW QUESTIONS

1. The diagnosis of lymphoma relies most heavily on all of the following *except*:
   a. Microscopic examination of affected lymph nodes
   b. Immunophenotyping using immunohistochemistry or flow cytometry
   c. Molecular/cytogenetic analysis
   d. Peripheral blood findings in a complete blood count

2. The most common lymphoma occurring in young adults is:
   a. Follicular lymphoma
   b. DLBCL
   c. Hodgkin lymphoma
   d. Mycosis fungoides

3. In a normal lymph node, the medulla includes predominantly:
   a. T cells
   b. B cells
   c. Tingible body macrophages
   d. Plasma cells

4. t(11;14) is the defining feature of:
   a. Follicular lymphoma
   b. Hodgkin lymphoma
   c. CLL
   d. Mantle cell lymphoma

5. The immunophenotype associated with mycosis fungoides is:
   a. Normal T cell immunophenotype
   b. Abnormal T cell immunophenotype with expression of CD4 and loss of CD7 antigen
   c. A mix of CD4+ and CD8+ T cells
   d. Abnormal T cell immunophenotype with expression of CD8 and loss of CD7 antigen

6. What is the major morphologic difference between Hodgkin and other B cell lymphomas?
   a. The extent of the lymph node involvement
   b. The presence of numerous reactive lymphocytes and only a few malignant cells in Hodgkin lymphoma
   c. The presence of numerous tingible body macrophages in Hodgkin lymphoma
   d. The preservation of normal lymph node architecture in Hodgkin lymphoma

7. Which morphologic diagnosis has to be confirmed with molecular studies for the presence of t(8;14)?
   a. Mantle cell lymphoma
   b. Burkitt lymphoma
   c. Follicular lymphoma
   d. Sézary Syndrome

8. What is the function of the germinal center?
   a. Generation of B cells producing immunoglobulins with the highest affinity for a particular antigen through the process of somatic mutations
   b. Production of plasma cells that secrete specific immunoglobulins following antigenic stimulation
   c. T cell maturation follwing their education in the thymus
   d. Generation of dendritic cells with unique antigen processing abilities

9. Marked paracortical expansion is most often associated with:
   a. Rheumatoid arthritis
   b. Syphilis
   c. Dermatopathic lymphadenopathy
   d. Follicular lymphoma

10. MGUS is best described as:
   a. The presence of monoclonal immunoglobulin in serum with only mild bone marrow plasmacytosis (<10% of plasma cells)
   b. The presence of monoclonal serum or urine immunoglobulin with significant bone marrow plasmacytosis
   c. The presence of significant bone marrow plasmacytosis in a patient with only a few clinical symptoms of plasma cell myeloma
   d. The presence of monoclonal immunoglobulin in a patient with a solitary mass composed of plasma cells

REFERENCES

1. Jaffe ES, Harris NL, Stein H, et al (eds): World Health Organization Classification of Tumours: Pathology and Genetics of Tumours of Haematopoietic and Lymphoid Tissues. Lyon: IARC Press, 2001.
2. MacLennan IC: Germinal centers. Annu Rev Immunol 1994;12:117-139.
3. Manser T: Textbook germinal centers? J Immunol 2004; 172:3369-3375.
4. Herman GE, Chlipala E, Bochenski G, et al: Zinc formalin fixative for automated tissue processing. J Histotechnol 1988;11:85-89.
5. Greenlee RT, Hill-Harmon MB, Murray T, et al: Cancer statistics, 2001. CA Cancer J Clin 2001;51:15-36.
6. Filipovich AH, Mathur A, Kamat D, et al: Primary immunodeficiencies: genetic risk factors for lymphoma. Cancer Res 1992;52(19 Suppl):5465s-5467s.
7. Mueller N: Overview of the epidemiology of malignancy in immune deficiency. J Acquir Immune Defic Syndr 1999;21 (Suppl 1):S5-S10.
8. Fisher SF, Fisher RI: The epidemiology of non-Hodgkin's lymphoma. Oncogene 2004;23:6524-6534.
9. The Non-Hodgkin's Lymphoma Classification Project: A clinical evaluation of the International Lymphoma Study Group Classification of Non-Hodgkin's Lymphoma. Blood 1997;89:3909-3918.
10. Pileri SA, Sabattini E, Agostinelli C, et al: Histopathology of B-cell chronic lymphocytic leukemia. Hematol Oncol Clin N Am 2004;18:807-826.
11. Stilgenbauer S, Bullinger L, Lichter P, et al: Review: genetics of chronic lymphocytic leukemia: genomic aberrations and VH gene mutation status in pathogenesis and clinical course. Leukemia 2002;16:993-1007.

12. Guidelines on the diagnosis and management of chronic lymphocytic leukaemia. Br J Haematol 2004;125:294-317.

13. Swerdlow SH, Williams ME: From centrocytic to mantle cell lymphoma: a clinicopathologic and molecular review of 3 decades. Hum Pathol 2002;33:7-20.

14. Horsman DE, Gascoyne RD, Coupland RW, et al: Comparison of cytogenetic analysis, southern analysis, and polymerase chain reaction for the detection of t(14;18) in follicular lymphoma. Am J Clin Pathol 1995;103:472-478.

15. Thieblemont C, Berger F, Coiffier B: Mucosa-associated lymphoid tissue lymphomas. Curr Opin Oncol 1995;7:415-420.

16. Parsonnet J, Isaacson P: Bacterial infection and MALT lymphoma. N Engl J Med 2004;350:213-215.

17. Dierlamm J, Baens M, Wlodarska I, et al: The apoptosis inhibitor gene AP12 and a novel 18q gene, MLT, are recurrently rearranged in the t(11;18)(q21;q21) associated with mucosa-associated lymphoid tissue lymphomas. Blood 1999;93:3601-3609.

18. Thieblemont C, Berger F, Dumontet C, et al: Mucosa-associated lymphoid tissue lymphoma is a disseminated disease in one third of 158 patients analyzed. Blood 2000;95:802-806.

19. Kyle RA, Therneau TM, Rajkumar SV, et al: Long-term follow-up of 241 patients with monoclonal gammopathy of undetermined significance: the original Mayo Clinic series 25 years later. Mayo Clin Proc 2004;79:859-866.

20. Kyle RA, Rajkumar SV: Multiple myeloma. N Engl J Med 2004;351:1860-1873.

21. Harris NL, Jaffe ES, Stein H, et al: A revised European-American classification of lymphoid neoplasms: a proposal from the International Lymphoma Study Group. Blood 1994;84:1361-1392.

22. Alizadeh AA, Eisen MB, Davis RE, et al: Distinct types of diffuse large B-cell lymphoma identified by gene expression profiling. Nature 2000;403:503-511.

23. Blum KA, Lozanski G, Byrd JC: Adult Burkitt leukemia and lymphoma. Blood 2004;104:3009-3020.

24. Cairo MS, Sposto R, Perkins SL, et al: Burkitt's and Burkitt-like lymphoma in children and adolescents: a review of the Children's Cancer Group experience. Br J Haematol 2003;120:660-670.

25. Clark DM, Boylston AW, Hall PA, et al: Antibodies to T cell antigen receptor beta chain families detect monoclonal T cell proliferation. Lancet 1986;2:835-837.

26. Fink-Puches R, Zenahlik P, Bäck B, et al: Primary cutaneous lymphomas: applicability of current classification schemes (European Organization for Research and Treatment of Cancer, World Health Organization) based on clinicopathologic features observed in a large group of patients. Blood 2002;99:800-805.

27. Escalon MP, Liu NS, Yang Y, et al: Prognostic factors and treatment of patients with T-cell non-Hodgkin lymphoma. Cancer 2005;103:2091-2098.

28. Foss HD, Anagnostopoulos I, Araujo I, et al: Anaplastic large-cell lymphomas of T-cell and null-cell phenotype express cytotoxic molecules. Blood 1996;88:4005-4011.

29. Braeuninger A, Kuppers R, Strickler JG, et al: Hodgkin and Reed-Sternberg cells in lymphocyte predominant Hodgkin disease represent clonal populations of germinal center-derived tumor B cells. Proc Natl Acad Sci U S A 1997;94:9337-9342.

30. Diehl V, Sextro M, Franklin J, et al: Clinical presentation, course, and prognostic factors in lymphocyte-predominant Hodgkin's disease and lymphocyte-rich classical Hodgkin's disease: report from the European Task Force on Lymphoma Project on Lymphocyte-Predominant Hodgkin's Disease. J Clin Oncol 1999;17:776-783.

31. Thomas RK, Re D, Wolf J, et al: Part I: Hodgkin's lymphoma—molecular biology of Hodgkin and Reed-Sternberg cells. Lancet Oncol 2004;5:11-18.

38

Pediatric and Geriatric Hematology

Roslyn McQueen

OUTLINE

Pediatric Hematology
Geriatric Hematology

OBJECTIVES

After completion of this chapter, the reader will be able to:

1. Describe the major differences in normal complete blood count values, reticulocytes, and nucleated red blood cells (NRBCs) among preterm newborns, full-term newborns, infants, children, adults, and elderly adults.
2. Explain the cause of physiologic anemia of infancy and the time frame in which it is expected.
3. Compare the RBC survival of preterm and full-term infants with that of adults.
4. Recognize and list factors affecting sample collection that can have an impact on the interpretation of newborn hematology values.
5. Compare and contrast the morphology of the lymphocytes of children and adults and reasons for differences.

6. State the general association of age with hemoglobin levels in the elderly.
7. Explain the clinical significance of anemia in the elderly.
8. Name the two most common anemias seen in the elderly and their common etiologies in this age group.
9. List other anemias affecting elderly individuals.
10. Compare the frequency of acute lymphocytic leukemias versus chronic lymphoblastic leukemias between children and the elderly.
11. Name malignancies of hematologic cells that are more common in the elderly than other age groups.

CASE STUDY

After studying this chapter, the reader should be able to respond to the following case study:

A full-term newborn infant in no apparent distress had a CBC performed as part of a panel of testing for infants born to mothers who received no prenatal care. Results included Hb 18.5 g/dL, HCT 55.5% and RBC 5.28×10^{12}/L. There were 7 NRBCs. RBC morphology was reported as macrocytic with slight to moderate polychromasia. The WBC count was 18×10^9/L with 50% neutrophils and 50% lymphocytes.

1. Are the results of the hemoglobin and hematocrit within limits expected for a newborn?
2. What is the significance of the elevated MCV, NRBCs, and polychromasia?
3. Comment on the WBC and differential count.

Hematologic values are fairly stable throughout adult life, but significant differences exist in the pediatric, and to some extent, in the geriatric populations. This chapter focuses on the more significant differences.

PEDIATRIC HEMATOLOGY

Children are not merely "small adults." The newborn infant, older child, and adult all exhibit profound hematologic dif-

ferences. Because children mature at different rates, it is inappropriate to use adult reference ranges for the assessment of pediatric blood values. Historically, pediatric reference values were inferentially assessed from adult data because of the limitations in attaining analyzable data. Pediatric procedures required large blood draws and tedious methodologies and lacked standardization. The implementation of child-friendly phlebotomy techniques and micropediatric procedures has revolutionized laboratory testing. Pediatric hematology has emerged as a specialized science with age-specific reference ranges that correlate the hematopoietic, immunologic, and chemical changes of a developing child.

Dramatic changes occur in the blood and bone marrow of the newborn infant during the first hours and days after birth, and there are rapid fluctuations in the quantities of all hematologic elements. There are significant hematologic differences between term and preterm infants and among newborns, infants, young children, and older children. Hematopoiesis is discussed in detail in Chapter 7. This chapter reviews neonatal hematopoiesis as a prerequisite to understanding the changes in pediatric hematologic reference ranges, morphologic features, and age-specific physiology.

Neonatal Hematopoiesis

Hematopoiesis, the formation and development of blood cells from stem cells, begins in the first weeks of embryonic development and proceeds systematically through three phases of development: mesoblastic (yolk sac), hepatic (liver), and myeloid (bone marrow). The first cells produced in the developing embryo are primitive erythroblasts formed in the yolk sac. These cells are particularly interesting because they do not develop into mature erythrocytes. They are erythropoietin insensitive and have the ability to differentiate into other cell lines on exposure to appropriate growth factors.[1-6]

By the second month of gestation, hematopoiesis ceases in the yolk sac, and the liver becomes the center for hematopoiesis, reaching its peak activity during the third and fourth gestational months. Leukocytes of each cell type systematically make their appearance. In week 9 of gestation, lymphocytes can be detected in the region of the thymus. They are subsequently found in the spleen and lymph nodes. During the fourth and fifth gestational months, the bone marrow emerges as a major site of blood cell production, and it becomes the major site by birth (Chapter 7).[1-6]

Hematopoiesis of the Newborn

Hematopoietically active bone marrow is referred to as *red marrow*, as opposed to inactive yellow (fatty) marrow. At the time of birth, the bone marrow is fully active and extremely cellular with all hematopoietic cell lineages undergoing cellular differentiation and amplification. In addition to the mature cells in fetal blood, there are significant numbers of circulating progenitor cells in cord blood.[7,8]

In a full-term infant, hepatic hematopoiesis has ceased except in widely scattered small foci that become inactive soon after birth.[1-6] Postembryonic extramedullary hematopoiesis is abnormal in a full-term infant. In a premature infant, foci of hematopoiesis are frequently seen in the liver and occasionally observed in the spleen, lymph nodes, or thymus.[1-10]

Pediatric Developmental Stages

Pediatric hematologic values change markedly in the first weeks and months of life. As a result, many variables influence the interpretation of what might be considered normal values at the time of birth. It is important to provide age-appropriate pediatric hematology values that span from neonatal life through adolescence. The pediatric population can be divided into three different developmental groups: (1) the neonatal period, which represents the first 4 weeks of life; (2) infancy, which incorporates the first year of life; and (3) childhood, which spans from age 1 to puberty (age 8-12 years).

Preterm, low-birth-weight infants are more apt to develop more health problems than other newborns. Since the 1990s, the rising quality of medical care in neonatal intensive care units has improved markedly the survival of smaller infants born at younger gestational ages with less mature hematopoietic systems.

Gestational Age and Birth Weight

Hematologic values obtained from full-term infants generally do not apply to preterm infants, and laboratory values for low-birth-weight preterm infants differ from ranges for extremely-low-birth-weight "micropreemies" (24-26 weeks' gestation).[11] A full-term infant is characterized as an infant who has completed 37 to 42 weeks of gestation. Infants born before 37 weeks are referred to as *premature* or *preterm*, whereas infants delivered after 42 weeks are considered *post-term*.[11,12] Infants can be subcategorized further by birth weights as (1) appropriate for gestational age; (2) small for gestational age, including low-birth-weight infants (≤2500 g); (3) very-low-birth-weight infants (≤1500 g); (4) extremely-low-birth-weight "micropreemies" (24-26 weeks' gestation with birth weight 500 g); and (5) large for gestational age (post-term infants).[11]

Hematologic Values at Birth

Neonatal hematologic values are affected by the gestational age of the infant, the age in hours after delivery, illness, and the level of support required. Other variables to be considered when evaluating laboratory data include site of sampling and technique (capillary versus venous, warm or un-warmed extremity), timing of sampling, and conditions such as the conduct of labor and the treatment of the umbilical vessels.[11,13,14]

As with all laboratory testing, each laboratory should establish reference intervals based on its instrumentation, methods, and patient population (Chapter 5). This section presents representative age-specific ranges and discusses significant morphologic features of erythrocytes, leukocytes, and platelets for full-term and preterm infants.

Red Blood Cell Count

Full-Term Infants.   At birth, the mean red blood cell (RBC) count for a full-term infant is 4.6×10^{12}/L to 6.1×10^{12}/L (Refer to the inside cover).[16]

Preterm/Premature Infants.   At day 3, the RBC range for preterm infants is 3.2×10^{12}/L to 5.3×10^{12}/L.[16]

Childhood to Adolescence.   At the end of the first year of life, the mean RBC count is 3.74×10^{12}/L to 4.94×10^{12}/L.[17] The adult mean values usually are attained by 14 years of age— 4.6×10^{12}/L to 6.0×10^{12}/L for males and 5.4×10^{12}/L for females (refer to the inside cover).

The RBC count increases during the first 24 hours of life, remains at this plateau for about 2 weeks, and then slowly declines. This elevation may be explained by the partial in utero anoxia that becomes more progressive as the fetus grows. Anoxia, the trigger for increased secretion of erythropoietin, stimulates erythropoiesis.[18,19] At birth, the physiologic environment changes, and the fetus makes the transition from its placenta-dependent oxygenation to the increased tissue oxygenation of the lungs.

After this brisk elevation, there is a continuous decline in the number of RBCs. The mechanism may be a decrease in the secretion of erythropoietin.[18-20] Studies show erythropoietin levels before birth equal to or greater than adult levels with gradual drops to near zero a few weeks after birth.[15,18-20] This corresponds with the physiologic anemia seen at 5 to 8 weeks of life. The life span of erythrocytes in full-term infants is shorter than that of adult erythrocytes; the life span of RBCs in premature infants is considerably shorter. The more immature the infant, the greater the degree of reduction.[1,18-22]

Erythrocyte Morphology of the Neonate

Early normoblasts are megaloblastic, hypochromic, and irregularly shaped.[1,2,13-18] During hepatic hematopoiesis, normoblasts are smaller than the megaloblasts of the yolk sac but are still macrocytic. Erythrocyte morphology remains macrocytic from the first 11 weeks of gestation until day 5 of postnatal life (Fig. 38-1).[1,2,13-18]

The macrocytic RBC morphology gradually changes to the characteristic normocytic, normochromic morphology.[1,2,13-16] Orthochromic normoblasts frequently are observed in the full-term infant on the first day of life but disappear within postnatal days 3 to 5. Nucleated RBCs (NRBCs) may persist longer than a week in immature infants. The average number of NRBCs ranges from 3 to 10 per 100 white blood cells (WBCs) for a normal full-term infant compared with 25 nucleated RBCs per 100 WBCs in a premature infant. The presence of nucleated RBCs for more than 5 days suggests hemolysis, hypoxic stress, or acute infection.[1,2,6,13-16,18-21]

Reticulocytes

An apparent reticulocytosis exists during gestation, decreasing from 90% reticulocytes at 12 weeks' gestation, to 15% at 6 months, and ultimately to 4% to 6% at birth. Reticulocytosis persists for about 3 days, then declines abruptly to 0.8% on postnatal days 4 to 7. At 2 months, the number of reticulocytes increases slightly, followed by a slight decline from 3 months to 2 years, when adult levels are attained.[1,2,6,13-16,18-21]

Premature Infants.   The reticulocyte counts of premature infants are inversely proportional to their gestational age, with a mean reticulocyte count of 5% at 32 weeks' gestation and 3.2% at term.[15] Significant polychromasia is seen on a Wright-stained blood smear, reflective of the postnatal reticulocytosis (Fig. 38-2).

Hemoglobin

Full-Term Infants.   Hemoglobin synthesis results from an orderly evolution of a series of embryonic, fetal, and adult hemoglobins. See Chapter 10 for an in-depth discussion of the ontogeny, structure, and types of hemoglobins. The hemoglobin level fluctuates dramatically in the weeks and months after birth as a result of physiologic changes, and various factors must be considered when analyzing pediatric hematologic values. The site of sampling, gestational age, and the time interval between delivery and clamping of the umbilical cord can influence the hemoglobin level in newborn infants.[1,2,6,9-11,13] There are significant differences between capillary and venous blood hemoglobin levels. Capillary samples in newborns generally have a higher hemoglobin concentration than venous samples, attributed to circulatory factors,.[11,13-19]

At birth, the average hemoglobin for a full-term infant is 11.5 to 21.5 g/dL; levels less than 14 g/dL are considered abnormal.[15,18] The hemoglobin value for a small-for-gestational-age preterm infant is 17.1 g/dL, much lower than in a full-term infant; hemoglobin values less than 13.7 g/dL are considered abnormal in preterm infants.[18]

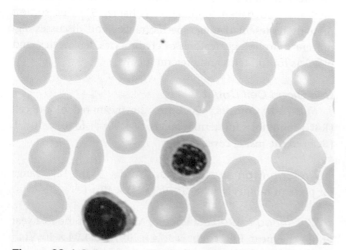

Figure 38-1 Peripheral blood film from a normal newborn demonstrating a normal lymphocyte, macrocytes, polychromasia and one nucleated RBC. (Peripheral blood ×1000).

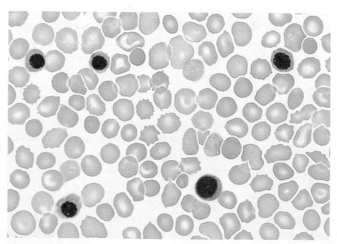

Figure 38-2 Blood film from a premature infant showing a normal lymphocyte pointer, four NRBCs, and increased polychromasia (peripheral blood, ×500).

Anemia of the Neonate. The hemoglobin concentration of term infants decreases during the first 5 to 8 weeks of life, a condition known as *physiologic anemia of infancy.* Infants born prematurely also experience a decrease in hemoglobin concentration, which is termed *physiologic anemia of prematurity.*[23-27] Additionally, the fetal RBC has a shorter life span than normal erythrocytes. Studies with chromium-labeled newborn RBCs, corrected for the elution rate of chromium from newborn cells, estimated a survival time of 60 to 80 days.[2] This physiologic anemia is not known to be associated with any abnormalities in the infant, however. The reasons for the shortened life span are unclear.

Along with hemoglobin, there is a reduction in the number of RBCs, a decrease in the reticulocyte percentages, and undetectable levels of erythropoietin (see Table 38-1). When the lungs replace the placenta as the source of oxygen, the increased oxygen saturation of the blood may generate a negative feedback response, slowing erythropoietin production[11,23-27] and erythropoiesis.[19,28,29] When the hemoglobin concentration decreases to approximately 11 g/dL, erythropoietic activity increases until it reaches its adult levels by 14 years of age.[11,23-29]

Premature Infants. The hemoglobin levels of premature infants are typically 1 g/dL or more below the values of full-term infants. Thereafter, a gradual recovery occurs, resulting in values approximating those of normal full-term infants by about 1 year of age.[15,20-25] The low-birth-weight infant (<1500 g) shows a progressive decline in hemoglobin, RBC count, mean cell volume (MCV), mean cell hemoglobin (MCH), and mean cell hemoglobin concentration (MCHC) and a slower recovery than other preterm and term infants.

Hematocrit

The average hematocrit in cord blood at birth for full-term infants is 55% (range 43% to 63%).[1,13,15,16] Frequently, newborns with increased hematocrits, especially values greater than 65%, experience hyperviscosity of the blood. This is problematic for the quality of peripheral blood smears.

The hematocrit usually increases during the first 48 postnatal hours, followed by a slow continuous decline to 46% to 62% at 2 weeks 33% to 50% between the second and fourth months. Normal adult values of 47% for males and 42% for females are achieved during adolescence.

Very-low-birth-weight preterm infants are frequently anemic at birth; many require transfusions or erythropoietin injections or both. Obladen et al[27] studied 562 very-low-birth-weight infants and showed median hematocrits of 47% on day 3, 44% on days 12 to 14, and 33% by 40 to 42 days of life (Table 38-1).

Red Blood Cell Indices

The RBC indices MCV, MCH, and MCHC provide a means for assessing and defining anemia (Chapter 18).

Mean Cell Volume. The erythrocytes of newborn infants are markedly macrocytic at birth. The average MCV for full-term infants is 110 ± 15 fL; however, a sharp decrease occurs during the first 24 hours of life. The MCV continues to decrease to 90 ± 12 fL in 3 to 4 months.[25,26] The more premature the infant, the higher the MCV. An MCV less than 94 fL in a newborn should be evaluated for α-thalassemia or iron deficiency.[1,30]

Mean Cell Hemoglobin. MCH in healthy neonates is 30 to 42 pg, and in premature infants, 27 to 41 pg.[25,26]

Mean Cell Hemoglobin Concentration. The average MCHC is the same for full-term infants, premature infants, and adults, approximately 33 g/dL.

Red Blood Cell Distribution Width. The RBC distribution width (RDW) is a measure of the variation of RBC volume, or anisocytosis. The RDW for normal full-term and preterm infants ranges from 15.2% to 18% (male) and 15.3% to 16.6% (female) compared with the normal adult range of 11.5% to 14.5%.[17]

White Blood Cell Values of the Newborn

Fluctuations in the number of WBCs are common at all ages but are greatest in infants. Leukocytosis is typical at birth for full-term and preterm infants with an average of 22×10^9/L ($9\text{-}30 \times 10^9$/L) at the first 12 hours of life.[31] There is an excess of polymorphonuclear neutrophils, bands, and occasional metamyelocytes with no evidence of disease. During the second day, the neutrophilic leukocyte count decreases progressively. By the first week, the WBC count declines to 12×10^9/L. The trend continues to 8×10^9/L to 10×10^9/L by the fourth year.[13-16]

Neutrophilic Leukocytes. Term and premature infants show a greater absolute neutrophil count than that found in older children, who characteristically maintain predominance of lymphocytes.

Full-Term Infant. Neutrophilic leukocytes account for 40% to 60% of the leukocytes at birth, decreasing to 40% by day 10, and 30% between the fourth and sixth months.[1,2,13-16] In the sixth year of life, adult values of 50% to 60% are attained (Table 38-2). The absolute number of segmented neutrophils

TABLE 38-1 Hematologic Values of Very-Low-Birth-Weight Infants During the First 6 Weeks of Life

Hematologic Value	AGE OF INFANT (DAYS)			
	3	**12-14**	**24-26**	**40-42**
Hemoglobin (g/dL)	15.6	14.4	12.4	10.6
Hematocrit (%)	47	44	39	33
RBC (10^{12}/L)	4.2	4.1	3.8	3.4
Reticulocytes (%)	7.1	1.7	1.5	1.8
Platelets (10^9/L)	203.5	318	338	357
WBC (10^9/L)	9.5	12.3	10.4	9.1

Modified from Obladen M, Diepold K, Maier RF, et al: Venous and arterial hematologic profiles of very low birth weight infants. Pediatrics 2000;106:707-711.

TABLE 38-2 Normal Leukocyte Counts for Newborn Infants*

Age	LEUKOCYTES Mean (Range)	TOTAL NEUTROPHILS Mean (Range)	%	LYMPHOCYTES Mean (Range)	%	MONOCYTES Mean	%	EOSINOPHILS Mean	%
Birth	18.1 (9.0-30.0)	11.0 (6.0-26.0)	61	5.5 (2.0-11.0)	31	1.1	6	0.4	2
12 h	22.8 (13.0-38.0)	15.5 (6.0-28.0)	68	5.5 (2.0-11.0)	24	1.2	5	0.5	2
24 h	18.9 (9.4-34.0)	11.5 (5.0-21.0)	61	5.8 (2.0-11.5)	31	1.1	6	0.5	2
1 wk	12.2 (5.0-21.0)	5.5 (1.5-10.0)	45	5.0 (2.0-17.0)	41	1.1	9	0.5	4
2 wk	11.4 (5.0-20.0)	4.5 (1.0-9.5)	40	5.5 (2.0-17.0)	48	1.0	9	0.4	3
1 mo	10.8 (5.0-19.5)	3.8 (1.0-9.0)	35	6.0 (2.5-16.5)	56	0.7	7	0.3	3
6 mo	11.9 (6.0-17.5)	3.8 (1.0-8.5)	32	7.3 (4.0-13.5)	61	0.6	5	0.3	3
1 y	11.4 (6.0-17.5)	3.5 (1.5-8.5)	31	7.0 (4.0-10.5)	61	0.6	5	0.3	3
2 y	10.6 (6.0-17.0)	3.5 (1.5-8.5)	33	6.3 (3.0-9.5)	59	0.5	5	0.3	3
4 y	9.1 (5.5-15.5)	3.8 (1.5-8.5)	42	4.5 (2.0-8.0)	50	0.5	5	0.3	3
6 y	8.5 (5.0-14.5)	4.3 (1.5-8.0)	51	3.5 (1.5-7.0)	42	0.4	5	0.2	3
8 y	8.3 (4.5-13.5)	4.4 (1.5-8.0)	53	3.3 (1.5-6.8)	39	0.4	4	0.2	2
10 y	8.1 (4.5-13.5)	4.4 (1.8-8.0)	54	3.1 (1.5-6.5)	38	0.4	4	0.2	2
16 y	7.8 (4.5-13.0)	4.4 (1.8-8.0)	57	2.8 (1.2-5.2)	35	0.4	5	0.2	3
21 y	7.4 (4.5-11.0)	4.4 (1.8-7.7)	59	2.5 (1.0-4.8)	34	0.3	4	0.2	3

*Numbers of leukocytes are in thousands per μL, ranges are estimates of 95% confidence limits, and percentages refer to differential counts. Neutrophils include band cells at all ages and a small number of metamyelocytes and myelocytes in the first few days of life.
From Dallman PR: In Rudolph AM (ed): Reference Ranges for Leukocyte Counts, Pediatrics, 16th ed. New York: Appleton-Century-Crofts, 1977:1178.

in full-term and preterm infants ranges from 3.5×10^9/L to 6×10^9/L at birth, which increases abruptly after 12 hours ($8.5\text{-}15 \times 10^9$/L) and returns to baseline by 48 hours (Table 38-3).[32-34]

Premature Infants. At birth, preterm infants exhibit a "left shift" with promyelocytes and myelocytes frequently observed. The trend to lymphocyte predominance occurs later than in term infants. Neutrophil counts in premature infants are similar to or slightly lower than the neutrophil counts in full-term infants during the first 5 days of life; however, the count gradually declines to 1.1×10^9/L to 6×10^9/L at 4 weeks.[32] There is no significant difference in the neutrophil count of infants by birth weight or gestational age; however, very-low-birth-weight infants have a significantly lower limit (1×10^9/L) compared with larger infants.[32-34] Nonetheless, a neutrophil count less than 1×10^9/L is considered to be abnormal in full-term and premature infants.

Neutropenia. *Neutropenia* is defined as a reduction in the number of circulating neutrophils less than 1.5×10^9/L. Neutropenia accompanied by bands and metamyelocytes is often associated with infection, particularly in preterm neonates. Neutropenia represents a decrease in neutrophil production or an increase in consumption.[35]

Neutrophilia. *Neutrophilia* refers to an increase in the number of neutrophils greater than 8×10^9/L. Morphologic changes associated with infection include Döhle bodies, vacuoles, and toxic granulation.[36]

TABLE 38-3 Polymorphonuclear Leukocyte and Band Counts in Newborns During the First 2 Days of Life*

Age	Absolute Neutrophil Count (per μL)	Absolute Band Count (per μL)
Birth	3500-6000	1300
12 h	8000-15,000	1300
24 h	7000-13,000	1300
36 h	5000-9000	700
48 h	3500-5200	700

*Normal values were obtained from the assessment of 3100 separate WBC counts obtained from 965 infants; 513 counts were from infants considered to be completely normal at the time the count was obtained and for the preceding and subsequent 48 hours. There was no difference in the normal ranges when infants were compared by birth weight or gestational age.
Modified from Monroe BL, Weinberg AG, Rosenfeld CR, et al: The neonatal blood count in health and disease: I. Reference values for neutrophilic cells. J Pediatr 1979;95:89-98; and Lubin BH: Reference values in infancy and childhood. In Nathan DG, Oski, FA (eds): Hematology of Infancy and Childhood, 4th ed. Philadelphia: Saunders, 1993.

Eosinophils and Basophils. The percentage of eosinophils and basophils remains consistent throughout infancy and childhood. Eosinophils range from 1% to 5% with an average of 3%. Basophils are rare and range from 0 to 1%.

Lymphocytes. Lymphocytes constitute about 30% of the leukocytes at birth and increase to 60% at 4 to 6 months. They decrease to 50% by 4 years, 40% by 6 years, and 30% by

8 years.[13-16] Lymphocytes of infants and children frequently appear reactive. Presumably, these differences between children and adults reflect intense immune system activity (Chapter 28).

Monocytes. The average monocyte count at birth is 6%. During infancy and childhood, an average of 5% is maintained except in the second and third week, when it increases to around 9%.

Platelets

Variable numbers of platelets have been reported for newborn infants (Table 38-4). The platelet count usually ranges from 100×10^9/L to 400×10^9/L for full-term and preterm infants.[14,36] Low normal platelet counts have been associated with birth trauma. After 2 weeks, the average platelet count is 300×10^9/L. Platelets of a newborn infant show great variation in size and shape. Adult reference ranges are achieved by 6 months of age. Neonatal thrombocytopenia is discussed in Chapter 43.

Very-Low-Birth-Weight Preterm Infant. The platelet count of very-low-birth-weight infants may be lower than in full-term infants, but the value increases gradually during the first month of life, regardless of birth weight.[13-16,36] Platelet counts of 100×10^9/L have been associated with high-risk infants with respiratory distress syndrome and newborns with trisomy syndromes.[14,36] Thrombocytopenia in premature infants should be considered abnormal, not physiologic.[13-16,36] A decrease to less than 50×10^9/L by 10 to 20 days of age in small (<1700 g) preterm infants is considered pathologic.

GERIATRIC HEMATOLOGY

The life expectancy and quality of life of the elderly have improved dramatically in recent decades. Global aging is occurring at a record-breaking rate. Although age 65 is considered the mean geriatric age, this number is constantly rising, with 122 as the upper limit. The World Health Organization reports that by 2050, one fifth of the global population will be adults 65 years and older.[37] The 85 and older age group is the fastest-growing segment of the elderly population. The number of centenarians will reach 1.1 million in less than 40 years.[37] The elderly can be roughly divided into three age categories: (1) the "young-old," age 65 to 74; (2) the "old-old," age 74 to 84; and (3) the "very old," age 85 and older.[38] The care of the elderly has become a growing concern as the life expectancy of the population continues to increase.

Disease and disabilities are not a function of age, although age may be a risk factor for many diseases. With the increase in the aging population, the incidence of age-related health conditions also is likely to increase.

Geriatric medicine is a rapidly growing branch of medicine. Inappropriate reference values may lead to unnecessary testing and investigations, or, more importantly, they may fail to detect a critical underlying disease. A growing concern about the interpretation of hematologic data in context with age is due partly to the tremendous heterogeneity of the aging process and partly to the difficulty in separating the effects of age per se from the effects of occult diseases that accompany aging.[39] This section focuses on hematologic changes in the elderly and presents hematologic reference ranges of various geriatric age groups and hematopathologic conditions associated with the geriatric population.

Aging and Hematopoiesis

The aging process is associated with the functional decline of several organ systems, such as cardiovascular, renal, musculoskeletal, pulmonary, and bone marrow reserve. Certain cells lose their ability to divide (e.g., nervous tissue, muscles), whereas others, such as bone marrow and the gastrointestinal mucosa, remain mitotic. Marrow cellularity begins at 80% to 100% in infancy and decreases to about 50% after 30 years, followed by a decline to 30% after age 65.[40-42] These changes may be due to a reduction in the volume of cancellous (spongy) bone along with an increase in fat, rather than a decrease in hematopoietic tissue.[42] Telomere shortening, which determines the number of divisions a cell undergoes, has not been associated with age-related bone marrow stem cell exhaustion.[43]

Hematologic Changes in the Elderly

In 1930, Wintrobe published hematologic normal ranges that are in use today. These were derived from healthy young adults, mostly medical students and nurses. What constitutes "normal" for elderly patients is a matter of considerable debate. There is controversy concerning the assignment of geriatric age-specific reference ranges, especially because aging is often accompanied by physiologic changes, and the prevalence of disease increases markedly. The baseline values for the elderly are the same reference values used for normal adults. For proper interpretation of hematologic data, however, there must be a complete understanding of the association of disease with the elderly. The next section highlights hematologic reference ranges from healthy, elderly individuals with and without evidence of underlying disease, and the subsequent section focuses on hematopathology in the elderly.

TABLE 38-4 Normal Platelet Counts for Full-Term and Preterm Infants

Age	Platelet Count/μL (mean ± 1 SD)
Preterm, 27-31 wk	275,000 ± 60,000
Preterm, 32-36 wk	290,000 ± 70,000
Term infants	310,000 ± 68,000
Normal child/adult	300,000 ± 50,000

Adapted from Oski FA, Naiman JL: Normal blood values in the newborn period. In: Hematologic Problems in the Newborn. Philadelphia: Saunders, 1982.

Assessment of Hematologic Parameters in Healthy Elderly Adults

Erythrocytes and Red Blood Cell Parameters

Most RBC parameters (e.g., RBC count and indices and RBC distribution width) for normal healthy elderly do not show significant deviations from younger adults. Most hematologic changes accompany anemia in combination with other pathologic diseases or disorders. There may be a gradual decline in hemoglobin starting at middle age, but the mean level decreases by less than 1 g/dL during the sixth through eighth decades.[44] Anemia frequently is found in the elderly. Males older than 60 have average hemoglobin levels of 12.4 to 15.3 g/dL, whereas males age 96 to 106 years have a mean hemoglobin level of 12.4 g/dL.[44,45] Males characteristically have higher hemoglobin levels than females, owing to the stimulating effect of androgens on erythropoiesis; however, the difference narrows with decreasing androgen levels in elderly males.[46] Elderly females have hemoglobin concentrations ranging from 11.7 to 13.8 g/dL. Characteristically, the lowest hemoglobin levels are generally found in the oldest patients (Table 38-5).

Leukocytes

In the healthy elderly with no underlying pathologic condition, there are no statistically significant differences in the total leukocyte count or WBC differential between the young-old and old-old compared with middle-aged adults.[45] Some investigators have reported, however, a lower leukocyte count, 3100/mm³ to 8500/mm³ ($3.1\text{-}8.5 \times 10^9$/L), in individuals older than age 65, owing primarily to a decrease in the lymphocyte count. Others have reported a decrease in the lymphocyte and the neutrophil counts in women, but not in men, older than age 50.[46]

Lymphocytes.   Immune senescence, age-related defects in lymphopoiesis, affects humoral and cellular immunity. The thymus disappears by early middle age, and adults depend on T lymphocyte response in the secondary tissue.[48,49] The number of naïve T cells decreases in the elderly, increasing the dependency on memory T cells. T cells of the elderly have impaired responsiveness to mitogens and antigens as a result of a decreased expression of costimulator CD28. B lymphocyte function depends on T cell interaction. When T cell inadequacies occur, there may be a decreased ability to generate an antibody response.[48-50]

Monocytes and Macrophages.   The aging process does not affect significantly the number and function of monocytes and macrophages, and there is little information on age-related changes in ability to process and present antigens.

Platelets.   The platelet count is not significantly changed with age. There have been reports of increased levels of β-thromboglobulin and platelet factor 4 in the α granules and decreased platelet membrane protein kinase C activity.[51,52] Thrombocytopenia may be drug induced or secondary to marrow infiltration of metastatic cancer, lymphoma, and leukemia. Thrombocytosis can be divided into primary and secondary causes. Primary thrombocytosis is a myeloproliferative disorder characterized by a sustained proliferation of megakaryocytes resulting in platelet counts of 600×10^9/L or greater (Chapter 34). Secondary thrombocytosis, or reactive thrombocytosis, is associated with infections, rheumatoid arthritis, chronic inflammatory bowel disease, iron deficiency anemia, sickle cell anemia, and postoperative splenectomy.[53-55]

Anemia and the Elderly

The etiology, characteristics, and classifications of the anemias are provided in other chapters of this textbook. This section emphasizes only the basic principles pertaining to geriatric hematology. The World Health Organization defines anemia as hemoglobin less than 13 g/dL in males and less than 12 g/dL in females.[56] Based on this definition, the prevalence of anemia in males older than 85 is approximately 44%.[54-60] It is unclear, however, if the low hemoglobin levels observed in the elderly are due to disease or normal changes related to aging. Most elderly individuals maintain a normal blood count, and elderly individuals with low hemoglobin levels have an underlying health problem.

The initial laboratory evaluation of anemia should include a complete blood count, a reticulocyte count, peripheral blood

TABLE 38-5 Hematologic Values in Ambulatory Healthy Adults

	84-98 years old	30-50 years old
RBC ($\times 10^{12}$/μL)		
Males	4.8 ± 0.4	5.1 ± 0.2
Females	4.5 ± 0.3	4.6 ± 0.3
Hemoglobin (g/dL)		
Males	14.8 ± 1.1	15.6 ± 0.7
Females	13.6 ± 1.0	14.0 ± 0.8
Hematocrit (%)		
Males	43.8 ± 3.3	45.3 ± 2.2
Females	40.7 ± 2.9	41.6 ± 2.3
MCV (fL)		
Males	91.3 ± 5.4	87.8 ± 2.8
Females	90.5 ± 4.1	90.5 ± 5.0
MCH (pg)		
Males	31.0 ± 2.0	30.1 ± 1.6
Females	30.2 ± 1.2	30.3 ± 2.1
MCHC (g/dL)		
Males	33.7 ± 1.5	34.2 ± 1.5
Females	33.4 ± 1.2	33.5 ± 1.5
WBC ($\times 10^9$/L)	7.6 ± 0.5	8.8 ± 0.4
Platelets ($\times 10^9$/L)	277 ± 2.1	361.0 ± 38.0
Neutrophils ($\times 10^9$/L)	4.5 ± 0.3	5.9 ± 0.3
Lymphocytes ($\times 10^9$/L)	1.9 ± 0.3	1.9 ± 0.8

Adapted from Zauber NP, Zauber AG: Hematologic data of healthy very old people. JAMA 1987;357:2181-2184; and Chatta, Lipschitz: Aging of the Hematopoietic System. 1999:894.

smear review, and chemistry panel, along with other diagnostic tools including iron studies (with ferritin), vitamin B_{12} and folate levels, and free erythrocyte protoporphyrin.

The variables contributing to anemia are a decrease in bone marrow function, a decline in physical activity, cardiovascular disease, and chronic inflammatory disorders. Iron deficiency anemia and anemia of chronic inflammation are the most common causes of anemia in the elderly. To a lesser extent, the elderly are prone to anemias such as sideroblastic, aplastic, hemolytic, myelophthisic, or anemia due to protein-calorie malnutrition.

Hypoproliferation or decreased production of RBCs is a common form of anemia in the elderly. Initially, this form of anemia was called *unexplained anemia, senile anemia,* and *anemia of senescence.* Hypoproliferative anemia often occurs secondary to iron deficiency, vitamin B_{12} or folate deficiency, renal failure, hypothyroidism, chronic inflammation, or endocrine disease.[57] Often the etiology of anemia in the elderly cannot be determined (Table 38-6).

Anemia of Chronic Disease. Anemia of chronic disease is also known as *anemia of chronic inflammation* (Chapter 19) because it frequently occurs with inflammatory disorders (e.g., rheumatoid arthritis, renal failure, liver disease), chronic infections, bedsores, collagen vascular disease, protein malnutrition, endocrine disorders, vitamin C deficiency, or neoplastic disorders.[57-65]

Morphology. Anemia of chronic inflammation is primarily due to decreased production of RBCs. The RBCs appear normocytic, normochromic with a normal RBC distribution width. Occasionally, a microcytic, hypochromic morphology can be observed, so differentiation from iron deficiency is necessary.

Laboratory Parameters. The anemia may be mild to moderate; however, rarely is the hemoglobin less than 10 g/dL.

TABLE 38-6 Classification of Geriatric Anemia with Mean Cell Volume and Red Cell Distribution Width (RDW) Indices

MCV	RDW	Anemia
Normal	Normal	Chronic inflammation (some) Hemorrhage Leukemia
Normal	High	Early iron deficiency anemia Mixed deficiency (e.g. vitamin B_{12} and iron) Sideroblastic anemia
Low	Normal	Chronic inflammation (some)
Low	High	Iron deficiency
High	Normal	Myelodysplastic syndrome
High	High	Vitamin B_{12} deficiency Folate deficiency Hemolytic

Reticulocytopenia is frequent. The serum iron and transferrin are decreased, but there are normal or elevated bone marrow iron stores and serum ferritin levels. Iron deficiency anemia and anemia of chronic inflammation can coexist in elderly patients.

Etiology. The major defect in anemia of chronic disease is an impairment of ferrokinetics. Hepcidin, an acute-phase reactant, is elevated during chronic inflammatory states. Hepcidin prevents absorption of iron in the intestine and its release from macrophages. To a lesser extent, erythropoiesis is impaired as a result of the action of proinflammatory cytokines, such as interleukin-1, tumor necrosis factor, and α and γ interferons.[66-72] In anemia of chronic inflammation, iron is unavailable for erythropoiesis, although it is present in reticuloendothelial cells. In cases of infection, the retention of iron in the reticuloendothelial cells prevents its availability to bacteria. Serum iron levels are low and unavailable for heme synthesis.[72,73] In addition, decreased erythrocyte survival and bone marrow suppression have been implicated in the etiology of anemia of chronic disease.

Iron Deficiency Anemia. Iron deficiency anemia is common in the elderly. Iron deficiency affects not only erythrocytes, but also the metabolic pathways in iron-dependent tissue enzymes.[62] Hemoglobin synthesis is reduced, and even a minimal decrease can cause profound functional disabilities in an elderly patient. The serum iron level decreases progressively with each decade of life, particularly in females. Nevertheless, healthy elderly adults usually have normal serum iron levels. When iron deficiency occurs in the elderly, it usually results from bleeding rather than poor nutrition or malabsorption. Serum iron levels also are known to decrease in the presence of infection, inflammation, or malignancy.

Morphology. The pathognomonic presentation of iron deficiency anemia is one of microcytic, hypochromic erythrocytes, anisocytosis, and a low reticulocyte count.

Laboratory Parameters. This anemia is characterized by a low serum iron level, high transferrin or total iron-binding capacity (TIBC) level, low transferrin saturation, low serum ferritin, and depleted bone marrow iron stores.[74-79] The serum ferritin is the most helpful and reliable test to diagnose iron deficiency anemia.[76] A serum ferritin level <15 ng/mL in a male and <10 ng/mL in a female and absence of iron from the bone marrow indicate iron deficiency. Overlapping values are observed in anemia of chronic disease. The serum ferritin level is elevated with chronic inflammation, and the elderly tend to have a higher baseline ferritin concentration.[76-82] It is possible that iron depletion can occur while the serum ferritin is still within the normal range. A normal ferritin reading does not exclude an iron-depleted state in a comorbidity situation.

Etiology. Iron deficiency anemia in the elderly often results from chronic gastrointestinal blood loss, not inadequate intake or absorption. Gastrointestinal conditions leading to blood loss include chronic nonsteroidal anti-inflammatory medication ingestion, gastritis, peptic ulcer disease, gastroesophageal reflux disease with esophagitis, colon cancer, and angiodysplasia.[76-82] It also may be due to poor diet of an elderly individual who has lost the taste or desire for food or is unable to prepare nutritious meals. Chapter 19 discusses iron disorders in detail.

Ineffective Erythropoiesis

Ineffective erythropoiesis has been attributed not only to maturation disorders such as vitamin B_{12} and folic acid deficiency, but also to sideroblastic anemia and thalassemia (abnormal globin synthesis). Sideroblastic anemias have impaired heme synthesis, and thalassemias have abnormal globin synthesis (Chapter 27). Megaloblastic anemia results from defective DNA synthesis (Chapter 20) with compromised cell division, but normal cytoplasmic development (i.e., asynchrony).[83-85] These megaloblastic cells are more prone to destruction in the bone marrow, resulting in "ineffective" erythropoiesis. Two causes of megaloblastic anemia are deficiencies of vitamin B_{12} and folate.

Vitamin B_{12} (Cobalamin) Deficiency.   Vitamin B_{12} (cobalamin) deficiency causes a megaloblastic disorder in 5% to 10% of the elderly.[57] It may be difficult to detect because anemia is present in only about 60% of the patients.[82] Pernicious anemia is a systemic disease characterized by megaloblastic hematopoiesis, neuropathy, or both.[86,87] In the absence of anemia, neurologic symptoms may be the only presentation. Even when anemia is present, it does not always manifest with the classic macrocytic and megaloblastic picture but may be normocytic or microcytic.

Morphology.   Megaloblastic anemia is characterized by the presentation of anemia, thrombocytopenia, oval macrocytes, hypersegmented neutrophils, leukopenia, and a bone marrow that shows megaloblastic erythrocyte precursors and giant metamyelocytes. Typically, the MCV is greater than 100 fL but may be normal, especially if the disease is complicated with iron deficiency or thalassemia. As mentioned previously, many elderly individuals have elevated MCV. The MCV increases slightly with age[88] and can be greater than 100 fL in heavy smokers; alcoholics; and individuals with chronic liver disease, hypothyroidism, or hemolysis.[84,87]

Laboratory Parameters.   Laboratory indications include elevated serum bilirubin and lactic dehydrogenase levels owing to intramedullary hemolysis.[62,89] Only 30% of patients with megaloblastic anemia present with low to normal serum vitamin B_{12} levels, however, because serum vitamin B_{12} levels do not always reflect tissue vitamin B_{12} concentrations. Two metabolites that accumulate in vitamin B_{12} deficiency are methylmalonic acid and homocysteine.[89-91] Elevated levels of methylmalonic acid and homocysteine have proven to be better diagnostic assessments for megaloblastic anemia than serum vitamin B_{12} levels, especially when serum vitamin B_{12} levels are normal in the presence of symptoms.

Etiology.   Vitamin B_{12} deficiency has been attributed to inadequate intestinal absorption, not inadequate intake. Pernicious anemia develops slowly and insidiously in patients when autoimmune antibodies destroy their parietal cells leaving them without intrinsic factor.[89] Inadequate vitamin B_{12}

absorption has been reported in other conditions, such as small bowel disorder, gastric resection, pancreatic insufficiency, resection of the terminal ileum, blind loop syndrome, and bacterial overgrowth. Pernicious anemia frequently is accompanied by a characteristic neurologic clinical disorder.[83-89] Neuropathy does not occur in all patients, however, and the extent of the neuropathy does not correlate with the severity of the hematologic picture. When intrinsic factor is absent or impaired, vitamin B_{12} injections are required. Treatment with vitamin B_{12} effectively corrects the anemia but may not reverse the neuropathy; early detection and treatment are important (Chapter 20).

Folate Deficiency.   A second megaloblastic anemia prevalent among the elderly results from folate deficiency. In contrast to vitamin B_{12} deficiency, folic acid deficiency usually develops in inadequate dietary intake because the body stores little folate.[87,88] Dietary folate is absorbed from the small intestine, especially in the proximal jejunum. Folic acid is reduced and methylated or formylated in the gut lumen.[87-89] Most serum folate is methyltetrahydrofolate, which is absorbed from the intestine and transferred to the bone marrow for incorporation into erythroid precursors and hepatocytes.

When elderly chronically ill patients present with hematologic or neuropsychiatric disorders, folate deficiency caused by poor diet may be present. Although certain studies support this, others conclude that folic acid has no effect on the progression of neurologic symptoms typical of a vitamin B_{12} deficiency.

Morphology.   The morphologic presentation of folic acid deficiency is similar to vitamin B_{12} deficiency.

Laboratory Parameters.   The RBC folate level is the diagnostic test for folic acid deficiency because tissue content is best estimated by RBC folate level. Serum homocysteine evaluation also can be useful because 90% of patients with folate deficiency have elevated homocysteine levels. If the serum methylmalonic acid level also is elevated, however, a diagnosis of vitamin B_{12} deficiency should be considered. The coexistence of folic acid and vitamin B_{12} deficiencies is important for treatment because vitamin B_{12}–deficient cell production improves with folate therapy, but not the neurologic component.[94]

Etiology.   Folate deficiency results from insufficient ingestion, absorption, and use or increased requirement, excretion, and destruction. The folate content of RBCs reflects liver stores, whereas the serum folate level depends on recent dietary changes and thus lacks a fixed criterion.[94] Alcoholic elderly patients are particularly prone to folic acid deficiency, especially because alcohol has a toxic effect on bone marrow and reduces folic acid absorption.[95]

Sideroblastic Anemia.   If an elderly individual presents with hypochromic anemia in the absence of iron deficiency or inflammation, the differential diagnosis is usually sideroblastic anemia. Sideroblastic anemias are a heterogeneous group of disorders characterized by impaired heme synthesis. The condition may be acquired or inherited (sex linked), with primary *acquired sideroblastic anemia* occurring more frequently in the elderly.[96,97] Sideroblastic anemia may occur secondary to alcohol use; drugs; toxins (especially lead); and numerous diseases, including infections, neoplasms (gastrointestinal, renal cell, and lymphomas), and inflammatory disorders (rheumatoid arthritis, systemic lupus erythematosus).

Morphology. The pathognomonic feature of sideroblastic anemia is the dimorphic morphology of microcytic and normocytic peripheral blood RBCs and ringed sideroblasts in the bone marrow. Other morphologic features include poikilocytosis, basophilic stippling, and Pappenheimer bodies.

Laboratory Parameters. In sideroblastic anemia, the MCV is low, normal, or high, but the reticulocyte count is always low. Serum iron, transferrin saturation, and ferritin levels are elevated, reflecting an iron overload. The bone marrow appears hypocellular, with 15% or more ringed sideroblasts, normoblasts that contain accumulations of iron surrounding the nucleus.

Etiology. Acquired sideroblastic anemia may signify myelodysplastic syndrome in the elderly. Idiopathic sideroblastic anemia is usually benign, however. Sideroblastic anemia often occurs as a consequence of hematologic malignant neoplasms, rheumatologic disorders, alcoholism, drugs, and toxins, especially lead.

Hemolytic Anemia. Hemolytic anemias are characterized by a shortened RBC survival time. There are three major types of hemolytic anemias: (1) immunologic; (2) intrinsic defects, such as RBC membrane defect, abnormal hemoglobins, or RBC enzyme defects; and (3) extrinsic factors, such as mechanical or lytic factors.[58,98] The elderly are at risk for drug-induced anemia because they may take multiple medications. Drug-induced hemolytic anemia has been associated with high doses of antibiotics (penicillin, chloramphenicol, cephalosporins), several nonsteroidal anti-inflammatory drugs, quinidine, phenacetin, and others. Hemolytic anemias in the elderly also can result from collagen vascular diseases, infections, and chronic lymphocytic leukemia.

Morphology. The hallmark of hemolytic anemia is reticulocytosis.

Laboratory Parameters. The presence of elevated lactate dehydrogenase and indirect bilirubin and a low haptoglobin suggests destruction of RBCs.[58,98] The direct antihuman globulin test, or Coombs test, is usually positive in autoimmune hemolytic anemia.

Hematologic Neoplasia in Older Individuals

Although hematologic malignancies may occur at any age, certain disorders are common in those older than 50 years. A brief overview of these is included in this chapter, with references to more detailed discussions.

Myelodysplastic Syndrome

Myelodysplastic syndromes, a heterogeneous group characterized by a defect in the hematopoietic stem cell that may affect multiple cell lineages, are diagnosed most frequently in the elderly.

Patients with myelodysplastic syndromes typically present with anemia, or pancytopenia. Dysplastic transformation occurs in RBCs, granulocytes, monocytes, and platelets. Marrow dyserythropoiesis includes ringed sideroblasts, bizarre nuclear shapes, dense chromatin, and megaloblastoid precursors. Peripheral blood RBC abnormalities include oval macrocytes and anisocytosis. Myeloid abnormalities include pseudo–Pelger-Huët cells and uneven cytoplasmic staining. The platelet count varies and giant platelets with bizarre morphology and micromegakaryocytes may be seen.[66,99,100] The marrow may have 5% to 20% blasts. In some patients, myelodysplastic syndrome terminates in acute leukemia (Chapter 35).

Myeloproliferative Disorders

Myeloproliferative disorders are monoclonal proliferations of hematopoietic stem cells with overaccumulation of RBCs, WBCs, or platelets in various combinations. Myeloproliferative disorders include chronic myelogenous leukemia, polycythemia vera, essential thrombocythemia, and chronic idiopathic myelofibrosis.

Chronic myelogenous leukemia and polycythemia vera express overproduction of erythrocytes, granulocytes, and platelets. The average age of patients with polycythemia vera is 60 years. The incidence of chronic myelogenous leukemia increases after age 50, with the frequency at age 80 of 1 in 10,000.[101]

Essential thrombocythemia manifests with increased megakaryocytopoiesis and peripheral blood thrombocytosis. It has been characterized as a disease of individuals older than age 50, but the diagnosis is now being made earlier because of the universal routine availability of platelet counts with the complete blood count.[101]

Chronic idiopathic myelofibrosis results in peripheral blood pancytopenia and may exhibit a combination of overproduction of hematopoietic cells and ineffective hematopoiesis. It is commonly diagnosed between age 50 and 70 years.[101] Myeloproliferative disorders are discussed further in Chapter 34.

Leukemia

Leukemia is a neoplastic disease characterized by a malignant proliferation of hematopoietic stem cells in the bone marrow, peripheral blood, and often other organs. Leukemia is classified on the basis of the cell type involved (lymphoid or nonlymphoid) and the stage of maturity (acute or chronic) of the leukemic cells. In the United States, the incidence of leukemia was 3.9 per 100,000 in 1940; in 2000, it was 1.4 per 100,000 for all age groups.[101-103] Although there has been an overall decrease in the incidence of leukemia, there has been a disproportionately greater incidence in leukemia in the elderly (Table 38-7). The peak incidence of leukemia seems to occur in the very young (age 1-4 years) and the very old (age ≥70, especially males). Acute myeloid leukemia (Chapter 36) and chronic lymphocytic leukemia (Chapter 37) have had the most dramatic age-related increase in incidence.

Approximately 13% of patients with acute leukemia initially present with previous hematologic disorders, such as

TABLE 38-7 SEER* incidence of Leukemia in the Elderly in the United States per 100,000 (2000-2003)

Age at diagnosis	All leukemias	ALL	CLL	AML	CML
65-69	35.0	1.3	14.3	11.0	4.1
70-74	46.4	1.5	17.9	15.3	5.5
75-79	63.0	1.6	24.5	19.8	8.0
80-84	73.4	1.2	27.8	23.1	9.4
≥85	80.3	2.0	30.8	21.4	9.7

ALL, acute lymphoblastic leukemia; CLL, chronic lymphocytic leukemia; AML, acute myeloid leukemia; CML, chronic myelogenous leukemia.

*Surveillance Epidemiology and End Results (SEER) rates are age-adjusted to the 2000 US Standard population census.

Ries LAG, Harkins D, Krapcho M, et al. (eds) *SEER Cancer Statistics Review*, 1975-2003. National Cancer Institute. Bethesda MD available at http://seer.cancer.gov/csr/1975_2003/.

myelodysplastic syndrome, hypoplastic bone marrow, polycythemia, or myelofibrosis. A geriatric patient is more likely than younger patients to succumb to toxicity of, or resistance to, chemotherapy.[101-103]

Chronic Lymphocytic Leukemia. Chronic lymphocytic leukemia is the most common cause of lymphocytosis in the elderly and constitutes 30% of all leukemias seen in Western countries.[104] It is a lymphoproliferative disorder characterized by a clonal expansion of mature but functionally deficient lymphocytes, predominantly of B cell origin. The onset is usually asymptomatic at a median age of 60 to 65 years, and it occurs twice as often in males as compared with females.[105] The peripheral smear shows a sustained lymphocytosis of at least 10×10^9/L with small, mature-appearing lymphocytes. The bone marrow is infiltrated by lymphocytes,[103] and immunophenotyping shows a characteristic pattern (Chapter 37).[105]

Multiple Myeloma

Multiple myeloma is a plasma cell cancer characterized by monoclonal gammopathy and multifocal destructive bone lesions throughout the skeleton. The neoplastic plasma cells secrete complete or incomplete immunoglobulins. Myeloma cells express not only plasma cell–associated antigens such as PCA-1 and CD10 (in some cells), but also myelomonocytic antigen CD33.[106] These findings suggest that multiple myeloma also may be a hematopoietic stem cell disease that arises from the transformation of stem cells that differentiate predominantly along the B cell–plasma cell pathway. Cytokines such as interleukin-1, interleukin-6, interleukin-11 and tumor necrosis factor-β are associated with disease aggressiveness, myeloma-cell proliferation, and poor prognosis.[107]

The age of peak incidence for multiple myeloma is 67 years, with 80% of cases occurring after 60.[103] It occurs at an equal frequency in males and females. A classic feature of multiple myeloma is serum immunoglobulin myeloma (M) protein, and urine free monoclonal light chains called *Bence-Jones protein*. Monoclonal immunoglobulin isotypes are IgG in 50% of patients and IgA in 25%; IgM, IgD, and IgE are rarely increased. Bence-Jones proteinuria or M-protein occurs in 60% to 70% of cases. The protein generates hyperviscosity with an increased sedimentation rate. Renal insufficiency, seen in 50% of patients, is second only to infections as a cause of death. The renal pathology is attributed to the Bence-Jones proteinuria, which is believed to be directly toxic to the tubular epithelial cells (Chapter 37).[106-108]

CHAPTER at a GLANCE

- The newborn infant, preadolescent child, and elderly adult all exhibit profound hematologic differences.
- Hematologic parameters continue to change and evolve over the first few days, weeks, and months of life. Data must be assessed in light of gestational age, birth weight, and developmental differences between newborns and older infants.
- The erythrocytes of newborn infants are markedly macrocytic at birth. A condition known as *physiologic anemia of infancy* occurs after the first weeks of life. Infants born prematurely also experience a decrease in hemoglobin concentration, which is termed *physiologic anemia of prematurity*.
- Fluctuations in the number of WBCs are common at all ages but are greatest in infants.
- Although common in elderly patients, anemia is not a normal occurrence of the aging process.
- The etiology of anemia may be multifactorial in elderly patients.

CHAPTER at a GLANCE—cont'd

- Anemia of chronic inflammation and iron deficiency anemia manifest with low serum iron and can be differentiated using serum ferritin.
- Vitamin B_{12} deficiency and folate deficiency are other common causes of anemia.
- Low normal levels of vitamin B_{12} may represent a clinically significant deficiency.
- The elderly experience an increased frequency of many neoplastic and malignant disorders, such as acute and chronic leukemia, myelodysplastic syndromes, and myeloproliferative disorders.

REVIEW QUESTIONS

1. The complete blood count values of children (age 3-12 years) differ from those of adults chiefly by:
   a. The presence of nucleated RBCs
   b. Notable polychromasia as evidence of increased reticulocytosis
   c. A lower platelet count
   d. A higher percentage of lymphocytes

2. Physiologic anemia of infancy results from:
   a. Iron deficiency from a milk-only diet during the early neonatal period
   b. Increased oxygenation of blood and decreased erythropoietin
   c. Replacement of active marrow with fat soon after birth
   d. Hemoglobin F and its diminished oxygen delivery to tissues

3. The complete blood count report on a 3-day-old neonate who was 6 weeks premature shows a decrease in hemoglobin compared with the value 2 days earlier. Which of the following should be considered as an explanation for this result when no apparent source of hemolysis or bleeding is evident?
   a. The sample was collected from a vein at the time an intravenous line was inserted.
   b. The sample was collected by heel puncture rather than finger puncture because of the infant's small size.
   c. The umbilical cord was clamped quickly to begin appropriate treatment for a preterm infant.
   d. The infant has become dehydrated.

4. The morphology of the lymphocytes of healthy children is:
   a. Similar to that seen in megaloblastic anemia
   b. Easily confused with leukemic blasts
   c. Often more "reactive" than healthy adult cells
   d. Similar to adult lymphocytes

5. With increasing age, the hemoglobin level of elderly adults is:
   a. Unchanged from that of middle-aged adults
   b. Increased owing to diminished respiration and poor tissue oxygenation
   c. Decreased for reasons that are unclear
   d. Comparable to that of newborns

6. Which of the following are the most common anemias in the elderly population?
   a. Megaloblastic and iron deficiency
   b. Sideroblastic and megaloblastic
   c. Myelophthisic and anemia of chronic disease
   d. Iron deficiency and anemia of chronic disease

7. When iron deficiency is recognized in an elderly individual, the etiology is usually:
   a. Iron-deficient diet
   b. Gastrointestinal bleeding
   c. Diminished absorption
   d. Impaired incorporation of iron into heme as a result of telomere loss

8. Which of the following conditions is *least likely* in an elderly individual?
   a. Acute lymphoblastic leukemia
   b. Multiple myeloma
   c. Myelodysplasia
   d. Chronic lymphocytic leukemia

REFERENCES

1. Brugnara C, Pratt OS: The neonatal erythrocyte and its disorders. In Nathan DG, Orkin SH, Ginsburg D, et al (eds): Nathan and Oski's Hematology of Infancy and Childhood, 6th ed. Philadelphia: Saunders, 2003:19-55.
2. Segal GB, Palis J: Hematology of the newborn. In Lichtman MA, Beutler E, Kipps TJ, et al (eds): Williams Hematology, 7th ed. New York: McGraw-Hill, 2006:81-98.
3. Hann IM, Bodger MP, Hoffbrand AV: Development of pluripotent hematopoietic progenitor cells in the human fetus. Blood 1983;62:118-123.
4. Forestier F, Daffos F, Catherine N, et al: Developmental hematopoiesis in normal human fetal blood. Blood 1991;77:2360-2363.
5. Ohls RK, Christensen RD: Development of the hematopoietic system. In Behrman RE, Kliegman R, Jenson HB (eds): Nelson Textbook of Pediatrics, 17th ed. Philadelphia: Saunders, 2004:1599-1602.
6. Christensen RD: Hematopoiesis in the fetus and neonate. Pediatr Res 1989;26:531-535.
7. Linch DC, Knott LJ, Rodeck CH, et al: Studies of circulating

hematopoietic progenitor cells in human fetal blood. Blood 1982;59:976-979.

8. Christensen RD: Circulating pluripotent hematopoietic progenitor cells in neonates. J Pediatr 1987;110:622-625.

9. Yoder MC: Embryonic hematopoiesis. In Christensen RD (ed): Hematologic Problems of the Neonate. Philadelphia: Saunders, 2002:3-20.

10. Tavassoli M: Embryonic and fetal hemopoiesis: an overview. Blood Cells 1991;1:269-281.

11. Stoll BJ, Kliegman RM: The high risk infant. In Behrman RE, Kleigman RN, Jenson HB (eds): Textbook of Pediatrics, 17th ed. Philadelphia: Saunders, 2004:547-559.

12. Peterec SM, Warshaw JB: The premature newborn. In McMillan JA (ed): Oski's Pediatrics, 4th ed. Philadelphia: Lippincott, Williams & Wilkins, 2006:220-235.

13. Miller DR: Normal blood values from birth through adolescence. In Miller DR, Baehner RL (eds): Blood Diseases of Infancy and Childhood: In the Tradition of CH Smith, 7th ed. St Louis: Mosby, 1995:3-53.

14. Oski FA, Naiman JL: Normal blood values in the newborn period. In Oski, FA, Naiman JL (eds): Hematologic Problems in the Newborn, 3rd ed. Philadelphia: Saunders, 1982:1-31.

15. Christensen RD: Expected hematologic values for term and preterm neonates. In Christensen RD (ed): Hematologic Problems of the Neonate. Philadelphia: Saunders, 2000:117-136.

16. Luchtman-Jones LL, Schwartz AL, Wilson DB: Hematologic problems in the fetus and neonate. In Martin RJ, Fanaroff AA, Walsh MC (eds): Neonatal-Perinatal Medicine, 8th ed. St Louis: Mosby, 2006:1287-1344,

17. Soldin S, Brugnara C, Wong EC (eds): Pediatric Reference Intervals, 5th ed. Washington, DC: AACC Press, 2005.

18. Zaizov R, Matoth Y: Red cell values on the first postnatal day during the last 16 weeks of gestation. Am J Hematol 1976;1:275-278.

19. Thomas RM, Canning CE, Cotes PM, et al: Erythropoietin and cord blood hemoglobin in the regulation of human fetal erythropoiesis. Br J Obstet Gynaecol 1983;90:795-800.

20. Pahal GS, Jauniaux E, Kinnon C, et al: Normal development of human fetal hematopoiesis between eight and seventeen weeks gestation. Am J Obstet Gynecol 2000;183:1029-1034.

21. Luchtman-Jones L, Schwartz AL, Wilson DB: The blood and hematopoietic system: diseases of the fetus and infant. In Fanaroff AA, Martin RJ, (eds). Neonatal-Perinatal Medicine, 6th ed. Philadelphia: Mosby, 1997:1201-1253.

22. Newborn Services Clinical Guideline: Normal haematological values. Available at: http://www.adhb.govt.nz/newborn/Guidelines/blood/haematologicalvalues.htm. Accessed July 10, 2006.

23. O'Brien RT, Pearson HA: Physiologic anemia of the newborn infant. J Pediatr 1971;79:132-138.

24. McIntosh N, Kempson C, Tyler RM: Blood counts in extremely low birth weight infants. Arch Dis Child 1988;63:74-76.

25. Geaghan SM: Hematologic values and appearances in the healthy fetus, neonate, and child. Clin Lab Med 1999;19:1-37.

26. Cavaliere TA: Red blood cell indices: implications for practice. NBIN 2004;4:231-239.

27. Obladen M, Diepold K, Maier RF: Venous and arterial hematologic profiles of very low birth weight infants. Pediatrics 2000;106:707-711.

28. Halvorsen S, Finne PH: Erythropoietin reduction in the human fetus and newborn. Ann N Y Acad Sci 1968;149:576-577.

29. Mann DL, Sites ML, Donati RM: Erythropoietic stimulating activity during the first ninety days of life. Proc Soc Exp Biol Med 1965;118:212-214.

30. Christensen RD, Ohls RK: Anemias unique to pregnancy and the perinatal period: anemias of the fetus and neonate. In Greer JP, Foerster J, Lukens J, et al (eds): Wintrobe's Clinical Hematology, 11th ed. Philadelphia: Lippincott, Williams & Wilkins, 2004:1467-1486.

31. Dallman PR: Reference ranges for leukocyte counts in children. In Rudolph AM (ed): Pediatrics, 16th ed. New York: Appleton-Century-Crofts, 1977:1178.

32. Mouzinho A, Rosenfeld CR, Sanchez PJ, et al: Revised reference ranges for circulating neutrophils in very-low-birth-weight neonates. Pediatrics 1994;94:76-82.

33. Alexander GR, Kogan M, Bader G, et al: US birth weight/gestational age-specific neonatal mortality: 1995-1997 rates for whites, Hispanics and blacks. Pediatrics 2003;111:e61-e66.

34. Monroe BL, Weinberg AG, Rosenfeld CR: The neonatal blood count in health and disease: I. Reference values for neutrophilic cells. J Pediatr 1976;95:89-98.

35. Dinauer MC: The phagocyte system and disorders of granulopoiesis and granulocyte function. In Nathan DG, Orkin SH, Ginsburg D, et al (eds): Nathan and Oski's Hematology of Infancy and Childhood, 6th ed. Philadelphia: Saunders, 2003:923-1010.

36. Ezekowitz RAB, Stockman JA III: Hematologic manifestations of systemic diseases. In Nathan DG, Orkin SH, Ginsburg D, et al (eds): Nathan and Oski's Hematology of Infancy and Childhood, 6th ed. Philadelphia: Saunders, 2003:1759-1809.

37. Federal Interagency Forum on Aging Related Statistics: Older Americans 2006: key indicators of well being. Available at: http://www.agingstats.gov. Accessed July 15, 2006.

38. Zauber NP, Zauber AG: Hematologic data of healthy old people. JAMA 1987;257:2181-2184.

39. Chatta GS, Dale DC: Aging and haemopoiesis: implications for treatment with haemopoietic growth factors. Drugs Aging 1996;9:37-47.

40. Lansdorp PM: Self-renewal of stem cells. Biol Blood Marrow Transplant 1997;3:171-178.

41. Hartstock RJ, Smith EB, Petty CS: Normal variation with aging of the amount of hematopoietic tissue in bone marrow from the anterior iliac crest. Am J Clin Pathol 1965;43:326-331.

42. Ricci C, Cova M, Kang Y, et al: Normal age-related pattern of cellular and fatty bone marrow distribution in the axial skeleton: MR imaging study. Radiology 1990;177:83-88.

43. Frenck RW Jr, Blackburn EH, Shannon KM: The rate of telomere sequence loss in human leukocyte varies with age. Proc Natl Acad Sci U S A 1998;95:5607-5610.

44. Myers AM, Saunders CR, Chalmers DG: The haemoglobin level of fit elderly people. Lancet 1968;2:261-263.

45. Salive ME, Cornoni-Huntley J, Guralnik JM, et al: Anemia and hemoglobin level in older persons: relationship with age, gender and healthy status. J Am Geriatr Soc 1992;40:489-496.

46. Allan RN, Alexander MK: A sex difference in the leukocyte count. J Clin Pathol 1965;21:691-694.

47. Zaino EC: Blood counts in the nonagenarian. N Y State J Med 1981;81:1199-1200.

48. Mangolas SC, Jilka RL: Bone marrow, cytokines and bone remodeling. N Engl J Med 1995;332:302-311.

49. Globerson A: T lymphocytes and aging. Int Arch Allergy Immunol 1995;107:491-497.

50. Song L, Kim YH, Chopra RK, et al: Age related effects in T cell activation and proliferation. Exp Gerontol 1993;28:313-321.

51. Sansoni P, Cossarizza A, Brianti V, et al: Lymphocyte subsets and natural killer cell activity in healthy old people and centenarians. Blood 1993;82:2767-2773.

52. Grubeck-Lobenstein B: Changes in the aging immune system. Biologicals 1997;25:205-208.

53. Zahavi J, Jones NA, Leyton J, et al: Enhances in vivo platelet "release reaction" in old healthy individuals. Thromb Res 1980;17:329-336.

54. Chong BH: Heparin-induced thrombocytopenia. Br J Haematol 1995;89:431-439.
55. Cortelazzo S, Finazzi G, Ruggeri M, et al: Hydroxyurea for patients with essential thrombocythemia and a high risk for thrombosis. N Engl J Med 1995;332:1132-1136.
56. World Health Organization/UNICEF/United Nations University: Indicators and Strategies for Iron Deficiency and Anaemia Programmes: Report of a Consultation, Geneva, 6-10 December 1993. Geneva: WHO, 1997.
57. Howe RB: Anemia in the elderly. Postgrad Med 1983;73:153-160.
58. Timiras ML, Brownstein H: Prevalence of anemia and correlation of hemoglobin with age in a geriatric screening clinic population. J Am Geriatr Soc 1987;35:639-643.
59. Ania BJ, Suman VJ, Fairbanks VF, et al: Prevalence of anemia in medical practice: community versus referral patients. Mayo Clin Proc 1994;69:730-735.
60. Smith D: Management and treatment of anemia in the elderly. Clin Geriatr 2002;10:8.
61. Daly MP: Anemia in the elderly. Am Fam Physician 1989;39:129-136.
62. Walsh JR: Hematologic problems. In Cassel CK, Cohen HJ, Larson EB, et al (eds): Geriatric Medicine, 3rd ed. New York: Springer Verlag, 1997:627-636.
63. Lipschitz DA: The anemia of chronic disease. J Am Geriatr Soc 1990;38:1258-1264.
64. Gardner LB, Benz EJ: Anemia of chronic disease. In Hoffman R, Benz EJ Jr, Shattil SJ, et al (eds): Hematology Basic Principles and Practices, 4th ed. Philadelphia: Saunders, 2006:465-472.
65. Cash J, Sears DA: The anemia of chronic disease: spectrum of associated disease in a series of unselected hospitalized patients. Am J Med 1989;87:638-644.
66. Dharmarajan TS, Bullecer ML, Bhagwati N: Hematologic disorders in older adults. In Dharmarajan TS, Norman RA (eds): Clinical Geriatrics. Boca Raton, FL: Parthenon Publishing, 2003:487-500.
67. Vreugdenhil G, Lowenberg B, Van Eijk HG, et al: Tumor necrosis factor alpha is associated with disease activity and the degree of anemia in patients with rheumatoid arthritis. Eur J Clin Invest 1992;22:488-493.
68. Casini-Raggi V, Kam L, Chong YJ, et al: Mucosal imbalance of IL-1 and IL-1 receptor antagonist in inflammatory bowel disease: a novel mechanism of chronic intestinal inflammation. J Immunol 1995;154:2434-2440.
69. Johnson RA, Waddelow TA, Caro J, et al: Chronic exposure to tumor necrosis factor in vivo preferentially inhibits erythropoiesis in nude mice. Blood 1989;74:130-138.
70. Wang CQ, Udupa KP, Lipschitz DA, et al: Interferon gamma exerts its negative regulatory effect primarily on the earliest stages of murine erythroid progenitor cell development. J Cell Physiol 1995;162:134-138.
71. Salleri C, Maciejewski JP, Sato T: Interferon-gamma constitutively expressed in the stromal microenvironment of human marrow cultures mediates potent hematopoietic inhibition. Blood 1996;87:4149-4157.
72. Ferguson BJ, Skikne BS, Simpson KM: Serum transferrin receptor distinguishes the anemia of chronic disease from iron deficiency anemia. J Lab Clin Med 1992;119:385-390.
73. Takala TI, Suominem P, Isoaho R, et al: Iron-replete reference intervals to increase sensitivity of hematologic and iron status laboratory tests in the elderly. Clin Chem 2002;48:1586-1589.
74. Guyatt GH, Patterson C, Ali M, et al: Diagnosis of iron deficiency anemia in elderly. Am J Med 1990;88:205-209.
75. Smieja MJ, Cook DJ, Hunt DL, et al: Recognizing and investigating iron deficiency anemia in hospitalized elderly people. Can Med Assoc J 1996;155:691-696.
76. Sharma JC, Roy SN: Value of serum ferritin as an index of iron deficiency in elderly anemic patients. Age Ageing 1984;13:248-250.
77. Pirrie R: The influence of age upon serum iron in normal subjects. J Clin Pathol 1952;5:10-15.
78. Garry PJ, Goodwin JS, Hunt WC: Iron status and anemia in the elderly: new findings and a review of previous studies. J Am Geriatr Soc 1983;31:389-399.
79. Patterson C, Turpie ID, Benger AM: Assessment of iron stores in anemic geriatric patients. J Am Geriatr Soc 1985;33:764-767.
80. Lynch SR, Finch CA, Monsen ER, et al: Iron status of elderly Americans. Am J Clin Nutr 1982;36:1032-1045.
81. Cook JD, Finch CA, Smith NJ: Evaluation of the iron status of a population. Blood 1976;48:449-455.
82. Powell DE, Thomas JH: The iron binding capacity of serum in elderly hospital patients. Gerontol Clin (Basel) 1969;11:36-47.
83. Pennypacker LC, Allen RH, Kelly JP, et al: High prevalence of cobalamin deficiency in elderly outpatients. J Am Geriatr Soc 1992;40:1197-1204.
84. Stabler SP: Vitamin B12 deficiency in older people: improving diagnosis and preventing disability. J Am Geriatr Soc 1998;46:1317-1319.
85. Nexo E, Hansen M, Rasmussen K, et al: How to diagnosis cobalamin deficiency. Scand J Clin Lab Invest Suppl 1994;219:61-76.
86. Lindenbaum J, Healton EB, Savage DG, et al: Neuropsychiatric disorders caused by cobalamin deficiency in the absence of anemia or macrocytosis. N Engl J Med 1988;318:1720-1728.
87. Karnaze DS, Carmel R: Low serum cobalamin levels in primary degenerative dementia. Arch Intern Med 1987;17:429-431.
88. Shayne M, Lichtman MA: Hematology in older persons. In Lichtman MA, Beutler E, Kipps TJ, et al (eds): Williams Hematology, 7th ed. New York: McGraw-Hill, 2006:111-121.
89. Carmel R: Prevalence of undiagnosed pernicious anemia in the elderly. Arch Intern Med 1996;1576:1097-1100.
90. Savage DG, Lindenbaum J, Stabler SP, et al: Sensitivity of serum methylmalonic acid and total homocysteine determinations for diagnosing cobalamin and folate deficiencies. Am J Med 1994;96:239-246.
91. Nimo RE, Carmel R: Increased sensitivity of detection of the blocking (type I) anti-intrinsic factor antibody. Am J Clin Pathol 1987;88:729-733.
92. Girdwood RH, Thompson AD, Williamson J: Folate status in the elderly. BMJ 1967;2:670-672.
93. Marcus DL, Freedman ML: Folic acid deficiency in the elderly. J Am Geriatr Soc 1985;33:552-558.
94. Webster SG, Leeming JT: Erythrocyte folate levels in young and old. J Am Geriatr Soc 1979;27:451-454.
95. Wu A, Chanarin I, Slavin G, et al: Folate deficiency in the alcoholic—its relationship to clinical and haematological abnormalities, liver disease and folate stores. Br J Haematol 1975;29:469-478.
96. Gardner FH: Refractory anemia in the elderly. Adv Intern Med 1987;32:155-175.
97. Cartwright GE, Deiss A: Sideroblasts, siderocytes, and sideroblastic anemia. N Engl J Med 1975;292:185-193.
98. Petz LD: Drug-induced immune haemolytic anaemia. Clin Haematol 1980;9:455-482.
99. Heaney ML, Golde DW: Myelodysplasia. N Engl J Med 1999;340:1649-1660.
100. Kouides PA, Bennett JM: Morphology and classification of myelodysplastic syndromes. Hematol Oncol Clin N Am 1992;6:485-499.
101. The Leukemia Lymphoma Society: Disease information.

Available at: http://www.leukemia-lymphoma.org. Accessed July 14, 2006.

102. National Cancer Institute: SEER Cancer Statistics Review 1975-2002, National Cancer Data Base, American College of Surgeons Commission on Cancer. Available at: http://seer.cancer.gov/csr/1975_2000/. Accessed July 14, 2006.

103. American Cancer Society: Available at: http://www.cancer.org/docroot/home/index/asp. Accessed July 14, 2006.

104. Lymphoma Information Network: Available at: http://www.lymphomainfo.net/nhl/type/sll.html. Accessed July 14, 2006.

105. Rozman C, Montserrat E: Chronic lymphocytic leukemia. N Engl J Med 1995;333:1052-1057.

106. Osserman EF, Merlini G, Butler VP Jr: Multiple myeloma and related plasma cell dyscrasias. JAMA 1987;258:2930-2937.

107. Klein B, Bataille R: Cytokine network in human myeloma. Hematol Oncol Clin North Am 1992;6:273-284.

108. Mandelli F, Avvisati G, Tribalto M: Biology and treatment of multiple myeloma. Curr Opin Oncol 1992;4:73-86.

Automated Cell Counting Instrumentation and Point of Care Testing

39

Sharral A. Longanbach, Deanne H. Chapman,
Karen Bourlier Waldron, and Martha K. Miers

OUTLINE

General Principles of
  Hematology
  Instrumentation
Principal Cell Counting
  Instruments
Automated Reticulocyte
  Counting
Limitations and
  Interferences
Clinical Utility of
  Automated Hematology
  Instrumentation
Point of Care Testing

OBJECTIVES

After completion of this chapter, the reader will be able to:

1. Explain the different principles of automated cell counting.
2. Describe how the general principles are used on the different instruments discussed.
3. Identify the hemogram parameters directly measured on the four analyzers presented.
4. Explain the derivation of calculated or indirectly measured hemogram parameters for the same four analyzers.
5. Explain the derivation of the white blood cell (WBC) differential count on the different instruments discussed.

6. Interpret and compare patient data, including WBC and red blood cell histograms or cytograms or both, from the major hematology instruments.
7. Explain the general principles of automated reticulocyte counting.
8. Identify sources of error in automated cell counting, and determine appropriate corrective action.
9. Discuss advantages and disadvantages of point of care testing as they apply to hematology tests.
10. Describe the principles of common instruments used for point of care testing for hemoglobin, hematocrit, WBC counts, and platelet counts.

utomation provides greater accuracy and greater precision than manual methods. Since the 1980s, instrumentation has virtually replaced manual cell counting, with the possible exception of phase platelet counting as a confirmatory procedure.[1] Hematology analyzers have been developed and are marketed by multiple instrument manufacturers. These analyzers typically provide the eight standard hematology parameters (complete blood count [CBC]) plus a three-part or five-part differential leukocyte count in less than 1 minute on 100 μL of whole blood. Automation allows for more efficient workload management and more timely diagnosis and treatment of disease.

GENERAL PRINCIPLES OF HEMATOLOGY INSTRUMENTATION

Despite the number of hematology analyzers available from different manufacturers and with varying levels of sophistication and complexity, only two basic principles of operation

are primarily used: electronic impedance (resistance) and optical scatter. *Electronic impedance*, or low-voltage direct current (DC) resistance, was developed by Coulter in the 1950s[2,3] and is the most common methodology used. *Radiofrequency* (RF), or alternating current resistance, is a modification sometimes used in conjunction with DC electronic impedance. Technicon Instruments (Tarrytown, N.Y.) introduced darkfield optical scanning in the 1960s, and Ortho Clinical Diagnostics, Inc. followed with a laser-based optical instrument in the 1970s.[3,4] *Optical scatter*, using both laser and nonlaser light, is frequently used on today's hematology instrumentation.

Electronic Impedance

The impedance principle of cell counting is based on the detection and measurement of changes in electrical resistance produced by cells as they traverse a small aperture. Cells suspended in an electrically conductive diluent such as saline are pulled through an aperture (orifice) in a glass tube. In the counting chamber, or transducer assembly, low-frequency electrical current is applied between an external electrode (suspended in the cell dilution) and an internal electrode (housed inside the aperture tube). Electrical resistance between the two electrodes, or impedance in the current, occurs as the cells pass through the sensing aperture, causing voltage pulses that are measurable (Fig. 39-1).[5,6] Oscilloscope screens on some instruments display the pulses that are generated by the cells as they interrupt the current. The number of pulses is proportional to the number of cells counted. The size of the voltage pulse is directly proportional to the size (volume) of the cell, allowing discrimination and counting of specific-sized cells through the use of threshold circuits. Pulses are collected and sorted (channelized) according to their amplitude by pulse height analyzers. The data are plotted on a frequency distribution graph, or *size distribution histogram*, with relative number on the *y* axis and size (channel number equivalent to specific size) on the *x* axis. The histogram produced depicts the volume distribution of the cells counted. Figure 39-2 illustrates the construction of a frequency distribution graph. Size thresholds separate the cell populations on the histogram, with the count being the cells enumerated between the lower and upper set thresholds for each population. Size distribution histograms may be used for the evaluation of one cell population or subgroups within a population.[6] The use of proprietary lytic reagents, as used on the older Coulter S-Plus IV, STKR, and Sysmex E-5000 to control shrinkage and lysis of specific cell types, allows for separation and quantitation of white blood cells (WBCs) into three populations (lymphocytes, mononuclear cells, and granulocytes) for the "three-part differential" on one size distribution histogram.[7-9]

Several factors may affect size or volume measurements in impedance or volume displacement instruments. Aperture diameter is crucial, with the red blood cell (RBC)/platelet

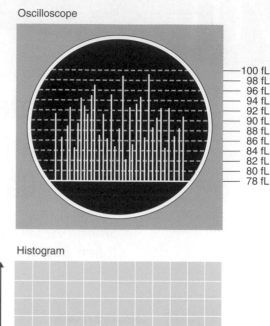

Oscilloscope

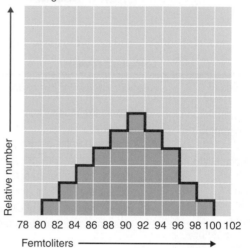

Histogram

Figure 39-2 Oscilloscope and histogram showing the construction of a frequency distribution graph. (Modified from Coulter Electronics, Inc.: Significant Advances in Hematology: Hematology Education Series, PN 4206115A. Hialeah, FL: Coulter Electronics, Inc., 1983.)

aperture smaller than the WBC aperture to increase platelet counting sensitivity. On earlier systems, protein buildup occurred, thereby decreasing the diameter of the orifice, slowing the flow of cells and increasing their relative electrical resistance. Protein buildup results in lower cell counts, which result in falsely elevated cell volumes. Impedance instruments once required frequent manual aperture cleaning, but current instruments incorporate "burn circuits" or other internal cleaning systems to prevent or slow down protein buildup.[7-10] Carryover of cells from one sample to the next also is minimized by these internal cleaning systems. Coincident passage of more than one cell at a time through the orifice causes artificially large pulses, resulting in falsely increased cell volumes and falsely decreased cell counts. This count reduction, or *coincident passage loss*, is statistically predictable (and mathematically correctable) because of its direct relationship to cell concentration and the size or effective volume of the aperture.[8-10] Coincidence correction typically is completed by the analyzer computer before final printout of cell counts from the instrument. Other factors affecting pulse height include

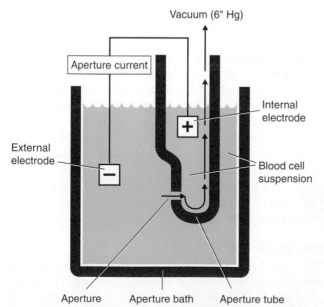

Figure 39-1 Coulter principle of cell counting. (From Coulter Electronics, Inc.: Coulter® STKR Product Reference Manual, PN 4235547E. Hialeah, FL: Coulter Electronics, Inc., 1988.)

orientation of the cell in the center of the aperture and deformability of the RBC, which may be altered by decreased hemoglobin (Hb) content.[11,12] Recirculation of cells back into the sensing zone creates erroneous pulses and falsely elevates cell counts. A back-wash or sweep-flow mechanism has been added to prevent recirculation of cells back into the sensing zone, and anomalously shaped pulses are edited out electronically.[7,8,10]

The use of hydrodynamic focusing avoids many of the potential problems inherent in a rigid aperture system. The sample stream is surrounded by a sheath fluid as it passes through the central axis of the aperture. Laminar flow allows the central sample stream to narrow sufficiently to separate and align the cells into single file for passage through the sensing zone.[13,14] The outer sheath fluid minimizes protein buildup and plugs, eliminates recirculation of cells back into the sensing zone with generation of spurious pulses, and reduces pulse height irregularity because off-center cell passage is prevented and better resolution of the blood cells is obtained. Coincident passage loss also is reduced because blood cells line up one after another in the direction of the flow.[15] Laminar flow and hydrodynamic focusing are discussed further in Chapter 33.

Radiofrequency

Low-voltage DC impedance, as described previously, may be used in conjunction with RF resistance, or high-voltage electromagnetic current flowing between both electrodes simultaneously. Although the total volume of the cell is proportional to the change in DC, the cell interior density (e.g., nuclear

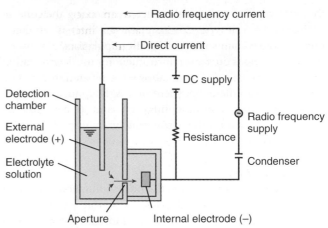

Figure 39-3 RF/DC detection method, showing simultaneous use of DC and RF in one measurement system on the Sysmex SE-9500. (From Toa Medical Electronics Co., Ltd.: Sysmex SE-9500 Operator's Manual [CN 461-2464-2]. Kobe, Japan: Toa Medical Electronics Co., Ltd., 1997.)

volume) is proportional to pulse size or change in the RF signal. *Conductivity*, as measured by this high-frequency electromagnetic probe, is attenuated by nuclear-to-cytoplasmic ratio, nuclear density, and cytoplasmic granulation. DC and RF voltage changes may be detected simultaneously and separated by two different pulse processing circuits.[15,16] Figure 39-3 illustrates the simultaneous use of DC and RF current.

Two different cell properties, such as impedance and conductivity, can be plotted against each other for the formation of a *two-dimensional distribution cytogram* or *scatterplot* (Fig. 39-4). Such plots display the cell populations as clusters, with

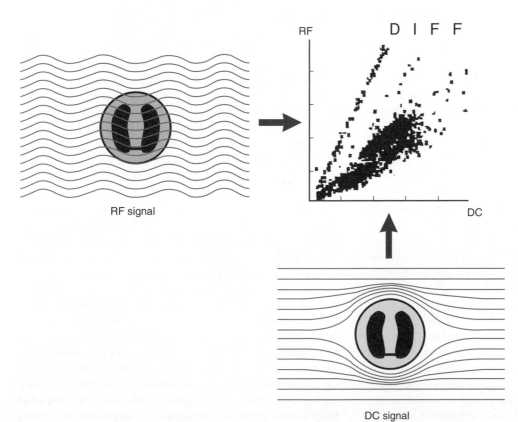

Figure 39-4 Illustration of cell size/volume measurement with DC voltage change versus the measure of cell nuclear volume/complexity with change in the RF signal. The two measurements can be plotted against each other for the formation of a two-dimensional distribution scatterplot. (From Toa Medical Electronics Co., Ltd.: Sysmex SE-9500 Operator's Manual [CN 461-2464-2]. Kobe, Japan: Toa Medical Electronics Co., Ltd., 1997.)

the number of dots in each cluster representing the concentration of that cell type. Computer cluster analysis can determine absolute counts for specific cell populations. The use of multiple methods on a given instrument for the determination of at least two cell properties allows the separation of WBCs into a five-part differential (neutrophils, lymphocytes, monocytes, eosinophils, and basophils). DC and RF detection are two methods used on the Sysmex analyzers to perform WBC differentials.[15,16]

Optical Scatter

Optical scatter may be used as the primary methodology or in combination with other methods. In optical scatter systems (flow cytometers), a hydrodynamically focused sample stream is directed through a quartz flow cell past a focused light source (see Fig. 33-3). The light source is generally a tungsten-halogen lamp or a helium-neon *laser* (*l*ight *a*mplification by *s*timulated *e*mission of *r*adiation). Laser light, termed *monochromatic light* because it is emitted as a single wavelength, differs from bright-field light in its intensity, its coherence (i.e., it travels in phase), and its low divergence or spread. These characteristics allow for the detection of interference in the laser beam and enable enumeration and differentiation of cell types.[13,17] Optical scatter may be used to study RBCs, WBCs, and platelets.[18]

As the cells pass through the sensing zone and interrupt the beam, light is scattered in all directions. Light scatter results from the interaction between the processes of absorption, diffraction (bending around corners or surface of cell), refraction (bending because of a change in speed), and reflection (backward rays caused by obstruction).[19] The detection and conversion of scattered rays into electrical signals is accomplished by photodetectors (photodiodes and photomultiplier tubes) at specific angles. Lenses fitted with blocker bars to prevent nonscattered light from entering the detector are used to collect the scattered light. A series of filters and mirrors separate the varying wavelengths and present them to the photodetectors. Photodiodes convert light photons to electronic signals proportional in magnitude to the amount of light collected. Photomultiplier tubes are used to collect the weaker signals produced at a 90-degree angle and multiply the photoelectrons into stronger, useful signals. Analogue-to-digital converters change the electronic pulses to digital signals for computer analysis.[13,17]

Forward-angle light scatter (0 degree) correlates with cell volume or size, primarily because of diffraction of light. Orthogonal light scatter (90 degrees), or side scatter, results from refraction and reflection of light from larger structures inside the cell and correlates with degree of internal complexity.[20] Forward low-angle scatter (2-3 degrees) and forward high-angle scatter (5-15 degrees) also correlate with cell volume and refractive index or with internal complexity.[21] Differential scatter is the combination of this low-angle and high-angle forward light scatter, primarily used on Bayer systems for cellular analysis. The angles of light scatter measured by the different flow cytometers are manufacturer and method specific.

Scatter properties at different angles may be plotted against each other for the generation of two-dimensional cytograms or scatterplots, as on the Abbott CELL-DYN instruments.[22,23] Optical scatter may also be plotted against absorption, as on the Bayer systems,[24,25] or against volume, as on the larger Coulter systems.[10] Computer cluster analysis of the cytograms may yield quantitative and qualitative information.

PRINCIPAL CELL COUNTING INSTRUMENTS

Overview

Hematology analyzers are produced by multiple manufacturers, including, but not limited to, Abbott Diagnostics (Abbott Park, Ill.),[26] Horiba ABX Diagnostics (Montpellier, France),[27] Bayer Diagnostics (Tarrytown, N.Y.),[28] Beckman Coulter, Inc. (Brea, Calif.),[29] and Sysmex Corporation (Kobe, Japan).[30] The following discussion is limited to instrumentation produced by four of these suppliers. Emphasis is not placed on sample size or handling, speed, level of automation, or comparison of instruments or manufacturers. Likewise, as technology continues to improve, the newest (or most recent) models produced by a manufacturer may not be mentioned. Instead, a detailed description of primary methods used by these manufacturers is given to show usage of, and clarify further, principles presented earlier and to enable the technologist to interpret patient data better, including instrument-generated histograms and cytograms, in the hematology laboratory. Table 39-1 summarizes methods used for hemogram determination on four major hematology instruments. Table 39-2 summarizes methods used for WBC differential determination on the same four analyzers.

Hematology analyzers have some common basic components, including hydraulics, pneumatics, and electrical systems. The hydraulics system includes aspirating unit, dispensers, diluters, mixing chambers, aperture baths or flow cells or both, and a hemoglobinometer. The pneumatics system includes vacuums and pressures required for operating the valves and moving the sample through the hydraulics system. The electrical system controls operational sequences of the total system and includes electronic analyzers and computing circuitry for processing the data generated. Some older-model instruments have oscilloscope screens that display the electrical pulses in real time as the cells are counted. A data display unit receives information from the analyzer and prints results, histograms, or cytograms.

Sample handling varies from instrument to instrument based on degree of automation, ranging from discrete analyzers to walkaway systems with "front-end load" capability. Computer functions also vary, with the larger instruments having extensive microprocessor and data management capabilities. Computer software capabilities include automatic start-up and shutdown, with internal diagnostic self-checks and some maintenance; quality control, with automatic review of quality control data, calculations, graphs, moving averages, and storage of quality control files; patient data storage and retrieval, with delta checks, panic or critical value flagging, and automatic verification of patient results based on user-defined algorithms; host query with laboratory/hospital information system to allow random access discrete testing

TABLE 39-1 Methods for Hemogram and Reticulocyte Count Determination on Four Major Hematology Instruments

Parameter	Coulter LH 750	Sysmex XE-2100	Abbott CELL-DYN 4000	Bayer ADVIA 2120
WBC	Impedance, hydrodynamic focusing	Hydrodynamic focusing, DC detection (Impedence)	Optical scatter (primary count), impedance (secondary count)	Hydrodynamic focusing, optical scatter and absorption
RBC	Impedance	Hydrodynamic focusing, DC detection (Impedence)	Impedance	Hydrodynamic focusing, laser low-angle (2-3 degrees) and high-angle (5-15 degrees) scatter
Hb	Modified cyanmethemoglobin (525 nm)	SLS-Hb (555 nm)	Modified cyanmethemoglobin (540 nm)	Modified cyanmethemoglobin (546 nm)
Hematocrit	$(RBC \times MCV) \div 10$	Cumulative pulse height detection	$(RBC \times MCV) \div 10$	$(RBC \times MCV) \div 10$
MCV	Mean of RBC volume distribution histogram	$(HCT \div RBC) \times 10$	Mean of RBC volume distribution histogram	Mean of RBC volume histogram
MCH	$(Hb \div RBC) \times 10$	$(Hb \div RBC) \times 10$	$(Hb \div RBC) \times 10$	$(Hb \div RBC) \times 10$
MCHC	$(Hb \div HCT) \times 100$	$(Hb \div HCT) \times 100$	$(Hb \div HCT) \times 100$	$(Hb \div HCT) \times 100$
Platelet count	Impedance (2-20 fL): least-squares fit of volume distribution histogram (0-70 fL)	Hydrodynamic focusing, DC detection (Impedence) ($\approx$2-30 fL)	Impedance ($\approx$2-30 fL)	Hydrodynamic focusing, laser low-angle (2-3 degrees) and high-angle (5-15 degrees) scatter (1-60 fL)
RDW	CV (%) of RBC histogram: $(SD \div MCV) \times 100$	RDW − SD (fL) or RDW − CV (%) available	Relative value, equivalent to CV	CV (%) of RBC histogram: $(SD \div MCV) \times 100$
Reticulocyte count	Supravital staining (new methylene blue); volume, conductivity, optical scatter (VCS technology)	Supravital staining (Auramine O); fluorescent detection	Proprietary stain (CD4K530), multiangle scatter, and fluorescent detection	Supravital staining (Oxazine 750); low-angle (2-3 degrees) and high-angle (5-15 degrees) optical scatter and absorbance

SLS, sodium lauryl sulfate.

TABLE 39-2 Methods for White Blood Cell Differential Determination on Four Major Hematology Instruments

Parameter	Coulter LH 750	Sysmex XE-2100	Abbott CELL-DYN 4000	Bayer ADVIA 2120
Neutrophils	VCS	DC/RF detection	MAPSS	Peroxidase staining, optical scatter and absorption
Lymphocytes	VCS	DC/RF detection	MAPSS	Peroxidase staining, optical scatter and absorption
Monocytes	VCS	DC/RF detection	MAPSS	Peroxidase staining, optical scatter and absorption
Eosinophils	VCS	Differential lysis, shrinkage; DC detection	MAPSS	Peroxidase staining, optical scatter and absorption
Basophils	VCS	Differential lysis, shrinkage; DC detection	MAPSS	Differential lysis, laser low-angle (2-3 degrees) and high-angle (5-15 degrees) scatter

MAPSS, multiangle polarized scatter separation; VCS, volume, conductivity, scatter.

capability; animal software; and even the ability to analyze body fluids.

Coulter Instrumentation

Beckman Coulter, Inc., manufactures an extensive line of hematology analyzers, including the smaller ONYX series that provide complete RBC, platelet, and WBC analysis with three-part differential; the larger MAXM and STKS that perform a CBC with five-part differential and reticulocyte analysis using an off-line sample preparation; and the GEN-S and the newer

LH 750, part of the LH 700 Series, that provide a fully automated on-line reticulocyte analysis.[29] Both systems additionally have the capability to perform CD4/CD8 counts.[31-33] Coulter instruments typically have two measurement channels in the hydraulics system for determining the hemogram data. The RBC and WBC counts and Hb determination are considered to be measured directly. The aspirated whole-blood sample is divided into two aliquots, and each is mixed with an isotonic diluent. The first dilution is delivered to the RBC aperture chamber, and the second is delivered to the WBC aperture chamber. In the RBC chamber, RBCs and platelets are counted and discriminated by electrical impedance as the cells are pulled through each of three sensing apertures (50-μm diameter, 60-μm length). Particles 2 to 20 fL are counted as platelets, and particles greater than 36 fL are counted as RBCs. In the WBC chamber, a reagent to lyse RBCs and release Hb is added before WBCs are counted simultaneously by impedance in each of three sensing apertures (100-μm diameter, 75-μm length). Alternatively, some models employ consecutive counts in the same RBC or WBC aperture. After counting cycles are completed, the WBC dilution is passed to the hemoglobinometer for determination of Hb concentration (light transmittance read at a wavelength of 525 nm). Electrical pulses generated in the counting cycles are sent to the analyzer for editing, coincidence correction, and digital conversion. Two of the three counts obtained in the RBC and the WBC baths must match within specified limits for the counts to be accepted by the instrument.[6,10] This multiple counting procedure prevents data errors resulting from aperture obstructions or statistical outliers and allows for excellent reproducibility on the Coulter instruments.

Pulse height is measured and categorized by pulse height analyzers; 256 channels are used for WBC and RBC analysis, and 64 channels are used for platelet analysis. Size-distribution histograms of WBC, RBC, and platelet populations are generated. The RBC mean cell volume (MCV) is the average volume of the RBCs taken from the size distribution data. The hematocrit (Hct), mean cell Hb (MCH), and mean cell Hb concentration (MCHC) are calculated from measured and derived values. The RBC distribution width (RDW) is calculated directly from the histogram as the coefficient of variation (CV) of the RBC volume distribution, with a reference range of 11.5% to 14.5%.[6] The RDW is an index of anisocytosis, but may be falsely skewed because it reflects the ratio of SD and MCV. That is, an RBC distribution histogram with normal divergence, but with a decreased MCV, may imply a high RDW, falsely indicating increased anisocytosis. MCV and RDW are used by the instrument to flag possible anisocytosis, microcytosis, and macrocytosis.[10]

Platelets are counted within the range of 2 to 20 fL, and a size-distribution histogram is constructed. If the platelet size distribution meets specified criteria, a statistical least-squares fit is applied to the raw data, fitting the data to a log-normal curve. The curve is extrapolated from 0 to 70 fL, and the final count is derived from this extended curve. This fitting procedure eliminates interfering particles in the noise region, such as debris, and in the larger region, such as small RBCs. The mean platelet volume (MPV), analogous to the RBC MCV, also is derived from the platelet histogram. Reference values for the MPV are about 7.8 to 11 fL, and the MPV increases slightly as the sample sits in the anticoagulant, ethylenediamine tetraacetic acid.[6]

Many older-model Coulter instruments, such as the STKR, and the newer smaller models, such as the ONYX, provide three-part leukocyte subpopulation analysis, which differentiates WBCs into lymphocytes, mononuclear cells, and granulocytes. In the WBC channel, a special lysing reagent causes *differential shrinkage* of the leukocytes, allowing the different cells to be counted and sized based on their impedance. A WBC histogram is constructed from the channelized data. Particles between approximately 35 and 90 fL are considered lymphocytes; particles between 90 and 160 fL, "mononuclears" (monocytes, blasts, immature granulocytes, and atypical lymphocytes); and particles between 160 and 450 fL, granulocytes, allowing the calculation of relative and absolute numbers for these three populations.[7] Proprietary computerized algorithms further allow flagging for increased eosinophils or basophils or both and interpretation of the histogram differential to include flagging for abnormal cells, such as atypical lymphocytes and blasts.[8] When cell populations overlap or a distinct separation of populations does not exist, a region alarm (R flag) may be triggered, indicating the area of interference on the size-distribution histogram. An R1 flag represents excess signals at the lower threshold region of the WBC histogram and a questionable WBC count. This interference is visualized as a "high takeoff" of the curve and may indicate the presence of nucleated RBCs, clumped platelets, unlysed RBCs, or electronic noise.[7,8] Figure 39-5 shows composite printouts from the Coulter STKR that include the "interpretive differential."

More recent Coulter instruments, the STKS, MAXM, GEN-S, and LH 750, generate hemogram data (including the WBC count) exactly as before but use Coulter's proprietary *VCS (volume, conductivity, scatter) technology* in a separate channel to evaluate WBCs for the determination of a five-part differential. The VCS technology includes the *v*olumetric sizing of cells by impedance, *c*onductivity measurements of cells, and laser light *s*catter, all performed simultaneously for each cell. After RBCs are lysed and WBCs are treated with a stabilizing reagent to maintain them in a "near-native" state, a hydrodynamically focused sample stream is directed through the flow cell past the sensing zone. Low-frequency DC measures size, while a high-frequency electromagnetic probe measures conductivity, an indicator of cellular internal content. The conductivity signal is corrected for cellular volume, yielding a unique measurement called *opacity*. Each cell also is scanned with monochromatic laser light that reveals information about the cell surface, such as structure, shape, and reflectivity. Coulter's unique rotated light scatter detection method, which covers a 10-degree to 70-degree range, allows for separation of cells with similar size, but different scatter characteristics. More than 8000 WBCs are analyzed in each sample.[32,35]

This combination of technologies provides a three-dimensional plot or cytograph of the WBC populations, which are separated by computer cluster analysis. Two-dimensional scatterplots of the three measurements represent different views of the cytograph. The discriminate function 1 (DF 1) scatterplot of volume (*y* axis) versus light scatter (*x* axis) shows clear separation of lymphocytes, monocytes, neutrophils, and eosinophils. Basophils are hidden behind the lymphocytes in this scatterplot but are separated by conductivity owing to their cytoplasmic granulation. The DF 2 scatterplot of volume (*y* axis) versus conductivity (*x* axis) shows lymphocytes, monocytes, and neutrophils as the prominant populations. When the neutrophil population is removed from the DF 2 scatter-

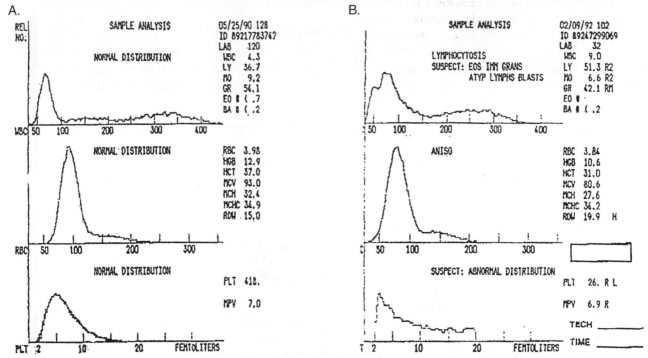

Figure 39-5 Printout from the Coulter STKR showing the "interpretive differential." **A,** Note the three distinct WBC populations, normal gaussian or bell-shaped distribution of RBCs, and right-skewed or log-normal distribution of platelets. **B,** Note the left shift in the WBC histogram with possible interference at the lower threshold region. R2 flag indicates interference and loss of valley owing to overlap or insufficient separation between the lymphocyte and mononuclear populations at the 90-fL region. RM flag indicates interference at more than one region. Eosinophil data have been suppressed. Also note the abnormal platelet size distribution with a low platelet count. Manual 200-cell differential counts: **A,** 42.5% neutrophils (37% segmented neutrophils, 5.5% bands), 41.5% lymphocytes, 4.5% monocytes, 1% basophils, 0.5% metamyelocytes, 9.5% myelocytes, 0.5% atypical lymphocytes; **B,** 51% neutrophils (23% segmented neutrophils, 28% bands), 12% lymphocytes, 9.5% monocytes, 1% metamyelocytes, 1.5% myelocytes, 25% atypical lymphocytes, and 17 nucleated RBCs/100 WBCs.

plot, the basophil population may be visualized on the Z axis (DF 3 display). DF 2 and DF 3 scatterplots are available at operator request. Single-parameter histograms of volume, conductivity, and light scatter also are available.[10,35] Figure 39-6 represents a standard patient printout from the Coulter LH 750 showing a DF 1 scatterplot.

Two types of WBC flags (alarms or indicators of abnormality) are generated on all hematology analyzers that provide a WBC differential count: (1) user defined, primarily set for distributional abnormalities, such as eosinophilia or lymphocytopenia (based on absolute eosinophil or lymphocyte counts); and (2) instrument specific, primarily suspect flags for morphologic abnormalities. For *distributional flags,* the user establishes reference ranges and programs the instrument to flag each parameter as high or low. *Suspect flags* indicating the possible presence of abnormal cells are triggered when cell populations fall outside expected regions or when specific statistical limitations are exceeded. Instrument-specific "suspect" flags on the Coulter LH700 Series include Immature Granulocytes/Bands, Blasts, Variant Lymphocytes, Nucleated Red Blood Cells, and Platelet Clumps. Inadequate separation of cell populations may disallow reporting of differential results by the instrument and may elicit a subsequent "Review Slide" message.[10,36]

On the LH 750, Coulter has added an IntelliKinetics application. This application is used to ensure consistency with the kinetic reactions. It provides the instrument the best signals for analysis independent of laboratory environment variations. As compared with earlier models Coulter IntelliKinetics provides better separation of cell populations for WBCs and the reticulocytes, enabling better analysis by the system algorithms.[36]

Sysmex Instrumentation

Sysmex Corporation, formerly TOA Medical Electronics Co., Ltd., manufactures a full line of hematology analyzers, including the small KX-21 and K-4500 that provide complete RBC, platelet, and WBC analysis with three-part differential; the larger SF-3000 and SE-9000 that perform a CBC with five-part differential; and the newer SE-9500/9000+RAM-1 or the XE-2100 systems that additionally provide a fully automated reticulocyte count.[30] The WBC, RBC, Hb, Hct, and platelet counts are considered to be measured directly. Three hydraulic subsystems are used for determining the hemogram: the WBC channel, RBC/platelet channel, and a separate Hb channel. In the WBC and RBC transducer chambers, diluted WBC and RBC samples are aspirated through the different apertures and counted using the impedance (DC detection) method for counting and sizing cells. Two unique features enhance the

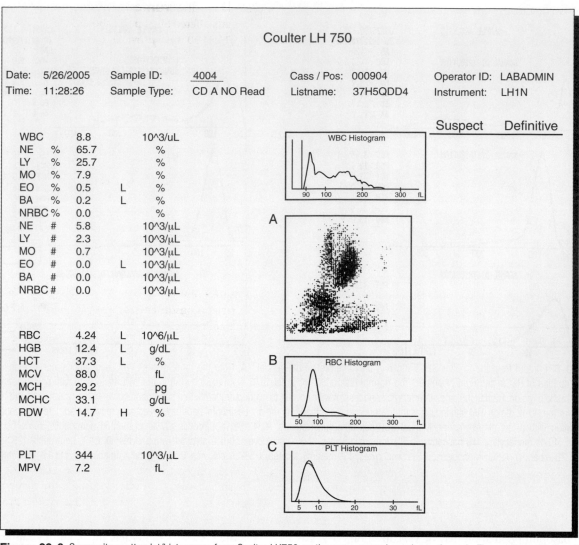

Coulter LH 750

Date: 5/26/2005   Sample ID: <u>4004</u>   Cass / Pos: 000904   Operator ID: LABADMIN
Time: 11:28:26   Sample Type: CD A NO Read   Listname: 37H5QDD4   Instrument: LH1N

Suspect   Definitive

WBC		8.8		10^3/uL
NE	%	65.7		%
LY	%	25.7		%
MO	%	7.9		%
EO	%	0.5	L	%
BA	%	0.2	L	%
NRBC	%	0.0		%
NE	#	5.8		10^3/µL
LY	#	2.3		10^3/µL
MO	#	0.7		10^3/µL
EO	#	0.0	L	10^3/µL
BA	#	0.0		10^3/µL
NRBC	#	0.0		10^3/µL

RBC	4.24	L	10^6/µL
HGB	12.4	L	g/dL
HCT	37.3	L	%
MCV	88.0		fL
MCH	29.2		pg
MCHC	33.1		g/dL
RDW	14.7	H	%

| PLT | 344 | | 10^3/µL |
| MPV | 7.2 | | fL |

WBC Histogram

A

B   RBC Histogram

C   PLT Histogram

Figure 39-6 Composite scatterplot/histograms from Coulter LH750 on the same normal specimen shown in Figures 39-7, 39-9 and 39-12. **A,** WBC two-dimensional scatterplot shows volume as determined by impedance on the *y* axis versus light scatter (DF 1) on the *x* axis. Computer-generated floating discriminators separate lymphocyte (LY), monocyte (MO), neutrophil (NE), and eosinophil (EO) regions. Data below the WBC threshold represent non-WBC debris. Large or clumped platelets, nucleated RBCs, WBC fragments, or unlysed RBCs in abnormal samples should fall below this threshold. DF 2 and DF 3 scatterplots (not shown) are derived from volume (*y* axis) versus conductivity (*x* axis). Basophils (BA) are best visualized on the DF 3 display, from which the neutrophil population has been removed. All two-dimensional scatterplots, single-parameter histograms, or the three-dimensional cytograph may be reviewed at operator request. The relative value (%) of each of the five WBC populations derived from this three-dimensional analysis is multiplied by the WBC count derived in a separate impedance channel for determination of the absolute counts (#). **B** and **C,** Relative number (*y* axis) versus volume distribution (*x* axis) histograms for RBCs and platelets (PLT). Note the normal gaussian or bell-shaped distribution of the RBCs in **B** and right-skewed or log-normal distribution of PLTs in **C.** The small population of larger RBCs on the right of the RBC curve represents coincident passage of doublets or triplets or both through the impedance aperture, creating larger pulses. This portion of the RBC curve is excluded from the calculation of the RDW. The MPV is analogous to the MCV.

impedance technology: (1) in the RBC/platelet channel, a sheathed stream with hydrodynamic focusing is used to direct cells through the aperture, reducing coincident passage, particle size distortion, and recirculation of blood cells around the aperture; and (2) in the WBC and RBC/platelet channels, "floating thresholds" are used to discriminate each cell population.[9,15,16]

As cells pass through the apertures, signals are transmitted in sequence to the analogue circuit and particle size distri-

bution analysis circuits for conversion to cumulative cell size distribution data. Particle size distribution curves are constructed, and optimal position of the autodiscrimination level (i.e., threshold) is set by the microprocessor for each cell population. The lower platelet threshold is automatically adjusted in the 2- to 6-fL volume range, and the upper threshold is adjusted in the 12- to 30-fL range, based on particle volume distribution. Likewise, the RBC lower and upper thresholds may be set in the 25- to 75-fL and 200- to 250-fL volume ranges. This "floating threshold" circuitry allows for discrimination of cell populations on a sample-by-sample basis. Cell counts include pulses between the lower and upper autodiscriminator levels, with dilution ratio, volume counted, and coincident passage error accounted for in the final computer-generated numbers. In the RBC channel, the floating discriminator is particularly useful in separating platelets from small RBCs. The Hct also is determined from the RBC/platelet channel, based on the principle that pulse height generated by the RBC is proportional to cell volume. The Hct is the RBC cumulative pulse height and is considered a true relative percentage volume of erythrocytes.[9,15] In the Hb flow cell, Hb is converted to oxyhemoglobin, which combines with sodium lauryl sulfate to become a sodium lauryl sulfate–Hb hemichrome molecule, with concentration measured as absorbance at 555 nm.[16,37]

The following indices are calculated in the microprocessor using directly measured or derived parameters: MCV, MCH, MCHC, RDW-SD, RDW-CV, MPV, and plateletcrit. RDW-SD is the RBC arithmetic distribution width measured at 20% of the height of the RBC curve, reported in femtoliters (fL) with a reference interval of 37 to 54 fL. RDW-CV is the RDW reported as a CV. Plateletcrit is the platelet volume ratio, analogous to the Hct. MPV is calculated from the plateletcrit and platelet count just as erythrocyte MCV is calculated from the Hct and RBC count. The proportion of platelets greater than 12 fL to the total platelet count may be an indicator of possible platelet clumping, giant platelets, or cell fragments.[9,15,16]

The SE-9000/9500 uses four detection chambers to analyze WBCs and obtain a five-part differential: the DIFF, IMI, EO, and BASO chambers. In the DIFF detection chamber, RBCs are hemolyzed and WBCs are analyzed simultaneously by low-frequency DC and high-frequency current *(DC/RF detection method)*. A scattergram of RF detection signals (*y* axis) versus DC detection signals (*x* axis) yields separation of the WBCs into lymphocytes, monocytes, and granulocytes. Floating discriminators determine the optimal separation between these populations. Granulocytes are analyzed further in the IMI detection chamber to determine "immature (leukocyte) information." RBCs are lysed, and WBCs other than immature granulocytes are selectively shrunk by temperature and chemically controlled reactions. Analysis of the treated sample using the DC/RF detection method allows separation of immature cells on the IMI scattergram. A similar differential shrinkage and lysis method is also used in the EO and BASO chambers. That is, eosinophils and basophils are counted by impedance (DC detection) in separate chambers in which the RBCs are lysed and WBCs other than eosinophils or basophils are selectively shrunk by temperature and chemically controlled reactions. Eosinophils and basophils are subtracted from the granulocyte count derived from the DIFF scattergram analysis for determination of the neutrophil count. User-defined distributional flags may be set, and instrument-specific suspect flags, similar to those described for the Coulter LH 700 Series, are triggered for the possible presence of morphologic abnormalities.[15,16] A POSITIVE or NEGATIVE interpretive message is displayed. Figure 39-7 is a patient report from the XE 2100 on the same patient sample represented in Figure 39-6.

CELL-DYN Instrumentation

Instruments offered by Abbott Laboratories include the smaller CELL-DYN 1700 that provides complete RBC, platelet, and WBC analysis with three-part differential; the larger CELL-DYN 3500R and 3700 that perform a CBC with five-part differential and reticulocyte analysis using an off-line sample preparation; and the CELL-DYN 4000 that provides fully automated, random-access reticulocyte analysis.[26] The CELL-DYN 4000 system has three independent measurement channels for determining the hemogram and differential: (1) an optical channel for WBC count and differential data, (2) an impedance channel for RBC and platelet data, and (3) an Hb channel for Hb determination.[22,23] An additional impedance channel for determining a WBC impedance count is used as an internal check against the primary WBC optical count. When the WBC impedance count and WBC optical count differ, an algorithm selects the most appropriate value for the reported WBC.[23] The WBC, RBC, Hb, and platelet counts are considered to be measured directly. A 60×70-μm aperture is used in the RBC/platelet transducer assembly for counting and sizing of RBCs and platelets by the electronic impedance method. A unique von Behrens plate is located in the RBC/platelet counting chamber to minimize the effect of recirculating cells. Pulses are collected and sorted in 256 channels according to their amplitude: particles between 1 and 35 fL are included in the initial platelet data, and particles greater than 35 fL are counted as RBCs. Floating thresholds are used to determine the best separation of the platelet population and to eliminate interference, such as noise, debris, or small RBCs, from the count. Coincident passage loss is corrected for in the final RBC and platelet counts. RBC pulse editing is applied before MCV derivation to compensate for aberrant pulses produced by nonaxial passage of RBCs through the aperture. The MCV is the average volume of the RBCs derived from RBC size distribution data. Hb is measured directly using a modified hemiglobin-cyanide method that measures absorbance at 540 nm. Hct, MCH, and MCHC are calculated from the directly measured or derived parameters. The RDW, equivalent to CV, is a relative value, derived from the RBC histogram by using the 20th and 80th percentiles. The platelet analysis is a two-dimensional optical platelet using fluorescent technology, the same technology used for direct nucleated RBC counting. Further analysis of platelets and platelet aggregates can be performed by using platelet-specific immunolabeling.[38-40] Other indices available include MPV and plateletcrit (analogous to Hct).[22,23]

The WBC count and differential are derived from the optical channel using CELL-DYN's patented multiangle polarized scatter separation (MAPSS). A hydrodynamically focused sample stream is directed through a quartz flow cell past a focused light source, an argon ion laser. Scattered light is measured at multiple angles: 0-degree forward light scatter is used for determination of cell size, 90-degree orthogonal light scatter is used for determination of cellular lobularity, 7-degree narrow angle scatter is used to correlate with cellular complexity, and 90-degree depolarized (90°D) light scattering is used for evaluation of cellular granularity. Orthogonal light scatter is split, with one portion directed to a 90-degree

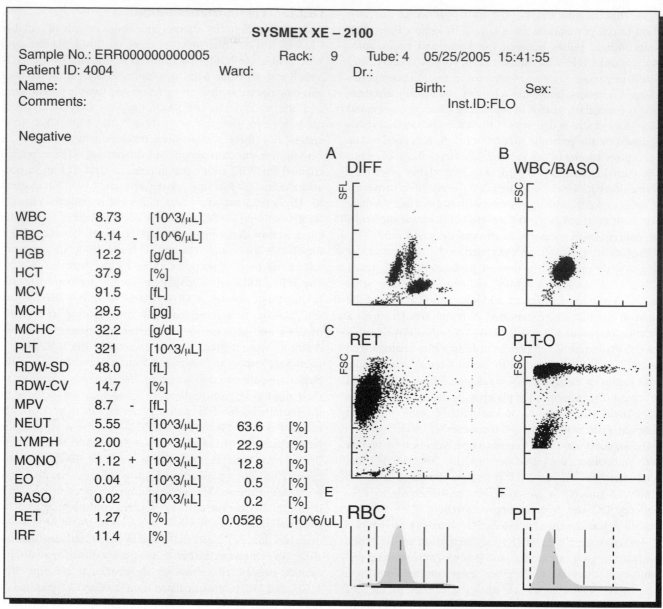

SYSMEX XE – 2100

Sample No.: ERR000000000005   Rack: 9   Tube: 4   05/25/2005 15:41:55
Patient ID: 4004   Ward: Dr.:
Name: Birth: Sex:
Comments: Inst.ID:FLO

Negative

WBC	8.73		[10^3/μL]		
RBC	4.14	-	[10^6/μL]		
HGB	12.2		[g/dL]		
HCT	37.9		[%]		
MCV	91.5		[fL]		
MCH	29.5		[pg]		
MCHC	32.2		[g/dL]		
PLT	321		[10^3/μL]		
RDW-SD	48.0		[fL]		
RDW-CV	14.7		[%]		
MPV	8.7	-	[fL]		
NEUT	5.55		[10^3/μL]	63.6	[%]
LYMPH	2.00		[10^3/μL]	22.9	[%]
MONO	1.12	+	[10^3/μL]	12.8	[%]
EO	0.04		[10^3/μL]	0.5	[%]
BASO	0.02		[10^3/μL]	0.2	[%]
RET	1.27		[%]	0.0526	[10^6/uL]
IRF	11.4		[%]		

A DIFF
B WBC/BASO
C RET
D PLT-O
E RBC
F PLT

Figure 39-7 Composite histograms/scatterplots from Sysmex XE-2100 on the same normal specimen shown in Figures 39-6, 39-9, and 39-12. In the DIFF scatterplot **(A)**, the *y* axis shows high-frequency current (RF) detection signals plotted against DC detection signals on the *x* axis. Floating discriminators determine optimal separation of lymphocytes (LYMPH), monocytes (MONO), and neutrophils (NEUT). In the WBC/BASO scatterplot, the total number of WBCs are optically counted, and a second count is performed, yielding the total number of basophils in the WBC count, illustrated on the WBC/BASO scatterplot **(B)**. BASO counts are determined by enumerating cells between the autodiscriminator level and an upper fixed discriminator position. The EO distribution histogram is not shown. The absolute neutrophil count (NEUT) ($\times 10^3$/μL) is computed by subtracting EO and BASO counts from the 10^3 result derived from the scatterplot analysis. Relative differential results (%) are computed by dividing absolute numbers by total WBC count. **C,** The reticulocyte channel is an optical count that measures mature RBCs, optical platelets, and reticulocytes, yielding a two-dimensional scatterplot analysis of the reticulocytes and the platelets. On the *x* axis, lateral fluorescent light scatter is plotted against the intensity of the forward light scatter on the *y* axis. This analysis also yields the optical platelet scatterplot as illustrated in **D. E** and **F,** Relative number (*y* axis) versus size distribution (*x* axis) histograms for RBCs and platelets (PLT). Note the bell-shaped RBC curve in **E** with little interference on the right side from coincident passage, minimized by hydrodynamic focusing in the RBC/PLT channel. The RDW (both RDW-SD and RDW-CV) is determined at the 20% relative height level, excluding any possible interference.
SFL, side fluorescence; FSC, forward scatter.

photomultiplier tube and the other portion directed through a polarizer to the 90°D photomultiplier tube. Light that has changed polarization (depolarized) is the only light that can be detected by the 90°D photomultiplier tube. Various combinations of these four measurements are used to differentiate and quantify the five major WBC subpopulations: neutrophils, lymphocytes, monocytes, eosinophils, and basophils.[22,41] Figure 39-8 illustrates Abbott's MAPSS technology.

The light scatter signals are converted into electrical signals, sorted into 256 channels on the basis of amplitude for each angle of light measured, and graphically presented as scatterplots. Scatter information from the different angles is

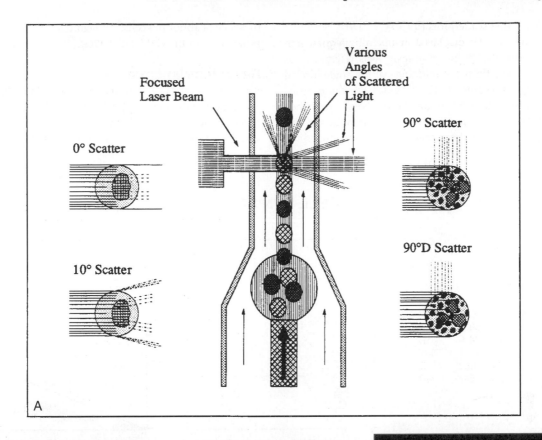

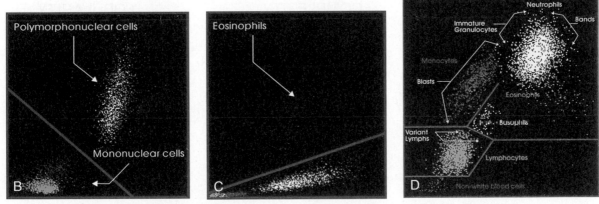

Figure 39-8 MAPSS technology showing the measurement and characterization of cells by looking at light scatter from four different angles. (From Abbott Laboratories: CELL-DYN® 3500 System Operator's Manual [LN 92722-05]. Abbott Park, Ill. Abbott Laboratories, 1996.) MAPPS, multiangle polarized scatter separation. 90° D, 90° depolarized.

plotted in various combinations: 90°/7°, or lobularity versus complexity; 0°/7°, size versus complexity; and 90°D/90°, granularity versus lobularity. Lobularity (*y* axis) plotted against complexity (*x* axis) yields separation of mononuclear (MONO) and polymorphonuclear (POLY) subpopulations. (Basophils cluster with the mononuclears in this analysis because the basophil granules dissolve in the sheath reagent, and the degranulated basophil is a less complex cell.) Each cell in the two clusters is identified as a MONO or POLY for further evaluation.

The MONO subpopulation is plotted on a 0°/7° scatterplot, with size on the *y* axis and complexity on the *x* axis. Three populations (lymphocytes, monocytes, and basophils) are seen clearly on this display. Nucleated RBCs, unlysed RBCs,

giant platelets, and platelet clumps fall below the lymphocyte cluster on this scatterplot and are excluded from the WBC count and differential. Information from the WBC impedance channel additionally is used in discriminating these particles.[23]

The POLY subpopulation is plotted on a 90°D/90° scatterplot, with granularity on the *y* axis and lobularity on the *x* axis. Because of the unique nature of eosinophil granules, eosinophils scatter more 90°D light, allowing clear separation of eosinophils and neutrophils on this display. Dynamic thresholds are used for best separation of the different populations in the various scatterplots. Each cell type is identified with a distinct color so that after all classifications are made and size (0°) is plotted against complexity (7°), each cell population can be visualized easily by the operator on the data terminal screen. Other scatterplots (90°/0°, 90°D/0°, 90°D/7°) are available and may be displayed at operator request. On earlier instruments, the 7° for complexity was referred to as the 10°. The change reflects the midrange of the angle instead of the end range; however, it still provides the same measurement and information.[42,43]As on the previously described instruments, user-defined distributional flags may be set, and instrument-specific suspect flags may alert the operator to the presence of abnormal cells.[22,42] Figure 39-9 represents a patient printout from the CELL-DYN 3700.

Bayer Instrumentation

Bayer Healthcare LLC manufactures the ADVIA 2120, the next generation of the ADVIA 120.[28,44] The ADVIA 2120 and 120 use much of the same technology as the older Technicon H-1, H-2, and H-3 Systems.[45] Bayer has simplified the hydraulics and

CELL-DYN 3700

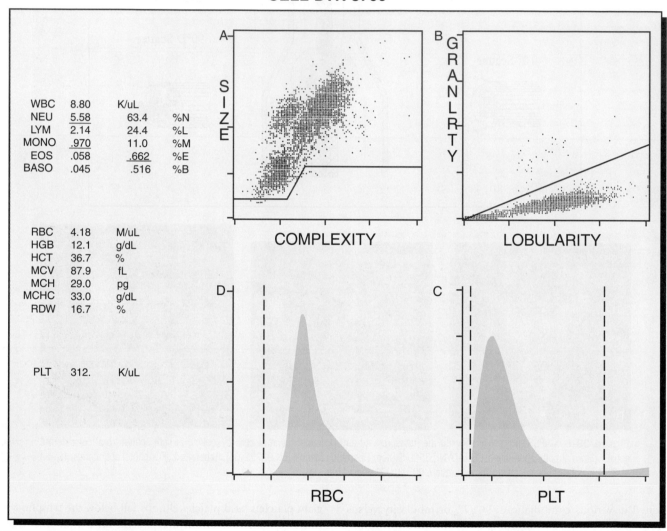

WBC	8.80	K/uL	
NEU	5.58	63.4	%N
LYM	2.14	24.4	%L
MONO	.970	11.0	%M
EOS	.058	.662	%E
BASO	.045	.516	%B

RBC	4.18	M/uL
HGB	12.1	g/dL
HCT	36.7	%
MCV	87.9	fL
MCH	29.0	pg
MCHC	33.0	g/dL
RDW	16.7	%
PLT	312.	K/uL

Figure 39-9 Composite scatterplots/histograms from CELL-DYN 3700 on the same normal sample shown in Figures 39-6, 39-7, and 39-12. **A,** WBC data derived by MAPSS. 0° forward light scatter, which correlates with volume (y axis), is plotted against 10° narrow-angle light scatter, which correlates with complexity (x axis). Neutrophil (NEU), monocyte (MONO), and lymphocyte (LYM) population clusters are indicated. Not shown: 90°/10° scatterplot that separates the leukocytes into mononuclear and polymorphonuclear cell populations and 0°/10° scatterplot that separates the mononuclear population into lymphocytes, monocytes, and basophils. (Basophils cluster with mononuclear cells because the cytoplasmic granules dissolve in the sheath fluid.) **B,** Separation of the polymorphonuclear population using 90° depolarized (90°D or Depol) light scatter (y axis) that correlates with granularity plotted against 90° orthogonal light scatter (x axis) that correlates with lobularity or internal complexity. Eosinophils, because of their unique granulation, scatter more 90°D light. A dynamic threshold is used to determine the best separation between the EOS and NEU populations. Computer algorithms determine the relative number (%) of each subpopulation. The absolute number (K/μL) is calculated by multiplying the percentage of each subpopulation by the WBC count. **C** and **D,** Platelet (PLT) and RBC data determined in the impedance channel. The small population of larger RBCs on the right of the RBC curve represents coincident passage of doublets or triplets or both through the aperture, creating larger pulses. The RDW is derived from the 20th and 80th percentiles of the RBC histogram, excluding these artificially large pulses from the calculation.

operations of the analyzer by replacing multiple complex hydraulic systems with a Unified Fluids Circuit (UFC) assembly, or Unifluidics technology. The ADVIA 2120 and 120 provide a complete hemogram and WBC differential while additionally providing a fully automated reticulocyte count.[24,25,44]

Four independent measurement channels are used in determining the hemogram and differential: (1) RBC/platelet channel, (2) Hb channel, (3) peroxidase (PEROX), and (4) basophil-lobularity (BASO) channels for WBC and differential data. WBC, RBC, Hb, and platelets are measured directly. Hb is determined using a modified cyanmethemoglobin method that measures absorbance in a colorimeter flow cuvette at approximately 546 nm. The RBC/platelet method uses flow cytometric light scattering measurements determined as cells pass through a sheath-stream flow cell past a laser optical assembly (laser diode light source). RBCs and platelets are isovolumetrically sphered before entering the flow cell to eliminate optical orientation noise. Laser light scattered at two different angular intervals (low angle [2-3 degrees], correlating with cell volume or size, and high angle [5-15 degrees], correlating with internal complexity [i.e., refractive index or Hb concentration]) is measured simultaneously (Fig. 39-10). This unique "differential scatter" technique, in combination with isovolumetric sphering, eliminates the adverse effect of variation in cellular Hb concentration on the determination of RBC volume (as seen by differences in cellular deformability affecting the pulse height generated on impedance instruments).[11,46] The Mie theory of light scatter of dielectric spheres[19] is used to plot scatter-intensity signals from the two angles against each other for a cell-by-cell RBC volume (y axis) versus Hb concentration (x axis) cytogram or RBC map

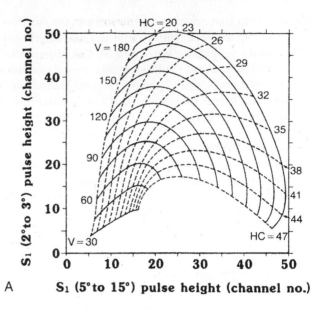

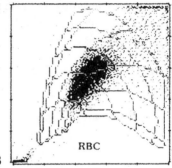

Figure 39-11 Cytograms or RBC maps showing the Mie theory of light scatter of dielectric spheres. **A,** Transformation between scatter angles (2-3 degrees and 5-15 degrees) and RBC volume (V) and Hb (HC). **B,** RBC map of patient sample. (From Groner W: New developments in flow cytochemistry technology. In Simson E [ed]: Proceedings of Technicon H-1 Hematology Symposium, October 11, 1985. Tarrytown, NY: Technicon Instruments Corporation, 1986:5.)

(Fig. 39-11).[21] Independent histograms of RBC volume and Hb concentration also are plotted. On the Technicon H-Systems, platelets are counted and sized from the high-angle signals only, and a platelet size-distribution histogram is generated.[24] The ADVIA 2120 and 120 use two-dimensional (low-angle and high-angle) platelet analysis, which allows better discrimination of platelets from interfering particles, such as RBC fragments and small RBCs. Larger platelets can be included in the platelet count.[25,44]

Several parameters and indices are derived from the measurements described in the previous paragraph. MCV and MPV are the mean of the RBC volume histogram and the platelet histogram. Hct, MCH, and MCHC are mathematically computed using RBC, Hb, and MCV values. RDW is calculated as the CV of the RBC volume histogram, whereas Hb distribution width (HDW), an analogous index, is calculated as the SD of the RBC Hb concentration histogram. The reference interval for HDW is 2.2 to 3.2 g/dL. Cell Hb concentration mean (CHCM), analogous to MCHC, is derived from cell-by-cell direct

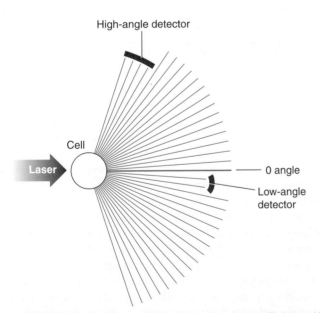

Figure 39-10 Differential scatter detection as used on the Technicon H Systems and ADVIA 120, showing forward high-angle (5-15 degrees) and forward low-angle (2-3 degrees) scatter detection for RBC and WBC analysis. (From Miles, Inc.: Technicon H Systems Training Guide. Tarrytown, NY: Miles, Inc., 1993.)

measure of Hb concentration. Interferences in the Hb colori-metric method, such as lipemia or icterus, affect the calculated MCHC but do not alter measured CHCM. CHCM generally is not reported as a patient result but is used by the instrument as an internal check against the MCHC and is available to the operator for back-calculation of Hb, if interferences are present. Unique RBC flags derived from CHCM include Hb concentration variance (HC VAR), hypochromia (HYPO), and hyperchromia (HYPER).[24,25]

Bayer hematology analyzers determine WBC count and a six-part WBC differential (neutrophils, lymphocytes, mono-cytes, eosinophils, basophils, and large unstained cells [LUCs]) by cytochemistry and optical flow cytometry, using the PEROX and BASO channels. LUCs include reactive or variant lym-phocytes and blasts.

Peroxidase (PEROX) Channel

In the PEROX channel, RBCs are lysed, and WBCs are stained for their peroxidase activity. The following reaction is catalyzed by cellular peroxidase, converting the substrate to a dark pre-cipitate in peroxidase-containing cells (neutrophils, mono-cytes, and eosinophils):

$$H_2O_2 + 4\text{-chloro-1-naphthol} \xrightarrow{\text{cellular peroxidase}} \text{dark precipitate}$$

A portion of the cell suspension is fed to a sheath-stream flow cell where a tungsten-halogen darkfield optics system is used in measuring absorbance (proportional to amount of peroxidase content in each cell) and forward scatter (proportional to size of each cell). Absorbance is plotted on the x axis of the cytogram, and scatter is plotted on the y axis.[24,25] A total WBC count (WBC-PEROX) is obtained from the optical signals in this channel and is used as an internal check against the primary WBC count obtained in the basophil-lobularity channel (WBC-BASO). If significant interference occurs in the WBC-BASO count, the instrument substitutes the WBC-PEROX.[25]

Computerized cluster analysis allows for classification of the different cell populations, including abnormal clusters such as nucleated RBCs and platelet clumps. Nucleated RBCs are analyzed on every sample using four counting algorithms, allowing the system to choose the most accurate count based on internal rules and conditions. Neutrophils and eosinophils contain the most peroxidase and cluster to the right of the cytogram. Monocytes stain weakly and cluster in the midre-gion of the cytogram. Lymphocytes, basophils, and LUCs (including variant or atypical lymphs and blasts) contain no peroxidase and appear on the left of the cytogram, with LUCs appearing above the lymphocyte area. Basophils cluster with the small lymphocytes and require further analysis for classification.[24,25,45,47]

Basophil-Lobularity (BASO) Channel

In the BASO channel, cells are treated with a reagent con-taining a nonionic surfactant in an acidic solution. Basophils are particularly resistant to lysis in this temperature-controlled reaction, whereas RBCs and platelets lyse and other leukocytes (nonbasophils) are stripped of their cytoplasm. Laser optics, using the same two-angle (2-3 degrees and 5-15 degrees) forward scattering system of the RBC/platelet channel, is used to analyze the treated cells. High-angle scatter (proportional to nuclear complexity) is plotted on the x axis, and low-angle scatter (proportional to cell size) is plotted on the y axis. Cluster analysis allows for identification and quantification of the individual cellular populations. The intact basophils are identifiable by their large low-angle scatter. The remaining nuclei are classified as mononuclear, polymorphonuclear, and blast cell nuclei based on their nuclear complexity (shape and cell density) and high-angle scatter.[24,25,45]

Basophils fall above a horizontal threshold on the cytogram. The stripped nuclei fall below the basophils, with polymor-phonuclears to the right and mononuclears to the left along the x axis. Blast cells uniquely cluster below the mononuclear cells. Lack of distinct separation between the polymorpho-nuclear and mononuclear nuclear clusters indicates WBC immaturity or suspected left shift. As indicated earlier, this channel provides the primary WBC count, the WBC-BASO. Relative differential results (%) are computed by dividing absolute numbers of the different cell classifications by the total WBC count.[24,25,45]

The nucleated RBC method is based on the physical characteristics of size and density of the nucleated RBC nuclei. These characteristics allow counting in both WBC channels on the ADVIA 2120, and algorithms are applied to enumerate the absolute number and percentage of nucleated RBCs. Information from the PEROX and BASO channels is used to generate differential morphology flags indicating the possible presence of atypical (reactive) lymphocytes, blasts, left shift, immature granulocytes, nucleated RBCs, or large platelets/platelet clumps.[24,25,47] Figure 39-12 is a patient printout from the ADVIA 120.

AUTOMATED RETICULOCYTE COUNTING

Reticulocyte counting is the last of the manual cell counting procedures to be automated and has been a primary focus of hematology analyzer advancement in recent years. The imprecision and inaccuracy in manual reticulocyte counting is due to multiple factors, including stain variability, slide distribution error, statistical sampling error, and interobserver error.[48] All of these potential errors, with the possible exception of stain variability, are correctable with automated reticulocyte counting. Increasing the number of RBCs counted dictates increased precision.[49] This was evidenced with the 1993 College of American Pathologists pilot reticulocyte proficiency survey (Set RT-A, Sample RT-01) on which the CV for the reported manual results was 35% compared with 8.3% for the flow cytometry method.[50] Precision of automated methods has continued to improve. The manual reticulocyte results for one sample in the 2000 Reticulocyte Survey Set RT/RT2-A showed a CV of 28.7% compared with 2.8% for one of the automated methods.[51] Automated reticulocyte analyzers may count 32,000 RBCs compared with 1000 cells counted by the routine manual procedure.[52]

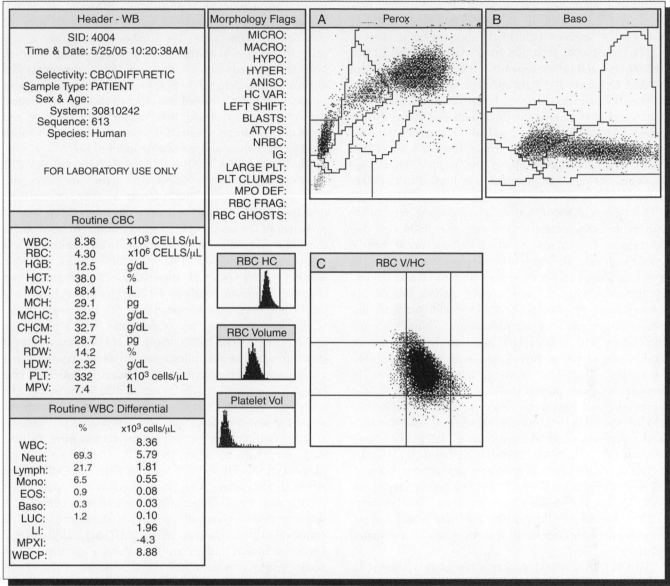

| Header - WB |
| SID: 4004 |
| Time & Date: 5/25/05 10:20:38AM |
| Selectivity: CBC\DIFF\RETIC |
| Sample Type: PATIENT |
| Sex & Age: |
| System: 30810242 |
| Sequence: 613 |
| Species: Human |
| FOR LABORATORY USE ONLY |

Morphology Flags

MICRO:
MACRO:
HYPO:
HYPER:
ANISO:
HC VAR:
LEFT SHIFT:
BLASTS:
ATYPS:
NRBC:
IG:
LARGE PLT:
PLT CLUMPS:
MPO DEF:
RBC FRAG:
RBC GHOSTS:

A Perox
B Baso
RBC HC
C RBC V/HC
RBC Volume
Platelet Vol

Routine CBC

WBC:	8.36	x10³ CELLS/µL
RBC:	4.30	x10⁶ CELLS/µL
HGB:	12.5	g/dL
HCT:	38.0	%
MCV:	88.4	fL
MCH:	29.1	pg
MCHC:	32.9	g/dL
CHCM:	32.7	g/dL
CH:	28.7	pg
RDW:	14.2	%
HDW:	2.32	g/dL
PLT:	332	x10³ cells/µL
MPV:	7.4	fL

Routine WBC Differential

	%	x10³ cells/µL
WBC:		8.36
Neut:	69.3	5.79
Lymph:	21.7	1.81
Mono:	6.5	0.55
EOS:	0.9	0.08
Baso:	0.3	0.03
LUC:	1.2	0.10
LI:		1.96
MPXI:		-4.3
WBCP:		8.88

Figure 39-12 Composite scatterplots/histograms from ADVIA 120 on the same normal specimen shown in Figures 39-6, 39-7, and 39-9. **A,** WBC data derived from the peroxidase (PEROX) channel in which the WBCs have been stained for their peroxidase activity. Darkfield optical scatter correlating with volume is plotted on the *y* axis against light absorbance proportional to staining intensity on the *x* axis. Computer cluster analysis separates the WBCs into neutrophils (NEUT), eosinophils (EOS), monocytes (MONO), lymphocytes (LYMPH), and large, unstained cells (LUCs) as indicated. Basophils cluster with small lymphocytes in the PEROX channel. **B,** WBC data derived from the laser-based basophil-lobularity (BASO) channel in which the cells have been treated with a differential lysis reagent. Low-angle (2-3 degrees) scatter that correlates with size is plotted on the *y* axis against high-angle (5-15 degrees) scatter that correlates with nuclear complexity (shape and cell density) on the *x* axis. Nonlysed basophils, which have large low-angle scatter, fall above the stripped nuclei (nonbasophils), which cluster into polymorphonuclear (PMN) and mononuclear (MN) populations. Blasts, when present, uniquely cluster below the MN population. Basophils are subtracted from the LYMPH count for the final absolute counts (× 10³/µL). Relative differential results (%) are computed by dividing absolute counts by the total WBC count. **C,** Platelet scatter cytogram, based on the Mie theory of light scatter, plots low-angle scatter (2-3 degrees) on the *y* axis versus high-angle scatter (5-15 degrees) on the *x* axis that correlate with cell volume and refractive index. This cell-by-cell analysis of volume and refractive index allows better discrimination of platelets, including large platelets, from interfering particles such as small RBCs and RBC fragments. **D,** RBCs also are analyzed using the Mie theory of light scatter. This RBC volume/Hb cytogram represents a linear plot of this RBC analysis. Volume (V) is plotted on the *y* axis versus Hb concentration (HC) on the *x* axis. The direct measure of Hb concentration allows classification of RBCs as macrocytic, normocytic, or microcytic and as hypochromic, normochromic, or hyperchromic. Single-parameter histograms for RBC Hb concentration (RBC HC), RBC volume, and platelet (PLT) volume are generated. The RBC histogram has markers at the 60 fL and 120 fL channels for visualization of microcytosis or macrocytosis or both. Likewise, the RBC HC curve has markers at the 28 g/dL and 41 g/dL channels for visualization of hypochromia and hyperchromia. HDW, analogous to the RDW, is derived from the Hb CONC histogram.

Available automated reticulocyte analyzers include flow cytometry systems such as the Becton Dickinson FACS or Coulter EPICS; Sysmex R-3500, R-500, and SE-9500/9000+RAM-1; CELL-DYN 3500R, 3700, and 4000 systems; Coulter GEN-S, STKS, MAXM, and LH750 systems; and Bayer ADVIA 2120 and 120 and Technicon H-3 RTC and RTX systems. All of these analyzers evaluate reticulocytes based on optical scatter or fluorescence after treating the RBCs with fluorescent dyes or nucleic acid stains to stain residual RNA in the reticulocytes.[16,24,25,36,42,43,52-55] Because neither the FACS nor EPICS system is generally available in the routine hematology laboratory, the remaining discussion is limited to the other analyzers.

The Sysmex R-3000/3500 is a stand-alone reticulocyte analyzer that uses auramine O, a supravital fluorescent dye, and measures forward scatter and side fluorescence as the cells pass through a sheath-stream flow cell past an argon laser. The signals are plotted on a scattergram with forward scatter intensity that correlates with size plotted against fluorescence intensity that is proportional to RNA content. Automatic discrimination separates the populations into mature RBCs and reticulocytes. The reticulocytes fall into low-fluorescence, middle-fluorescence, or high-fluorescence regions, with the less mature reticulocytes showing higher fluorescence. The *immature reticulocyte fraction* (IRF) is the sum of the middle-fluorescence and high-fluorescence ratios and indicates the ratio of immature reticulocytes to total reticulocytes in a sample. Platelets, which also are counted, fall below a lower discriminator line.[53] The Sysmex SE-9500/9000+RAM-1 module uses the same flow cytometry methodology for reticulocyte counting as the R-3500.[16] Off-line sample preparation is not required. The smaller Sysmex R-500 uses flow cytometry with a semiconductor laser as the light source and polymethine supravital fluorescent dye to provide automated reticulocyte counts.[30]

The CELL-DYN 3500R performs reticulocyte analysis by measuring 10-degree and 90-degree scatter in the optical channel (MAPSS technology) after the cells have been isovolumetrically sphered to eliminate optical orientation noise. The RBCs are stained with the thiazine dye new methylene blue N in an off-line sample preparation before the sample is introduced to the instrument. The operator simply must change computer functions on the instrument before aspiration of the reticulocyte preparation.[42] The CELL-DYN 4000 also uses MAPSS technology but adds fluorescent detection to allow for fully automated, random access reticulocyte testing.[26,43] The RBCs are stained with a proprietary, membrane-permeable fluorescent dye (CD4K530) that binds stoichiometrically to nucleic acid and emits green light as the cells pass through a sheath-stream flow cell past an argon-ion laser. Platelets and reticulocytes are separated based on intensity of green fluorescence (scatter measured at 7 degrees and 90 degrees), and the reticulocyte count along with the IRF is determined.[43,56]

Beckman Coulter also has incorporated reticulocyte methods into its primary cell counting instrumentation—the GEN-S, STKS, and MAXM and LH700 Series systems. Off-line

staining preparations are required for the STKS and MAXM, but the same laser optics employed in cell counting are used for reticulocyte enumeration. The Coulter method uses a new methylene blue stain and the VCS technology described earlier. Volume is plotted against light scatter (DF 5 scatterplot) and against conductivity (DF 6 scatterplot), correlating with opacity of the RBC. Stained reticulocytes show greater optical scatter and greater opacity than mature RBCs. Relative and absolute reticulocyte counts are reported, along with mean reticulocyte volume and maturation index or IRF.[52]

The Bayer ADVIA 2120 and 120 and Technicon H-3 RTC or RTX systems enumerate reticulocytes in the same laser optics flow cell used in the RBC/platelet and BASO channels described earlier. The H-3 systems require an off-line sample preparation. The reticulocyte reagent isovolumetrically spheres the RBCs and stains the reticulocytes with oxazine 750, a nucleic acid–binding dye. Three detectors measure low-angle scatter (2-3 degrees), high-angle scatter (5-15 degrees), and absorbance simultaneously as the cells pass through the flow cell. Three cytograms are generated: (1) high-angle scatter versus absorption, (2) low-angle scatter versus high-angle scatter (Mie cytogram or RBC map), and (3) volume versus Hb concentration. The absorption cytogram allows separation and quantitation of reticulocytes, with additional subdivision into low-absorbing, medium-absorbing, and high-absorbing cells based on amount of staining. The sum of the medium-absorbing and high-absorbing cells reflects the IRF. Volume and Hb concentration for each cell are derived from the RBC map using Mie scattering theory.[25,57] Unique reticulocyte indices (MCVr, CHCMr, RDWr, HDWr, CHr, and CHDWr) are provided. Hb content (CHr) of each cell is calculated as the product of the cell volume and the cell Hb concentration. A single-parameter histogram of CHr is constructed, with a corresponding distribution width (CHDWr) calculated.[24,25] These reticulocyte indices are not available on the routine patient printout but are available to the operator. Figure 39-13 is a reticulocyte printout from an ADVIA 120, showing the cytograms and reticulocyte indices.

Automation of reticulocytes has allowed for increased precision and accuracy and greatly expanded the analysis of immature RBCs, providing new parameters and indices that may be useful in the diagnosis and treatment of anemias. The IRF is a reliable indicator of changes in erythropoietic activity and may prove to be a valuable therapeutic monitoring tool in patients with chronic renal failure.[58,59] The reticulocyte maturity measurements also may be useful in evaluating bone marrow suppression during chemotherapy, monitoring hematopoietic regeneration after bone marrow or stem cell transplantation, monitoring renal transplant engraftment, and monitoring efficacy of anemia therapy.[58-64] The additional reticulocyte indices derived on the ADVIA 2120 and 120 seem valuable in following erythropoietin therapy response, and CHr in particular has proved useful in the early detection and diagnosis of iron-deficient erythropoiesis in children.[60,64,65] Widespread use of the new parameters may be limited by instrumentation availability.

ADVIA 120

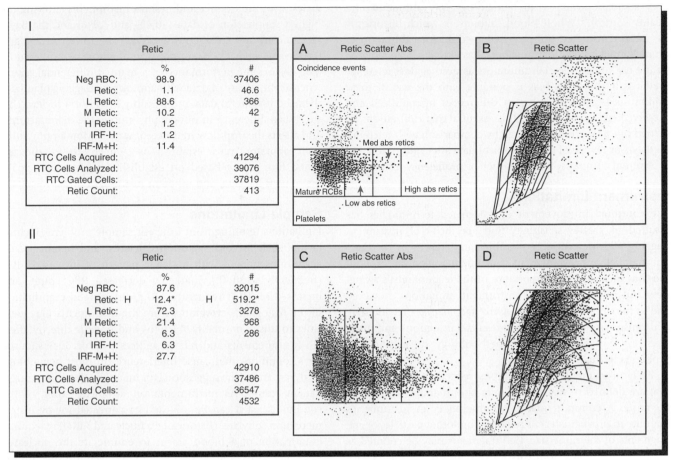

Figure 39-13 Composite cytograms from the ADVIA 120. *I*, Normal reticulocyte count. *II*, High reticulocyte count with a large immature reticulocyte fraction (IRF). *I-A* and *II-C*, Reticulocyte scatter/absorption cytograms show high-angle (5-15 degrees) scatter on the *y* axis versus absorption on the *x* axis, allowing separation of low-absorbing, medium-absorbing, and high-absorbing cells based on the amount of staining with nucleic acid–binding dye (oxazine 750). *I-B* and *II-D*, Reticulocyte scatter cytograms represent low-angle (2-3 degrees) scatter on the *y* axis versus high-angle (5-15 degrees) scatter on the *x* axis (RBC map). Because the RBCs are evaluated by the instrument on a cell-by-cell basis, unique reticulocyte indices can be derived.

LIMITATIONS AND INTERFERENCES

Establishing automation in the hematology laboratory requires critical evaluation of the instrument's methods, limitations, and performance goals for the individual laboratory. The Clinical Laboratory and Standards Institute (formerly National Committee for Clinical Laboratory Standards) has approved a standard for performance goals for the internal quality control of multichannel hematology analyzers.[66] This standard provides guidelines for instrument calibration and assessment of performance criteria, including accuracy, precision, linearity, sensitivity, and specificity. The clinical accuracy (sensitivity and specificity) of the methods should be such that the instrument appropriately identifies patients who have disease and patients who do not have disease.[67] Quality control systems should reflect the laboratory's established performance goals and provide a high level of assurance that the instrument is working within its specified limits.

Calibration

Calibration is crucial in defining the accuracy (as contrasted with precision; Chapter 5) of the data produced. Calibration, or the process of electronically correcting an instrument for analytical bias (numerical difference from the "true" value), may be accomplished by appropriate use of reference methods, reference materials, or commercially prepared calibrators.[66] Because few instruments are precalibrated by the manufacturer, calibration must be performed at initial installation and verified at least every 6 months under Clinical Laboratory Improvement Act (CLIA) of 1988 requirements.[68] Periodic recalibration may be required after major instrument repair requiring optical alignment or part replacement.

Whole-blood calibration using fresh whole-blood specimens requires the use of reference methods, materials, and procedures to determine "true" values.[2,69,70] The International Committee for Standards in Hematology has established guidelines for selecting a reference blood cell counter for this purpose,[2] but the cyanmethemoglobin method remains the only standard available in hematology for calibration and quality control.[71] Whole-blood calibration, which historically has been considered the preferred method for calibration of multichannel hematology analyzers, has virtually been replaced by the use of commercial calibrators assayed against reference methods. Calibration bias is possible with the use of these calibrators because of inherent differences in stabilized and preserved cell suspensions.[72] It is essential that calibrations be carried out properly and verified by comparison with reference methods or review of quality control data after calibration and by external comparison studies such as proficiency testing.[2,73]

Instrument Limitations

The continual improvement of automated technologies has resulted in greater sensitivity and specificity of instrument flagging with detection of possible interferences in the data. The parallel improvement in instrument walk-away capabilities has increased the importance of the technologist's awareness and understanding of instrument limitations, however, and of his or her ability to recognize factors that may interfere and cause erroneous laboratory results. Limitations and interferences may be related to methodology or to inherent problems in the blood sample.

Each instrument has limitations related to methodology that are defined in instrument operation manuals and in the literature. A common method limitation is an instrument's inability to distinguish cells reliably from other particles or cell fragments of the same size. Cell fragments may be counted as platelets in samples from chemotherapy-treated patients with increased WBC fragility.[1,2] Likewise, schistocytes or small RBCs may interfere in the platelet count. Larger platelet clumps may be counted as WBCs, resulting in a falsely decreased platelet count and potentially increasing the WBC count. Micromegakaryocytes may be counted as nucleated RBCs or WBCs. RBCs containing variant Hbs such as Hb S or Hb C are often resistant to lysis, with the unlysed cells being falsely counted as nucleated RBCs or WBCs and interfering in the Hb reaction.[74] This phenomenon has become more apparent with the gentler diluent and lysing reagents of the analyzers with automated WBC differential technology. Nonlysis also may be seen in severe liver disease, with chemotherapy treatment, and in neonates (increased levels of Hb F) on the older Sysmex instruments[15] and with markedly elevated serum urea nitrogen levels on the Technicon H instruments.[24] The Technicon H Systems are able to provide a correct WBC count from the BASO channel (i.e., the WBC-BASO) with its stronger lysing reagent. The ADVIA 2120 and 120 reports the WBC-BASO as the primary WBC count.[25] An extended lyse cycle may be used on the CELL-DYN 3500, and the newer instruments are able to provide a correct WBC impedance count when lyse-resistant RBCs are present.[23,53] The Sysmex SE-9000 and Sysmex SE-9500 also have an additional WBC impedance channel.[16,75]

Suppression of automated data, particularly WBC differential data, may occur when internal instrument checks fail or cast doubt on the validity of the data. Some manufacturers release results with specific error codes or flagging for further review. The rejection rate of the different instruments varies, with the Coulter and Sysmex instruments showing the highest suppression of data (10.4% and 18%) and the Bayer (Technicon) and CELL-DYN analyzers the lowest (1.2% and 0%) in one study.[76] The suppression of automated differential data ensures the performance of a manual differential count, whereas the release of data with appropriate flagging mandates the need for careful data and possibly blood film review. This suggests a difference in philosophy among the manufacturers and affects the workflow in different ways.[76] More importantly, each laboratory must establish its own criteria for directed blood film review based on established performance goals, instrument flagging, and inherent instrument limitations.[77]

Sample Limitations

Limitations resulting from inherent sample problems include factors such as cold agglutinins, icterus, and lipemia. Cold agglutinins present with a classic pattern of increased MCV (frequently >130 fL), markedly decreased RBC count, and increased MCHC (frequently >40 g/dL). Careful examination of the histograms/cytograms from the instruments may yield clues to this abnormality.[78] Icterus and lipemia directly affect Hb measurements and related indices.[74] Table 39-3 summarizes conditions that cause interference on most hematology analyzers and offers suggestions for manually obtaining correct patient results. As instrumentation advances, some of the conditions listed can be adjusted or corrected for by instrumentation software. Historically, a nucleated RBC flag required examination of a blood smear to enumerate the nucleated RBCs and correct the WBC. All four major vendors offer online nucleated RBC enumeration and WBC correction, although the laboratory must validate the results. Lipemia interferes with the Hb reading by falsely elevating the Hb and associated indices. The Bayer technology uses direct measurement of the CHCM parameter, allowing back-calculation of the Hb unaffected by lipemia and thus eliminating the need for manual method of saline replacement in lipemic samples. These two examples of nucleated RBCs and lipemia show instrument advances, and continued future advances in technology will eliminate or decrease the need for manual intervention to obtain accurate results.

Sample age and improper sample handling can have profound effects on the reliability of hematology test results. These factors have even greater significance as hospitals move toward more "off-site" testing by large reference laboratories. Specific problems with older samples include increased WBC fragility, swelling and possible lysis of RBCs, and the deterioration of platelets.[15] Stability studies should be performed before use of an instrument, and specific guidelines should be established for specimen handling and rejection.

CLINICAL UTILITY OF AUTOMATED HEMATOLOGY INSTRUMENTATION

Automated cell counting analyzers have directly affected the availability, accuracy, and clinical usefulness of the CBC and WBC differential count. Some parameters available on hema-

TABLE 39-3 Conditions That Cause Interference on Most Hematology Analyzers

Condition	Parameters Affected*	Rationale	Instrument Indicators	Corrective Action
Cold agglutinins	RBC ↓, MCV ↑, MCHC ↑, grainy appearance	Agglutination of RBCs	Dual RBC population on RBC map, or right shift on RBC histogram	Warm sample to 37° C and rerun
Lipemia icterus chylomicrons	Hb ↑, MCH ↑	↑ Turbidity affects spectrophotometric reading	Hb × 3 ≠ HCT ± 3, abnormal histogram/cytogram[†]	Plasma replacement[‡]
Hemolysis	RBC ↓, HCT ↓	RBCs lysed and not counted	Hb × 3 ≠ HCT ± 3, may show lipemia pattern on histogram/cytogram[†]	Request new sample
Lysis-resistance RBCs with abnormal Hbs	WBC ↑, Hb ↑	RBCs with Hb S, C, or F may fail to lyse and be counted as WBCs	Interference at noise-WBC interface on histogram/cytogram	Manual dilutions, allowing incubation time for lysis
Microcytosis or schistocytes	RBC ↓	Size of RBCs or RBC fragments < lower RBC threshold	Left shift on RBC histogram, MCV flagged if below limits	Smear review
Nucleated RBCs, megakaryocyte fragments or micromegakaryoblasts	WBC ↑	Nucleated RBCs or micromegakaryoblasts counted as WBCs	Nucleated RBC flag resulting from interference at noise-lymphocyte interface on histogram/cytogram	Count nucleated RBCs or micromegakaryoblasts per 100 WBCs and correct[§]
Platelet clumps	PLT ↓, WBC ↑	Large clumps counted as WBCs	Platelet clumps/N flag, interference at noise-lymphocyte interface on histogram/cytogram	Redraw specimen in sodium citrate, multiply result by 1.1
WBC >100,000/µL	Hb ↑, RBC ↑, HCT incorrect, abnormal indices	↑ Turbidity on Hb, WBCs counted with RBC count	Hb × 3 ≠ HCT ± 3, WBC count may be above linearity	Spun hematocrit, manual Hb (spin/read supernatant),[‡] correct RBC count, recalculate indices; if above linearity, dilute for correct WBC count
Leukemia, especially with chemotherapy	Spurious WBC ↓, spurious PLT ↑	Fragile WBCs, fragments counted as platelets	Inconsistent platelet count with previous results	Smear review, phase platelet count
Old specimen	MCV ↑, MPV ↑, PLT ↓, automated differential may be incorrect	RBCs swell as sample ages, platelets swell and degenerate, WBCs affected by prolonged exposure to EDTA	Abnormal clustering on WBC histogram/cytogram	Establish stability and sample rejection criteria

*Manufacturer's labeling.
[†]Lipemia shows signature pattern on Bayer ADVIA 120 and Technicon H cytograms.
[‡]Hb can be back-calculated from directly measured MCHC on Bayer ADVIA 120 and Technicon H cytograms.
[§]Small nucleated RBCs thresholded out of WBC count on Sysmex SE-9000 and CELL-DYN 3500; correction for nucleated RBCs may not be necessary. CELL-DYN 4000 and the Sysmex XE-2100 directly measure nucleated RBCs, which are gated out of the WBC count.[30,43] Semiautomated Sysmex instruments have adjustable lower thresholds to allow inclusion of all nucleated cells in the WBC count.[79]
EDTA, ethylenediamine tetraacetic acid.

tology instrumentation, but not available manually, have provided further insight into various clinical conditions. The RDW, a quantitative estimate of erythrocyte anisocytosis, has been used with the MCV in anemia classification. Various discriminants (mathematical formulas or discriminant functions) using these two values have been proposed for the differentiation of iron deficiency from thalassemia minor,

based on the typical pattern of iron deficiency having a low MCV with a high RDW and β-thalassemia minor having a low MCV with a normal RDW (Chapter 16).[80-84] RDW has been shown to be unreliable as a sole discriminator of microcytic anemias.[85] The direct measure of RBC Hb concentration on the Bayer systems has proved to be a valuable tool in the early detection of iron deficiency anemia and in the discrimination of iron deficiency from thalassemia minor.[86,87] Directly measured Hb concentration also has been used in the detection of iron-deficient erythropoiesis in iron-replete subjects treated with recombinant erythropoietin.[88] The MPV may be useful in detecting whether or not the bone marrow is working correctly. A low MPV may indicate marrow hypoproduction, whereas a high MPV may be suspicious of an abnormal myeloproliferative disorder.[89] Methodology, anticoagulation, and storage time all influence the MPV, however, making the parameter less useful.[90]

The automated WBC differential has had a significant impact on the laboratory workflow because of the labor-intensive nature of the manual differential count. The "three-part differential" available on earlier instruments generally proved suitable as a screening leukocyte differential to identify samples that required further workup or a manual differential count.[91-93] It has been shown, however, that partial differential counts do not substitute for a complete differential in abnormal populations.[94-96] The five-part automated differentials available on the larger instruments have been evaluated extensively and seem to have acceptable clinical sensitivity and specificity for detection of distributional and morphologic abnormalities.[39,40,97-104] Abnormal cells such as blasts and nucleated RBCs in low concentration may not be detected by the instruments but likewise may be missed by the routine 100-cell manual/visual differential count.[105,106] The CELL-DYN 4000, with its added fluorescent detection technology, has been shown to have high sensitivity and specificity for flagging nucleated RBCs and platelet clumps.[46,107] As technology continues to improve, blood smear review to confirm the presence of platelet clumps or nucleated RBCs and correct leukocyte counts for interference from platelet clumps or nucleated RBCs is becoming unnecessary.[40,56,107]

Instrument evaluations based on the CLSI H20-T or H20-A Standard (Reference Leukocyte Differential Count [Proportional] and Evaluation of Instrumental Methods)[108] using an 800-cell or a 400-cell manual leukocyte differential count as the reference method have shown acceptable correlation coefficients for all WBC types, with the possible exception of monocytes.[40,76,109-111] Further studies using monoclonal antibodies as the reference method for counting monocytes suggest that automated analyzers yield a more accurate assessment of monocytosis than do manual methods.[112,113]

Histograms and cytograms along with instrument flagging provide valuable information in the diagnosis and treatment of RBC and WBC disorders. Multiple reports indicate the efficacy of histograms and cytograms in the characterization of various abnormal conditions, including RBC disorders such as cold agglutination and WBC diseases such as leukemias and myelodysplastic disorders.[78,114-116] The major instrument manufacturers have published case study books with histograms and cytograms to aid the technologist in the interpretation of instrument data.[34,117-120]

Manufacturers are developing integrated hematology workstations for the greatest automation and laboratory efficiency. The Sysmex Total Hematology Automation System (HST series) robotically links the SE-9000, R-3500 (automated reticulocyte analyzer), and SP-100 (automatic slide maker and stainer). The HST line links two XE2100 and one SP-100 for complete automation or systemization of hematology testing. The SE-Alpha is a smaller version that links the SE-9000 and SP-100.[30] The Bayer ADVIA Lab Cell links the ADVIA 2120 to the track, and the Autoslide (automatic slide maker stainer) links to the ADVIA 2120. The other manufacturers have or are developing similar automation systems.[121,122] Finally, as a result of increasing customer needs, manufacturers are adding body fluid counting to their high-end instrumentation. The Beckman LH 750 counts WBCs and RBCs on body fluids, and the ADVIA 2120/120 counts WBCs and RBCs on cerebrospinal fluids and performs a differential.[123,124]

Selection of a hematology analyzer for an individual laboratory requires careful evaluation of the laboratory's needs and scrutiny of several probing instrument questions and issues, including instrument specifications and system requirements, methods, training requirements, maintenance, reagent usage, data management, staff response, and short-term and long-term expenditures.[125] All instruments claim to improve laboratory efficiency through increased automation resulting in improved workflow and faster turnaround time or by adding new parameters that may have clinical efficacy. The instrument selected should "fit" the workload and patient population and positively affect patient outcomes.[126] The instrument selected for a cancer center may be different from one chosen for a community hospital.[127] Ultimately, the instrument decision may be swayed by individual preferences, however.[76]

POINT OF CARE TESTING

Definition

This section provides a brief overview of point of care testing in hematology. For a more complete discussion, the reader is referred to the "Additional Resources" at the end of the chapter.

Point of care testing is defined as diagnostic laboratory testing at or near the site of patient care. CLIA introduced the concept of "testing site neutrality," meaning that it does not matter where the diagnostic testing is performed or who performs the test; all testing sites must follow the same regulatory requirements based on the "complexity" of the test. Under CLIA, testing is classified as waived, moderately complex (including physician-performed microscopy), and highly complex. Tests are classified as waived if they are determined to be "simple tests with an insignificant risk of an erroneous result." Most, but not all, point of care testing is waived. Originally, there were 8 tests in the waived category; to date, that category has expanded to 76 tests. Examples of waived tests performed at the point of care are glucose, Hb, Hct, pregnancy, and urine regent strip testing. Nonwaived point of care testing includes coagulation testing (activated clotting time, prothrombin time, and activated partial thromboplastin time), blood gases, and various chemistry tests. Point of care testing commonly is performed in hospital inpatient units, outpatient clinics and surgery centers, emergency departments, long-term care facilities, and dialysis units. Facilities performing waived testing are required to obtain a certificate of waiver, pay the appropriate fees, and follow the manufacturers' testing instructions.

Point of care testing has become popular with advances in technology allowing for whole-blood analysis at the bedside. The speed and miniaturization of biosensor technology has led to the development of instruments that can detect abrupt changes in the patient's status in the minimum amount of time. In addition, some point of care tests do not rely on an instrument and are simple to perform with minimal steps and short testing times.

Advantages and Disadvantages

Fast test results speed up the medical decision-making process that is essential for immediate treatment. Centralized laboratories may not be able to support a protocol that requires a diagnostic test result within 5 minutes. Direct patient samples such as whole blood or urine are used to support that short turnaround time and are not compromised by time delays, transportation delays, temperature, or manipulation. Point of care testing has been challenged to address the continuing pressures of cost containment, reducing hospital and clinic stays and preventing unnecessary admissions.

The cost, usage, and oversight of point of care testing often have been cited as disadvantages. The cost per test is often higher than tests performed in the central laboratory. Increased usage of the tests because they are so readily available and simple to use would only add to that cost burden. That is where oversight comes into play. Appropriate use of point of care testing along with method selection, training, and policies and procedures would ensure quality testing protocols. Laboratorians often are involved in the oversight of point of care testing sites because they are the most familiar with clinical laboratory regulations and requirements.

Quality Assurance for Point of Care Testing

As with any laboratory test, consideration of the accuracy and precision of the results is crucial. Manufacturers have robust quality systems in place to ensure that the test performs within their published specifications. Testing personnel must evaluate these specifications in their own testing environment on their patient population and challenge such systems to meet their diagnostic needs. Quality control and calibration protocols must be simple to perform and have limited handling and preparation steps. The quality control systems need to perform in a variety of environments and appropriately assess the performance of the instrument or method. Storage and handling requirements must be simplified because some testing areas may have limited storage and refrigeration.

Methods

The most common hematology tests performed at the point of care is the Hb and Hct. The point of care clinical application for the Hb/Hct focuses on transfusion therapy and acute hemodilution during surgery, particularly during cardiac bypass surgery.

Hematocrit

Centrifuge-based microhematocrits have been around for years and correlate well with the standard cell counters. Inexperienced operators may not be aware of the common sources of error that may be introduced with the inadequate time, insufficient time, and inaccurate reading of the microhematocrit tube (Chapter 14).[128] Examples include Hematastat II (Separation Technology Inc., Altamonte Springs, FL) and STAT-Crit (Wampole Laboratories, Cranbury, N.J.).

Conductivity-based microhematocrits measure the resistance of RBCs to electrical conduction in a sample. This method may be found in stand-alone instruments or multiparameter blood gas and electrolyte analyzers. Hct results may be falsely decreased by low levels of protein, as in intraoperatively salvaged autologous blood, and by elevated concentrations of sodium and chloride. Examples include:

I-Stat (Abbott Diagnostics, Abbott Park, Ill.)
ABL 77 (Radiometer America, Westlake, Ohio)
IRMA (ITC, subsidiary of Thoratec Corporation, Edison, N.J.)
Gem Premier (Instrumentation Laboratory Company, Lexington, Mass.)

Hemoglobin

In point of care testing, Hb is measured by modified hemoglobinometers or by oximeters integrated with a blood gas analyzer. The HemoCue hemoglobinometer (HemoCue, Inc., Lake Forest, Calif.) uses a small cuvette that contains a lysing agent and reagents to form an Hb azide, which is measured by a photometer. It compares well with reference methods, but the major source of error is involved with mixture of blood with tissue juices during specimen collection. The Hb-Quick hemoglobinometer (Avox Systems, Inc, San Antonio, Tex.) measures total Hb by a spectrophotometric method. The STAT-Site M^{Hgb} Meter (Stanbio Laboratory, Boerne, Tex.) uses reflectance photometry to measure reflected light in the test area. The test card is composed of molded plastic with a fluid well that contains numerous pads impregnated with specific chemical reagents. A drop of whole blood is applied to the center of the well and reacts with the chemicals in the pads to produce a specific color that is measured from the bottom of the card.[129]

Cell Counts/Platelets

Traditional cell counting principles can be employed at the point of care for the analysis of WBCs, RBCs, and platelets. The Ichor Hematology Analyzer (Helena Laboratories, Beaumont, Tex.) performs a CBC along with a platelet aggregation. Another option for cell quantitation and differentiation employs a buffy coat analysis method. The quantitative buffy coat analysis (QBCII) from QBC Diagnostics, Inc. (State College, Penn.), involves centrifugation in specialized capillary tubes designed to expand the buffy coat layer. The layers (platelets, mononuclear cells, and granulocyte) can be measured with the assistance of fluorescent dyes and a measuring device.[130]

- Automation provides greater accuracy and greater precision than manual cell counting methods.
- The primary principles of operation, electronic impedance and optical scatter, are used on most automated hematology analyzers. Radiofrequency is sometimes used in conjunction with electronic impedance.
- The electronic impedance method detects and measures changes in electrical resistance between two electrodes as cells pass through a sensing aperture. The measurable voltage changes are plotted on frequency distribution graphs, or histograms, which allow the evaluation of cell populations based on size.
- Radiofrequency resistance uses high-voltage electromagnetic current. Measurable changes in the RF signal are proportional to cell interior density, or conductivity. Impedance and conductivity can be plotted against each other on a two-dimensional distribution cytogram or scatterplot, which allows the evaluation of cell populations using cluster analysis.
- Optical scatter systems (flow cytometers) use detection of interference in a laser beam or light source to enumerate and differentiate cell types.
- Major manufacturers of hematology instrumentation include Beckman Coulter, Inc., Sysmex Corporation, Abbott Laboratories, and Bayer Corporation. Beckman Coulter primarily uses the impedance method of counting and sizing cells; Sysmex, a combination of impedance and RF; Abbott, impedance and optical measurements; and Bayer, optical flow cytometry.
- Reticulocyte analysis has been incorporated into the primary cell counting instrumentation of all major manufacturers. All use either fluorescent dyes or nucleic acid stains to stain reticulocytes before the cells are counted using fluorescence or absorbance.
- Each instrument has limitations related to methodology that may result in instrument flagging of specific results or suppression of automated data. Likewise, inherent sample problems may result in instrument flagging that indicate possible rejection of automated results.
- Automation has had a significant impact on laboratory workflow, particularly automation of the WBC differential. Additionally, newer parameters, such as RDW, IRF, and CHr have documented clinical utility.
- Point of care testing is defined as diagnostic laboratory testing at or near the site of patient care.
- The Clinical Laboratory Improvement Act of 1988 introduced the concept of "testing site neutrality," which means it does not matter where the diagnostic testing is performed or who performs the test; all testing sites must follow the same regulatory requirements based on the "complexity" of the test.
- Tests are classified as waived if they are determined to be "simple tests with an insignificant risk of an erroneous result." Most, but not all, point of care testing is waived.
- There are now more than 76 tests in the waived category.
- The most common hematology tests performed at the point of care are the Hb and HCT. Some point of care testing devices also perform a CBC.

REVIEW QUESTIONS

Examine the histograms/scatterplots from four major instruments on the same patient sample (Fig. 39-14). Compare the results, and respond to the questions.

1. How does the numerical data for the hemogram WBC and differential compare among the four instruments?
   a. They appear to be comparable, with each instrument flagging the results for further scrutiny.
   b. The Sysmex did not detect the irregularities detected by the other instruments.
   c. The Coulter did not detect the irregularities detected by the other instruments.
   d. The Advia did not detect the irregularities detected by the other instruments.

2. The manual differential showed the presence of nucleated RBCs and blasts. Which was the only instrument to flag for the possible presence of blasts?
   a. Advia
   b. CELL-DYN
   c. Coulter
   d. Sysmex

3. Which instrument was the only one *failing* to alert to the possibility of nucleated RBCs?
   a. Advia
   b. CELL-DYN
   c. Coulter
   d. Sysmex

4. What do you suspect is the cause of the variance in platelet flags? The instruments' reporting flags:
   a. Have higher levels of sensitivity
   b. All use the same principle for counting platelets
   c. Are susceptible to false-positive platelet flags under certain conditions
   d. Have higher values for the lower limit of the reference range

5. Should a manual differential be performed? Explain.

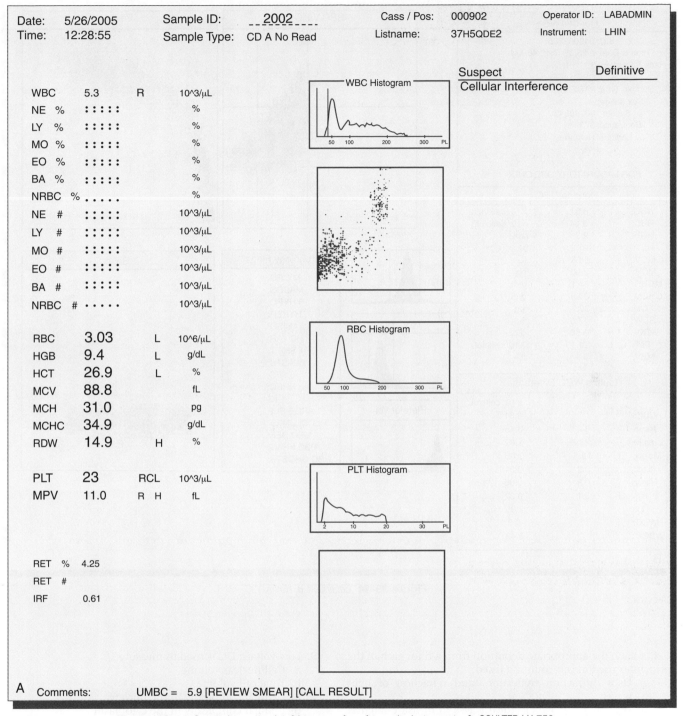

| Date: | 5/26/2005 | | Sample ID: | 2002 | | Cass / Pos: | 000902 | Operator ID: | LABADMIN |
| Time: | 12:28:55 | | Sample Type: | CD A No Read | | Listname: | 37H5QDE2 | Instrument: | LHIN |

Suspect   Definitive
Cellular Interference

WBC	5.3	R	10^3/µL
NE %	: : : : :		%
LY %	: : : : :		%
MO %	: : : : :		%
EO %	: : : : :		%
BA %	: : : : :		%
NRBC %	. . . . .		%
NE #	: : : : :		10^3/µL
LY #	: : : : :		10^3/µL
MO #	: : : : :		10^3/µL
EO #	: : : : :		10^3/µL
BA #	: : : : :		10^3/µL
NRBC #	. . . . .		10^3/µL

WBC Histogram

RBC	3.03	L	10^6/µL
HGB	9.4	L	g/dL
HCT	26.9	L	%
MCV	88.8		fL
MCH	31.0		pg
MCHC	34.9		g/dL
RDW	14.9	H	%

RBC Histogram

| PLT | 23 | RCL | 10^3/µL |
| MPV | 11.0 | R H | fL |

PLT Histogram

RET %	4.25
RET #	
IRF	0.61

A   Comments: UMBC = 5.9 [REVIEW SMEAR] [CALL RESULT]

Figure 39-14 Composite scatterplots/histograms from four major instruments. **A,** COULTER LH 750.

Continued

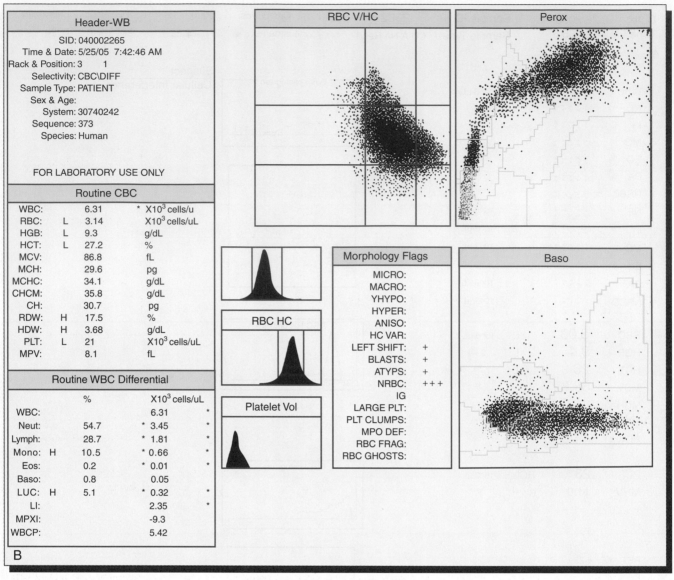

Figure 39-14 *Continued.* **B,** ADVIA 120.

6-8. Match the appropriate definition from a-d for each of the principles used in cell counting listed.
   a. Uses diffraction, reflection, and refraction of light waves
   b. Uses high-voltage electrical waves to measure internal complexity of cells
   c. Based on detection and measurement of changes in electrical current between two electrodes
   d. Uses the variation in electrical charges applied to cells based on their surface markers

6. Impedance

7. Radiofrequency

8. Optical scatter

9. Low-voltage DC is used to measure:
   a. Cell nuclear volume
   b. Total cell volume
   c. Cellular complexity in the nucleus
   d. Cellular complexity in the cytoplasm

10. Orthogonal light scatter is used to measure:
   a. Cell volume or size
   b. Internal complexity
   c. Granularity
   d. Nuclear density

11. On the Coulter instruments, Hct is a calculated value. Which of the following directly measured parameters is used in the calculation of that value?
   a. RDW
   b. Hb
   c. MCV
   d. MCHC

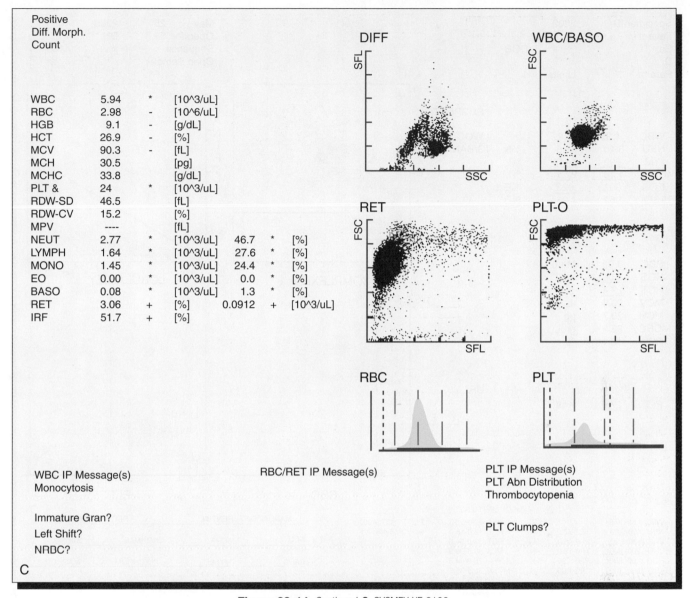

Positive Diff. Morph. Count						
WBC	5.94	*	[10^3/uL]			
RBC	2.98	-	[10^6/uL]			
HGB	9.1	-	[g/dL]			
HCT	26.9	-	[%]			
MCV	90.3	-	[fL]			
MCH	30.5		[pg]			
MCHC	33.8		[g/dL]			
PLT &	24	*	[10^3/uL]			
RDW-SD	46.5		[fL]			
RDW-CV	15.2		[%]			
MPV	----		[fL]			
NEUT	2.77	*	[10^3/uL]	46.7	*	[%]
LYMPH	1.64	*	[10^3/uL]	27.6	*	[%]
MONO	1.45	*	[10^3/uL]	24.4	*	[%]
EO	0.00	*	[10^3/uL]	0.0	*	[%]
BASO	0.08	*	[10^3/uL]	1.3	*	[%]
RET	3.06	+	[%]	0.0912	+	[10^3/uL]
IRF	51.7	+	[%]			

WBC IP Message(s)
Monocytosis

Immature Gran?
Left Shift?
NRBC?

RBC/RET IP Message(s)

PLT IP Message(s)
PLT Abn Distribution
Thrombocytopenia

PLT Clumps?

C

Figure 39-14 *Continued.* **C,** SYSMEX XE 2100.

12-15. Match the following technologies used for determining WBC differentials with the instrument on which they are used.
  a. Abbott CELL-DYN
  b. Bayer Healthcare
  c. Sysmex
  d. Coulter LH750

12. VCS technology

13. MAPSS technology

14. Peroxidase, optical scatter, and absorbance

15. RF/DC detection

16. Point of care instruments that are essentially hemoglobinometers measure Hb by reaction of the blood with a chemical agent and subsequent quantitation by:
  a. Spectrophotometry
  b. Buffy coat expansion
  c. Fluorometry
  d. Electrical impedance

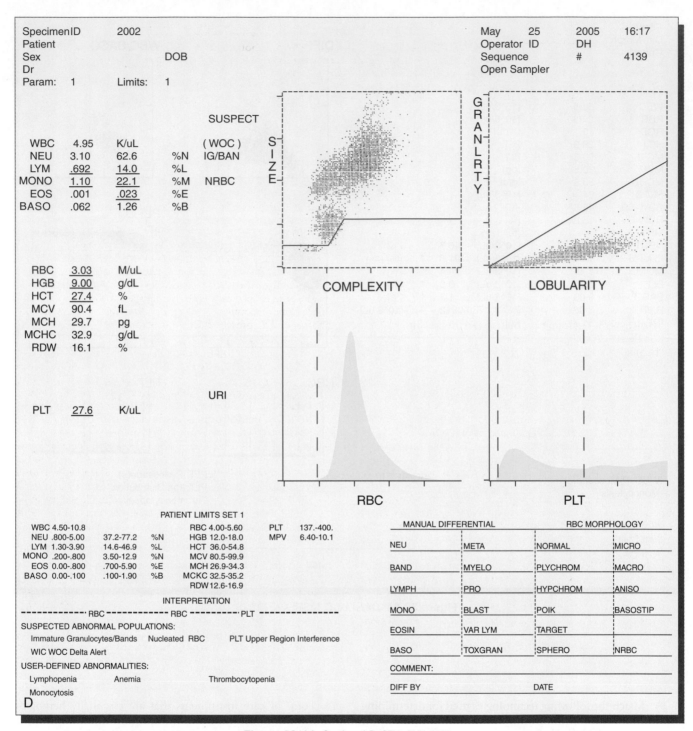

SpecimenID   2002

Patient

Sex   DOB

Dr

Param: 1   Limits: 1

May   25   2005   16:17
Operator ID   DH
Sequence   #   4139
Open Sampler

SUSPECT

(WOC)

IG/BAN

NRBC

WBC	4.95	K/uL	
NEU	3.10	62.6	%N
LYM	.692	14.0	%L
MONO	1.10	22.1	%M
EOS	.001	.023	%E
BASO	.062	1.26	%B

RBC	3.03	M/uL
HGB	9.00	g/dL
HCT	27.4	%
MCV	90.4	fL
MCH	29.7	pg
MCHC	32.9	g/dL
RDW	16.1	%

| PLT | 27.6 | K/uL |

SIZE

COMPLEXITY

GRANLRTY

LOBULARITY

URI

RBC

PLT

PATIENT LIMITS SET 1

WBC 4.50-10.8			RBC 4.00-5.60	PLT 137.-400.
NEU .800-5.00	37.2-77.2	%N	HGB 12.0-18.0	MPV 6.40-10.1
LYM 1.30-3.90	14.6-46.9	%L	HCT 36.0-54.8	
MONO .200-.800	3.50-12.9	%N	MCV 80.5-99.9	
EOS 0.00-.800	.700-5.90	%E	MCH 26.9-34.3	
BASO 0.00-.100	.100-1.90	%B	MCKC 32.5-35.2	
			RDW 12.6-16.9	

INTERPRETATION

------------ RBC ---------- RBC -------- PLT -------------

SUSPECTED ABNORMAL POPULATIONS:

Immature Granulocytes/Bands   Nucleated RBC   PLT Upper Region Interference

WIC WOC Delta Alert

USER-DEFINED ABNORMALITIES:

Lymphopenia   Anemia   Thrombocytopenia

Monocytosis

D

MANUAL DIFFERENTIAL		RBC MORPHOLOGY	
NEU	META	NORMAL	MICRO
BAND	MYELO	PLYCHROM	MACRO
LYMPH	PRO	HYPCHROM	ANISO
MONO	BLAST	POIK	BASOSTIP
EOSIN	VAR LYM	TARGET	
BASO	TOXGRAN	SPHERO	NRBC
COMMENT:			
DIFF BY		DATE	

Figure 39-14 *Continued.* **D,** CELL-DYN 4000.

ACKNOWLEDGMENTS

The authors wish to thank Emily Mabry, MT (HEW), Hematology Supervisor at Maury Regional Hospital in Columbia, Tenn., for developing the cases and coordinating the samples, and the Hematology Laboratories at Maury Regional Hospital in Columbia, the Veterans Administration Hospital in Nashville, Bedford County Medical Center in Shelbyville, and Marshall Medical Center in Lewisburg, Tenn., for their assistance in analyzing the specimens presented in this chapter on the different instruments.

REFERENCES

1. Morris MW, Davey FR: Basic examination of blood. In Henry JB (ed): Clinical Diagnosis and Management by Laboratory Methods, 20th ed. Philadelphia: Saunders, 2001:479-519.

2. Koepke JA: Quantitative blood cell counting. In Koepke JA (ed): Practical Laboratory Hematology. New York: Churchill Livingstone, 1991:43-60.

3. Stiene-Martin EA: Introduction to hematologic automation. In Stiene-Martin EA, Lotspeich-Steininger CA, Koepke JA (eds): Clinical Hematology: Principles, Procedures, Correlations. Philadelphia: Lippincott-Raven, 1998:515-518.

4. Dotson MA: Multiparameter hematology instruments. In Stiene-Martin EA, Lotspeich-Steininger CA, Koepke JA (eds): Clinical Hematology: Principles, Procedures, Correlations. Philadelphia: Lippincott-Raven, 1998:519-551.

5. Coulter WH: High speed automatic blood cell counter and cell size analyzer. Proc Natl Electron Conf 1956;12:1034.

6. Coulter Electronics, Inc.: Significant Advances in Hematology: Hematology Education Series, PN 4206115 A. Hialeah, FL: Coulter Electronics, Inc., 1983.

7. Coulter Electronics, Inc.: Coulter Counter Model S-Plus IV with Three-Population Differential: Product Reference Manual, PN 423560B. Hialeah, FL: Coulter® Electronics, Inc., 1983.

8. Coulter Electronics, Inc.: Coulter STKR Product Reference Manual, PN 4235547E. Hialeah, FL: Coulter Electronics, Inc., 1988.

9. Toa Medical Electronics Co., Ltd.: Sysmex Model E-5000 Operator's Manual (CN 461-2104-2). Kobe, Japan: Toa Medical Electronics Co., Ltd., 1985.

10. Coulter Corporation: Coulter® STKS Operator's Guide, PN 423592811. Hialeah, FL: Coulter Corporation, 1992.

11. Mohandas N, Clark MR, Kissinger S, et al: Inaccuracies associated with the automated measurement of mean cell hemoglobin concentration in dehydrated cells. Blood 1980;56:125-128.

12. Arnfred T, Kristensen SD, Munck V: Coulter counter model S and model S-plus measurements of mean erythrocyte volume (MCV) are influenced by the mean erythrocyte haemoglobin concentration (MCHC). Scand J Clin Lab Invest 1981;41:717-721.

13. Johnson KL: Basics of flow cytometry. Clin Lab Sci 1992;5:22-24.

14. Louie J, Parker JW: Flow cytometry. In Stiene-Martin EA, Lotspeich-Steininger CA, Koepke JA (eds): Clinical Hematology: Principles, Procedures, Correlations. Philadelphia: Lippincott-Raven, 1998:552-562.

15. Toa Medical Electronics Co., Ltd.: Sysmex NE-8000 Operator's Manual (CN 461-2326-5). Kobe, Japan: Toa Medical Electronics Co., Ltd., 1990.

16. Sysmex Corporation: Sysmex XE-2100 Operator's Manual. Kobe, Japan: Sysmex Corporation, 1999.

17. Shapiro HM: How a flow cytometer works. In Shapiro HM (ed): Practical Flow Cytometry, 2nd ed. New York: Alan R Liss, 1988:21-86.

18. Paraskevas F: Clinical flow cytometry. In Greer JP, Foerster J, Lukens J, et al (eds): Wintrobe's Clinical Hematology, 11th ed. Philadelphia: Lippincott, Williams & Wilkins, 2004:99-117.

19. Jovin TM, Morris SJ, Striker G, et al: Automatic sizing and separation of particles by ratios of light scattering intensities. J Histochem Cytochem 1976;24:269-283.

20. McCoy JP, Lovett EJ: Basic principles in clinical flow cytometry. In Keren DF (ed): Flow Cytometry in Clinical Diagnosis. Chicago: ASCP Press, 1989:12-40.

21. Tycko DH, Metz MH, Epstein EA, et al: Flow-cytometric scattering measurement of red blood cell volume and hemoglobin concentration. Appl Opt 1985;24:1395-1364.

22. Abbott Laboratories: CELL-DYN 3000 System Operator's Manual (LN 92420-01). Abbott Park, IL: Abbott Laboratories, 1993.

23. Abbott Laboratories: CELL-DYN 3500 System Operator's Manual (LN 92722-05). Abbott Park, IL: Abbott Laboratories, 1996.

24. Miles Inc.: Technicon H-3 RTX/RTC System: System Reference Guide, PN TK9-2823-10. Tarrytown, NY: Miles, Inc., 1993.

25. Bayer Corporation: ADVIA120 Operator's Guide, V1.03.00B. Tarrytown, NY: Bayer Diagnostics, 1998.

26. Abbott Diagnostics Division: Diagnostic products. Available at: www.abbott.com. Accessed August 13, 2006.

27. HORIBAABX Hematology: The product line. Available at: www.abx.com. Accessed August 13, 2006.

28. Bayer Diagnostics: Laboratory testing products. Available at: www.bayerdiag.com. Accessed August 12, 2006.

29. Beckman Coulter: Hematology systems. Available at: www.beckman.com. Accessed August 13, 2006.

30. Sysmex Corporation: Hematology products. Available at: www.sysmex.co.uk. Accessed August 12, 2006.

31. Beckman Coulter: GenS.series. Available at: http://www.beckman.com/products/instrumetn/hematology/gens_analyzer.asp. Accessed August 14, 2006.

32. Beckman Coulter: Technical Application Information. Coulter® 3-D VCS technology. Available at: http://www.beckman.com/resourcecenter/literature/DiagLit/ClinLitList.asp?ProductCategoryID=HEMA. Accessed August 12, 2006.

33. Beckman Coulter: LH750. Available at: http://www.beckman.com/products/instrumetn/hematology/lh750_analyzer.asp. Accessed August 14, 2006.

34. Bessman D, Williams U, Gilmer PR: Mean platelet volume: the inverse relation of platelet size and count in normal subjects and an artifact of other particles. Am J Clin Pathol 1981;76:289.

35. Coulter Electronics, Inc.: Coulter® VCS Technology Casebook, PN 4206281-2A. Hialeah, FL: Coulter Electronics, Inc., 1989.

36. Beckman Coulter Inc.: Coulter LH700 Series Operator's Guide. Fullerton, CA: Beckman Coulter Inc., 2003.

37. Sysmex Corporation: System XE-2100 Operator's Guide. Kobe, Japan, 1999.

38. Matzdorff AC, Kühnel G, Scott S, et al: Comparison of flow cytometry and the automated blood analyzer system CELL-DYN 4000® for platelet analysis. Lab Hematol 1998;4:163-168.

39. Bowden KL, Procopio N, Wystepek E, et al: Platelet clumps, nucleated red cells, and leukocyte counts: a comparison between the Abbott CELL-DYN® 4000 and Coulter® STKS. Lab Hematol 1998;4:7-16.

40. Jones RG, Faust A, Glazier J, et al: CELL-DYN® 4000: utility within the core laboratory structure and preliminary comparison of its expanded differential with the 400-cell manual differential count. Lab Hematol 1998;4:34-44.

41. Abbott Diagnostics: CELL-DYN® Rainbow™ Classification Program, PN 97-9427/R3-20. Abbott Park, IL: Abbott Diagnostics, September 1992.

42. Abbott Laboratories: CELL-DYN® 3500 System Operator's Manual: Reticulocyte Package (9140293D). Abbott Park, IL: Abbott Laboratories, 1999.

43. Abbott Laboratories: CELL-DYN® 4000 Operator's Manual. Santa Clara, CA: Abbott Laboratories, 1997.

44. Bayer Healthcare: Bayer® ADVIA 2120 Operator's Guide. Tarrytown, NY: Bayer Healthcare Inc., 2003, 2005.

45. Groner W: New developments in flow cytochemistry technology. In Simson E (ed): Proceedings of the Technicon H-1 Hematology Symposium, October 11, 1985. Tarrytown, NY: Technicon Instruments Corporation, 1986:1-8.

46. Mohandas N, Kim YR, Tycko DH, et al: Accurate and independent measurement of volume and hemoglobin concentration of individual red cells by laser light scattering. Blood 1986;68:506-513.

47. Harris N, Jou JM, Devoto G, et al: Performance evaluation of the ADVIA 2120 hematology analyzer: an international multicenter clinical trial. Lab Hematol 2005;11:62-70.

48. Koepke J: Current limitations in reticulocyte counting: implications for clinical laboratories. In Porstmann B (ed): The Emerging Importance of Accurate Reticulocyte Counting. New York: Caduceus Medical, 1993:18-22.

49. Clinical and Laboratory Standards Institute (formerly NCCLS): Methods for Reticulocyte Counting (Flow Cytometry and Supravital Dyes): Approved Guideline. CLSI document H44-A-2. Wayne, PA: Clinical and Laboratory Standards Institute, 2004.

50. College of American Pathologists: CAP Surveys: Reticulocyte (Pilot) Survey Set RT-A, 1993. Northfield, IL: College of American Pathologists, 1993.

51. College of American Pathologists: CAP Surveys: Reticulocyte Survey Set RT/RT2-A, 2000. Northfield, IL: College of American Pathologists, 2000.

52. Coulter Corporation: Introducing a new reticulocyte methodology using Coulter® VCS technology on Coulter STKS and MAXM hematology systems: Product Brochure TC93003201. Miami, FL: Coulter Corporation, 1993.

53. Toa Medical Electronics Co., Ltd.: Sysmex R-3000 Automated Reticulocyte Analyzer: Product Brochure Lit. No. SP-9620. Los Alamitos, CA: Toa Medical Electronics (USA), Inc., 1991.

54. Coulter Corporation: Coulter® STKS with Reticulocyte Analysis Operator's Guide (PN 4237188). Miami, FL: Coulter Corporation, 1993.

55. Beckman Coulter: Technical Application information: Coulter® VCS reticulocyte method. Available at: http://www.beckman.com/resourcecenter/literature/DiagLit/ClinLitList.asp?ProductCategoryID=HEMA. Accessed August 13, 2006.

56. Bowen KL, Glazier J, Mattson JC: Abbott CELL-DYN® 4000 automated red blood cell analysis compared with routine red blood cell morphology by smear review. Lab Hematol 1998;4:45-47.

57. Colella G: Technical advancements of the H-3 hematology analyzer. In Baizac F, Chapman S, Verderese C (eds): Conference Proceedings: H-3 New Perspectives for Hematology. New York: Caduceus Medical, 1993:28-29.

58. Davis BH, Bigelow NC, van Hove L, et al: Evaluation of automated reticulocyte analysis with immature reticulocyte fraction as a potential outcomes indicator of anemia in chronic renal failure patients. Lab Hematol 1998;4:169-175.

59. Fourcade C, Jary L, Belaouni H: Reticulocyte analysis provided by the Coulter GEN.S: significance and interpretation in regenerative and non-regenerative hematologic conditions. Lab Hematol 1999;5:153-158.

60. Goldberg M: Recombinant erythropoietin therapy and the detection of iron-deficient erythropoiesis in iron-replete individuals. In Baizac F, Chapman S, Verderese C (eds): Conference Proceedings: H-3 New Perspectives for Hematology. New York: Caduceus Medical, 1993:16-18.

61. d'Onofrio G: Simultaneous H-3 RBC and reticulocyte measurement: is it clinically useful? In Balzac F, Chapman S, Verderese C (eds): Conference Proceedings: H-3 New Perspectives for Hematology. New York: Caduceus Medical, 1993:23-27.

62. Davis BH, Bigelow NC: Automated reticulocyte analysis: clinical practice and associated new parameters. Hematol Oncol Clin N Am 1994;8:617-630.

63. Kessler C, Campbell P, Bolufe V, et al: Immature reticulocyte fraction and reticulocyte maturity index. Technical application information. Available at: http://www.beckman.com/resourcecenter/literature/DiagLit/ClinLitList.asp?ProductCategoryID=HEMA; available at: www.coulter.com/coulter/Hematology/Retic-Literature-Review/default.asp). Accessed August 13, 2006.

64. Brugnara C, Zurakowski D, DiCanzio J, et al: Reticulocyte hemoglobin content to diagnose iron deficiency in children. JAMA 1999;281:2225-2230.

65. Ullrich C, Wu A, Armbsy C, et al: Screening healthy infants for iron deficiency using reticulocyte hemoglobin content. JAMA 2005;294:924-930.

66. Clinical and Laboratory Standards Institute: Performance Goals for the Internal Quality Control of Multichannel Hematology Analyzers: Approved Standard. CLSI Publication H26-A. Wayne, PA: Clinical and Laboratory Standards Institute, 1996.

67. Clinical and Laboratory Standards Institute: Assessment of the Clinical Accuracy of Laboratory Tests Using Receiver Operating Characteristics (ROC) Plots: Approved Guideline. CLSI Document GP1O-A. Wayne, PA: Clinical and Laboratory Standards Institute, 1995.

68. Clinical Laboratory Improvement Amendments Brochure #3: Calibration and calibration verification. Available at: http://www.cms.hhs.gov/CLIA/05_CLIA_Brochures.asp. Accessed August 12, 2006.

69. Gilmer PR, Williams U, Koepke JA, et al: Calibration methods for automated hematology instruments. Am J Clin Pathol 1977;68:185-190.

70. Koepke JA: The calibration of automated instruments for accuracy in hemoglobinometry. Am J Clin Pathol 1977;68:180-184.

71. International Committee for Standardization in Haematology: Recommendations for reference method for haemoglobinometry in human blood (ICSH Standard 1995) and specifications for international haemiglobincyanide standard (4th ed). J Clin Pathol 1996;49:271-274.

72. Savage RA: Calibration bias and imprecision for automated hematology analyzers: an evaluation of significance of short-term bias resulting from calibration of an analyzer with S Cal. Am J Clin Pathol 1985;84:186-190.

73. College of American Pathologists: Laboratory General: CAP Checklist, 1999 edition. Northfield, IL: College of American Pathologists, 1998.

74. Cornbleet J: Spurious results from automated hematology cell counters. Lab Med 1983;14:509-514.

75. Tsuda I, Tatsumi N: Evaluation of detection of immature WBC by the new Sysmex SE-9000 automated hematology analyzer. Poster presentation, International Society for Laboratory Hematology 7th International Symposium on Technology Innovations in Laboratory Hematology, Lake Tahoe, NV, April 7-10, 1994.

76. Bentley SA, Johnson A, Bishop CA: A parallel evaluation of four automated hematology analyzers. Am J Clin Pathol 1993;100:626-632.

77. Miers MK, Exton MG, Hurlbut TA, et al: White blood cell differentials as performed by the Technicon® H-1: evaluation and implementation in a tertiary care hospital. Lab Med 1991;22:99-106.

78. Strobel SL, Panke TW, Bills GL: Cold erythrocyte agglutination and infectious mononucleosis. Lab Med 1993;24:219-221.

79. Culp NB, Fritsma G: New approaches to nucleated RBC correction of WBC counts. Clin Lab Sci 1990;4:3.

80. Bessman JD, Feinstein DI: Quantitative anisocytosis as a discriminant between iron deficiency and thalassemia minor. Blood 1979;53:288-293.

81. Bessman JD, Gilmer PR, Gardner FH: Improved classification of anemias by MCV and RDW. Am J Clin Pathol 1983;80:322-326.

82. Fossat C, Sainty D, David M, et al: Value of new parameters and histograms in erythrocyte counting for anemia classification. XXII Congress of the International Society of Hematology, 1988, 11.

83. Green R, King R: A new red cell discriminant incorporating volume dispersion for differentiating iron deficiency anemia from thalassemia minor. Blood Cells 1989;15:481-495.

84. Fernandes B, Houwen B: A new algorithm for classification of microcytic anaemias. Paper presented at the International Society for Laboratory Hematology 7th International Symposium on Technology Innovations in Laboratory Hematology, Lake Tahoe, NV, April 7-10, 1994.

85. Duca D, Green R: Red cell distribution width is a poor discriminator for distinguishing iron deficiency anemia from thalassemia minor or the anemia of chronic disease [abstract]. Poster presentation: 1993 Fall Meeting of the American Society of Clinical Pathologists (ASCP) and the College of American Pathologists (CAP), Orlando, FL, October 16-22, 1993.

86. Green R, King R, Greenbaum A, et al: Early detection of iron deficiency by direct measurement of red cell hemoglobin concentration: sequential studies in phlebotomized normal volunteers. Blood 1990;76(Suppl):122.

87. Mohandas N, Greenbaum A, Green R: Variability in cell hemoglobin content of individual red cells can be used to discriminate iron deficiency from thalassemia minor. Blood 1990;76:155.

88. Brugnara C, Chambers LA, Malynn E, et al: Red blood cell regeneration induced by subcutaneous recombinant erythropoietin: iron-deficient erythropoiesis in iron-replete subjects. Blood 1993;81:956-964.

89. Coulter Electronics: Proceedings of the Coulter Automated Differential International Symposium, September 26, 1986. Hialeah, FL: Coulter Electronics, 1987.

90. Reardon DM, Hutchinson D, Preston FE, et al: The routine measurement of platelet volume: a comparison of aperture-impedance and flow cytometric systems. Clin Lab Haematol 1985;7:251-257.

91. Allen JK, Batjer ID: Evaluation of an automated method for leukocyte differential counts based on electronic volume analysis. Arch Pathol Lab Med 1985;109:534-539.

92. Pierre RV, Payne BA, Lee WK, et al: Comparison of four leukocyte differential methods with the National Committee for Clinical Laboratory Standards (NCCLS) reference method. Am J Clin Pathol 1987;87:201-209.

93. Payne BA, Pierre RV, Lee WK: Evaluation of the TOA E-5000® automated hematology analyzer. Am J Clin Pathol 1987; 88:51-57.

94. Ross DW, Watson JS, Davis PH, et al: Evaluation of the Coulter three-part differential screen. Am J Clin Pathol 1985;84:481-484.

95. Cornbleet J, Kessinger S: Evaluation of Coulter S-Plus three-part differential in population with a high prevalence of abnormalities. Am J Clin Pathol 1985;84:620-626.

96. Miers MK, Fogo AB, Federspiel CF, et al: Evaluation of the Coulter S-Plus IV differential as a screening tool in a tertiary care hospital. Am J Clin Pathol 1987;87:745-751.

97. Ross DW, Bentley SA: Evaluation of an automated hematology system (Technicon® H-1). Arch Pathol Lab Med 1986;110:803-808.

98. Bollinger PB, Drewinko B, Brailas CD, et al: The Technicon H-1: an automated hematology analyzer for today and tomorrow. Am J Clin Pathol 1987;87:71-78.

99. Watson JS, Davis RA: Evaluation of the Technicon® H-1 hematology system. Lab Med 1987;18:316-322.

100. Warner BA, Reardon DM: A field evaluation of the Coulter STKS®. Am J Clin Pathol 1991;95:207-217.

101. Hallawell R, O'Malley C, Hussein S, et al: An evaluation of the Sysmex NE-8000 hematology analyzer. Am J Clin Pathol 1991;96:594-601.

102. Cornbleet PJ, Myrick D, Judkins S, et al: Evaluation of the CELL-DYN® 3000 differential. Am J Clin Pathol 1992;98:603-614.

103. Cornbleet PJ, Myrick D, Levy R: Evaluation of the Coulter STKS five-part differential. Am J Clin Pathol 1993;99:72-81.

104. Brigden ML, Page NE, Graydon C: Evaluation of the Sysmex NE-8000 automated hematology analyzer in a high-volume outpatient laboratory. Am J Clin Pathol 1993;100:618-625.

105. Rumke CL: The statistically expected variability in differential leukocyte counting. In Koepke JA (ed): Differential Leukocyte Counting. Skokie, IL: College of American Pathologists, 1978.

106. Koepke JA, Dotson MA, Shifman MA: A critical evaluation of the manual/visual differential leukocyte counting method. Blood Cells 1985;11:173-181.

107. Paterakis G, Kossivas L, Kendall R, et al: Comparative evaluation of the erythroblast count generated by three-color fluorescence flow cytometry, the Abbott CELL-DYN® 4000 hematology analyzer, and microscopy. Lab Hematol 1998;4:64-70.

108. Clinical Laboratory and Standards Institute: Reference leukocyte differential count (proportional) and evaluation of instrumental methods: approved standard. CLSI Document H20-A. Wayne, PA: Clinical Laboratory and Standards Institute, 1992.

109. Warner BA, Reardon DM, Marshall DP: Automated haematology analysers: a four-way comparison. Med Lab Sci 1990; 47:285-296.

110. Swaim WR: Laboratory and clinical evaluation of white blood cell differential counts: comparison of the Coulter® VCS, Technicon® H-1, and 800-cell manual method. Am J Clin Pathol 1991;95:381-388.

111. Buttarello M, Gadotti M, Lorenz C, et al: Evaluation of four automated hematology analyzers: a comparative study of differential counts (imprecision and inaccuracy). Am J Clin Pathol 1992;97:345-352.

112. Goossens W, Hove LV, Verwilghen RL: Monocyte counting: discrepancies in results obtained with different automated instruments. J Clin Pathol 1991;44:224-227.

113. Seaberg R, Cuomo J: Assessment of monocyte counts derived from automated instrumentation. Lab Med 1993;24:222-224.

114. Watson JS, Ross DW: Characterization of myelodysplastic syndromes by flow cytochemistry with the Technicon® H-1. J Med Tech 1987;4:18-20.

115. Krause JR, Costello RT, Krause J, et al: Use of the Technicon H-1 in the characterization of leukemias. Arch Pathol Lab Med 1988;112:889-894.

116. Penchansky L, Krause JR: Flow cytochemical study of acute leukemia of childhood with the Technicon® H-1. Lab Med 1991;22:184-189.

117. Walters JG, Garrity PF: Case Studies in the New Morphology. McGraw Park, IL: American Scientific Products, 1987.

118. Simson E, Ross DW, Kocher WD: Atlas of Automated Cytochemical Hematology. Tarrytown, NY: Technicon Instruments Corporation, 1988.

119. Hinchliffe RF, Helliwell MM: Red Cells in Children: An H-1 Atlas. Tarrytown, NY: Bayer Diagnostics, 1993.

120. Beckman Coulter, Inc.: Coulter® Gen-S™ System: Clinical Case Studies, PN 9914978. Brea, CA: Beckman Coulter, Inc., 1996.

121. Sysmex Corporation: Laboratory testing products. Available at: www.sysmex.com/usa/ourproducts/our_products_detail. cfm?p_id=34. Accessed August 13, 2006.

122. Bayer Diagnostics: Laboratory testing products. Available at: www.labnews.de/en/ne_lib/bp_det.php?id=119&search. Accessed August 13, 2006.

123. Harris N, Kunicka J, Kratz A: The ADVIA 2120 hematology system: flow cytometry-based analysis of blood and body fluids in the routine hematology laboratory. Lab Hematol 2005;11:47-61.

124. Body Fluid Analysis Made Simple—and Automated. www.beckmancoulter.com/products/instrument/hematology/body-fluid-application.asp. Accessed August 13, 2006.

125. Camden TL: How to select the ideal hematology analyzer. Medical Laboratory Observer 1993;25:29-33.

126. van Hove L: Guest editorial: which hematology analyzer do you need? Lab Hematol 1998;4:32-33.

127. Albitar M, Dong Q, Saunder D, et al: Evaluation of automated leukocyte differential counts in a cancer center. Lab Hematol 1999;5:10-14.

128. Baer D: Hematology Testing at the Bedside. Lab Med 1995; 26:48-51.

129. Wu J, Peterson J, Mohammad A, et al: Point-of-care hemoglobin measurement by Stat-Site MHgb Reflectance Meter. Point of Care 2003;March:8-11.

130. Santrach PJ: Point of Care Hematology, Hemostasis and Thrombolysis Testing: Principles and Practice of Point-of-Care Testing. Philadelphia: Lippincott, Williams & Wilkins, 2002:157-158.

ADDITIONAL RESOURCES

Centers for Medicare and Medicaid Services. Available at: http://www.cms.hhs.gov/clia/.

College of American Pathologists. Available at: http://www.cap.org.

Howerton D, Anderson N, Bosse D, Granade S. Good laboratory practices for waived testing sites. MMWR Morb Mortal Wkly Rep 2005;54:1-37.

Joint Commission on Accreditation of Healthcare Organizations. Available at: http://www.jcaho.org.

Kost J (ed): Principles and Practice of Point-of-Care Testing. Philadelphia: Lippincott, Williams & Wilkins, 2002.

Point of Care: The Journal of Near-Patient Testing and Technology. Philadelphia: Lippincott, Williams & Wilkins

Point of Care.net. Available at: http://www.pointofcare.net.

Normal Hemostasis and Coagulation

40

Margaret G. Fritsma and George A. Fritsma

OBJECTIVES

After completion of this chapter, the reader will be able to:

1. List the systems that interact to provide hemostasis.
2. Establish the properties of the vascular intima in the initiation and regulation of hemostasis and fibrinolysis.
3. List the functions of the blood cells, especially platelets, in hemostasis.
4. Describe the relationships among platelet function, von Willebrand factor, and fibrinogen and their impact on hemostasis.
5. Describe the nature, origin, and function of each of the tissue and plasma factors necessary for normal coagulation.
6. Explain the role of vitamin K in the production and function of plasma clotting factors in the prothrombin group.

7. Diagram fibrinogen structure, fibrin formation, fibrin polymerization, and fibrin cross-linking.
8. Distinguish between serine proteases and cofactors in the coagulation pathway.
9. Describe the tissue factor pathway, amplification pathway, and contact activation in coagulation.
10. Show how tissue factor pathway inhibitor, the protein C pathway, and the serine protease inhibitors function to regulate coagulation and prevent thrombosis.
11. Describe the fibrinolytic pathway and its products.

CASE STUDY

After studying the material in this chapter, the reader should be able to respond to the following case study:

A newborn boy bled excessively after circumcision. His prothrombin time test results and platelet count were normal, but his activated partial thromboplastin time test was prolonged. A bleeding time test was not performed.

1. What is the likely disorder?
2. How should this infant be treated?

Blood is a fluid while in the body, but it transforms itself to a sturdy gel a few minutes after it is removed. Hemostasis is a combination of cellular and biochemical events that function in harmony to keep blood liquid within the veins and arteries, prevent blood loss from injuries by the formation of thrombi, and re-establish blood flow during the healing process.[1] When hemostasis systems are out of balance, thrombosis (clotting) or hemorrhage (bleeding) is life-threatening. Clinical laboratory scientists, hematopathologists, and hematologists investigate all of the major hemostasis systems—the blood vessels, blood cells, and plasma proteins—to prevent, predict, diagnose, and manage hemostatic disease.

OVERVIEW OF HEMOSTASIS

The cellular elements of hemostasis are the vascular intima, blood platelets, erythrocytes, neutrophils, and monocytes. The coagulation and fibrinolysis mechanisms are the enzyme systems of hemostasis.[2]

Primary and Secondary Hemostasis

Many hematologists and clinical laboratory scientists speak of primary and secondary hemostasis (Table 40-1). Primary hemostasis mechanisms are activated by small injuries to blood vessels or by the commonplace *desquamation* of dying or damaged endothelial cells. In primary hemostasis, the blood vessel contracts to seal the wound, and platelets fill the open space to form a plug. The insults that trigger primary hemostasis mechanisms seem trivial, but primary system defects such as thrombocytopenia, platelet disorders, or von Willebrand disease (VWD) cause debilitating, sometimes fatal chronic hemorrhage.

Secondary hemostasis is triggered directly or by primary hemostasis and is necessary to control bleeding from large wounds incurred through trauma, surgery, or dental procedures. The coagulation system, a series of enzymes and enzyme cofactors, accomplishes secondary hemostasis by producing a fibrin thrombus. Although the vascular intima and platelets usually are associated with primary hemostasis, and coagulation and fibrinolysis are associated with secondary hemostasis, all systems interact in early and late hemostatic events.

Vascular Intima in Hemostasis

The innermost lining of blood vessels is a contiguous layer of cells called *endothelial cells* (Box 40-1; Fig. 40-1).[3] These form a smooth, unbroken surface that promotes the fluid passage of

> ### BOX 40-1 Vascular Intima
>
> **Innermost Vascular Lining**
> Endothelial cells (endothelium)
>
> **Supporting the Endothelial Cells**
> Internal elastic lamina, composed of elastin and collagen, surrounds endothelium
>
> **Subendothelial Connective Tissue**
> Collagen and fibroblasts in veins
> Collagen, fibroblasts, and smooth muscle cells in arteries

blood and prevents turbulence that otherwise may activate platelets and coagulation enzymes. An elastin-rich internal elastic lamina and its surrounding layer of connective tissues support the endothelial cells. In all blood vessels, fibroblasts occupy the connective tissue layer and produce collagen. Smooth muscle cells, intermixed with fibroblasts in arteries and arterioles but not in the walls of veins, venules, or capillaries, contract during primary hemostasis.

Procoagulant Properties of Vascular Intima

Intimal cells and their environment play a premier role in hemostasis.[4] The function of the vascular intima is to promote coagulation when damaged. First, any harmful local stimulus, be it mechanical or chemical, induces vasoconstriction in arteries and arterioles (Table 40-2). Smooth muscle cells contract, the vascular lumen narrows or closes, and blood flow to the injured site is minimized. Second, the subendothelial connective tissues of arteries and veins are rich in collagen, a flexible, elastic structural protein that binds and activates platelets. Third, endothelial cells secrete von Willebrand factor (VWF), a 600,000-D to 20,000,000-D glycoprotein that is necessary for platelets to adhere to exposed subendothelial collagen in arterioles.[5] Fourth, on activation, endothelial cells secrete and coat themselves with P-selectin, an adhesion molecule that promotes platelet and leukocyte binding.[6] Endothe-

TABLE 40-1 Primary and Secondary Hemostasis

Primary Hemostasis	Secondary Hemostasis
Desquamation and small injuries to blood vessels	Large injuries to blood vessels and surrounding tissues
Involves vascular intima and platelets	Involves platelets and coagulation system
Rapid, short-lived response	Delayed, long-term response
Damaged or activated endothelial cells	Tissue factor is exposed on cell membranes

Figure 40-1 Normal blood flow in intact vessels. Smooth, rhomboid endothelial surfaces promote even flow. Larger cells are focused toward the center. The endothelium provides several hemostasis-suppressing materials.

EC: Endothelial cell
SMC: Smooth muscle cell
FB: Fibroblast
IEL: Internal elastic lamina
RBC: Red blood cell
PLT: Platelet
Lines: Collagen

Normal intimal layer suppresses hemostasis:
• Smooth surface
• Prostacyclin
• Heparan sulfate
• Tissue factor pathway inhibitor
• Thrombomodulin

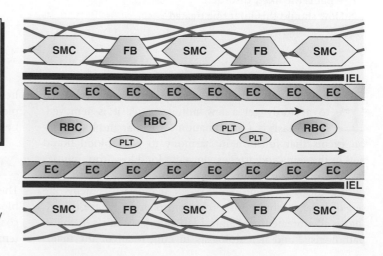

TABLE 40-2 Procoagulant Properties of the Vascular Intima

Structure	Procoagulant Property
Smooth muscle cells in arterioles and arteries	Induce vasoconstriction
Exposed subendothelial collagen	Binds VWF and platelets
Damaged or activated endothelial cells	Secrete VWF
	Secrete adhesion molecules: P-selectin, ICAMs, PECAMs
Exposed smooth muscle cells and fibroblasts	Tissue factor exposed on cell membranes
Endothelial cells in inflammation	Tissue factor is induced by inflammation

ICAMs, intercellular adhesion molecules; PECAMs, platelet endothelial cell adhesion molecules; VWF, von Willebrand factor.

lial cells also secrete immunoglobulin-like adhesion molecules called *intercellular adhesion molecules* and *platelet endothelial cell adhesion molecules* that promote leukocyte binding.[7] Finally, subendothelial cells (i.e., smooth muscle cells and fibroblasts) support a constitutive surface protein called *tissue factor.*[8] Exposed tissue factor activates the coagulation system through factor VII. Tissue factor also appears on the surface of endothelial cells and on blood-borne monocytes during inflammation.[9]

Anticoagulant Properties of Vascular Intima

Although damaged vessels have procoagulant properties, the intact intima prevents intravascular thrombosis by several mechanisms (Box 40-2). First, endothelial cells are rhomboid and contiguous, providing a smooth inner surface that evens the blood flow and prevents turbulence. Endothelial cells synthesize prostacyclin, a platelet activation inhibitor produced from the eicosanoid synthesis pathway. Prostacyclin prevents unnecessary or undesirable platelet activation in undamaged vessels.[10]

Nitric oxide is synthesized in endothelial cells, vascular smooth muscle cells, neutrophils, and macrophages. Nitric oxide counteracts vasoconstriction and maintains healthy arterioles.[11] *Heparan sulfate* is an intimal glycosaminoglycan that retards coagulation by activating antithrombin, a coagulation regulatory protein.[12] *Heparin* is a pharmaceutical, manufactured from porcine gut tissues, that resembles heparan sulfate.

BOX 40-2 Anticoagulant Properties of Intact Endothelium

Cells are rhomboid, presenting a smooth, contiguous surface
Secretes eicosanoid platelet inhibitor *prostacyclin*
Secretes vascular "relaxing" factor *nitric oxide*
Secretes anticoagulant glycosaminoglycan *heparan sulfate*
Secretes coagulation extrinsic pathway regulator *TFPI*
Maintains cell membrane *thrombomodulin,* protein C coagulation control system activator

Heparin is used extensively as a therapeutic to prevent propagation of the thrombi that cause coronary thrombosis, strokes, deep vein thromboses, and pulmonary thrombotic emboli.[13]

Another important endothelial cell anticoagulant is tissue factor pathway inhibitor (TFPI), which inactivates coagulation factor VIIa in the presence of factor Xa and controls the tissue factor or extrinsic coagulation pathway. Finally, endothelial surface membranes anchor and support *thrombomodulin,* a protein that activates the protein C pathway. The protein C pathway regulates the coagulation mechanism by digesting activated coagulation factors V and VIII.

Fibrinolytic Properties of Vascular Intima

Endothelial cells support fibrinolysis with the secretion of tissue plasminogen activator (TPA). During thrombus formation, TPA binds polymerized fibrin and triggers the activation of nearby fibrin-bound plasminogen to form plasmin that ultimately digests the thrombus and restores blood flow. Endothelial cells also may secrete plasminogen activator inhibitor-1 (PAI-1) together with other cells, a TPA control protein.[14]

Although the significance of the vascular intima in hemostasis is well recognized, clinical laboratory scientists possess few valid measures of blood vessel disorders.[15] In the future, new laboratory protocols may enable us to assess effectively the integrity of endothelial cells, smooth muscle cells, fibroblasts, and their collagen matrix.[16]

Platelets

Platelets are produced from the cytoplasm of bone marrow megakaryocytes (Chapter 13).[17] Although platelets are only 2 to 3 μm in diameter on a fixed, stained peripheral blood film, they are complex, metabolically active cells that interact with their environment, initiate, and control hemostasis.[18]

Platelets adhere, aggregate, and secrete (Table 40-3).[19] Adhesion is the property of binding to nonplatelet surfaces such as subendothelial collagen or VWF (Figs. 40-2 and 40-3), whereas aggregation is interplatelet attachment (Fig. 40-4).[20] Secretion of platelet granule contents occurs during adhesion and aggregation, although most secretion occurs late in the

TABLE 40-3 Platelet Function

Platelet Function	Characteristics
Adhesion: platelets roll and cling to nonplatelet surfaces	Reversible; seals endothelial gaps, some secretion of growth factors, in arterioles VWF is necessary for adhesion
Aggregation: platelets adhere to each other	Irreversible; platelet plugs form, secretion of all platelet contents, requires fibrinogen
Secretion: platelets discharge the contents of their granules	Irreversible; occurs during aggregation, essential to coagulation

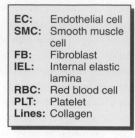

Figure 40-2 Platelet adhesion. On endothelial cell desquamation, platelets adhere to the subendothelium and fill in until new endothelial cells grow.

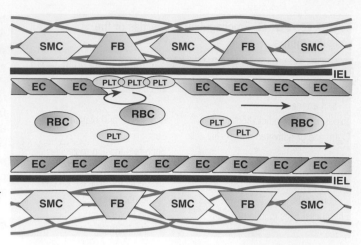

EC: Endothelial cell
SMC: Smooth muscle cell
FB: Fibroblast
IEL: Internal elastic lamina
RBC: Red blood cell
PLT: Platelet
Lines: Collagen

Damaged intima support hemostasis:
• Vasoconstriction
• Exposure of tissue factor
• von Willebrand factor
• Tissue factor
• P-selectin

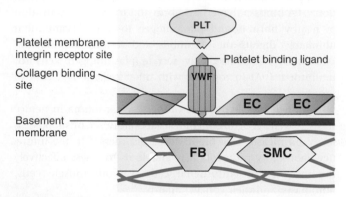

Platelet membrane integrin receptor site
Platelet binding ligand
Collagen binding site
Basement membrane

Figure 40-3 Platelet adhesion. Platelet, VWF, and collagen interaction. In arterioles and arteries, where blood moves rapidly, platelets adhere by binding VWF. The larger VWF multimers form a fibrillar carpet on which the platelets assemble.

TABLE 40-4 Platelet Granule Contents

Platelet α Granules	Platelet δ Granules (Dense Bodies)
Large molecules	Small molecules
β-thromboglobulin	ADP (activates neighboring platelets)
Factor V	ATP
Factor XI	Calcium
Protein S	Serotonin (vasoconstrictor)
Fibrinogen	
VWF	
Platelet factor 4 (heparin inhibitor)	
Platelet-derived growth factor	

platelet activation process.[21] See Chapter 13 for a description of these properties and Table 40-4 for a summary of platelet granule contents.[22]

Other Blood Cells

Erythrocytes, monocytes, and lymphocytes also participate in hemostasis. Erythrocytes add bulk and structural integrity to the fibrin clot; there is a tendency to bleed when the hematocrit is less than 30%. In inflammation, monocytes and lymphocytes provide surface-borne tissue factor that triggers coagulation. Leukocytes also have a series of membrane integrins and selectins that bind adhesion molecules and help stimulate the production of inflammatory materials that promote the wound healing process.[23]

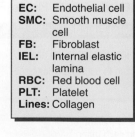

Figure 40-4 Platelet aggregation. In severe vascular damage, platelets aggregate to form a platelet plug.

EC: Endothelial cell
SMC: Smooth muscle cell
FB: Fibroblast
IEL: Internal elastic lamina
RBC: Red blood cell
PLT: Platelet
Lines: Collagen

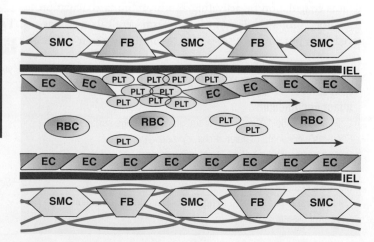

Coagulation

Blood plasma transports at least 16 glycoproteins, mostly trypsin-like enzymes called *serine proteases* that function in harmony to form a fibrin clot. Control proteins regulate each step of the process. The coagulation system, similar to other humoral amplification mechanisms, is complex because it must translate a diminutive physical or chemical stimulus into a profound lifesaving event.[24] The absence of a single plasma procoagulant may doom the individual to lifelong anatomic hemorrhage, chronic inflammation, and transfusion dependence.

Fibrinolysis

The final stage of hemostasis is fibrinolysis, the slow digestion and removal of the fibrin clot as healing occurs.[25] Plasminogen is bound to fibrin during coagulation and is activated by TPA to the serine protease, plasmin. Plasmin systematically degrades the fibrin clot into fragments called *fibrin degradation products*. The remainder of this chapter examines normal coagulation, coagulation control, and fibrinolysis in detail.

COAGULATION SYSTEM

Nomenclature of Procoagulants

Plasma transports at least 16 procoagulants, also called *coagulation factors* or *clotting factors*. Nearly all are glycoproteins synthesized in the liver, although a few are made by monocytes, endothelial cells, and megakaryocytes (Table 40-5; Fig. 40-5). Eight are enzymes that circulate in an inactive form called *zymogens*; six others are *cofactors* that bind and stabilize their respective enzymes. During clotting, the procoagulants become activated and produce a localized thrombus. At least seven additional plasma glycoproteins are controls that regulate the coagulation process.

In 1958 the International Committee for the Standardization of the Nomenclature of the Blood Clotting Factors officially named the plasma procoagulants using Roman numerals in the order of their initial description or discovery.[26] When a procoagulant becomes activated, a lower-case "a" appears behind the numeral; activated factor VII is VIIa. Zymogens and cofactors become activated in the coagulation process.

We customarily call factor I *fibrinogen* and factor II *prothrombin*, although occasionally they are identified by their numerals. The numeral III was given to tissue thromboplastin, a crude mixture of tissue factor and phospholipid. Now that the precise structure of tissue factor has been described, the numeral is seldom used. The numeral IV identifies the plasma cation calcium (Ca^{2+}); however, no one refers to calcium by the numeral, only by its name or chemical symbol. The numeral VI was assigned to a procoagulant that later was determined to be activated factor V; VI was withdrawn from the naming system

TABLE 40-5 Sixteen Plasma Procoagulants, Their Function, Molecular Weight, Plasma Half-Life, and Plasma Concentration

Factor	Customary Name	Function	Molecular Weight (D)	Half-Life (h)	Mean Plasma Concentration
I*	Fibrinogen	Thrombin substrate, polymerizes to form fibrin	340,000	100-150	200-400 mg/dL
II*	Prothrombin	Serine protease	71,600	60	10 mg/dL
III*	Tissue factor	Cofactor	44,000	Insoluble	None
IV*	Ionic calcium	Mineral	40	NA	8-10 mg/dL
V	Labile factor	Cofactor	330,000	24	1 mg/dL
VII	Stable factor	Serine protease	50,000	6	0.05 mg/dL
VIII	Antihemophilic factor	Cofactor	330,000	12	0.01 mg/dL
	VWF	Factor VIII carrier and platelet adhesion	600,000-20,000,000	24	1 mg/dL
IX	Christmas factor	Serine protease	57,000	24	0.3 mg/dL
X	Stuart-Prower factor	Serine protease	58,800	48-52	1 mg/dL
XI	Plasma thromboplastin antecedent (PTA)	Serine protease	143,000	48-84	0.5 mg/dL
XII	Hageman factor	Serine protease	84,000	48-70	3 mg/dL
Prekallikrein	Fletcher factor, PK	Serine protease	85,000	35	35-50 µg/mL
High-molecular-weight kininogen	Fitzgerald factor, HMWK	Cofactor	120,000	156	5 mg/dL
XIII	Fibrin-stabilizing factor (FSF)	Transglutaminase	320,000	150	2 mg/dL
Platelet factor 3	Phospholipids, phosphatidyl serine, PF3	Assembly molecule	—	Released by platelets	—

*These factors are customarily identified by name rather than Roman numeral.
From Greenberg DL, Davie EW: The blood coagulation factors: their complementary DNAs, genes, and expression. In Colman RW, Marder VJ, Clowes, AM, et al (eds): Hemostasis and Thrombosis, 5th ed. Lippincott, Williams & Wilkins, 2006: 21-58.

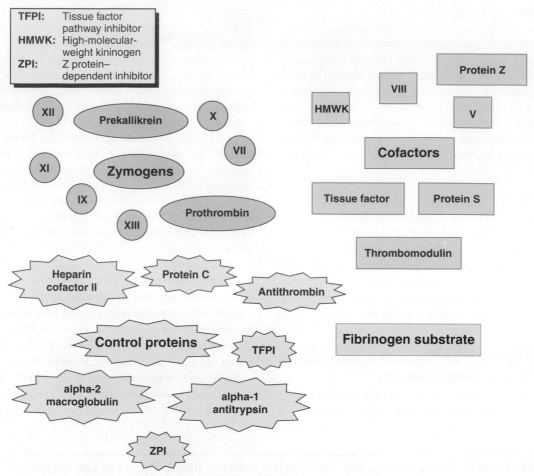

Figure 40-5 Plasma procoagulants and anticoagulants.

and never reassigned. Prekallikrein (pre-K), also called *Fletcher factor,* and high-molecular-weight kininogen (HMWK), also called *Fitzgerald factor,* have never received Roman numerals because they belong to the kallikrein and kinin systems, and their primary functions lie within these systems. Platelet phospholipids, particularly phosphatidylserine, are essential to the coagulation process but are given no Roman numeral; instead they were called collectively *platelet factor 3.* The molecular weights, plasma concentrations, and plasma half-lives of the procoagulants are given in Table 40-5. These essential pieces of clinical information help us to interpret laboratory tests and to design effective replacement therapies in deficiency-related hemorrhagic diseases.

Classification of Procoagulants
Physiologic Function of Procoagulants

The plasma procoagulants may be serine proteases or cofactors.[27] Serine proteases are proteolytic enzymes of the trypsin family and include the procoagulants thrombin (IIa); factors VIIa, IXa, Xa, XIa, and XIIa; and pre-K.[28] Each member has a reactive seryl amino acid residue in its active site and acts on its substrate by hydrolyzing peptide bonds, digesting the

primary backbone and producing small polypeptide fragments. Serine proteases are synthesized as inactive zymogens, consisting of a single peptide chain (Table 40-6). Activation occurs when the zymogen is cleaved at one or more specific sites by the action of another protease during the coagulation process. Activation is a localized cell-surface process, limited to the site of injury. Generalized plasma activation of zymogens is called *disseminated intravascular coagulation.* When acute, disseminated intravascular coagulation is a morbid, often fatal condition (Chapter 42).

The coagulation cofactors are tissue factor (a noncirculating constitutive protein of the subendothelium), factor V, factor VIII, and HMWK. Each cofactor binds its particular serine protease. When bound, serine proteases gain stability and increased reactivity (Table 40-7).[29]

The remaining components of the coagulation pathway are factor XIII, fibrinogen, calcium, VWF, and phospholipids (Box 40-3). Factor XIIIa is a transglutaminase that catalyzes the transfer of amino acids among the γ chains of fibrin polymers. This reaction cross-links fibrin polymers to provide physical strength to the fibrin clot. Factor XIIIa reacts with other plasma and cellular structural proteins and is essential to wound

TABLE 40-6 Plasma Procoagulant Serine Proteases

Inactive Zymogen	Active Protease	Cofactor	Substrate
Prothrombin (II)	Thrombin (IIa)	—	Fibrinogen
VII	VIIa	Tissue factor	IX, X
IX	IXa	VIIIa	X
X	Xa	Va	Prothrombin
XI	XIa	—	IX
XII	XIIa	HMWK	XI
Pre-K	Kallikrein	HMWK	XI

TABLE 40-7 Plasma Procoagulant Cofactors

Inactive Form	Active Form	Binds
Tissue factor	Exposed tissue factor	VIIa
V	Va	Xa
VIII	VIIIa	IXa
HMWK	Kinin	XIIa, Pre-K

BOX 40-3 Other Plasma Procoagulants

Fibrinogen
Factor XIII
Phospholipids
Calcium
VWF

---

healing and tissue integrity. Factor XIII is a heterodimer whose α subunit is produced mostly from megakaryocytes and monocytes. The β subunit is produced in the liver.[30]

Coagulation occurs on the surface of platelet or endothelial cell membrane phospholipids and not in fluid phase. Serine proteases bind to negatively charged phospholipid surfaces, mostly phosphatidyl serine, through positively charged calcium ions, so calcium is involved in most of the coagulation pathway reactions. Any fluid phase reaction is reduced by the coagulation control proteins.

Fibrinogen is the ultimate substrate of the coagulation pathway. When hydrolyzed by thrombin, fibrinogen polymerizes to form the primary structural protein of the fibrin clot.[31] VWF is a large glycoprotein that participates in platelet adhesion and transports the procoagulant factor VIII. VWF is synthesized in megakaryocytes and endothelial cells.[32]

Biochemical Nature of Several Procoagulants

Fibrinogen Structure and Fibrin Formation.
Fibrinogen is the primary substrate of thrombin. It is a 340,000-D glycoprotein synthesized in the liver. The normal plasma concentration of fibrinogen ranges from 200 to 400 mg/dL, the most concentrated of all the plasma procoagulants. Platelet α-granules absorb, transport, and release abundant fibrinogen.[33]

The fibrinogen molecule is a mirror-image dimer, each half consisting of three nonidentical polypeptides, designated α, β, and γ, united by disulfide bonds (Fig. 40-6). The six N-termini assemble to form a bulky central region called the *E domain*. The carboxyl termini assemble at the two ends of the molecule to form two *D domains*.[34]

Thrombin cleaves fibrinopeptides A and B from the protruding N-termini of each of the two α and β chains, reducing the overall molecular weight by 10,000 D. The cleaved fibrinogen is called *fibrin monomer*. The exposed fibrin monomer α and β chain ends have an immediate affinity for portions of the D domain of neighboring monomers, a union that forms an insoluble fibrin polymer (Fig. 40-7).

Factor XIIIa catalyzes the formation of covalent bonds between the carboxyl terminals of γ chains from adjacent D domains. These bonds link the ε-amino acid of lysine moieties and the γ-amide group of glutamine units. Multiple cross-links form to provide an insoluble meshwork of fibrin polymers. Cross-linking also covalently incorporates fibronectin, a plasma protein involved in cell adhesion, and α_2-antiplasmin, rendering the fibrin mesh resistant to fibrinolysis. Plasminogen, the primary serine protease of the fibrinolytic system, also becomes covalently bound via lysine moieties, as does TPA, a serine protease that ultimately hydrolyzes and activates bound plasminogen to initiate fibrinolysis.

von Willebrand Factor/Factor VIII Complex.
VWF is a multimeric glycoprotein composed of multiple subunits of 240,000 D each.[35] The subunits are produced by endothelial cells and megakaryocytes, where they combine to form molecules that range from 600,000 to 20,000,000 D (Fig. 40-8). VWF molecules are stored in platelet α-granules and in endothelial cells, where their storage sites are called *Weibel-Palade bodies*. The molecules are released from storage into the plasma, where they circulate at a concentration of 7 to 10 μg/mL.

VWF provides receptor sites for platelets and collagen. The primary platelet receptor site binds a platelet surface receptor, glycoprotein Ib/IX/V, and fills the space between the platelet and exposed subendothelial collagen during platelet

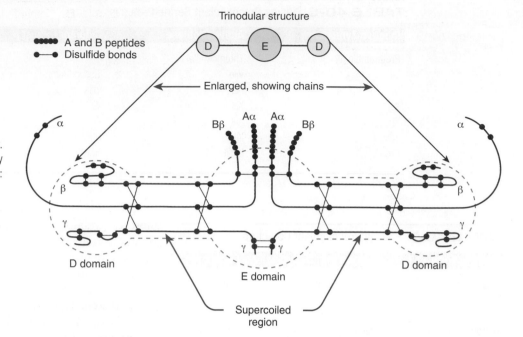

Figure 40-6 Structure of fibrinogen. (From McKenzie SB: Clinical Laboratory Hematology. Upper Saddle River, N.J.: Prentice Hall, 2004:688.)

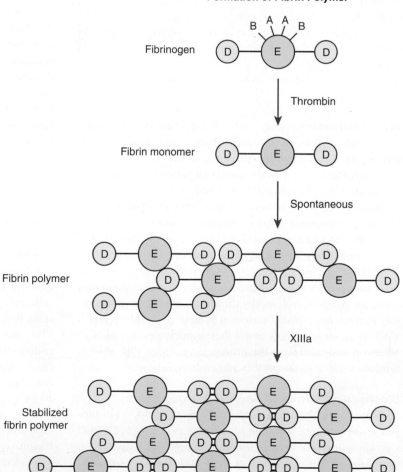

Figure 40-7 Formation of a stabilized fibrin mesh. Fibrin monomers polymerize by affinity of thrombin-cleaved E domain to adjacent D domains. Factor XIIIa catalyzes the cross-linking of γ chains of adjacent D domains to form a urea-insoluble stable fibrin clot. (Modified from McKenzie SB: Clinical Laboratory Hematology. Upper Saddle River, N.J.: Prentice Hall, 2004:689.)

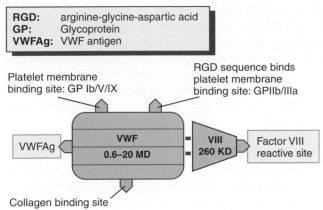

Figure 40-8 VWF–factor VIII complex. VWF binds platelet glycoprotein (GP) Ib/V/IX to provide platelet adhesion. RGD sequences bind GP IIb/IIIa ($\alpha_{IIb}\beta_3$) to promote platelet aggregation. GP IIb/IIIa also binds RGD sequences of fibrinogen. A third VWF site binds collagen. VWF also provides a binding site for coagulation factor VIII.

adhesion.[36] Arginine-glycine-aspartic acid (RGD) sequences bind a second platelet integrin, glycoprotein IIb/IIIa. A third site binds the plasma procoagulant cofactor, factor VIII.

Factor VIII is produced by hepatocytes and other tissues. It is one of two plasma procoagulants whose production is sex-linked, the other being factor IX. Factor VIII has a molecular mass of 260 KD and circulates bound to VWF. Free factor VIII is unstable except during coagulation and cannot be detected in plasma.

Factor VIII is labile and deteriorates over hours in stored blood despite being bound to VWF. Males with hemophilia A have diminished factor VIII activity but normal VWF levels.[37] Because factor VIII depends on VWF for stability, individuals with VWD have diminished VWF and diminished factor VIII activity levels. Typically, factor VIII levels decrease to hemorrhagic levels (<30%) only in severe VWD.

Vitamin K–Dependent Prothrombin Group. Prothrombin; factors VII, IX, and X; and the regulatory proteins, protein C, protein S, and protein Z, are vitamin K dependent (Table 40-8). These are named the *prothrombin group* because of their structural resemblance to prothrombin; all seven proteins have 10 to 12 glutamic acid units near their N-termini. Vitamin K is a quinone found in green leafy vegetables, fish, and liver and is produced by the intestinal organisms *Bacteroides fragilis* and *Escherichia coli*. Vitamin K catalyzes an essential post-translational modification of the prothrombin group proteins: γ-carboxylation of N-terminal glutamic acids (Fig. 40-9). Glutamic acid is modified to γ-carboxyglutamic acid when a second carboxyl group is added to the γ-carbon. With two ionized carboxyl groups, the γ-carboxyglutamic acids gain a net negative charge, enabling them to bind ionic calcium (Ca^{2+}). The bound calcium enables the vitamin K–dependent proteins to bind negatively charged phospholipids, such as phosphatidylserine. Phospholipid binding is essential to coagulation reactions.

TABLE 40-8 Vitamin K–Dependent Coagulation Factors

Procoagulants	Regulatory Proteins
Prothrombin	Protein C
Factor VII	Protein S
Factor IX	Protein Z
Factor X	

In vitamin K deficiency or in the presence of warfarin, a vitamin K antagonist, the vitamin K–dependent procoagulants are released from the liver with diminished γ-carboxylation. These are called *des-γ-carboxyl proteins* or *proteins in vitamin K antagonism*, and they cannot participate in the coagulation reaction. Vitamin K antagonism is the basis for oral anticoagulant therapy.

Tissue Factor Pathway

Tissue factor, a membrane receptor for factor VIIa, is present on vascular cells that are not normally in contact with blood, such as fibroblasts. Coagulation is triggered by the exposure of tissue factor to plasma proteins on injury.[38] Factor VIIa binds to tissue factor in the presence of phospholipid and calcium and triggers the activation of the zymogens, beginning with factors IX and X. Factor IXa binds VIIIa on phospholipid surfaces; this complex also activates factor X (Fig. 40-10).

Factor Xa binds factor Va on phospholipid surfaces (Figs. 40-11 and 40-12). This factor Xa–factor Va complex activates prothrombin in a multistep hydrolytic process that releases a peptide fragment from prothrombin called *prothrombin 1+2*. Activated prothrombin is termed *thrombin*. Thrombin cleaves fibrinopeptides A and B from plasma fibrinogen, causing the formation of fibrin polymer. Fibrin polymer is stabilized by the cross-linking action of factor XIIIa (see Fig. 40-7).

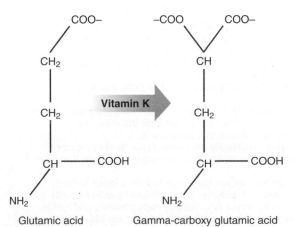

Figure 40-9 Vitamin K catalyzes the addition of a second carboxyl group to the γ carbon of glutamic acid residues near the N-terminus of factors II, VII, IX, and X. The γ-carboxylation provides a pocket for a calcium ion that promotes phospholipid binding.

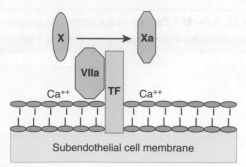

Figure 40-10 Activated factor VII and tissue factor activate factor X.

The tissue factor pathway is characterized by multimolecular complex formations. The first complex is composed of tissue factor, factor VIIa, phospholipid, and Ca^{2+}. The second is composed of factor IXa, factor VIIIa, phospholipid, and Ca^{2+}, sometimes called *tenase*. The third complex is composed of factor Xa, factor Va, phospholipid, and Ca^{2+} and is often called *prothrombinase* (Table 40-9).

Factor XI Activation Pathway

Thrombin also activates factor XI. Factor XIa activates factor IX, and the reaction proceeds as described previously. This pathway is essential to normal coagulation, as evidenced by moderate-to-severe hemorrhage in individuals with Rosenthal syndrome, or factor XI deficiency.

Contact Factors

The "contact factor" complex, composed of factor XIIa, HMWK (Fitzgerald), and prekallikrein (Fletcher), activates factor XI. Factor XIIa transforms prekallikrein, a glycoprotein that circulates bound to HMWK, into its active form kallikrein, which cleaves HMWK into bradykinin. Deficiencies of XII, HMWK, or prekallikrein do not cause bleeding but may prolong laboratory tests. Factor XII is activated in vitro by contact with negatively charged surfaces, such as nonsiliconized glass or the ellagic acid in the activated partial thromboplastin time (APTT) reagent. In vivo, foreign materials such as stents or valve prostheses may activate contact factors to cause thrombosis.

Thrombin

The primary function of thrombin is to cleave fibrinopeptides A and B from the α and β chains of the fibrinogen molecule, triggering fibrin polymerization (see Fig. 40-7). In addition, thrombin amplifies the coagulation mechanism by activating cofactors V and VIII and factor XI. Thrombin also activates factor XIII, the fibrin-stabilizing factor. Factor XIIIa forms covalent bonds between the D domains of the fibrin polymer to cross-link and stabilize the fibrin clot. Thrombin also initiates aggregation of platelets, activates the protein C pathway to control coagulation, and activates thrombin activatable fibrinolysis inhibitor (TAFI) to control fibrinolysis. Because of its multiple autocatalytic functions, thrombin is considered the chief protease of the coagulation pathway.

Extrinsic, Intrinsic, and Common Pathways

Before 1992, most coagulation experts identified the activation of factor XII as the primary step in coagulation because it could be found in blood, whereas tissue factor could not. Consequently, the reaction system that begins with factor XII and culminates in fibrin polymerization has been called the *intrinsic pathway*. The coagulation factors of the intrinsic pathway, in order of reaction, were XII, pre-K, HMWK, XI, IX, VIII, X, V, prothrombin, and fibrinogen (Figs. 40-11 and 40-12).

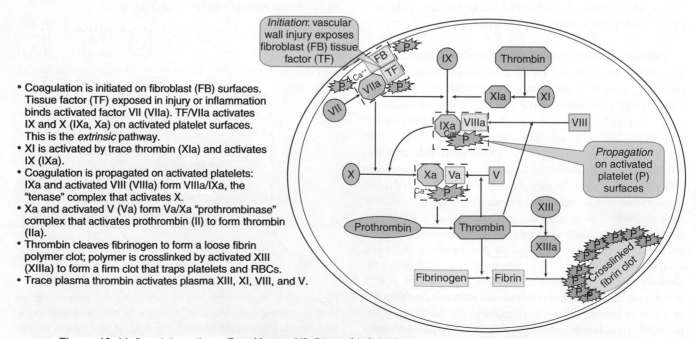

- Coagulation is initiated on fibroblast (FB) surfaces. Tissue factor (TF) exposed in injury or inflammation binds activated factor VII (VIIa). TF/VIIa activates IX and X (IXa, Xa) on activated platelet surfaces. This is the *extrinsic* pathway.
- XI is activated by trace thrombin (XIa) and activates IX (IXa).
- Coagulation is propagated on activated platelets: IXa and activated VIII (VIIIa) form VIIIa/IXa, the "tenase" complex that activates X.
- Xa and activated V (Va) form Va/Xa "prothrombinase" complex that activates prothrombin (II) to form thrombin (IIa).
- Thrombin cleaves fibrinogen to form a loose fibrin polymer clot; polymer is crosslinked by activated XIII (XIIIa) to form a firm clot that traps platelets and RBCs.
- Trace plasma thrombin activates plasma XIII, XI, VIII, and V.

Figure 40-11 Coagulation pathway. (From Marques MB, Fritsma GA: Quick Guide to Coagulation. Washington, DC: AACC Press, 2006.)

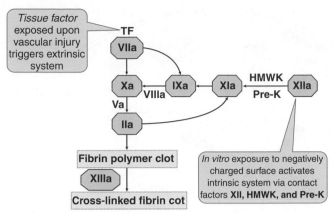

Figure 40-12 Simplified coagulation pathway. Exposed tissue factor activates factor VII, which activates factors IX and X. Factor IX/VIII complex also activates factor X, and the factor X/V complex activates prothrombin (II). The resulting thrombin (IIa) cleaves fibrinogen to form fibrin polymer and cross-linked fibrin. Thrombin also activates factor XI, which activates factor IX, and the pathway proceeds as before. In vitro exposure to negatively charged particles or surfaces activates factor XII (XIIa) in the presence of Pre-K (Fletcher factor) and HMWK (Fitzgerald factor). Fletcher, Fitzgerald, and XII are the contact factors that trigger the intrinsic mechanism.

TABLE 40-9 Coagulation Cascade Complexes

	Components	Function
First complex	VIIa, tissue factor, phospholipid, and Ca^{2+}	Cleaves IX and X
Second complex	IXa, VIIIa, phospholipid, and Ca^{2+}	Cleaves X, called *tenase*
Third complex	Xa, Va, phospholipid, and Ca^{2+}	Cleaves prothrombin, called *prothrombinase*

The tissue factor pathway has been called the *extrinsic pathway* and includes the factors VII, X, V, prothrombin, and fibrinogen. Neither factor VIII nor factor IX is included in the extrinsic pathway because their contribution was bypassed in the prothrombin time test, the test used to measure the integrity of the extrinsic pathway. Because tissue factor is itself external to coagulation, the term *extrinsic* still applies. The two pathways had in common factor X, factor V, prothrombin, and fibrinogen (Table 40-10); this portion of the coagulation pathway is often called the *common pathway*. Although the terms *intrinsic pathway, extrinsic pathway,* and *common pathway* have been largely supplanted by the current cell-based coagulation model, they are used extensively to identify the coagulation factors, particularly in laboratory testing.

Cell-Based Coagulation

In vivo, coagulation factors become activated on the surface of platelets and cells that carry tissue factor.[39] Factor X is activated by the TF:VIIa complex on the tissue factor–bearing cell surface and forms the prothrombinase complex. This complex gener-

TABLE 40-10 Factors of the Intrinsic and Extrinsic Pathways in Order of Reaction

Intrinsic Pathway	Extrinsic Pathway
XII	
Pre-K	
HMWK	
XI	
IX	
VIII	
	VII
X	X
V	V
Prothrombin	Prothrombin
Fibrinogen	Fibrinogen

ates a small amount of thrombin before being neutralized by TFPI. Although not enough thrombin is produced on tissue factor–bearing cells to form a fibrin clot, there is enough to activate platelets and factors V, VIII, and XI. Activated platelets release factor V from their α-granules, which is activated by thrombin to factor Va on the platelet surface. Thrombin also activates factor VIII, which is freed from VWF and binds to the platelet surface.

Factor IXa, activated by the TF:VIIa complex, binds to factor VIIIa on the platelet surface and activates factor X. Factor IXa is not as readily degraded by plasma inhibitors and continues to activate factor X. Factor Xa binds to factor Va on the platelet and activates prothrombin, producing enough thrombin to cleave fibrinogen and produce a fibrin clot. Coagulation reactions that occur on cell and platelet surfaces generally are confined to the site of injury.

COAGULATION REGULATORY MECHANISMS

Figure 40-13 illustrates coagulation mechanism regulatory points. The coagulation regulatory proteins are summarized in Table 40-11.

Tissue Factor Pathway Inhibitor

Factor VIIa and tissue factor combine to activate factors IX and X in the tissue factor pathway. Factor Xa reacts with the factor VIIa–tissue factor complex to bind a coagulation regulatory protein, TFPI (Fig. 40-14). TFPI inactivates factor VIIa. Because of the action of TFPI, the tissue factor–factor VIIa reaction is short-lived; coagulation pathway amplification occurs primarily through factor XI.[40]

Protein C Regulatory System

During thrombosis, thrombin propagates the clot as it cleaves fibrinogen and activates factors V, VIII, XI, and XIII. In intact normal vessels, where coagulation would be inexpedient, thrombin binds the endothelial cell membrane protein *thrombomodulin* and triggers an essential coagulation regulatory

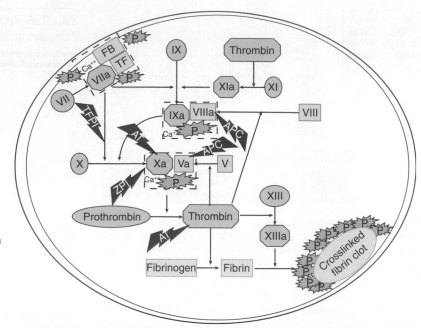

- Tissue factor pathway inhibitor (TFPI) binds the TF/VIIa complex and prevents formation of free Xa.
- Protein Z-dependent protease inhibitor (ZPI) and antithrombin (AT) inactivate Xa.
- AT inactivates thrombin.
- Activated protein C (APC) inactivates VIIIa and Va.

Figure 40-13 The coagulation pathway, showing regulatory points. (From Marques MB, Fritsma GA: Quick Guide to Coagulation. Washington, DC: AACC Press, 2006.)

TABLE 40-11 Coagulation Regulatory Proteins

Name	Function	Molecular Mass (D)	Half-Life (h)	Mean Plasma Concentration
TFPI	With Xa, binds tissue factor VIIa	33,000	Unknown	60-80 ηg/mL
Thrombomodulin	Endothelial cell surface receptor for thrombin	450,000	Does not circulate	None
Protein C	Serine protease	62,000	7-9	2-6 μg/mL
Protein S	Cofactor	75,000	Unknown	20-25 μg/mL
Antithrombin	SERPIN	58,000	68	24-40 mg/dL
Heparin cofactor II	SERPIN	65,000	60	30-70 μg/mL
α_1-antitrypsin	SERPIN	60,000	Unknown	250 mg/dL
α_2-macroglobulin	SERPIN	725,000	60	150-400 mg/dL

SERPIN, serine protease inhibitor.

system called the *protein C system*.[41] The thrombin-thrombomodulin complex activates the plasma zymogen protein C (Fig. 40-15). Activated protein C (APC) binds free plasma protein S. The stabilized APC–protein S complex hydrolyzes and inactivates factors Va and VIIIa.

Protein S, the cofactor that binds and stabilizes APC, is synthesized in the liver and circulates in the plasma in two forms: free and covalently bound to the complement control protein, C4b-binding protein. Bound protein S cannot participate in the protein C anticoagulant pathway; only free plasma protein S can serve as the APC cofactor. Protein S–C4b binding is of particular interest in inflammatory conditions because C4b-binding protein is an acute-phase reactant. When the plasma C4b level increases, additional protein S is bound,

and free protein S levels become proportionally decreased. Chronic congenital protein C or protein S deficiency may be associated with recurrent venous thromboembolic disease, underscoring the importance of the protein C regulatory system.

Serine Protease Inhibitors

Antithrombin is a serine protease inhibitor (SERPIN) that binds and neutralizes thrombin and factors IXa, Xa, XIa, and XIIa. Antithrombin was the first of the coagulation regulatory proteins to be identified and the first to be assayed routinely in the clinical hemostasis laboratory.[42] Other members of the SERPIN family are heparin cofactor II, α_1-antitrypsin, α_2-macroglobulin, and protein Z–dependent protease inhibitor (ZPI).[43] ZPI covalently binds protein Z and factor Xa in a

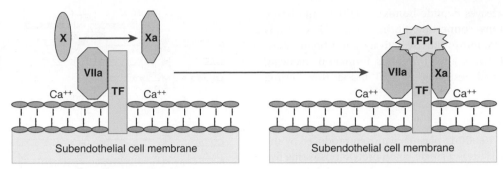

Figure 40-14 TFPI binds the complex of tissue factor, VIIa, and Xa.

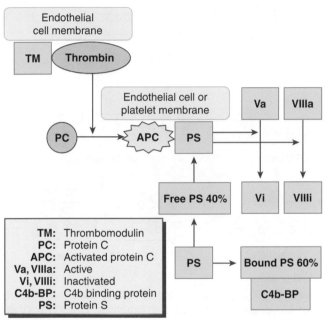

Figure 40-15 Protein C pathway. After binding thrombomodulin, thrombin activates protein C. Free protein S binds and stabilizes APC. The APC/protein S complex digests and inactivates active factors V and VIII.

complex with Ca^{++} and phospholipid to inhibit factor Xa–induced thrombin formation.[44] Similar to protein S, protein Z is nonproteolytic; however, ZPI undergoes cleavage and the loss of a peptide fragment on binding factor Xa. ZPI inhibits factor XIa independent of protein Z, phospholipid, and Ca^{++}. The anti-XIa property of ZPI is proportional to the dosage of unfractionated heparin.[45]

Antithrombin and heparin cofactor II require heparin for effective anticoagulant activity. Heparin cofactor II is a SERPIN that inactivates primarily thrombin in the presence of heparin. α_1-antitrypsin and α_2-macroglobulin are able to inhibit serine proteases reversibly.

Unfractionated therapeutic heparin is a heterogeneous glycosaminoglycan composed of 15 to 30 saccharide units. Unfractionated heparin increases antithrombin's ability to neutralize thrombin and factors IXa, Xa, XIa, and XIIa by 1000-fold. Any heparin molecule of 17 or more saccharide units simultaneously binds antithrombin and thrombin. The anti-

thrombin covalently binds and inactivates a thrombin molecule, forming an inactive thrombin-antithrombin complex, which is released from the heparin molecule. Unfractionated heparin's catalytic effect is to "approximate" thrombin with antithrombin, meaning to bring the two molecules into proximity with each other, and to induce allostery, or change in steric conformation, of the antithrombin molecule (Fig. 40-16). Heparin fractions of less than 17 saccharide units, such as are found in therapeutic *low-molecular-weight heparin,* are able to bind antithrombin or thrombin but cannot bring them into the necessary spatial configuration. Nevertheless, the allosteric changes of the antithrombin make it capable of inactivating factor Xa and other serine proteases. Endothelial cells secrete heparan sulfate, a natural glycosaminoglycan, which also activates antithrombin, although not to the same intensity as unfractionated heparin.

FIBRINOLYSIS

Fibrinolysis, the final stage of coagulation, begins a few hours after fibrin polymerization and cross-linking. Fibrinolysis is the systematic, accelerating hydrolysis of fibrin polymers by bound

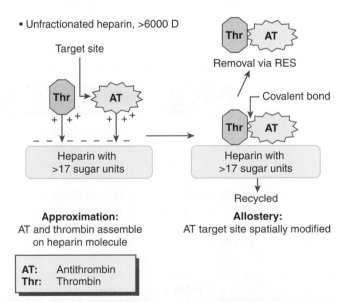

Figure 40-16 Unfractionated heparin potentiates antithrombin-thrombin reaction.

plasmin, which cleaves peptide bonds at arginine and lysine moieties in regions connecting fibrin's D and E domains (Fig. 40-17).[46] TPA and urokinase activate fibrin-bound plasminogen several hours after thrombus formation, reducing thrombus bulk and restoring normal blood flow during vascular repair.

Plasminogen

Plasminogen is a 90,000-D plasma zymogen produced by the liver (Table 40-12).[47] It is a single-chain protein possessing five glycosylated loops termed *kringles*. Kringles enable plasminogen to bind fibrin lysine residues during polymerization; this binding is essential to fibrinolysis. Plasminogen likewise binds plasma α_2-antiplasmin, the major fibrinolysis control protein, collagen, kininogen, and cell-surface receptors. Fibrin-bound plasminogen becomes converted to a two-chain active plasmin molecule when cleaved at Arg561-Val562 by neighboring bound TPA or urokinase. Plasmin is a serine protease that systematically digests fibrin polymer by hydrolysis of arginine-related and lysine-related peptide bonds. As fibrin becomes digested, the exposure of carboxy-terminal lysine residues binds additional plasmin, incrementally accelerating clot digestion. Plasmin is capable of digesting fluid-phase fibrinogen and factors V and VIII; however, localization to fibrin through lysine binding prevents systemic activity. Plasma α_2-antiplasmin rapidly binds and inactivates free plasmin. Several amino-carboxalic acids have affinity for plasminogen's kringles, accounting for the antifibrinolytic properties of therapeutic tranexamic acid and ε-aminocaproic acid.

Plasminogen Activation

Tissue Plasminogen Activator

Endothelial cells secrete TPA, which hydrolyzes fibrin-bound plasminogen and initiates fibrinolysis. TPA, with two glycosylated kringle regions, forms covalent lysine bonds with fibrin during polymerization and segregates at the surface of the thrombus with plasminogen, where it begins the digestion

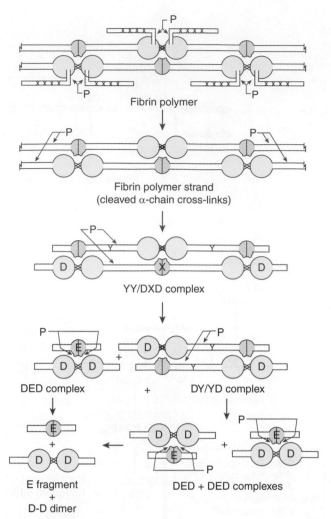

Figure 40-17 Degradation of fibrin by plasmin. (From Thompson AR, Harker LA: Manual of Hemostasis and Thrombosis. Philadelphia: Davis, 1983:1-19.)

TABLE 40-12 Proteins of the Fibrinolysis Pathway

Name	Function	Molecular Mass (D)	Half-Life (h)	Mean Plasma Concentration
Plasminogen	Plasma serine protease	90,000	24-26	15-21 mg/dL
TPA	Secreted by activated endothelium, serine protease	68,000	Unknown	4-7 µg/dL
Urokinase	Secreted by kidney, serine protease activates plasminogen	54,000	Unknown	—
PAI-1	Secreted by endothelium, inhibits tissue plasminogen activator	52,000	1	14-28 mg/dL
α_2-antiplasmin	Inhibits plasmin	51,000	Unknown	7 mg/dL

TPA, Tissue plasminogen activator; PAI-1, Plasminogen activator inhibitor-1.

process by cleaving the plasminogen at Arg561-Val562. Free TPA circulates bound to inhibitors such as PAI-1 and is cleared from plasma. Synthetic recombinant TPAs mimic intrinsic TPA and are a family of drugs used to dissolve pathologic clots that form in venous and arterial thrombotic disease.

Urokinase

Urinary tract epithelial cells, monocytes, and macrophages secrete another intrinsic plasminogen activator called *urokinase*. Urokinase circulates in plasma at 2 to 4 ηg/mL and becomes incorporated into the mix of fibrin-bound plasminogen and TPA at the time of thrombus formation. Urokinase has only one kringle region, does not bind firmly to fibrin, and has a relatively minor physiologic effect. The action of urokinase is independent of fibrin; however, leading to the conclusion that urokinase may have its primary function in degrading the extracellular matrix. Similar to TPA, purified urokinase preparations are used to dissolve thrombi in heart attacks, strokes, and deep vein thrombosis.

Plasminogen Activator Inhibitor-1

TPA and urokinase are prevented from activating free, fluid-phase plasminogen by a plasma inhibitor, PAI-1. Probable sources of PAI-1 include the endothelium, adipocytes, megakaryocytes, and hepatocytes. Platelets store a pool of PAI-1, accounting for more than half of its availability and for its delivery to the fibrin clot. PAI-1 is present in excess to the TPA concentration, and circulating TPA normally is bound to PAI-1. Only at times of endothelial cell activation, such as after trauma, does the level of TPA secretion exceed that of PAI-1 to initiate fibrinolysis. Plasma PAI-1 levels vary widely. PAI-1 deficiency has been associated with chronic mild bleeding; excess PAI-1 may be associated with thrombophilia.

α₂-antiplasmin

Bound plasmin digests clots and restores blood vessel patency. Free plasmin digests plasma fibrinogen, factor V, factor VIII, and fibronectin, causing a potentially fatal *primary fibrinolysis*. α₂-antiplasmin is a plasma protein that rapidly and irreversibly binds free plasmin. α₂-antiplasmin also becomes cross-linked through lysine bonds to fibrin kringles during polymerization. There it renders fibrin resistant to digestion by plasmin.

Thrombin-Activatable Fibrinolysis Inhibitor

TAFI is a plasma procarboxypeptidase that becomes activated by the thrombin-thrombomodulin complex. This is the same complex that activates the protein C pathway; however, the two functions are independent. Activated TAFI inhibits fibrinolysis by cleaving exposed carboxy-terminal lysine residues from partially degraded fibrin, preventing the binding of TPA and plasminogen and blocking the formation of plasmin. TAFI is a link between the coagulation and fibrinolytic systems. In coagulation factor–deficient states, decreased thrombin production may reduce the activation of TAFI, resulting in increased fibrinolysis that contributes to bleeding. Conversely, in thrombotic disorders, increased thrombin generation may increase the activation of TAFI. The resulting decreased fibrinolysis may contribute further to thrombosis. TAFI also may play a role in regulating inflammation and wound healing.[48]

Fibrin Degradation Products and D-Dimer

Fibrinolysis produces a series of identifiable fibrin fragments, X, Y, D, E, and D-D.[49] Several of these fragments inhibit hemostasis and contribute to hemorrhage by preventing platelet activation and by hindering fibrin polymerization. The various fragments may be detected by quantitative or semiquantitative immunoassay, revealing fibrinolytic activity. The D-D fragment, called *D-dimer,* is separately detectable by a quantitative monoclonal antibody immunoassay. D-dimer is a specific marker for thrombosis; its immunoassay is used to identify chronic and acute disseminated intravascular coagulation and to rule out venous thromboembolism in suspected cases of deep venous thrombosis or pulmonary embolism.

CHAPTER at a GLANCE

- The vascular intima, the platelets (plus red blood cells and white blood cells), and the coagulation system are the three systems that interact to provide hemostasis.
- The vascular intima initiates and regulates hemostasis and fibrinolysis.
- Platelets function in primary and secondary hemostasis through adhesion, aggregation, and secretion of granular contents.
- Platelets adhere to collagen through VWF and use fibrinogen to aggregate.
- Most coagulation factors originate in the liver.
- The plasma factors of the "prothrombin" group require vitamin K in their production.
- Fibrinogen is acted on by thrombin to form first fibrin monomer, then fibrin polymer, and then, when acted on by factor XIIIa, cross-linked fibrin.

- Coagulation factors circulate as trypsin-like enzymes called serine proteases or as cofactors that stabilize the proteases.
- The coagulation pathway is initiated by tissue factor and amplified through factor XI.
- The coagulation pathway is regulated by TFPI, the SERPINs, and APC. These pathways prevent thrombosis.
- The fibrinolytic pathway digests the thrombus.

Now that you have completed this chapter, go back and read again the case study at the beginning and respond to the questions presented.

REVIEW QUESTIONS

1. What intimal cell synthesizes and stores VWF?
   a. Smooth muscle cell
   b. Endothelial cell
   c. Fibroblast
   d. Platelet

2. What subendothelial structural protein triggers coagulation through activation of factor VII?
   a. Thrombomodulin
   b. Nitric oxide
   c. Tissue factor
   d. Thrombin

3. What coagulation plasma protein should be assayed when platelets fail to aggregate properly?
   a. Factor VIII
   b. Fibrinogen
   c. Thrombin
   d. VWF

4. What role does vitamin K play for the prothrombin group factors?
   a. Carboxylates the factors to allow calcium binding
   b. Provides a surface on which the proteolytic reactions of the factors occur
   c. Protects them from inappropriate activation by compounds such as thrombin
   d. Accelerates the binding of the serine proteases and their cofactors

5. What is the source of fibrinopeptides A and B?
   a. Plasmin proteolysis of fibrin
   b. Thrombin proteolysis of fibrinogen
   c. Proteolysis of prothrombin by factor Xa
   d. Plasmin proteolysis of cross-linked fibrin

6. What serine protease forms a complex with factor VIIIa, and what is the substrate of this complex?
   a. Factor IXa, factor X
   b. Factor VIIa, factor X
   c. Factor Va, prothrombin
   d. Factor Xa, prothrombin

7. Amplification of the coagulation pathway, initiated through the tissue factor pathway, probably occurs through which of the following?
   a. Contact activation
   b. Factor XII
   c. Factor VII
   d. Factor XI

8. What two regulatory proteins form a complex that digests activated factors V and VIII?
   a. TFPI and SERPIN
   b. Antithrombin and protein C
   c. APC and protein S
   d. α_2-macroglobulin and α_1-antitrypsin

9. Coagulation factor VIII circulates bound to:
   a. VWF
   b. Factor IX
   c. Platelets
   d. Factor V

10. Most coagulation factors are synthesized in:
    a. The liver
    b. Monocytes
    c. Endothelial cells
    d. Megakaryocytes

REFERENCES

1. Corriveau DM: Major elements of hemostasis. In Corriveau DM, Fritsma GA (eds): Hemostasis and Thrombosis in the Clinical Laboratory. Philadelphia: Lippincott, 1988:1-33.
2. Colman RW, Clowes AW, George JN, et al: Overview of hemostasis. In Colman RW, Marder VJ, Clowes AM, et al (eds): Hemostasis and Thrombosis, 5th ed. Philadelphia: Lippincott, Williams & Wilkins, 2006:437-442.
3. Ruggeri ZM: Von Willebrand factor, platelets and endothelial cell interactions. J Thromb Haemost 2003;1:1335-1342.
4. Furie B, Furie BC: Molecular and cellular biology of blood coagulation. N Engl J Med 1992;326:800-806.
5. Haberichter SL, Montgomery RS: Structure and function of von Willebrand factor. In Colman RW, Marder VJ, Clowes AM, et al (eds): Hemostasis and Thrombosis, 5th ed. Philadelphia: Lippincott, Williams & Wilkins, 2006:707-722.
6. Bevilacqua MP, Nelson RM: Selectins. J Clin Invest 1993; 91:379-387.
7. Kansas GS: Selectins and their ligands: current concepts and controversies. Blood 1996;88:3259-3287.
8. Morrissey JH, Mutch NJ: Tissue factor structure and function. In Colman RW, Marder VJ, Clowes AM, et al (eds): Hemostasis and Thrombosis, 5th ed. Philadelphia: Lippincott, Williams & Wilkins, 2006:91-106.

9. Hathaway WE, Goodnight SH: Mechanisms of hemostasis and thrombosis. In Hathaway WE, Goodnight SH (eds): Disorders of Hemostasis and Thrombosis, 2nd ed. New York: McGraw-Hill, 2001;1:3-19.
10. Ruggeri ZM, Savage B: Platelet-vessel wall interactions in flowing blood. In Colman RW, Marder VJ, Clowes AM, et al (eds): Hemostasis and Thrombosis, 5th ed. Philadelphia: Lippincott, Williams & Wilkins, 2006:723-736.
11. Moncada SP, Palmer RMJ, Higgs AJ: Nitric oxide: physiology, pathophysiology and pharmacology. Pharmacol Rev 1991; 43:109-142.
12. Huntington JA: Mechanisms of glycosaminoglycan activation of the serpins in hemostasis. J Thromb Haemost 2003;1:1535-1549.
13. Francis CW, Berkowitz SD: Antithrombotic and thrombolytic agents. In Kitchens CS, Alving BM, Kessler CM (eds): Consultative Hemostasis and Thrombosis. Philadelphia: Saunders, 2002;24:375-93.
14. Dellas C, Loskutoff DJ: Historical analysis of PAI-1 from its discovery to its potential role in cell motility and disease. Thromb Haemost 2005;93:631-640.
15. Polgar J, Matuskova J, Wagner DD: The P-selectin, tissue factor, coagulation triad. J Thromb Haemost 2005;3:1590-1596.

16. Thompson AR, Harker LA: Manual of Hemostasis and Thrombosis, 3rd ed. Philadelphia: Davis, 1983.

17. Cramer EM, Vainchenker W: Platelet production: cellular and molecular regulation. In Colman RW, Marder VJ, Clowes AM, et al (eds): Hemostasis and Thrombosis, 5th ed. Philadelphia: Lippincott, Williams & Wilkins, 2006:443-462.

18. Fritsma GA: Platelet production and structure. In Corriveau DM, Fritsma GA (eds): Hemostasis and Thrombosis in the Clinical Laboratory. Philadelphia: Lippincott, 1988:206-228.

19. George JN, Colman RW: Overview of platelet structure and function. In Colman RW, Marder VJ, Clowes AM, et al (eds): Hemostasis and Thrombosis, 5th ed. Philadelphia: Lippincott, Williams & Wilkins, 2006:437-442.

20. Ruggeri ZM: New insights into the mechanism of platelet adhesion and aggregation. Semin Hematol 1994;31:229-239.

21. Brace LD: Platelet physiology. In Corriveau DM, Fritsma GA (eds): Hemostasis and Thrombosis in the Clinical Laboratory. Philadelphia: Lippincott, 1988:229-277.

22. Walsh PN: Role of platelets in blood coagulation. In Colman RW, Marder VJ, Clowes AM, et al (eds): Hemostasis and Thrombosis, 5th ed. Philadelphia: Lippincott, Williams & Wilkins, 2006:605-616.

23. Carlos TM, Harlan JM: Leukocyte-endothelial adhesion molecules. Blood 1994;84:2068-2101.

24. Aird WC: Hemostasis and irreducible complexity. J Thromb Haemost 2003;1:227-230.

25. Collen D, Lijnen HR: Tissue-type plasminogen activator: a historical perspective and personal account. J Thromb Haemost 2004;2:541-546.

26. Sherry S: The founding of the International Society on Thrombosis and Haemostasis: how it came about. Thromb Haemost 1990;64:188-191.

27. Saito H: Normal hemostatic mechanisms. In Ratnoff OD, Forbes CD (eds): Disorders of Hemostasis, 3rd ed. Philadelphia: Saunders, 1996:23-52.

28. Coughlin SR: Protease-activated receptors in hemostasis, thrombosis and vascular biology. J Thromb Haemost 2005;3:1800-1814.

29. Lane DA, Philippou H, Huntington JA: Directing thrombin. Blood 2005;106:2605-2612.

30. Lorand L: Factor XIII and the clotting of fibrinogen: from basic research to medicine. J Thromb Haemost 2005;3:1337-1348.

31. Mosesson MW: Fibrinogen and fibrin structure and functions. J Thromb Haemost 2005;3:1894-1904.

32. Blann AD: Plasma von Willebrand factor, thrombosis, and the endothelium: the first 30 years. Thromb Haemost 2006;95:49-55.

33. Harrison P, Wilborn B, Devilli N, et al: Uptake of plasma fibrinogen into the α granules of human megakaryocytes and platelets. J Clin Invest 1989;84:1320-1324.

34. Mosesson MW: Fibrinogen and fibrin structure and functions. J Thromb Haemost 2005;3:1894-1904.

35. Sadler JE: Von Willebrand factor. J Biol Chem 1991;266:22777-22780.

36. Kunicki TJ: Platelet glycoprotein polymorphisms and relationship to function, immunogenicity, and disease. In Colman RW, Marder VJ, Clowes AM, et al (eds): Hemostasis and Thrombosis, 5th ed. Philadelphia: Lippincott, Williams & Wilkins, 2006:493-506.

37. Jacquemin M, De Maeyer M, D'Oiron R, et al: Molecular mechanisms of mild and moderate hemophilia A. J Thromb Haemost 2003;1:456-463.

38. Broze GJ: Tissue factor pathway inhibitor and the revised theory of coagulation. Ann Rev Med 1995;46:103-112.

39. Hoffman M: Remodeling the blood coagulation cascade. J Thromb Thrombolysis 2003;16:17-20.

40. Golino P: The inhibitors of the tissue factor:factor VII pathway. Thromb Res 2002;106:V257-V265.

41. Dahlback B: The protein C anticoagulant system: inherited defects as basis for venous thrombosis. Thromb Res 1995;77:1-43.

42. de Moerloose P, Bounameaux HR, Mannucci PM: Screening test for thrombophilic patients: which tests, for which patient, by whom, when, and why? Semin Thromb Hemost 1998;24:321-327.

43. Broze GJ Jr: Protein Z-dependent regulation of coagulation. Thromb Haemost 2001;86:8-13.

44. Broze GJ: Protein Z and protein Z-dependent protease inhibitor. In Colman RW, Marder VJ, Clowes AM, et al (eds): Hemostasis and Thrombosis, 5th ed. Philadelphia: Lippincott, Williams & Wilkins, 2006:215-220.

45. Al-Shanqeeti A, van Hylckama VA, Berntorp E, et al: Protein Z and protein Z-dependent protease inhibitor: determinants of levels and risk of venous thrombosis. Thromb Haemost 2005;93:411-413.

46. Kolev K, Machovich R: Molecular and cellular modulation of fibrinolysis. Thromb Haemost 2003;89:610-621.

47. Bennett B, Ogston D: Fibrinolytic bleeding syndromes. In Ratnoff OD, Forbes CD (eds): Disorders of Hemostasis, 3rd ed. Philadelphia: Saunders, 1996:296-322.

48. Bouma BN, Mosnier LO: Thrombin activatable fibrinolysis inhibitor (TAFI) at the interface between coagulation and fibrinolysis. Pathophysiol Haemost Thromb 2003/2004;33:375-381.

49. Lowe GD: Circulating inflammatory markers and risks of cardiovascular and non-cardiovascular disease. J Thromb Haemost 2005;3:1618-1627.

50. Greenberg DL, Davie EW: The blood coagulation factors: their complementary DNAs, genes, and expression. In Colman RW, Marder VJ, Clowes AM, et al (eds): Hemostasis and Thrombosis, 5th ed. Philadelphia: Lippincott, Williams & Wilkins, 2006:21-58.

41

Hemorrhagic Coagulation Disorders

Marisa B. Marques and George A. Fritsma

OBJECTIVES

After completion of this chapter, the reader will be able to:

1. Distinguish among the causes of localized versus generalized, soft tissue versus mucocutaneous, and acquired versus congenital bleeding.
2. List laboratory tests to differentiate among acquired hemorrhagic disorders of liver disease, vitamin K deficiency, and kidney failure, and interpret results when given.
3. Interpret laboratory assays to diagnose and subtype von Willebrand disease.
4. Use the results of laboratory tests to identify and monitor the treatment of congenital single

coagulation factor deficiencies, such as, but not limited to, hemophilias A, B, and C.
5. Compare the relative frequency of acquired and inherited bleeding disorders, and note the most frequent cause of each.
6. Explain the principle and rationale for the use of each laboratory test for the detection and monitoring of hemorrhagic disorders.
7. Discuss treatments for hemorrhagic disorders.

CASE STUDY

After studying this chapter, the reader should be able to respond to the following case study:

A 55-year-old man presents to the emergency department with severe epistaxis. He reports that he has a congenital bleeding abnormality and has had multiple episodes of bleeding into his joints (hemarthroses). Physical examination reveals mild jaundice and enlarged liver and spleen. The complete blood count was abnormal owing to anemia and thrombocytopenia (74,400/μL or 74.4 × 10⁹/L). The pro-

thrombin time was 18 seconds (reference range 12-14 seconds), and the partial thromboplastin time was 43 seconds (reference range 25-35 seconds).

1. What is the most likely diagnosis or diagnoses?
2. What treatment does he need?

SYMPTOMS OF HEMORRHAGIC COAGULATION DISORDERS

Hemorrhage is severe bleeding that requires intervention. Hemorrhage may be *localized* or *generalized, acquired* or *congenital.* To establish the cause of a bleeding event or a tendency to bleed, the clinician must obtain a complete patient and family history and do a thorough physical examination before ordering diagnostic laboratory tests.[1]

Localized versus Generalized Hemorrhage

Bleeding from a single location commonly indicates trauma, infection, tumor, or an isolated blood vessel defect. A surgical

site that bleeds excessively because of inadequate cauterization or an ineffective suture is an example of localized bleeding. Localized bleeding seldom implies a defect of vessels, platelets, or the coagulation cascade.[2] Bleeding from multiple sites, spontaneous and recurring, or bleeding that requires intervention and transfusion is potential evidence for a disorder of primary (blood vessels or platelets) or secondary (coagulation factor deficiency) hemostasis.

Soft Tissue and Joint Hemorrhage versus Mucocutaneous Hemorrhage

Generalized bleeding may adhere to a soft tissue (anatomic) or a mucocutaneous pattern. Soft tissue hemorrhage is seen in acquired or congenital *plasma procoagulant* deficiencies. Examples of anatomic bleeding include recurrent or excessive bleeding after minor trauma, dental extraction, or a surgical procedure; such bleeding may suggest a disorder of secondary hemostasis. In such cases, hemorrhage may immediately follow a traumatic event but is often delayed or recurs after the initial blood flow is stopped. In other patients, bleeding episodes are spontaneous. Most anatomic bleeds are internal, such as into joints, body cavities, or the central nervous system, and may have few visible signs. Because joint bleeds (hemarthroses) cause swelling and acute pain, they may not be immediately recognized as hemorrhages. Repeated hemarthroses cause permanent cartilage damage that impairs function. Bleeds into soft tissues, such as muscle or fat, may cause nerve compression and subsequent temporary or permanent loss of function.[3] When the bleeding involves body cavities, it causes symptoms related to the organ that is affected. Bleeding into the central nervous system may cause headache, confusion, seizures, and coma and must be managed as a medical emergency. Bleeds into the kidney may present as hematuria and potentially may be associated with acute kidney failure.

Mucocutaneous hemorrhage may manifest as purpura, which are purple lesions of the skin caused by extravasated red blood cells.[4] Petechiae and ecchymoses are purpura of less than or greater than 3 mm, and more than one such lesion may indicate a disorder of primary hemostasis. Other symptoms of primary hemostasis defects are menorrhagia (increased menstrual flow), bleeding from the gums, hematemesis (vomiting blood), and epistaxis (nosebleeds). Although nosebleeds are common, especially among children, they suggest a hemostatic defect when they occur repeatedly, last longer than 10 minutes, issue from both nostrils, or require medical treatment.[5]

Mucocutaneous hemorrhage tends to be associated with *thrombocytopenia, qualitative platelet disorders, mild or severe von Willebrand disease (VWD), or vascular disorders such as scurvy or telangiectasia*. A careful history and physical examination should distinguish between soft tissue and mucocutaneous bleeding, and the distinction helps direct investigative testing profiles and treatment.

Whenever a soft tissue or mucocutaneous generalized hemostatic disorder is suspected, hemostasis laboratory testing is essential. Emergency department physicians often must treat acute hemorrhage as a medical emergency, however, before taking a history or waiting for the results of laboratory assays. In this instance, fresh frozen plasma (FFP) may be used to correct procoagulant deficiencies, and platelet transfusions may be used for thrombocytopenia.[6,7] Box 41-1 lists symptoms that suggest generalized hemorrhagic disorders.

Acquired versus Congenital Bleeding Disorders

Liver disease, kidney failure, chronic infections, autoimmune disorders, obstetric complications, dietary deficiencies, and inflammatory disorders may be associated with generalized bleeding. If the clinical manifestation first occurs during adulthood, is associated with another disease, and is not found in relatives, it is probably an acquired, not a congenital,

---

> **BOX 41-1** Generalized Bleeding Signs Heralding a Possible Hemostatic Defect
>
> - Hematemesis (vomiting blood)
> - Menorrhagia (menstrual hemorrhage)
> - Recurrent or excessive bleeding from trauma, surgical site, or dental extraction
> - Purpura—recurrent, chronic bruising in multiple locations
> - Repeated nosebleeds (epistaxis) or episodes that last more than 10 minutes
> - Simultaneous hemorrhage from several sites

---

condition. When an adult patient presents with generalized hemorrhage, the physician first looks for an underlying disease, takes a personal and family history and drug exposures, and orders laboratory tests to assess hemostasis (Table 41-1). The initial hemostasis profile should consist of a complete blood count that includes a platelet count, prothrombin time (PT), partial thromboplastin time (PTT), fibrinogen, and sometimes thrombin time.[8] These tests take on clinical significance when the history and physical examination already have established the existence of abnormal bleeding.[2,9]

Congenital hemorrhagic disorders are uncommon, occurring in 1 in 100 individuals, and are usually diagnosed in infants or young children who often have relatives with similar symptoms. Congenital bleeding disorders lead to repeated hemorrhages that may be spontaneous or follow minor injury or may occur in unexpected locations, such as joints, body cavities, retinal veins and arteries, or the central nervous system. Patients with mild congenital hemorrhagic disorders may have no symptoms until they reach adulthood or experience some physical challenge such as trauma, dental extraction, or a surgical procedure. The most common congenital deficiencies are VWD, factor VIII and IX deficiencies, and platelet function disorders. Inherited fibrinogen, prothrombin, and factor V, VII, X, XI, and XIII deficiencies also exist but are rare (Box 41-2).

ACQUIRED HEMORRHAGIC DISORDERS

More patients have acquired bleeding disorders secondary to a chronic disease process than have congenital or inherited conditions. Common examples of secondary hemostatic

TABLE 41-1 Screening Tests for a Generalized Hemostatic Disorder

Test	Assesses for
Hemoglobin, hematocrit; reticulocyte count	Anemia associated with chronic bleeding; bone marrow response
Platelet count	Thrombocytopenia
PT	Deficiencies of fibrinogen, prothrombin, factors V, VII, or X
Activated PTT	Deficiencies of all factors except VII and XIII
Thrombin time	Hypofibrinogenemia and dysfibrinogenemia

disorders are liver disease, vitamin K deficiency, and renal failure. Tests performed in the clinical hemostasis laboratory are helpful to confirm the diagnosis and help guide the management of some acquired hemorrhagic disorders.[10]

Liver Disease

The bleeding associated with liver disease may be generalized or localized. Mucocutaneous bleeding occurs in thrombocytopenia and decreased platelet function. Soft tissue bleeding is associated with procoagulant dysfunction and deficiency, with or without the presence of enlarged vessels (varices) in the esophagus, a long-term complication of cirrhosis.

Procoagulant Deficiency in Liver Disease

The liver produces nearly all of the plasma coagulation factors and regulatory proteins. Hepatitis, cirrhosis, obstructive jaundice, cancer, poisoning, or congenital disorders of bilirubin metabolism may suppress the synthetic function of hepatocytes reducing the concentrations or activities of the plasma procoagulants to below hemostatic levels (usually <30%).

Liver disease particularly affects production of the vitamin K–dependent factors prothrombin (factor II), VII, IX, and X and proteins C, S, and Z. These are produced in their *des-γ-carboxyl* form that cannot participate in coagulation. Factor VII, with a plasma half-life of 3 to 5 hours, is typically the first procoagulant to exhibit decreased activity. Because the PT is particularly sensitive to factor VII activity, it is typically prolonged in mild liver disease, serving as a sensitive early marker.[11,12] Vitamin K deficiency produces a similar effect.

Declining factor V level is a more specific marker of liver disease because factor V is non–vitamin K dependent. Factor V activity assay may be used to distinguish liver disease from vitamin K deficiency.[13]

Fibrinogen is an acute-phase reactant that usually is elevated in early or mild liver disease, although it also may be abnormal. The moderately diseased liver produces fibrinogen with excessive sialic acid residues, a condition called *dysfibrinogenemia*. Dysfibrinogenemia causes mild soft tissue bleeding associated with a prolonged thrombin time and an exceptionally prolonged reptilase time.[14] In end-stage liver disease, the fibrinogen level may decrease to less than 100 mg/dL, which is a mark of liver failure.[15]

von Willebrand factor (VWF) and factors VIII and XIII are acute-phase reactants that may be unaffected or elevated in mild-to-moderate liver disease.[16-19] In contrast to the others, VWF is produced from endothelial cells and megakaryocytes and is stored in endothelial cells and platelets.

Platelet Abnormalities in Liver Disease

Moderate *thrombocytopenia* occurs in one third of patients with liver disease. Platelet counts less than $100,000/\mu L$ $(100 \times 10^9/L)$ may be the result of shortened platelet survival and sequestration associated with portal hypertension and hepatosplenomegaly. In alcoholism-related hepatic cirrhosis, alcohol toxicity also suppresses platelet production. Platelet aggregation and secretion properties are often abnormal, and platelet aggregometry and lumiaggregometry results are affected. Aggregometry may be used to predict bleeding risk but is too complex to be used for diagnostic screening in liver disease.[20]

Disseminated Intravascular Coagulation in Liver Disease

Chronic or compensated disseminated intravascular coagulation (DIC) is a significant outcome of liver disease that is caused by the decreased production of regulatory antithrombin, protein C, or protein S and by the release of activated procoagulants from degenerating liver cells. In addition, the failing liver does not clear activated procoagulants that are normally produced from abdominal organs and present in the portal circulation. In primary or metastatic liver cancer, hepatocytes also may produce procoagulant substances that trigger chronic DIC, leading to ischemic complications.

If the DIC is acute, the PT, PTT, and thrombin time are expected to be prolonged; the fibrinogen level is less than 100 mg/dL and fibrin degradation products, including D-dimers, are significantly increased. If the DIC is chronic and compensated, the only abnormal test may be the D-dimer, a hallmark for unregulated coagulation and fibrinolysis.[21] Although DIC can be corrected only by removing its underlying cause, the hemostatic deficiencies temporarily correct with FFP, platelets, activated protein C, or antithrombin concentrates.[22,23]

Hemostasis Laboratory Tests in Liver Disease

The PT, PTT, thrombin time, fibrinogen assay, platelet count, and D-dimer concentration are useful in characterizing the hemostatic abnormalities in liver disease (Table 41-2). Factor V and VII assays in combination differentiate liver disease from vitamin K deficiency.

Plasminogen deficiency, a shortened euglobulin lysis time, and increased D-dimer or fibrin degradation product assays confirm systemic fibrinolysis. The *reptilase time* occasionally may be useful to confirm dysfibrinogenemia. This test duplicates the thrombin time test, except that venom of *Bothrops atrox* is substituted for thrombin reagent. The venom triggers fibrin polymerization by removing fibrinopeptide A, but not fibrinopeptide B, from the fibrinogen molecule. The subsequent polymerization is slowed by structural defects, prolonging the test. The reptilase time test is insensitive to heparin and can be useful to assess fibrinogen function even when there is heparin contamination in the sample.

TABLE 41-2 Hemostasis Laboratory Tests in Liver Disease

Test	Interpretation
Fibrinogen assay	>400 mg/dL in early, mild liver disease; <200 mg/dL in moderate-to-severe liver disease or dysfibrinogenemia
Thrombin time	Prolonged owing to dysfibrinogenemia, fibrinogen deficiency, or elevated fibrin degradation products
Reptilase time	Prolonged in hypofibrinogenemia, significantly prolonged in dysfibrinogenemia
PT	Prolonged even in mild liver disease owing to des-γ-carboxyl factors VII, X and prothrombin; use seconds, not INR
PTT	Mildly prolonged in severe liver disease owing to DIC or des-γ-carboxyl factors IX, and prothrombin
Platelet count	Mild thrombocytopenia, platelet count <100,000 $\times$ 10^9/L
Platelet aggregometry	Mild suppression of platelet aggregation and secretion, but test is not clinically predictive of bleeding
Fibrin degradation products	>0.25 mg/mL by semiquantitative immunoassay
D-dimer	>240 ng/mL by quantitative assay
Euglobulin lysis time	Lysis in <2 hours in primary or secondary systemic fibrinolysis

INR, international normalized ratio.

Hemostatic Treatment to Relieve Liver Disease–Related Hemorrhage

Vitamin K therapy may correct the bleeding associated with des-γ-carboxyl prothrombin and factors VII, IX, and X, although its therapeutic effect is less effective than in vitamin K deficiency owing to the impaired synthetic ability of the liver. In severe liver disease, transfusion with FFP provides all the coagulation factors in hemostatic concentrations. A unit of FFP consists of 200 to 280 mL of plasma. The typical dose is 2 units in adults, but it varies widely depending on the indication and the ability of the patient to handle extra volume. Circulatory overload is likely to occur at 30 mL/kg, but it may occur even with smaller volume in patients with compromised cardiac function. Owing to the small concentration and short half-life of factor VII, FFP is unlikely to return the PT to within the normal range except for a brief period after the transfusion.

If the fibrinogen level is less than 50 mg/dL, the risk of spontaneous bleeding is imminent, and cryoprecipitate is preferred for its smaller volume and high fibrinogen concentration. FFP and cryoprecipitate present a small risk of virus transmission, as do other single-donor blood products. Allergic transfusion reactions are much more common with plasma-containing products. Other therapeutic options in patients with liver disease–related bleeding are platelets, prothrombin complex, activated protein C, antithrombin concentrate, and recombinant activated factor VII.

Renal Failure and Hemorrhage

Chronic renal failure of any cause is associated with *platelet dysfunction* and *mild-to-moderate mucocutaneous bleeding*. Acute renal failure also may be associated with acute gastrointestinal bleeding caused by specific anatomic lesions.[24] Platelet adhesion and aggregation are suppressed, perhaps because of platelet coating by guanidinosuccinic acid or dialyzable phenolic compounds.[25] Decreased red blood cell and platelet mass contribute to the bleeding and may be corrected with dialysis, erythropoietin or red blood cell transfusions, and interleukin-11 therapy.[26]

Hemostasis activation syndromes that deposit fibrin in the renal microvasculature often affect the glomeruli. Examples of these syndromes include DIC, hemolytic-uremic syndrome, and thrombotic thrombocytopenic purpura. Although these are not hemorrhagic disorders, they cause thrombocytopenia, which may lead to bleeding. Fibrin also may be deposited during renal transplant rejection and during the glomerulonephritis syndrome of systemic lupus erythematosus; this may be associated with an increase in the quantitative plasma D-dimer, thrombin-antithrombin, prothrombin fragment 1+2, or fibrin degradation products.[27]

Laboratory tests for bleeding in renal disease provide only modest information with little predictive or management value. The bleeding time may be prolonged but is too unreliable to provide an accurate diagnosis or to monitor treatment.[28] Platelet aggregometry test results vary, and coagulation tests such as the PT and PTT are expected to be normal.

Management of renal failure–related bleeding typically focuses on the severity of the hemorrhage without reliance on laboratory tests. Renal dialysis improves platelet function, particularly when anemia is well controlled.[29] Desmopressin acetate (DDAVP) may be administered intravenously or intranasally to increase the plasma concentration of high-molecular-weight multimers of VWF, also aiding platelet adhesion and aggregation. Renal failure patients should not take aspirin, clopidogrel, or other platelet inhibitors because these drugs increase the risk of hemorrhage.

Nephrotic Syndrome and Hemorrhage

Nephrotic syndrome is a state of increased glomerular permeability associated with a variety of conditions, such as chronic glomerulonephritis, diabetic glomerulosclerosis, systemic lupus erythematosus, amyloidosis, or renal vein thrombosis.[30] In nephrotic syndrome, low-molecular-weight proteins are lost through the glomerulus into the urine. Procoagulants such as prothrombin and factors VII, IX, X, and XII have been detected in the urine, as have the regulatory proteins antithrombin and protein C. In 25% of cases, loss of regulatory proteins takes precedence over loss of procoagulants and leads to a tendency toward venous thrombosis.[31]

Vitamin K Deficiency

Vitamin K is ubiquitous in foods, and the daily requirement is small, so pure dietary deficiency is rare. Body stores are limited, however, and become exhausted when the diet is interrupted, as when patients are fed only with parenteral nutrition for an extended period. Also, because vitamin K is fat soluble and requires bile salts for absorption, biliary duct obstruction or atresia, fat malabsorption, and chronic diarrhea may cause vitamin K deficiency. Broad-spectrum antibiotics that disrupt normal flora may cause a slight reduction in vitamin K absorption, although this is insignificant when the diet is otherwise normal.

Hemorrhagic Disease of the Newborn Caused by Vitamin K Deficiency

Because of their sterile intestine and the minimal vitamin K passage through human milk, newborns are vitamin K deficient.[32] Hemorrhagic disease of the newborn was common in the United States before routine administration of vitamin K to infants was legislated in the 1960s, but it still occurs in developing countries. Normal newborns' levels of prothrombin and factors VII, IX, and X are lower than in adults, and premature infants have even lower concentrations of these factors.[33] Breastfeeding prolongs the deficiency because passively acquired maternal antibodies delay establishment of gut flora.

Vitamin K Antagonists

The γ-carboxylation cycle of coagulation factors is interrupted by warfarin-type oral anticoagulants that disrupt the vitamin K epoxide reductase and vitamin K quinone reductase reactions (Fig. 41-1). In deficient γ-carboxylation, the liver releases dysfunctional des-γ-carboxyl prothrombin; factors VII, IX, and X; and proteins C, S, and Z—known as *proteins in vitamin K antagonism*. Therapeutic overdose or the accidental or felonious administration of warfarin-containing compounds such as rat poisons may result in moderate-to-severe hemorrhage because of the lack of functional factors. The effect of "superwarfarins," often used as rodenticides, lasts for weeks to months and requires repeated administration of vitamin K with follow-up PT monitoring.[34]

Detecting Vitamin K Deficiency or Proteins in Vitamin K Antagonism

Clinical suspicion of vitamin K deficiency is supported by a prolonged PT with or without a prolonged PTT. If normal plasma is mixed with patient plasma, the mixture yields normal PT and PTT results, indicating factor deficiencies as the cause of the prolonged screening tests. Specific single-factor assays always detect low factor VII because of its short half-life, followed by decreases in factors IX and X and prothrombin. Therapy for vitamin K deficiency employs the administration of oral or (in an emergency) parenteral vitamin K. Because synthesis of functional factors requires at least 3 hours, in the case of severe bleeding, FFP or a prothrombin complex concentrate may be administered. All preparations of prothrombin

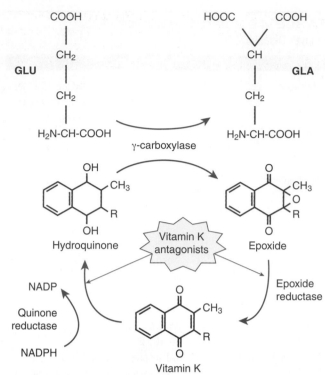

Figure 41-1 Glutamic acid (GLU) catalyzed by γ-carboxylase gains a carboxyl group to become γ-carboxy-glutamic acid (GLA). This post-translational modification enables the vitamin K–dependent coagulation factors II, VII, IX, and X and proteins C, S, and Z to bind ionic calcium necessary for normal coagulation. Vitamin K donates the carboxyl group through the quinone reductase pathway. Antagonists such as warfarin inactivate quinone reductase and epoxide reductase to prevent carboxylation.

complex concentrate are moderately purified plasma-derived products containing varying proportions of prothrombin and factors VII, IX, and X.

Autoanti-VIII Inhibitor and Acquired Hemophilia

Acquired autoantibodies that specifically inhibit prothrombin; factors V, VIII, IX, and XIII; and VWF have been described in nonhemophiliac patients. Anti-VIII is the most common. Patients with the highest risk of developing an autoantibody to factor VIII, diagnostic of acquired hemophilia, are usually older than age 60 and have no apparent underlying disease. It also may occur in women 2 to 5 months after pregnancy. In some cases, it is associated with rheumatoid arthritis, inflammatory bowel disease, systemic lupus erythematosus, or lymphoproliferative disease. Inhibitors that develop after pregnancy typically disappear with or without immunosuppression. Acquired hemophilia has an incidence of 1 in 1 million individuals per year; patients present with sudden and severe bleeding in soft tissues or from gastrointestinal or genitourinary sources. Although most patients recover, it is fatal in at least 20% of cases. Autoantibodies to other procoagulants are less frequent but may create similar symptoms.[35]

Clot-Based Studies in Acquired Hemophilia

PT, PTT, and thrombin time are recommended for any patient with sudden onset of anatomic hemorrhage resembling acquired hemophilia. The PTT should be prolonged, whereas the PT and thrombin time should be normal. A factor assay reveals the factor VIII level to be less than 30% and often undetectable.

The inhibitor is confirmed with clot-based mixing studies. The PTT prolongation may be corrected initially by the addition of normal plasma to the test specimen in a 1:1 ratio but again becomes prolonged on incubation of the mixture of the patient's plasma and normal plasma at 37° C. The lack of correction after incubation occurs because factor VIII autoantibodies are usually of the IgG isotype, time and temperature dependent. Consequently, the inhibitor effect may be evident only after the patient's inhibitor is allowed to interact with the factor VIII in the normal plasma for 1 to 2 hours at 37° C before testing. A few high-avidity inhibitors may cause immediate prolongation of the PTT, and an incubated mixing study is unnecessary.

The in vitro kinetics of factor VIII neutralization is nonlinear. Although there is early rapid loss of factor VIII activity, residual activity remains, indicating an intermediate equilibrium. This is called *type II kinetics* (Fig. 41-2). In contrast, alloantibodies to factor VIII, which develop in 20% to 25% of severe hemophiliacs in response to factor VIII therapy, exhibit type I kinetics. In the latter, there is linear in vitro neutralization of factor VIII activity over 1 to 2 hours, which results in complete inactivation. Type I kinetics provides for relatively accurate in vitro measurement, whereas in type II kinetics the titration of inhibitor activity is semiquantitative.[36]

Quantitation of autoanti-VIII inhibitor is accomplished by the Bethesda assay, which is ordinarily employed in hemophiliacs with alloantibodies to factor VIII. Titer results help the clinician choose the proper therapy to control bleeding. Repeat titers are used to follow the response to immunosuppressive drugs but are not needed for management of the bleeding symptoms.

Other Factor Inhibitors

Antiprothrombin antibodies, detectable by immunoassay, develop in approximately 30% of patients with lupus anticoagulant.[37] Although lupus anticoagulant is associated with thrombosis, some patients with antiprothrombin antibody have bleeding and a prolonged PT. A low prothrombin activity level and a positive test for lupus anticoagulant make the diagnosis. Non–lupus anticoagulant–associated anti-prothrombin is rare. Factor V and XIII inhibitors have been documented in patients receiving isoniazid treatment for tuberculosis.[38,39] Antibodies to thrombin and factor V may follow exposure to topical bovine thrombin or fibrin glue.[40] Autoanti-X is rare; however, X deficiency in amyloidosis may be caused by what seems to be an absorptive mechanism.[41] In many acquired inhibitors, mixing studies show uncorrected prolongation without incubation (immediate mixing study), and their titers may be determined by the Bethesda procedure.

Management of Acquired Hemophilia

During acute bleeding, activated prothrombin complex concentrates or recombinant activated factor VII may bypass the inhibitor and control bleeding. Patients with low-titer inhibitor may respond to DDAVP or factor VIII concentrates, but close monitoring of their response to therapy with factor VIII levels is warranted. Plasma exchange may be used in severe cases, but the response is unreliable. When bleeding is controlled, immunosuppressive therapy may reduce the inhibitor titer.[42]

Acquired von Willebrand Disease

Acquired VWF deficiency, with symptoms similar to the congenital form, has been described in association with hypothyroidism, autoimmune, lymphoproliferative or myeloproliferative disorders, benign monoclonal gammopathies, Wilms tumor, intestinal angiodysplasia, congenital heart disease, pesticide exposure, and hemolytic-uremic syndrome.[43,44] The pathogenesis of acquired VWD varies and may involve decreased production, an autoantibody, or adsorption of VWF to abnormal cell surfaces, as seen in association with lymphoproliferative disorders.

Acquired VWD manifests with moderate-to-severe mucocutaneous bleeding and may be suspected in any patient with recent onset of bleeding without significant past medical history. Although the PT is not prolonged, the PTT may be abnormal if the deficiency of VWF is severe enough to cause a deficiency of factor VIII. As in congenital VWD, the diagnosis is based on diminished VWF activity (ristocetin cofactor) and VWF antigen by immunoassay. It may be difficult to differentiate between mild, previously asymptomatic congenital VWD and the acquired form.

If the patient presents with bleeding, DDAVP or plasma-derived factor VIII/VWF concentrates such as Humate-P or Alphanate are effective to control symptoms. Cryoprecipitate is no longer recommended for treatment of VWD because it has not undergone viral inactivation.

Disseminated Intravascular Coagulation

DIC, although often identified through hemorrhagic symptoms, is classified as a thrombotic disorder and is described in Chapter 42.

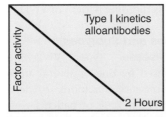
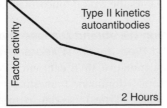

Figure 41-2 In type I linear kinetics, the inhibitor inactivates the factor in vitro. In type II kinetics, the inhibitor and factor reach equilibrium. In general, acquired inhibitors exhibit type II kinetics; their laboratory measurement is less accurate.

CONGENITAL HEMORRHAGIC DISORDERS

von Willebrand Disease

VWD is a mucocutaneous bleeding disorder caused by a quantitative or structural abnormality of VWF. Both abnormalities lead to decreased platelet adhesion to the injured vessel wall (impaired primary hemostasis). VWD is the most prevalent of the congenital bleeding disorders, affecting approximately 1% of the population and both sexes (autosomal dominant inheritance). The diagnosis of VWD is confounded, however, by ABO blood group because VWF levels are normally lowest in group O individuals and highest in group AB individuals.[45]

Molecular Biology and Functions of von Willebrand Factor

VWF is a diverse glycoprotein with a range of molecular masses from 800,000 to 20,000,000 D. Its plasma concentration is 0.5 to 1 mg/dL, but a great deal more is readily available on demand from storage organelles. VWF is synthesized in endothelial cells and megakaryocytes and stored in endothelial cells, Weibel-Palade bodies, and platelets' α-granules; Weibel-Palade bodies and α-granules release it in response to a variety of stimuli.[46]

The gene for VWF spans 178 kb with 52 exons on chromosome 12.[47] The translated protein is a monomer of 2813 amino acids that, after glycosylation, forms dimers that are transferred to storage organelles, where they polymerize. At the time of storage, a signal sequence and a propolypeptide, also known as *VWF antigen II*, are cleaved so that the mature monomers, already polymerized, consist of 2050 amino acids.[48]

Each VWF monomer has four functional domains that bind factor VIII, platelet glycoprotein Ib/V/IX, platelet glycoprotein IIb/IIIa, and collagen.[49] On release from intracellular stores, VWF forms a complex with factor VIII named *VIII/VWF* (Fig. 41-3). VWF protects factor VIII from proteolysis, prolonging its plasma half-life from a few minutes to 8 to 12 hours. Table 41-3 lists the nomenclature for the structural and functional components of the factor VIII/VWF molecule.

Although VWF serves as the factor VIII carrier molecule, its primary function is to mediate platelet adhesion to subendothelial collagen in areas of high flow rate and high shear force, as in capillaries and arterioles. VWF first binds fibrillar collagen exposed during the desquamation of endothelial cells. Subsequently, platelets adhere through their glycoprotein Ib/V/IX receptor to the VWF "carpet." The largest VWF multimers are best equipped to serve the adhesion function. When VWF binds glycoprotein Ib/V/IX, platelets become activated and express a second VWF binding site, glycoprotein IIb/IIIa. This receptor binds VWF and fibrinogen to mediate irreversible platelet-to-platelet aggregation.

Pathophysiology of von Willebrand Disease

Structural (qualitative) or quantitative VWF abnormalities reduce platelet adhesion, leading to mucocutaneous hemorrhage of variable severity. Severe quantitative VWF deficiency creates factor VIII deficiency owing to the inability to protect

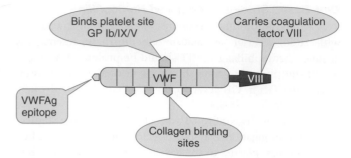

Figure 41-3 Large VWF multimers bind intimal collagen on blood vessel injury and expand to form a "carpet" to which platelets adhere through glycoprotein Ib/V/IX binding sites. VWF stabilizes factor VIII and presents epitopes that serve as sites for immunoassay.

TABLE 41-3 Nomenclature for the VIII/VWF Complex

Term	Meaning
VIII/VWF	Customary term for the plasma combination of factor VIII and VWF
VWF	600,000 to 20,000,000 D multimers that participate in platelet adhesion to injured vessels and transport factor VIII
VWF:Ag	Epitope that is the antigenic basis for the VWF immunoassay
VWFR:Co	Ristocetin cofactor activity, also called the *VWF activity assay;* VWF activity is measured by the ability of ristocetin to cause agglutination of reagent platelets by the patient's VWF
VIII	Procoagulant factor VIII, the protein transported on VWF; it binds activated factor IX and the complex of VIIIa-IXa digests and activates factor X; factor VIII deficiency is called *hemophilia A*
VIII:C	Factor VIII coagulant activity as measured in a factor-specific clot-based assay

factor VIII from proteolysis. Most VWD patients have VWF levels in the 30% to 50% range, maintaining a factor VIII level sufficient for competent coagulation. When factor VIII levels decrease to less than 30%, anatomic soft tissue bleeding accompanies the typical mucocutaneous bleeding pattern of VWD.

von Willebrand Disease Types and Subtypes

Type 1 von Willebrand Disease. Type 1 VWD is a quantitative VWF deficiency caused by one of several autosomal dominant frameshifts, nonsense mutations, or deletions.[50] Type 1 is seen in more than 70% of patients with VWD.[51,52] The levels of VWF and factor VIII are variably, although proportionally, reduced. There is mild-to-moderate bleeding, usually following a hemostatic challenge such as dental extraction or surgery.[53] In women, menorrhagia is a common complaint that leads to the diagnosis of VWD.

Type 2 von Willebrand Disease.   Type 2 VWD comprises a variety of qualitative VWF abnormalities. VWF levels may be normal or mildly decreased, but VWF function is abnormal.

Subtype 2A von Willebrand Disease.   Ten to 20% of VWD patients have subtype 2A, which arises from well-characterized autosomal dominant point mutations in the A2 structural domain of VWF. These mutations render VWF more susceptible to proteolysis with consequent predominance of small-molecular-weight multimers in the plasma. The latter have lower activity than the larger forms of the molecule. Patients with VWD subtype 2A have normal or slightly reduced VWF antigen levels, with more markedly decreased VWF activity as a result of the loss of the high-molecular-weight and intermediate-molecular-weight multimers essential for platelet adhesion.

Subtype 2B von Willebrand Disease.   Rare mutations within the A1 domain increase the affinity of VWF to platelet glycoprotein Ib/V/IX in subtype 2B. Large VWF multimers spontaneously bind resting platelets and are unavailable for normal platelet adhesion. Consequently, the electrophoretic multimer pattern is characterized by the lack of the high-molecular-weight multimers but the presence of intermediate-molecular-weight multimers. There also may be moderate thrombocytopenia caused by chronic platelet activation.

A platelet mutation that increases glycoprotein Ib/V/IX affinity for normal VWF multimers creates a clinically similar disorder called *platelet-type* or *pseudo-VWD.* In this instance, the large multimers also are lost from the plasma, and platelets are activated (Fig. 41-4). Clinically and in the laboratory, the two entities are indistinguishable.

Subtype 2M von Willebrand Disease.   Subtype 2M is a qualitative variant of VWF, with decreased platelet receptor binding with a normal multimeric pattern. The distinguishing feature of subtype 2M that separates it from type 1 is a discrepancy between the concentration of VWF antigen and its measured activity.

von Willebrand Disease Normandy Variant, Subtype 2N, or Autosomal Hemophilia.   A rare autosomal missense VWF mutation impairs its factor VIII binding site. This condition results in factor VIII deficiency despite normal VWF antigen concentration and activity and a normal multimeric pattern. This disorder also is known as *autosomal hemophilia* because it can affect men and women, and its manifestations are indistinguishable from hemophilia. Subtype 2N is suspected when a woman is diagnosed with hemophilia after soft tissue bleeding symptoms. In men, this condition is suspected when a misdiagnosed hemophilia A patient fails to respond to factor VIII concentrate therapy because the factor has a plasma half-life of mere minutes when unable to bind VWF. The diagnosis of VWD subtype 2N is made by a molecular assay that detects the specific mutation responsible for the abnormal factor VIII binding to VWF.

Type 3 von Willebrand Disease.   Autosomal recessive translation or deletion mutations of the VWF gene produce severe mucocutaneous and anatomic hemorrhage in compound heterozygotes or, in consanguinity, homozygotes. In this rare disorder, VWF is absent or nearly absent. Factor VIII levels also are proportionally diminished or absent, and primary and secondary hemostasis is impaired.

Pitfalls in the Diagnosis of von Willebrand Disease

Varying penetrance, ABO blood group, hormones, age, exercise, and physical stress influence VWF production and plasma concentration. Increased estrogen during pregnancy normalizes the plasma VWF level even in moderate deficiency; however, VWF levels decrease rapidly after delivery and may lead to acute postpartum hemorrhage. Because VWF is an acute-phase reactant, levels increase in acute inflammation and stress. Consequently, individuals experience fluctuation in disease severity over time, and the clinical manifestations of the disease vary from individual to individual within families despite possessing, presumably, the same mutation. Overall, however, individuals with abnormal VWF activity report easy bruising. When the clinical presentation suggests VWD, testing should be repeated until it is conclusive.[54]

Laboratory Detection and Classification of von Willebrand Disease

Although laboratory assays are essential, definitive diagnosis depends on a combination of personal or family history of mucocutaneous bleeding and decreased VWF activity.[55] A complete blood cell count also is necessary to rule out thrombocytopenia as the cause for mucocutaneous bleeding, whereas PT and activated PTT assess the coagulation system. The standard VWD evaluation includes a quantitative VWF assay by enzyme immunoassay or automated immunoassay such as the LIA test; the VWF activity test that determines the factor's ability to bind to platelets, also known as *ristocetin cofactor activity assay;* and a factor VIII activity level.

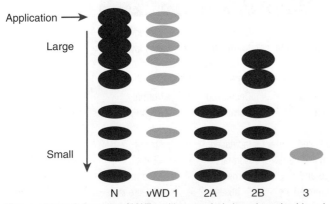

Figure 41-4 Schematic of VWF multimer analysis by polyacrylamide gel electrophoresis shows diminished concentration but normal ratios in type 1, absence of large and intermediate multimers in subtype 2A, absence of large forms in subtype 2B, and absence of all multimers in type 3.

When the VWF activity (ristocetin cofactor) assay result is significantly lower than the VWF antigen concentration, qualitative or type 2 VWD is suspected. Additional tests are needed to define the subtype. Low-dose ristocetin–induced platelet aggregometry, also called the *ristocetin response curve,* identifies subtype 2B. In this instance, the patient's VWF binds to platelets at concentrations too low to induce such binding in control plasma. VWF multimer analysis by sodium dodecyl-sulfate-polyacrylamide gel electrophoresis further differentiates between VWD type 2A and 2B. Multimer analysis is technically demanding and performed mainly in reference laboratories for differentiation of these subtypes. Table 41-4 displays the expected test results for all VWD types and subtypes.

Clinical laboratory physicians and scientists must communicate that the patient's current condition, such as inflammation, acute stress, or pregnancy, is likely to increase the levels of VWF even in patients with VWD. A negative profile does not exclude it as a possibility, and a repeat positive test in the patient or kindred or both may be necessary to yield a definitive diagnosis.

Because acquired VWD may present as any one of the subtypes, results of laboratory workup are not helpful to differentiate it from the inherited condition. Review of the clinical history with emphasis on age at onset of bleeding, comorbid conditions, and family history may signal acquired disease versus the congenital form.

Treatment of von Willebrand Disease

Mild bleeding may resolve with the use of local measures, such as limb elevation, pressure, and ice packs.[56] Moderate bleeding may respond to estrogen and DDAVP, which trigger the release of VWF from storage organelles. Therapeutic dosages are managed through serial VWF antigen concentration assays. DDAVP is consistently effective in type 1 disease and mostly useful in subtype 2A. It is contraindicated in subtype 2B, however, because it causes the release of abnormal VWF with increased affinity for platelet receptors, which may intensify thrombocytopenia and lead to platelet activation and thrombosis. Aminocaproic acid inhibits fibrinolysis and may control bleeding when used alone or in conjunction with DDAVP.

In severe VWD (type 3) and in subtype 2B, commercial preparations containing VWF and factor VIII from human plasma fractionation replace both factors. The calculation of the proper dose follows principles similar to those used for hemophilia A provided in the next section. Laboratory monitoring is essential to determine whether the given amount reached the target VWF level and to follow its degradation between doses. Recombinant and affinity-purified factor VIII preparations contain no VWF and cannot be used to treat VWD. Cryoprecipitate and FFP are less desirable alternatives because the risk of virus transmission is higher than for the purified preparations, and the necessary volume per dose may cause fluid overload. In an emergency, however, before the availability of the concentrate, a dose of cryoprecipitate may be lifesaving. Therapy for bleeding secondary to acquired VWD follows the same principles as delineated previously plus treatment of the primary disease, if applicable. Therapeutic recommendations are summarized in Table 41-5.

Hemophilia A–Factor VIII Deficiency

The hemophilias are congenital single-factor deficiencies marked by anatomic soft tissue bleeding. Second to VWD in prevalence among congenital bleeding disorders, hemophilias occur in 1 in 10,000 individuals. Of these, 85% are deficient in factor VIII, 14% are deficient in factor IX, and 1% are deficient in factor XI or one of the other coagulation factors, such as prothrombin, V, VII, X, or XIII. Congenital deficiency of factor VIII is called *classic hemophilia* or *hemophilia A.*[57]

Factor VIII

Factor VIII is a two-chain, 285,000-D protein translated from the X chromosome. When the coagulation cascade is activated, thrombin cleaves circulating factor VIII and releases

TABLE 41-4 Laboratory Detection and Classification of von Willebrand Disease*

Laboratory Test	Type 1	Type 2A	Type 2B	Type 3
VWF activity	Low	Low	Low	Very low
VWF antigen	Low	Normal to slight decrease	Normal to slight decrease	Very low
CBA/VWF antigen ratio	>0.5	<0.5	<0.5	NA
Platelet count	Normal	Normal	Decreased	Normal
PTT	Normal to slightly prolonged	Normal	Normal	Prolonged
RIPA	Decreased	Decreased	Increased	Absent
Factor VIII activity	Mildly low	Normal	Normal	<5%
VWF multimers	Normal pattern	Large and intermediate forms absent	Large forms absent	All forms decreased

*Expected results are given, but results vary over time and within affected kindred.
CBA, collagen binding assay; NA, not applicable; RIPA, ristocetin-induced platelet aggregometry using 1 mg/mL ristocetin.

TABLE 41-5 Therapeutic Strategies in von Willebrand Disease

Type	Primary Approach	Other Options
1	Estrogen, DDAVP, EACA	Factor VIII/VWF concentrate
2A	Estrogen, DDAVP, EACA	Factor VIII/VWF concentrate
2B	Factor VIII/VWF concentrate	EACA
2N	Factor VIII/VWF concentrate	EACA
3	Factor VIII/VWF concentrate	Platelet transfusions

EACA, ε-aminocaproic acid.
DDAVP, desmopressin acetate.

a large polypeptide called the *B domain* that dissociates from the molecule. This leaves behind a calcium-dependent heterodimer that detaches from its VWF carrier molecule to bind phospholipid and factor IXa. The VIIIa-IXa complex, sometimes called *tenase,* cleaves and activates factor X at a rate 10,000 times faster than free IXa can cleave the substrate. Consequently, factor VIII deficiency significantly slows the coagulation pathway's production of thrombin and leads to hemorrhage. In vitro, factor VIII deteriorates at about 5% per hour at room temperature.[58]

Hemophilia A Genetics

The gene for factor VIII spans 186 kb of the X chromosome and is the site of various deletions, stop codons, and nonsense and mis-sense mutations. Most of these mutations result in quantitative disorders in which the factor VIII coagulant activity and antigen concentration levels are in agreement, but rare cases result in low activity despite normal antigen levels. The latter possess qualitative or "structural" factor VIII abnormalities commonly known as *cross-reacting material positive.*

Male hemizygotes, whose sole X chromosome contains a factor VIII gene mutation, experience anatomic bleeding, but female heterozygotes, who are carriers do not. Female carriers who have children with an unaffected man may bear children with the following chances of hemophilia inheritance: 25% of a normal daughter, 25% of a carrier daughter, 25% of a normal son, and 25% of a hemophilic son. All sons of hemophiliac men are normal, whereas all daughters are carriers of the disease. In addition, approximately 30% of newly diagnosed cases arise as a result of spontaneous germline mutations and have a negative family history of hemophilia. Rarely, the symptoms of hemophilia A may be seen in females. This phenomenon could be due to true homozygosity or double heterozygosity, such as in the female offspring of a hemophiliac father and a carrier mother. Other possibilities include a spontaneous germline mutation in the otherwise normal allele of a heterozygous female, or a disproportional inactivation of the X chromosome with the normal gene, termed *extreme lyonization.* Finally, VWD of the Normandy subtype may present as mild hemophilia A in males and females.[59]

Clinical Manifestations of Hemophilia A

Hemophilia A causes anatomic bleeds, with deep muscle and joint hemorrhages; hematomas; wound oozing after trauma or surgery; and bleeding into the central nervous system, peritoneum, retroperitoneum, gastrointestinal tract, and kidneys. Acute joint bleeds are extremely painful and cause temporary immobilization. Chronic joint bleeds cause inflammation and eventual permanent loss of mobility, whereas bleeding into muscles may cause nerve compression injury, with first temporary and then lasting disability. Cranial bleeds lead to severe, debilitating, often serious and durable neurologic symptoms, such as loss of memory, paralysis, seizures, and coma, and may be rapidly fatal. Onset of bleeding may be immediate after a triggering event or may become manifest after a delay of several hours. Some bleeding seems to be spontaneous.

The diagnosis of hemophilia A begins with laboratory testing after the birth of an infant to a mother who has a family history of hemophilia. In the absence of family history, abnormal bleeding in the neonatal period, which may appear as easy bruising, bleeding from the umbilical stump, postcircumcision bleeding, hematuria, or intracranial bleeding, is considered suspicious for hemophilia. Severe hemophilia usually is diagnosed in the first year of life, whereas mild hemophilia may not become apparent until a triggering event such as trauma, surgery, or dental extraction occurs in late childhood, adolescence, or adulthood.

The laboratory diagnosis of coagulopathies in the newborn or older infant is complicated by the requirement for an unhemolyzed specimen of at least 2 mL volume from tiny veins and by the typically low newborn levels of some coagulation factors. It is expected that the PT and PTT would be prolonged because of physiologically low levels of prothrombin and factors VII, IX, and X even in full-term infants. Factor VIII levels are similar to the levels in adults, even in infants who are born prematurely, allowing skillful laboratory staff to provide the correct diagnosis of hemophilia A using the factor VIII activity assay.

The severity of hemophilia A symptoms is inversely proportional to factor VIII activity. Hematologists classify an activity level of less than 1% as severe, associated with spontaneous or exaggerated bleeding in the neonatal period. Levels of 1% to 5% are seen in moderate hemophilia, which is usually diagnosed in early childhood after symptoms become apparent. In mild hemophilia, with activity levels 5% to 20%, hemorrhage follows significant trauma and becomes a risk factor mainly in surgery or dental extractions, and patients may go for long periods without symptoms.

Hemophilia A Complications

As a result of frequent bleeds, hemophiliac patients often have debilitating and progressive musculoskeletal lesions, deformities, and neurologic deficiencies after intracranial hemorrhage. In addition, other effects of chronic diseases, such as limited productivity, low self-esteem, poverty, drug dependency, and depression, are common problems. Before the advent of sterilized factor concentrates, chronic hepatitis often resulted from repeated exposure to blood products. Consequently, 70% of hemophiliacs treated before 1984 are human immunodeficiency virus (HIV) positive or have died from acquired immune deficiency syndrome (AIDS).[60]

Laboratory Diagnosis of Hemophilia A

The laboratory workup for a suspected congenital single coagulation factor deficiency starts with the PT, PTT, and thrombin time and continues with factor assays based on the results of the screening tests. Before the physician initiates laboratory testing, however, a clear history of the patient's hemorrhagic symptoms must be recorded. In hemophilia A, the PT and thrombin time are normal, and the PTT is prolonged, provided that the test system is sensitive to deficiencies at or less than the 30% plasma level. Table 41-6 lists the expected results for each clot-based screening assay in any single-factor deficiency associated with bleeding, including deficiencies of fibrinogen; prothrombin; and factors V, VII, VIII, IX, X, and XI.[42] Contact factor deficiencies (factor XII, high-molecular-weight kininogen, and prekallikrein) have no relationship to bleeding and do not appear in Table 41-6.

Hemophilia A Carrier Detection

Approximately 90% of female carriers of hemophilia A are detected using the ratio of factor VIII activity to VWF antigen (VIII/VWF). The ratio is useful because VWF production is unaffected by factor VIII deficiency. Using a ratio rather than a factor VIII assay alone normalizes for some of the physiologic variations that affect factor VIII activity and VWF antigen assays, such as estrogens, inflammation, stress, or exercise.

The laboratory scientist establishes a reference interval for the VIII/VWF ratio using plasmas from 30 or more normal women. If the test subject's ratio is below the lower limit of the interval, she is likely to be a carrier. These results may be influenced by extreme lyonization, variation in VWF production, and analytical variables; consequently, if carrier status is suspected, and the VIII/VWF ratio is greater than the lower limit of the reference range, genetic testing may be used to detect many of the polymorphisms associated with factor VIII deficiency.[61,62]

Hemophilia A Treatment

The goal of hemophilia A treatment is to increase the patient's factor VIII activity to hemostatic levels whenever he or she

TABLE 41-6   Results of Clot-Based Screening Assays in Congenital Single-Factor Deficiencies*

Deficient Factor	Prothrombin Time	Partial Thromboplastin Time	Thrombin Time	Reflex Test
Fibrinogen	Prolonged	Prolonged	Prolonged	Fibrinogen assay
Prothrombin	Prolonged	Prolonged	Normal	Prothrombin and factors V, VII, and X assays
V	Prolonged	Prolonged	Normal	Prothrombin and factors V, VII, and X assays
VII	Prolonged	Normal	Normal	Factor VII assay
VIII	Normal	Prolonged	Normal	Factors VIII, IX, and XI assays
IX	Normal	Prolonged	Normal	Factors VIII, IX, and XI assays
X	Prolonged	Prolonged	Normal	Prothrombin and factors V, VII, and X assays
XI	Normal	Prolonged	Normal	Factors VIII, IX, and XI assays
XIII	Normal	Normal	Normal	Factor XIII quantitative assay (urea solubility)

*Results are valid when no anticoagulants are in use.

experiences or suspects a bleeding episode or anticipates a hemostatic challenge such as a surgical procedure. The target activity level depends on the nature of the bleeding, is seldom greater than 75%, and should be maintained until the threat is resolved. In the case of hemarthrosis or another localized bleed, the sooner the target factor level is reached, the less painful is the episode, and the less likely the patient is to experience side effects of inflammation, nerve compression, or anemia. Because factor VIII has a half-life of 8 to 12 hours, infusions are required at least twice per day. Many hemophiliacs maintain themselves on a steady prophylactic dose designed to keep the factor VIII level greater than 1%.[63] Although initially more expensive, the prophylactic approach saves downstream resources by ameliorating the adverse effects of repeated hemorrhages and their long-term consequences.

Many hemophiliacs respond to the administration of intranasal or intramuscular DDAVP alone or in combination with an antifibrinolytic such as aminocaproic acid (Amicar). When DDAVP treatment proves ineffective, intravenous factor VIII concentrates are the next option. High-purity factor VIII concentrates are produced from mammalian cells using recombinant DNA technology or from human plasma using factor VIII–specific monoclonal antibodies and column separation.[64] Intermediate-purity concentrates are prepared by chemical fractionation of human plasma and contain, in addition to factor VIII, VWF, fibrinogen, and noncoagulant proteins. All plasma-derived concentrates undergo viral inactivation steps, and since 1985, none has transmitted lipid-envelope viruses such as HIV, hepatitis B, or hepatitis C. Plasma-derived factor VIII concentrates may transmit nonlipid viruses such as parvovirus B19 and hepatitis A.[65,66] Recombinant products may use human albumin in the manufacturing process, introducing the theoretical risk of transmission of Creutzfeld-Jakob disease; however, distributors more recently have developed products free of all human protein.[65]

Hematologists treating a hemophiliac patient base their factor VIII concentrate dose calculations on the definition of a unit of factor activity, known as the amount present in 1 mL of normal plasma and synonymous with 100% activity. They further calculate the desired increase after factor VIII concentrate infusion by subtracting the patient's preinfusion factor level from the target level. The desired increase is multiplied by the patient's plasma volume to compute the dosage. The patient's plasma volume may be estimated from his or her blood volume and hematocrit. The blood volume is approximately 65 mL/kg of body weight, and the plasma volume is the plasmacrit (100% − hematocrit %), as in the following formulas:

$$\text{Plasma volume} = \text{weight in kilograms} \times 65 \text{ mL/kg} \times (1 - \text{hematocrit})$$

$$\text{Factor VIII concentrate dose} = \text{plasma volume} \times (\text{target factor VIII level} - \text{initial factor VIII level})$$

Overdosing seems to confer no thrombotic risk, but it wastes resources. Regardless of the dose administered, laboratory monitoring and close clinical observation are essential

to prevent or halt bleeding and its complications. Repeat dosing is done on an 8- to 12-hour schedule, reflecting the half-life of factor VIII. The second administration of factor VIII uses half the concentration of the first dose.

Hemophilia A and Factor VIII Inhibitors

Alloantibody inhibitors of factor VIII arise in response to treatment in 30% of severe and 3% of moderately hemophiliac patients. An inhibitor is suspected when bleeding persists or when the plasma factor VIII activity fails to increase to the target after appropriate concentrate administration. Most factor VIII inhibitors are IgG_4, non–complement-fixing, warm-reacting antibodies. It is impossible to predict which patients are likely to develop inhibitors based on their genetics, demographics, or the type of concentrate used.[66]

The first step in inhibitor detection is a factor VIII assay. If the activity level exceeds 30%, no inhibitor is present. If the level is less than 30%, the laboratory scientist proceeds to mixing studies. When the test plasma from the bleeding patient has a prolonged PTT, it is mixed 1:1 with normal plasma with a factor VIII activity near 100%. If no inhibitor is present, the mixture should produce a normal or near-normal PTT result because the mixture contains excess (at least 50%) factor VIII activity from the normal plasma. If an inhibitor is present, however, the factor VIII from the normal plasma is partially neutralized, and the mixture's PTT remains prolonged or "uncorrected." Because factor VIII inhibitors are warm-reacting antibodies, the mixture must be incubated at 37° C for 1 to 2 hours before performing the PTT.

If mixing studies and the clinical picture suggest a factor VIII inhibitor, a Bethesda assay is used to quantitate the inhibitor. Normal plasma with 100% factor activity is mixed at increasing dilutions in a series of tubes with the full-strength test plasma. Factor VIII assays are performed on each mixture, and the operator compares the results of the various dilutions and expresses the titer as Bethesda units. One Bethesda unit is the reciprocal of the dilution that caused neutralization of 50% of the factor VIII from the normal control plasma. The same assay is employed to measure factor VIII inhibitors in acquired hemophilia. Although the complex kinetics of acquired autoantibodies diminishes the accuracy of the results, this method is adequate to monitor therapy.

Hemophiliacs with inhibitors may be low or high responders. Low responders have titers of 5 Bethesda units or fewer, and their titers do not increase significantly after factor VIII administration. High responders have inhibitors that exceed 5 Bethesda units, and the titer increases anamnestically after therapy.[67] Each laboratory may choose to maintain a database of hemophilia patients with inhibitors because previous titers may predict behavior after therapy in the future.

Treatment of Hemophilia A Patients with Inhibitors

Every hemophiliac with an inhibitor needs an individualized treatment plan to control bleeding episodes. Low responders often stop bleeding on administration of large doses of factor VIII concentrate and may be so maintained. High responders may gain no benefit and instead are treated with plasma-derived concentrates of activated vitamin K–dependent factors, called *activated prothrombin complex concentrates.* These generate thrombin in the presence of factor VIII inhibitors. Dosing of the most commonly used activated prothrombin complex concentrate, factor VIII inhibitor bypassing activity (Feiba VH Immuno, Baxter Healthcare, Deerfield, Ill.), depends on the degree of bleeding but should not exceed 200 U/kg of body weight/day, distributed in two to four injections, because the activated factors may trigger DIC. Recombinant activated factor VII (VIIa) also bypasses the physiologic factor VIII requirement because it promotes thrombin formation through the tissue factor pathway.[68]

Hemophilia B–Factor IX Deficiency

Hemophilia B, also called *Christmas disease,* represents approximately 14% of hemophilia cases in the United States, although its incidence in India nearly equals that of hemophilia A. Hemophilia B is caused by deficiency of factor IX, one of the vitamin K–dependent serine proteases. Factor IX is a substrate for factors XI and VII because it is cleaved by either to form dimeric factor IXa (Fig. 41-5). Subsequently, factor IXa complexes with factor VIIIa to cleave and activate its substrate, factor X. Factor IX deficiency reduces thrombin production and causes soft tissue bleeding indistinguishable from hemophilia A. It also is a sex-linked, markedly heterogeneous disorder with more than 220 separate mutations resulting in a range of mild-to-severe bleeding manifestations. Determination of the carrier status of hemophilia B is less successful than in hemophilia A because of the large number of factor IX mutations and the lack of a linked molecule such as VWF to be used as a normalization index. DNA analysis occasionally may be used to establish carrier status when hemophilia B has been diagnosed and its specific mutation identified in a relative.

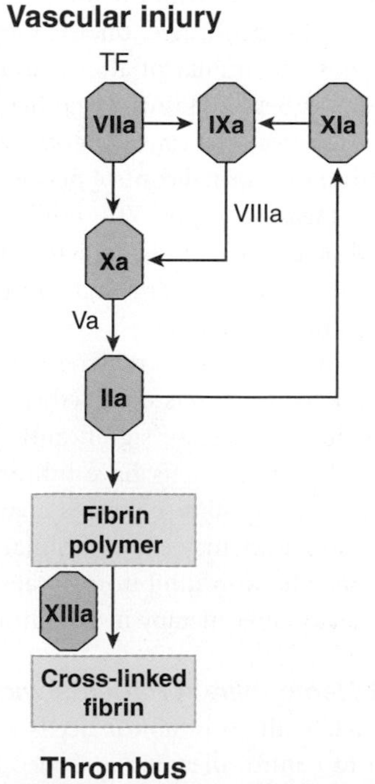

In the laboratory diagnosis of hemophilia B, the PTT typically is prolonged, whereas the PT is normal.[69] In the case of suspicious clinical symptoms, the factor assay should be performed despite a normal PTT result because the PTT reagent may be insensitive to mild factor IX deficiency.

Recombinant or monoclonal antibody column-purified plasma-derived factor IX concentrates are used to treat hemophilia B. Dosing is calculated as for factor VIII concentrates with the difference that the calculated initial dose is doubled to compensate for factor IX distribution to the extravascular space. Repeat doses of factor IX are given every 24 hours, reflecting the half-life of the factor. The second and subsequent doses, if needed, are half the initial dosage, provided that factor assays determine the target level of factor IX was achieved.

Inhibitors to factor IX arise in only 3% of hemophilia B patients. Such alloantibodies react rapidly with factor IX and may be detected using the Bethesda assay. Treatment of bleeding in the presence of inhibitors is accomplished as for patients with factor VIII inhibitors, with activated prothrombin complex concentrates or recombinant factor VIIa concentrate.

Hemophilia C–Rosenthal Syndrome, Factor XI Deficiency

Factor XI deficiency is an autosomal dominant hemophilia with mild-to-moderate bleeding symptoms. More than half of the cases have been described in Ashkenazi Jews, but individuals of any ethnic group may be affected. The frequency and severity of bleeding episodes do not correlate with factor XI levels, and laboratory monitoring of treatment serves little purpose after the diagnosis is established. The physician treats hemophilia C with frequent infusions of FFP during times of hemostatic challenge.[70]

Other Congenital Single-Factor Deficiencies

The remaining congenital single-factor deficiencies listed in Table 41-7 are rare, caused by autosomal recessive mutations, and often associated with consanguinity. The PT, PTT, and thrombin time may be employed to distinguish among these disorders, as shown in Table 41-6. In addition, immunoassays may be performed to distinguish among the more prevalent quantitative and the less prevalent qualitative abnormalities. In qualitative disorders, often called *dysproteinemias,* such as dysfibrinogenemia or dysprothrombinemia, the ratio of factor activity to antigen is less than 0.7. The bleeding symptoms in the dysproteinemias may be more severe than in quantitative deficiencies, but the risk of inhibitor formation is theoretically lower. The clot-based measurement of prothrombin and factor X may be supplemented by more reproducible chromogenic substrate assays. Fibrinogen is usually measured using the Clauss assay, a modification of the thrombin time, but may be measured turbidimetrically or by immunoassay.

Vascular injury

Figure 41-5 Simplified coagulation cascade mechanism showing positions of all factors whose absence may cause hemorrhage.

TABLE 41-7 Rare Congenital Single-Factor Deficiencies

Deficiency	Factor Levels	Symptoms	Therapy
Afibrinogenemia	No measurable fibrinogen	Severe anatomic bleeding	Cryoprecipitate to increase to >100 mg/dL
Hypofibrinogenemia	Fibrinogen activity assay <100 mg/dL	Moderate systemic bleeding	Cryoprecipitate to increase to >100 mg/dL
Dysfibrinogenemia	Fibrinogen activity assay <100 mg/dL	Mild systemic bleeding	Cryoprecipitate to increase to >100 mg/dL
Prothrombin deficiency	Factor II <30%	Mild systemic bleeding	PCC to increase level to 75%
Factor V deficiency	Factor V <30%	Mild systemic bleeding	FFP to increase factor to 75%
Factor VII deficiency	Factor VII <30%	Moderate to severe anatomic bleeding	FFP, activated factor VII concentrate
Factor X deficiency	Factor X <30%	Severe anatomic bleeding	PCC to increase level to 75%
Factor XI deficiency	Factor XI <50%	Anatomic bleeding	FFP to increase factor to 75%
Factor XIII deficiency	Factor XIII <1%	Moderate to severe systemic bleeding, poor wound healing	FFP or cryoprecipitate every 3 wk

PCC, prothrombin complex concentrate; FFPs, fresh frozen plasma.

Because platelets transport about 20% of circulating factor V, the platelet function in *factor V deficiency* may be diminished, reflected in a prolonged bleeding time but normal platelet aggregation.[71] The PT and PTT are prolonged. A combined factor V and VIII deficiency may be caused by a genetic defect traced to chromosome 18 that affects transport of both factors by a common protein in the Golgi apparatus.[72]

Factor VII deficiency causes moderate-to-severe anatomic hemorrhage that does not necessarily reflect the factor VII activity level. The half-life of factor VII is less than 6 hours, affecting the frequency of therapy. Prothrombin complex concentrate and activated factor VIIa preparations are effective and may provide a target level of 10% to 30%. Many factor VII deficiencies are dysproteinemias.[73] Only the PT is prolonged in factor VII deficiency.

Factor X deficiency causes moderate-to-severe anatomic hemorrhage that may be treated with FFP or prothrombin complex concentrate to reach therapeutic levels of 10% to 40%.[74] The half-life of factor X is 24 to 40 hours. Acquired factor X deficiency has been described in amyloidosis, in paraproteinemia, and in association with antifungal drugs. The hemorrhagic symptoms are severe and life-threatening. The PT and PTT are prolonged in factor X deficiency. The Russell viper venom time test, which activates the coagulation mechanism at the level of factor X, is prolonged in deficiencies of factors X and V, prothrombin, and fibrinogen. This test may be useful in distinguishing a factor VII deficiency, which does not affect it, from deficiencies in the common pathway, although specific factor assays are the standard approach.

Plasma factor XIII is a tetramer of paired α and β monomers. The intracellular form is a homodimer (two α chains) and is stored in platelets, monocytes, the placenta, the prostate, and the uterus. The α chain contains the active enzyme site, and the β chain is a binding and stabilizing portion. Factor XIII deficiency occurs in three forms related to the affected chain, as shown in Table 41-8. Patients with factor XIII deficiency have normal PT, PTT, and thrombin time despite anatomic bleeds and poor wound healing. They form weak (non–cross-linked) clots that dissolve within 2 hours when suspended in a 5 M urea solution, the standard factor XIII screening assay. To confirm factor XIII deficiency, factor activity may be measured accurately using a chromogenic substrate assay.

Finally, autosomal deficiencies of the fibrinolytic regulatory proteins α_2-antiplasmin and plasminogen activator inhibitor-1 have been reported to cause moderate to severe bleeding. Both are rare and may be diagnosed using chromogenic substrate assays.

TABLE 41-8 Factor XIII Deficiency

Type of Deficiency	Incidence	Factor XIII Activity	β-Protein	α-Protein
I	Rare	Absent	Absent	Absent
II	Frequent	Absent	Normal	Low
III	Rare	Low	Absent	Low

CHAPTER at a GLANCE

- Hemorrhage can be classified as localized versus generalized, acquired versus congenital, and anatomic soft tissue versus mucocutaneous.
- Acquired hemorrhagic disorders that are diagnosed in the hemostasis laboratory include thrombocytopenia of various etiologies, liver and renal disease, vitamin K deficiency, scurvy, acquired hemophilia or VWD, and DIC.
- VWD is the most common congenital bleeding disorder, and the diagnosis and classification of the type and subtypes require a series of clinical laboratory assays.

- The hemophilias are congenital single-factor deficiencies that cause moderate to severe anatomic hemorrhage. The clinical laboratory plays a key role in the diagnosis, classification, and treatment monitoring of the hemophiliac patient.

Now that you have completed this chapter, go back and read again the case study at the beginning and respond to the questions presented.

REVIEW QUESTIONS

1. What is the most common acquired bleeding disorder?
   a. VWD
   b. Vitamin K deficiency
   c. Liver disease
   d. Hemophilia

2. To what factor deficiency is the PT most sensitive?
   a. Prothrombin
   b. VII
   c. VIII
   d. IX

3. Which of the following conditions causes a prolonged thrombin time?
   a. Prothrombin deficiency
   b. Antithrombin deficiency
   c. Hypofibrinogenemia
   d. Warfarin therapy

4. In hemophilia A, which of the following statements about cross-reacting material positive (CRM$^+$) and cross-reacting material negative (CRM$^-$) status is correct?
   a. CRM$^+$ means a qualitative factor defect.
   b. CRM$^+$ means a quantitative factor deficiency.
   c. CRM$^-$ means a qualitative factor defect.
   d. CRM$^-$ means the ratio of quantitative assay to qualitative assay is less than 1.

5. The typical treatment for vitamin K deficiency when the patient is bleeding is Vitamin K and:
   a. FFP
   b. Factor VIIa concentrate
   c. Factor VIII concentrate
   d. Prothrombin complex concentrate

6. If a patient has anatomic soft tissue bleeding and poor wound healing, but the PT, PTT, thrombin time, platelet count, and platelet functional assay results are normal, what factor deficiency could exist?
   a. Fibrinogen
   b. Prothrombin
   c. Factor XII
   d. Factor XIII

7. What therapy may be used for a hemophilic boy who is bleeding and who has a high-titer factor VIII inhibitor?
   a. Cryoprecipitate
   b. FFP
   c. Factor VIII concentrate
   d. Activated prothrombin complex concentrate

8. A patient with suspected VWD has a normal level of VWF antigen but reduced VWF activity. This pattern of test results is consistent with which subtype?
   a. Type 1
   b. Type 2A
   c. Type 3
   d. Type 2N (Normandy)

9. Which of the following assays can be used to distinguish vitamin K deficiency from liver disease?
   a. Factor V assay
   b. Prothrombin time
   c. Factor VII assay
   d. Protein C assay

10. Mucocutaneous hemorrhage is typical of:
    a. Acquired hemorrhagic disorders
    b. Localized hemorrhagic disorders
    c. Defects in primary hemostasis
    d. Defects in fibrinolysis

REFERENCES

1. Hathaway WE, Goodnight SH: Evaluation of bleeding tendency in the outpatient child and adult. In Hathaway WE, Goodnight SH (eds): Disorders of Hemostasis and Thrombosis. New York: McGraw-Hill, 2001:52-60.
2. Liu MC, Kessler CM: A systematic approach to the bleeding patient. In Kitchens CS, Alving BM, Kessler CS (eds): Consultative Hemostasis and Thrombosis. Philadelphia: Saunders, 2002:27-40.
3. Miller R, Beeton K, Goldman E, et al: Counseling guidelines for managing musculoskeletal problems in haemophilia in the 1990s. Haemophilia 1977;3:9-13.
4. Kitchens CS: Purpura and related hematovascular lesions. In Kitchens CS, Alving BM, Kessler CS (eds): Consultative Hemostasis and Thrombosis. Philadelphia: Saunders, 2002:149-164.
5. Bowie EJ, Owen CA: Clinical and laboratory diagnosis of hemorrhagic disorders. In Ratnoff OD, Forbes CD (eds): Disorders of Hemostasis, 3rd ed. Philadelphia: Saunders, 1996:53-78.
6. Cattaneo M, Bettega D, Lombardi R, et al: Sustained correction of the bleeding time in an afibrinogenaemic patient after infusion of fresh frozen plasma. Br J Haematol 1992;82:388-390.
7. Friedberg RC, Donnelly SF, Boyd JC, et al: Clinical and blood bank factors in the management of platelet refractoriness and alloimmunization. Blood 1993;81:3428-3434.
8. Hathaway WE, Goodnight SH: Screening tests of hemostasis. In Hathaway WE, Goodnight SH (eds): Disorders of Hemostasis and Thrombosis. New York: McGraw-Hill, 2001:41-51.
9. McKinley L, Wrenn K: Are baseline prothrombin time/partial thromboplastin time values necessary before instituting anticoagulation? Ann Emerg Med 1993;22:697-702.
10. Weiss AE: Acquired coagulation disorders. In Corriveau DM, Fritsma GA (eds): Hemostasis and Thrombosis in the Clinical Laboratory. Philadelphia: Lippincott, 1988:169-205.
11. Robert A, Chazouilleres O: Prothrombin time in liver failure: time, ratio, activity percentage, or international normalized ratio? Hepatology 1996;24:1392-1394.
12. Glueck HI, Will RM, McAdams AJ: Measurement of prothrombin: a neglected liver function test in infancy and childhood. J Pediatr 1970;76:914-922.
13. Ragni MV: Liver disease, organ transplantation, and hemostasis. In Kitchens CS, Alving BM, Kessler CS (eds): Consultative Hemostasis and Thrombosis. Philadelphia: Saunders, 2002:481-491.
14. Ratnoff OD: Hemostatic defects in liver and biliary tract disease and disorders of vitamin K metabolism. In Ratnoff OD, Forbes CD (eds): Disorders of Hemostasis, 3rd ed. Philadelphia: Saunders, 1996:422-442.
15. Dymock IW, Tucher JS, Woolf IL, et al: Coagulation studies as a prognostic index in acute liver failure. Br J Haematol 1975;29:385-395.
16. Lechner K, Niessner H, Thaler E: Coagulation abnormalities in liver disease. Semin Thromb Hemost 1977;4:40.
17. Walls WE, Losowsky MS: The hemostatic defect of liver disease. Gastroenterology 1971;60:108-119.
18. Green G, Poller L, Thomson JM, et al: Factor VII as a marker of hepatocellular synthetic function in liver disease. J Clin Pathol 1976;29:971.
19. Wilson DB, Salen H, Mruk J, et al: Biosynthesis of coagulation factor V by a human hepatocellular carcinoma line. J Clin Invest 1984;73:654-657.
20. Bovill EG: Liver diseases. In Hathaway WE, Goodnight SH (eds): Disorders of Hemostasis and Thrombosis, 2nd ed. New York: McGraw-Hill, 2001:226-236.
21. Elias A, Aptel I, Huc B, et al: D-dimer test and diagnosis of deep vein thrombosis: a comparative study of 7 assays. Thromb Haemost 1996;76:518-522.
22. Schwartz RS, Bauer KA, Rosenberg, RD, et al: Clinical experience with antithrombin III concentrate in treatment of congenital and acquired deficiency of antithrombin. Am J Med 1989;87(Suppl 3b):53S-60S.
23. Dettenmeier P, Swindell B, Stroud M, et al: Role of activated protein C in the pathophysiology of severe sepsis. Am J Crit Care 2003;12:518-524.
24. Saito H: Alterations of hemostasis in renal disease. In Ratnoff OD, Forbes CD (eds): Disorders of Hemostasis, 3rd ed. Philadelphia: Saunders, 1996:443-456.
25. Rabiner SF: Uremic bleeding. Prog Hemost Thromb 1972; 1:233-250.
26. Leng SX, Elias JA: Interleukin-11. Int J Biochem Cell Biol 1997;29:1059-1062.
27. Ambuhl PM, Wuthrich RP, Korte W, et al: Plasma hypercoagulability in haemodialysis patients: impact of dialysis and anticoagulation. Nephrol Dial Transplant 1997;12:2355-2364.
28. Lind SE: The bleeding time does not predict surgical bleeding. Blood 1991;77:2547-2552.
29. Akizawa T, Kinugasa E, Kitaoka T, et al: Effects of recombinant human erythropoietin and correction of anemia on platelet function in hemodialysis patients. Nephron 1991;58:400-406.
30. Brunzel NA: Renal and metabolic disease. In Fundamentals of Urine and Body Fluid Analysis, 2nd ed. Philadelphia: Saunders, 2002:271-310.
31. Kauffmann R, Veltkamp J, van Tilburg N, et al: Acquired antithrombin III deficiency and thrombosis in the nephrotic syndrome. Am J Med 1978;298:562-571.
32. Bleyer WA, Hakami N, Shepard TH: The development of hemostasis in the human fetus and newborn infant. J Pediatr 1971;79:838-853.
33. Zipursky A, Desa D, Hsu E, et al: Clinical and laboratory diagnosis of hemostatic disorders in newborn infants. Am J Pediatr Hematol Oncol 1979;1:217-226.
34. Friedman PA: Vitamin K-dependent proteins. N Engl J Med 1984;310:1458-1460.
35. Green D: Spontaneous inhibitors to coagulation factors. Clin Lab Haematol 2000;22 (Suppl 1):21-25.
36. Biggs R, Austen DEG, Denson DWE, et al: The mode of action of antibodies which destroy factor VIII: II. antibodies which give complex concentration graphs. Br J Haematol 1972; 23:137.
37. Miesbach W, Matthias T, Scharrer I: Identification of thrombin antibodies in patients with antiphospholipid syndrome. Ann N Y Acad Sci 2005;1050:250-256.
38. Krumdieck R, Shaw DR, Huang ST, et al: Hemorrhagic disorder due to an isoniazid-associated acquired factor XIII inhibitor in a patient with Waldenstrom's macroglobulinemia. Am J Med 1991;90:639-645.
39. Shapiro SS, Hultin M: Acquired inhibitors to the blood coagulation factors. Semin Thromb Hemost 1975;1:336-385.
40. Israels SJ, Israels ED: Development of antibodies to bovine and human factor V in two children after exposure to topical bovine thrombin. Am J Pediatr Hematol Oncol 1994;16:249-254.
41. Barker B, Altuntas F, Paranjape G, et al: Presurgical plasma exchange is ineffective in correcting amyloid associated factor X deficiency. J Clin Apheresis 2004;19:208-210.
42. von Depka M: Immune tolerance therapy in patients with acquired hemophilia. Hematology 2004;9:245-257.
43. Zimmerman TS, Ruggeri ZM: von Willebrand disease. Clin Haematol 1983;12:175-200.
44. Kumar S, Pruthri RK, Nichols WL: Acquired von Willebrand disease. Mayo Clin Proc 2002;77:181-187.

45. Gill JC, Endres-Brooks J, Bauer PJ, et al: The effect of ABO blood group on the diagnosis of von Willebrand disease. Blood 1987;69:1691-1695.

46. Sadler JE: von Willebrand factor. J Biol Chem 1991;266:22777-22780.

47. Miller JL: von Willebrand disease. Hematol Oncol Clin N Am 1990;4:107-123.

48. Ginsburg D, Sadler JE: von Willebrand disease: a database of point mutations, insertions and deletions. For the Consortium on von Willebrand Factor Mutations and Polymorphisms, and the Subcommittee on von Willebrand Factor of the Scientific and Standardization Committee of the International Society of Thrombosis and Haemostasis. Thromb Haemost 1993; 69:177-184.

49. Ginsburg D, Bowie EJW: Molecular genetics of von Willebrand disease. Blood 1992;79:2507-2519.

50. Lee CA, Abdul-Kadir R: von Willebrand disease and women's health. Semin Hematol 2005;42:42-48.

51. Rosenfeld SJ, Gralnick HR: von Willebrand's disease. In Ratnoff OD, Forbes CD (eds): Disorders of Hemostasis. Philadelphia: Saunders, 1996:186-207.

52. Sadler JE: A revised classification of von Willebrand disease. Thromb Haemost 1994;71:520-525.

53. Schneppenheim R, Budde U: Phenotypic and genotypic diagnosis of von Willebrand disease: a 2004 update. Semin Hematol 2005;42:15-28.

54. Sadler JE, Rodeghiero F, on behalf of the ISTH SSC Subcommittee on von Willebrand Factor: Provisional criteria for the diagnosis of VWD type 1. J Thromb Haemost 2005;3:775-777.

55. Favaloro EJ, Bonar R, Kershaw G, et al; Royal College of Pathologists of Australasia Quality Assurance Program in Haematology: Laboratory diagnosis of von Willebrand disorder: use of multiple functional assays reduces diagnostic error rates. Lab Hematol 2005;11:91-97.

56. Rodeghiero F, Castaman G: Treatment of von Willebrand disease. Semin Hematol 2005;42:29-35.

57. DiMichelle DM: Hemophilia A (FVIII deficiency). In Hathaway WE, Goodnight SH (eds): Disorders of Hemostasis and Thrombosis, 2nd ed. New York: McGraw-Hill, 2001:127-139.

58. Forbes CD: Clinical aspects of the genetic disorders of coagulation. In Ratnoff OD, Forbes CD (eds): Disorders of Hemostasis. Philadelphia: Saunders, 1996:138-185.

59. Weiss AE: The hemophilias. In Corriveau DM, Fritsma GA (eds): Hemostasis and Thrombosis in the Clinical Laboratory. Philadelphia: Lippincott, 1988:128-168.

60. Lusher JM, Warrier I: Hemophilia A. Hematol Oncol Clin N Am 1992;6:1021-1033.

61. Peake IR, Lillicrap DP, Boulyjenkov V, et al: Hemophilia: strategies for carrier detection and prenatal diagnosis. Bull World Health Organization 1993;71:429-458.

62. Rossetti LC, Radic CP, Larripa IB, et al: Genotyping the hemophilia inversion hotspot by use of inverse PCR. Clin Chem 2005;51:1154-1158.

63. Nilsson IN, Berntop E, Lofqvist T, et al: Five years experience of prophylactic treatment in severe hemophilia A and B. J Intern Med 1992;232:25-32.

64. Lusher JM, Arkin S, Abildgaard CF, et al: Recombinant factor VIII for the treatment of previously untreated patients with hemophilia A. N Engl J Med 1993;328:453-457.

65. Kessler CM, Gill JC, White GC, et al: B-domain deleted recombinant factor VIII preparations are bioequivalent to a monoclonal antibody purified plasma-derived factor VIII concentrate: a randomized, three-way crossover study. Haemophilia 2005;11:84-91.

66. Bray GL, Gomperts ED, Courter S, et al: A multicenter study of recombinant factor VIII (Recombinate): safety, efficacy, and inhibitor risk in previously untreated patients with hemophilia A. Blood 1994;83:2428-2437.

67. McMillan EW, Shapiro SS, Whitehurst D, et al: The natural history of factor VIII inhibitors in patients with hemophilia A: a national cooperative study: II. Observations on the initial development of factor VIII inhibitors. Blood 1988;71:344-348.

68. Franchini M, Zaffanello M, Veneri D: Recombinant factor VIIa: an update on its clinical use. Thromb Haemost 2005;93:1027-1035.

69. Kessler CM, Mariani G: Clinical manifestations and therapy of the hemophilias. In Colman RW, Marder VJ, Clowes AW, et al (eds): Hemostasis and Thrombosis, 5th ed. Philadelphia: Lippincott Williams & Wilkins, 2006: 887-905.

70. Walsh PN, Gailani D: Factor XI. In Colman RW, Marder VJ, Clowes AW, et al (eds): Hemostasis and Thrombosis, Basic Principles and Clinical Practice, 5th ed. Philadelphia: Lippincott, Williams & Wilkins, 2006:221-35.

71. Miletich JP, Majerus DW, Majerus PW: Patients with congenital factor V deficiency have decreased factor Xa binding sites on their platelets. J Clin Invest 1978;62:824-831.

72. Nichols WC, Seligsohn U, Zivelin A, et al: Linkage of combined factors V and VIII deficiency to chromosome 18q by homozygosity mapping. J Clin Invest 1997;596-601.

73. Chaing S, Clarke B, Sridhara S, et al: Severe factor VII deficiency caused by mutations abolishing the cleavage site for activation and altering binding to tissue factor. Blood 1994; 83:3524-3535.

74. Fair DS, Edgington TS: Heterogeneity of hereditary and acquired factor X deficiencies by combined immunochemical and functional analyses. Br J Haematol 1985;59:235-248.

Thrombosis Risk Testing

42

George A. Fritsma and Marisa B. Marques

OBJECTIVES

After completion of this chapter, the reader will be able to:

1. Describe the prevalence of thrombotic disease in developed countries.
2. Define thrombophilia.
3. Distinguish between venous and arterial thrombosis.
4. Discern among acquired thrombosis risk factors related to lifestyle and disease and congenital risk factors, noting which can be assessed in the hemostasis laboratory.
5. Discuss in relative terms, such as "most common" or "uncommon," the frequency with which ethnic groups are affected by various heritable risk factors.
6. Show how a hemostasis laboratory scientist may communicate with clinicians on the use of thrombosis risk profiles and screens.
7. List and employ the predictors of arterial thrombotic disease, such as high-sensitivity C-reactive protein, homocysteine, fibrinogen, lipoprotein (a), and factor assays to assess thrombotic risk.
8. Offer a sequence of lupus anticoagulant antibody testing that provides the greatest diagnostic validity, and interpret the results of the testing.
9. Develop, perform, and report an antithrombin testing protocol.
10. List and employ tests of the protein C pathway, including protein C and protein S activity and concentration, activated protein C resistance, and the factor V Leiden assay, to assess thrombotic risk.
11. Explain the molecular test for prothrombin 20210A mutation and its relationship to venous thrombosis, and interpret given test results.
12. Describe the causes and pathophysiology of disseminated intravascular coagulation (DIC).
13. List and employ a primary test profile for diagnosis and management of DIC in an acute care facility.
14. Discuss the value of quantitative D-dimer assays.
15. Describe the efficacy of the localized thrombosis monitors prothrombin fragment 1+2, fibrinopeptide A, and thrombin-antithrombin complex.
16. Describe the cause and clinical significance of heparin-induced thrombocytopenia (HIT).
17. Describe the clinical diagnosis, laboratory diagnosis, and management of HIT.

CASE STUDY

After studying the material in this chapter, the reader should be able to respond to the following case study:

A 42-year-old woman with no significant past medical history developed sudden onset of shortness of breath and chest pain. She was taken to an emergency department where she was diagnosed with a pulmonary embolism. After admission, she was treated with intravenous heparin and given a hypercoagulability workup.

1. What conditions can be tested for while she is in the hospital?
2. What is the most common acquired risk factor for thrombosis?
3. What is the implication of the possibility of diagnosing a congenital risk factor for thrombosis in this patient?

DEVELOPMENTS IN THROMBOSIS TESTING

Before 1992, clinical laboratory scientists assayed only three proven venous thrombosis risk factors: antithrombin, protein C, and protein S deficiencies.[1] Taken together, these three markers accounted for no more than 7% of cases of recurrent venous thrombotic disease and bore no relationship to arterial thrombosis. Since the report by Dahlback et al[2] of activated protein C (APC) resistance in 1993 and the characterization by Bertina et al[3] of the factor V Leiden (FVL) mutation as its cause in 1994, efforts devoted to thrombosis prediction and evaluation have redefined the hemostasis laboratory. The list of new tests includes APC resistance, FVL mutation, prothrombin 20210A mutation, factor VIII activity, and lupus anticoagulant (LA) and anticardiolipin (ACL) antibodies for venous thrombosis and tissue plasminogen activator (TPA), plasminogen activator inhibitor 1 (PAI-1), high-sensitivity C-reactive protein, lipoprotein (a), plasma homocysteine, and tests for platelet activity such as urinary 11-dehydro thromboxane B_2 for arterial thrombosis. The past decade also has seen technical improvements in the diagnostic accuracy of integrated LA identification kits and D-dimers and tests for coagulation activation markers, such as prothrombin fragment 1+2 (PF 1+2) and thrombin-antithrombin (TAT) complex.[4] In addition, old tests, such as the fibrinogen assay and the factor VIII assay, have been applied to prediction of venous and arterial thrombotic risk.

INTRODUCTION TO THROMBOSIS

Etiology of Thrombosis

Thrombosis is a multifaceted disorder resulting from abnormalities in blood flow such as stasis, the coagulation system, platelet function, leukocyte activation molecules, and the blood vessel wall. Thrombosis is the inappropriate formation of platelet or fibrin clots that obstruct blood vessels. These obstructions cause ischemia and necrosis.[5] Thrombophilia is the predisposition to thrombosis secondary to a congenital or acquired disorder. The theoretical causes of thrombophilia are the following:

- Physical, chemical, or biologic events such as chronic or acute inflammation that release prothrombotic mediators from damaged blood vessels or suppress blood vessel production of normal antithrombotic substances
- Inappropriate and uncontrolled platelet activation
- Uncontrolled triggering of the plasma coagulation system
- Inadequate control of coagulation-impaired fibrinolysis

Prevalence of Thrombosis

At least 30% of the world's people are expected to die of a thrombotic condition, and 25% of initial thrombotic events are fatal.[6] Many fatal thromboses go undiagnosed before autopsy.

Prevalence of Venous Thrombosis

The annual incidence of venous thrombosis in the unselected U.S. population is 1 in 1000.[7,8] This includes the comparatively innocent thrombosis of superficial leg veins and the more dangerous deep vein thrombosis that form in the iliac, popliteal, and femoral veins of the upper legs and calves.[9] Large occlusive thrombi also may form, although less often, in the veins of the upper extremities, liver, spleen, intestines, brain, and kidneys. The symptoms of thrombosis include the sensation of heat, localized pain, redness, and swelling. In deep vein thrombosis, the entire leg swells.

Fragments, called *emboli*, may separate from the proximal end of a venous thrombus, move swiftly through the right chambers of the heart, and lodge in the arterial pulmonary vasculature, causing ischemia and death of lung tissue.[10] Nearly 95% of these pulmonary emboli arise from thrombi in the deep leg and calf veins. Of the 250,000 cases of pulmonary emboli that occur in the United States annually, 10% to 15% of the victims die within 3 months. Many pulmonary emboli go undiagnosed because of the uncertainty of the symptoms. Coagulation system imbalances, such as inappropriate activation, gain of coagulation factor function, inadequate control, or fibrinolysis, are the mechanisms most often implicated in venous thrombosis.[11]

Prevalence of Arterial Thrombosis

Cardiovascular disease causes 500,000 premature deaths annually in the United States; 500,000 cerebrovascular accidents result in 100,000 stroke-related deaths. About 80% of heart attacks and 85% of strokes are caused by thrombi that block coronary arteries or carotid end arteries of the vertebrobasilar system.[12] Transient ischemic attacks and peripheral arterial occlusions are more frequent than strokes and coronary artery disease and, although not fatal, may cause substantial morbidity.

One important mechanism for arterial thrombosis is the well-described atherosclerotic plaque formation in the vessel walls. Activated platelets, monocytes, and macrophages embed the plaque within the endothelial lining, suppressing the normal release of antithrombotic molecules such as nitric oxide and exposing prothrombotic substances such as tissue factor. Small unstable plaques rupture, occluding arteries and releasing thrombotic mediators to trigger thrombotic events. Activated platelets also form arterial platelet plugs with minimal fibrin, the "white thrombi" that cause death of surrounding tissue.

The hemostasis-related lesions we associate with arterial thrombosis are blood vessel wall destruction and platelet activation. Often these are inseparable. Researchers currently are examining new thrombosis markers that capture pathologic events in platelets and endothelial cells before a thrombotic event occurs.

THROMBOSIS RISK FACTORS

Acquired Thrombosis Risk Factors

In life, individuals acquire a legion of habits and conditions that may maintain or damage their hemostasis systems. Their multiplicity makes it difficult to pinpoint precisely the factors that contribute to thrombosis or to determine which have the greatest influence. These factors seem to contribute to venous and arterial thrombosis in varying degrees. Table 42-1 lists the nondisease risk factors implicated in thrombosis.[13]

Thrombosis Risk Factors Associated with Systemic Diseases

In addition to life events, several conditions threaten individuals with thrombosis. Some are listed in Table 42-2, with reference to the laboratory's diagnostic contribution.[14]

Together, transient and chronic antiphospholipid (APL) antibodies may be detected in 1% of the unselected population. Chronic APL antibodies confer a risk of venous or arterial thrombosis—a condition called the *antiphospholipid syndrome* (APS). Chronic APL antibodies often accompany autoimmune connective tissue disorders, such as lupus erythematosus; some appear in patients without any apparent underlying morbidity.

Malignancies often are implicated in venous thrombosis. One mechanism is tumor production of tissue factor analogues that trigger chronic low-grade disseminated intravascular coagulation (DIC).[15] In addition, stasis and inflammatory effects increase the risk of thrombosis. Migratory thrombophlebitis, or Trousseau syndrome, is a sign of occult adenocarcinoma such as cancer of the pancreas or colon.[16]

Myeloproliferative disorders such as essential thrombocythemia and polycythemia vera may trigger thrombosis, probably through platelet hyperactivity. A cardinal sign of acute promyelocytic leukemia is DIC secondary to the release of procoagulant granules from the malignant promyelocytes. DIC can intensify during therapy at the time of vigorous cell lysis.[17]

Paroxysmal nocturnal hemoglobinuria is a stem cell mutation that seems to destroy membrane-anchored platelet activation suppressors. Venous or arterial thromboses occur in at least 40% of cases.[18]

Chronic inflammatory diseases cause thrombosis through a variety of mechanisms, such as elevated fibrinogen and factor VIII, decreased fibrinolysis, promotion of atherosclerotic plaque formation, or reduced free protein S activity secondary to increased C4b-binding protein (C4bBP). Diabetes mellitus is a particularly dangerous chronic inflammatory condition, increasing the risk of cardiovascular disease sixfold. Conditions associated with venous stasis, such as congestive heart failure, also are common risk factors for venous thrombosis. Untreated atrial fibrillation increases the risk of ischemic strokes due to clot formation in the right atrium and embolization to the brain.[19] Nephrotic syndrome creates protein imbalances that lead to thrombosis through loss of plasma procoagulants.

Congenital Thrombosis Risk Factors

Congenital thrombophilia is suspected when a thrombotic event occurs in young adults; occurs in unusual sites such as the mesenteric, renal, or axillary veins; is recurrent; or occurs in a patient who has a positive family history (Table 42-3).[20] Because thrombosis is multifactorial, however, even patients with congenital thrombophilia are most likely to experience thrombotic disease because of a combination of constitutional and acquired conditions.[21]

TABLE 42-1 Nondisease, or Lifestyle, Risk Factors That Contribute to Thrombotic Disease

Risk Factor	Comment	Contribution to Thrombosis	Laboratory Diagnosis
Age	Thrombosis after age 50	Risk doubles by decade	—
Immobilization	Distance driving, air travel, wheelchair, bedrest, obesity	Decreased blood flow	—
Diet	Fatty foods; inadequate folate, vitamin B_6, and vitamin B_{12}	Homocysteinemia: relative risk of 2-7× for arterial or venous thrombosis	Plasma homocysteine, vitamin levels, and lipid profile
Lipid metabolism imbalance	Hyperlipidemia, hypercholesterolemia, dyslipidemia, lipoprotein (a) elevation, HDL-C decreased, LDL-C elevated	Varied risk: moderate thrombosis association with hypercholesterolemia alone; may be congenital	Lipid profiles: total cholesterol, HDL-C, LDL-C, triglycerides, and lipoprotein (a)
Oral contraceptives	30 µg, formulation with progesterone	4-6×	—
Pregnancy	—	3-5×	—
Hormone replacement therapy	—	2-4×	—
Femoral and tibial fractures	—	80% incidence of thrombosis if not treated with anticoagulant	—
Hip, knee, gynecologic, prostate surgery	—	50% incidence of thrombosis if not treated with anticoagulant	—
Smoking	—	Depends on degree	hsCRP, fibrinogen
Inflammation	Chronic or acute	Arterial thrombosis	hsCRP, fibrinogen
Central venous catheter	Endothelial injury and activation	33% of children with central venous lines develop venous thrombosis	—

hsCRP, high-sensitivity C-reactive protein.

TABLE 42-2 Diseases with Thrombotic Risk Components

Disease	Comment	Contribution to Thrombosis	Laboratory Diagnosis
Antiphospholipid syndrome	Chronic antiphospholipid antibody often secondary to autoimmune disorders	1.6-3.2× risk when chronic: stroke, myocardial infarction, recurrent spontaneous abortion, venous thrombosis	Mixing studies, lupus anticoagulant profile, anticardiolipin antibody and anti-β_2-GPI immunoassay
Myeloproliferative disorders	Essential thrombocythemia, polycythemia vera	Plasma viscosity, platelet activation	Platelet counts and aggregometry
Hepatic and renal disorders	Diminished production or loss of control proteins	Deranged coagulation pathways	Protein C, protein S, and antithrombin assays; factor assays
Cancer	Trousseau syndrome, low-grade chronic DIC	20× risk of thrombosis; 10-20% of people with idiopathic venous thrombosis have cancer	DIC profile including platelet count, D-dimer, fibrinogen assay
Leukemia	Acute promyelocytic leukemia (M3), acute monocytic leukemia (M4-M5)	Chronic DIC	DIC profile including platelet count, D-dimer, fibrinogen assay
Paroxysmal nocturnal hemoglobinuria	Platelet-related thrombosis	DVT, PE, DIC	Flow cytometry phenotyping, DIC profile
Chronic inflammation	Diabetes, infections, autoimmune disorders, smoking	—	Factor VIII assay, fibrinogen, hsCRP

DVT, deep vein thrombosis; hsCRP, high-sensitivity C-reactive protein; PE, pulmonary embolism; DIC, disseminated intravascular coagulation.

TABLE 42-3 Congenital Thrombosis Risk Factors and Their Odds for Predicting Thrombosis

Risk Factor	Comment	Risk of Thrombosis	Laboratory Tests
Antithrombin deficiency	Antithrombin inhibits the serine proteases thrombin and factors IXa, Xa, and XIa. Antithrombin function is enhanced by heparin	Heterozygous: 10-20×	Clot-based and chromogenic antithrombin assays and immunoassay for antithrombin concentration
Protein C deficiency	APC is a serine protease that hydrolyzes factors Va and VIIIa; requires protein S as cofactor	Homozygous: 100%, rarely reported Heterozygous: 2-5×	Clot-based and chromogenic protein C activity assays and immunoassay
Free protein S deficiency	Cofactor for APC; 40% is free, 60% bound to C4bBP	Homozygous: 100%, causing neonatal purpura fulminans Heterozygous: 1.6-11.5×	Clot-based free protein S activity assays, free and total protein S immunoassays
APC resistance	FVL (R506Q) mutation gain of function renders factor V resistant to APC	Homozygous purpura fulminans: 100% but rarely reported Heterozygous: 3×	APTT-based APC resistance test and confirmatory molecular assay
Prothrombin G20210A	Mutation in the gene's untranslated 3′ promoter region creates moderate prothrombin activity elevation	Homozygous: 18× Heterozygous: 1.6-11.5×	Molecular assay only. Phenotypic assay provides no specificity
Dysfibrinogenemia and fibrinogenemia	Association with arterial thrombosis	Under investigation: acute-phase reactant	Fibrinogen clotting assay, thrombin time, reptilase time
Plasminogen mutations	Rare cases described	—	Chromogenic substrate
TPA deficiency, PAI-1 elevation	PAI-1 increase may be common	—	Chromogenic substrate assays

APTT, activated partial thromboplastin time; TPA, tissue plasminogen activator; PAI-1, plasminogen activator inhibitor-1; APC, activated protein C.

The antithrombin test (previously called the *AT III test*) has been available since 1972, and protein C and protein S activity assays became available in the mid-1980s. The 1990s have brought us the APC resistance assay; the confirmatory FVL mutation molecular assay; prothrombin 20210A by molecular assay; and tests for dysfibrinogenemia, plasminogen deficiency, plasma TPA, and plasma PAI-1.

APC resistance exists in 3% to 8% of Caucasians. Prevalence extends to Arabs and Hispanics, but the mutation is absent from African or East Asian populations (Table 42-4).[22] APC resistance may exist in the absence of the FVL mutation and occasionally is acquired in pregnancy and oral contraceptive therapy.

The prothrombin G20210A gene mutation is the second most common inherited thrombophilic tendency in patients with a personal and family history of deep vein thrombosis.[23] Taken together, protein C, protein S, and antithrombin deficiencies are found in 0.2% to 1% of the world population. The incidences of dysfibrinogenemia and the various forms of abnormal fibrinolysis (plasminogen deficiency, TPA deficiency, or PAI-1 excess) are under investigation.

Double Hit

Thrombosis often is associated with a combination of genetic defects, diseases, and lifestyle influences. The fact that an individual may possess protein C, protein S, or antithrombin deficiency does not mean thrombosis is inevitable. Many heterozygotes may experience no thrombotic event during their lifetime, whereas others clot only when two or more risk factors converge. A young woman with heterozygous FVL mutation has a 35-fold increase in thrombosis risk on starting oral contraceptives. In the Physician's Health Study, homocysteinemia tripled the risk of idiopathic venous thrombosis, and the FVL mutation doubled it. When both were present, the risk of venous thrombosis was increased 10-fold.[24]

LABORATORY APPROACH TO THROMBOSIS EVALUATION

When thrombophilia is suspected, it is important to assess all known risk factors because it is the combination of positive results that determine the patient's cumulative risk of thrombosis.[25] The presence or absence of laboratory-detected risk factors does not affect treatment, however, when a thrombosis is present. Anticoagulant therapy and thrombotic events that have occurred in the recent past affect the interpretation of antithrombin, protein C, protein S, factor VIII, and LA testing. These assays should be performed 10 to 14 days after anticoagulant therapy is withdrawn (Table 42-5).

Antiphospholipid Antibodies

APL antibodies are a family of immunoglobulins that bind protein-phospholipid complexes.[26] APL antibodies include LAs, detected by clot-based profiles, and immunoassay-detected ACL antibodies and anti-β_2-glycoprotein I (β_2-GPI) antibody. Chronic autoimmune APL antibodies are associated with APS, which includes transient ischemic attacks, strokes, coronary and peripheral artery disease, venous thromboembolism, and repeated pregnancy complications.[27,28]

APL antibodies arise as IgM, IgG, or IgA isotypes. Because they may bind a variety of protein-phospholipid complexes, they are called *nonspecific inhibitors*. Their name reflects that they previously were thought to bind phospholipids directly; however, their target antigens are the proteins assembled on anionic phospholipid surfaces.[29] The plasma protein most often bound by APL antibodies is β_2-GPI, although annexin V and prothrombin sometimes are implicated. APL antibodies probably develop in response to newly formed protein-phospholipid complexes, and investigators still are learning exactly how they cause thrombosis.[30,31]

TABLE 42-4 Prevalence of Congenital Thrombosis Risk Factors in the General Population and in Patients with Recurrent Thrombotic Disease

Factor	Unselected Population	People with at Least One Thrombotic Event
APC resistance, FVL mutation	3-8% of Caucasians, none in Asians or Africans	20-25%
Prothrombin G20210A	2-3% of Caucasians	4-8%
Antithrombin deficiency	1 in 2000-5000	1-1.8%
Protein C deficiency	1 in 300	2.5-5%
Protein S deficiency	Unknown	2.8-5%
Hyperhomocysteinemia associated with *MTHFR* mutations	11%	13.1-26.7%
Dysfibrinogenemia	Unknown	1%
Abnormal fibrinolysis	Unknown	2%

TABLE 42-5 Complete Thrombophilia Laboratory Test Profile

Assay	Reference Results	Comment
APC resistance	Ratio ≥1.8	Clot-based screen based on PTT
FVL mutation	Wild-type	Molecular assay performed in follow-up to APC resistance assay <1.8
Prothrombin G20210A	Wild-type	Molecular assay. There is no phenotypic assay for prothrombin G20210A
Lupus anticoagulant profile*	Negative for lupus anticoagulant	Minimum of two clot-based assays, such as PTT, DRVVT, or dilute prothrombin time with phospholipid neutralization test for immunoglobulins of the antiphospholipid antibody family
ACL antibody	IgG: <12 GPL IgM: <10 MPL	Immunoassay for immunoglobulins of the antiphospholipid antibody family
Anti-β_2-GPI antibody	<20 G units	Immunoassay for an immunoglobulin of the antiphospholipid antibody family. β_2-GPI is the key phospholipid-binding protein in the family
Antithrombin activity*	78-126%	Serine protease inhibitor suppresses factors Xa and IIa. When consistently below reference limit, follow up with antithrombin antigen assay
Protein C activity*	70-140%	Digests factors VIIIa and Va. When consistently below reference limit, follow up with protein C antigen assay
Protein S activity*	65-140%	Protein C cofactor. When consistently below reference limit, follow up with total and free protein S antigen assay, C4bBP
Factor VIII activity	50-186%	Confirm elevated factor VIII
Fibrinogen	220-498 mg/dL	Clot-based assay. Elevation may be associated with arterial thrombosis
PAI-1	<30 IU/mL	Elevation may be associated with venous thrombosis

*Inaccurate during active thrombosis or anticoagulant therapy. Perform 14 days after anticoagulant therapy is discontinued.
GPL, IgG anticardiolipin antibody unit; MPL, IgM anticardiolipin antibody unit; GPI, glycoprotein-I; DRVVT, dilute Russell viper venom time; PAI-1, plasminogen activator inhibitor-1.

Clinical Consequences of Antiphospholipids

One to 2% of unselected individuals of both sexes and all races and 5% to 15% of individuals with recurrent venous or arterial thrombotic disease have APL antibodies.[32] Most APL antibodies arise in response to a bacterial, viral, fungal, or parasitic infection or in numerous drug regimens (Box 42-1) and disappear within 12 weeks. Such transient alloimmune APL antibodies have no clinical consequences.[33] Nevertheless, the laboratory scientist must follow up any positive APL assay to determine persistence.

Autoimmune APL antibodies are part of the family of autoantibodies that arise in collagen vascular diseases; 50% of patients with systemic lupus erythematosus have autoimmune APL antibodies. Autoimmune APL antibodies are also detected in rheumatoid arthritis and Sjögren syndrome but may arise spontaneously, a situation called *primary APS*. Autoimmune APL antibodies may persist, and 30% are associated with arterial and venous thrombosis. A chronic APL antibody without a known autoimmune disorder confers a 1.8-fold to 3.2-fold risk of thrombosis.

Detecting and Confirming Antiphospholipids

Clinicians suspect APS in unexplained venous or arterial thrombosis, thrombocytopenia, or recurrent fetal loss.[34] Specialized clinical hemostasis laboratories offer APL detection systems that include clot-based assays for LA and immunoassays for ACL and β_2-GPI. Occasionally, an LA is suspected because of an unexplained prolonged partial thromboplastin time (PTT) that does not correct when the test is repeated in mixing studies.[35,36]

Lupus Anticoagulant

Test systems that employ low reagent phospholipid concentrations are sensitive to LA.[37] There are four such systems, at least two of which are required to comprise an LA profile. The need for multiple test systems arises from the multiplicity of LA reaction characteristics, and a confirmed positive result in one system is conclusive despite a negative result in another. The four available systems are PTTs formulated with low reagent phospholipid levels, the dilute Russell viper venom time (DRVVT), the kaolin clotting time (KCT), and the dilute thromboplastin time (DTT).[38] As illustrated in Figure 42-1, the KCT and PTT trigger coagulation at the level of factor XII; DRVVT, at factor X; and DTT, at factor VII (Chapter 45). The

> **BOX 42-1** Drugs Known to Induce Antiphospholipid Antibodies
>
> - Various antibiotics
> - Phenothiazine
> - Hydralazine
> - Quinine and quinidine
> - Calcium channel blockers
> - Procainamide
> - Phenytoin
> - Cocaine
> - Elevated estrogens

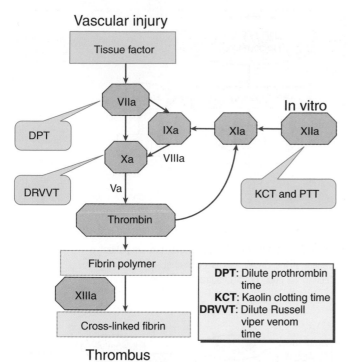

Figure 42-1 The coagulation mechanism illustrating that KCT and PTT trigger coagulation at the level of factor XII; DRVVT, at factor X; and DPT, at factor VII.

1. Prolonged phospholipid-dependent clot formation using a screen such as the low phospholipid PTT, DRVVT, KCT, or DTT
2. Failure to correct the prolonged clot formation by mixing with normal platelet-poor plasma and repeating test (mixing study)
3. Shortening or correction of the prolonged screen by addition of excess phospholipids
4. Exclusion of other coagulopathies

In performing mixing studies, it is essential to use only platelet-poor plasma (plasma centrifuged so that it has a platelet count <10,000/μL). Platelet-poor plasma avoids neutralization of LA by the platelet membrane. Platelet fragments formed during freezing and thawing can neutralize LA and lead to a false-negative LA result.

Performing the Clot-Based Lupus Anticoagulant Mixing Study

When the PTT or DRVVT is prolonged and anticoagulant therapy is ruled out, a new aliquot of patient plasma is mixed 1:1 with pooled normal platelet-poor plasma, and the assay is repeated on the mixture using the same test system (immediate mix). Some LAs are time and temperature dependent, so if the result of the mixture has corrected to within 10% or 5 seconds of the normal platelet-poor plasma result, the test should be repeated again after incubating the mix at 37°C for 1 to 2 hours. Each laboratory manager or director must decide what degree of shortening constitutes correction. Many use the Rosner index, which defines correction as a mixture result within 10% of the result of the platelet-poor normal plasma.[40]

most common combination in U.S. specialty or reference laboratories is the low phospholipid PTT and the DRVVT (Figs. 42-2 and 42-3). This combination of assays fulfills the following LA requirements of the International Society on Thrombosis and Haemostasis[39]:

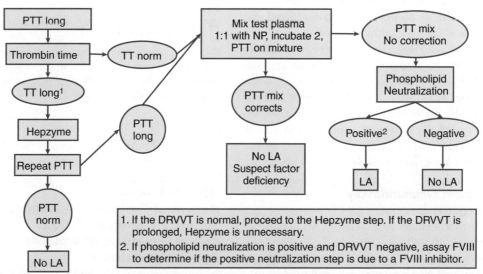

Figure 42-2 Lupus anticoagulant (LA) detection scheme using an LA-sensitive partial thromboplastin time (PTT) detection system. Perform in conjunction with the DRVVT (see Fig. 42-3). If the LA-sensitive PTT is prolonged but the Dilute Russell viper venom time (DRVVT) is normal, perform a thrombin time to detect heparin. If the thrombin time is prolonged, treat the plasma with Hepzyme, and repeat the LA-sensitive PTT. If the PTT is still prolonged, or if no heparin was present, mix the patient plasma with normal plasma, incubate 1 to 2 hours, and repeat. If the PTT mix is normal, suspect a factor deficiency and confirm. If the PTT mix is prolonged, proceed to the phospholipid neutralization step to confirm LA. If the phospholipid neutralization result is positive but the DRVVT is negative, perform a factor VIII assay to determine if the phospholipid neutralization step result is due to a factor VIII inhibitor.

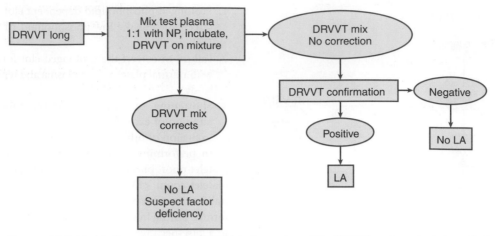

Figure 42-3 LA detection scheme using DRVVT detection systems. If the DRVVT is prolonged, mix the patient plasma with normal plasma, incubate 1 to 2 hours, and repeat. If the DRVVT mix is normal, suspect a factor deficiency and confirm. If the DRVVT mix is prolonged, proceed to the phospholipid neutralization step to confirm.

If either test remains prolonged (is uncorrected), LA is presumed, and confirmation is necessary. Confirmatory tests employ the same assay that was originally prolonged, adding a phospholipid reagent. If LA was the cause of prolongation, the high-phospholipid test result shortens (corrects).[41]

Anticardiolipin Antibody Immunoassay

LA and ACL coexist in 60% of cases, and both may be found in APS.[42] The ACL test is an immunoassay that may be normalized among laboratories and is not affected by heparin, oral anticoagulants, current thrombosis, or factor deficiencies.

The manufacturer coats microplate wells with bovine heart cardiolipin and blocks with a bovine serum solution containing β_2-GPI. Test sera or plasmas are serially diluted and pipetted to the wells along with calibrators and controls. ACL binds the cardiolipin-β_2-GPI target and cannot be washed from the wells. Enzyme-labeled antihuman IgG, IgM, or IgA conjugates are added. A color-producing substrate follows, and a color change indicates ACL. Patient and control color intensity are compared with the calibrator curve. Results are expressed using GPL, MPL, or APL units, where 1 unit is equivalent to 1 µg/mL of an affinity-purified standard IgG, IgM, or IgA specimen.[43] Reference limits are established in each laboratory.

Anti-β_2-Glycoprotein I Immunoassay

IgM and IgG anti-β_2-GPI immunoassays are performed as a part of the profile that includes ACL assays.[44] An anti-β_2-GPI result of greater than 20 GPL or MPL units correlates with thrombosis more closely than ACL. Any positive ACL or β_2-GPI assay should be repeated on a new specimen collected after 12 weeks to distinguish a transient alloantibody from a chronic autoantibody (Fig. 42-4).

Antiphosphatidylserine Immunoassay

In instances where an APL antibody is suspected but the routine LA, ACL, and β_2-GPI assay results are negative, the clinician may wish to order the antiphosphatidylserine immunoassay

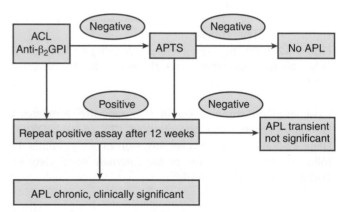

Figure 42-4 A reflexive immunoassay sequence for antiphospholipid (APL) antibodies. If the IgM or IgG anti-cardiolipin (ACL) antibody or the IgM or IgG anti-β_2-GPI test is positive, confirm after 12 weeks for chronicity. If either is positive, the patient has a clinically significant APL. If the initial ACL and anti-β_2-GPI are negative, but an APL antibody is suspected, perform the antiphosphatidylserine antibody immunoassay. If positive, repeat after 12 weeks to establish chronicity.

to detect APL antibodies specific for phosphatidylserine.[45] A result greater than or equal to 16 G or 22 M antiphosphatidylserine units is considered positive.

Activated Protein C Resistance and Factor V Leiden Mutation
Clinical Importance of Activated Protein C Resistance

Activated factors V (Va) and VIII (VIIIa) are inactivated by the APC–protein S complex. A mutation in the factor V gene substitutes glutamine for arginine at position 506 (V R506Q) of the factor V molecule. The arginine is a cleavage site for APC, so the substitution slows or prevents hydrolysis of the factor V molecule (Fig. 42-5). Resistant factor Va remains active and increases the production of thrombin. The factor V R506Q mutation is named for the city in which it was first described,

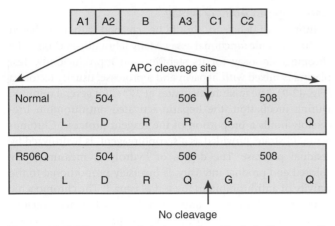

Figure 42-5 FVL mutation. A single mutation of the factor V gene results in the substitution of glutamine for arginine at position 506 (R506Q) of the factor V molecule. The normal arginine at position 506 is a cleavage site for APC, so the substitution slows or prevents cleavage of the factor V molecule.

Leiden (FVL mutation). Three to 8% of Northern European Caucasians possess FVL (see Table 42-4).[46] Owing to its prevalence and threefold thrombosis risk (18-fold when homozygous), the acute care hemostasis laboratory must provide APC resistance detection to screen for FVL.[47]

Activated Protein C Resistance Clot-Based Assay

Patient plasma is mixed 1:4 with factor V–depleted plasma.[48] PTT reagent is added to 2 aliquots of the mixture and incubated for 3 minutes (Fig. 42-6). A solution of calcium chloride is pipetted to one mixture, and the clot formation is timed. A solution of calcium chloride with APC is added to the second

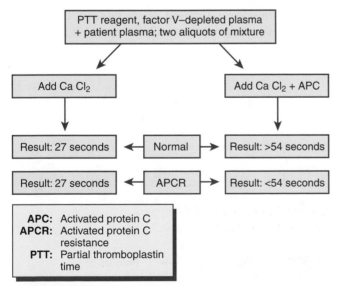

Figure 42-6 Example of an APC resistance test with factor V–depleted plasma. Patient plasma is mixed 1:4 with factor V–depleted plasma and PTT reagent. This mixture is mixed with calcium chloride with and without APC. The mixture with APC should give a clot time at least twice as long as the mixture without APC. A ratio less than 2 implies APC resistance.

mixture and timed. The normal ratio of PTT results between the two assays is 1.8 or greater. In APC resistance, the ratio is less than 1.8.[49]

Performance Characteristics for the Activated Protein C Resistance Test

Factor V–depleted plasma compensates for potential factor deficiencies and for oral anticoagulant therapy by providing procoagulant cofactors. The scientist uses platelet-poor plasma in the APC resistance test to prevent loss of sensitivity caused by the abundant release of platelet factor V. Most APC resistance reagent kits contain polybrene to neutralize heparin. LA affects the test system adversely, however.[50] If LA is present, the molecular test for FVL is indicated.[51]

Factor V Leiden Mutation Assay

Most laboratories confirm the APC resistance diagnosis using the molecular FVL mutation test. The determination of zygosity is important to predict the risk for thrombosis.

Prothrombin G20210A

A G-to-A mutation at base 20210 of the 3' untranslated region of the prothrombin (factor II) gene has been associated with mildly elevated plasma prothrombin levels, averaging 130%.[52] The reason the mutation increases the risk of thrombosis seems to be related to the elevated prothrombin activity.[53] The prevalence of this mutation among individuals with familial thrombosis is 5% to 18%, whereas prevalence worldwide is 0.3% to 2.4%, depending on race.[54] The risk of venous thrombosis in heterozygotes is only two to three times the baseline risk. Although the mutation may cause a slight elevation, a prothrombin activity assay provides little diagnostic value because there is considerable overlap between normal prothrombin levels and the levels in the mutation.

Antithrombin Assay

Antithrombin is a serine protease inhibitor (SERPIN) that neutralizes thrombin and factors IXa, Xa, XIa, and XIIa. Antithrombin activity is enhanced by unfractionated and low-molecular-weight heparin (Figs. 42-7 and 42-8). Antithrombin was the first of the plasma coagulation control proteins to be identified and the first to be assayed routinely in the clinical hemostasis laboratory.[55] Other members of the SERPIN family are heparin cofactor II, α_2-macroglobulin, α_2-antiplasmin, and α_1-antitrypsin. Typically, hemostasis specialty laboratories or reference laboratories are the only places that offer SERPIN assays other than antithrombin.

Antithrombin Deficiency

Acquired antithrombin deficiency occurs in liver disease, in nephrotic syndrome, with prolonged heparin therapy, with asparaginase therapy, with use of oral contraceptives, and in DIC, where antithrombin is rapidly consumed. Congenital deficiency is present in 1 in 2000 to 5000 of the general population and accounts for 1% to 1.8% of recurrent venous thromboembolic disease.[56] About 90% of antithrombin deficiency is quantitative, or type 1; the remainder of cases are

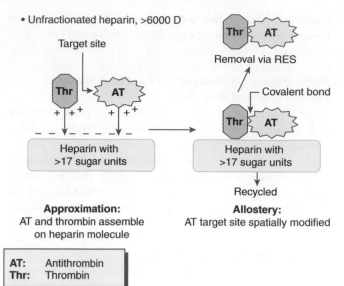

Approximation:
AT and thrombin assemble
on heparin molecule

Allostery:
AT target site spatially modified

AT:	Antithrombin
Thr:	Thrombin

Figure 42-7 Antithrombin activity is enhanced by its reaction with unfractionated heparin. Unfractionated heparin provides molecules that are greater than 17 sugar moieties in length or greater than 6000 D molecular weight. Antithrombin and its substrate, such as thrombin or factor Xa, assemble on the surface of the heparin molecule (approximation). The antithrombin becomes sterically modified (allostery), and the covalent reaction proceeds.

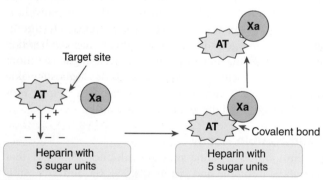

Figure 42-8 Low-molecular-weight heparin enhances antithrombin activity through allostery alone. Low-molecular-weight heparin binds antithrombin and induces its steric modification. Modified antithrombin then bonds with factor Xa. This reaction, in the absence of approximation, favors the antithrombin–factor Xa reaction over the thrombin-antithrombin reaction.

caused by mutations creating structural abnormalities in the protease binding site or the heparin binding site.

Antithrombin Reference Ranges

Adult plasma antithrombin activity levels range from 78% to 126% when measured by clot-based or chromogenic assay. Antithrombin antigen levels range from 22 to 39 mg/dL by latex microparticle immunoassay, and the plasma biologic half-life is 72 hours. Adult levels are reached by 3 months of age and remain steady throughout adult life except during periods of physiologic challenge, such as pregnancy. Antithrombin levels decrease with age.

Antithrombin Activity Assay

Antithrombin deficiency should be screened with a clot-based or chromogenic functional assay. Many laboratories choose the chromogenic assay for its stability and reproducibility. Test plasma is mixed with heparin and a protease, usually factor Xa (Fig. 42-9). The mixture incubates at 37° C for several minutes. During incubation, the heparin-activated antithrombin irreversibly binds a proportion of the reagent protease. Chromogenic substrate, provided as a second reagent, is hydrolyzed by residual protease. The degree of hydrolysis, measurable by colored end product intensity, is inversely proportional to the activity of antithrombin in the test plasma.[57] The chromogenic substrate test for plasma antithrombin activity detects quantitative and qualitative antithrombin deficiencies and detects mutations affecting the proteolytic site, but not the heparin binding site.

Antithrombin Antigen Assay

Antithrombin concentration is measured in a turbidometric microparticle immunoassay using a suspension of latex microbeads coated with antibody. In the absence of antithrombin, the wavelength of incident monochromatic light exceeds the latex microparticle diameter, so the light passes through unabsorbed. In the presence of antithrombin, the particles form larger aggregates. The antithrombin concentration is directly proportional to the rate of light absorption change.[58] Antithrombin antigen levels are diminished in quantitative (type 1), but not qualitative (type 2) antithrombin deficiency. Oral anticoagulant warfarin therapy may increase the antithrombin level and mask mild deficiency. The antithrombin level remains decreased for 10 to 14 days after surgery or a thrombotic event, so the assay should not be used in this period to establish a congenital deficiency.

Heparin Resistance Affecting the Antithrombin Assay

Antithrombin may be decreased during prolonged or intense heparin therapy and may be totally consumed if the patient

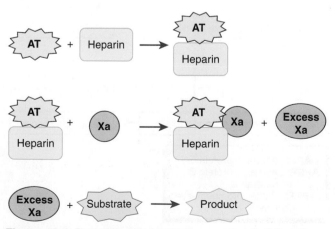

Figure 42-9 The antithrombin functional assay principle. Patient plasma is mixed with reagent heparin and a measured substrate, usually coagulation factor Xa, and allowed to react. Excess factor Xa reacts with a chromogenic substrate to produce a colored solution. The intensity of color is inversely proportional to antithrombin activity in the original specimen.

has a congenital antithrombin deficiency. In this instance, heparin may be administered in therapeutic or higher dosages, but it neither exerts an anticoagulant effect nor is detected by the PTT. This is heparin resistance. In this instance, an antithrombin assay is necessary to confirm antithrombin deficiency. Antithrombin deficiency may be treated with antithrombin concentrate (Thrombate III; Alecris Biotherapeutics, Inc., Research Triangle Park, N.C.).

Assays of the Protein C Control Pathway

Thrombin is an important coagulation factor because it cleaves fibrinogen and activates platelets and factors V, VIII, XI, and XIII. In the intact vessel where clotting would be inexpedient, thrombin binds endothelial cell membrane thrombomodulin and becomes an anticoagulant.[59] How does this happen? The thrombin-thrombomodulin complex activates plasma protein C; APC binds free plasma protein S (Fig. 42-10). The stabilized APC–protein S complex hydrolyzes factors Va and VIIIa to slow coagulation. Recurrent venous thrombosis is the potential consequence of any deficiency in this complex pathway.

Protein S, the cofactor that binds and stabilizes APC, circulates in the plasma in two forms: free and covalently bound to the complement control protein C4bBP. Bound protein S cannot participate in the protein C anticoagulant pathway; only free plasma protein S is available to serve as the APC cofactor. Protein S–C4bBP binding is of particular interest in inflammatory conditions, where the plasma C4bBP level becomes elevated, binding additional protein S. Free protein S levels are proportionally decreased.

Protein C and Protein S Reference Ranges

Heterozygous deficiency of protein C or protein S leads to a 1.6-fold to 11.5-fold increased risk of recurrent deep vein thrombosis and pulmonary embolism.[60] Protein S deficiency also has been implicated in transient ischemic attacks and strokes, particularly in the young. The reference interval for protein C and protein S activity and antigen levels is 65% to 140%, and levels ordinarily remain between 30% and 65% for heterozygotes.

Proteins C and S and prothrombin and factors VII, IX, and X are vitamin K dependent. Because protein C's half-life is 6 hours, its level decreases as rapidly as that of factor VII when warfarin therapy is started. In heterozygous protein C deficiency, protein C activity may decrease to a thrombotic level (<65%) more rapidly than the other procoagulant factors reach an anticoagulant level (<10%). Consequently, a patient may experience warfarin-induced skin necrosis, a paradoxical situation in which the early stage of oral anticoagulant therapy brings on thrombosis of the dermal vessels. This complication is suspected when the patient presents with painful necrotic lesions that are preceded by itching. The necrosis may require surgical débridement. To avoid this risk, heparin is recommended with oral anticoagulants until a satisfactory and stable international normalized ratio is reached (Chapter 46).

Levels of protein C and protein S remain below normal for 10 to 14 days after cessation of oral anticoagulants. Similarly, for several days after surgery or a thrombotic event, these proteins are diminished even without oral anticoagulants. Their activities are depressed in liver or renal disease, vitamin K deficiency, and DIC. Protein C and protein S assays cannot be used to establish a congenital deficiency soon after thrombosis, warfarin therapy, or under a variety of pathologic conditions.

Homozygous protein C or protein S deficiency results in neonatal purpura fulminans, a condition that is rapidly fatal when left untreated. Treatment includes factor concentrates and lifelong oral anticoagulant therapy.

Protein C Assays

Functional assays detect quantitative and qualitative protein C deficiencies. Chromogenic or clottable assays are available for this purpose. In the former, the patient's plasma is mixed with venom from *Agkistrodon contortrix contortrix*, which activates protein C. Subsequently, a chromogenic substrate is added, and its hydrolysis by APC is measured by the amount of colored product. The intensity of color is proportional to the activity of protein C in the test plasma (Fig. 42-11). The assay detects abnormalities that affect the molecule's proteolytic properties, but it misses the rare mutations that affect protein C's phospholipid or protein S binding sites. In the instance where the protein C chromogenic assays and immunoassays are normal but the clinical condition indicates possible protein C deficiency, a clot-based protein C assay may detect abnormalities at these additional sites on the molecule. The clottable assay is based on the effect of APC to prolong the PTT. Test plasma is mixed with protein C–depleted normal plasma to ensure normal levels of all factors but protein C. A solution of

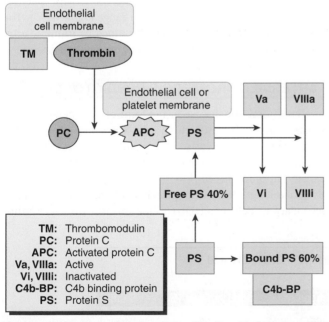

Figure 42-10 The protein C pathway. The thrombin-thrombomodulin complex assembles on endothelial cell membrane phospholipid and activates protein C. APC forms a complex with protein S on another phospholipid surface, typically platelet membrane phospholipid. The complex hydrolyzes active factors V and VIII.

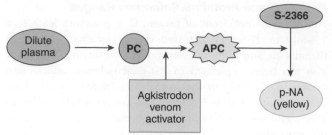

Figure 42-11 Chromogenic protein C assay principle. Protein C in plasma is activated by *Agkistrodon contortrix contortrix* venom. The APC acts on a chromogenic substrate to produce a colored product. The intensity of color is proportional to protein C activity.

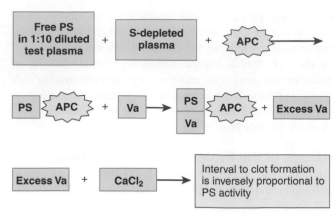

Figure 42-12 Clottable protein S assay principle. Patient plasma is diluted and mixed with protein S–depleted plasma and APC. A measured amount of activated factor V is added and allowed to react with the APC–protein S complex. Excess factor Va is clotted with calcium chloride. The interval to clot formation is proportional to protein S activity.

Agkistrodon contortrix contortrix venom with particulate activators is added, followed by calcium chloride, and the interval to clot formation is measured. Prolongation is proportional to plasma protein C activity. The clottable protein C activity assay may be performed using an automated coagulation analyzer. Therapeutic heparin levels greater than 1 IU/mL leads to overestimation of protein C. APC resistance, LA, and factor VIII levels greater than 150%, as may appear in inflammation, all may cause errors in the clot-based protein C activity levels.

Enzyme immunoassay is used to measure protein C antigen when the functional activity is low and acquired causes have been ruled out. Microtiter plates coated with rabbit antihuman protein C are used to capture test plasma protein C, and the amount of antigen is quantitated by color development after the sequential addition of peroxidase-conjugated antihuman protein C and orthophenylenediamine substrate. The protein C antigen concentration assay detects most acquired deficiencies and quantitative congenital deficiencies but does not detect qualitative congenital abnormalities.

Protein S Assays

As with antithrombin and protein C, protein S deficiency screening requires a functional assay. A clot-based assay is performed by mixing the patient's plasma with protein S–depleted normal plasma to ensure normal levels of all other factors. APC and bovine factor Va are added, followed by calcium chloride, and the interval to clot formation is measured. The more prolonged the test result, the lower the protein S activity (Fig. 42-12).

Calibration is necessary with each run of assays because the interassay coefficient of variation may exceed 5%. Therapeutic heparin levels greater than 1 IU/mL lead to overestimation of protein S activity. APC resistance, LA, and factor VIII levels greater than 150% all may cause underestimation of protein S activity. Factor VII activation may occur during prolonged plasma storage at 4° C to 6° C; this also may cause underestimation of protein S activity. When there is clinical suspicion of primary protein S deficiency based on low activity level, an enzyme immunoassay is employed to measure total and free protein S antigen. These assays detect most quantitative congenital deficiencies and aid in the diagnosis of qualitative type II congenital deficiencies characterized by normal antigen but decreased activity of protein S. In type III deficiency, the amount of free antigen protein S and its activity, but not the total result, are below the normal range (Table 42-6). The concentration of plasma C4bBP determined by immunoassay aids in the classification of the types of protein S deficiency.

ARTERIAL THROMBOSIS PREDICTORS

Arterial thrombotic disease in the form of peripheral vascular disease, myocardial infarction, and cerebrovascular disease arises from atherosclerosis. The traditional predictors of risk for arterial thrombosis are elevated total cholesterol and low-density lipoprotein cholesterol (LDL-C), or a high total cholesterol:high-density lipoprotein cholesterol (HDL-C) ratio secondary to deficient HDL-C. One third of primary cardio-

TABLE 42-6 Anticipated Protein S Test Results in Qualitative and Quantitative Deficiencies

Type of Deficiency		Activity (%)	Free Antigen (%)	Total Antigen (%)	C4bBP
I	Quantitative	<65	<65	<65	Normal
II	Qualitative	<65	>65	>65	Normal
III	Inflammation	<65	<65	>65	Elevated

C4b BP, C4b-Binding protein.

vascular and cerebrovascular events occur in patients whose lipid profiles are normal, however.[61] Half of individuals with lipid risk factors never experience a thrombotic event.

Researchers have sought additional arterial thrombosis predictors by analyzing lipoprotein subtypes and by performing prospective randomized observations on markers of inflammation. The results of these studies have led to numerous markers of arterial thrombosis risk (Table 42-7), as detailed in this section. The fibrinolytic pathway markers plasminogen, α_2-antiplasmin, and PAI-1 also are useful markers. Other proteins, such as TPA, show marked diurnal variation and require a specialized phlebotomy protocol to prevent in vitro elevation.[62] Homocysteine, fibrinogen, and high-sensitivity C-reactive protein (CRP) are well-established assays with considerable predictive ability.

High-Sensitivity C-Reactive Protein

There is a clear correlation between the acute-phase reactant CRP and myocardial infarction and stroke.[63]

High-Sensitivity C-Reactive Protein Measurement

Plasma CRP increases several hundred–fold in response to acute inflammatory stimuli. The increase remains stable over several days in vivo, and the protein is resistant to in vitro degradation.[64] Conventional flocculation assays used for CRP measurement in acute or chronic inflammatory illness detect only gross elevations. The monoclonal antibody–based high-sensitivity CRP enzyme immunoassay, or its automatable rapid counterpart, the monoclonal latex microparticle assay, detects normal or slightly elevated CRP concentrations. Consequently,

the high-sensitivity CRP assay is an established clinical tool to evaluate low-level systemic inflammation and predict cardiovascular or cerebrovascular disease.[65,66]

Data from at least 10 studies involving tens of thousands of individuals show that mild chronic elevations of CRP may point to atherosclerosis 6 or more years before myocardial infarction or stroke.[67] The high-sensitivity CRP procedure enhances cardiac risk assessment independently and in conjunction with lipid profile markers and is available on automated coagulation analyzers.

High-Sensitivity C-Reactive Protein Reference Range and Relative Risk Ratios

The high-sensitivity CRP mean for individuals with no coronary artery disease by angiography is 0.87 mg/L. In contrast, the mean for patients with three affected arteries is 1.43 mg/L. Using the high-sensitivity CRP assay, CRP levels may predict the risk of stroke independent of lipid concentrations, as shown in Table 42-8. CRP levels serve as strong predictors of risk of myocardial infarction when combined with total cholesterol (Table 42-9) or with the total cholesterol:HDL-C ratio (Table 42-10).[68]

Plasma Homocysteine

Homocysteine is a naturally occurring, sulfur-containing amino acid formed in the metabolism of dietary methionine.[69,70] Homocysteine circulates in the form of various disulfides, altogether called *total homocysteine*. Homocysteine's concentration in plasma depends primarily on adequate protein intake, vitamins B_6 and B_{12}, and folate. Its concentration is

---

TABLE 42-7 Markers of Arterial Thrombosis Risk

Marker	Reference Interval	Comments
hsCRP	<0.55 mg/L	Marker of inflammation; report in relative risk ranges; stable, reproducible
Fibrinogen	200-400 mg/dL	>300 mg/dL increases thrombotic risk; high correlation with risk; inadequate reproducibility with numerous test platforms
Homocysteine	4.6-12.1 μmol/L	Normals and predictive values vary with population; may be reduced through vitamin B_6, B_{12}, and folate supplement
Total cholesterol	<200 mg/dL	Reproducible; some relationship with diet; risk prediction is not independent of inflammation
Total cholesterol:HDL-C ratio	<10	Reproducible; elevated ratio has some relationship with diet and exercise; risk prediction is not independent of inflammation
LDL-C	<130 mg/dL	Reproducible; may be significantly lowered with statin therapy
Lipoprotein (a)	2.2-49.4 mg/dL	Varies with race and age; may be lowered with statin therapy; inadequate reproducibility
Plasminogen, TPA, PAI-1, α_2-antiplasmin	—	Available from hemostasis reference laboratories

hsCRP, high-sensitivity C-reactive protein; TPA, tissue plasminogen activator; PAI-1, plasminogen activator inhibitor-1; HDL-C, high density lipoprotein cholesterol; LDL-C, low density lipoprotein cholesterol.

TABLE 42-8 Relative Risk for Myocardial Infarction (MI) or Stroke: Males and Females at Four C-Reactive Protein Quartile Levels Independent of Lipids

Quartile	CRP (mg/L)	RELATIVE RISK OF MI OR STROKE	
		Males	Females
1	≤0.55	1.0	1.0
2	0.56-1.14	1.8	2.9
3	1.15-2.10	2.5	3.5
4	≥2.11	2.9	5.5

regulated by three enzymes: cystathionine β-synthase, which converts homocysteine to cystathionine in the presence of vitamin B_6; 5,10-methylenetetrahydrofolate reductase (MTHFR), required for the remethylation of homocysteine to methionine in the folic acid cycle; and methionine synthase, which requires vitamin B_{12} (Fig. 42-13). Vitamin deficiencies and a functional mutation in the MTHFR gene or an inherited deficiency of cystathionine β-synthase or methionine synthase result in increased levels of plasma homocysteine.[71] Although cystathionine β-synthase or methionine synthase deficiencies are rare, 50% of the North American population is heterozygous for the MTHFR polymorphism.

Clinical Significance of Homocysteinemia

Fasting homocysteinemia is an independent risk factor for arterial thrombosis with relative ratios of 1.7 for coronary artery disease, 2.5 for cerebrovascular disease, and 6.8 for peripheral artery disease. Mild elevations of homocysteine are an independent risk factor for occlusive arterial disease.[72,73] Homozygous MTHFR G677T is associated with homocysteinemia but is not an independent thrombosis risk factor. Several

theories link homocysteinemia with coronary artery disease, most involving damage to the endothelial cell.[74]

Homocysteine Test Principles

High-performance liquid chromatography has been a common approach to homocysteine analysis. The plasma is first treated with a reducing agent to convert all disulfide forms to homocysteine, which becomes bound to fluorescein to form a detectable fluorescent derivative. High-performance liquid chromatography methods are not standardized among clinical laboratories.

An enzyme immunoassay procedure is available from several distributors. In the Abbott Axsym assay, plasma disulfides are reduced, the homocysteine is converted to S-adenosylhomocysteine, and the S-adenosylhomocysteine is bound to an antibody conjugated to a fluorescein tracer. This method provides for automated analysis.

When blood is collected for homocysteine, the serum or plasma must be separated from the red blood cells within minutes to avoid red blood cell release of homocysteine. The serum or plasma must be kept cold and protected from light. Plasma homocysteine increases by 10% per hour if blood is kept intact at room temperature after collection. Plasma collection may be accomplished using heparin, sodium citrate, or ethylenediamine tetraacetic acid anticoagulants.

Homocysteine Reference Range and Therapy

The reference ranges for homocysteine differ between males and females, and they increase with age, as shown in Table 42-11. Therapy usually includes administration of the appropriate vitamin (folate, vitamin B_6, and vitamin B_{12}) to correct for the dietary deficiency or the abnormal methionine metabolism. Folate supplementation of grain in the United States, instituted in January 1999 to prevent fetal neural tube defects, may

TABLE 42-9 Relative Risk for Myocardial Infarction: Three C-Reactive Protein Levels Related to Total Cholesterol

CRP	TOTAL CHOLESTEROL		
	Low (≤191 mg/dL)	Medium (192-223 mg/dL)	High (≥224 mg/dL)
Low (≤0.72 mg/L)	1.0	1.4	2.3
Medium (0.73-1.69 mg/L)	1.2	1.5	4.3
High (≥1.70 mg/L)	1.1	2.3	5.3

TABLE 42-10 Relative Risk for Myocardial Infarction: Three C-Reactive Protein Levels Related to Total Cholesterol:High-Density Lipoprotein Cholesterol (TC:HDL-C) Ratio

CRP	TC:HDL-C RATIO		
	Low (≤3.78)	Medium (3.79-5.01)	High (≥5.02)
Low (≤0.72 mg/L)	1.0	1.2	2.8
Medium (0.73-1.69 mg/L)	1.1	2.5	3.4
High (≥1.70 mg/L)	1.3	2.8	4.4

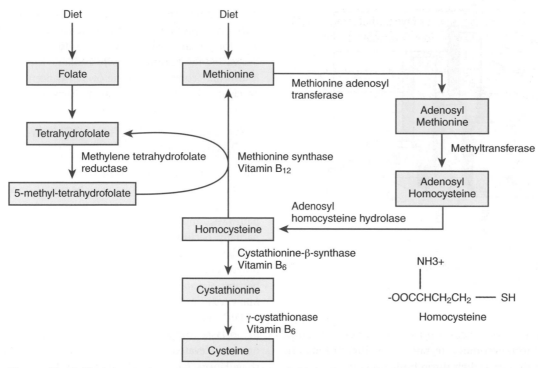

Figure 42-13 The homocysteine metabolic pathway. Dietary methionine is converted to homocysteine. Homocysteine is remethylated via methionine synthase to form methionine in the presence of vitamin B_{12}. This reaction requires 5-methyl tetrahydrofolate, which is supplied through dietary folate. Homocysteine also is metabolized via cystathionine β-synthase and γ-cystathionase to cysteine, which is excreted in urine or reused in protein metabolism. Cysteine production requires vitamin B_6. Deficiencies of vitamin B_6, vitamin B_{12}, or folate and mutations in methionine synthase, methylene tetrahydrofolate reductase, or cystathionine β-synthase result in hyperhomocysteinemia.

TABLE 42-11 Homocysteine Reference Ranges Using Enzyme Immunoassay

Population	Reference Range (μmol/L)
Female	
<60 y	4.6-12.1
>60 y	6.6-14.1
Male	
<60 y	5.0-15.6
>60 y	7.0-17.6

TABLE 42-12 Relative Risk of Coronary Events According to Concentration of Fibrinogen*

Fibrinogen Concentration Quintile	Relative Risk of Coronary Event
1	1.0
2	1.89
3	2.33
4	2.56
5	2.89

*The relative risks are shown for each of five quintiles of subjects defined according to the concentrations of each factor from 1, the group with the lowest concentration, to 5, the group with the highest. Relative risks have been adjusted for all confounding factors. The group with the lowest values serves as the reference group.

reduce the need for vitamin therapy and may shift the reference ranges. Whether such intervention will result in positive clinical outcomes has not been determined, however.

Fibrinogen Activity Assay

Fibrinogen may be measured using the clot-based method of Clauss and predicts cardiovascular risk.[75] Fibrinogen levels have a positive correlation to relative risk of myocardial infarction in patients with angina pectoris, as shown in Table 42-12. The relative risk triples between the first and fifth quintiles, and even high-normal levels predict increased risk. This predictive capacity is reflected in healthy individuals and patients with angina.[76] There is a relationship between fibrinogen and total cholesterol levels (Fig. 42-14). High fibrinogen concentrations can be used to predict hypercholesterolemia and identify patients who are at high risk for new coronary events. In contrast, low fibrinogen levels are associated with low risk of cardiovascular events, even in patients with high total cholesterol levels.

Elevated fibrinogen makes blood more viscous, favoring coagulation, platelet activation, and formation of atherothrombotic lesions. It directly promotes platelet activation by

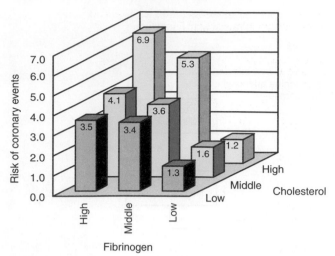

Figure 42-14 Tertiles of fibrinogen by total cholesterol predict relative risk of coronary events.

binding to the glycoprotein IIb/IIIa membrane receptors. Because fibrinogen becomes integrated into atherothrombotic lesions, it contributes to their thrombotic potential.

Although fibrinogen is a strong predictor of arterial thrombosis, the use of its assay for this purpose is limited. There are no independent therapeutic regimens that specifically lower fibrinogen, and no clinical trials suggest that reduction of fibrinogen concentrations in blood reverses the odds of thrombosis. Further, fibrinogen assays are not standardized. Clinical hemostasis laboratories may use the clot-based Clauss assay, immunoassay, or nephelometry, all yielding variant results. Nevertheless, statin (cholesterol-lowering) therapy, smoking cessation, and exercise lower fibrinogen levels along with LDL-C and total cholesterol, and the assay parallels the results of the other members of the risk prediction profile.

Lipoprotein (a)

Lipoprotein (a) is an LDL with noteworthy thrombosis risk prediction characteristics. The plasma level is measured by enzyme immunoassay, and its reference ranges are shown in Table 42-13. Although lipoprotein (a) concentrations in African Americans are higher than in Caucasians, the level is a stronger predictor of thrombosis in Caucasians, and its measurement may be considered to be a part of an arterial thrombosis prediction profile.[77]

TABLE 42-13 Normal Ranges for Lipoprotein (a) by Race and Sex

Race	Males	Females
African Americans	4.7-71.8 mg/dL	4.4-75 mg/dL
Caucasians	2.2-49.4 mg/dL	2.1-57.3 mg/dL

Lipoprotein (a) may contribute to thrombosis by its antifibrinolytic property. The molecule competes with plasminogen for binding sites on newly formed fibrin polymer, decreasing the plasmin activity available for clot degradation. It also may contribute to the overall concentration of LDL-C. Levels may be lowered with statin drugs, as are LDL-C levels.

DISSEMINATED INTRAVASCULAR COAGULATION

DIC is generalized activation of hemostasis secondary to a systemic disease and involving all hemostatic systems: vascular intima, platelets, leukocytes, coagulation, coagulation control pathways, and fibrinolysis.[78] In DIC, fibrin microthrombi partially occlude small vessels and lead to consumption of platelets, coagulation factors and control proteins, and fibrinolytic enzymes.[79] Consequently, fibrin degradation products become elevated and interfere with normal fibrin formation.[80] Many toxic and inflammatory processes are set loose.[81]

DIC may be acute and uncompensated, with multiple hemostasis component deficiencies, or chronic, with normal or even elevated clotting factor levels. In chronic DIC, liver coagulation factor production and bone marrow platelet production compensate for increased consumption.

Although DIC is a thrombotic process, the thrombi that form are small and ineffective, so systemic hemorrhage is often the first or most apparent symptom. Acute DIC is often fatal and requires immediate medical intervention. The diagnosis relies heavily on the hemostasis laboratory, and scientists often perform a DIC laboratory profile under medical emergency circumstances. *Defibrination syndrome* and *consumption coagulopathy* are alternate names for DIC.

Causes of Disseminated Intravascular Coagulation

Any disorder that contributes hemostatic molecules or promotes their endogenous secretion may cause DIC. Although any attempt to classify and list all the causes of DIC is hopeless, the major triggering mechanisms and examples of each are listed in Table 42-14.

The more acutely ill the patient, the more dangerous the symptoms. Chronic DIC may be associated with vascular tumors, tissue necrosis, liver disease, renal disease, chronic inflammation, prosthetic devices, and adenocarcinoma. The malignancies most associated with DIC are pancreatic, prostatic, ovarian, and lung cancers; multiple myeloma; and myeloproliferative diseases. Acute DIC is seen in association with obstetric emergencies, intravascular hemolysis, septicemia, viremia, burns, acute inflammation, crush injuries, dissecting aortic aneurysms, and cardiac disorders.

Pathophysiology

Triggering events may activate coagulation at any point in the pathway. When triggered, DIC proceeds in a standard sequence of events. Circulating thrombin is the primary culprit because it activates platelets, catalyzes fibrin formation, and consumes

TABLE 42-14 Disorders Associated with Disseminated Intravascular Coagulation Grouped According to Mechanism

Mechanism	Example Disorders
Release of tissue factor into circulation through endothelial cell damage or monocyte activation	Physical trauma such as crush or brain injuries, surgery
	Thermal injuries such as burns or cold
	Ischemia and infarction such as myocardial infarction
	Adenocarcinoma
	Degradation of muscle, rhabdomyolysis
Exposure of subendothelial tissue factor in vasodilation	Asphyxia and hypoxia
	Hypovolemic and hemorrhagic shock
	Heatstroke
	Vasculitis
	Malignant hypertension
Endotoxins with activation of cytokines	Bacterial, protozoal, fungal, and viral infections
	Toxic shock syndrome
Circulating immune complexes	Bacterial and viral infections
	Allergic reactions and anaphylaxis
	Acute hemolytic transfusion reactions
	Heparin-induced thrombocytopenia with thrombosis
	Drugs that trigger an immune response
	Graft rejection
Particulate matter from tissue injury	Abruptio placentae
	Amniotic fluid embolism
	Eclampsia, preeclampsia, HELLP syndrome
	Retained dead fetus or missed abortion
	Rupture of uterus
	Tubal pregnancy
	Fat embolism
	Heatstroke
Infusion of activated clotting factors	Activated prothrombin complex concentrate
Secretion of proteolytic enzymes	Acute promyelocytic or myelomonocytic leukemia
	Bacterial, protozoal, fungal, and viral infections
	Pancreatitis
Toxins that trigger coagulation	Snake or spider venom
	Pancreatitis
Thrombotic disease or thrombogenic conditions	Deep vein thrombosis, pulmonary embolus
	Thrombotic thrombocytopenic purpura, hemolytic-uremic syndrome
	Coagulation control system deficiencies
	Purpura fulminans, skin necrosis
	Pregnancy, postpartum period, estrogen treatments
Severe hypoxia or acidosis	Diabetes
	Chronic inflammation
Platelet activation	Vascular tumors
	Aortic aneurysm
	Vascular surgery, coronary artery bypass surgery
	Vascular prostheses
	Thrombocytosis, thrombocythemia, polycythemia

HELLP, hemolysis, elevated liver enzymes, and low platelet count.

control proteins. The fibrinolytic system may become activated at the level of plasminogen or TPA subsequent to fibrin formation, and endothelial cells may be damaged, releasing coagulation active substances. Finally, leukocytes, particularly monocytes, may be induced to secrete tissue factor by the cytokines released during inflammation.

Thrombin cleaves fibrinogen, creating fibrin monomers. In normal hemostasis, fibrin monomers spontaneously polymerize to form an insoluble gel. The polymer becomes strengthened through cross-linking, binding plasminogen as it forms. In DIC, a percentage of fibrin monomers fail to polymerize and circulate in plasma as soluble fibrin monomers. The monomers coat platelets and coagulation proteins, creating an anticoagulant effect (Fig. 42-15).

Soluble fibrin monomers, fibrin polymer, and cross-linked fibrin all activate plasminogen. Normally, the active form of plasminogen, plasmin, acts locally to digest only the solid fibrin clot to which it is bound. In DIC, plasmin circulates in the plasma and digests all forms of fibrin.[82] Consequently, fibrin degradation products labeled X, Y, D, E, and D-dimer are detectable in the plasma in concentrations exceeding 20,000 ηg/mL (Fig. 42-16). D-dimer arises only from cross-linked fibrin polymer, whereas the other fibrin degradation products may be produced from fibrinogen or fibrin monomers or polymers.[83]

Platelets become enmeshed in the fibrin polymer or are exposed to thrombin; both events trigger platelet activation, which drives the coagulation system and produces thrombo-

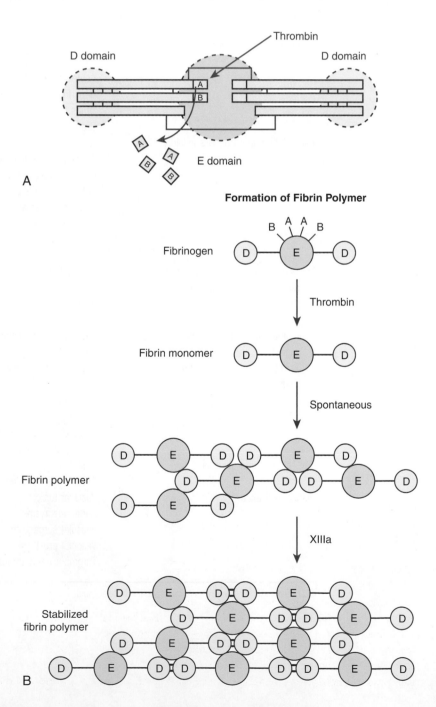

Figure 42-15 Normal fibrinogen polymerization. **A,** Thrombin cleaves fibrinopeptides A and B from the α and β chains of fibrinogen, creating fibrin monomer with D and E domains. **B,** Fibrin monomer normally polymerizes and becomes cross-linked by the action of factor XIIIa. When excess fibrin degradation products are present, the fibrin monomer fails to polymerize normally, causing increased plasma fibrin monomer.

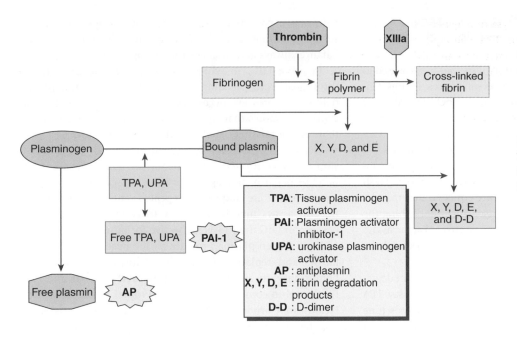

Figure 42-16 Fibrinolysis produces the fibrin degradation products X, Y, D, and E and D-dimer. The D-dimer is produced from cross-linked fibrin.

cytopenia. At the same time, control of the coagulation pathway is lost as protein C, protein S, and antithrombin are consumed. The combination of thrombin activation, circulating plasmin, loss of control, and thrombocytopenia contribute to the overall hemorrhagic outcomes of DIC.

Plasmin digests factors V, VIII, IX, and XI and other plasma proteins. Plasmin also may trigger complement, leading to hemolysis, and the kinin system, leading to inflammation, hypotension, and shock. In fibrinolytic therapy, amyloidosis, and some cases of liver disease, plasminogen is activated independent of the coagulation pathway. This condition, called *systemic fibrinolysis*, produces laboratory-measurable fibrin degradation products and prolonged prothrombin time (PT) and PTT with a normal platelet count.[84]

Symptoms of Disseminated Intravascular Coagulation

The symptoms signaling DIC frequently are masked by the symptoms of the underlying disorder and may be chronic, acute, or fulminant. Thrombosis in the microvasculature of major organs may produce symptoms of organ failure, such as renal function impairment, adult respiratory distress syndrome, and central nervous system manifestations. Skin, bone, and bone marrow necrosis may be seen. Purpura fulminans is seen in meningococcemia, chickenpox, and spirochete infections.

Laboratory Diagnosis

DIC is a clinical diagnosis that requires laboratory confirmation (Chapter 45). The primary profile includes a platelet count, blood film examination, PT, PTT, D-dimer, and fibrinogen assays. Anticipated DIC results are shown in Table 42-15. Prolonged PT and PTT reflect coagulation factor consumption. Fibrinogen levels may decrease in DIC, but because fibrinogen is an acute-phase reactant that increases in inflammation, the

TABLE 42-15 Anticipated Results of Disseminated Intravascular Coagulation Primary Laboratory Profile

Test	Normal Range	DIC
Platelet count	$200\text{-}400 \times 10^9/L$	$<200 \times 10^9/L$
Prothrombin time	11-14 s	>14 s
Partial thromboplastin time	25-35 s	>35 s
D-dimer	0-100 ηg/mL	>500 ηg/mL
Fibrinogen	200-400 mg/dL	<200 mg/dL

fibrinogen level alone provides little information and may exceed 400 mg/dL. The peripheral blood film confirms thrombocytopenia in nearly all cases, and the presence of schistocytes may help establish the diagnosis of DIC in about 50%.[85,86] An elevated D-dimer assay is essential to the diagnosis. D-dimer also may be elevated in inflammatory conditions, localized thrombosis, or renal disease in the absence of DIC; the PT, PTT, platelet count, blood film examination, and other laboratory assays must be provided with the D-dimer to rule out these disorders.[87]

The D-dimer reference limit is typically 250 ηg/mL, although the interval varies with location and technology. In 85% of DIC cases, D-dimers reach 10,000 to 20,000 ηg/mL. A normal D-dimer assay rules out localized venous thrombosis such as deep vein thrombosis or pulmonary emboli where levels increase to greater than 500 ηg/mL.[88] D-dimer levels typically are elevated in inflammation, sickle cell crisis, pregnancy, and renal disease, so an abnormal result cannot be used to diagnose venous thromboembolism definitively.[89] The judicious use of the D-dimer assay reduces the requirement for invasive diagnostic tests such as pulmonary angiography when pulmonary embolism is suspected.[90]

Specialized Laboratory Tests That May Aid in the Diagnosis of Disseminated Intravascular Coagulation

Table 42-16 lists specialized laboratory tests that may be used to diagnose and classify DIC in special circumstances. Results consistent with DIC and clinical comments are included. Many of these tests are available in acute care facilities but are not routinely applied to DIC diagnoses. Others are available only in tertiary care facilities and hemostasis reference laboratories.[91-93]

Protein C, protein S, and antithrombin typically are consumed in DIC, and their assay adds little to the diagnosis. Fresh frozen plasma, APC, or antithrombin concentrates may be used to treat DIC. These assays are useful in establishing the necessity for therapy and monitoring its effect. Factor assays may clarify PT and PTT results. The thrombin time and the reptilase time also are sensitive DIC screens.

Tests of the fibrinolytic pathway include serum fibrin degradation products, chromogenic plasminogen activity assay, TPA and PAI-1 immunoassays, and the euglobulin clot lysis time test, a time-honored, clot-based assay. These tests are seldom offered in the acute care hemostasis laboratory because they require careful specimen management, but they may help in the diagnosis of primary fibrinolysis, sometimes seen after fibrinolytic therapy.

Treatment of Disseminated Intravascular Coagulation

To arrest DIC, the physician must diagnose and treat the underlying disorder. Surgery, anti-inflammatory agents, antibiotics, or obstetric procedures as appropriate may normalize hemostasis, particularly in chronic DIC. Supportive therapy, such as maintenance of nutrition and fluid and electrolyte balance, always accompanies the management.

In acute DIC, in which multiorgan failure from microthrombosis and bleeding threatens the life of the patient, heroic measures are necessary. Treatment falls into two categories: therapies that slow the clotting process and therapies that replace missing platelets and coagulation factors.

Heparin may be used for its antithrombotic properties to stop the uncontrolled activation of the coagulation cascade. Because heparin may aggravate bleeding, careful observation and support are required. Repeated anti-Xa chromogenic heparin assays may be necessary to control heparin dosage because in DIC the PTT is ineffective for monitoring heparin.

Fresh frozen plasma provides all the necessary coagulation factors and replaces blood volume lost during acute DIC hemorrhage. Its effects are best monitored with PTs and PTTs. Prothrombin complex concentrate (Proplex T complex; Baxter Healthcare Corporation, Glendale, Calif.) is rarely needed but may be an alternative if plasma expansion must be avoided. Fibrinogen is often of paramount concern, and cryoprecipitate supplies it at high concentrations and low volume, along with factor VIII. Repeated fibrinogen assays, PTs, and PTTs are necessary to confirm cryoprecipitate effectiveness. Platelet transfusions are necessary if thrombocytopenia is severe. Effectiveness and platelet consumption are monitored with platelet counts and computation of corrected platelet count increments (Chapter 45). Red blood cells are used as necessary to respond to the resulting anemia. Antifibrinolytic therapy is contraindicated in all but proven systemic fibrinolysis.[94]

TABLE 42-16 Specialized Hemostasis Laboratory Assays Useful in Disseminated Intravascular Coagulation Diagnosis and Classification

Assay	DIC Results	Characteristics
Serum FDP	>10 µg/mL	Obsolete, replaced by quantitative D-dimer
Soluble fibrin monomer	Positive	Hemagglutination assay provides a valid predictive index. Avoid obsolete tests such as protamine sulfate solubility or ethanol gelation
Thrombus precursor protein	>3.5 µg/mL	Immunoassay with no interference from fibrinogen or FDPs
Protein C, protein S, and antithrombin activity assays	<50%	Useful in monitoring therapy, especially antithrombin and activated protein C concentrates
Factor assays: prothrombin and factors V, VIII, X	<50%	Factors V and VIII are increased in inflammation and may give misleading results
Thrombin time, reptilase time	Prolonged	Fibrinogen levels <80 mg/dL, elevated FDPs, and soluble fibrin monomer all cause prolongation
Plasminogen, tissue plasminogen activator	Decreased	May be useful for further analyzing systemic fibrinolysis. Specimen management protocol must be strictly observed
Euglobulin clot lysis time	<2 h or >12 h	End point is clot dissolution. A shortened ELT indicates increased fibrinolysis, a lengthened ELT indicates deficiency; both may occur in DIC
Peripheral blood film examination	Anemia with schistocytes, thrombocytopenia	Schistocytes (microangiopathic hemolytic anemia) present in 50% of cases; leukocytosis is common
Localized thrombosis markers: prothrombin 1+2, thrombin-antithrombin	Elevated	Most useful in diagnosis of localized thrombotic events but may be used to monitor DIC therapy. Useful for clinical trials

ELT, euglobulin lysis time; FDP, fibrin degradation products.

LOCALIZED THROMBOSIS MONITORS

In addition to D-dimer, several peptides and coagulation factor complexes are released into the plasma during coagulation. One complex, TAT, and one peptide, PF 1+2, may be assayed as a means to detect and monitor localized venous or arterial thromboses. TAT and PF 1+2 immunoassays are sensitive but nonspecific because, in addition to thrombosis, they become elevated in DIC, septicemia, eclampsia, pancreatitis, leukemia, liver disease, and trauma.[95] They are of particular value in clinical trials.

PF 1+2 is released from prothrombin at the time of its conversion to thrombin by the prothrombinase complex (Fig. 42-17). It has a plasma half-life of 90 minutes and a reference range of 0.3 to 1.5 ηmol/L. Elevated PF 1+2 may be seen in venous thromboembolism. Heparin or oral anticoagulant therapy reduces its plasma concentration.

The TAT covalent complex is formed when antithrombin neutralizes thrombin. This reaction is enhanced by the presence of heparin. TAT has a half-life of 3 minutes and a normal range of 0.5 to 5 ηg/mL. To avoid in vitro release or activation of PF 1+2 or TAT, plasma specimens collected in 3.2% sodium citrate are centrifuged and separated within minutes of collection, and the plasma is frozen until ready for assay.

HEPARIN-INDUCED THROMBOCYTOPENIA

Heparin-induced thrombocytopenia (HIT), also called *heparin-induced thrombocytopenia with thrombosis*, is an adverse effect of unfractionated heparin therapy.

Cause and Clinical Significance of Heparin-Induced Thrombocytopenia

One to 5% of patients receiving unfractionated heparin for more than 5 days develop an IgG antibody to heparin–platelet factor 4 complexes. In 30% to 50%, the immune complex that is formed binds platelet Fc receptors, leading to platelet activation, thrombocytopenia, and formation of microvascular thrombi.[96,97] HIT occurs in intravenous and subcutaneous heparin administrations at prophylactic and therapeutic dosages, although it is more frequent with therapeutic levels.[98] Venous thrombosis predominates 5:1, but arterial thrombosis accounts for the most disturbing symptoms. Patients may have pulmonary emboli, limb gangrene requiring amputation, stroke, and myocardial infarction. HIT is often a medical emergency, and the mortality rate is 20%.[99]

Platelet Count in Heparin-Induced Thrombocytopenia

Patients receiving heparin must have platelet counts performed daily. A decrease in platelet count during heparin administration is a recognized signal for HIT, but the interpretation of the thrombocytopenia is confounded by the fact that 30% of patients receiving heparin develop an immediate, benign, and limited thrombocytopenia, sometimes called *HIT type I.*[100] This benign form of thrombocytopenia usually develops in 1 to 3 days, whereas immune-mediated HIT, sometimes called *HIT type II,* develops after about 5 days. There is significant overlap in patients previously exposed to heparin. In HIT, the decrease in platelet count may exceed 40%, whereas in benign thrombocytopenia, the decrease is relatively small; however, in both cases, the platelet count may remain within the normal range.

Laboratory Tests

Because at least 10% of hospitalized patients receive heparin, the acute care laboratory must provide a procedure to confirm HIT and differentiate it from benign thrombocytopenia. The heparin-induced antibody immunoassay is available in most acute care facility laboratories, although seldom as a STAT assay (Chapter 45).[101] The assay may become positive before clinical signs of HIT are evident and is more sensitive than aggregometry.[102] It may be negative, however, in a few patients, possibly because peptides other than platelet factor 4 also may form complexes with heparin to cause HIT. Microbial contamination, lipemia, or hemolysis may invalidate the test results. The presence of immune complexes or immunoglobulin aggregates in the patient specimen may cause increased nonspecific binding and produce false-positive results.

Many laboratories provide aggregometry or lumiaggregometry for the diagnosis of HIT (Chapter 45).[103] Aggregometry is technically demanding and is only 50% sensitive for HIT. The reference method is the ^{14}C serotonin washed platelet release assay, provided in reference laboratories that possess radionuclide licenses.

Heparin-Induced Thrombocytopenia Therapy

When heparin-induced antibodies are detected, the administration of heparin must be discontinued immediately, and an alternate form of anticoagulation must be considered. Complete removal of anticoagulant therapy is risky because additional thrombotic events are likely to occur. Although low-molecular-weight heparin causes HIT in less than 1% of cases in which it is the sole anticoagulant, it is contraindicated when HIT already has been induced during unfractionated heparin

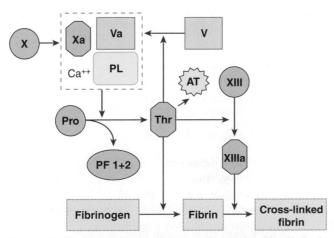

Figure 42-17 PF 1+2 is cleaved during activation of prothrombin by the Xa-Va complex. TAT is a complex formed on the generation of thrombin. Plasma antithrombin covalently reacts with thrombin to form the TAT complex. PF, prothrombin fragment; TAT, thrombin-antithrombin.

therapy. Likewise, oral anticoagulant therapy is discouraged because this may precipitate a potentially fatal warfarin-induced skin necrosis syndrome.

Recombinant lepirudin (Refludan; Hoechst Marion Roussel, Bridgewater, N.J.) is a direct thrombin inhibitor modeled after leech saliva that binds the reactive site of thrombin. Lepirudin is administered as a continuous infusion and may be monitored using the PTT or Ecarin (Pentapharm, Basel, Switzerland) prothrombin assay based on the snake venom reagent from *Echis carinatus*, available only from reference laboratories. Argatroban, another direct thrombin inhibitor, also may be monitored using the PTT.

SUMMARY

The importance of laboratory diagnosis has become evident in all forms of thrombotic disease—chronic and acute, arterial and venous, primary and secondary. The most promising current area of development is the prediction of risk of cardiovascular and cerebrovascular disease. It is hoped that the future will give us markers of endothelial cell disease, measures of leukocyte adhesion, and more specific markers of inflammation and platelet activity.

CHAPTER at a GLANCE

- Thrombosis is the most prevalent condition in developed countries and accounts for most illnesses and premature deaths.
- Thrombosis may be arterial, causing peripheral artery disease, heart disease, and stroke, or venous, causing deep vein thrombosis and pulmonary emboli.
- Most thrombosis occurs as a result of lifestyle habits and aging, but many thrombotic disorders are related to congenital risk factors.
- Thrombosis risk profiles may be offered to clinicians for screening purposes in high-risk populations.
- The main hemostasis predictors of arterial thrombotic disease are high-sensitivity CRP, homocysteine, fibrinogen, lipoprotein (a), and elevated coagulation factors.
- APL antibody testing requires a series of essential hemostasis laboratory assays, both clot based and immunoassays.
- Antithrombin may be assayed using chromogenic substrate and enzyme immunoassay analyses.

- The tests of the protein C pathway include protein C and protein S activity and concentration, APC resistance, FVL assay, and the C4b-binding protein assay.
- The molecular test for prothrombin 20210A mutation predicts the risk of venous thrombosis.
- DIC is a clinical diagnosis confirmed by a series of assays in the acute care facility.
- Chronic thrombosis may be determined using the PF 1+2, thrombin-antithrombin complex, and quantitative D-dimer assay.
- The laboratory provides confirmatory tests in HIT with thrombosis.

Now that you have completed this chapter, go back and read again the case study at the beginning and respond to the questions presented.

REVIEW QUESTIONS

1. What is the prevalence of venous thrombosis in the United States?
   a. 0.001
   b. 0.01
   c. 10% to 15%
   d. 500,000/y

2. What is thrombophilia?
   a. Predisposition to thrombosis secondary to a congenital or acquired disorder
   b. Inappropriate triggering of the plasma coagulation system
   c. A condition in which clots form uncontrollably
   d. Inadequate fibrinolysis

3. What acquired thrombosis risk factor is measured in the hemostasis laboratory?
   a. Smoking
   b. Immobilization
   c. Body mass index
   d. LA

4. Trousseau syndrome, a low-grade chronic DIC, is often associated with what type of disorder?
   a. Renal disease
   b. Hepatic disease
   c. Adenocarcinoma
   d. Chronic inflammation

5. What is the most common heritable thrombosis risk factor in Caucasians?
   a. Prothrombin 20210A mutation
   b. APC resistance
   c. Antithrombin deficiency
   d. Protein S deficiency

6. What test is *not* routinely used in the lupus anticoagulant profile?
   a. Dilute Russell viper venom time
   b. Low-phospholipid PTT
   c. Dilute PT
   d. D-dimer

7. A patient with venous thrombosis is tested for protein S deficiency. The protein S activity, antigen, and free antigen all are less than 65%, and the C4b-binding protein level is normal. What type of deficiency is likely?
   a. I
   b. II
   c. III
   d. No deficiency is indicated because the reference range includes 25%.

8. What fibrinolysis system assay is associated with arterial thrombotic risk?
   a. PAI-1
   b. Lipoprotein (a)
   c. Factor VIIa
   d. Factor XII

9. How does lipoprotein (a) cause thrombosis?
   a. It causes elevated factor VIII levels.
   b. It coats the endothelial lining of arteries.
   c. It contributes additional phospholipid in vivo for formation of the Xase complex.
   d. It substitutes for plasminogen or TPA in the forming clot.

10. What test may be used to confirm the presence of LA?
    a. Bethesda titer
    b. PT
    c. Antinuclear antibody
    d. PTT using high phospholipid reagent

11. What DNA-based test may be used to confirm APC resistance?
    a. Prothrombin 20210A
    b. FVL
    c. MTHFR 1298
    d. MTHFR 677

12. What therapy may occasionally cause DIC?
    a. Factor VIII
    b. Factor VIIa
    c. Antithrombin concentrate
    d. Activated prothrombin complex concentrate

13. Which of the following tests for the integrity of the entire fibrinolytic system?
    a. Euglobulin lysis
    b. Soluble fibrin monomer
    c. 5 M urea solubility assay
    d. Fibrinogen degradation products

14. What is the most important application of the quantitative D-dimer test?
    a. Diagnose primary fibrinolysis
    b. Diagnose liver and renal disease
    c. Rule out deep venous thrombosis
    d. Diagnose acute myocardial infarction

REFERENCES

1. Francis JL: Laboratory investigation of hypercoagulability. Semin Thromb Hemost 1998;24:111-126.
2. Dahlback B, Carlsson M, Svensson PJ: Familial thrombophilia due to a previously unrecognized mechanism characterized by poor anticoagulant response to activated protein C: prediction of a cofactor to activated protein C. Proc Natl Acad Sci U S A 1993;90:1004-1008.
3. Bertina RM, Koeleman BPC, Koster T, et al: Mutation in blood coagulation factor V associated with resistance to activated protein C. Nature 1994;369:64-67.
4. Nieuwdorp M, Stroes ES, Meijers JC, et al: Hypercoagulability in the metabolic syndrome. Curr Opin Pharmacol 2005;5:155-159.
5. Kitchens CS, Alving BM, Kessler CM: Consultative Hemostasis and Thrombosis. Philadelphia: Saunders, 2002.
6. Thom T, Haase N, Rosamond W: Heart disease and stroke statistics—2006 update: a report from the American Heart Association statistics committee and stroke statistics subcommittee. Circulation 2006;105:85-151.
7. Goldhaber SZ: Pulmonary embolism. N Engl J Med 1998;339:93-104.
8. Anderson FA, Wheeler HB, Goldberg RJ, et al: A population-based perspective of the hospital incidence and case-fatality rate of deep-vein thrombosis and pulmonary embolism. The Worcester DVT study. Arch Intern Med 1991;151:933-938.
9. Jensen R: The interface of the physician and the laboratory in the detection of venous thrombotic risk—part I. Clin Hemost Rev 1997;11:1-4.
10. Blanchette VS, Al-Musa A, Stain AM, et al: Central venous access catheters in children with haemophilia. Blood Coagul Fibrinolysis 1996;7:S39-S42.
11. Rosendaal FR: Risk factors for venous thrombotic disease. Thromb Haemost 1999;82:610-619.
12. Lowe GDO: Acute stroke. In Hull R, Pineo GF (eds): Disorders of Thrombosis. Philadelphia: Saunders, 1996:116-125.
13. Heit JA: Epidemiology of venous thromboembolism. In Colman RW, Clowes AM, Goldhaber SZ, et al (eds): Hemostasis and Thrombosis: Basic Principles and Clinical Practice, 5th ed. Philadelphia: Lippincott, 2006:1227-1234.
14. Rosenberg RD, Bauer KA: New insights into hypercoagulable states. Hosp Pract 1986;21:131-138.
15. Fritsma GA: Laboratory measurement of hemorrhage and thrombosis. In Rodak B (ed): Diagnostic Hematology. Philadelphia: Saunders, 1995:549-584.
16. Rak J, Milsom C, May L, et al: Tissue factor in cancer and angiogenesis: the molecular link between genetic tumor progression, tumor neovascularization, and cancer coagulopathy. Semin Thromb Hemost 2006;32:54-70.
17. De Stefano V, Sora F, Rossi E, et al: The risk of thrombosis in patients with acute leukemia: occurrence of thrombosis at diagnosis and during treatment. J Thromb Haemost 2005;3:1985-1992.
18. Rosse WF, Ware RE: The molecular basis of paroxysmal nocturnal hemoglobinuria. Blood 1995;86:3277-3286.
19. Wolf PA, Dawber TR, Thomas HE, et al: Epidemiologic assessment of chronic atrial fibrillation and risk of stroke: the Framingham study. Neurology 1978;28:973-977.
20. Lane DA, Mannuci PM, Bauer KA, et al: Inherited thrombophilia: part 2. Thromb Haemost 1996;76:824-834.
21. Johnson CM, Mureebe L, Silver D: Hypercoagulable states: a review. Vasc Endovasc Surg 2005;39:123-133.
22. Itakkura H: Racial disparities in risk factors for thrombosis. Curr Opin Hematol 2005;12:364-369.

23. Brown K, Luddington R, Williamson D, et al: Risk of venous thromboembolism associated with a G to A transition at position 20210 in the 3'-untranslated region of the prothrombin gene. Br J Haematol 1997;98:907-909.

24. Ridker PM, Hennekens CH, Selhub J, et al: Interrelation of hyperhomocysteinemia, factor V Leiden, and risk of future venous thromboembolism. Circulation 1997;95:1777-1782.

25. Heit JA, O'Fallon WM, Petterson TM, et al: Relative impact of risk factors for deep vein thrombosis and pulmonary embolism: a population-based study. Arch Intern Med 2002;162:1245-1248.

26. Alarcon-Segovia D, Cabral AR: The concept and classification of antiphospholipid/cofactor syndromes. Lupus 1996;5:364-367.

27. Lim W, Crowther MA, Eikelboom JW: Management of antiphospholipid antibody syndrome: a systematic review. JAMA 2006;295:1050-1057.

28. Miyakis S, Locksin T, Atsumi T, et al: International consensus statement on an update of the classification criteria for defining antiphospholipid syndrome (APS). J Thromb Haemost 2006;4:295-306.

29. Kandiah DA, Sheng YH, Krilis SA: Beta-2 glycoprotein I: target antigen for autoantibodies in the "antiphospholipid syndrome." Lupus 1996;5:381-386.

30. Lie JT: Vasculopathy of the antiphospholipid syndromes revisited: thrombosis is the culprit and vasculitis the consort. Lupus 1966;5:368-371.

31. Lopez-Pedrera C, Buendia P, Barbarroja N, et al: Anti-phospholipid-mediated thrombosis: interplay between anticardiolipin antibodies and vascular cells. Clin Appl Thromb Hemost 2006;12:41-45.

32. Hughes GRV: The antiphospholipid syndrome. Lupus 1996;5:345-346.

33. Triplett DA: Antiphospholipid antibodies. In Hathaway WE, Goodnight SH (eds): Disorders of Hemostasis and Thrombosis, 2nd ed. New York: McGraw-Hill, 2001:405-419.

34. Hughes GRV: An immune mechanism in thrombosis. QJM 1988;258P:753-754.

35. Mannucci PM, Canciani MT, Mari D, et al: The varied sensitivity of partial thromboplastin and prothrombin-reagents in the demonstration of lupus-like anticoagulants. Scand J Haematol 1979;22:423-432.

36. Comp PC: Congenital and acquired hypercoagulable states. In Hull R, Pineo GF (eds): Disorders of Thrombosis. Philadelphia: Saunders, 1996:339-347.

37. Kaczor DA, Bickford NN, Triplett DA: Evaluation of different mixing study reagents and dilution effect in lupus anticoagulant testing. Am J Clin Pathol 1991;95:408-411.

38. Sato K, Kagami K, Asai M, et al: Detection of lupus anticoagulant using a modified diluted Russell's viper venom test. Rinsho Byori (KIV) 1995;43:263-268.

39. Brandt JT, Triplett DA, Alving B, et al: Criteria for the diagnosis of lupus anticoagulants: an update. Thromb Haemost 1995;74:1185-1190.

40. Devreese KM: Interpretation of normal plasma mixing studies in the laboratory diagnosis of lupus anticoagulants. Thromb Res 2006, Accessed Online May 15, 2006.Epub ahead of print.

41. Rauch J, Tannenbaum H, Janoff AS: Distinguishing plasma lupus anticoagulants from anti-factor antibodies using hexagonal (II) phase phospholipids. Thromb Haemost 1989;62:892-896.

42. Triplett DA: Laboratory diagnosis of lupus anticoagulants. Semin Thromb Hemost 1990;16:182-192.

43. Walker TS, Triplett DA, Javed N, et al: Evaluation of lupus anticoagulants: antiphospholipid antibodies, endothelium associated immunoglobulin, endothelial prostacyclin secretion, and antigenic protein S levels. Thromb Res 1988;51:267-281.

44. Koike T, Matsuura E: What is the true antigen for anticardiolipin antibodies? Lancet 1991;337:671-672.

45. Colaco CB, Male DK: Anti-phospholipid antibodies in syphilis and a thrombotic subset of SLE: distinct profiles of epitope specificity. Clin Exp Immunol 1985;59:449-456.

46. Samaha M, Trossaert M, Conard J, et al: Prevalence and patient profile in activated protein C resistance. Am J Clin Pathol 1995;104:450-454.

47. Rosen S, Johansson K, Lindberg B, et al: Multicenter evaluation of a kit for activated protein C resistance on various coagulation instruments using plasmas from healthy individuals. Thromb Haemost 1994;72:255-260.

48. Dahlback B, Hildebrand B: Inherited resistance to activated protein C is corrected by anticoagulant cofactor activity found to be a property of factor V. Proc Natl Acad Sci U S A 1994;91:1396-1400.

49. De Ronde H, Bertina RM: Laboratory diagnosis of APC-resistance: a critical evaluation of the test and the development of diagnostic criteria. Thromb Haemost 1994;72:880-886.

50. Ragland BD, Reed CE, Eiland BM, et al: The effect of lupus anticoagulant in the second-generation assay for activated protein C resistance. Am J Clin Pathol 2003;119:66-71.

51. Ts'ao C, Neofotistos D, Oropeza M, et al: Modified APC-resistance test: variable ratios with respect to source of factor V-deficient plasma. Am J Hematol 1997;54:214-218.

52. Poort SR, Rosendaal FR, Reitsma PY, et al: A common genetic variation in the 3' untranslated region of the prothrombin gene is associate with elevated plasma prothrombin levels and an increase in venous thrombosis. Blood 1996;88:3698-3703.

53. Danckwardt S, Hartmann K, Gehring NH, et al: 3' end processing of the prothrombin mRNA in thrombophilia. Acta Haematol 2006;115:192-197.

54. Naeem MA, Anwar M, Ali W, et al: Prevalence of prothrombin gene mutation (G-A 20210 A) in general population: a pilot study. Clin Appl Thromb Hemost 2006;12:223-226.

55. Thaler E, Lechner K: Antithrombin III deficiency and thromboembolism. Clin Haematol 1981;10:369-390.

56. Wu O, Robertson L, Twaddle S, et al: Screening for thrombophilia in high-risk situations: systematic review and cost-effectiveness analysis. The Thrombosis: Risk and Economic Assessment of Thrombophilia Screening (TREATS) study. Health Technol Assess 2006;10:1-110.

57. Rosen S: Chromogenic methods in coagulation diagnostics. Hamostaseologie 2005;25:259-266.

58. Laroche P, Plassart V, Amiral J: Rapid quantitative latex immuno assays for diagnosis of thrombotic disorders. XIIth Congress of the International Society on Thrombosis and Hemostasis [abstract]. Thromb Haemost 1989;62:379.

59. Dahlback B: The protein C anticoagulant system: inherited defects as basis for venous thrombosis. Thromb Res 1995;77:1-43.

60. Bick RL: Hypercoagulability and thrombosis. Med Clin North Am 1994;78:635-665.

61. Morrow DA, Ridker PM: High sensitivity C-reactive protein (hs-CRP): a novel risk marker in cardiovascular disease. Prev Cardiol 1999;1:13-16.

62. Ridker PM: Evaluating novel cardiovascular risk factors: can we better predict heart attacks? Ann Intern Med 1999;130:933-937.

63. Ridker PM: Fibrinolytic and inflammatory markers for arterial occlusion: the evolving epidemiology of thrombosis and hemostasis. Thromb Haemost 1997;78:53-59.

64. Pepys MB, Baltz ML: Acute phase proteins with special refer-

ence to C-reactive protein and related proteins (pentaxins) and serum amyloid A proteins. Adv Immunol 1983;34:141-212.

65. Wilkins J, Gallimore R, Moore E, et al: Rapid automated high sensitivity enzyme immunoassay of C-reactive protein. Clin Chem 1998;44:1358-1361.

66. Ledue T, Weiner D, Sipe J: Analytical evaluations of particle-enhanced immunonephelometric assays for C-reactive protein, serum amyloid A and mannose-binding protein in human serum. Ann Clin Biochem 1998;35:745-753.

67. Ridker PM, Cushman M, Stampfer MJ, et al: Inflammation, aspirin, and the risk of cardiovascular disease in apparently healthy men. N Engl J Med 1997;336:973-979.

68. Ridker PM, Glynn RJ, Hennekens CH: C-reactive protein adds to the predictive value of total and HDL cholesterol in determining risk of first myocardial infarction. Circulation 1998;97:2007-2011.

69. Williams RH, Maggiore JA: Hyperhomocysteinemia pathogenesis, clinical significance, laboratory assessment, and treatment. Lab Med 1999;30:468-474.

70. Homocysteinemia. In Hathaway WE, Goodnight SH (eds): Disorders of Hemostasis and Thrombosis, 2nd ed. New York: McGraw-Hill, 2001:397-401.

71. Boers GHJ: Hyperhomocysteinemia as a risk factor for arterial and venous disease: a review of evidence and relevance. Thromb Haemost 1997;78:520-522.

72. Guba SC, Fonseca V, Fink LM: Hyperhomocysteinemia and thrombosis. Semin Thromb Hemost 1999;25:291-309.

73. Refsum H, Ueland PM, Nygard O, et al: Homocysteine and cardiovascular disease. Annu Rev Med 1998;49:31-62.

74. D'Angelo A, Selhub J: Homocysteine and thrombotic disease. Blood 1997;90:1-11.

75. Thompson SG, Kienast J, Pyke SD, et al: Hemostatic factors and the risk of myocardial infarction or sudden death in patients with angina pectoris. N Engl J Med 1995;332:635-641.

76. Meade TW, Mellows S, Brozovic M, et al: Haemostatic function and ischaemic heart disease: principal results of the Northwick Park Heart Study. Lancet 1986;2:533-537.

77. Deb A, Caplice NM: Lipoprotein(a): new insights into mechanisms of atherogenesis and thrombosis. Clin Cardiol 2004;27:258-264.

78. Bick RL, Scates SM: Disseminated intravascular coagulation. Lab Med 1992;23:161-166.

79. Bauer KA, Rosenberg RD: The pathophysiology of the prethrombotic state in humans: insights gained from studies using markers of hemostatic system activation. Blood 1987;70:343-350.

80. Giles AR: Disseminated intravascular coagulation. In Bloom AL, Forbes CD, Thomas DP, et al (eds): Haemostasis and Thrombosis. New York: Churchill Livingstone, 1994:969-986.

81. Marder VJ, Feinstein DI, Colman RW, et al: Consumptive thrombohemorrhagic disorders. In Colman RW, Clowes AM, Goldhaber SZ, et al (eds): Hemostasis and Thrombosis: Basic Principles and Clinical Practice, 5th ed. Philadelphia: Lippincott, 2006:1571-1600.

82. Vaughan DE, Declerck PJ: Regulation of Fibrinolysis. In Loscalzo J, Schafer AI (eds): Thrombosis and Hemorrhage. Philadephia: Lippincott, Williams & Wilkins, 2003:105-120.

83. Jensen R: The diagnostic use of fibrin breakdown products. Clin Hemost Rev 1998;12:1-2.

84. Hersch SL, Kunelis T, Francis RB Jr: The pathogenesis of accelerated fibrinolysis in liver cirrhosis: a critical role for tissue plasminogen activator inhibitor. Blood 1987;69:1315-1319.

85. Brain MC, Dacie JV, Hourihane DOB: Microangiopathic haemolytic anaemia; the possible role of vascular lesions in pathogenesis. Br J Haematol 1962;8:358-374.

86. Nieuwenhuizen W: Plasma assays for derivatives of fibrin and of fibrinogen, based on monoclonal antibodies. Fibrinolysis 1988;2:1-5.

87. Bick RL, Baker WF: Diagnostic efficacy of the D-dimer assay in disseminated intravascular coagulation (DIC). Thromb Res 1992;65:785-790.

88. Janssen MC, Sollersheim H, Verbruggen B, et al: Rapid D-dimer assays to exclude deep venous thrombosis and pulmonary embolism: current status and new developments. Semin Thromb Hemost 1998;24:393-400.

89. Wada H, Wakita Y, Nakase T, et al: Hemostatic molecular markers before the onset of disseminated intravascular coagulation. Am J Hematol 1999;60:273-278.

90. Francalance I, Comeglio P, Liotta AA, et al: D-dimer concentrations during normal pregnancy, as measured by ELISA. Thromb Res 1995;80:89-92.

91. Gaffney PJ, Perry MJ: Unreliability of current serum fibrin degradation product (FDP) assays. Thromb Haemost 1985; 53:301-302.

92. Saito H: Normal hemostatic mechanisms. In Ratnoff OD, Forbes CS (eds): Disorders of Hemostasis. Philadelphia: Saunders, 1991:18-47.

93. Carville DGM, Dimitrijevic N, Walsh M, et al: Thrombus precursor protein: marker of thrombosis early in the pathogenesis of myocardial infarction. Clin Chem 1996;42:1537-1541.

94. Avvisati G, Ten Cate JW, Buller HR, et al: Tranexamic acid for control of haemorrhage in acute promyelocytic leukemia. Lancet 1989;2:122-124.

95. Speiser W, Mallek R, Koppensteiner R, et al: D-dimer and TAT measurement in patients with deep venous thrombosis: utility in diagnosis and judgment of anticoagulant treatment effectiveness. Thromb Haemost 1990;64:196-201.

96. Brace LD: Testing for heparin-induced thrombocytopenia by platelet aggregometry. Clin Lab Sci 1992;5:80-81.

97. Vermylen J, Hoylaerts MF, Arnout J: Antibody-mediated thrombosis. Thromb Haemost 1997;78:420-426.

98. George JN: Heparin-associated thrombocytopenia. In Hull R, Pineo GF (eds): Disorders of Thrombosis. Philadelphia: Saunders, 1996:359-373.

99. Eby CS: Heparin induced thrombocytopenia. Clin Lab Sci 1999;12:365-369.

100. Warkentin TE: Heparin-induced thrombocytopenia. In Colman RW, Clowes AM, Goldhaber SZ, et al (eds): Hemostasis and Thrombosis: Basic Principles and Clinical Practice, 5th ed. Philadelphia: Lippincott, 2006:1649-1662.

101. Amiral J, Bridey F, Dreyfus M, et al: Platelet factor 4 complexed to heparin is the target for antibodies generated in heparin-induced thrombocytopenia. Blood 1986;67:27-30.

102. Sheridan D, Carter C, Kelton JG: A diagnostic test for heparin-induced thrombocytopenia. Blood 1986;67:27-30.

103. Isenhaart CE, Brandt JT: Platelet aggregation studies for the diagnosis of heparin-induced thrombocytopenia. Am J Clin Pathol 1993;99:324-330.

43

Thrombocytopenia and Thrombocytosis

Larry D. Brace

OBJECTIVES

After completion of this chapter, the reader will be able to:

1. Define thrombocytopenia and thrombocytosis, and state their associated platelet counts.
2. Compare and contrast the clinical symptoms of platelet disorders and clotting factor deficiencies.
3. Explain the primary pathophysiologic processes of thrombocytopenia.
4. Name and list the unique diagnostic features of at least four disorders included in congenital hypoplasia of the bone marrow and their inheritance patterns.
5. Differentiate between acute and chronic immune thrombocytopenia.
6. Describe immunologic and nonimmunologic mechanisms by which drugs may induce thrombocytopenia.
7. Differentiate between neonatal isoimmune thrombocytopenia and neonatal autoimmune thrombocytopenia.
8. Explain the laboratory findings and pathophysiology associated with thrombotic thrombocytopenic purpura and hemolytic-uremic syndrome.
9. Paraphrase the pathophysiology of thrombotic complications in heparin-induced thrombocytopenia, and describe the sequence of treatment options.
10. Given clinical history and laboratory test results for patients with thrombocytopenia or thrombocytosis, suggest a diagnosis that is consistent with the information provided.

CASE STUDY

After studying the material in this chapter, the reader should be able to respond to the following case study:

An 18-month-old African-American girl sustained severe burns over 40% to 50% of her body, including both lower extremities. Within 1 month, she underwent a below-knee amputation of the left lower extremity. Over the next several years, she underwent skin-grafting surgeries, central venous line placement, and other burn-related surgeries. During these surgeries, the patient was exposed to heparinized saline irrigation. Four years after the burn injury, a thrombosis was noted in the right femoral artery during a grafting surgery. Unfractionated heparin was used during the surgery. Surgeons were unable to save the leg and an above-knee amputation was necessary. At this time, hypercoagulability studies were ordered.

	Patient Results	Reference Range
Protein C antigen	78%	70-137%
Protein S antigen	120%	63-156%
Antithrombin activity	111%	76-136%

The patient was normal when tested for the factor V Leiden and prothrombin A20210G mutations and did not have antiphospholipid antibody syndrome. Her platelet count had been decreasing steadily for 7 days before surgery but was still within the reference range.

1. Is the heparin used during the grafting surgeries significant in this patient's case?
2. What test should be ordered next?

Bleeding disorders resulting from platelet abnormalities, whether quantitative or qualitative, usually are manifested by bleeding into the skin or mucous membranes or both (mucocutaneous bleeding). Common presenting symptoms include petechiae, purpura, ecchymoses, epistaxis, and gingival bleeding. Similar findings also are seen in vascular disorders, but vascular disorders (e.g., Ehlers-Danlos syndrome, hereditary hemorrhagic telangiectasia) are relatively rare. In contrast, deep tissue bleeding, such as hematoma and hemarthrosis, is associated with clotting factor deficiencies.

THROMBOCYTOPENIA: DECREASE IN CIRCULATING PLATELETS

Although the reference range for the platelet count varies among laboratories, it is generally considered to be approximately 150,000 to 450,000/μL (150,000-450,000/mm^3 or 150-450 $\times$ 10^9/L). Thrombocytopenia (platelet count <100,000/μL) is the most common cause of clinically important bleeding. The primary pathophysiologic processes that result in thrombocytopenia are decreased platelet production, accelerated platelet destruction, and abnormal platelet distribution (sequestration) (Box 43-1).

Small vessel bleeding in the skin attributed to thrombocytopenia is manifested by hemorrhages of different sizes (Fig. 43-1). *Petechiae* are small pinpoint hemorrhages about 3 mm in diameter, *purpura* are about 1 cm in diameter and generally round, and *ecchymoses* are 3 cm or larger and usually irregular in shape. Ecchymosis corresponds with the lay term *bruise*. Clinical bleeding varies and often is not closely correlated with the platelet count. It is unusual for clinical bleeding to occur when the platelet count is greater than 50,000/μL, but the risk of clinical bleeding increases progressively as the platelet count decreases from 50,000/μL. Patients with platelet counts 20,000/μL or sometimes lower may have little or no bleeding symptoms. In general, patients with platelet counts less than 10,000/μL are considered to be at high risk for a serious hemorrhagic episode.

Impaired or Decreased Platelet Production

Abnormalities in platelet production may be divided into two categories: One type is associated with megakaryocyte hypoplasia in the bone marrow, and the other type is associated with ineffective thrombopoiesis, as may be seen in disordered proliferation of megakaryocytes.

Congenital Hypoplasia

Lack of adequate bone marrow megakaryocytes (megakaryocytic hypoplasia) is seen in a wide variety of congenital disorders, including Fanconi anemia (pancytopenia), thrombocytopenia with absent radii (TAR syndrome), Wiskott-Aldrich syndrome, Bernard-Soulier syndrome, May-Hegglin anomaly, and several other, less common disorders. Although thrombocytopenia is a feature of Bernard-Soulier syndrome and Wiskott-Aldrich syndrome, the primary abnormality in these disorders is a qualitative defect, and they are discussed in Chapter 44.

BOX 43-1   Classification of Thrombocytopenia

Impaired or Decreased Production of Platelets

Congenital
   May-Hegglin anomaly
   Bernard-Soulier syndrome
   Fechtner syndrome
   Sebastian syndrome
   Epstein syndrome
   Montreal platelet syndrome
   Fanconi anemia
   Wiskott-Aldrich syndrome
   Thrombocytopenia with absent radii (TAR)
   Congenital amegakaryocytic thrombocytopenia
   Autosomal dominant and X-linked thrombocytopenia
Neonatal
Viral
Drug-induced
Acquired

Increased Platelet Destruction

Immune
   Acute and chronic immune thrombocytopenia purpura
   Drug-induced: immunologic
   Heparin-induced thrombocytopenia
   Neonatal alloimmune (isoimmune neonatal) thrombocytopenia
   Neonatal autoimmune thrombocytopenia
   Post-transfusion isoimmune thrombocytopenia
   Secondary autoimmune thrombocytopenia
Nonimmune
   Thrombocytopenia in pregnancy and pre-eclampsia
   Human immunodeficiency virus
   Hemolytic disease of the newborn
   Thrombotic thrombocytopenia purpura
   Disseminated intravascular coagulation
   Hemolytic uremic syndrome
   Drugs: nonimmune mechanisms of platelet destruction

Disorders Related to Distribution or Dilution

Splenic sequestration
Kasabach-Merritt syndrome
Hypothermia
Loss of platelets: massive blood transfusions, extracorporeal circulation

Data from Colvin[29] and Thompson and Harker.[32]

May-Hegglin anomaly is a rare autosomal dominant disorder; the exact frequency is unknown. Large platelets (20 μm in diameter) are present on the peripheral blood film, and Döhle bodies are present in neutrophils (Fig. 43-2) and occasionally monocytes. Other than an increase in size, platelet morphology is normal. Thrombocytopenia is present in about one third to one half of affected patients. Platelet function in response to platelet activating agents is usually normal. In

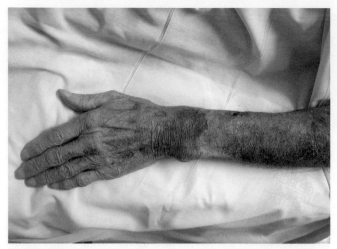

Figure 43-1 Purpura and petechiae indicate systemic (mucocutaneous) hemorrhage. (From Kitchens CS, Alving BM, Kessler CM: Consultative Hemostasis and Thrombosis. Philadelphia, Saunders, 2002.)

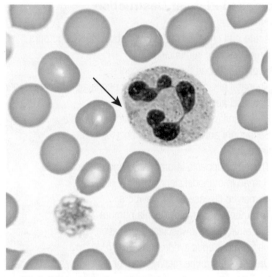

Figure 43-2 Döhle body in polymorphonuclear neutrophil and giant platelets associated with May-Hegglin anomaly (peripheral blood, ×1000). (From Carr JH, Rodak BF: Clinical Hematology Atlas, ed 2. Philadelphia: Saunders, 2004.)

some patients, megakaryocytes are increased in number and have abnormal ultrastructure. Mutations in the *MYH9* gene that encodes for nonmuscle myosin heavy chain (a cytoskeletal protein in platelets) have been reported.[1] This mutation may be responsible for the abnormal size of platelets in this disorder. Most patients are asymptomatic, unless severe thrombocytopenia is present, but bleeding times may be prolonged in some patients in the absence of bleeding complications.

Two other disorders involving mutations of the *MYH9* gene have been reported: Sebastian syndrome and Fechtner syndrome.[2] Sebastian syndrome is inherited as an autosomal dominant disorder characterized by large platelets, thrombocytopenia, and granulocytic inclusions. Similar abnormalities are observed in Fechtner syndrome and are accompanied by

deafness, cataracts, and nephritis. In another large platelet syndrome, Epstein syndrome, large platelets are associated with deafness, ocular problems, and glomerular nephritis, although the genetic defect has not been established conclusively.[3]

TAR syndrome is a rare autosomal recessive disorder characterized by neonatal thrombocytopenia and congenital absence or extreme hypoplasia of the radial bones of the forearms with absent, short, or malformed ulnae. In addition, patients tend to have cardiac lesions and a high incidence of transient leukemoid reactions with elevated white blood cell counts (sometimes with counts >100,000/μL) in 90% of patients.[4] Other bony abnormalities also may exist. Platelet counts are usually 10,000 to 30,000/μL. The defects are presumed to occur as a result of a specific type of fetal injury at about 8 weeks of gestation. TAR syndrome is one of the inherited, impaired DNA repair disorders. Because exposure to radiation causes cellular DNA damage, it is also considered to be a radiation sensitivity syndrome.[5]

Although thrombocytopenia is one characteristic of Fanconi anemia, the abnormalities are extensive and include bony abnormalities, abnormalities of visceral organs, and pancytopenia. Chapter 21 contains a more detailed description.

Congenital Amegakaryocytic Thrombocytopenia

Congenital amegakaryocytic thrombocytopenia is an autosomal recessive disorder reflecting bone marrow failure.[6] Affected infants usually have platelet counts less than 20,000/μL at birth, have petechiae and evidence of bleeding, and frequently have physical anomalies. About half of the infants develop aplastic anemia in the first year of life, and there are reports of myelodysplasia and leukemia later in childhood. Stem cell transplantation is considered curative for infants with clinically severe disease or aplasia.[7] It has been shown that this disorder is caused by mutations in the *c-mlp* gene resulting in complete loss of *c-mlp* (thrombopoietin receptor) function. This loss of function results in reduced megakaryocyte progenitors and high thrombopoietin levels.[8]

Autosomal Dominant and X-Linked Thrombocytopenia

Autosomal dominant and X-linked thrombocytopenia are well documented. In autosomal dominant thrombocytopenia, bleeding is usually mild, platelet function is normal, and the megakaryocytes seem to be normal in number and morphology.[9,10] X-linked thrombocytopenia can result from mutations in WASP (Wiskott-Aldrich syndrome protein) or mutations in the *GATA-1* gene.[11-13] X-linked thrombocytopenias range from mild thrombocytopenia to macrothrombocytopenia with severe bleeding.

Neonatal Hypoplasia

Causes of neonatal megakaryocytic hypoplasia include infection with cytomegalovirus (CMV), *Toxoplasma*, rubella, and human immunodeficiency virus (HIV) and in utero exposure to certain drugs, particularly chlorothiazide diuretics and the oral hypoglycemic, tolbutamide. CMV is the most common infectious agent causing congenital thrombocytopenia at an overall incidence of 0.5% to 1% of all births,[14] but only 10% to 15% of infected infants have symptomatic disease,[15] suggesting that the incidence of significant neonatal thrombocytopenia caused by CMV is about 1 in 1000 infants. Although the mechanism of thrombocytopenia is not well understood, reports suggest that CMV inhibits megakaryocytes and their precursors, resulting in impaired platelet production.[16] About 1 in 1000 to 1 in 3000 infants are affected by congenital toxoplasmosis. About 40% of such infants develop thrombocytopenia.[17] Although congenital rubella is now rare in countries with organized immunization programs,[18,19] persistent thrombocytopenia is a prominent feature of infants with congenital rubella syndrome. Thrombocytopenia also is a feature of maternal transmission of HIV to the neonate and is a sign of intermediate to severe disease.[20]

Maternal ingestion of chlorothiazide diuretics or tolbutamide can have a direct cytotoxic effect on the fetal marrow megakaryocytes. Thrombocytopenia may be severe, with platelet counts of 70,000/μL and sometimes lower. Bone marrow examination reveals a marked decrease or absence of megakaryocytes. The thrombocytopenia develops gradually and is slow to regress when the drug is stopped. Recovery usually occurs within a few weeks after birth.[10,21,22]

Acquired Hypoplasia

Drugs. A wide array of chemotherapeutic agents used for the treatment of hematologic and nonhematologic malignancies suppresses bone marrow megakaryocyte production and the production of other hematopoietic cells. Examples include the commonly used agents methotrexate, busulfan, cytosine arabinoside, cyclophosphamide, and cisplatin. The resulting thrombocytopenia may lead to hemorrhage, and the platelet count should be monitored closely. Drug-induced thrombocytopenia is often the dose-limiting factor for many chemotherapeutic agents. Recombinant interleukin-11 has been approved for treatment of chemotherapy-induced thrombocytopenia, and thrombopoietin may prove to be useful for this purpose.[23-25] Zidovudine used for the treatment of HIV infection also is known to cause myelotoxicity and severe thrombocytopenia.[26]

Several drugs specifically affect megakaryocytopoiesis without significantly affecting other marrow elements. Although its mechanism of action is unknown, anagrelide is one such agent. This effect has made anagrelide useful for treating the thrombocytosis of patients with essential thrombocythemia and other myeloproliferative disorders.[27]

Ethanol ingestion for long periods (months to years) may result in persistent severe thrombocytopenia. Although the mechanism is unknown, studies indicate that alcohol can inhibit megakaryocytopoiesis in some individuals. Mild thrombocytopenia is a common finding in alcoholic patients in whom other causes, such as portal hypertension, splenomegaly, and folic acid deficiency, have been excluded. The platelet count usually returns to normal within a few weeks of alcohol withdrawal but may persist for longer periods. A transient, rebound thrombocytosis may develop when alcohol ingestion is stopped.[10]

Interferon therapy commonly causes mild to moderate thrombocytopenia, although under certain circumstances, the thrombocytopenia can be severe and life-threatening. Interferon-α and interferon-γ inhibit stem cell differentiation and proliferation in the bone marrow, but the mechanism of action is unclear.[28]

Thrombocytopenia presumably caused by megakaryocyte suppression also has been reported to follow the administration of large doses of estrogen or estrogenic drugs such as diethylstilbestrol. Other drugs, such as certain antibacterial agents (e.g., chloramphenicol), tranquilizers, and anticonvulsants, also have been associated with thrombocytopenia caused by bone marrow suppression.[29-31]

Ineffective Thrombopoiesis

Thrombocytopenia is a usual feature of the megaloblastic anemias (pernicious anemia, folic acid deficiency, and vitamin B_{12} deficiency). Quantitative studies indicate that, similar to erythrocyte production in these disorders, platelet production is ineffective. Although the bone marrow generally contains an increase in the number of megakaryocytes, the total number of platelets released into the circulation is decreased. Thrombocytopenia is caused by impaired DNA synthesis, and the bone marrow may contain grossly abnormal megakaryocytes with deformed, dumbbell-shaped nuclei, sometimes in large numbers. Stained peripheral blood smears reveal large platelets that may have a decreased survival time and may have abnormal function. Thrombocytopenia is usually mild, and there is evidence of increased platelet destruction. Patients typically respond to vitamin replacement within 1 to 2 weeks.[22,32-34]

Miscellaneous

Viruses are known to cause thrombocytopenia by acting on megakaryocytes or circulating platelets, either directly or in the form of viral antigen-antibody complexes. Live measles vaccine can cause degenerative vacuolization of megakaryocytes 6 to 8 days after vaccination. Some viruses interact readily with platelets by means of specific platelet receptors. Other viruses associated with thrombocytopenia include CMV, varicella, rubella, Epstein-Barr virus (infectious mononucleosis), and the virus that causes Thai hemorrhagic fever.[10]

Certain bacterial infections commonly are associated with the development of thrombocytopenia. This may be the result of toxins of bacterial origin, direct interactions between bacteria and platelets in the circulation, or extensive damage to the endothelium, as in meningococcemia. Many cases of thrombocytopenia in childhood result from infection. Purpura may occur in many infectious diseases in the absence of thrombocytopenia, presumably because of vascular damage (Chapter 44).[10,35]

A common cause of unexplained thrombocytopenia is infiltration of the bone marrow by malignant cells with a progressive decrease in marrow megakaryocytes as the abnormal cells replace normal marrow elements. Inhibitors of thrombopoiesis may be produced by these abnormal cells and may help to account for the thrombocytopenia associated with conditions such as myeloma, lymphoma, metastatic cancer, and myelofibrosis.[22,32,36]

Increased Platelet Destruction

Thrombocytopenia as a result of increased platelet destruction can be separated into two categories: increased platelet destruction caused by immunologic responses and increased destruction caused by mechanical damage or consumption or both. Regardless of the process, increased production is required to maintain a normal platelet count, and the patient becomes thrombocytopenic only when production capacity is no longer able to compensate for the increased rate of destruction.

Immune Mechanisms of Platelet Destruction

Immune (Idiopathic) Thrombocytopenic Purpura: Acute and Chronic. The term *idiopathic thrombocytopenic purpura* (ITP) was used to describe cases of thrombocytopenia arising without apparent etiology or underlying disease state. Although the acronym for the disorder remains the same, the word *idiopathic* has been replaced by *immune* with the realization that acute and chronic ITP are immunologically mediated.

Acute ITP is primarily a disorder of children, although a similar picture is seen occasionally in adults. The disorder is characterized by abrupt onset of bruising, petechiae, and sometimes mucosal bleeding (e.g., epistaxis) in a previously healthy child. The primary hematologic feature is thrombocytopenia, which frequently occurs 1 to 3 weeks after an infection.

The infection is most often a nonspecific upper respiratory or gastrointestinal virus, but acute ITP also may occur after rubella, rubeola, chickenpox, or other viral illnesses and may follow live virus vaccination.[37] The incidence of acute ITP is estimated to be 4 per 100,000 children, with a peak frequency between 2 and 5 years of age. There is no sex predilection. In about 10% to 15% of the children initially thought to have acute ITP, the thrombocytopenia persists for 6 months or more, and these children are reclassified as having chronic ITP.[38] The observation that acute ITP often follows a viral illness suggests that some children produce antibodies and immune complexes against viral antigens, and that platelet destruction may result from the binding of these antibodies or immune complexes to the platelet surface.

The diagnosis of acute ITP in a child with severe thrombocytopenia almost always can be made without bone marrow examination. If the child has onset of bleeding signs and symptoms, an otherwise normal complete blood count (all red blood cell [RBC] and white blood cell parameters and morphology), and a normal physical examination (except for signs of bleeding), there is a high likelihood that the child has ITP. In addition, if the bleeding symptoms develop suddenly and there is no family history of hemorrhagic abnormalities or thrombocytopenia, the diagnosis of ITP is almost certain. There is, at present, no specific test that is diagnostic of acute or chronic ITP.

In mild cases of acute ITP, patients may have only scattered petechiae. In most cases of acute ITP, however, patients develop fairly extensive petechiae and some ecchymoses and may have hematuria or epistaxis or both. About 3% to 4% of acute ITP cases are considered severe and typically have generalized purpura, often accompanied by gastrointestinal bleeding, hematuria, mucous membrane bleeding, and retinal hemorrhage. Of the "severe" cases, 25% to 50% are considered to be at risk for intracranial hemorrhage, which is the primary complication that contributes to the overall 1% to 2% mortality rate for patients with acute ITP.[38] Most patients with life-threatening hemorrhage have a platelet count of less than 4000/μL.[39] Hemorrhage is rarely experienced by patients whose platelet count exceeds 10,000/μL.

Most patients with acute ITP recover with or without treatment. Most patients recover within 3 weeks, although for some, recovery may take 6 months. In a few children, recurrent episodes of acute ITP are seen occasionally after complete recovery from the first episode.[40] Most patients with acute ITP have relatively mild symptoms, and no treatment is needed. The most severe cases may need to be treated, however, and intravenous immunoglobulin (IVIG), platelet transfusions, and splenectomy (or some combination of these) seem to offer the most immediate benefit.[37,38]

Chronic ITP can be found in patients of any age, although most cases are found in patients between 20 and 50 years old. Females with this disorder outnumber males 2:1 to 3:1, with the highest incidence occurring in women between 20 and 40 years old. The incidence of chronic ITP ranges from 3.2 to 6.6 cases/100,000/yr.[41] Chronic ITP usually begins insidiously, with platelet counts that are variably decreased and sometimes normal for periods. Presenting symptoms are those of mucocutaneous bleeding, with menorrhagia, recurrent epistaxis, or easy bruising (ecchymoses) being most common.

Platelet destruction in chronic ITP is the result of an immunologic process. The offending antibodies attach to platelets, and as a result, the antibody-labeled platelets are removed from the circulation by reticuloendothelial cells, primarily in the spleen. In addition, cytotoxic T cell–mediated lysis of platelets has been shown in vitro using $CD3^+/CD8^+$ lymphocytes from patients with active chronic ITP.[42] Overall, the life span of the platelet is shortened from 7 to 10 days to a few hours, and the rapidity with which platelets are removed from the circulation correlates with the degree of thrombocytopenia. If plasma from a patient with ITP is infused into the circulation of a normal recipient, the recipient develops thrombocytopenia. The thrombocytopenia-producing factor in the plasma of the ITP patient is an IgG antibody that can be removed from serum by adsorption with normal human platelets. Epitopes on platelet glycoprotein (GP) IIb and GP IIIa ($\alpha IIb/\beta_3$) are most often the target of autoantibodies in ITP, although epitopes on GP Ib and several other platelet membrane glycoproteins also have been identified as targets.[43,44] Because megakaryocytes also express GP IIb/IIIa and GP Ib/IX on their membranes, these cells are obvious targets of the antibodies. Platelet turnover studies have shown impaired platelet production in ITP.

The only abnormalities in the peripheral blood of patients with ITP are related to platelets. In most cases, platelets number between 30,000/µL and 80,000/µL. Patients with ITP undergo periods of remission and exacerbation, however, and their platelet counts may range from near-normal to less than 20,000/µL during these periods (Fig. 43-3). Morphologically, platelets appear normal, although larger in size than usual. This is reflected in an increased mean platelet volume as measured by electronic cell counters. The marrow typically is characterized by megakaryocytic hyperplasia. Megakaryocytes are increased in size, and young forms with a single nucleus, smooth contour, and diminished cytoplasm are commonly seen. In the absence of bleeding, infection, or other underlying disorder, erythrocyte and leukocyte precursors are normal in number and morphology. Coagulation test abnormalities include tests dependent on normal platelet function, such as the bleeding time and clot retraction. Although platelet-associated IgG levels are increased in most patients,[10,21,46] it has not been shown conclusively that any method of testing for platelet antibodies is sensitive or specific for ITP.

The initial treatment of chronic ITP depends on the urgency for increasing the platelet count. ITP patients with a platelet count greater than 30,000/µL who receive no treatment can expect a mortality rate equal to that of the general population. Unless there are additional risk factors, ITP patients with platelet counts greater than 30,000/µL should not be treated. If additional risk factors, such as old age, coagulation defects, recent surgery, trauma, or uncontrolled hypertension, exist, the platelet count should be kept at 50,000/µL or higher depending on the clinical situation. In patients in whom the need is considered urgent, IVIG remains the treatment of choice. For most patients, however, the initial treatment of chronic ITP consists principally of prednisone. About 70% to 90% of patients respond with an increase in platelet count and a decrease in hemorrhagic episodes. Although reported response rates vary widely, about 50% of patients have a long-term beneficial effect from corticosteroid treatment.[37] If the response to corticosteroids is inadequate, steroid therapy can be supplemented with IVIG or, in some cases, anti-D

immunoglobulin.[48,49] For patients in whom prednisone becomes ineffective, splenectomy is necessary. Splenectomy eliminates the primary site of platelet removal and destruction, but it also removes an organ containing autoantibody-producing lymphocytes. Splenectomy is the most effective treatment for adult chronic ITP, with 88% of patients showing improvement and 66% having a complete and lasting response.[50] In the most severe refractory cases, immunosuppressive (chemotherapeutic) agents such as azathioprine given alone or with steroids may be necessary. In such patients, platelet transfusions may be of transient benefit in treating severe hemorrhagic episodes but should not be given routinely.[46] IVIG given alone or just before platelet transfusion also may be beneficial.[37,46]

Chronic ITP occurring in association with HIV infection, with hemophilia, and with pregnancy presents special problems in diagnosis and therapy. Unexplained thrombocytopenia in otherwise healthy members of high-risk populations may be an early manifestation of acquired immune deficiency syndrome (AIDS).[36,46]

Differentiation of Acute versus Chronic Idiopathic Thrombocytopenic Purpura. The differences between acute and chronic ITP are summarized in Table 43-1. Acute ITP occurs most frequently in children 2 to 9 years old and in young adults, whereas chronic ITP occurs in patients of all ages, although most commonly in adults 20 to 50 years old and more commonly in women. Of patients with acute ITP, 60% to 80% have a history of infection, usually viral (rubella, rubeola, chickenpox, and nonspecific respiratory tract infection), occurring 2 to 21 days before onset. Acute ITP also may occur after immunization with live vaccine for measles, chickenpox, mumps, and smallpox.

Acute ITP usually is self-limited, and spontaneous remissions occur in 80% to 90% of patients, although the duration of the illness may range from days to months. In chronic ITP, there is typically a fluctuating clinical course, with episodes of bleeding that last a few days or weeks, but spontaneous remissions are uncommon and usually incomplete.[46]

Symptoms of acute ITP vary, but petechial hemorrhages, purpura, and often bleeding from the gums and gastrointestinal or urinary tract typically begin suddenly, sometimes over a few hours. Hemorrhagic bullae in the oral mucosa are often prominent in patients with severe thrombocytopenia of acute onset. Usually the severity of bleeding is correlated with the degree of thrombocytopenia.[46] In contrast, presenting symptoms of chronic ITP begin with a few scattered petechiae or other minor bleeding manifestations. Occasionally, a bruising tendency, menorrhagia, or recurrent epistaxis is present for months or years before diagnosis. Platelet counts range from 5000/µL to 75,000/µL and are generally higher than those in acute ITP. Giant platelets are commonly seen. Platelet-associated immunoglobulin levels are elevated in most patients, but the test lacks sensitivity and specificity.[46]

Treatment also varies for acute and chronic ITP. In chronic ITP, initial therapy often consists of glucocorticoids (corticosteroids), which interfere with splenic and hepatic macrophages to increase platelet survival time. If the patient does not respond to corticosteroids or cannot tolerate them because of

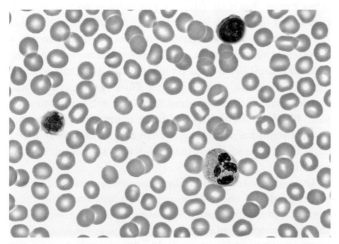

Figure 43-3 Typical peripheral blood cell morphology in ITP. Note scarce platelets and increased platelet size but normal RBC and leukocyte morphology (peripheral blood, ×500).

TABLE 43-1 Clinical Picture of Acute and Chronic Immune Thrombocytopenic Purpura

Characteristics	Acute	Chronic
Age at onset	2-6 y	20-50 y
Sex predilection	None	Female over male, 3:1
Prior infection	Common	Unusual
Onset of bleeding	Sudden	Gradual
Platelet count	<20,000/μL	30,000-80,000/μL
Duration	2-6 wk	Months to years
Spontaneous remission	90% of patients	Uncommon
Seasonal pattern	Higher incidence in winter and spring	None
Therapy		
Steroids	70% response rate	30% response rate
Splenectomy	Rare	<45 y, 90% response; >45 y, 40% response

Data from Triplett,[21] Quick,[35] and Bussel and Cines.[37]

the resultant immunosuppression and toxicity, splenectomy may be necessary. In acute ITP, treatment for all but the most severely thrombocytopenic and hemorrhagic patients is contraindicated. When necessary, a good response to IVIG or corticosteroids or both usually can be obtained, and splenectomy is rarely required.[37,38]

Immunologic Drug-Induced Thrombocytopenia. As can be seen in Box 43-2, many drugs can induce acute thrombocytopenia. Drug-induced immune-mediated thrombocytopenia can be divided into several types based on interaction of the antibody with the drug and platelets. Mechanisms of drug/antibody binding are shown in Figure 43-4.

One type is typified by quinidine/quinine-induced thrombocytopenia and has been recognized for more than 100 years. The antibody induced by drugs of this type interacts with platelets only in the presence of the drug. Many drugs can induce such antibodies, but quinine, quinidine, and sulfonamide derivatives do so more often than other drugs. When antibody production has begun, the platelet count falls rapidly and often may be less than 10,000/μL. Patients may have abrupt onset of bleeding symptoms. If this type of drug-induced thrombocytopenia develops in a pregnant woman, she and her fetus may be affected. Quinine previously was used to facilitate labor but is no longer used for this purpose.

The initial studies of quinidine-induced thrombocytopenia suggested that the drug first combines with the antibody, and the antigen-antibody (immune) complex then attaches to the platelet in an essentially nonspecific manner (the "innocent bystander" hypothesis). It now seems clear, however, that the antibodies responsible for drug-induced thrombocytopenia bind to the platelets by their Fab regions, rather than by attaching "nonspecifically" as immune complexes. The "innocent bystander" and "immune complex" concepts for this type of drug-induced thrombocytopenia should be abandoned. The

Fab portion of the antibody binds to a platelet membrane constituent, usually the GP Ib/IX complex or the GP IIb/IIIa complex, only in the presence of drug.[51,52] The mechanism by which the drug promotes binding of a drug-dependent antibody to a specific target on the platelet membrane without covalently linking to the target or the antibody remains to be determined, however. Because the Fc portion of the immunoglobulin is not involved in binding to platelets, it is still available to the Fc receptors on phagocytic cells. This situation may contribute to the rapid onset and relatively severe nature of the thrombocytopenia. Most drug-induced platelet antibodies are of the IgG class, but in rare instances, IgM antibodies are involved.[46]

A second mechanism of drug-induced thrombocytopenia is induction of hapten-dependent antibodies. Some drug molecules are too small by themselves to trigger an immune response, but they may act as a hapten and combine with a larger carrier molecule (usually a plasma protein or protein constituent of the platelet membrane) to form a complex that can act as a complete antigen.[46] Penicillin and penicillin derivatives constitute the primary offending agents causing drug-induced thrombocytopenia by this mechanism. Drug-induced thrombocytopenia of this type is often severe. The initial platelet count may be less than 10,000/μL and sometimes less than 1000/μL. The number of bone marrow megakaryocytes is usually normal to elevated.[46] Bleeding is often severe and rapid in onset, and hemorrhagic bullae in the mouth may be prominent.

Drug-induced autoantibodies represent a third mechanism of drug-induced thrombocytopenia. In this case, the drugs stimulate the formation of an autoantibody that binds to a specific platelet membrane glycoprotein with no requirement for the presence of free drug. Gold salts and procainamide are two examples of such drugs. Levodopa also may cause

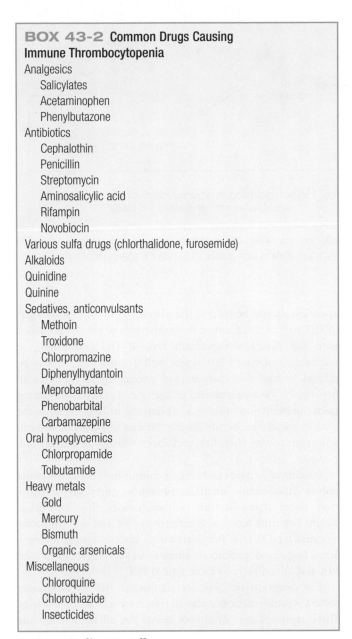

BOX 43-2 Common Drugs Causing Immune Thrombocytopenia

Analgesics
 Salicylates
 Acetaminophen
 Phenylbutazone
Antibiotics
 Cephalothin
 Penicillin
 Streptomycin
 Aminosalicylic acid
 Rifampin
 Novobiocin
Various sulfa drugs (chlorthalidone, furosemide)
Alkaloids
Quinidine
Quinine
Sedatives, anticonvulsants
 Methoin
 Troxidone
 Chlorpromazine
 Diphenylhydantoin
 Meprobamate
 Phenobarbital
 Carbamazepine
Oral hypoglycemics
 Chlorpropamide
 Tolbutamide
Heavy metals
 Gold
 Mercury
 Bismuth
 Organic arsenicals
Miscellaneous
 Chloroquine
 Chlorothiazide
 Insecticides

Data from Triplett[21] and Quick.[35]

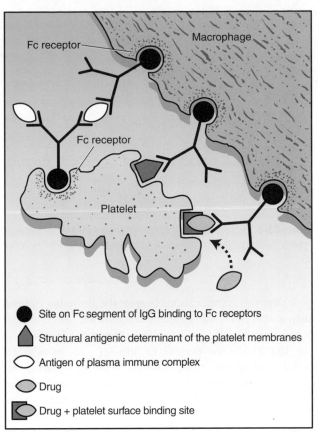

- Site on Fc segment of IgG binding to Fc receptors
- Structural antigenic determinant of the platelet membranes
- Antigen of plasma immune complex
- Drug
- Drug + platelet surface binding site

Figure 43-4 Immunoglobulin binds a platelet membrane antigen or antigen and drug combination. Macrophage Fc receptors bind the Fc portion of the immunoglobulin. This may result in platelet removal and thrombocytopenia. (From Rapaport SI: Introduction to Hematology, 2nd ed. Philadelphia: JB Lippincott, 1987:489.)

thrombocytopenia in the same way. The precise mechanism by which these drugs induce autoantibodies against platelets is not known with certainty.

Heparin-induced thrombocytopenia (HIT) is a good example of another type of drug-induced thrombocytopenia. Heparin binds to platelet factor 4 (PF4), a heparin-neutralizing protein made and released by platelets (Fig. 43-5). Binding of heparin by plasma PF4 or platelet membrane–expressed PF4 causes a conformational change of PF4, resulting in the exposure of neoepitopes. Exposure of these neoepitopes ("new antigens") stimulates the immune system of some individuals, leading to the production of an antibody to one of the neoepitopes. In HIT, heparin and PF4 form a complex on the platelet surface or circulating free complexes to which the antibody

binds. The Fab portion of the immunoglobulin molecule binds to an exposed neoepitope in the PF4 molecule, leaving the Fc portion of the IgG free to bind with the platelet FcγR receptor, causing platelet activation.[53,54] Because the Fc portions of the IgG molecules are involved in binding to platelet FcγR receptors, they are not available to the Fc receptors of the cells of the reticuloendothelial system. This may explain the less severe nature of this thrombocytopenia. That does not mean, however, that the thrombocytopenia is less serious. The opposite may be true. Because platelets are activated by occupancy of their FcγR receptors, in vivo platelet aggregation with thrombosis is possible. HIT sometimes is referred to as *heparin-induced thrombocytopenia and thrombosis*. Heparin binding to PF4 is required to expose the neoepitope to which the antibody binds. The treatment for HIT is to discontinue heparin treatment and replace it with another suitable anticoagulant. Low-molecular-weight heparin should not be used as a heparin replacement for this purpose because the antibody cross-reacts with low-molecular-weight heparin and PF4 to result in platelet activation and aggregation.[55]

HIT is a relatively common side effect of unfractionated heparin administration, with about 1% to 5% of patients

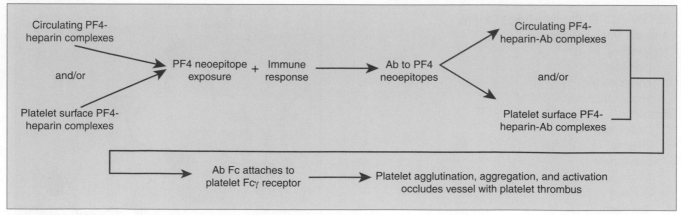

Figure 43-5 Heparin-induced thrombocytopenia (HIT) with thrombosis. An antibody binds the heparin-PF4 complex in plasma or on the platelet surface. The Fc portion binds platelet Fc receptors and activates the platelet. The activated platelets aggregate to form platelet thrombi in the arterial circulation.

developing this complication. Despite the thrombocytopenia, patients with HIT usually are not at significant risk of bleeding because their platelet count typically does not decrease to less than 40,000/μL. Ten percent to 30% of patients with HIT develop thrombotic complications, however. Patients who develop HIT should be removed from heparin therapy as soon as the diagnosis is made because continued heparin therapy can lead to significant morbidity and mortality, including gangrene of the extremities, amputation, and death. After discontinuation of heparin, the platelet count begins to increase and should return to normal within a few days.[56]

Because the immune system is involved in the development of HIT, it is typically 7 to 14 days (the time necessary to mount an immune response on first exposure to an antigen) after the institution of heparin therapy until the clinical signs of HIT are seen. If the patient has been exposed to heparin previously, however, symptoms of HIT may be seen in 1 to 3 days. Because the platelet count may fall sharply in 1 day, it is recommended that patients receiving unfractionated heparin therapy have daily platelet counts. One other sign of impending HIT is that some patients develop heparin resistance. This is the clinical situation in which a patient who had been adequately anticoagulated at a certain heparin dosage suddenly requires increasing amounts of heparin to maintain the same level of anticoagulation. This situation can result from in vivo activation of platelets and release of PF4 and β-thromboglobulin from platelet α granules. Both of these substances neutralize heparin, resulting in a normalization of the partial thromboplastin time test that is used to monitor heparin therapy. Heparin resistance often is seen before the development of thrombocytopenia.[57]

A common benign form of HIT that occurs on heparin administration is type I (nonimmune mediated). It is important to distinguish benign type I from type II. Type I is associated with a decrease in the platelet count rapidly after administration of heparin, but the thrombocytopenia is mild (the platelet count rarely decreases to <100,000/μL) and transient, and there is a rapid return of the platelet count to the preheparin level even if heparin therapy is continued. Careful

attention should be paid to the platelet count and other signs of HIT so that this form of thrombocytopenia is not confused with the clinically significant type II HIT. Although the mechanism of type I HIT is not well documented, it may be related to the well-documented proaggregatory effects of heparin.[55,58] Because activated or aggregated platelets are cleared from the circulation, this may explain the mild decrease in the platelet count that occurs during the first few days of heparin administration. This has not been clearly documented, however.

Binding of heparin and related compounds depends on the polysaccharide chain length, composition, and degree of sulfation. Short chain heparin polysaccharides (low-molecular-weight heparin) have lower affinity to PF4 and are less prone to cause type II HIT. Pentasaccharide and its synthetic derivatives (e.g., fondaparinux or idraparinux) do not seem to bind PF4 and are unlikely to cause type II HIT.

The detection of clinically significant HIT by laboratory testing is problematic because all tests have a lack of sensitivity. Three methods are commonly used, but all depend on the presence of free heparin-induced antiplatelet antibodies in the patient's serum or plasma in sufficient quantity to cause a positive test. HIT can be detected by a platelet aggregation technique.[59] In this method, serum from the patient is added to platelet-rich plasma from normal donors, heparin is added to the mixture, and platelet aggregation is monitored for typically 20 minutes. The specificity of the method is excellent (near 100%), but the sensitivity is quite low, typically about 50%. The sensitivity of the test can be improved but requires the use of several heparin concentrations and of platelet-rich plasma from two or more blood donors, preferably of the same ABO blood type as the patient. In addition, the individuals donating blood for platelet-rich plasma must be free of aspirin for 10 to 14 days before donation because platelets from donors who have ingested aspirin produce a false-negative test for HIT.[55] In this regard, in the author's experience, patients who develop HIT while on aspirin therapy rarely develop thrombotic complications, and the drop in their platelet count is less precipitous, gradually decreasing over the course of several days (unpublished observations). Given the efficacy of aspirin in primary and secondary prevention of myocardial infarction and thrombotic stroke, it is increasingly difficult to find a sufficient pool of suitable (and willing) blood donors. Although time-consuming, reasonable sensitivity can be obtained with sufficient attention to the details of the technique.[27]

Dense granules of platelets contain serotonin, and platelets have an active mechanism for rapid uptake of serotonin with storage in platelet-dense granules. This property of platelets is used in another test for HIT in which washed normal platelets are incubated with radioactive serotonin (Fig. 43-6).[61] Radioactive serotonin is taken up rapidly and stored in the dense granules of the donor platelets, which are washed and resuspended. In the presence of heparin-dependent anti-platelet antibody and heparin, the donor platelets become activated and release the contents of their dense granules when the concentration of heparin in the test suspension is near the therapeutic range. The reappearance of radioactive serotonin in the plasma indicates the presence of a heparin-dependent antiplatelet antibody (i.e., HIT). Under these same conditions, supratherapeutic concentrations of heparin do not activate platelets, however, and if platelets release the contents of dense granules at therapeutic and subtherapeutic concentrations of heparin, the test is not positive for HIT. A similar phenomenon is observed in the test using platelet aggregometry.[55,60] This method is commonly called the *serotonin release assay* and, before the development of enzyme-linked immunosorbent assays for HIT, was considered the "gold standard" for detection of HIT. Its major drawback is the requirement for radio-labeled serotonin. Most clinical laboratories no longer use isotopic techniques; this test is performed only in a few specialized centers. In addition, it has some of the same methodologic drawbacks as the platelet aggregation technique; in particular, the use of drug-free donor platelets. Nonetheless, when properly performed, this technique seems to have similar specificity and superior sensitivity compared with the platelet aggregation method.

More recently, an enzyme-linked immunosorbent assay has been developed based on the knowledge that the antigenic target of the heparin-dependent antiplatelet antibody is a PF4-heparin complex (Fig. 43-7). In this assay, PF4 (or a related compound) is coated to the surface of microplate wells. Heparin and the serum or plasma from the patients suspected to have HIT are added to wells of the microtiter plate. If the antibody is present, it adheres to the PF4 in the presence of heparin or heparin-like compounds. The plate wells are washed, and an enzyme-labeled monoclonal antibody against human IgG is added. After an appropriate incubation period, the plate is washed, and a chromogenic substrate for the enzyme is added. Color development in the assay well indicates the presence of the heparin-dependent antiplatelet antibody in the patient plasma.[62] This assay has greater sensitivity than the platelet aggregation method and similar sensitivity to the serotonin release assay, but it has lower specificity than the serotonin release assay or the platelet aggregation method. The enzyme-linked immunosorbent assay method is considerably less labor intensive, does not require blood from healthy drug-free donors, and can be performed in most laboratories.

For patients who develop type II HIT, it is essential that heparin therapy be withdrawn immediately. It is not prudent, however, to withdraw anticoagulant/antithrombotic therapy without a suitable alternative. It is clear from the literature that under these circumstances, withdrawal of heparin treatment without replacement anticoagulant therapy results in an unacceptably high rate of thrombotic events. In the recent past, good alternatives were not available. Today, several alternative agents are suitable substitutes (although considerably more expensive) for heparin, including direct thrombin inhibitors such as hirudin and its analogues, argatroban and related synthetic direct thrombin inhibitors, and fondaparinux (Arixtra) and related synthetic pentasaccharides (e.g., idraparinux). The pentasaccharide-derived products represent the antithrombin binding site on heparin and heparin-derived agents such as low-molecular-weight heparins.

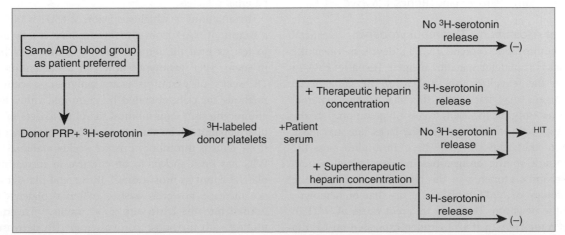

Figure 43-6 The serotonin release assay for heparin-induced thrombocytopenia (HIT). Donor platelets in platelet-rich plasma are labeled with tritiated (^{3}H) serotonin, washed, and suspended in patient plasma. Heparin in therapeutic and saturating doses is added to 2 aliquots. Release of radioactive serotonin in the therapeutic aliquot in combination with no release in the supratherapeutic system indicates HIT.

Figure 43-7 Enzyme immunoassay for HIT. The solid-phase target antigen is a complex of PF4 and heparin or a heparin surrogate. Antiheparin/PF4 in patient serum binds the antigen and is bound by enzyme-labeled anti-human antibody, a "sandwich" assay. The enzyme catalyzes the release of a chromophore from its substrate.

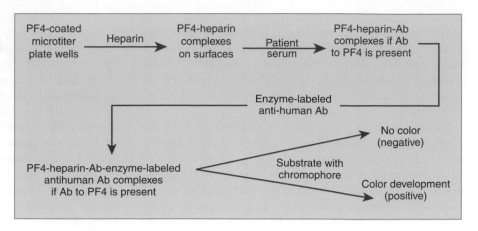

Treatment for any drug-induced thrombocytopenia is first to identify the offending drug, immediately discontinue its use, and substitute another suitable therapeutic agent. This is often difficult to accomplish. Many patients are taking multiple drugs, and it is not always easy to determine which of the drugs is at fault. Under these conditions, identifying the causative agent may be a trial-and-error procedure by eliminating the most likely drugs one at a time. Second, even if the patient is taking only one agent, there may not be a suitable replacement, or there may be a prolonged period required for the alternative drug to become effective. Drugs usually are cleared from the circulation rapidly, but dissociation of drug-antibody complexes may require longer periods, perhaps 1 to 2 weeks.[10] In some cases, such as that observed with gold salts, thrombocytopenia may persist for months. Platelet transfusions may be necessary for patients with life-threatening bleeds. Although it is true that the transfused platelets are destroyed rapidly, they may function to halt bleeding effectively before they are destroyed. In addition, high-dose IVIG may be used because it is a generally effective treatment for most drug-induced immune thrombocytopenias. Laboratory testing to identify the specific drug involved is usually beyond the capabilities of most laboratories. This type of testing is performed by many reference laboratories, however.

Neonatal Alloimmune Thrombocytopenia. Neonatal alloimmune thrombocytopenia (NAIT) develops when the mother lacks a platelet-specific antigen (usually HPA-1a [P1^{A1}]) that the fetus has inherited from the father. Fetal platelet antigens may pass from the fetal to the maternal circulation as early as the 14th week of gestation.[63] If the mother is exposed to a fetal antigen she lacks, she may make antibodies to that fetal antigen. These antibodies cross the placenta, attach to the antigen-bearing fetal platelets, and result in thrombocytopenia in the fetus. In this regard, the pathophysiology of NAIT is the same as that of hemolytic disease of the newborn. The most frequent cause of NAIT in caucasians is the HPA-1a (P1^{A1}) antigen expressed on GP IIIa of the surface membrane GP IIb/IIIa complex, followed by HPA-5b (Br^a). The antigen HPA-3a (Bak^a) is present on GP IIb and is an important cause of neonatal thrombocytopenia in

Asians. Platelet antigen HPA-4 (Penn and Yuk) accounts for a few affected neonates. Clinically significant thrombocytopenia develops in an estimated 1 in 1000 to 2000 newborns.[64] With the first pregnancy, about 50% of neonates are affected, whereas with subsequent pregnancies the risk is 75% to 97%.[64] The incidence of intracranial hemorrhage or death or both is about 25%, and about half of the intracranial hemorrhages occur in utero in the second trimester. Affected infants may appear normal at birth but soon manifest scattered petechiae and purpuric hemorrhages. In many infants with NAIT, serious hemorrhage does not develop, however, and the infants recover over a 1- to 2-week period as the passively transferred antibody levels decrease.[10,38] In symptomatic cases, platelet levels are usually less than 30,000/μL and may diminish even further in the first few hours after birth.

The diagnosis of NAIT is one of exclusion of other causes of neonatal thrombocytopenia, including maternal ITP and maternal ingestion of drugs known to be associated with drug-induced thrombocytopenia. The presence of thrombocytopenia in a neonate with a P1^{A1}-negative mother or a history of the disorder in a sibling is strong presumptive evidence in favor of the diagnosis. Confirmation should include platelet typing of both parents and evidence of a maternal antibody directed at paternal platelets.[37]

In situations in which suspicion of NAIT is high or there is a history of NAIT from a first pregnancy, it may be necessary to test or treat the fetus to prevent intracranial hemorrhage in utero. Fetal genotypes now can be determined at 10 to 18 weeks of gestation using polymerase chain reaction methods on cells obtained by chorionic villus sampling or amniocentesis.[65] Periumbilical sampling to determine the fetal platelet count can be performed at about 20 weeks of gestation. If the fetus is thrombocytopenic, weekly maternal infusion of IVIG has been shown to be effective in increasing the fetal platelet count in most cases.[66] If the fetal platelet count does not increase, however, washed maternal platelets have been infused into the fetus with good results.[67] Treatment of the mother with high-dose corticosteroids (to decrease maternal antibody production) is not recommended because of potential fetal toxicity. In situations in which the diagnosis of NAIT is known or highly suspected, delivery should be by cesarean section to avoid fetal trauma associated with vaginal delivery. After delivery, the affected infant may be treated with transfusion of the appropriate antigen-negative platelets (usually maternal). In addition, IVIG can be used alone or in combination with platelet transfusion. IVIG should not be used as the sole treatment in a bleeding infant because responses usually take 1 to 3 days.[64]

Neonatal Autoimmune Thrombocytopenia. The diagnosis of ITP or systemic lupus erythematosus in the mother is a prerequisite for the diagnosis of neonatal autoimmune thrombocytopenia. Neonatal autoimmune thrombocytopenia is due to passive transplacental transfer of antibodies from mothers with ITP or, occasionally, systemic lupus erythematosus. The neonate does not have an ongoing autoimmune process per se, but rather is an incidental target of the mother's autoimmune process. During pregnancy, relapse is relatively common for women with ITP in complete or partial remission; this has been attributed to the facilitation of reticuloendothelial phagocytosis by the high estrogen levels in pregnant women. Women commonly develop chronic ITP during pregnancy. ITP in the mother tends to remit after delivery. Corticosteroids are the primary treatment for pregnant women with ITP, and, at the doses used, there is a relatively low incidence of adverse fetal side effects.[68] Neonatal autoimmune thrombocytopenia occurs in only about 10% of pregnant women with autoimmune thrombocytopenia, and intracranial hemorrhage occurs in 1% or less. It is no longer recommended that high-risk infants be delivered by cesarean section to avoid the trauma of vaginal delivery and accompanying risk of hemorrhage for the infant regardless of the maternal platelet count.[69]

Affected newborns may have normal to decreased platelets at birth and have a progressive decrease in the platelet count for about 1 week before the platelet count begins to increase. It has been speculated that the falling platelet count is associated with maturation of the infant's reticuloendothelial system and accelerated removal of antibody-labeled platelets by cells of the reticuloendothelial system. Neonatal thrombocytopenia typically persists for about 1 to 2 weeks but sometimes lasts for several months and usually does not require treatment. Severely thrombocytopenic infants usually respond quickly to IVIG treatment. If an infant develops hemorrhagic symptoms, platelet transfusion, IVIG, or corticosteroids should be started immediately.[37]

Post-Transfusion Purpura. Post-transfusion purpura (PTP) is a relatively rare disorder that typically develops about 1 week after transfusion of platelet-containing blood products, including fresh or frozen plasma, whole blood, and packed or washed RBCs. PTP is manifested by the rapid onset of severe thrombocytopenia and moderate to severe hemorrhage that may be life-threatening. Plasma from the recipient contains alloantibodies to antigens on the platelets or platelet membranes of the transfused blood product and directed against an antigen the recipient does not have. In more than 90% of cases, the antibody is directed against the HPA-1a (P1^{A1}) antigen, and

most of the remaining cases have antibodies directed against P1^{A2} or epitopes on GP IIb/IIIa.[37] Involvement of other alloantigens, such as HPA-3a (Bak), HPA-4 (Penn), and HPA-5b (Br), has been reported. The mechanism by which the recipient's own platelets are destroyed is not unknown. Most patients with this type of thrombocytopenia are multiparous middle-aged women. Almost all other patients have a history of prior blood transfusion. PTP seems to be exceedingly rare in men who have never been transfused or women who have never been pregnant or transfused.[73] PTP seems to require prior exposure to "foreign" platelet antigens and behaves in many respects similar to an anamnestic immune response.

No clinical trials have been conducted for the treatment of PTP, primarily because of the small number of cases. If PTP is untreated or treatment is ineffective, mortality rates may approach 10%.[74] In addition, untreated or unresponsive patients have a protracted clinical course, with thrombocytopenia typically lasting 3 weeks but in some cases, 4 months. Plasmapheresis and exchange transfusion have been used with some success in the past, but the treatment of choice is now IVIG. Many patients with PTP respond to a 2-day course of IVIG, generally within the first 2 to 3 days, although a second course occasionally may be necessary.[74] IVIG also is much easier to use, and the response rates are higher than for plasmapheresis or exchange transfusion. Corticosteroid therapy used alone is not particularly efficacious but may be beneficial in combination with other, more effective treatments.[37]

Secondary Thrombocytopenia, Presumed to Be Immune Mediated. Severe thrombocytopenia has been observed in patients receiving biologic response modifiers such as interferons, colony-stimulating factors, and interleukin-2.[75-77] The thrombocytopenia associated with these substances is reversible and, at least for interferon, may be immune mediated because increased levels of platelet-associated IgG have been measured. Immune thrombocytopenia develops in about 5% to 10% of patients with chronic lymphocytic leukemia and in a smaller percentage of patients with other lymphoproliferative disorders.[78,79] Thrombocytopenia also is noted in 14% to 26% of patients with systemic lupus erythematosus.[80] The clinical picture is similar to that of ITP: The bone marrow has a larger than normal number of megakaryocytes, and increased levels of platelet-associated IgG frequently are found.[36] Parasitic infections also are known to cause thrombocytopenia. Malaria is the most studied in this group and is regularly accompanied by thrombocytopenia, the onset of which corresponds to first appearance of antimalarial antibodies, a decrease in serum complement, and control of parasitemia. There is evidence for the adsorption of microbial antigens to the platelet surface and subsequent antibody binding via the Fab terminus.[81] Immune destruction of platelets seems to be the most likely mechanism for the thrombocytopenia.

Nonimmune Mechanisms of Platelet Destruction

Nonimmune platelet destruction may result from exposure of platelets to nonendothelial surfaces, from activation of the coagulation process, or from platelet consumption by endovascular injury without measurable depletion of coagulation factors.[36]

Thrombocytopenia in Pregnancy and Preeclampsia

Incidental Thrombocytopenia of Pregnancy. Incidental thrombocytopenia of pregnancy also is known as *pregnancy-associated thrombocytopenia* and *gestational thrombocytopenia*. This disorder is the most common cause of thrombocytopenia in pregnancy. Random platelet counts in pregnant and postpartum women are slightly higher than normal, but about 5% of pregnant women develop a mild thrombocytopenia (100,000-150,000/μL) with 98% of such women having platelet counts greater than 70,000/μL. These women are healthy and have no prior history of thrombocytopenia. They do not seem to be at increased risk for bleeding or neonatal thrombocytopenia. The cause of this type of thrombocytopenia is unknown. Maternal platelet counts return to normal within several weeks of delivery. These women commonly experience recurrence in subsequent pregnancies.

Preeclampsia and Other Hypertensive Disorders of Pregnancy. Approximately 20% of cases of thrombocytopenia of pregnancy are associated with hypertensive disorders. These disorders include the classifications preeclampsia, preeclampsia-eclampsia, preeclampsia with chronic hypertension, chronic hypertension, and gestational hypertension. Preeclampsia complicates about 5% of all pregnancies and typically occurs at about 20 weeks of gestation. The disorder is characterized by the onset of hypertension and proteinuria and may include abdominal pain, headache, blurred vision, or mental function disturbances.[83] Thrombocytopenia occurs in 15% to 20% of patients with preeclampsia, and about 40% to 50% of patients progress to eclampsia (hypertension, proteinuria, and seizures).[84,85]

Some patients with preeclampsia have microangiopathic hemolysis, elevated liver enzymes, and a low platelet count—HELLP syndrome. HELLP syndrome affects an estimated 4% to 12% of patients with severe preeclampsia[46,86,87] and seems to be associated with higher rates of maternal and fetal complications. This disorder may be difficult to differentiate from thrombotic thrombocytopenic purpura (TTP), hemolytic-uremic syndrome (HUS), and disseminated intravascular coagulation (DIC).

The development of thrombocytopenia in these patients is thought to be via increased platelet destruction. The mechanism of platelet destruction is unclear, however. Some evidence (elevated D-dimer) suggests that these patients have an underlying low-grade DIC.[88] Elevated platelet-associated immunoglobulin is commonly found in these patients, however, suggesting immune involvement.[89] Early reports suggested that there may be a component of in vivo platelet activation because low-dose aspirin has been shown to prevent preeclampsia in high-risk patients.[90,91] When aspirin is used to prevent preeclampsia, however, there is only a 15% reduction in risk.

The treatment of preeclampsia is delivery of the infant whenever possible. After delivery, the thrombocytopenia usually resolves in a few days. In cases in which delivery is not possible (e.g., the infant would be too premature), bed rest and aggressive treatment of the hypertension may help to increase the platelet count in some patients. Such treatments include magnesium sulfate and other antiepileptic therapies to inhibit eclamptic seizures.

Hemolytic Disease of the Newborn.
Thrombocytopenia, usually moderate in degree, occurs frequently in infants with hemolytic disease of the newborn. Although the RBC destruction characteristic of this disorder is antibody induced, the antigens against which the antibodies are directed are not expressed on platelets. Platelets may be destroyed as the result of their interaction with products of RBC breakdown, rather than their direct participation in an immunologic reaction.[36]

Other Causes of Thrombocytopenia During Pregnancy. As has been discussed previously, ITP is a relatively common disorder in women of childbearing age, and pregnancy does nothing to ameliorate the symptoms of this disorder. ITP should be a part of the differential diagnosis of thrombocytopenia in a pregnant woman. There is little or no correlation between the level of maternal autoantibodies and the fetal platelet count. Other causes of thrombocytopenia during pregnancy include HIV, systemic lupus erythematosus, antiphospholipid syndromes, TTP, and HUS. Of women with ITP, 10% to 25% have their first manifestation of the disease during pregnancy or the postpartum period, and TTP tends to recur in subsequent pregnancies.[92,93] Plasmapheresis is the treatment of choice, and the maternal mortality is 90% or greater without such treatment.

Thrombotic Thrombocytopenic Purpura.
TTP, sometimes referred to as *Moschcowitz syndrome*, is characterized by the triad of microangiopathic hemolytic anemia, thrombocytopenia, and neurologic abnormalities.[94] In addition, fever and renal dysfunction (the pentad) are often present. Additional symptoms are present in most patients at the time of diagnosis and include diarrhea, anorexia, nausea, weakness, and fatigue. TTP is uncommon but not rare, and its incidence may be increasing. About twice as many women as men are affected, and it is most common in women 30 to 40 years old.[34,95] About half of the patients who develop TTP have a history of a viral-like illness several days before the onset of TTP.

There seem to be at least four types of TTP. In most patients, TTP occurs as a single acute episode, although a small fraction of these may have recurrence at seemingly random intervals. Recurrent TTP occurs in 11% to 28% of TTP patients.[96,97] A third type of TTP is drug induced. The primary agents involved are the purinoreceptor (adenosine diphosphate) blocking agents ticlopidine (Ticlid) and clopidogrel (Plavix) used for inhibition of platelet function. Ticlopidine seems to cause TTP in about 0.025% of patients, whereas the incidence of clopidogrel-induced TTP is approximately four times less frequent.[95] Another type is chronic relapsing TTP, a rare form of TTP in which episodes occur at intervals of approximately 3 months starting in infancy.[98,99]

Although it is unclear what triggers their deposition, hyaline thrombi are found in the end arterioles and capillaries. These hyaline thrombi are composed of platelets and von Willebrand factor (VWF) but contain very little fibrin or fibrinogen. As these platelet-VWF thrombi are deposited, thrombocytopenia develops. The degree of thrombocytopenia is directly related to the extent of microvascular platelet aggregation. RBCs flowing under arterial pressure are prone to fragmentation and hemolysis when they encounter the strands of these thrombi.

Hemolysis is usually quite severe, and most patients have less than 10 g/dL hemoglobin at the time of diagnosis. Examination of the peripheral blood smear reveals a marked decrease in platelets, RBC polychromasia, and RBC fragmentation (microspherocytes, schistocytes, keratocytes), a triad of features characteristic of microangiopathic hemolytic anemias (Fig. 43-8). Nucleated RBC precursors also may be present

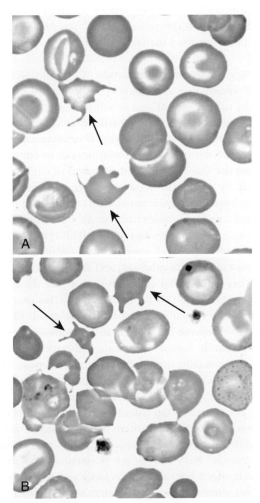

Figure 43-8 Microangiopathic hemolytic anemia in thrombotic thrombocytopenia purpura (TTP). Abundant schistocytes reflect platelet clots in microvasculature. (From Carr JH, Rodak BF: Clinical Hematology Atlas, ed 2. Philadelphia: Saunders, 2004.)

depending on the degree of hemolysis. Other laboratory evidence of intravascular hemolysis includes reduction of haptoglobin, hemoglobinuria, hemosiderinuria, increased serum unconjugated bilirubin, and increased lactate dehydrogenase activity. Bone marrow examination reveals erythroid hyperplasia and a normal to increased number of megakaryocytes. The partial thromboplastin time, prothrombin time, fibrinogen, fibrin degradation products, and D-dimer tests are usually normal and may be useful in differentiating this disorder from DIC.

The thrombotic lesions also give rise to the other characteristic manifestations of TTP because they are deposited in the vasculature of all organs. The thrombi occlude blood flow and lead to organ ischemia. Symptoms depend on the severity of ischemia in each organ. Neurologic manifestations range from headache to paresthesia and coma. Visual disturbances may be of neurologic origin or may be due to thrombi in the choroid capillaries of the retina or hemorrhage into the vitreous. Renal dysfunction is common and present in more than half of patients.[96,97] Symptoms of renal dysfunction include proteinuria and hematuria. Overwhelming renal damage with anuria and fulminant uremia usually does not occur, however, helping to distinguish TTP from HUS.[10] Gastrointestinal bleeding occurs frequently in severely thrombocytopenic patients, and abdominal pain is occasionally present and caused by occlusion of the mesenteric microcirculation.

ADAMTS 13 and Thrombotic Thrombocytopenic Purpura. The development of TTP seems to be directly related to the accumulation of unusually large von Willebrand factor (ULVWF) multimers in the plasma of patients with TTP. VWF multimers are made by megakaryocytes and endothelial cells. The primary source of plasma VWF seems to be endothelial cells. Endothelial cells secrete VWF into the subendothelium and plasma and store it in Weibel-Palade bodies (storage granules). Endothelial cells and megakaryocytes make even larger VWF multimers (ULVWF) than those found in plasma, and these are even more effective than the normal plasma VWF multimers at binding platelet GP Ib-IX or GP IIb-IIIa complexes under fluid shear stresses (Fig. 43-9).[98] In the plasma, the ULVWF multimers are rapidly cleaved into the smaller VWF multimers normally found in the plasma by a VWF-cleaving metalloprotease, also called "a disintegrin-like and metalloprotease domain with thrombospondin type I motifs" (ADAMTS 13). The metalloprotease seems to be more effective when VWF multimers are partially unfolded by high shear stress.[100,101]

Familial chronic relapsing TTP is a form characterized by recurrent episodes of thrombocytopenia with or without ischemic organ damage. In this type of TTP, the VWF-cleaving metalloprotease is completely deficient. The more common form of TTP (usually not familial) does not tend to recur, but the patients also are deficient in the metalloprotease. In this more common form of TTP, the metalloprotease deficiency is through removal of the enzyme (or blockade of its function) by a specific autoantibody that is present during TTP but disappears during remission.[102,103] An assay to measure the

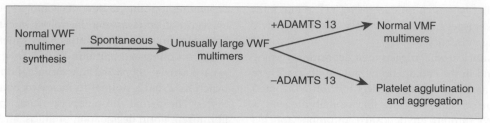

Figure 43-9 Mechanism for TTP. ULVWF multimers are normally digested by von Willebrand cleaving protease, ADAMTS13 (see text for full name). In TTP, the absence of ADAMTS13 allows release of ULVWF, triggering platelet activation. TTP, thrombotic thrombocytopenic purpura; ULVW, unusually large von Willebrand factor.

VWF-cleaving enzyme has been introduced.[104] This test may be useful in the rapid diagnosis of TTP if it can be adapted for use in the clinical laboratory. At present, the assays lack sensitivity and specificity for TTP.

In patients with TTP, ULVWF multimers tend to be present in the plasma at the beginning of the episode. These ULVWF multimers and usually the normal-sized plasma multimers disappear as the TTP episode progresses and the thrombocytopenia worsens. Platelets and VWF are consumed during the deposition of microvascular "hyaline" thrombi characteristic of this disorder.[105] If the patient survives an episode of TTP and does not relapse, the plasma VWF multimers are normal after recovery. If ULVWF multimers are found in the plasma after recovery, however, it is likely that the patient will have recurrent episodes of TTP. The episodes may be infrequent and at irregular intervals (intermittent TTP) or frequent and at regular intervals, as is often the case when TTP episodes occur in early childhood or infancy.

The most effective treatment for TTP is plasma exchange using fresh frozen plasma or cryoprecipitate-poor (lacking most of the fibrinogen, fibronectin, and VWF) plasma.[106] Either of these approaches may produce dramatic effects within a few hours. Because plasmapheresis is not available in all centers, the patient should be given corticosteroids and infusions of fresh frozen plasma immediately. Plasma exchange should be arranged as quickly as possible. Plasmapheresis and replacement/infusion of plasma is effective on two fronts. First, some of the ULVWF multimers may be removed by apheresis, and plasma (fresh frozen plasma or cryoprecipitate-poor plasma) supplies the deficient protease, which is able to degrade the ULVWF multimers in the blood of the patient. Because some patients with TTP have recovered while receiving immunosuppressive treatment (corticosteroids) alone, it is recommended that all patients with TTP receive high-dose corticosteroids in addition to plasma exchange. Plasma exchange typically is continued over a 5-day period. If the patient does not respond within 5 days, or the condition of the patient worsens in the first few days of plasma exchange, additional treatment is instituted. Additional treatments include vincristine or azathioprine (or other immunosuppressive agents), splenectomy, or passing the patient's plasma over a staphylococcal A column to remove immune complexes. The use of antiplatelet agents, prostacyclin, heparin, or fibrinolytic agents is controversial and has not been clearly shown to be helpful. Platelet transfusions should be avoided unless intracranial or other serious hemorrhagic problems arise.[46]

Before 1990, TTP was fatal in more than 80% of patients. With rapid diagnosis and the advent of exchange plasmapheresis, 80% of patients who are treated early can be expected to survive. Because patients are known to relapse, however, the platelet count should be monitored on a regular basis until they are in remission. The detection of ULVWF multimers in patient samples after complete remission has predicted relapse accurately in 90% of the patients tested[107]; this may prove to be useful in the long-term management of TTP.

Hemolytic-Uremic Syndrome. Clinically, HUS resembles TTP except that it is found predominantly in children 6 months to 4 years old and is self-limiting. Approximately 90% of cases are caused by *Shigella dysenteriae* serotypes or enterohemorrhagic *Escherichia coli* OH serotypes, particularly O157:H7.[108] These organisms sometimes can be cultured from stool samples. The bloody diarrhea typical of childhood HUS is caused by colonization of the large intestine with the offending organism, which causes erosive damage to the colon. *S. dysenteriae* produces Shiga toxin, and the enterohemorrhagic *E. coli* produce either Shiga-like toxin-1 (SLT-1) or SLT-2, which can be detected in fecal samples from patients with HUS. The toxins enter the bloodstream and attach to renal glomerular capillary endothelial cells, which become damaged and swollen and release ULVWF multimers.[108,109] This process leads to formation of hyaline thrombi in the renal vasculature and the development of renal failure, thrombocytopenia, and microangiopathic hemolytic anemia, although the RBC fragmentation is usually not as severe as that seen in TTP. The extent of renal involvement correlates with the rate of recovery. In more severely affected children, renal dialysis may be needed. The mortality rate associated with HUS in children is much less than in TTP, but there is often residual renal dysfunction that may lead to renal hypertension and severe renal failure. Because HUS in children is essentially an infectious disorder, it affects boys and girls equally and is often found in geographic clusters of cases rather than random distribution.

The adult form of HUS is associated most often with exposure to immunosuppressive agents or chemotherapeutic agents or both, but it also may occur during the postpartum period. Usually the symptoms of HUS do not appear until weeks or months after exposure to the offending agent.[110] This disorder most likely results from direct renal arterial endothelial damage caused by the drug or one of its metabolic products. The damage to endothelial cells results in release of VWF (including ULVWF multimers), turbulent flow in the arterial system with increased shear stresses on platelets, and VWF-mediated platelet aggregation in the renal arterial system. Compared with childhood HUS, the renal impairment in adults seems to be more severe, and dialysis is usually required. The cause of HUS associated with pregnancy or oral contraceptive use is unclear but may be related to development of an autoantibody to endothelial cells. In outbreaks of HUS associated with consumption of E. coli–contaminated water, children and adults have developed HUS.

The cardinal signs of HUS are hemolytic anemia, renal failure, and thrombocytopenia. The thrombocytopenia is usually mild to moderate in severity. Renal failure is reflected in elevated blood urea nitrogen and creatinine levels. The urine nearly always contains RBCs, protein, and casts. The hemolytic process is shown by a hemoglobin level of less than 10 g/dL, elevated reticulocyte count, and the presence of schistocytes in the peripheral blood.

Differentiating the adult form of HUS from TTP may be difficult. The lack of neurologic symptoms, the presence of renal dysfunction, and the absence of other organ involvement suggest HUS. Also, in HUS, the thrombocytopenia tends to be mild to moderate (platelet consumption occurs primarily in the kidneys), whereas the thrombocytopenia in TTP is usually severe. Similarly, fragmentation of RBCs and the resultant anemia tend to be milder than that observed in TTP because RBCs are being fragmented primarily in the kidneys. In some cases of HUS, other organs become involved, and the differentiation between HUS and TTP becomes less clear. In such cases, it is prudent to treat as though the patient has TTP.

Disseminated Intravascular Coagulation. A common cause of destructive thrombocytopenia is activation of the coagulation cascade (by a variety of agents or conditions), resulting in a consumptive coagulopathy that entraps platelets in intravascular fibrin clots. This disorder is described in more detail in Chapter 42 but is included here briefly for the sake of completeness. DIC has many similarities to TTP, including microangiopathic hemolytic anemia and deposition of thrombi in the arterial circulation of most organs. In DIC, however, the thrombi are composed primarily of platelets and fibrinogen, whereas in TTP the thrombi are composed primarily of platelets and VWF.

One form of DIC is acute with rapid platelet consumption and results in severe thrombocytopenia. In addition, levels of factor V, factor VIII, and fibrinogen are decreased as a result of in vivo thrombin generation. The test for D-dimer (a breakdown product of stabilized fibrin) is almost always positive. This form of DIC is life-threatening and must be treated immediately.

In chronic DIC, there is an ongoing, low-grade consumptive coagulopathy. Clotting factors may be slightly reduced or normal, and compensatory thrombocytopoiesis results in a moderately low to normal platelet count.[34] D-dimer may not be detectable or may be slightly to moderately increased. Chronic DIC is not generally life-threatening, and treatment usually is not urgent. Chronic DIC is almost always due to some underlying condition. If that condition can be corrected, the DIC usually resolves without further treatment. Chronic DIC should be followed carefully, however, because it can transition to the life-threatening acute form.

Drugs. A few drugs directly interact with platelets to cause thrombocytopenia. Ristocetin, an antibiotic no longer in clinical use, facilitates the interaction of VWF with platelet membrane GP Ib and results in in vivo platelet agglutination and thrombocytopenia. Hematin, used for treatment of acute intermittent porphyria, may be followed by a transient thrombocytopenia that seems to be caused by stimulation of platelet secretion and aggregation. Protamine sulfate and bleomycin may induce thrombocytopenia by a similar mechanism.[46]

Disorders Related to Distribution or Dilution

An abnormal distribution of platelets also may cause thrombocytopenia. The normal spleen sequesters approximately one third of the total platelet mass. Mild thrombocytopenia may be present in any of the "big spleen" syndromes. The total body platelet mass is often normal in these disorders, but numerous platelets are sequestered in the enlarged spleen, and consequently the venous blood platelet count is low. Disorders such as Gaucher disease, Hodgkin disease, sarcoidosis, lymphomas, cirrhosis of the liver, and portal hypertension may result in splenomegaly and lead to thrombocytopenia.

Lowering the body temperature to less than 25° C, as is routinely done in cardiovascular surgery, results in a transient but mild thrombocytopenia secondary to platelet sequestration in the spleen and liver. An associated transient defect in function also occurs with hypothermia. Platelet count and function return to baseline values on return to normal body temperature.[32]

Thrombocytopenia often follows surgery involving extracorporeal circulatory devices, as a consequence of damage and partial activation of platelets in the pump. In a few cases, severe thrombocytopenia, marked impairment of platelet function, and activation of fibrinolysis and intravascular coagulation may develop.[46]

The administration of massive amounts of stored whole blood may produce a temporary thrombocytopenia. This phenomenon is explained by the fact that stored blood contains platelets whose viability is severely impaired by the effects of storage and temperature. Under these conditions, the dead or damaged platelets are rapidly sequestered by the reticuloendothelial system of the patient. If encountered, this problem may be minimized by the use of platelet concentrates or units of fresh whole blood along with the stored blood. This situation is only rarely encountered, however, because the practice of transfusing whole blood has been replaced almost completely by the use of specific components. Finally, mild thrombocytopenia may be encountered in patients with chronic renal failure, severe iron deficiency, megaloblastic anemias, postcompression sickness, and chronic hypoxia.

THROMBOCYTOSIS

Thrombocytosis is defined as an abnormally high platelet count, typically more than 450,000/μL. The term *reactive thrombocytosis* is used to describe an elevation in the platelet count secondary to inflammation, trauma, or other underlying and seemingly unrelated conditions. In reactive thrombocytosis, the platelet count is elevated for a limited period and usually does not exceed 800,000/μL, although platelet counts greater than 1 million/μL are occasionally seen (Fig. 43-10). A marked and persistent elevation in the platelet count is a hallmark of myeloproliferative disorders such as polycythemia vera, chronic myelocytic leukemia, or myelofibrosis with myeloid metaplasia. In these conditions, the platelet count often exceeds 1 million/μL. Although the terms *thrombocythemia* and *thrombocytosis* are often used interchangeably, in this text, the term *thrombocythemia* is used only as part of the description of the myeloproliferative disorder known as *essential thrombocythemia* (Fig. 43-11). In essential thrombocythemia, platelet counts typically exceed 1 million/μL and may reach levels of several million.[34,111,112] Processes resulting in thrombocytosis are summarized in Box 43-3.

Reactive (Secondary) Thrombocytosis

Platelet counts between 450,000/μL and 800,000/μL with no change in platelet function can result from acute blood loss; postsplenectomy; childbirth; and tissue necrosis secondary to surgery, chronic inflammatory disease, infection, exercise, iron deficiency anemia, hemolytic anemia, renal disorders, or

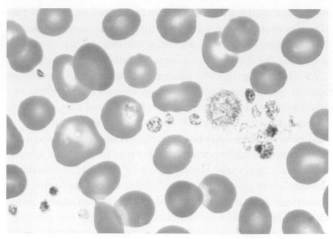

Figure 43-11 Peripheral blood smear morphology in essential thrombocythemia. Note increased platelet number and wide variation in platelet size characteristic of essential thrombocythemia. RBC and white blood cell morphology is characteristically normal. (From Carr JH, Rodak BF: Clinical Hematology Atlas, ed 2. Philadelphia: Saunders, 2004.)

BOX 43-3 Processes Resulting in Thrombocytosis

Reactive Thrombocytosis
Associated with blood loss and surgery
Postsplenectomy thrombocytosis
Iron deficiency anemia
Inflammation and disease
Stress or exercise

Thrombocytosis Associated with Myeloproliferative Disorders
Polycythemia vera
Chronic myelogenous leukemia
Myelofibrosis with myeloid metaplasia
Thrombocythemia: essential or primary

Data from Colvin[29] and Thompson and Harker.[32]

---

malignancy. Occasionally, patients manifest a platelet count of 1 to 2 million/μL (see Fig. 43-10). In reactive thrombocytosis, platelet production remains responsive to normal regulatory stimuli (e.g., thrombopoietin, a humoral factor that is produced in the kidney parenchyma), and morphologically normal platelets are produced at a moderately increased rate. This is in contrast to essential thrombocythemia, which is characterized by unregulated or autonomous platelet production and platelets of variable size.[111,112]

Examination of the bone marrow from patients with reactive thrombocytosis reveals a normal to increased number of megakaryocytes that are normal in morphology. Results of platelet function tests, including aggregation induced by various agents, and the bleeding time are usually normal in

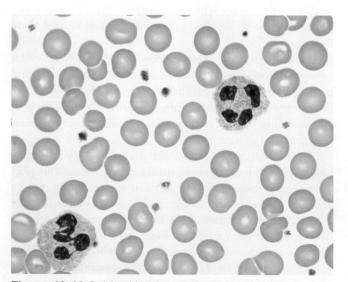

Figure 43-10 Peripheral blood smear morphology of reactive thrombocytosis. Note the increased number of platelets but reasonably normal platelet morphology, characteristic of reactive thrombocytosis.

reactive thrombocytosis but also may be normal in patients with elevated platelet counts accompanying myeloproliferative disorders.

Reactive thrombocytosis is not associated with thrombosis, hemorrhage, or abnormal thrombopoietin levels. It seldom produces symptoms per se and disappears when the underlying disorder is brought under control.[111,112]

Reactive Thrombocytosis Associated with Hemorrhage or Surgery

After acute hemorrhage, the platelet count may be low for 2 to 6 days (unless platelets have been transfused) but typically rebounds to elevated levels for several days before returning to the prehemorrhage level. A similar pattern of thrombocytopenia and thrombocytosis is seen after major surgical procedures in which there is significant blood loss. In both cases, the platelet count typically returns to normal 10 to 16 days after the episode of blood loss.

Postsplenectomy Thrombocytosis

Removal of the spleen typically results in platelet counts that can reach or exceed 1 million/µL regardless of the reason for splenectomy. The spleen normally sequesters about one third of the circulating platelet mass. After splenectomy, one would expect an initial increase in the platelet count of approximately 30% to 50%. The platelet count, however, far exceeds levels that could result from equilibration of the splenic platelet pool into the circulating platelet pool. The cause of the accelerated platelet production is unknown. In contrast to blood loss from hemorrhage or other types of surgery, the platelet count reaches a maximum 1 to 3 weeks after splenectomy and remains elevated for 1 to 3 months. In some patients who undergo splenectomy for chronic anemia, the count can remain elevated for several years.

Iron Deficiency Anemia

Mild iron deficiency anemia secondary to chronic blood loss is associated with thrombocytosis in about 50% of cases. Thrombocytosis can be seen in severe iron deficiency anemia, but thrombocytopenia also has been reported. In some cases of iron deficiency, the platelet count may be 2 million/µL. After iron therapy is started, the platelet count usually returns to normal within 7 to 10 days. It is believed that iron plays some role in regulating thrombopoiesis because treatment of the iron deficiency with iron replacement has resulted in a normalization of the platelet count in thrombocytopenic patients and has been reported to induce thrombocytopenia in patients with normal platelet counts. Not enough research has been done, however, to elucidate the role of iron in thrombopoiesis.

Inflammation and Disease

Similar to elevated C-reactive protein, fibrinogen, VWF, and other acute-phase reactants, thrombocytosis may be an indication of inflammation. Thrombocytosis may be found in association with rheumatoid arthritis, rheumatic fever,

osteomyelitis, ulcerative colitis, acute infections, and malignancy. In rheumatoid arthritis, the presence of thrombocytosis can be correlated with activation of the inflammatory process.

Kawasaki disease (Kawasaki syndrome) is an acute febrile illness of infants and young children. It is a self-limited acute vasculitic syndrome of unknown origin, although an infectious etiology has been suspected. Although the disease is self-limiting, there can be lifelong sequelae, including coronary artery thrombosis and aneurysms. The acute febrile stage of the disease lasts 2 weeks or longer with fever of 104° F or higher and is unresponsive to antibiotics. The longer the fever exists, the higher the risk of cardiovascular complications. The subacute phase lasts an additional week to 10 days. During this phase, the platelet count usually is elevated, and counts of 2 million/µL have been reported. In addition, acute-phase reactants such as C-reactive protein and sedimentation rate are elevated. The white blood cell count can be moderately to markedly elevated with a left shift, and many patients develop a mild normochromic/normocytic anemia. During this phase, cardiovascular complications and aneurysms develop. The higher the platelet count, the higher the risk of cardiovascular complication. After the subacute phase, the convalescent phase occurs, during which all signs of illness disappear and the acute-phase reactants subside to normal. The highest incidence of Kawasaki disease is found in Japan and in individuals of Japanese descent, although the disease seems to be found in most, if not all, ethnic groups. The treatment for Kawasaki disease is antiplatelet agents and immunoglobulin.

An elevated platelet count also may be early evidence of a tumor (e.g., Hodgkin disease) and various carcinomas. Finally, hemophilic patients often have platelet counts above normal limits, even in the absence of active bleeding.

Exercise-Induced Thrombocytosis

Strenuous exercise is a well-known cause of relative thrombocytosis and is likely due to release of platelets from the splenic pool or hemoconcentration by transfer of plasma water to the extravascular compartment or both. Normally, the platelet count returns to its pre-exercise baseline level 30 minutes after completion of exercise.

Rebound Thrombocytosis

Thrombocytosis often follows the thrombocytopenia caused by marrow-suppressive therapy. "Rebound" thrombocytosis usually reaches a peak 10 to 17 days after withdrawal of the offending drug (e.g., alcohol or methotrexate) or after institution of therapy for the underlying condition with which thrombocytopenia is associated (e.g., vitamin B_{12} deficiency).[46]

Thrombocytosis Associated with Myeloproliferative Disorders

Primary or autonomous thrombocytosis is a typical finding in four chronic myeloproliferative disorders: polycythemia vera, chronic myelocytic leukemia, myelofibrosis with myeloid metaplasia, and essential thrombocythemia. Depending on the duration and stage of the myeloproliferative disorder at the time of diagnosis, it may be difficult to differentiate among these disorders. Chapter 34 provides a more complete description of these disorders. In the other types of myeloproliferative disorders, the platelet count seldom reaches the extreme values characteristic of essential thrombocythemia. Diagnosis of essential thrombocythemia should not be based on the platelet count alone but should be combined with physical examination, history, and other laboratory data.[34,112]

Essential (Primary) Thrombocythemia

Essential thrombocythemia is a clonal disorder related to other chronic myeloproliferative diseases and is the most common cause of primary thrombocytosis. It is characterized by peripheral blood platelet counts exceeding 1 million/μL and uncontrolled proliferation of marrow megakaryocytes. Although the platelet count may (or may not) be markedly elevated in other myeloproliferative disorders, persistent marked elevation of the platelet count is an absolute requirement for the diagnosis of essential thrombocythemia (see Fig. 43-11). There is evidence that essential thrombocythemia is caused by a clonal proliferation of a single abnormal pluripotential stem cell that eventually crowds out normal stem cells. As with most myeloproliferative disorders, essential thrombocythemia is neither congenital nor hereditary, is prevalent in middle-aged and older patients, and affects equal numbers of men and women. In contrast to other myeloproliferative disorders, however, the other marrow cell lines are not involved at the time of diagnosis.

The clinical manifestations of essential thrombocythemia are hemorrhage, platelet dysfunction, and thrombosis. Bleeding times are usually normal. There is no specific clinical sign, symptom, or laboratory test that establishes the diagnosis of essential thrombocythemia. The diagnosis must be made by ruling out the other myeloproliferative disorders and systemic illnesses that produce reactive thrombocytosis.

Thrombosis in the microvasculature is relatively common in essential thrombocythemia, and the incidence at the time of diagnosis is 10% to 20%. This thrombosis can lead to digital pain, digital gangrene, or erythromyalgia (throbbing, aching, and burning sensation in the extremities, particularly in the palms and soles).[112] The symptoms of erythromyalgia can be explained by arteriolar inflammation and occlusive thrombosis mediated by platelets and are relieved for several days by a single dose of aspirin.[113] Thrombosis of large veins and arteries also may occur in essential thrombocythemia. The most common arteries involved are those in the legs, the coronary arteries, and the renal arteries, but involvement of the mesenteric, subclavian and carotid arteries is not uncommon (in fact, neurologic complications are relatively common). Venous thrombosis may involve the large veins of the legs and pelvis, hepatic veins, or splenic veins.[114] The platelets of some patients who have had thrombotic episodes have been shown to have increased binding affinity for fibrinogen and to generate more than the usual quantities of thromboxane B_2, and these patients have elevated levels of thromboxane B_2 and β-thromboglobulin in the blood. These findings suggest enhanced in vivo platelet activation and perhaps an expla-

nation for the thrombotic tendencies of patients with essential thrombocythemia. The primary cause of death for patients with essential thrombocythemia seems to be thrombosis. Hemorrhagic episodes occur less frequently than thrombotic episodes in patients with essential thrombocythemia.

As with bleeding secondary to platelet function disorders, the hemorrhagic manifestations of essential thrombocythemia are mucocutaneous in nature, with gastrointestinal tract bleeding occurring most frequently. Other sites of bleeding include the mucous membranes of the nose and mouth, the urinary tract, and the skin. Symptoms may be aggravated by aspirin use. In most cases of thrombocythemia, patients experience no clotting disorders. In an occasional patient with essential thrombocythemia, there is a paradoxical combination of thromboembolic (clotting) and hemorrhagic episodes associated with this condition. A patient with essential thrombocythemia who has had a thrombotic event may have a hemorrhagic event later.[115]

The bleeding manifestations may be related to a variety of qualitative abnormalities in the platelets, including deficiencies in epinephrine receptors and ultrastructural defects in granules, mitochondria, and microfilaments. Platelets may be agranular or hypogranular and have a clear, light-blue appearance on a routine Wright-stained smear of the peripheral blood. Although their size is heterogeneous, giant and bizarre-shaped platelets are characteristic of myeloproliferative diseases, and megakaryocyte fragments or nuclei are commonly encountered in the peripheral blood. Platelets may be notably clumped on blood smears, exhibiting marked variation in size and shape. The number and volume of megakaryocytes are increased in the bone marrow, and they are predominantly large, show some cellular atypia, and tend to form clusters. Often the platelets are functionally defective when tested in vitro. Aggregation is usually absent in response to epinephrine and may be decreased with adenosine diphosphate but is usually normal with collagen. An absent epinephrine response may help to differentiate essential thrombocythemia from reactive thrombocytosis because this response is usually normal in reactive thrombocytosis but absent in most cases of essential thrombocythemia. Platelet adhesion also may be decreased.[112]

The degree of thrombocytosis has not been found to predict hemorrhagic or thrombotic events reliably. The role of lowering platelet counts as a prophylactic treatment in this disease is not established. The risks from exposure to mutagenic alkylating agents used to decrease the platelet count may be greater than the risk of thrombosis or hemorrhage. When deemed necessary because of thrombotic tendencies or splenomegaly, a variety of myelosuppressive agents (e.g., melphalan, busulfan, hydroxyurea, or even radioactive phosphorus) can be used.[112] In patients with life-threatening hemorrhage or thrombosis and an extremely high platelet count, platelet apheresis may be used to reduce the platelet count rapidly. In these situations, a myelosuppressive agent is added for longer-term control of the platelet count.[116] Interferon-α has been used to treat essential thrombocythemia with approximately 60% complete remissions, although 28%

of patients given the drug could not tolerate the doses required.[117-119] A newer agents that has shown great promise in the treatment of essential thrombocythemia is anagrelide. The drug acts by inhibiting megakaryocyte maturation and platelet release.[120] In one large study, anagrelide decreased the platelet count in 93% of patients.[121] Many patients cannot tolerate anagrelide, however, and in these patients, other, more traditional chemotherapeutic agents seem to be more effective. Despite the newer treatments for essential thrombocythemia, whether a patient with essential thrombocythemia and an elevated platelet count who is asymptomatic should or should not be treated remains controversial.

Patients with essential thrombocythemia have a low incidence of transformation to acute leukemia or fatal thrombotic or hemorrhagic complications. Therapy to prevent thrombotic complications seems to be effective in preventing morbidity but does not seem to improve survival, at least in high-risk patients.

CHAPTER at a GLANCE

- Thrombocytopenia is the most common cause of clinically significant bleeding.
- Thrombocytopenia may be a result of decreased platelet production, increased destruction, or abnormal distribution of platelets and manifests with small vessel bleeding in the skin.
- Decreased production of platelets can be attributed to megakaryocyte hypoplasia, ineffective thrombopoiesis, or marrow replacement by abnormal cells.
- Patients experiencing an increased amount of platelet destruction become thrombocytopenic only when the rate of production of their platelets no longer can compensate.
- Pathologic destruction of platelets is the result of immunologic and nonimmunologic mechanisms.
- Acute ITP commonly occurs in children after a viral illness, and there are usually spontaneous remissions. Chronic ITP more commonly is seen in women and requires treatment if the platelet count decreases to less than 30,000/μL.

- Treatment of drug-induced thrombocytopenia must begin with identification of the causative drug and discontinuation of its use.
- TTP presents with the triad of symptoms of microangiopathic hemolytic anemia, thrombocytopenia, and neurologic abnormalities that can be accompanied by fever and renal dysfunction.
- Abnormal distribution of platelets can be caused by splenic sequestration.
- Reactive thrombocytosis is secondary to inflammation, trauma, or a variety of underlying conditions. Platelet counts are increased for a limited time. Thrombocytosis seen in myeloproliferative disorders is marked and persistent.

Now that you have completed this chapter, go back and read again the case study at the beginning and respond to the questions presented.

REVIEW QUESTIONS

1. The autosomal dominant abnormality associated with decreased platelet production is:
   a. Fanconi anemia
   b. TAR syndrome
   c. May-Hegglin anomaly
   d. Wiskott-Aldrich anomaly

2. Which of the following is *not* a hallmark of ITP?
   a. Petechiae
   b. Thrombocytopenia
   c. Large overactive platelets
   d. Megakaryocyte hypoplasia

3. The specific antigen most commonly responsible for the development of NAIT is:
   a. Bak
   b. Pl^{A1}
   c. GP Ib
   d. Lewis antigen a

4. A 2-year-old child with an unexpected platelet count of 15 $\times 10^9$/L and a recent history of a viral infection most likely has:
   a. HIT
   b. NAIT
   c. Acute ITP
   d. Chronic ITP

5. What is the first step in treatment of HIT?
   a. Start low-molecular-weight heparin therapy.
   b. Stop heparin infusion immediately.
   c. Switch to warfarin (Coumadin) immediately.
   d. Initiate a platelet transfusion.

6. A defect in primary hemostasis (platelet response to an injury) often results in:
   a. Musculoskeletal bleeding
   b. Mucosal bleeding
   c. Hemarthroses
   d. None of the above

7. When a drug acts as a hapten to induce thrombocytopenia, an antibody forms against:
   a. Typically unexposed, new platelet antigens
   b. The combination of the drug bound to a platelet membrane protein
   c. The drug alone in the plasma, but the immune complex then binds the platelet membrane
   d. The drug alone, but only when it is bound to the platelet membrane

8. *TAR* refers to:
   a. Abnormal platelet morphology in which the radial striations of the platelets are missing
   b. Abnormal appearance of the iris of the eyes with missing radial striations
   c. Abnormal bone formation including hypoplasia of the forearms
   d. Neurologic defects affecting the root (radix) of spinal nerves

9. Neonatal autoimmune thrombocytopenia occurs when:
   a. The mother lacks a platelet antigen that the infant possesses, and she builds antibodies to that antigen, cross the placenta.
   b. The infant develops an autoimmune process such as ITP secondary to in utero infection.
   c. The infant develops an autoimmune disease such as lupus erythematosus before birth.
   d. The mother has an autoimmune antibody to her own platelets, which crosses the placenta and reacts with the infant's platelets.

10. HUS in children is related to:
   a. Diarrhea secondary to *Shigella* sp.
   b. Meningitis secondary to *Haemophilus* sp.
   c. Pneumonia secondary to *Mycoplasma* sp.
   d. Pneumonia secondary to respiratory viruses

REFERENCES

1. Kelley MJ, Jawien W, Ortel TL, et al: Mutations of MYH9, encoding for non-muscle myosin heavy chain A, in May Hegglin anomaly. Nat Genet 2000;26:106-108.
2. The May Hegglin/Fechtner syndrome consortium: mutations in MHY9 result in May-Hegglin anomaly, and Fechtner and Sebastian syndromes. Nat Genet 2000;26:103-105.
3. Mhawech P, Saleem A: Inherited giant platelet disorders: classification and literature review. Am J Clin Pathol 2000;113:176-190.
4. Hall JG: Thrombocytopenia and absent radius (TAR) syndrome. J Med Genet 1987;24:79-83.
5. Symonds RP, Clark BJ, George WD, et al: Thrombocytopenia with absent radii (TAR) syndrome: a new increased cellular radiosensitivity syndrome. Clin Oncol (R Coll Radiol) 1995;7:56-58.
6. Freedman MH, Doyle JJ: Inherited bone marrow failure syndromes. In Lilleyman JS, Hann IM, Branchette VS (eds): Pediatric Hematology. London: Churchill Livingstone, 1999:23-49.
7. Lackner A, Basu M, Bierings M, et al: Haematopoietic stem cell transplantation for amegakaryocytic thrombocytopenia. Br J Haematol 2000;109:773-775.
8. van den Oudenrijn SM, Bruin M, Folman CC, et al: Mutations in the thrombopoietin receptor, Mlp, in children with congenital amegakaryocytic thrombocytopenia. Br J Haematol 2000;110:441-448.
9. Stormorken H, Hellum B, Egeland T, et al: X-linked thrombocytopenia and thrombocytopathia: attenuated Wiscott-Aldrich syndrome: functional and morphological studies of platelets and lymphocytes. Thromb Haemost 1991;65:300-305.
10. Thorup OA: Leavell and Thorup's Fundamentals of Clinical Hematology, 5th ed. Philadelphia: Saunders, 1987.
11. Villa AL, Notarangelo P, Maachi E, et al: X-linked thrombocytopenia and Wiskott-Aldrich syndrome are allelic diseases with mutations in the WASP gene. Nat Genet 1999;9:414-417.
12. Mehaffey MG, Newton AL, Gandhi MJ, et al: X-linked thrombocytopenia caused by a novel mutation of GATA-1. Blood 2001;98:2681-2688.
13. Freson KK, Devriendt G, Matthijs G, et al: Platelet characteristics in patients with X-linked macrothrombocytopenia because of a novel GATA-1 mutation. Blood 2001;98:85-92.
14. Casteels AA, Naessens F, Cordts L, et al: Neonatal screening for congenital cytomegalovirus infections. J Perinat Med 1999;27:116-121.
15. Brown HL, Abernathy MP: Cytomegalovirus infection. Semin Perinatol 1998;22:260-266.
16. Crapnell KED, Zanfani A, Chaudhuri JL, et al: In vitro infection of megakaryocytes and their precursors by human cytomegalovirus. Blood 2000;95:487-493.
17. McAuley J, Boyer D, Patel D, et al: Early and longitudinal evaluations of treated infants and children and untreated historical patients with congenital toxoplasmosis: the Chicago Collaborative Treatment Trial. Clin Infect Dis 1994;18:38-72.
18. Sullivan EM, Burgess MA, Forrest JM: The epidemiology of rubella and congenital rubella in Australia, 1992-1997. Commun Dis Intell 1999;23:209-214.
19. Tookey PA, Peckham CS: Surveillance of congenital rubella in Great Britain, 1971-96. BMJ 1999;318:769-770.
20. Tovo PA, de-Martino M, Gabiano C, et al: Prognostic factors and survival in children with perinatal HIV-1 infection. The Italian Register for HIV Infections in Children. Lancet 1992;339:1249-1253.
21. Triplett DA (ed): Platelet Function: Laboratory Evaluation and Clinical Application. Chicago: American Society of Clinical Pathologists, 1978.
22. Brown BA: Hematology: Principles and Procedures, 6th ed. Philadelphia: Lea & Febiger, 1993.
23. Aster R: Drug-induced thrombocytopenia. In Michelson AD (ed): Platelets. New York: Elsevier Science, 2002:593-606.
24. Vadhan-Raj S: Clinical experience with recombinant human thrombopoietin in chemotherapy-induced thrombocytopenia. Semin Hematol 2000;37:28-34.
25. Basser RL, Underhill C, Davis MD, et al: Enhancement of platelet recovery after myelosuppressive chemotherapy by recombinant human megakaryocyte growth and development factor in patients with advanced cancer. J Clin Oncol 2000;18:2852-2861.
26. Koch MA, Volberding PA, Lagakos SW, et al: Toxic effects of zidovudin in asymptomatic human immunodeficiency virus-infected individuals with CD4+ cell counts of 0.5×10^9/L or less: detailed and updated results from Protocol 019 of the AIDS Clinical Trials Group. Arch Intern Med 1992;152:2286-2292.
27. Silverstein MN, Tefferi A: Treatment of essential thrombocythemia with anagrelide. Semin Hematol 1999;36:23-25.
28. Martin TG, Shuman MA: Interferon-induced thrombocytopenia: is it time for thrombopoietin? Hepatology 1998;28:1430-1432.

29. Colvin BT: Thrombocytopenia. Clin Haematol 1985;14:661-681.

30. Sata M, Yano Y, Yoshiyama, et al: Mechanisms of thrombocytopenia induced by interferon therapy for chronic hepatitis B. J Gastroenterol 1997;32:206-221.

31. Trannel TJ, Ahmed I, Goebert D: Occurrence of thrombocytopenia in psychiatric patients taking valproate. Am J Psychiatry 2001;158:128-130.

32. Thompson AR, Harker LA: Manual of Hemostasis and Thrombosis, 3rd ed. Philadelphia: Davis, 1983.

33. Taghizadeh M: Megaloblastic anemias. In Harmening DM (ed): Clinical Hematology and Fundamentals of Hemostasis, 3rd ed. Philadelphia: Davis, 1997:116-134.

34. Corriveau DM, Fritsma GA: Hemostasis and Thrombosis in the Clinical Laboratory. Philadelphia: Lippincott, 1988.

35. Quick AJ: Hemorrhagic Diseases and Thrombosis, 2nd ed. Philadelphia: Lea & Febiger, 1966.

36. Davis GL: Quantitative and qualitative disorders of platelets. In Stiene-Martin EA, Lotspeich-Steininger C, Koepke JA (eds): Clinical Hematology: Principle, Procedures, Correlations, 2nd ed. Philadelphia: Lippincott, 1998:717-734.

37. Bussel J, Cines D: Immune thrombocytopenia, neonatal alloimmune thrombocytopenia, and post-transfusion purpura. In Hoffman R, Benz EJ, Shattil SJ, et al (eds): Hematology Basic Principles and Practice, 3rd ed. New York: Churchill Livingstone, 2000:2096-2114.

38. Kessler CM, Acs P, Mariani G: Acquired disorders of coagulation: the immune coagulopathies. In Colman RW, Hirsh J, Marder VJ, et al (eds): Hemostasis and Thrombosis: Basic Principles and Clinical Practice, 5th ed. Philadelphia: Lippincott, 2006:1061-1085.

39. Woerner SJ, Abildgaard CF, French BN: Intracranial hemorrhage in children with idiopathic thrombocytopenic purpura. Pediatrics 1981;67:453-460.

40. Dameshek W, Ebbe S, Greenberg L, et al: Recurrent acute idiopathic thrombocytopenic purpura. N Engl J Med 1963;269:647-653.

41. Stasi R, Provan D: Management of immune thrombocytopenic purpura in adults. Mayo Clin Proc 2004;79:504-522.

42. Olsson B, Andersson P, Jernas M, et al: T-cell-mediated cytotoxicity toward platelets in chronic idiopathic thrombocytopenic purpura. Nat Med 2003;9:1123-1124.

43. Kunicki TJ, Newman PJ: The molecular immunology of human platelet proteins. Blood 1992;80:1386-1404.

44. Beer JH, Rabaglio M, Berchtold P, et al: Autoantibodies against the platelet glycoproteins (GP) IIb/IIIa, Ia/IIa, and IV and partial deficiency in GPIV in a patient with a bleeding disorder and a defective platelet collagen interaction. Blood 1993;82:820-829.

45. Baleem PJ, Segal GM, Stratton JR, et al: Mechanisms of thrombocytopenia in chronic autoimmune thrombocytopenic purpura: evidence of both impaired platelet production and increased platelet clearance. J Clin Invest 1987;80:33-40.

46. George JN, Kojouri K: Immune thrombocytopenic purpura. In Colman RW, Marder VJ, Clowes AW, et al (eds): Hemostasis and Thrombosis, 5th ed. Philadelphia: Lippincott, Williams & Wilkins, 2006:1085-1094.

47. Chong BH, Ho S-J: Autoimmune thrombocytopenia. J Thromb Haemost 2005;3:1763-1772.

48. Jacobs P, Wood L, Novitzky N: Intravenous gammaglobulin has no advantages over oral corticosteroids as primary therapy for adults with immune thrombocytopenia: a prospective randomized clinical trial. Am J Med 1994;1:55-59.

50. Kourik J, Vesely SK, Terrell DR, et al: Splenectomy for adult patients with ITP. Blood 2004;104:2623-2634.

51. Smith ME, Reid DM, Jones CE, et al: Binding of quinine- and quinidine-dependent drug antibodies to platelets is mediated by the Fab domain of the immunoglobulin G and is not Fc dependent. J Clin Invest 1987;79:912-917.

52. Pfueller SL, Bilsont RA, Logan D, et al: Heterogeneity of drug-dependent platelet antigens and their antibodies in quinine- and quinidine-induced thrombocytopenia: involvement of glycoproteins Ib, IIb, IIIa, and IX. Blood 1988;11:190-198.

53. Chong BH, Fawaz I, Chesterman CN, et al: Heparin-induced thrombocytopenia: mechanism of interaction of the heparin-dependent antibody with platelets. Br J Haematol 1989;73:235-240.

54. Amiral J, Bridley F, Dreyfus M, et al: Platelet factor 4 complexed to heparin is the target for antibodies generated in heparin-induced thrombocytopenia [letter]. Thromb Haemost 1992;68:95.

55. Brace LD, Fareed J, Tomeo J, et al: Biochemical and pharmacological studies on the interaction of PK 10169 and its subfractions with human platelets. Haemostasis 1986;16:93-105.

56. Warkentin TE: Heparin-induced thrombocytopenia. In Colman RW, Marder VJ, Clowes AW, et al (eds): Hemostasis and Thrombosis, 5th ed. Philadelphia: Lippincott, Williams & Wilkins, 2006:1649-1663.

57. Rhodes GR, Dixon RH, Silver D: Heparin-induced thrombocytopenia: eight cases with thrombotic-hemorrhagic complications. Am Surg 1977;186:752-758.

58. Brace LD, Fareed J: An objective assessment of the interaction of heparin and its subfractions with human platelets. Semin Thromb Hemost 1985;11:190-198.

59. Fratantoni JC, Pollet R, Gralnick HR: Heparin-induced thrombocytopenia: confirmation by in vitro methods. Blood 1975;45:395-401.

60. Brace LD: Testing for heparin-induced thrombocytopenia by platelet aggregometry. Clin Lab Sci 1992;5:80-81.

61. Sheridan D, Carter C, Kelton JG: A diagnostic test for heparin-induced thrombocytopenia. Blood 1986;67:27-30.

62. Collins JL, Aster RH, Moghaddam M, et al: Diagnostic testing for heparin-induced thrombocytopenia (HIT): an enhanced platelet factor 4 complex enzyme linked immunosorbent assay (PF4 ELISA). Blood 1997;90(Suppl 1):461.

63. Gruel Y, Boizard B, Daffos F, et al: Determination of platelet antigens and glycoproteins in the human fetus. Blood 1986;68:488-92.

64. Mueller-Eckhardt C, Kiefel V, Grubert A, et al: 348 cases of suspected neonatal alloimmune thrombocytopenia. Lancet 1989;1:363-366.

65. McFarland JG, Aster RH, Bussel JB, et al: Prenatal diagnosis of neonatal alloimmune thrombocytopenia using allele-specific oligonucleotide probes. Blood 1991;78:2276-2282.

66. Levin AB, Berkowitz RL: Neonatal alloimmune thrombocytopenia. Semin Perinatol 1991;15(Suppl 2):35-40.

67. Kaplan C, Daffos F, Forestier F, et al: Management of alloimmune thrombocytopenia: antenatal diagnosis and in utero transfusion of maternal platelets. Blood 1988;72:340-343.

68. Rayburn WF: Glucocorticoid therapy for rheumatic diseases: maternal, fetal, and breast-feeding considerations. Am J Reprod Immunol 1992;28:138-140.

69. Clerc JM: Neonatal thrombocytopenia. Clin Lab Sci 1989;2:42-47.

70. Simon TL, Collins J, Kunicki TJ, et al: Posttransfusion purpura associated with alloantibody specific for the platelet antigen, Pen[a]. Am J Hematol 1988;29:38-40.

71. Kickler TS, Herman JH, Furihata K, et al: Identification of Bak[a], a new platelet-specific antigen associated with post-transfusion purpura. Blood 1988;71:894-898.

72. Christie DJ, Pulkrabek S, Putnam JL, et al: Posttransfusion purpura due to an alloantibody reactive with glycoprotein Ia/IIa (anti-HPA-5b). Blood 1991;77:2785-2789.

73. Mueller-Eckhardt C: Post-transfusion purpura. Br J Haematol 1986;64:419-424.

74. Vogelsang G, Kickler TS, Bell WR: Post-transfusion purpura: a report of five patients and a review of the pathogenesis and management. Am J Hematol 1986;21:259-267.

75. McLaughlin P, Talpaz M, Quesada JR, et al: Immune thrombocytopenia following α-interferon therapy in patients with cancer. JAMA 1985;254:1353-1354.

76. Yoshida Y, Hirashima K, Asano S, et al: A phase II trial of recombinant human granulocyte colony-stimulating factor in the myelodysplastic syndromes. Br J Haematol 1991;78:378-384.

77. Paciucci PA, Mandeli J, Oleksowicz L, et al: Thrombocytopenia during immunotherapy with interleukin-2 by constant infusion. Am J Med 1990;89:308-312.

78. Fink K, Al-Mondhiry H: Idiopathic thrombocytopenic purpura in lymphoma. Cancer 1976;37:1999-2004.

79. Carey RW, McGinnis A, Jacobson BM, et al: Idiopathic thrombocytopenic purpura complicating chronic lymphocytic leukemia: management with sequential splenectomy and chemotherapy. Arch Intern Med 1976;136:62-66.

80. Miller MH, Urowitz MB, Gladman DD: The significance of thrombocytopenia in systemic lupus erythematosus. Arthritis Rheum 1983;26:1181-1186.

81. Kelton JG, Keystone J, Moore J, et al: Immune-mediated thrombocytopenia of malaria. J Clin Invest 1983;71:832-836.

82. Burrows RF, Kelton JG: Fetal thrombocytopenia and its relation to maternal thrombocytopenia. N Engl J Med 1993; 329:1463-1466

83. Barron WM: The syndrome of preeclampsia. Gastroenterol Clin North Am 1992;21:851-872.

84. Schindler M, Gatt S, Isert P, et al: Thrombocytopenia and platelet function defects in pre-eclampsia: implications for regional anesthesia. Anaesth Intensive Care 1990;18:169-174.

85. Gibson W, Hunter D, Neame PB, et al: Thrombocytopenia in preeclampsia and eclampsia. Semin Thromb Hemost 1982;8:234-247.

86. Martin JN Jr, Blake PG, Perry KG Jr, et al: The natural history of HELLP syndrome: patterns of disease progression and regression. Am J Obstet Gynecol 1991;164:1500-1509.

87. Green D: Diagnosis and management of bleeding disorders. Compr Ther 1988;14:31-36.

88. Trofatter KF Jr, Howell ML, Greenberg CS, et al: Use of the fibrin D-dimer in screening for coagulation abnormalities in preeclampsia. Obstet Gynecol 1989;73:435-440.

89. Burrows RF, Hunter DJS, Andrew M, et al: A prospective study investigating the mechanism of thrombocytopenia in preeclampsia. Obstet Gynecol 1987;70:334-338.

90. Benigni A, Gregorini G, Frusca T, et al: Effect of low-dose aspirin on fetal and maternal generation of thromboxane by platelets in women at risk for pregnancy-induced hypertension. N Engl J Med 1989;321:357-362.

91. Schiff E, Peleg E, Goldenberg M, et al: The use of aspirin to prevent pregnancy-induced hypertension and lower the ratio of thromboxane A2 to prostacyclin in relatively high risk pregnancies. N Engl J Med 1989;321:351-356.

92. Ezra Y Rose M, Eldor A: Therapy and prevention of thrombotic thrombocytopenic purpura during pregnancy: a clinical study of 16 pregnancies. Am J Hematol 1996;51:1-6.

93. Dashe JS,Ramin SM, Cunningham FG: The long-term consequences of thrombotic microangiopathy (thrombotic thrombocytopenic purpura and hemolytic uremic syndrome) in pregnancy. Obstet Gynecol 1998;91:662-668.

94. Moschcowitz E: An acute febrile pleiochromic anemia with hyaline thrombosis of the terminal arterioles and capillaries: a hitherto undescribed disease. Arch Intern Med 1925;36:89-93.

95. Moake JL: Thrombotic thrombocytopenic purpura and hemolytic uremic syndrome. In Michelson AD (ed): Platelets. Academic Press/Elsevier, 2002:607-620.

96. Bell WR, Braine HG, Ness PM, et al: Improved survival in thrombotic thrombocytopenic purpura-hemolytic uremic syndrome: clinical experience in 108 patients. N Engl J Med 1991;325:398-403.

97. Rock GA, Shumak KH, Buskard NA, et al: Comparison of plasma exchange with plasma infusion in the treatment of thrombotic thrombocytopenic purpura. N Engl J Med 1991;325:393-397.

98. Moake JL, Turner NA, Stathopoulos NA, et al: Involvement of large plasma von Willebrand factor (VWF) multimers and unusually large VWF forms derived from endothelial cells in shear-stress induced platelet aggregation. J Clin Invest 1986;78:1456-1461.

99. Furlan M, Robles R, Solenthaler M, et al: Deficient activity of von Willebrand factor-cleaving protease in chronic relapsing thrombotic thrombocytopenic purpura. Blood 1997;89:3097-3103.

100. Furlan M, Robles R, Lammle B: Partial purification and characterization of a protease from human plasma cleaving von Willebrand factor to fragments produced by in vivo proteolysis. Blood 1996;87:4223-4234.

101. Tsai HM: Physiologic cleaving of von Willebrand factor by a plasma protease is dependent on its conformation and requires calcium ion. Blood 1996;87:4235-4244.

102. Tsai HM, Lian ECY: Antibodies to von Willebrand factor-cleaving protease in acute thrombotic thrombocytopenic purpura. N Engl J Med 1998;339:1585-1594.

103. Furlan M, Lammle B: von Willebrand factor in thrombotic thrombocytopenic purpura. Thromb Haemost 1999;82:592-600.

104. Gerritsen HE, Turecek PL, Schwarz HP, et al: Assay of von Willebrand factor (VWF)-cleaving protease based on decreased collagen binding affinity of degraded VWF: a tool for the diagnosis of thrombotic thrombocytopenic purpura (TTP). Thromb Haemost 1999;82:1386-1389.

105. Moake JL, McPherson PD: Abnormalities of von Willebrand factor multimers in thrombotic thrombocytopenic purpura and the hemolytic uremic syndrome. Am J Med 1989;87: 3-9.

106. Byrnes JJ, Moake JL, Klug P, et al: Effectiveness of the cryosupernatant fraction of plasma in the treatment of refractory thrombotic thrombocytopenic purpura. Am J Hematol 1990;34:169-174.

107. Kwaan HC, Soff GA: Management of thrombotic thrombocytopenic purpura and hemolytic uremic syndrome. Semin Hematol 1997;34:159-166.

108. Karmali MA: The association of verotoxins and the classical hemolytic uremic syndrome. In Kaplan BS, Trompeter RS, Moake JL (eds): Hemolytic-Uremic Syndrome and Thrombotic Thrombocytopenic Purpura. New York: Marcel Dekker, 1992:199-212.

109. Obrig TG: Pathogenesis of Shiga toxin (verotoxin)-induced endothelial cell injury. In Kaplan BS, Trompeter RS, Moake JL (eds): Hemolytic-Uremic Syndrome and Thrombotic Thrombocytopenic Purpura. New York: Marcel Dekker, 1992:405-419.

110. Charba D, Moake JL, Harris MA, et al: Abnormalities of von Willebrand factor multimers in drug-associated thrombotic microangiopathies. Am J Hematol 1993;42:268-277.

111. Santhosh-Kumar CR, Yohannon MD, Higgy KE, et al: Thrombocytosis in adults: analysis of 777 patients. J Intern Med 1991;229:493-495.

112. Mitus AJ, Schafer AI: Thrombocytosis and thrombocythemia. Hematol Oncol Clin N Am 1990;4:157-178.

113. Michiels JJ, Ten Cate FJ: Erythromyalgia in thrombocythemia of various myeloproliferative disorders. Am J Hematol 1992;39:131-136.

114. Hoffman R: Primary thrombocythemia. In Hoffman R, Benz EJ, Shattil SJ, et al (eds): Hematology Basic Principles and Practice, 3rd ed. New York: Churchill Livingstone, 2000:1188-1204.

115. Schafer AI: Bleeding and thrombosis in the myeloproliferative disorders. Blood 1984;64:1-12.

116. Panlilio AL, Reiss RF: Therapeutic plateletpheresis in thrombocythemia. Transfusion 1979;19:147-152.

117. Middelhoff G, Boll I: A long term trial of interferon alpha-therapy in essential thrombocythemia. Ann Hematol 1992;64:207-209.

118. Lazzarino M, Vitale A, Morra E, et al: Interferon alpha-2b as treatment for Philadelphia-negative myeloproliferative disorders with excessive thrombocytosis. Br J Haematol 1989; 72:173-177.

119. Giles FJ, Singer CRJ, Gray AG, et al: Alpha interferon for essential thrombocythemia. Lancet 1988;2:70-72.

120. Petitt RM, Silverstein MN, Petrone ME: Anagrelide for control of thrombocythemia in polycythemia and other myeloproliferative disorders. Semin Hematol 1997;34:51-54.

121. Tefferi A, Silverstein MN, Petitt RM, et al: Anagrelide as a new platelet-lowering agent in essential thrombocythemia: mechanism of action, efficacy, toxicity, current indications. Semin Thromb Hemost 1997;23:379-383.

44

Qualitative Disorders of Platelets and Vasculature

Larry D. Brace

OBJECTIVES

After completion of this chapter, the reader will be able to:

1. Describe the effect of aspirin on the cyclooxygenase pathway.
2. Describe the defect in each of the following hereditary disorders: storage pool disease, gray platelet syndrome, Glanzmann thrombasthenia, and Bernard-Soulier syndrome (BSS).
3. Discuss general mechanisms of action for antiplatelet drugs.
4. Explain the effects of paraproteins on platelet function.
5. Compare and contrast Glanzmann thrombasthenia and BSS.
6. Recognize the clinical presentation of patients with dysfunctional platelets.
7. Distinguish among the following types of inherited platelet disorders: membrane receptor abnormality, secretion disorder, and storage pool deficiency.
8. For each of the inherited platelet disorders listed, name useful laboratory tests, and recognize diagnostic results.
9. Identify the most common type of hereditary platelet defect.
10. Discuss the mechanism of the platelet defects associated with myeloproliferative diseases, uremia, and liver disease.
11. Recognize conditions associated with acquired vascular disorders.

CASE STUDY

After studying the material in this chapter, the reader should be able to respond to the following case study:

A 19-year-old Caucasian woman with a chief complaint of easy bruising, occasional mild nosebleeds, and heavy periods was examined by her physician. At the time of her examination, she had a few small bruises on her arms and legs, but no other problems. Initial laboratory data revealed a prolonged bleeding time of 10 minutes, a normal prothrombin time, and a normal partial thromboplastin time. A complete blood count, including platelet count and morphology, was normal.

A detailed history revealed that her bleeding problems occurred most frequently after aspirin ingestion. Her mother and one of her brothers also had some of the same symptoms. Blood was drawn for platelet function studies, and platelet aggregation tests were performed. Aggregation induced by adenosine diphosphate was near-normal, arachidonic acid–induced aggregation was absent, epinephrine induced only primary aggregation, and collagen-induced aggregation was decreased, although a near-normal aggregation response could be obtained with high collagen concentration. Spontaneous aggregation was not observed.

1. What are three possible explanations for the test results so far?
2. Given the bleeding history in her family, which of the three explanations seems most likely?

A quantitative test for adenosine triphosphate (ATP) release was performed using the firefly luciferin-luciferase bioluminescence assay. The result of this test showed a marked decrease in the amount of ATP released when platelets were stimulated with thrombin.

3. Based on the ATP test results, what is the likely cause of her bleeding symptoms?

Clinical manifestations of bleeding disorders can be divided into two broad, rather poorly defined groups: (1) superficial bleeding (e.g., petechiae, epistaxis, or gingival bleeding), usually associated with a platelet defect or vascular disorder; and (2) deep tissue bleeding (e.g., hematomas or hemarthrosis), usually associated with plasma clotting factor deficiencies.[1] This chapter describes platelet and vascular disorders. Bleeding problems resulting from defects in the coagulation mechanism are described in Chapter 41.

QUALITATIVE PLATELET DISORDERS

Excessive bruising, superficial (mucocutaneous) bleeding, and a prolonged bleeding time in a patient whose platelet count is normal suggest an acquired or a congenital disorder of platelet function. Congenital disorders have been described as a result of abnormalities of each of the major phases of platelet function: adhesion, aggregation, and secretion. Rapid progress in this field began in the 1960s, mostly as a result of the development of instruments and test methods for measuring platelet function.[2] Qualitative disorders are summarized in Box 44-1.

Disorders of Adhesion Receptors
Bernard-Soulier (Giant Platelet) Syndrome

Bernard-Soulier syndrome (BSS) is a rare syndrome that is usually manifested in infancy or childhood with hemorrhage characteristic of defective platelet function: ecchymoses, epistaxis, and gingival bleeding. Hemarthroses and expanding hematomas are only rarely seen. BSS is inherited as an autosomal recessive disorder in which the glycoprotein (GP) Ib/IX/V complex is missing from the platelet surface or exhibits abnormal function. Heterozygotes who have about 50% of normal levels of GP Ib, GP V, and GP IX have normal or near-normal platelet function. Homozygotes have a moderate to severe bleeding disorder characterized by a prolonged bleeding time, enlarged platelets, thrombocytopenia, and usually decreased platelet survival. Platelet counts usually range from 40,000/μL to near-normal.[3] On peripheral blood smears, platelets typically are 5 to 8 μm in diameter, but can be 20 μm (Fig. 44-1). Viewed by electron microscopy, BSS platelets contain a larger number of cytoplasmic vacuoles and membrane complexes, and these observations extend to megakaryocytes, where the appearance of the demarcation membrane system is irregular.[2,4-7]

Four glycoproteins are required to form the GP Ib/IX/V complex: GP Ibα, GP Ibβ, GP IX, and GP V. In the complex, these proteins are present in the ratio of 2:2:2:1. The gene for GP Ibα is located on chromosome 17, the gene for GP Ibβ is located on chromosome 22, and the genes for GP IX and GP V are located on chromosome 3. For surface expression of the GP Ib/IX complex, it seems that synthesis of three proteins, GP Ibα, GP Ibβ, and GP IX, is required. Only GP V can be expressed alone in significant quantities on the surface of platelets, but the expression seems to be enhanced if the rest of the complex is present. The most frequent forms of BSS involve defects in GP Ibα synthesis or expression. The presence of GP Ibα is essential to normal function because it contains

---

BOX 44-1 Qualitative Abnormalities: Changes in Platelet Function (Thrombocytopathy)

Disorders of platelet adhesion
  Bernard-Soulier syndrome (giant platelet syndrome)
  von Willebrand disease
  Acquired defects of platelet adhesion
    Myeloproliferative and lymphoproliferative disorders and
      dysproteinemias
    Antiplatelet antibodies
    Cardiopulmonary bypass
    Chronic liver disease
    Drug-induced membrane modification
Disorders of primary aggregation
  Glanzmann thrombasthenia (congenital)
  Hereditary afibrinogenemia
  Acquired
    Acquired von Willebrand disease
    Uremia
Disorders of platelet secretion (release reactions)
  Storage pool diseases
  Dense granule deficiencies
    Hermansky-Pudlak syndrome
    Wiskott-Aldrich syndrome
    Thrombocytopenia with absent radii syndrome
    Chédiak-Higashi syndrome
  α granule deficiencies
    Gray platelet syndrome
  Thromboxane pathway disorders: aspirin-like defects
  Hereditary aspirin-like defects
    Cyclooxygenase or thromboxane synthetase deficiency
  Drug inhibition of the prostaglandin pathways
    Drug inhibition of platelet phosphodiesterase activity
Hyperactive prethrombotic platelets

Data from Thompson AR, Harker LA: Manual of Hemostasis and Thrombosis, 3rd ed. Philadelphia: Davis, 1983; and Colvin BT: Thrombocytopenia. Clin Haematol 1985;14:661-681.

---

binding sites for von Willebrand factor (VWF) and thrombin. Defects in the GP Ibβ and GP IX genes also are known to result in BSS, however.[8-10]

BSS platelets have normal aggregation responses to adenosine diphosphate (ADP), epinephrine, collagen, and arachidonic acid but do not respond to ristocetin or botrocetin and have diminished response to thrombin.[2,4,6] The lack of response to ristocetin or botrocetin is due to the lack of GP Ib/IX/V complexes and the inability of BSS platelets to bind VWF. Lack of binding to VWF also accounts for the inability of platelets to adhere to exposed subendothelium and the resultant bleeding characteristic of this disorder. This defect in adhesion shows the importance of initial platelet attachment in primary hemostasis. In many respects, this disorder resembles the defect seen in von Willebrand disease (VWD). In contrast to VWD, this abnormality cannot be corrected by the addition of normal plasma or cryoprecipitate, consistent with a defect that resides in the platelets.

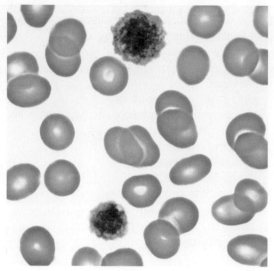

Figure 44-1 Giant platelets in Bernard-Soulier syndrome (peripheral blood, ×1000). (Modified from Carr JH, Rodak BF: Clinical Hematology Atlas, 2nd ed. Philadelphia: Saunders, 2004.)

Several unusual variants of BSS have been described in which all or most of the GP Ib/IX/V complex is present, but the mutations affect binding domains, affect interactions between elements of the complex, or result in truncation of a specific protein in the complex. In these cases, the complex fails to bind VWF or does so poorly.[9]

Platelet-type VWD (pseudo-VWD) is associated with a gain of function and spontaneous binding of plasma VWF. GP Ibα mutations that give rise to platelet-type VWD are Gly233Val or Ser and Met239Val.[11,12] Loss of residues 421-429 in GP Ibα also has been reported to result in platelet-type VWD.[13]

There is no specific treatment for BSS. Platelet transfusions are the treatment of choice, but patients invariably develop alloantibodies and become refractory to further platelet transfusion. BSS patients tend to do better if apheresis platelets are used for transfusion because this tends to limit the number of donors to which the patient is exposed, and the rate of alloimmunization tends to be lower.[4,6] Other treatments that have been used include desmopressin acetate (DDAVP) and, more recently, recombinant factor VIIa.

Glanzmann Thrombasthenia

Glanzmann thrombasthenia originally was described as a bleeding disorder associated with abnormal in vitro clot retraction and a normal platelet count. It is inherited as an autosomal recessive disorder and is seen most frequently in populations with a high degree of consanguinity. Heterozygotes are clinically normal, whereas homozygotes have serious bleeding problems. This rare disorder manifests itself clinically in the neonatal period or infancy, occasionally with bleeding after circumcision and frequently with epistaxis and gingival bleeding. Hemorrhagic manifestations include petechiae, purpura, menorrhagia, gastrointestinal bleeding, and hematuria. There are wide variations in the clinical symptoms. Some patients may have minimal symptoms, whereas others may have frequent and serious hemorrhagic compli-

cations. The severity of the bleeding episodes seems to decrease with age.[14,15]

The biochemical lesion responsible for the disorder is a deficiency or abnormality of the platelet membrane GP IIb/IIIa (α_{IIb}/β_3) complex, a membrane receptor capable of binding fibrinogen, VWF, fibronectin, and other adhesive ligands. Typically, the platelets of homozygous individuals lack surface-expressed GP IIb/IIIa, whereas the GP IIb/IIIa content of the platelets from heterozygotes has been found to be 50% to 60% of normal.[4,16] Binding of fibrinogen to the GP IIb/IIIa complex mediates normal platelet aggregation responses. Failure of such binding results in a profound defect in hemostatic plug formation and the serious bleeding characteristic of thrombasthenia.[2,4,6,17-19]

More than 70 mutations are known to give rise to Glanzmann thrombasthenia.[20-22] The α_{IIb} and β_3 genes are present on chromosome 17, and genetic defects are distributed widely over the two genes. α_{IIb} is synthesized in megakaryocytes as pro-α_{IIb} which complexes β_3 in the endoplasmic reticulum. The complex is transported to the Golgi body where α_{IIb} is cleaved to heavy and light chains to form the complete complex. Uncomplexed α_{IIb} and β_3 are not processed in the Golgi body. Similar to the GP Ib/IX/V complex, it is necessary for both proteins of the GP IIb/IIIa complex to be produced and assembled into a complex for the complex to be expressed on the platelet surface. Gene defects that lead to the absence of production of either protein lead to absence of the complex on the platelet surface. Defects that interfere with or prevent complex formation or affect complex stability have the same effect.

Numerous variants of Glanzmann thrombasthenia have been described in which the GP IIb/IIIa complex is qualitatively abnormal. α_{IIb} and β_3 are produced, form a complex, and are processed normally. One or more functions of the complex (e.g., fibrinogen binding or signal transduction) are abnormal, however. Bleeding in these patients ranges from mild to severe.

One component of the α_{IIb}/β_3 integrin, β_3, is a component of the vitronectin receptor, α_V/β_3, found on endothelial cells, osteoclasts, fibroblasts, monocytes, and activated B lymphocytes, where it acts as a receptor for a variety of adhesive protein ligands. Patients who have β_3 gene defects that result in absence of the α_{IIb}/β_3 integrin also lack the vitronectin receptor. These patients do not seem to have a more severe form of Glanzmann thrombasthenia.[23,24] The vitronectin receptor is thought to play a role in vascularization, but so far no evidence for abnormal blood vessel development has been documented in individuals lacking the vitronectin receptor. It also is unclear whether platelet vitronectin receptors play any significant role in platelet functional processes.[20]

The typical laboratory features of Glanzmann thrombasthenia are a markedly prolonged bleeding time, a normal platelet count and normal platelet morphology, poor in vitro clot retraction, and a lack of platelet aggregation in response to all platelet-activating agents (including ADP, collagen, thrombin, and epinephrine).[2,4,6,18] If the stimulating agent is strong enough (e.g., thrombin), the platelets undergo the release/secretion reaction, even in the absence of aggregation.

Ristocetin-induced binding of VWF to platelets and the resulting platelet agglutination are normal. The results of the complete blood count are usually normal, unless there is another underlying disorder or the patient has had a recent hemorrhagic episode. Tests for platelet procoagulant activity, previously called *platelet factor 3*, are usually diminished.[2,16,25] There seem to be several reasons for this. When normal platelets are activated, procoagulant microvesicles are shed from the platelet surface, and coagulation factors assemble on the microvesicle surfaces during activation of the coagulation cascade. In Glanzmann thrombasthenia, markedly fewer microvesicles are produced. Second, prothrombin binds directly to GP IIb/IIIa. Because this complex is missing in Glanzmann thrombasthenia, significantly less thrombin is generated in response to tissue factor. Finally, Glanzmann thrombasthenia platelets are not as activated by thrombin as are normal platelets.[26-29]

A subdivision of Glanzmann thrombasthenia into cases with absent (type 1) and subnormal (type 2) in vitro clot retraction has been proposed. In general, type 2 individuals have more residual GP IIb/IIIa complexes (10% to 20% of normal) compared with type 1 (0% to 5% of normal), although there is considerable variability in each subdivision.[30,31]

Thrombasthenia is one of the few forms of platelet dysfunction in which hemorrhage is severe and disabling. Bleeding of all types, including epistaxis, ecchymoses, hemarthrosis, subcutaneous hematomas, menorrhagia, and gastrointestinal and urinary tract hemorrhage, has been reported. Treatment of bleeding episodes in patients with Glanzmann thrombasthenia requires the transfusion of normal platelets. In Glanzmann thrombasthenia, the defective platelets may interfere with the normal transfused platelets, and it may be necessary to infuse more donor platelets than expected to control bleeding. As in BSS or any situation in which repeated transfusions are required, patients with Glanzmann thrombasthenia may become alloimmunized. Strategies to reduce alloimmunization include use of single-donor platelet apheresis products, human leukocyte antigen–matched donor platelets, or ABO-matched donor platelets.[32]

A variety of treatments have been used successfully to control or prevent bleeding alone or in combination with platelet transfusion. To a large extent, the site of hemorrhage determines these therapeutic approaches. Hormonal therapy (norethindrone acetate) has been used to control menorrhagia. If the patient is treated with oral contraceptives, excessive bleeding should be reduced. Menorrhagia at the onset of menses is uniformly severe and can be life-threatening, leading some to suggest that birth control pills be started before menarche. Also, antifibrinolytic (aminocaproic acid or tranexamic acid) therapy can be used to control gingival hemorrhage or excessive bleeding after tooth extraction.[31] Recombinant factor VIIa has proved to be useful to treat severe bleeding in patients with isoantibodies to α_{IIb}/β_3 and for patients undergoing invasive procedures.[33] Recombinant factor VIIa is thought to enhance thrombus formation at the site of a lesion by stimulating tissue factor–independent thrombus generation and fibrin formation.[34]

Rarely, a thrombasthenia-like state can be acquired. Such conditions include autoantibodies against GP IIb/IIIa, multiple myeloma in which the paraprotein is directed against GP IIIa, and afibrinogenemia. A thrombasthenic-like state also can be induced in individuals with otherwise normal platelet function by the antiplatelet therapeutic drugs ticlopidine and clopidogrel.[15,18]

Disorders of Platelet Secretion (Release Reactions)

Of the hereditary platelet function defects, disorders involving storage pool defects and the release reaction are the most common. The clinical features of this group of disorders are mucocutaneous hemorrhage and hematuria, epistaxis, and easy and spontaneous bruising. Petechiae are less common than in other qualitative platelet disorders. Hemorrhage is rarely severe but may be exacerbated by aspirin or other antiplatelet agents. In most of these disorders, the platelet count is normal, and the bleeding time is usually, although not always, prolonged. Platelet aggregation abnormalities are usually seen but vary depending on the disorder.[2,4,35,36]

Storage Pool Diseases

Dense Granule Deficiencies. The inheritance of dense granule deficiency does not follow a single mode, and it is likely that a variety of genetic abnormalities lead to the development of this disorder. Dense granule deficiencies can be subdivided into deficiency states associated with albinism and those in otherwise normal individuals (nonalbinos). In the platelets of nonalbinos, there is evidence for the presence of dense granule membranes in normal to near-normal numbers, suggesting that the disorder arises from an inability to package the dense granule contents.[37,38] In this regard, serotonin accumulates in normal dense granules by an active uptake mechanism in which plasma serotonin is transported by a specific carrier-mediated system across the plasma membrane into the cytoplasm, and a second carrier-mediated system in the dense granule membrane transports serotonin from the cytoplasm to the interior of the dense granules.[39] These transport mechanisms are used in the serotonin release assay employed to detect heparin-dependent antiplatelet antibodies (Chapter 43). In addition to serotonin transport mechanisms, a nucleotide transporter MRP4 (ABCC4) that is highly expressed in platelets and dense granules has been identified. It would be expected that mutations in the gene for this transporter could affect nucleotide accumulation in dense granules.[40]

As an isolated abnormality, dense granule deficiency is not typically a serious hemorrhagic problem. Bleeding is usually mild and most often is limited to easy bruisability. Dense granule deficiency affects the results of platelet aggregation tests. Platelet-dense (δ) granules are intracellular storage sites for ADP, adenosine triphosphate, calcium, pyrophosphate, and serotonin. The contents of these granules are extruded when platelet secretion is induced, and secreted ADP plays a major role in propagation of platelet activation, recruitment, and aggregation and growth of the hemostatic plug. In platelet-rich plasma of patients with dense granule deficiency, addition of arachidonic acid fails to induce an aggregation response. Epinephrine and low-dose ADP induce a primary wave of aggregation, but a secondary wave is missing. Responses to low concentrations of collagen are decreased to absent, but a high concentration of collagen may induce a near-normal aggregation response.[36,39] This aggregation pattern is caused by the lack of ADP secretion and is almost identical to the pattern observed in patients taking aspirin.

In addition to being found as an isolated problem, dense granule deficiency is found in association with several disorders. Hermansky-Pudlak syndrome is an autosomal recessive disorder characterized by tyrosinase-positive oculocutaneous albinism, defective lysosomal function in a variety of cell types, cereoid-like deposition in the cells of the reticuloendothelial system, and a profound platelet δ granule deficiency.[41] Several of the genes responsible for Hermansky-Pudlak syndrome have been mapped to chromosome 19. At least seven genes individually can give rise to Hermansky-Pudlak syndrome. These genes encode for proteins involved in intracellular vesicular trafficking and active in the biogenesis of organelles.[42] Although bleeding associated with most dense granule deficiencies is rarely severe, Hermansky-Pudlak syndrome seems to be an exception. Although most bleeding episodes in Hermansky-Pudlak syndrome are not severe, lethal hemorrhage has been reported, and in one series hemorrhage accounted for 16% of deaths in patients with Hermansky-Pudlak syndrome. A unique morphologic abnormality has been described in the platelets of four families with Hermansky-Pudlak syndrome. This abnormality consists of marked dilation and tortuosity of the surface-connecting tubular system (the so-called "Swiss cheese platelet").[2,6,25,43]

Chédiak-Higashi syndrome is a rare autosomal recessive trait characterized by partial oculocutaneous albinism, frequent pyogenic bacterial infections, and giant lysosomal granules in cells of hematologic (see Fig. 28-5) and nonhematologic origin, platelet δ granule deficiency, and hemorrhage. The Chédiak-Higashi syndrome protein gene is located on chromosome 13, and a series of nonsense and frameshift mutations all result in a truncated Chédiak-Higashi syndrome protein that gives rise to a disorder of generalized cellular dysfunction involving fusion of cytoplasmic granules. The disorder progresses to an accelerated phase in 85% of Chédiak-Higashi syndrome patients and is marked by lymphocytic proliferation in the liver, spleen, and marrow and macrophage accumulation in tissues. During this stage, the pancytopenia worsens, resulting in hemorrhage and ever-increasing susceptibility to infection, leading to death at an early age. Initially, the bleeding time is increased because of δ granule deficiency and consequent defective platelet function. During the accelerated phase, however, the thrombocytopenia also contributes to the prolonged bleeding time. Bleeding episodes vary from mild to moderate but worsen as the platelet count decreases.[6,25]

Wiskott-Aldrich syndrome is an X-linked recessive disease characterized by the triad of severe eczema, recurrent infections owing to immune deficiency, and life-threatening thrombocytopenia. Bleeding episodes are typically moderate to severe. A milder form without immune deficiency is known as hereditary X-linked thrombocytopenia (Chapter 43). In Wiskott-Aldrich syndrome, a combination of ineffective thrombocytopoiesis and increased platelet sequestration and destruction accounts for the thrombocytopenia. Similar to all X-linked recessive disorders, it is found primarily in males.[6,9,16,25,44] The Wiskott-Aldrich syndrome gene encodes for a 502-amino acid protein, WASP, that is found exclusively in hematopoietic cells. WASP is primarily involved in signal transduction.

Wiskott-Aldrich platelets are structurally abnormal. The number of α granules and dense bodies is decreased, and the platelets are small, a feature of diagnostic importance. Diminished levels of stored adenine nucleotides are reflected in the lack of dense bodies observed on transmission electron micrographs. The platelet aggregation pattern in Wiskott-Aldrich syndrome is typical of a storage pool deficiency. The platelets show a decreased aggregation response to ADP, collagen, and epinephrine and lack a secondary wave of aggregation to these agonists. The response to thrombin is normal, however.[6,25] The most effective treatment for the thrombocytopenia seems to be splenectomy, which would be consistent with peripheral destruction of platelets. Bone marrow transplantation also has been attempted with some success.[25,45]

Thrombocytopenia with absent radii syndrome (Chapter 43) is a rare autosomal recessive disorder characterized by the congenital absence of the radial bones (the most pronounced skeletal abnormality), numerous cardiac and other skeletal abnormalities, and thrombocytopenia (90% of cases). It is mentioned here because the platelets have structural defects in dense granules with corresponding abnormal aggregation responses. Marrow megakaryocytes may be decreased, immature, or normal.[6,46]

α Granule Deficiency: Gray Platelet Syndrome.

Alpha granules are the storage site for proteins produced by the megakaryocyte (e.g., platelet-derived growth factor, thrombospondin, and platelet factor 4) or present in plasma and taken up by platelets and transported to α granules for storage (e.g., albumin, IgG, and fibrinogen). There are 50 to 80 α granules per platelet that are primarily responsible for the granular appearance of platelets on stained blood films. This rare disorder was first described in 1971 and results from the specific absence of morphologically recognizable α granules in platelets. The disorder is inherited in an autosomal recessive fashion. Clinically, gray platelet syndrome is characterized by lifelong mild bleeding tendencies, prolonged bleeding time, moderate thrombocytopenia, fibrosis of the marrow, and large platelets whose gray appearance on a Wright-stained blood film is the source of the name for this disorder.[2,4,6,47]

In electron photomicrographs of platelets and megakaryocytes, the platelets appear to have virtually no α granules, although they do contain vacuoles and small α granule precursors that stain for VWF and fibrinogen. The other types of granules are present in normal numbers. The membranes of the vacuoles and the α granule precursors have P-selectin (CD62) and GP IIb/IIIa, and these proteins can be translocated to the cell membrane on stimulation with thrombin. This indicates that these structures are α granules that cannot store the typical α granule proteins. This may provide an explanation for the observation that, in gray platelet syndrome, the plasma levels of platelet factor 4 and β-thromboglobulin are increased. Most patients develop early-onset myelofibrosis, which can be attributed to the inability of megakaryocytes to store newly synthesized platelet-derived growth factors.[38]

Treatment of severe bleeding episodes may require platelet transfusions. Few other treatments are available for these patients. Cryoprecipitate has been used to control bleeding. DDAVP was found to shorten the bleeding time and has been used as successful prophylaxis in a dental extraction procedure. Some authors believe that DDAVP should be the initial therapy of choice.[2,4,38,48,49]

A rare disorder in which both types of granules are deficient is known as *α-δ storage pool deficiency*. It seems to be inherited as an autosomal dominant characteristic. In these patients, other membrane abnormalities also have been described.[9]

Quebec platelet disorder is an autosomal dominant bleeding disorder that results from a deficiency of multimerin (a multimeric protein that is stored complexed with factor V in α granules) and shows protease-related degradation of many α granule proteins even though α granule structure is maintained. Although not a consistent feature, thrombocytopenia may be present.[9]

Thromboxane Pathway Disorders: Aspirin-like Effects

Platelet secretion requires the activation of several biochemical pathways. One such pathway is the one leading to thromboxane formation. A series of phospholipases catalyze the release of arachidonic acid and several other compounds from membrane phospholipids. Arachidonic acid is converted to intermediate prostaglandins by cyclooxygenase and to thromboxane A_2 by thromboxane synthase. Thromboxane A_2 and other substances generated during platelet activation cause mobilization of ionic calcium from internal stores into the cytoplasm, occupancy of several activation receptors, and a cascade of events resulting in secretion and aggregation of platelets (Chapter 13).[50]

Several acquired or congenital disorders of platelet secretion are traced to structural and functional modifications of arachidonic acid pathway enzymes. Inhibition of cyclooxygenase occurs on ingestion of drugs such as aspirin and ibuprofen. As a result, the amount of thromboxane A_2 produced from arachidonic acid depends on the degree of inhibition. Thromboxane A_2 is required for storage granule secretion and maximal platelet aggregation in response to epinephrine, ADP, and low concentrations of collagen.[6,14,25,51]

Hereditary absence or abnormalities of the components of the thromboxane pathway are usually termed *aspirin-like defects* because the clinical and laboratory manifestations resemble those that follow aspirin ingestion. Platelet aggregation responses are similar to those in δ storage pool disorders (see earlier). In contrast to storage pool disorders, however, ultrastructure and granular contents are normal. Deficiencies

of the enzymes cyclooxygenase and thromboxane synthase are well documented, and dysfunction or deficiency of thromboxane receptors is known.[38]

Inherited Disorders of Other Receptors and Signaling Pathways

The $α_2β_1$ (GP Ia/IIa) integrin is one of the collagen receptors in the platelet membrane. A deficiency of this receptor has been reported in a patient who lacked an aggregation response to collagen, whose platelets did not adhere to collagen and who had a lifelong mild bleeding disorder.[52] A deficiency in another collagen receptor, GP VI, also has been reported in patients with mild bleeding. The platelets of these patients failed to aggregate in response to collagen, and adhesion to collagen also was impaired.[53] A family with gray platelet syndrome and defective collagen adhesion has been described. Affected members of the family have a severe deficiency of GP VI.[54]

Platelets seem to contain at least three receptors for ADP. $P2X_1$ is linked to an ion channel that facilitates calcium ion influx. $P2Y_1$ and $P2Y_{12}$ ($P2T_{AC}$) are members of the seven-transmembrane domain (STD) family of G protein–linked receptors. $P2Y_1$ is thought to mediate calcium mobilization and shape change in response to ADP. Pathology of the $P2Y_1$ receptor has not yet been reported. $P2Y_{12}$ is thought to be responsible for macroscopic platelet aggregation and is coupled to adenylate cyclase through a G-inhibitory (G_i) protein complex.[55] Some patients have been reported to have decreased platelet aggregation in response to ADP but normal platelet shape change and calcium mobilization. These patients have an inherited deficiency of the $P2Y_{12}$ receptor.[56-58] Bleeding problems seem to be relatively mild in these patients, but the only treatment for severe bleeding is platelet transfusion.

Congenital defects of the $α_2$-adrenergic (epinephrine) receptor associated with decreased platelet activation and aggregation in response to epinephrine are known. The receptors that mediate aggregation in response to epinephrine, ADP, and collagen are STD receptors, as are the protease-activated receptors (PARs) for thrombin. So far, defects in the PAR receptors have not been described.[9]

A group of intracellular defects that affect platelet function include defects in which all elements of the thromboxane pathway are normal, but insufficient calcium is released from the dense tubular system, and the cytoplasmic concentration of ionic calcium in the cytoplasm never reaches high enough levels to support secretion. This group of disorders is often referred to as *calcium mobilization defects*. These represent a heterogeneous group of disorders in which the defects reside in the various intracellular signaling pathways, including defects in G protein subunits and phospholipase C isoenzymes.[25,59,60]

Finally, Scott syndrome is a rare autosomal recessive disorder in which platelets secrete and aggregate normally but do not transport phosphatidylserine and phosphatidylethanolamine from the inner leaflet to the outer leaflet of the plasma membrane. This phospholipid "flip" normally occurs during platelet activation and is essential for the binding of vitamin K–dependent clotting factors. In the membrane of resting platelets, phosphatidylserine and phosphatidylethanolamine are restricted to the inner leaflet of the plasma membrane, and phosphatidylcholine is expressed on the outer leaflet. This asymmetry is maintained by the enzyme aminophospholipid translocase.[61] When platelets are activated, the asymmetry is lost, and phosphatidylserine and phosphatidylethanolamine "flip" to the outer leaflet and facilitate the assembly of clotting factor complexes. The phospholipid "flip" is mediated by a calcium-dependent enzyme, scramblase.[62] In Scott syndrome, platelet plug formation (including adhesion, aggregation, and secretion) occurs normally, but clotting factor complexes do not assemble on the activated platelet surface, and thrombin generation is absent or much reduced. Because lack of thrombin generation leads to inadequate fibrin, the platelet plug is not stabilized, and a bleeding diathesis results.[63,64]

Lastly, Stormorken syndrome is a condition in which platelets are always in an "activated" state and express phosphatidylserine on the outer leaflet of the membrane without prior activation. It has been postulated that these patients have a defective aminophospholipid translocase.[65]

Acquired Defects of Platelet Function
Drugs

Inhibitors of the Prostaglandin Pathway.   The most common cause of acquired platelet dysfunction is through drug ingestion, with aspirin and other drugs that inhibit the platelet prostaglandin synthetic pathways being the most common. A single 200-mg dose of acetylsalicylic acid (aspirin) can irreversibly acetylate 90% of the platelet cyclooxygenase (see Fig. 13-19). The acetylated enzyme is completely inactive. Platelets lack a nucleus and cannot synthesize new enzymes. The inhibitory effect is permanent for the circulatory life span of the platelet (7-10 days). Endothelial cells synthesize new cyclooxygenase, and endothelial cell cyclooxygenase seems to be less sensitive to aspirin than the platelet enzyme, at least at low doses. This has led to the concept that low-dose aspirin may be better than higher doses of aspirin because platelet thromboxane production is inhibited while endothelial cells recover prostacyclin production. Others argue that inhibition of platelet function is the more important effect, and higher doses of aspirin are better for this purpose. For these reasons, there are wide-ranging opinions as to the optimal dose of aspirin. What is lost in these arguments is that endothelial cells also produce another potent platelet inhibitor, nitric oxide (NO), and its production is not affected by aspirin. Although aspirin may inhibit a proaggregatory mechanism (thromboxane production) and an antiaggregatory mechanism (prostacyclin production), the NO platelet inhibitory mechanism is not affected. It may be necessary to define a test system to determine the optimal dose of aspirin on an individual basis because some patients have, or develop, aspirin resistance, and a dose that previously was sufficient to inhibit platelet function effectively is no longer able to produce that effect. Finally, in contrast to almost all other therapeutic agents, a single dose of aspirin is usually prescribed in a "one dose fits all" fashion (e.g., 325 mg) without regard to the patient's weight, age, health status, or other measurable parameters. This prescription is based on the assumption that the biologic effect would be the same in all patients. Evidence is emerging, however, that there is considerable interindividual response to a single dose of aspirin.[5,25,66-68] One study has shown that patients who do not respond well to aspirin have worse outcomes than patients who respond well.[69]

Individuals known to have a defect in their hemostatic mechanism, such as storage pool deficiency, thrombocytopenia, vascular disorders, or VWD, may experience a marked increase in bleeding time on aspirin ingestion, and such individuals should be advised to avoid the use of aspirin and related agents.[25]

The list of drugs affecting the prostaglandin pathway that converts arachidonic acid to thromboxane is long and beyond the scope of this chapter. Many of these drugs inhibit cyclooxygenase, but, in contrast to aspirin and closely related compounds, the inhibition is reversible. These drugs are said to be competitive inhibitors of cyclooxygenase, and as the blood concentration of the drug decreases, platelet function is recovered. This group of drugs includes ibuprofen and related compounds, such as ketoprofen and fenprofen, naproxen, and sulfinpyrazone. In contrast to aspirin, most of the agents have little effect on the bleeding time test. Except for their potential to irritate the gastric mucosa, these drugs have not been reported to cause clinically important bleeding.[14,17,25,70]

The association of chronic alcohol consumption with thrombocytopenia is well known. Chronic, periodic, and even acute alcohol consumption may result in a transient decrease in platelet function, however, and the inhibitory effect seems to be more pronounced when alcohol is consumed in excess. These effects are well known, and most patients who are scheduled for any medical procedure in which there may be hemostatic challenge are advised to abstain from alcohol consumption for about 3 days before the procedure. Impaired platelet function seems to be related at least in part to inhibition of thromboxane synthesis. A reduced platelet count and impaired platelet function may contribute to the increased incidence of gastrointestinal hemorrhage associated with chronic excessive alcohol intake.[14,25,71,72]

Drugs That Inhibit Membrane Function.   Many drugs interact with the platelet membrane and cause a clinically significant platelet function defect that may lead to hemorrhage. Some of these drugs are useful antiplatelet agents, whereas for many other drugs, their effects on the platelet membrane are an adverse side effect.[50]

The thienopyridine derivatives clopidogrel and its predecessor ticlopidine are antiplatelet agents used to treat patients with arterial occlusive disease for prevention of myocardial infarction, to decrease the risk of thrombotic stroke in patients with cerebrovascular disease, and for patients who are intolerant of aspirin. In contrast to aspirin, the effect of these agents does not reach a steady state for 3 to 5 days, although a steady state can be reached sooner with a loading dose. As prophylactic agents, they have been shown to be as efficacious as aspirin. The mechanism of action seems to be interference with the binding of ADP to a platelet membrane STD receptor, $P2Y_{12}$.[56] The major effect seems to be inhibition of stimulus-response coupling between the platelet ADP receptor and fibrinogen binding to GP IIb/IIIa. As a consequence, platelet activation and aggregation induced by ADP are markedly inhibited, and responses to other aggregating agents, such as collagen, are reduced. Clopidogrel has more effect on the bleeding time than aspirin, although there is little difference in the risk of bleeding.[73] Clopidogrel and ticlopidine can produce major side effects in some patients, including long-lasting neutropenia, aplastic anemia, thrombocytopenia, gastrointestinal distress, and diarrhea. Clopidogrel has the same clinical efficacy as ticlopidine, but the incidence and severity of these side effects are much lower.[14,74] Clopidogrel has become the drug of choice for this class of antiplatelet agents. Clopidogrel and aspirin are increasingly being used in combination to prevent arterial thrombosis primarily based on the synergistic action of these two drugs that inhibit platelet function by different mechanisms. Similar to aspirin, the effects of the thienopyridines are not readily reversible; platelet function after cessation of drug intake is about 50% of normal at 3 days, and complete recovery of function occurs at 7 days.[75]

A newer group of antiplatelet agents targets the platelet membrane GP IIb/IIIa (α_{IIb}/β_3) receptor, interfering with the ability of this receptor to bind fibrinogen and inhibiting platelet aggregation to all of the usual platelet aggregating agents. Platelet function studies on platelets from patients receiving therapeutic doses of these drugs essentially mimic a mild form of Glanzmann thrombasthenia. Two different types of agents are included in this group. The first such agent approved for clinical use in the United States was the Fab fragment of the mouse/human chimeric monoclonal antibody 7E3 (c7E3 Fab; abciximab [RheoPro]) that binds to GP IIb/IIIa, prevents the binding of fibrinogen, and prevents platelet aggregation. Numerous studies have shown the efficacy of this drug as an antiplatelet and antithrombotic agent. The second type of agent in this group targets a GP IIb/IIIa recognition site for an Arg-Gly-Asp (RGD) sequence found in fibrinogen and several adhesive proteins. These agents bind to the recognition site, prevent the binding of fibrinogen, and consequently prevent platelet aggregation. These compounds are relatively easily synthesized and contain the RGD sequence recognized by the receptor or a structure that mimics the RGD sequence and are bound by the RGD recognition site on GP IIb/IIIa. When the receptor site is occupied by the drug, GP IIb/IIIa is no longer functional as the aggregation receptor. The goal of therapy with these drugs is to induce a controlled thrombasthenia-like state. Currently, the use of these agents is limited by the need to administer them by constant intravenous infusion. An orally active agent of this type is in development and clinical trials.[76-78]

Dipyridamole is an inhibitor of platelet phosphodiesterase, the enzyme responsible for converting cyclic adenosine monophosphate (cAMP) to AMP (see Fig. 13-20). Because elevated cytoplasmic cAMP is inhibitory to platelet function, inhibition of phosphodiesterase would allow the accumulation of cAMP in the cytoplasm. Dipyridamole alone does not inhibit platelet aggregation to the usual platelet agonists, but promotes the inhibitory effect of agents that stimulate cAMP formation, such

as prostacyclin, stable analogues of prostacyclin, and NO. At one time, dipyridamole, alone or in combination with aspirin, was widely used. By the 1990s, interest in dipyridamole had waned. There has been a resurgence of interest in dipyridamole, however, as an agent compounded with aspirin (Aggrenox).

Antibiotics are well known for their ability to interfere with platelet function. Most of these drugs contain the β-lactam ring and are either a penicillin or a cephalosporin (Fig. 44-2). These drugs can prolong the bleeding time, but this effect is seen only in patients receiving large parenteral doses and is a problem only for hospitalized patients. One postulated mechanism for the antiplatelet effect of these drugs is that they associate with the membrane via a lipophilic reaction and block receptor-agonist interactions or stimulus-response coupling. They also may inhibit calcium influx in response to thrombin stimulation, reducing the ability of thrombin to activate platelets. Although these drugs may prolong the bleeding time and in vitro aggregation responses to certain agonists, the association with a hemostatic defect severe enough to cause clinical hemorrhage is uncertain and is not predicted by the bleeding time test.[5,17,51,74]

Nitrofurantoin is an antibiotic that is not related to the β-lactam drugs but may prolong the bleeding time test and inhibit platelet aggregation when high concentrations are present in the blood. This drug is not known to cause clinical bleeding, however.[74]

The dextrans, another class of commonly used drugs, can increase the bleeding time, inhibit platelet aggregation, and impair platelet procoagulant activity when given as an intravenous infusion. These drugs have no effect on platelet function, however, when added directly to platelet-rich plasma. Dextrans are partially hydrolyzed, branched-chain polysaccharides of glucose. The two most commonly used are dextran 70 (molecular mass of 70,000-75,000 D) and dextran 40 (molecular mass of 40,000 D), also known as *low-molecular-weight* dextran. Both drugs are effective plasma expanders and

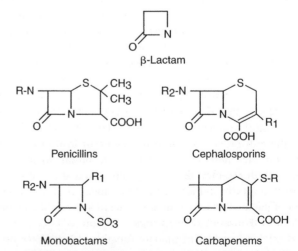

Figure 44-2 Chemical structure of major classes of β-lactam antibiotics. (From Mahon CR, Lehman DE, Manuselis G: Textbook of Diagnostic Microbiology, 3rd ed. Philadelphia: Saunders, 2007.)

are commonly used for this purpose. Because of their effects on platelets, they have been extensively used as antithrombotic agents. There does not seem to be any increased risk of hemorrhage associated with the use of these agents, but their efficacy in preventing postoperative pulmonary embolism is equal to that of low-dose subcutaneous heparin.[14,44,71,74]

Hydroxyethyl starch, or hetastarch, is a synthetic glucose polymer with a mean molecular mass of 450,000 D that also is used as a plasma expander. It has effects similar to the dextrans. The mechanism of action of these drugs is not clearly elucidated but is presumed to involve interaction with the platelet membrane.[14,44,71]

Miscellaneous Drugs That Inhibit Platelet Function. The following agents are of diverse chemical structure and function, but all are known to inhibit platelet function. The mechanisms by which they induce platelet dysfunction are largely unknown. Nitroglycerin, nitroprusside, propranolol, and isosorbide dinitrate are drugs used to regulate cardiovascular function that seem to be able to cause a decrease in platelet secretion and aggregation. Patients taking phenothiazine or tricyclic antidepressants may have decreased secretion and aggregation responses, but these effects are not associated with an increased risk for hemorrhage. Local and general anesthetics may impair in vitro aggregation responses. The same is true of antihistamines. Finally, some radiographic contrast agents are known to inhibit platelet function.[74]

Disorders That Affect Platelet Function

Myeloproliferative Disorders. Chronic myeloproliferative disorders (MPDs) include polycythemia vera, chronic myeloid leukemia, essential thrombocythemia, and myelofibrosis with myeloid metaplasia (Chapter 34). Platelet dysfunction is a common finding in patients with these disorders. Hemorrhagic complications occur in about one third, thrombosis occurs in another third, and although uncommon, some patients develop both. These complications are serious causes of morbidity and mortality. Although the occurrence of hemorrhage or thrombosis in MPD patients is largely unpredictable, certain patterns have emerged. Hemorrhage and thrombosis are less common in chronic myeloid leukemia than the other MPDs. Bleeding seems to be more common in myelofibrosis with myeloid metaplasia, but thrombosis is more common in the other MPDs. Abnormal platelet function has been postulated as a contributing cause. This postulate is supported by the observation that bleeding is usually mucocutaneous in nature, and thrombosis may be arterial or venous. In patients with these disorders, thrombosis may occur in unusual sites, including the mesenteric, hepatic, and portal circulations. Patients with essential thrombocythemia may develop digital artery thrombosis and ischemia of the fingers and toes, occlusions of the microvasculature of the heart, and cerebrovascular occlusions that result in neurologic symptoms.[74]

In MPDs, a variety of platelet function defects have been described, but their clinical importance is uncertain. Platelets have been reported to have abnormal shapes, decreased procoagulant activity, and a decreased number of secretory gran-

ules. In essential thrombocythemia, platelet survival may be shortened. The bleeding time is prolonged in only a few patients, and hemorrhage can occur in patients with a normal bleeding time. The risk of thrombosis or hemorrhage correlates poorly with the elevation of the platelet count.

The most common abnormalities are decreased aggregation and secretion in response to epinephrine, ADP, and collagen.[79] Possible causes of the platelet dysfunction include loss of platelet surface membrane α-adrenergic (epinephrine) receptors, impaired release of arachidonic acid from membrane phospholipids in response to stimulation by agonists, impaired oxidation of arachidonic acid by the cyclooxygenase and lipoxygenase pathways, a decrease in the contents of dense granules and α granules, and loss of a variety of platelet membrane receptors for adhesion and activation. There seems to be no correlation between a given MPD and the type of platelet dysfunction observed, with the exception that most patients with essential thrombocythemia are lacking an in vitro platelet aggregation response to epinephrine. This observation may be helpful in the differential diagnosis.[14,17,74,80]

Multiple Myeloma and Waldenström Macroglobulinemia. Platelet dysfunction is observed in approximately one third of patients with IgA myeloma or Waldenström macroglobulinemia, a much smaller percentage of patients with IgG multiple myeloma, and only occasionally in patients with monoclonal gammopathy of undetermined significance (Chapter 37). Platelet dysfunction results from coating of the platelet membranes by paraprotein and does not depend on the type of paraprotein present. In addition to the interaction of the protein with platelets, the paraprotein may interfere with fibrin polymerization and the function of other coagulation proteins. Almost all patients with malignant paraprotein disorders have clinically significant bleeding, but thrombocytopenia is still the most likely cause of bleeding in these patients. Other causes of bleeding include hyperviscosity syndrome, complications of amyloidosis (e.g., acquired factor X deficiency), and, in rare instances, a circulating heparin-like anticoagulant or fibrinolysis.[16,71,74]

Cardiopulmonary Bypass Surgery. Cardiopulmonary bypass induces thrombocytopenia and a severe platelet function defect that assumes major importance in surgical bleeding after bypass. The function defects most likely result from platelet activation and fragmentation in the extracorporeal circuit. Causes of platelet activation include adherence and aggregation of platelets to fibrinogen (adsorbed onto the surfaces of the bypass circuit material), mechanical trauma and shear stresses, blood conservation devices, bypass pump-priming solutions, hypothermia, complement activation, and exposure of platelets to the blood-air interface in bubble oxygenators. Some degree of platelet degranulation typically is found after bypass surgery, indicating platelet activation and secretion has occurred during the operation. Platelet membrane fragments or "microparticles" are found consistently in the blood of bypass patients, providing additional evidence of the severe mechanical stress encountered by platelets during bypass procedures. The severity of the platelet function defect closely correlates with the length of time on bypass. After an uncomplicated bypass procedure, normal platelet function returns in about 1 hour, although the platelet count does not return to normal for several days. Thrombocytopenia is caused by hemodilution, accumulation of platelets on the surfaces of the bypass materials, sequestration or removal of damaged platelets by the liver and reticuloendothelial system, and consumption associated with normal hemostatic processes after surgery.[71,74]

Liver Disease.   Moderate to severe liver disease is reported to be associated with a variety of hemostatic abnormalities, including reduction in clotting proteins, reduction of proteins in the natural anticoagulant pathways, dysfibrinogenemia, and excessive fibrinolysis. Mild to moderate thrombocytopenia is seen in approximately one third of patients with chronic liver disease in association with hypersplenism or as a result of alcohol toxicity.[4,74]

Abnormal platelet function tests found in patients with chronic liver disease include reduced platelet adhesion; abnormal platelet aggregation to ADP, epinephrine, and thrombin; abnormal platelet factor 3 availability; and reduced procoagulant activity. An acquired storage pool deficiency also has been suggested. The prolonged bleeding time in these patients may respond to infusion of DDAVP. It is unclear whether DDAVP provides a benefit in preventing bleeding in these patients or is simply correcting an abnormal laboratory test result.

In chronic alcoholic cirrhosis, the thrombocytopenia and platelet abnormalities may result from the direct toxic effects of alcohol on bone marrow megakaryocytes. The severe bleeding diathesis associated with end-stage liver disease has many causes, such as markedly decreased or negligible coagulation factor production, excessive fibrinolysis, dysfibrinogenemia, thrombocytopenia, and (occasionally) disseminated intravascular coagulation. Upper gastrointestinal bleeding is a relatively common feature of cirrhosis, particularly alcoholic cirrhosis, and recombinant factor VIIa has been shown to be effective for some patients.[81]

Uremia.   Uremia is commonly accompanied by bleeding caused by platelet dysfunction. In uremia, guanidinosuccinic acid (GSA) is present in the circulation in higher than normal levels as a result of inhibition of the urea cycle. GSA is dialyzable, and dialysis (peritoneal dialysis or hemodialysis) is usually effective in correcting the prolonged bleeding time and the abnormal platelet function characteristic of uremia. NO diffuses into platelets; activates soluble guanylate cyclase; and inhibits platelet adhesion, activation, and aggregation.[82] Because GSA is an NO donor, NO is present in the circulation at higher than normal levels. Abnormal platelet function in uremic patients is far more common than clinically significant bleeding.[2,50,52]

Platelet aggregation pattern abnormalities are not uniform, and any combination of defects may be seen. There is evidence of a deficient release reaction, such as lack of primary ADP-induced aggregation, and subnormal platelet procoagulant activity. The bleeding time is characteristically prolonged in uremia and seems to correlate with the severity of renal failure in these patients. There does not seem to be any significant correlation, however, between the bleeding time test and the risk of clinically significant bleeding. Anemia is an independent cause of a prolonged bleeding time, and the severity of anemia in uremic patients correlates with the severity of renal failure. Many uremic patients are treated with recombinant erythropoietin to increase their hematocrit. Maintenance of the hematocrit at greater than 30% also may help to normalize the bleeding times.[2,71,73]

Bleeding is uncommon in uremic patients and is seen more often in patients who are concurrently taking drugs that interfere with platelet function or in association with heparin used for hemodialysis. Platelet concentrates often are used for severe hemorrhagic episodes in patients with uremia but usually do not correct the bleeding. Other therapies that are sometimes effective include cryoprecipitate, DDAVP, and conjugated estrogen.[2,71,73]

Hereditary Afibrinogenemia.   Hereditary afibrinogenemia has been documented in more than 150 families. Although this is not truly a platelet function disorder, platelets do not exhibit normal function in the absence or near-absence of fibrinogen. In most patients, the bleeding time is prolonged, and because fibrinogen is essential for normal platelet aggregation, platelet aggregation test results are abnormal. Abnormalities in platelet retention/adhesion studies involving the use of glass beads also have been documented. In addition, all clot-based tests (including the partial thromboplastin time, prothrombin time, reptilase time, thrombin time, and whole-blood clotting time) are abnormal. Addition of fibrinogen to samples or infusion of fibrinogen into the patient results in correction of the abnormal test results.[2,83]

A high incidence of hemorrhagic manifestations is found in patients with afibrinogenemia (or severe hypofibrinogenemia). Bleeding is the cause of death in about one third of such patients. Cryoprecipitate or fibrinogen concentrates can be used to treat bleeding episodes. Some patients develop antibodies to fibrinogen, and this treatment then becomes ineffective.[83]

Hyperaggregable Platelets

Patients with a variety of disorders associated with thrombosis or increased risk for thrombosis, including hyperlipidemia, diabetes mellitus, peripheral arterial occlusive disease, acute arterial occlusion, myocardial infarction, and stroke, have been reported to have increased platelet reactivity. Platelets from these patients tend to aggregate at lower concentrations of aggregating agents than platelets from "normal" individuals. Spontaneous aggregation (aggregation in response to stirring only) is also an index of abnormally increased platelet reactivity and often accompanies increased sensitivity to platelet agonists. The presence of spontaneous aggregation by itself is considered to be consistent with the presence of a hyperaggregable state. Because participation of platelets is necessary for the development of arterial thrombosis, the presence of hyperaggregable platelets is often an indication that an antiplatelet agent should be used as part of a therapeutic or prophylactic regimen for arterial thrombosis.[71,84,85]

Acquired platelet function defects are seen occasionally in patients with autoimmune disorders, including systemic lupus erythematosus, rheumatoid arthritis, scleroderma, and the immune thrombocytopenias, such as immune thrombocytopenic purpura.[74]

Purified fibrin degradation products can induce platelet dysfunction in vitro. The pathophysiologic relevance of this observation is uncertain because the concentrations of fibrin degradation products required are unlikely to be reached in vivo. Patients with disseminated intravascular coagulation may have reduced platelet function, however, as a result of in vivo stimulation by thrombin and other agonists, resulting in in vivo release of granule contents. This has been called *acquired storage pool disease*; the term *exhausted platelets* may be more appropriate.[86]

VASCULAR DISORDERS

The pathophysiology of disorders of vessels and their supporting tissues is obscure. Laboratory studies of platelets and blood coagulation usually yield normal results. The diagnosis is often based on medical history and is made by ruling out other sources of bleeding disorders. The usual clinical sign is the tendency to bruise easily or to bleed spontaneously, especially from mucosal surfaces. Vascular disorders are summarized in Box 44-2.

Hereditary Vascular Disorders
Hereditary Hemorrhagic Telangiectasia (Rendu-Weber-Osler Syndrome)
The mode of inheritance of hereditary hemorrhagic telangiectasia is autosomal dominant. The vascular defect of this disorder is characterized by thin-walled blood vessels with a discontinuous endothelium, inadequate smooth muscle, and inadequate or missing elastin in the surrounding stroma. Telangiectasias (dilated, superficial blood vessels that create small, focal red lesions) occur throughout the body but are most obvious on the face, lips, tongue, conjunctiva, nasal mucosa, fingers, toes, and trunk and under the tongue. The lesions blanch when pressure is applied. The disorder usually becomes manifest by puberty and progresses throughout life. Telangiectasias are fragile and prone to rupture. Epistaxis is an almost universal finding, and symptoms almost always worsen with age. The age at which nosebleeds begin is a good gauge of the severity of the disorder. Although the oral cavity, gastrointestinal tract, and urogenital tract are common sites of bleeding, bleeding can occur in virtually every organ.[87]

The laboratory features relate to the severity of the hemorrhagic tendencies. The bleeding time is usually normal, and the tourniquet test result may be normal or show increased capillary fragility. The diagnosis of hereditary hemorrhagic telangiectasia is based on the characteristic skin or mucous membrane lesions, a history of repeated hemorrhage, and a family history of a similar affliction. Patients with hereditary hemorrhagic telangiectasia do well despite the lack of specific therapy and the seriousness of their hemorrhagic manifestations.[2,6,87] There are several other disorders and conditions in which telangiectasias are present, including cherry-red hemangiomas (common in older men and women), ataxia-telangiectasia (Louis-Bar syndrome), and chronic actinic telangiectasia and in association with chronic liver disease and pregnancy.[87]

Hemangioma-Thrombocytopenia Syndrome (Kasabach-Merritt Syndrome)
Kasabach and Merritt originally described the association of a giant cavernous hemangioma (vascular tumor), thrombocytopenia, and a bleeding diathesis. The hemangiomas are visceral or subcutaneous, but rarely both. External hemangiomas may become engorged with blood and resemble hematomas. Other well-recognized features of Kasabach-Merritt syndrome include acute or chronic disseminated intravascular coagulation and microangiopathic hemolytic anemia. A hereditary basis for this syndrome has not been established, but the condition is present at birth. Several treatment modalities are available for the tumors and the coagulopathy and range from corticosteroid therapy to surgery.[6,88]

Ehlers-Danlos Syndrome and Other Genetic Disorders
Ehlers-Danlos syndrome may be transmitted as an autosomal dominant, recessive, or X-linked trait. It is manifested by hyperextensible skin; hypermobile joints; joint laxity; fragile tissues; and a bleeding tendency, primarily subcutaneous hematoma formation. Eleven distinct varieties of the disorder are recognized. The severity of bleeding ranges from easy bruisability to arterial rupture. The disorder generally can be ascribed to defects in collagen production, structure, or cross-linking, with resulting inadequacy of the connective tissues. Platelet abnor-

---

BOX 44-2 Vascular Disorders

Hereditary vascular disorders
  Hereditary hemorrhagic telangiectasia (Rendu-Weber-Osler syndrome)
  Hemangioma-thrombocytopenia syndrome (Kasabach-Merritt syndrome)
  Ehlers-Danlos syndrome and other genetic disorders
Acquired vascular disorders
  Allergic purpura (Henoch-Schönlein purpura)
  Senile purpura
  Paraproteinemia and amyloidosis
  Drug-induced vascular purpuras
  Vitamin C deficiency (scurvy)
Purpuras of unknown origin
  Purpura simplex (easy bruisability)
  Psychogenic purpura

From Thompson AR, Harker LA: Manual of Hemostasis and Thrombosis, 3rd ed. Philadelphia: Davis, 1983.

malities have been reported in some patients. Common laboratory abnormalities include a positive tourniquet test and prolonged bleeding time.[6]

Other inherited vascular disorders include pseudoxanthoma elasticum and homocystinuria (autosomal recessive disorders) and Marfan syndrome and osteogenesis imperfecta (autosomal dominant disorders). In addition to vascular defects, Marfan syndrome is characterized by skeletal and ocular defects.[6]

Acquired Vascular Disorders
Allergic Purpura (Henoch-Schönlein Purpura)
The term *allergic purpura* or *anaphylactoid purpura* generally is applied to a group of nonthrombocytopenic purpuras characterized by apparently allergic manifestations, including skin rash and edema. Allergic purpura has been associated with certain foods, drugs, cold, insect bites, and vaccinations. The term *Henoch-Schönlein purpura* is applied when the condition is accompanied by transient arthralgia, nephritis, abdominal pain, and purpuric skin lesions frequently confused with the hemorrhagic rash of immune thrombocytopenic purpura.[2,6,44]

General evidence implicates autoimmune vascular injury, but the pathophysiology of the disorder is unclear. Preliminary evidence indicates that the vasculitis is mediated by immune complexes containing IgA antibodies. It has been suggested that allergic purpura may represent autoimmunity to components of vessel walls.[2,6]

Henoch-Schönlein purpura is primarily a disease of children, occurring most commonly in children 3 to 7 years old. It is relatively uncommon among individuals younger than age 2 years and older than age 20. Twice as many boys as girls are affected. The onset of the disease is sudden, often following an upper respiratory infection. The organism may damage the endothelial lining of blood vessels, resulting in vasculitis. Attempts have been made to implicate a specific infectious agent, particularly beta-hemolytic streptococcus.[2,6]

Malaise, headache, fever, and rash may be the presenting symptoms. The delay in the appearance of the skin rash often poses a difficult problem in differential diagnosis. The skin lesions are urticarial and gradually become pinkish, then red, and finally hemorrhagic. The appearance of the lesions may be very rapid and accompanied by itching. The lesions have been described as "palpable purpura," in contrast to the perfectly flat lesions of thrombocytopenia and most other forms of vascular purpura. These lesions are most commonly found on the feet, elbows, knees, buttocks, and chest. Ultimately, a brownish-red eruption is seen. Petechiae also may be present.[2,6]

As the disease progresses, abdominal pain, polyarthralgia, headaches, and renal disease may develop. Renal lesions are present in 60% of patients during the second to third week of the course of the disorder. Proteinuria and hematuria are commonly present.[2,4,6]

The platelet count is normal. Tests of hemostasis, including the bleeding time, tourniquet test, and tests of blood coagulation, usually yield normal results in patients with allergic purpura. Anemia usually is not present, unless the hemorrhagic manifestations have been severe. The white blood cell count and the erythrocyte sedimentation rate are usually elevated. The disease must be distinguished from other forms of nonthrombocytopenic purpura. Numerous infectious diseases that may be associated with purpura also must be considered in the differential diagnosis. Drugs or chemicals sometimes may be implicated.[2,6]

In the pediatric age group, the average duration of the initial attack is about 4 weeks. Relapses are frequent, usually after a period of apparent well-being. Except for patients in whom chronic renal disease develops, the prognosis is usually good. Occasionally, death from renal failure has occurred. Treatment is primarily symptomatic because there currently is no effective treatment. Corticosteroids sometimes have been helpful in alleviating symptoms. Most patients recover without treatment.[2,6]

Paraproteinemia and Amyloidosis
Platelet function can be inhibited by myeloma proteins. Abnormalities in platelet aggregation, secretion, clot retraction, and procoagulant activity correlate with the concentration of the plasma paraprotein and are likely due to coating of the platelet membrane with the paraprotein. Under these conditions, platelet adhesion and activation receptor functions are inhibited, and the paraprotein coating also inhibits assembly of clotting factors on the platelet surface. High concentrations of paraprotein can cause severe hemorrhagic manifestations as a result of a combination of hyperviscosity and platelet dysfunction. About one third of patients with IgA myeloma and Waldenström macroglobulinemia and approximately 5% of patients with IgG myeloma (usually IgG_3) exhibit platelet function abnormalities. Finally, the paraprotein may contribute further to bleeding by inhibiting fibrin polymerization. In these patients, there is poor correlation between abnormal laboratory tests (e.g., prothrombin time, activated partial thromboplastin time, thrombin time, bleeding time) and evidence of clinical bleeding. Treatment for the bleeding complications of these disorders is primarily reduction in the level of the paraprotein. This can be accomplished quickly, albeit transiently, by plasmapheresis. Longer-term treatment is usually chemotherapy for the underlying plasma cell malignancy.[74,89]

Amyloid is a fibrous protein consisting of rigid, linear, nonbranching, aggregated fibrils approximately 7.5 to 10 nm wide and of indefinite length. Amyloid is deposited extracellularly and may lead to damage of normal tissues. Various proteins can serve as subunits of the fibril, including monoclonal light chains (λ more frequently than κ). Amyloidosis, the deposition of abnormal quantities of amyloid in tissues, may be primary or secondary and localized or systemic. A discussion of the clinical spectrum of amyloidosis is beyond the scope of this chapter. Purpura, hemorrhage, and thrombosis may be a part of the clinical presentation of patients with amyloidosis, however. Thrombosis and hemorrhage have been ascribed to amyloid deposition in the vascular wall and surrounding tissues. Platelet function has been shown to be abnormal in a few cases, and in rare cases patients may have thrombocytopenia. Current treatments for amyloidosis are not effective.[90]

Senile Purpura

Senile purpura occurs more commonly in elderly men than women and is due to a lack of collagen support for small blood vessels and loss of subcutaneous fat and elastic fibers. The number of cases increases with advancing age. The dark blotches are flattened, are about 1 to 10 mm in diameter, do not blanch with pressure, and resolve slowly, often leaving a brown stain in the skin (age spots). The lesions are limited mostly to the extensor surfaces of the forearms and backs of the hands and occasionally occur on the face and neck. With the exception of increased capillary fragility, results of laboratory tests are normal, and no other bleeding manifestations are present.[2,6]

Drug-Induced Vascular Purpuras

Purpura associated with drug-induced vasculitis occurs in the presence of functionally adequate platelets. A variety of drugs are known to cause vascular purpura, including aspirin, warfarin (Coumadin), barbiturates, diuretics, digoxin, methyldopa, and several antibiotics. Sulfonamides and iodides have been implicated most frequently. The lesions vary from a few petechiae to massive, generalized petechial eruptions. Mechanisms include development of antibodies to vessel wall components, development of immune complexes, and changes in vessel wall permeability. As soon as the disorder is recognized, the offending drug should be discontinued. No other treatment is necessary.[6]

Miscellaneous Causes of Vascular Purpura

Insufficient dietary intake of vitamin C (ascorbic acid) results in scurvy and decreased synthesis of collagen, with weakening of capillary walls and the appearance of purpuric lesions.[6] A diagnosis of purpura simplex (simple vascular purpura) or vascular fragility is made when a cause for purpura cannot be found. The ecchymoses are superficial, bleeding is usually mild, and laboratory test results are most often normal.[6] Cutaneous bleeding and bruising through intact skin has been observed in patients in whom no vascular or platelet dysfunction can be detected. Most such cases involve women with emotional problems, and the bruising is often accompanied by nausea, vomiting, or fever. Evidence of a psychosomatic origin is equivocal. Laboratory test results are invariably normal.[6]

CHAPTER at a GLANCE

- Inherited qualitative platelet disorders can cause bleeding disorders ranging from mild to severe.
- BSS is caused by the lack of expression of GP Ib/IX/V complexes on the platelet surface. This receptor complex is responsible for platelet adhesion, and its absence results in a severe bleeding disorder.
- Glanzmann thrombasthenia is caused by the lack of expression of GP IIb/IIIa complexes on the platelet surface. This complex is known as the *platelet aggregation receptor*, and its absence is associated with a severe bleeding disorder.
- Storage pool disorders result from the absence of intraplatelet α granules, dense granules, or both. Platelet dysfunction associated with these disorders is generally mild; bleeding symptoms also are usually mild.
- Aspirin-like defects result from defects in elements of the arachidonic acid metabolic pathway. Platelet dysfunction mimics that seen after aspirin ingestion.
- Deficiencies of several of the receptors for platelet-activating substances have been documented, and bleeding symptoms of varying severity are associated with these deficiencies.

- Drugs are the most common cause of acquired platelet dysfunction, and aspirin is the most frequent cause. Several new classes of antiplatelet agents with different effects than aspirin are now available and gaining in popularity.
- A variety of pathologic conditions can result in platelet dysfunction and range from hematologic malignancies to kidney disease and liver disease.
- Vascular disorders that result in bleeding are uncommon. There are a few well-recognized inherited disorders, however, such as Ehlers-Danlos syndrome and hereditary hemorrhagic telangiectasia that can result in substantial blood loss.
- Vascular disorders can be acquired, and this is much more common than inherited disorders. Causes range from the effects of aging to drug effects to allergic reaction.

Now that you have completed this chapter, go back and read again the case study at the beginning and respond to the questions presented.

REVIEW QUESTIONS

1. The clinical presentation of platelet-related bleeding may include all of the following *except*:
   a. Bruising
   b. Nosebleeds
   c. Gastrointestinal bleeding
   d. Bleeding into the joints (hemarthroses)

2. A defect in GP IIb/IIIa causes:
   a. Glanzmann thrombasthenia
   b. BSS
   c. Gray platelet syndrome
   d. Storage pool disease

3. Aspirin ingestion blocks the synthesis of:
   a. Thromboxane A_2
   b. Ionized calcium
   c. Collagen
   d. ADP

4. Patients with BSS have which of the following laboratory test findings?
   a. Abnormal platelet response to arachidonic acid
   b. Abnormal platelet response to ristocetin
   c. Abnormal platelet response to collagen
   d. Thrombocytosis

5. Which of the following is the most common of the hereditary platelet function defects?
   a. Glanzmann thrombasthenia
   b. BSS
   c. Storage pool defects
   d. Multiple myeloma

6. A mechanism of antiplatelet drugs targeting GP IIb/IIIa function is:
   a. Interference with platelet adhesion to the subendothelium by blocking the collagen binding site
   b. Inhibition of transcription of the GP IIb/IIIa gene
   c. Direct binding to GP IIb/IIIa
   d. Interference with platelet secretion

7. The impaired platelet function in myeloproliferative disorders results from:

   a. Abnormally shaped platelets
   b. Extended platelet life span
   c. Increased procoagulant activity
   d. Decreased numbers of α and dense granules

8. Which is a *congenital* qualitative platelet disorder?
   a. Senile purpura
   b. Ehlers-Danlos syndrome
   c. Henoch-Schönlein purpura
   d. Waldenström macroglobulinemia

9. In uremia, platelet function is impaired by higher than normal levels of:
   a. Urea
   b. Uric acid
   c. Creatinine
   d. Nitric oxide

10. The platelet defect associated with increased paraproteins is:
    a. Impaired membrane activation owing to protein coating
    b. Hypercoagulability owing to antibody binding and membrane activation
    c. Impaired aggregation because the hyperviscous plasma prevents platelet-endothelial interaction
    d. Hypercoagulability because the increased proteins bring platelets closer together, leading to inappropriate aggregation

REFERENCES

1. Triplett DA: How to evaluate platelet function. Lab Med Pract Phys 1978;July/Aug:37-43.
2. Thorup OA: Leavell and Thorup's Fundamentals of Clinical Hematology, 5th ed. Philadelphia: Saunders, 1987.
3. Geddis AE, Kaushansky K: Inherited thrombocytopenias: toward a better molecular understanding of disorders of platelet production. Curr Opin Pediatr 2004;16:15-24.
4. Coller BS, Mitchell WB, French DL: Hereditary qualitative platelet disorders. In Lichtman MA, Beutler E, Kipps TJ, et al (eds): Williams Hematology, 7th ed. New York: McGraw-Hill, 2006:1795-1832.
5. Thompson AR, Harker LA: Manual of Hemostasis and Thrombosis, 3rd ed. Philadelphia: Davis, 1983.
6. Powers LW: Diagnostic Hematology: Clinical and Technical Principles. St Louis: Mosby, 1989.
7. Nurden P, Nurden A: Giant platelets, megakaryocytes and the expression of glycoprotein Ib-IX complexes. C R Acad Sci III 1996;319:717-726.
8. Clementson KJ: Platelet GP Ib-V-IX complex. Thromb Haemost 1997;78:266-270.
9. Nurden AT: Inherited abnormalities of platelets. Thromb Haemost 1999;82:468-480.
10. Lopez JA, Andrews RK, Afshar-Kharghan V, et al: Bernard-Soulier syndrome. Blood 1998;91:4397-4418.
11. Takahashi H, Murata M, Moriki T, et al: Substitution of Val for Met at residue 239 of platelet glycoprotein Ib alpha in Japanese patients with platelet-type von Willebrand disease. Blood 1995;85:727-733.
12. Matsubara Y, Murata M, Sugita K, et al: Identification of a novel point mutation in platelet glycoprotein Ibα, Gly to Ser at residue 233, in a Japanese family with platelet-type von Willebrand disease. J Thromb Haemost 2003;1:2198-2205.
13. Othman M, Elbatarny HS, Notley C, et al: Identification and functional characterization of a novel 27bp deletion in the macroglycopeptide-coding region of the GPIbα gene resulting in platelet-type von Willebrand disease [abstract 1023]. Blood 2004;104.
14. George JN, Shattil SJ: The clinical importance of acquired abnormalities of platelet function. N Engl J Med 1991;324:27-39.
15. Caen JP: Glanzmann's thrombasthenia. Baillieres Clin Haematol 1989;2:609-623.
16. Triplett DA (ed): Platelet Function: Laboratory Evaluation and Clinical Application. Chicago: American Society of Clinical Pathologists, 1978.
17. Rapaport SI: Introduction to Hematology, 2nd ed. Philadelphia: Lippincott, 1987.
18. Meyer M, Kirchmaier CM, Schirmer A, et al: Acquired disorder of platelet function associated with autoantibodies against membrane glycoprotein IIb-IIIa complex: 1. Glycoprotein analysis. Thromb Haemost 1991;65:491-496.
19. Tarantino MD, Corrigan JJ Jr, Glasser L, et al: A variant form of thrombasthenia. Am J Dis Child 1991;145:1053-1057.
20. Friedlander M, Brooks PC, Shaffer RW, et al: Definition of two angiogenic pathways by distinct a_v integrins. Science 1995;270:1500-1502.
21. Nurden AT, George JN: Inherited disorders of the platelet membrane: Glanzmann thrombasthenia, Bernard-Soulier syndrome and other disorders. In Colman RW, Clowes AW, Goldhaber SZ, et al (eds): Hemostasis and Thrombosis: Basic Principles and Clinical Practice, 5th ed. Philadelphia: Lippincott, Williams & Wilkins, 2006:987-1010.
22. Nurden AT: Qualitative disorders of platelets and megakaryocytes. J Thromb Haemost 2005;3:1773-1782.

23. Coller BS, Cheresh DA, Asch E, et al: Platelet vitronectin receptor expression differentiates Iraqi-Jewish from Arab patients with Glanzmann thrombasthenia in Israel. Blood 1991;77:75-83.

24. French DL: The molecular genetics of Glanzmann's thrombasthenia. Platelets 1998;9:5-20.

25. Corriveau DM, Fritsma GA: Hemostasis and Thrombosis in the Clinical Laboratory. Philadelphia: Lippincott, 1988.

26. Rosa JP, Artcanuthurry V, Grelac F, et al: Reassessment of protein tyrosine phosphorylation in thrombasthenic platelets: evidence that phosphorylation of cortactin and a 64 kD protein is dependent on thrombin activation and integrin aIIbb$_3$. Thromb Haemost 1997;89:4385-4392.

27. Byzova TV, Plow EF: Networking in the hemostatic system: integrin aIIbb$_3$ binds prothrombin and influences its activation. J Biol Chem 1997;272:27183-27188.

28. Gemmell CH, Sefton MV, Yeo EL: Platelet-derived microparticle formation involves glycoprotein IIb-IIIa: inhibition by RGDs and a Glanzmann's thrombasthenia defect. J Biol Chem 1993;268:14586-14589.

29. Reverter JC, Beguin S, Kessels H, et al: Inhibition of platelet-mediated tissue factor-induced thrombin generation by the mouse/human chimeric 7E3 antibody: potential implications for the effect of c7E3 Fab treatment on acute thrombosis and "clinical restenosis." J Clin Invest 1996;98:863-874.

30. Caen JP: Glanzmann's thrombasthenia. Clin Hematol 1972;1:383-392.

31. George JN, Caen JP, Nurden AT: Glanzmann's thrombasthenia: the spectrum of clinical disease. Blood 1990;75:1383-1395.

32. Jennings LK, Wang WC, Jackson CW, et al: Hemostasis in Glanzmann's thrombasthenia (GT): GT platelets interfere with the aggregation of normal platelets. Am J Pediatr Hematol Oncol 1991;13:84-90.

33. Poon MC, d'Oiron R, Von Depka M, et al: International Data Collection on Recombinant Factor VIIa and Congenital Platelet Disorders Study Group: prophylactic and therapeutic recombinant factor VIIa administration to patients with Glanzmann's thrombasthenia: results of an international survey. J Thromb Haemost 2004;2:1096-1103.

34. Lisman T, Adelmaier J, Heijnen HFG, et al: Recombinant factor VIIa restores aggregation of αIIb/β$_3$-deficient platelets via tissue factor-independent fibrin generation. Blood 2004;103:1720-1727.

35. Pati H, Saraya AK: Platelet storage pool disease. Indian J Med Res 1986;84:617-620.

36. Rao AK: Hereditary disorders of platelet secretion and signal transduction. In Colman RW, Clowes AW, Goldhaber SZ, et al (eds): Hemostasis and Thrombosis: Basic Principles and Clinical Practice, 5th ed. Philadelphia: Lippincott, Williams & Wilkins, 2006:961-974.

37. Weiss HJ, Lages B, Vicic W, et al: Heterogeneous abnormalities of platelet dense granule ultrastructure in 20 patients with congenital storage pool deficiency. Br J Haematol 1993;83:282-295.

38. Bennett JS: Hereditary disorders of platelet function. In Hoffman R, Benz EJ Jr, Shattil SJ, et al (eds): Hematology: Basic Principles and Practice, 4th ed. New York: Churchill Livingstone, 2005:2327-2345.

39. Abrams CS, Brass LF: Platelet signal transduction. In Colman RW, Clowes AW, Goldhaber SZ, et al (eds): Hemostasis and Thrombosis: Basic Principles and Clinical Practice, 5th ed. Philadelphia: Lippincott, Williams & Wilkins, 2006:617-630.

40. Jedlitschky G, Tirwschmann K, Lubenow LE, et al: The nucleotide transporter MRP4 (ABCC4) is highly expressed in human platelets and present in dense granules, indicating a role in mediator storage. Blood 2004;104:3603-3610.

41. Spritz RA: Molecular genetics of the Hermansky-Pudlak and Chediak-Higashi syndromes. Platelets 1998;9:21-29.

42. Dell'Angellica EC, Aguilar RC, Wolins N, et al: Molecular characterization of the protein encoded by the Hermansky-Pudlak syndrome type 1 gene. J Biol Chem 2000;275:1300-1306.

43. White JG: Inherited abnormalities of the platelet membrane and secretory granules. Hum Pathol 1987;18:123-139.

44. Quick AJ: Hemorrhagic Diseases and Thrombosis, 2nd ed. Philadelphia: Lea & Febiger, 1966.

45. Cleary AM, Insel RA, Lewis DB: Disorders of lymphocyte function. In Hoffman R, Benz EJ Jr, Shattil SJ, et al (eds): Hematology: Basic Principles and Practice, 4th ed. New York: Churchill Livingstone, 2005:831-855.

46. de Alarcon PA, Graeve JA, Levine RF, et al: Thrombocytopenia and absent radii syndrome: defective megakaryocytopoiesis-thrombocytopoiesis. Am J Pediatr Hematol Oncol 1991;13:77-83.

47. Raccuglia G: Gray platelet syndrome: a variety of qualitative platelet disorder. Am J Med 1971;51:818-828.

48. Berrebi A, Klepfish A, Varon D, et al: Gray platelet syndrome in the elderly. Am J Hematol 1988;28:270-272.

49. Pfueller SL, Howard MA, White JG, et al: Shortening of the bleeding time by 1-deamino-8-arginine vasopressin (DDAVP) in the absence of platelet von Willebrand factor in gray platelet syndrome. Thromb Haemost 1987;58:1060-1063.

50. Brace LD, Venton DL, Le Breton GC: Thromboxane A2/prostaglandin H2 mobilizes calcium in human blood platelets. Am J Physiol 1985;249:H1-H7.

51. Moake JL, Funicella T: Common bleeding problems. Clin Symp 1983;35:1-32.

52. Nieuwenhuis HK, Sakariassen KS, Houdijk WPM, et al: Deficiency of platelet membrane glycoprotein Ia associated with a decreased platelet adhesion to subendothelium: a defect in platelet spreading. Blood 1986;68:692-695.

53. Moroi M, Jung SM, Okuma M, et al: A patient with platelets deficient in glycoprotein VI that lack both collagen-induced aggregation and adhesion. J Clin Invest 1989;84:1440-1445.

54. Nurden P, Jandrot-Perrus M, Combrie R, et al: Severe deficiency of glycoprotein VI in a patient with gray platelet syndrome. Blood 2004;104:107-114.

55. Cattaneo M: Inherited platelet-based bleeding disorders. J Thromb Haemost 2003;1:1628-1636.

56. Daniel JL, Dangelmaier C, Jin J, et al: Molecular basis for ADP-induced platelet activation: I. Evidence for three distinct ADP receptors on human platelets. J Biol Chem 1998;273:2024-2029.

57. Nurden P, Savi P, Heilmann E, et al: An inherited bleeding disorder linked to a defective interaction between ADP and its receptor on platelets. J Clin Invest 1995;95:1612-1622.

58. Cattaneo M, Zighetti ML, Lombardi R, et al: Molecular basis of defective signal transduction in the platelet P2Y12 receptor of a patient with congenital bleeding. Proc Natl Acad Sci U S A 2003;100:1978-1983.

59. Rao AK: Congenital disorders of platelet function: disorders of signal transduction and secretion. Am J Med Sci 1998;316:69-76.

60. Rao AK: Inherited defects in platelet signaling mechanisms. J Thromb Haemost 2003;1:671-681.

61. Zhou Q, Sims PJ, Wiedmer T: Expression of proteins controlling transbilayer movement of plasma membrane phospholipids in B lymphocytes from a patient with Scott syndrome. Blood 1998;92:1707-1712.

62. Zhou Q, Zhao J, Stout JG, et al: Molecular cloning of human plasma membrane phospholipid scramblase: a protein mediating transbilayer movement of plasma membrane phospholipids. J Biol Chem 1997;272:18240-18244.

63. Zwaal RF, Comfurius P, Bevers EM: Scott syndrome, a bleeding disorder caused by a defective scrambling of membrane phospholipids. Biochim Biophys Acta 2004;1636:119-128.

64. Sims P, Wiedmer T: Unraveling the mysteries of phospholipid scrambling. Thromb Haemost 2001;86:266-275.

65. Stormorken H, Holmsen H, Sund R, et al: Studies on the haemostatic defect in a complicated syndrome: an inverse Scott syndrome platelet membrane abnormality? Thromb Haemost 1995;74:1244-1251.

66. Helgason CM, Bolin KM, Hoff JA, et al: Development of aspirin resistance in persons with previous ischemic stroke. Stroke 1994;25:2331-2336.

67. Helgason CM, Tortorice KL, Winkler SR, et al: Aspirin response and failure in cerebral infarction. Stroke 1993;24:345-350.

68. Beardsley DS: Hemostasis in the perinatal period: approach to the diagnosis of coagulation disorders. Semin Perinatol 1991;15(Suppl 2):25-34.

69. Eikelboom JW, Hirsch J, Weitz J, et al: Aspirin-resistant thromboxane biosynthesis and the risk of myocardial infarction, stroke, or cardiovascular death in patients at high risk for cardiovascular events. Circulation 2002;105:1650-1655.

70. Green D: Diagnosis and management of bleeding disorders. Compr Ther 1988;14:31-36.

71. Bick RL, Scates SM: Qualitative platelet defects. Lab Med 1992;23:95-103.

72. Haut MJ, Cowan DH: The effect of ethanol on hemostatic properties of human blood platelets. Am J Med 1974;56:22-33.

73. Wilhite DB, Comerota AJ, Schmieder FA, et al: Managing PAD with multiple platelet inhibitors: the effect of combination therapy on bleeding time. J Vasc Surg 2003;38:710-713.

74. Lopez J, Thiagarajan P: Acquired disorders of platelet function. In Hoffman R, Benz EJ Jr, Shattil SJ (eds): Hematology: Basic Principles and Practice, 4th ed. New York: Churchill Livingstone, 2005:2347-2367.

75. Schleinitz MD, Heidenreich PA: A cost-effectiveness analysis of combination antiplatelet therapy of high-risk acute coronary syndromes: clopidogrel plus aspirin versus aspirin alone. Ann Intern Med 2005;142:251-259.

76. Coller BS: GPIIb/IIIa antagonists: pathophysiologic and therapeutic insights from studies of c7E3 Fab. Thromb Haemost 1997;78:730-735.

77. Tcheng JE: Platelet glycoprotein IIb/IIIa integrin blockade: recent clinical trials in interventional cardiology. Thromb Haemost 1997;78:205-209.

78. Van de Werf F: Clinical trials with glycoprotein IIb/IIIa receptor antagonists in acute coronary syndromes. Thromb Haemost 1997;78:210-213.

79. Landolfi R, Marchioli R, Patrono C: Mechanisms of bleeding and thrombosis in myeloproliferative disorders. Thromb Haemost 1997;78:617-621.

80. Swart SS, Pearson D, Wood JK, et al: Functional significance of the platelet alpha2-adrenoreceptor: studies in patients with myeloproliferative disorders. Thromb Res 1984;33:531-541.

81. Bosch J, Thabut D, Bendtsen F, et al: Recombinant factor VIIa for upper gastrointestinal bleeding in patients with cirrhosis: a randomized, double-blind trial. Gastroenterology 2004;127:1123-1130.

82. Boccardo P, Remuzzi G, Galbusera M: Platelet dysfunction in renal failure. Semin Thromb Hemost 2004;30:579-589.

83. Martinez J, Ferber A: Disorders of fibrinogen. In Hoffman R, Benz EJ Jr, Shattil SJ, et al (eds): Hematology: Basic Principles and Practice, 4th ed. New York: Churchill Livingstone, 2005:2097-2109.

84. Eldrup-Jorgensen J, Flanigan DP, Brace LD, et al: Hypercoagulable states and lower limb ischemia in young adults. J Vasc Surg 1989;9:334-341.

85. Helgason CM, Hoff JA, Kondos GT, et al: Platelet aggregation in patients with atrial fibrillation taking aspirin or warfarin. Stroke 1993;24:1458-1461.

86. Pareti FI, Capitanio A, Mannucci L, et al: Acquired dysfunction due to circulation of "exhausted" platelets. Am J Med 1980;69:235-240.

87. Coller BS, Schneiderman PI: Clinical evaluation of hemorrhagic disorders: the bleeding history and differential diagnosis of purpura. In Hoffman R, Benz EJ Jr, Shattil SJ, et al (eds): Hematology: Basic Principles and Practice, 4th ed. New York: Churchill Livingstone, 2006:1824-1840.

88. Maceyko RF, Camisa C: Kasabach-Merritt syndrome. Pediatr Dermatol 1991;8:133-136.

89. Brace LD: The multiple myelomas: a review of selected aspects. Allied Health Behav Sci 1981;3:47-61.

90. Gertz MA, Lacy MQ, Dispenzieri A: Amyloidosis. In Hoffman R, Benz EJ Jr, Shattil SJ, et al (eds): Hematology: Basic Principles and Practice, 4th ed. New York: Churchill Livingstone, 2005:1537-1560.

45

Laboratory Evaluation of Hemostasis

George A. Fritsma

OBJECTIVES

After completion of this chapter, the reader will be able to:

1. Describe proper hemostasis specimen collection, management, and centrifugation, and recognize descriptions of situations that violate these standards.
2. Describe criteria for acceptability of hemostasis specimens, and recognize descriptions of unacceptable specimens.
3. Predict the effect on hemostasis tests of unacceptable specimens, and recommend corrective actions.
4. Calculate the amount of anticoagulant needed to collect samples from patients with elevated hematocrits.
5. Describe the principle of platelet function tests to determine the source of platelet deficiency–based hemorrhage, and interpret the results when given.
6. Diagnose and monitor treatment of von Willebrand disease through the judicious selection and interpretation of laboratory tests.
7. Diagnose and monitor heparin-induced thrombocytopenia with thrombosis.

8. Describe the principle, appropriately select, and interpret clot-based coagulation screening tests, including activated coagulation time, prothrombin time, partial thromboplastin time, and thrombin clotting time.
9. Interpret screening test results collectively to narrow the diagnosis for a patient and recommend additional tests to confirm diagnoses.
10. Describe the principle, appropriate selection, and interpretation of mix studies to detect factor deficiencies, lupus anticoagulants, and specific factor inhibitors.
11. Describe the principle, appropriately select, and interpret coagulation factor assays and Bethesda titers.
12. Describe the principle, appropriately select, and interpret tests of fibrinolysis, including fibrin degradation products, D-dimer, plasminogen, and plasminogen activators.
13. Recognize standard abbreviations for the aforementioned tests.

CASE STUDY

After studying the material in this chapter, the reader should be able to respond to the following case study:

A 54-year-old woman experienced a pulmonary embolism on September 26 and was placed on oral anticoagulants. Monthly prothrombin times were collected to monitor therapy. From October through January, her international normalized ratio (INR) was stable at 2.4, but on February 1 her INR was 1.3. The reduced INR was reported to her physician.

On questioning, she reported that there had been no change in her warfarin (Coumadin) dosage or in her diet. She recalled, however, that the phlebotomist had used a tube with a red and gray stopper. She had thought this to be out of the ordinary and had remarked about it to the phlebotomist, who made no response. The clinical laboratory scientist who had performed the prothrombin time re-examined the blood specimen and saw that it was in a blue-stoppered tube.

1. What did the phlebotomist do?
2. What was the consequence of this action?
3. What else could cause an unexpectedly short prothrombin time?

HEMOSTASIS SPECIMEN COLLECTION

Most hemostasis laboratory procedures require plasma from a whole-blood specimen collected by venipuncture and mixed 9:1 with a 3.2% solution of sodium citrate anticoagulant. Phlebotomists, clinical laboratory scientists, and other personnel who collect blood specimens are required to adhere closely to published protocols for specimen collection, transport, and management. The supervisor is responsible for the current validity of specimen collection and handling protocols and insures that personnel employ approved techniques[1] (Chapter 3).

Managing the Patient When Collecting Hemostasis Specimens

Patients need not fast for hemostasis testing, and little special preparation is required before collection of hemostasis laboratory specimens. There are many drugs that may affect the outcomes of coagulation tests, however; for example, aspirin suppresses most platelet function assays. Phlebotomists may manage patients by standard protocols. If there is a reason to anticipate a bleeding disorder (e.g., if the patient has multiple bruises or mentions a tendency to bleed), the phlebotomist should observe the venipuncture site for several minutes and should apply a pressure bandage before dismissing the patient.

Hemostasis Specimen Collection Tubes

Most hemostasis specimens are collected in plastic blue stoppered sterile blood collection tubes containing a measured volume of 0.105 to 0.109 mol/L (3.2%) of buffered sodium citrate anticoagulant.[2] Tubes of uncoated soda-lime glass are unsuitable because their negative surface charge activates platelets and plasma procoagulants.

The phlebotomist must observe certain rules in hemostasis specimen collection, as follows:

- If the hemostasis specimen is part of a series of tubes from a single venipuncture site, it must be collected first or immediately after a nonadditive tube. The hemostasis tube may not immediately follow tubes that contain heparin, ethylenediamine tetraacetic acid (EDTA), sodium fluoride, or clot-promoting materials as are found in plastic red stopper or in serum separator (gel, red and gray stopper) tubes. These additives may transfer to the hemostasis specimen on the stopper needle and invalidate all hemostasis test results.[3]
- The ratio of whole blood to anticoagulant should be 9:1. Evacuated tubes are designed so that the vacuum draws the correct volume of blood. Collection tube manufacturers indicate the allowable range of collection volume error. In most cases, the volume of blood collected must be within 90% of the calibrated volume. A "short draw" (i.e., a specimen smaller than the volume specified) generates erroneously prolonged clot-based coagulation test results because the relative excess anticoagulant neutralizes test reagent calcium.[4] Smaller tubes provide less tolerance for short draws.
- When specimens are collected using winged needle "butterfly" sets, the phlebotomist must compensate for the internal volume of the tubing, usually 0.5 mL. If a single

tube is collected using a needle set, the phlebotomist should collect a nonadditive discard tube first. This ensures that the needle set tubing is filled before the hemostasis specimen is collected.
- Clotted specimens are useless for hemostasis testing, even if the clot is small. A few seconds after collection the phlebotomist must gently invert the specimen at least six times to mix the blood and anticoagulant and prevent clot formation. The clinical laboratory scientist must visually examine for clots again just before centrifugation and testing.
- Excessive specimen agitation causes hemolysis, procoagulant activation, and platelet activation. The phlebotomist must never shake the tube.
- The test results from visibly hemolyzed specimens are unreliable, and the specimen must be recollected (Table 45-1).
- Excess manipulation of the needle may promote release of procoagulant substances from the skin and connective tissue, contaminating the specimen and causing clotting factor activation. Consequently, test results from specimens collected during a "traumatic" venipuncture may be factitiously shortened and unreliable.
- Specimens that are lipemic or icteric may give erroneous results when the laboratory employs optical coagulometers for clot-based testing. When specimens are cloudy or highly colored, the clinical laboratory scientist employs an alternative mechanical detection system. Lipemia and icterus may cause a recollect.[5]
- Slowed or stopped venous circulation is stasis. Stasis causes local concentration of factor VIII/von Willebrand factor (VWF), which may result in false shortening of clot-based coagulation test results. When collecting blood, the phlebotomist must remove the tourniquet within 1 minute of its application to avoid stasis.[6]

Managers of many hemostasis specialty laboratories insist that specimens from patients who are difficult to draw and specimens for specialized tests such as platelet aggregometry be collected by syringe, as described in the following sections. Many hemostasis laboratories employ clinical laboratory scientists and phlebotomists who are specially trained for specimen collection to ensure the integrity of the specimen.

TABLE 45-1 Hemostasis Specimen Collection Errors Requiring Recollects

Short draw	Whole-blood volume <90% of required volume
Clot in specimen	Each specimen must be visually inspected before centrifugation
Visible hemolysis	Hemolysis indicates factitious activation of coagulation mechanism and platelets
Lipemia or icterus	Optical instruments may not measure clots in cloudy or highly colored specimens. The scientist reflexes to a mechanical instrument
Prolonged tourniquet application	Stasis elevates concentration of VWF and factor VIII and shortens clot-based tests

Hemostasis Specimen Collection with Syringes and Winged Needle Sets

Although impractical for high-volume hemostasis screening, the syringe occasionally is used in place of evacuated blood collection units. Syringes are especially useful for collecting hemostasis specimens from patients whose veins are small or fragile or scarred by repeated venipunctures. The use of syringes presents additional needle-stick risk to the phlebotomist, however, so careful training and handling are essential.

The phlebotomist selects sterile syringes of 20 mL capacity or less with nonthreaded "Luer-slip" hubs. The phlebotomist assembles the syringes: a winged needle set (Fig. 45-1), a

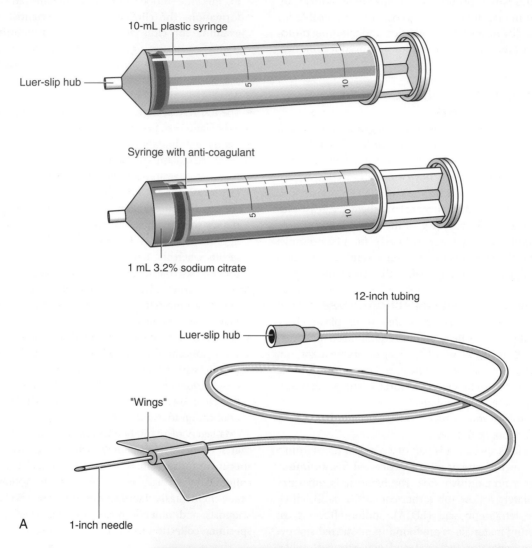

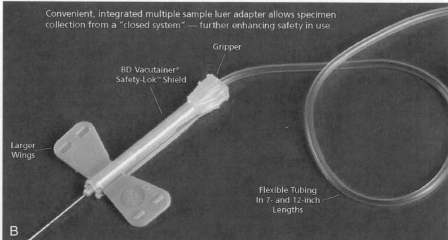

Figure 45-1 A, Syringes and winged needle set for collecting special hemostasis specimens. **B,** Winged needle set illustrating safety interlock.

tubing clamp, and standard venipuncture materials. The phlebotomist then uses the following protocol:

1. Attach the syringe to the needle set hub.
2. Prepare the patient for venipuncture, and then insert the winged needle. Immobilize the needle set tubing by loosely taping it to the arm about 2 inches from the needle.
3. Fill the syringe.
4. Place the syringe on a clean surface, and clamp the tubing near the hub.
5. Attach a second syringe if needed; release the clamp and fill the syringe.
6. Replace the clamp, and remove the needle set.
7. Immediately activate the needle cover.

Having seen to the patient's welfare, the phlebotomist cautiously transfers the blood specimen to sealed evacuated tubes by affixing a 19 gauge needle to each syringe and by gently pushing the needle through the stopper. To avoid needle-stick injury, the tube must be placed in a rack, not hand-held, before the puncture is made. The specimen is allowed to flow gently down the side. The specimen is not pushed forcibly into the tube because agitation causes hemolysis and platelet activation. The transfer must be accomplished within a few seconds of the time the syringe is filled, and the tube must be gently inverted at least six times. The specimen volume must be correct.

Choosing Needles for Hemostasis Specimens

Whether using evacuated collection tubes or syringes, the bore of the needle should be sufficient to prevent activation of platelets and plasma procoagulants. If the overall specimen is 25 mL, a 20 gauge or 21 gauge thin-wall needle is used (Table 45-2). For a larger specimen, a 19 gauge needle is required. A 23 gauge needle is acceptable for pediatric patients or patients whose veins are small.

Collecting Hemostasis Specimens from Indwelling Catheters

Blood specimens may be drawn from central or peripheral lines. Before collecting blood for hemostasis testing, the line must be flushed with 5 mL of saline, and the first 5 mL of blood, or six times the internal volume of the catheter, must be collected and discarded. Avoid flushing with heparin. Blood is collected into a syringe and transferred to an evacuated tube as described in the section on hemostasis specimen collection with syringes and winged needle sets.

Collecting Hemostasis Specimens by Capillary Puncture

Several near-patient testing instruments offer clot-based coagulation screens using 10 to 50 μL of whole capillary blood, including the following:

- I-stat and I-stat 1 (Abbott Point of Care, Inc., East Windsor, N.J.)
- INRatio PT/INR (Hemosense, Inc., San Jose, Calif.)
- Gem PCL Plus (Instrumentation Laboratory, Inc, Lexington, Mass.)
- Hemochron Jr. Signature Microcoagulation System, the Hemochron Jr. II Microcoagulation System, and the Protime Microcoagulation System (International Technidyne, Edison, N.J.)
- CoaguCheck and CoaguCheck Plus diagnostic coagulation systems (Roche Diagnostics/Boehringer Mannheim Corporation, Indianapolis, Ind)

These instruments are designed to perform prothrombin time (PT) and activated partial thromboplastin time (PTT) tests. Portable instrument results adequately correspond with laboratory plasma-based techniques[7] and provide the capability for point of care testing, self-testing, and neonatal testing.[8] The capillary puncture must be free flowing at the time the blood is captured in the instrument cartridge.

Anticoagulants Used for Hemostasis Specimens

Buffered Sodium Citrate (Primary Hemostasis Anticoagulant)

The anticoagulant used for hemostasis testing is buffered 3.2% (0.105-0.109M) sodium citrate, $Na_3C_6H_5O_7 \cdot 2H_2O$, molecular weight 294.10. Sodium citrate binds calcium ions to prevent coagulation. The buffer stabilizes specimen pH as long as the stopper remains in place.[9]

The anticoagulant solution is mixed with blood to produce a 1:10 ratio; 1 part anticoagulant to 10 parts final solution (9 parts blood). In most cases, 0.3 mL of anticoagulant is mixed with 2.7 mL of whole blood, the volumes in the most commonly used evacuated collection tubes, but any volumes are valid, provided that the 1:10 ratio is maintained. The ratio yields a final citrate concentration of 10.5 to 10.9 mMol/L of anticoagulant in whole blood.[10]

Adjusting Sodium Citrate Volume for High Hematocrits

The 1:10 ratio is effective provided that the hematocrit is 55% or less. In polycythemia, the decrease in plasma volume relative to whole blood unacceptably increases the anticoagulant-to-plasma ratio, causing falsely prolonged clot-based coagulation test results. The phlebotomist provides a tube with a relatively

TABLE 45-2 Choosing Needles for Hemostasis Specimen Collection

Application	Preferred Needle Gauge and Length
Adult with good veins, specimen ≤25 mL	20 gauge or 21 gauge thin-wall, 1 or 1.25 inches
Adult with good veins, specimen ≥25 mL	19 gauge, 1 or 1.25 inches
Adult with small veins or child	23 gauge but apply minimal pressure
Transfer blood from syringe to tube	19 gauge
Syringe with winged needle set	20 gauge or 21 gauge thin-wall. Use only for small, friable, or hardened veins or special coagulation testing

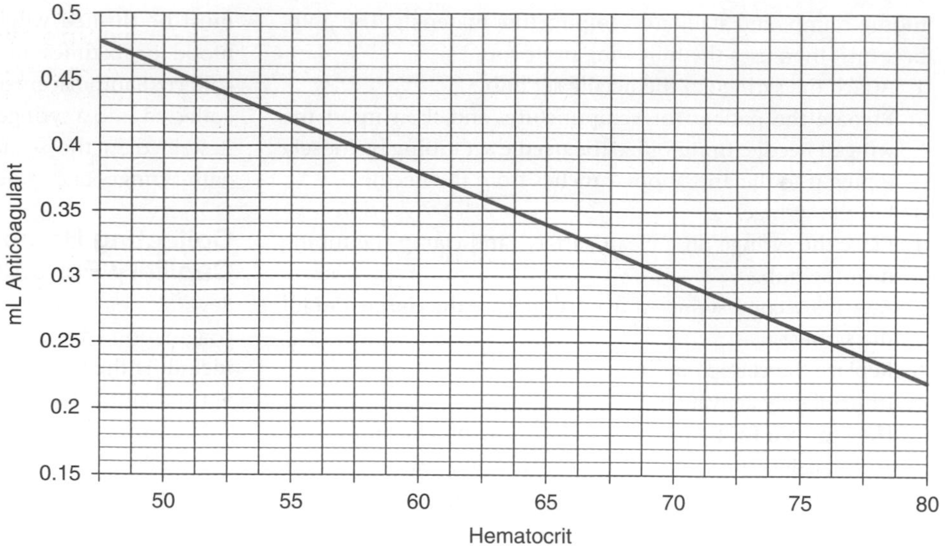

Figure 45-2 Graph for computing the volume of anticoagulant in a 5-mL specimen when the patient's hematocrit is 55%. (From Ingram GIC, Brozovic M, Slater NGP: Bleeding Disorders, Investigations, and Management, 2nd ed. Oxford: Blackwell, 1982:244-245.)

reduced anticoagulant volume for collecting blood from a patient whose hematocrit is known to be 55%. The amount of anticoagulant needed may be computed for a 5-mL total volume specimen from the graph in Figure 45-2 or by using the following formula, which may be used for any total volume:

$$C = (1.85 \times 10^{-3})(100 - H)V$$

Where C is volume of sodium citrate in milliliters, V is volume of whole blood–sodium citrate solution in milliliters, and H is hematocrit in percent. There is no evidence suggesting a need for increasing the volume of anticoagulant in anemia, even when the hematocrit is less than 20%.

Hemostasis Applications of Ethylenediamine Tetraacetic Acid and Heparin Anticoagulated Specimens

Few data support the use of EDTA anticoagulated specimens for coagulation testing, although one comparison study indicates EDTA specimens may be used for PT monitoring of oral anticoagulant therapy.[11] EDTA is used for complete blood counts, including platelet counts, and may be required for specimens used for molecular genetic testing, such as testing for factor V Leiden mutation or the prothrombin 20210 mutation. Heparinized specimens have never been validated for coagulation testing; however, other anticoagulant formulations, such as in vitro hirudin, are in trials.[12]

HEMOSTASIS SPECIMEN MANAGEMENT

Hemostasis Specimen Transport and Storage
Hemostasis Specimen Storage Temperature
Sodium citrate whole-blood specimens are kept stoppered to maintain pH and retained in a vertical position with the stopper uppermost. Specimens collected for platelet aggregometry are maintained at 18° C to 24° C, never at refrigerator

temperatures (2° C to 4° C) (Table 45-3). Specimens collected for the PT may be maintained at 18° C to 24° C and the PTT at 2° C to 4° C or 18° C to 24° C during transport but should never be stored at temperatures greater than 24° C. Heat destroys the activity of coagulation factor VIII. Specimens collected for PT testing are held at 18° C to 24° C and tested within 24 hours of the time of collection.[13]

Hemostasis Specimen Storage Time
Specimens collected for PT testing may be held at either 18° C to 24° C or 2° C to 4° C and tested within 24 hours of the time of collection. Specimens collected for PTT testing also may be held at 18° C to 24° C or 2° C to 4° C, but must be tested within 4 hours of the time of collection, provided that the specimen does not contain unfractionated heparin anticoagulant. If a patient is receiving unfractionated heparin therapy, specimens for PTT testing must be centrifuged within 1 hour of the time of collection, and the plasma, which should be platelet-poor plasma (PPP), must tested within 4 hours of the time of collection.[14]

Preparation of Hemostasis Specimens for Assays
Whole-Blood Specimens Used for Platelet Aggregometry
Blood for whole-blood platelet aggregometry or lumiaggregometry must be collected with 3.2% sodium citrate and held at 18° C to 24° C until testing. Chilling destroys platelet activity. Aggregometry may be started immediately and must be completed within 3 hours of specimen collection. The scientist mixes the specimen by gentle inversion, checks for clots just before testing, and rejects specimens with clots. Most specimens for whole-blood aggregometry are mixed 1:1 with normal saline before testing, although if the platelet count is less than $200 \times 10^9/L$, the specimen is tested undiluted.[15]

TABLE 45-3 Hemostasis Specimen Storage Times and Temperatures

Application	Temperature (°C)	Time
PT with no unfractionated heparin present in specimen	18-24	24 h
PTT with no unfractionated heparin present in specimen	2-4 or 18-24	4 h
PTT for unfractionated heparin therapy	2-4 or 18-24	Separate within 1 h, test within 4 h
PT when unfractionated heparin is present in specimen	2-4 or 18-24	Separate within 1 h, test within 4 h
Factor assays except factor VII	2-4 or 18-24	4 h
Factor VII assay	18-24	4 h
Optical platelet aggregometry using PRP	18-24	Wait 30 min, test within 3 h
Whole-blood aggregometry	18-24	Test within 3 h
Storage for 2 wk	−20	2 wk
Storage for 6 mo	−70	6 mo

Platelet-Rich Plasma Specimens Used for Platelet Aggregometry

Optical platelet aggregometers are designed to test platelet-rich plasma (PRP), plasma with a platelet count of 200 to 300 × 10^9/L. Sodium citrate–anticoagulated blood first is checked visually for clots, then centrifuged at 50g for 30 minutes with the stopper in place to maintain the pH. The supernatant plasma is transferred by plastic pipette to a clean plastic tube, and the tube is sealed and stored at 18° C to 24° C until the test is begun. PRP aggregometry is initiated 30 minutes after the specimen is centrifuged and completed within 3 hours of the time of collection. An aliquot of the plasma is counted to ensure the platelet count is between 200 and 300 × 10^9/L. To produce sufficient PRP, the original specimen must measure 9 to 12 mL of whole blood.

Platelet-Poor Plasma Required for Most Clot-Based Testing

Most clot-based plasma coagulation tests require PPP. PPP is plasma with a platelet count of less than 10 × 10^9/L.[16] Sodium citrate–anticoagulated whole blood is centrifuged at 1500g for 15 minutes with the stopper in place to maintain the pH and prevent aerosolization of the specimen during centrifugation. The hemostasis laboratory manager may choose alternate forces and times, provided that the resulting specimen is consistently platelet poor.

The presence of greater than 10 × 10^9/L platelets may affect clot-based test results. Platelets may release the membrane phospholipid phosphatidylserine that neutralizes lupus anticoagulant if present. Platelets secrete fibrinogen, factors V and VIII, and VWF (Chapter 13). These may shorten or desensitize PTs, PTTs, and clot-based coagulation assays. Finally, platelets release platelet factor 4 (PF4), a protein that binds and neutralizes therapeutic heparin in vitro, factitiously shortening the PTT.

The clinical laboratory scientist routinely counts coagulation plasmas to ensure they are platelet poor and inspects the PPP for hemolysis, lipemia, and icterus. Visible hemolysis implies platelet or coagulation pathway activation, so the specimen is rejected, and a new specimen is collected. Lipemia and icterus may affect the end point results of optical coagulation instruments. The operator should maintain a separate mechanical end point coagulometer to substitute for the optical instrument if the specimen is too cloudy for optical determinations.

Long-Term Hemostasis Specimen Storage Requires Freezing

If the hemostasis test cannot be completed within the prescribed interval, the laboratory scientist must centrifuge the specimen at a force and time sufficient to yield PPP. The supernatant PPP must be transferred by plastic pipette to a plastic tube, stoppered, quick-frozen, and stored at −20° C for 2 weeks or less or −70° C for 6 months or less. At the time the test is performed, the specimen must be thawed rapidly at 37° C, mixed well, and tested within 1 hour of the time it is removed from the freezer. If it cannot be tested immediately, the specimen may be stored at 2° C to 4° C for 2 hours after thawing.

PLATELET FUNCTION TESTS

A platelet count is performed, and the blood film is reviewed before beginning platelet function tests because thrombocytopenia is a common cause of mucocutaneous hemorrhage (Chapter 43).[17] Qualitative platelet abnormalities are suspected only when systemic hemorrhagic symptoms such as easy bruising, petechiae, purpura, or epistaxis are present, and the platelet count exceeds 50 × 10^9/L (Chapter 44). Although hereditary platelet function disorders are rare, acquired disorders, associated with hemorrhage and thrombosis, are common. Acquired defects often are associated with liver disease, renal disease, myeloproliferative disorders, myelodysplastic syndromes, myeloma, uremia, autoimmune disorders, anemias, and drug therapy (Chapter 44). Platelet morphology is often a clue; Bernard-Soulier syndrome is associated with mild thrombocytopenia and large gray platelets (see Fig. 44-1). The presence of large platelets with an elevated mean platelet volume often indicates rapid platelet turnover, such as in immune thrombocytopenic purpura or thrombotic thrombocytopenic purpura. Giant or bizarre platelets are seen in myeloproliferative disorders, acute leukemia, and myelodysplastic syndromes.

Bleeding Time Test for Platelet Function

The bleeding time test is occasionally helpful for diagnosing an unexplored bleeding disorder, although it fails as a screen.[18] Recording the duration of bleeding from a controlled puncture wound imperfectly assesses the adhesion and aggregation components of platelet function. Results also are prolonged in vascular disease such as scurvy or vasculitis.

Bleeding time tests were first described by Duke in 1910[19] and Ivy[20] in 1941. These tests failed to correct for the critical nonplatelet variables of intracapillary pressure, skin thickness at the puncture site, and size and depth of the wound, all of which interfere with the accurate interpretation of the test.

In the current bleeding time method, the clinical laboratory scientist places a blood pressure cuff on the upper arm and inflates it to 40 mm Hg to control intracapillary pressure in the forearm. A site on the volar surface of the forearm near the antecubital crease is selected and prepared. The skin thickness in this area varies only slightly from one individual to another, so the results are comparable, provided that the area is free of superficial blood vessels, rashes, hair, and scar tissue. A spring-loaded bleeding time lancet that produces a standard wound 5 mm long and 1 mm deep is placed firmly on the site parallel to the long axis of the arm and triggered. Simplate (Organon Teknika Corp., Durham, N.C.) and Surgicutt (International Technidyne Corp., Edison, N.J.) are suitable bleeding time lancets. A stopwatch is started at the same moment the lancet is triggered.[21] The clinical laboratory scientist safely discards the lancet and blots the wound with filter paper every 30 seconds, taking care that the paper contacts only the blood and not the wound. Touching the wound dislodges the platelet clot and prolongs the result. Blotting continues until the bleeding stops, then the watch is stopped, and the interval is recorded. The clinical laboratory scientist must place a pressure or "butterfly" bandage over the site to reduce scarring.

The reference range for the standardized lancet bleeding time is 2-9 minutes. The bleeding time is prolonged in thrombocytopenia, hereditary and acquired platelet dysfunction, von Willebrand disease, afibrinogenemia, severe hypofibrinogenemia, and vascular disorders. A single dose of aspirin causes a measurable prolongation of the bleeding time in about 50% of normal individuals.[22] Many other drugs may give prolonged results. Owing to its poor predictive value for bleeding and its tendency to scar the forearm, the bleeding time assay is falling into disuse.

Platelet Aggregometry and Lumiaggregometry

Functional platelets adhere to subendothelial collagen, aggregate with each other, and secrete the contents of their α granules, lysosomes, and dense bodies. Normal adhesion requires intact platelet membranes and plasma VWF. Normal aggregation requires that platelet membranes are intact, the plasma fibrinogen level is normal, and normal secretions come from platelet organelles. Platelet adhesion, aggregation, and secretion are assessed using in vitro platelet aggregometry.

An aggregometer is an instrument designed to measure platelet aggregation in a suspension of citrated whole blood or PRP. The specimen is collected and managed in compliance with standard laboratory protocol and maintained at 18° C to 24° C until testing begins. Specimens for aggregometry may first stand 30 minutes after collection while the platelets regain their responsiveness and must be tested within 3 hours of collection to avoid deterioration of labile plasma and platelet procoagulants. After electronically calibrating the instrument in accordance with manufacturer instructions, the operator pipettes the specimens to instrument-compatible cuvettes, drops in plasticized stir bars, and allows the specimens to warm to 37° C for 10 minutes in incubation wells before testing. The operator transfers the first cuvette, containing specimen and stir bar, to the instrument's reaction well and starts the stirring device and recording device, often a desktop computer. The stirring device turns the stir bar at 800 to 1200 rpm, keeping the platelets in suspension. After a few seconds, an agonist (aggregating agent) is pipetted forcibly into the specimen to start the reaction. Aggregation is complete in 6 to 10 minutes. The operator prepares to retest the next specimen cuvette with another agonist.

Platelet Aggregometry Using Platelet-Rich Plasma

PRP aggregometry is performed using an aggregometer that is a specialized photometer (PACKS-4; Helena Laboratories, Beaumont, Tex.). PRP is prepared and adjusted, if necessary, to a count of 200 to 300 × 10^9/L by mixing with PPP. The adjusted PRP is placed in a cuvette equipped with a stir bar, warmed to 37° C, and transferred to the reaction well. The instrument directs focused light through the sample cuvette to a photomultiplier (Fig. 45-3). As the PRP is stirred, the recorder first stabilizes to form the baseline, near 0% transmission. In a normal specimen, after the agonist is added, the platelets' shape changes from discoid to spherical. The intensity of the transmitted light increases slightly in proportion to the degree of shape change. Percent transmittance is monitored continuously and recorded on the chart (Fig. 45-4). As platelet aggregates form, more light passes through the PRP, and the recorder begins to move toward 100% light transmission. Abnormalities are reflected in diminished or absent shape change and diminished aggregation.

Whole-Blood Platelet Aggregometry

In whole-blood aggregometry, platelet aggregation is measured using electrical impedance in a saline-diluted, whole-blood suspension. Parallel electrodes that produce a small direct

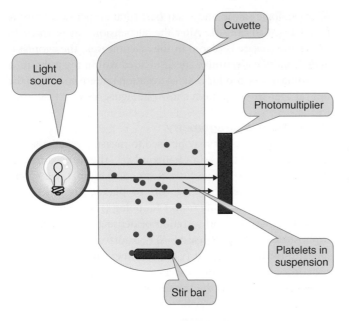

Figure 45-3 Platelet-rich plasma in an optical aggregometer. Platelet count is approximately $200 \times 10^9/L$, and platelets are maintained in suspension by a magnetic stir bar turning at 1000 rpm. (Courtesy of Kathy Jacobs, Chronolog, Inc., Havertown, Penn.)

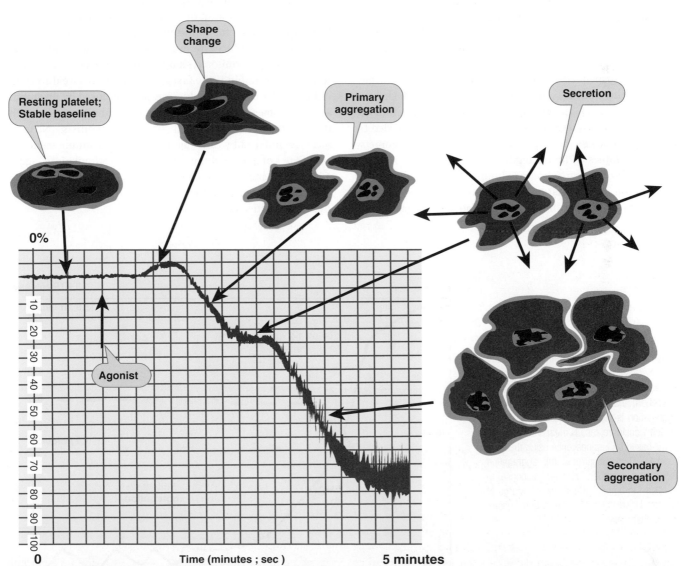

Figure 45-4 Optical aggregometry occurs in five phases: baseline at 0% aggregation, shape change after addition of agonist, primary aggregation, ADP and ATP release, and second-wave aggregation that forms large aggregates. (Courtesy of Kathy Jacobs, Chronolog, Inc., Havertown, Penn.)

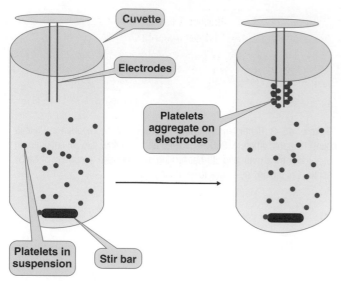

Figure 45-5 The aggregating platelets form a layer on the electrodes, and current is impeded by the platelet layer. Resistance (Ω) is proportional to aggregation, providing a tracing that resembles optical aggregometry. (Courtesy of Kathy Jacobs, Chronolog, Inc., Havertown, Penn.)

current are suspended within the blood suspension. As aggregation occurs, platelets collect on the electrodes, reducing the current (Fig. 45-5). The change is directly proportional to the level of platelet aggregation and is amplified and recorded by the aggregometer's circuitry. A whole-blood aggregometry tracing resembles a PRP tracing.

Whole-blood aggregometry eliminates the need for PRP preparation. The operator pipettes an aliquot of properly mixed whole blood to the cuvette and adds an equal volume of physiologic saline and a stir bar. Total suspension volume may be 300 to 500 μL. After the suspension has warmed to 37° C, the cuvette is placed in the reaction well, the agonist is added, and the electrodes are suspended within the mixture. A recording device produces an aggregation pattern similar to the optical aggregation pattern shown in Figure 45-4.

Platelet Lumiaggregometry

The lumiaggregometer may be used to measure platelet aggregation and secretion simultaneously.[23] The procedure for lumiaggregometry differs little from conventional aggregometry and simplifies the diagnosis of platelet dysfunction.[24] The instrument, available from Chronolog (Havertown, Penn.) records aggregation and secretion of dense granule adenosine triphosphate (ATP). Released ATP oxidizes a firefly-derived luciferin-luciferase reagent (Chrono-lume; Chronolog) to give proportional chemiluminescence. The instrument detects, amplifies, and records the light emission.[25]

Lumiaggregometry may be performed using whole blood or PRP.[26] To perform lumiaggregometry, the operator adds an ATP standard to the first aliquot of specimen, then adds luciferin-luciferase and tests for full luminescence. A second aliquot is prepared with the luciferin-luciferase, an agonist is added, and the specimen is monitored simultaneously for aggregation and secretion. Thrombin is the first agonist used because thrombin induces full secretion. The luminescence induced by thrombin addition is measured, recorded, and used for comparison with the luminescence produced by other agonists. Normal secretion induced by other agonists produces luminescence at about 50% of that resulting from thrombin stimulation. Figure 45-6 depicts simultaneous aggregation and secretion responses to thrombin; Figure 45-7 is a scanning electron micrograph of resting and activated platelets.

Figure 45-6 Normal lumiaggregometry tracing *(solid line)*, illustrating monophasic aggregation curve with superimposed release (secretion, *dashed line*) reaction curve. Aggregation is measured in ohms (Ω) using the left Y scale; release is measured in μmol/L ATP based on luminescence using the right Y scale. Curve illustrates full aggregation *(solid)* and secretion *(dashed)* response to 1 U/mL thrombin. (Courtesy of Margaret Fritsma, University of Alabama at Birmingham, Birmingham, Ala.)

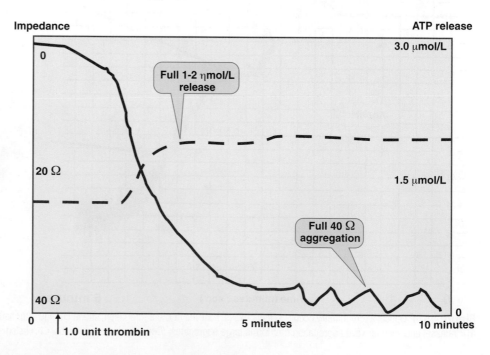

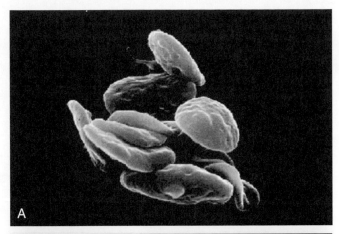
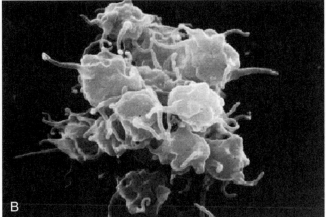

Figure 45-7 Scanning electron micrograph of resting **(A)** and activated **(B)** platelets.

TABLE 45-4 Platelet Aggregometry Agonists, Reaction Concentrations, and Platelet Receptors

Agonist	Typical Concentration	Receptors
Thrombin	1 U/mL	Protease activatable receptor 1 (PAR-1) and PAR-4; GP Ibα and GP V
ADP	1-10 μmol/L	P2Y$_1$, P2Y$_{12}$
Epinephrine	2-10 μmol/L	α$_2$-adrenergic receptor
Collagen	1-5 μg/mL	GP Ia/IIa, GP VI
Arachidonic acid	500 μmol/L	TPα, TPβ
Ristocetin	1 mg/mL	GP Ib/V/IX in association with VWF

Platelet Agonists (Activating Agents) Used in Aggregometry

The agonists used most in clinical practice are thrombin adenosine diphosphate (ADP), epinephrine, collagen, arachidonic acid, and ristocetin. Table 45-4 lists representative concentrations and platelet activation pathways tested by each agonist. Small volumes (2-5 mL) of concentrated agonist are used so that their dilutional effect in the reaction system is negligible.

Thrombin.   Thrombin cleaves two platelet membrane protease-activatable receptors (PAR), PAR-1 and PAR-2, both members of the seven-transmembrane repeat receptor family (Chapter 13). Thrombin also cleaves glycoprotein (GP) 1bα and GP V. Activation involves G proteins and the eicosanoid and the diacyglyceryl pathways and results in full secretion and aggregation. In lumiaggregometry, the operator ordinarily begins with 1 U/mL of thrombin to determine full secretion. Normally, thrombin induces the release of 1 to 2 M of ATP, detected by the firefly luciferin-luciferase luminescence assay. Other agonists, such as 1 to 5 μg/mL of collagen, induce the release of 0.5 to 1 ηmol/L of ATP. Thrombin-induced secretion may be diminished to less than 1 M in severe storage pool disorders but is relatively unaffected by membrane disorders or pathway enzyme deficiencies. Reagent thrombin is stored dry

at −20° C and reconstituted with physiologic saline before use. Leftover reconstituted thrombin may be aliquotted, refrozen, and reused.

Adenosine Diphosphate.   ADP binds P2Y$_1$ and P2Y$_{12}$, also members of the seven-transmembrane repeat receptor family. ADP-induced platelet activation relies on the G protein response and the eicosanoid synthesis pathway to suppress adenyl cyclase activity and induce calcium mobilization to the platelet cytosol. The resulting increase in cytosolic free calcium mediates platelet activation and induces secretion of dense granule stored ADP, which activates neighboring platelets.

ADP has been the most commonly used agonist, particularly in systems that measure only aggregation. When testing normal specimens, the ADP concentration may be adjusted to between 1 μmol/L and 10 μmol/L to induce "biphasic" aggregation (see Fig. 45-4). At ADP concentrations near 1 μmol/L, platelets achieve primary aggregation, followed in seconds by disaggregation, a deflection from baseline that lasts 1 to 2 minutes and returns to baseline. Primary aggregation involves shape change with formation of microaggregates, both reversible. Secondary aggregation is full aggregate formation after release of platelet ADP. At ADP concentrations near 10 μmol/L, there is simultaneous irreversible shape change, secretion, and formation of aggregates, resulting in a monophasic curve and full deflection of the tracing. In a biphasic tracing, reagent ADP induces shape change that is followed by a brief flattening of the curve called *lag phase* just before secretion of endogenous ADP begins.

Clinical laboratory scientists make some effort to reach the correct ADP concentration that is able to generate the elusive biphasic curve. This enables them to use aggregometry alone to distinguish between membrane-associated platelet defects and storage pool or release defects. This effort grows ephemeral with the advent of lumiaggregometry, which provides a more direct measure of platelet secretion. Aggregation to ADP (usually at 5 μmol/L) is diminished in platelet membrane disorders, cyclooxygenase pathway enzyme deficiencies, nonsteroidal anti-inflammatory drug (NSAID) and aspirin therapy, or storage pool disorders. ADP is stored at −20° C, reconstituted with physiologic saline, and used immediately. Leftover reconstituted ADP subsequently may be aliquotted and refrozen for later use.

Epinephrine. Epinephrine binds the α-adrenergic receptor, identical to muscle receptors, and activates the platelet through the same metabolic pathways as exogenous ADP. The results of epinephrine-induced aggregation match those of ADP except that epinephrine cannot induce aggregation in storage pool disorder or release defects, no matter how high its concentration. For unknown reasons, the platelets of about 10% of normal individuals do not respond to epinephrine. Epinephrine is stored at 2° C to 5° C, reconstituted with distilled water, and used. Leftover reconstituted epinephrine may be aliquotted and frozen for later use.

Collagen. Collagen binds GP Ia/IIa and GP VI but induces no primary wave. After a lag of 30 to 60 seconds, aggregation begins, and a monophasic curve develops. Collagen-induced aggregation using collagen at 1 to 5 μg/mL depends on intact membrane receptors, membrane G protein integrity, and normal eicosanoid pathway function. Loss of collagen-induced aggregation may indicate a membrane abnormality, storage pool disorder, release defect, or effects of aspirin and other NSAIDs. Most managers purchase lyophilized fibrillar collagen preparations such as Chrono-Par Collagen. Collagen is stored at 2° C to 5° C and used without further dilution. Collagen may not be frozen.

Arachidonic Acid. Arachidonic acid assesses the viability of the platelet eicosanoid pathway. Free acid at 500 ηmol/L is added to the specimen to induce a monophasic aggregometry curve with virtually no lag phase. Aggregation is independent of membrane integrity. Deficiencies in eicosanoid pathway enzymes, including suppressed cyclooxygenase, result in reduced aggregation and secretion. Arachidonic acid is readily oxidized and must be stored at −20° C in the dark. The clinical laboratory scientist dilutes arachidonic acid with a solution of bovine albumin for immediate use. Aliquots of bovine albumin–dissolved arachidonic acid may be thawed and refrozen three times.

Ristocetin: Ristocetin-Induced Platelet Aggregation Test. Although this test is called the *ristocetin-induced platelet aggregation* test, ristocetin actually induces an *agglutination* reaction because there is no platelet shape change and little secretion. A normal result implies that VWF is present and the platelets possess a functional VWF receptor, GP Ib/V/IX (Chapter 13).[27]

Ristocetin induces a monophasic aggregation tracing from a normal specimen. Specimens from patients with von Willebrand disease (except subtype 2b) produce a reduced or absent ristocetin reaction to 10 mg/mL of ristocetin, although all other agonists generate normal tracings (Table 45-5). Exogenous VWF from normal plasma restores the ristocetin aggregation reaction, confirming the diagnosis. In patients

TABLE 45-5 Typical Normal Ranges in Platelet Aggregometry

Agonist	Concentration	Aggregation Impedance	ATP Secretion
Thrombin	1 U	Not recorded	1-2 ηmol/L
Collagen	1 μg/mL	15-27 Ω	0.5-1.7 ηmol/L
	5 μg/mL	15-31 Ω	0.9-1.7 ηmol/L
ADP	5 μmol/L	1-17 Ω	0.0-0.7 ηmol/L
	10 μmol/L	6-24 Ω	0.4-1.7 ηmol/L
Arachidonic acid	500 μmol/L	5-17 Ω	0.6-1.4 ηmol/L
Ristocetin	1 mg/mL	>10 Ω	Not recorded

with Bernard-Soulier syndrome, a congenital abnormality of the GP Ib or IX portion of the GP Ib/V/IX receptor results in diminished ristocetin reaction that is not corrected by addition of VWF.

In subtype 2b von Willebrand disease, a VWF gain-of-function mutation, aggregation occurs even when reduced concentrations of ristocetin (1 mg/mL) are added. This response illustrates the increased affinity of large VWF multimers for platelet receptors.

Any discussion of von Willebrand disease must register the expected variation in laboratory results from one patient to another in the same kindred and from time to time in one patient. The ristocetin-induced platelet aggregation test result is diagnostic in only about 70% of cases. Consequently, the clinical laboratory scientist must add the ristocetin cofactor test, the immunometric VWF antigen assay, the collagen binding assay, and the coagulation factor VIII activity assay to the von Willebrand disease profile. Ultimate confirmation and characterization of von Willebrand disease is based on sodium dodecyl sulfate-polyacrylimide gel (SDS-PAGE) immunoelectrophoresis to characterize VWF monomers.[28]

Ristocetin Cofactor Assay for von Willebrand Factor. One essential refinement of ristocetin aggregometry is the substitution of formalin-fixed or lyophilized normal "reagent" platelets for patient's platelets.[29] When reagent platelets are used, the test is called the *ristocetin cofactor* or *VWF activity assay*. The clinical laboratory scientist prepares the patient's PPP; mixes it with reagent platelets; adds ristocetin; and performs optical, not impedance, aggregometry. The ristocetin cofactor assay yields a proportional relationship between VWF activity and the aggregometry response of the reagent platelets. Comparison of the aggregation results of patients' PPP with standard dilutions of normal PPP permits a quantitative expression of the VWF activity level. The ristocetin cofactor test also is available as an automated assay on the Dade-Behring (Deerfield, Ill.) BCT or the BCS instrument.

Summary of Agonist Responses in Various Platelet Disorders. Thrombin produces maximum ATP release through at least two membrane binding sites. Arachidonic acid

TABLE 45-6 Anticipated Aspirin Ranges and Aspirin-like Disorder in Platelet Aggregometry

Agonist	Concentration	Aggregation Impedance	ATP Secretion
ADP	5 μmol/L	1-13 Ω	<0.1 ηmol/L
Collagen	1 μg/mL	10-18 Ω*	0.2-0.4 ηmol/L
	5 μg/mL	21-25 Ω*	0.3-0.7 ηmol/L
Collagen	1 μg/mL	10-18 Ω†	0.2-0.4 ηmol/L
	5 μg/mL	10-18 Ω†	0.2-0.4 ηmol/L
Arachidonic acid	500 μmol/L	< 0.5 Ω§	< 0.1 ηmol/L

*Aspirin suppresses the 1 μg/mL collagen aggregation ≥50% compared to the 5 μg/mL collagen response.
†Aspirin-like disorder suppresses both collagen responses proportionally.
§Arachidonic acid does not distinguish aspirin effect from aspirin-like disorder.

tests for cyclooxygenase deficiencies. Collagen, ADP, and epinephrine test for abnormalities in their respective membrane binding site and the eicosanoid synthesis pathway. Ristocetin checks for abnormalities of plasma VWF in von Willebrand disease. The following conditions may be detected through platelet lumiaggregometry.

Nonsteroidal Anti-inflammatory Drugs and Platelet Aggregometry. NSAIDs such as aspirin, ibuprofen, indomethacin, and sulfinpyrazone permanently inactivate or temporarily inhibit cyclooxygenase; prevent secretion of dense granule serotonin, ADP, and ATP; and suppress secondary aggregation. Secretion and aggregation in response to the agonists ADP, epinephrine, and in particular collagen and arachidonic acid are reduced, although thrombin produces a normal secretion response. Ristocetin induces normal aggregation; secretion is not measured in the ristocetin reaction. The physician or clinical laboratory scientist must instruct the patient to avoid all drugs (if possible) for 1 week before blood is collected for aggregometry and particularly to avoid NSAIDs.

Platelet Release Defects: Deficient Eicosanoid Pathway Enzymes and Aggregometry. Congenital or acquired deficiencies of cyclooxygenase, thromboxane synthase, protein kinase C, or any enzyme in the eicosanoid activation pathway prevent secretion. Thrombin produces normal responses, but secretion and aggregation are diminished in response to the agonists ADP, epinephrine, collagen, and arachidonic acid. Because the aggregation responses resemble the responses seen after the use of NSAIDs, release defects are often called *aspirin-like* disorders. Aggregation to collagen at 1 μg/mL is reduced by NSAIDs and aspirin-like disorder; however, collagen aggregation at 5 μg/mL is reduced in platelet release defects, but not NSAIDs. A differential aggregation of 50% or greater between 1 μg/mL and 5 μg/mL of collagen may distinguish aspirin from aspirin-like disorder (Table 45-6).[30] Ristocetin induces the expected normal aggregation pattern.

Platelet Storage Pool Defects and Aggregometry. In a storage pool defect, ATP release in response to thrombin is reduced, as it is to ADP, epinephrine, arachidonic acid, and collagen (Table 45-7). Ristocetin induces normal aggregation.

Platelet Membrane Defects: Thrombasthenia and Aggregometry. Glanzmann thrombasthenia, a membrane

TABLE 45-7 Expected Results for Storage Pool Disorder for a Variety of Agonists

Agonist	Concentration	Aggregation Impedance	ATP Secretion
Thrombin	1 U/mL	Not recorded	<0.1 ηmol/L
Collagen	5 μg/mL	20 Ω	<0.1 ηmol/L
Arachidonic acid	500 μmol/L	12 Ω	<0.1 ηmol/L

defect characterized by dysfunction or loss of the GP IIb/IIIa receptor site, may be diagnosed by its characteristically diminished secretion and aggregation responses to all agonists except a modest response to arachidonic acid and full, but nondiagnostic, aggregation to ristocetin.

Acquired Platelet Disorders and Aggregometry. Platelets are defective in acquired hematologic and systemic disorders, such as acute leukemias, aplastic anemias, myeloproliferative disorders, myelodysplastic syndromes, myeloma, uremia, liver disease, and ethanol abuse. These disorders are investigated in any case where aggregation is abnormal and no other explanation is available. Platelet aggregometry may be used to predict the risk of bleeding or thrombosis in these disorders.[31]

Testing for Heparin-Induced Thrombocytopenia with Thrombosis

One percent to 5% of patients receiving unfractionated porcine heparin for more than 5 days develop heparin-dependent anti-PF4 antibodies that seem to cause thrombocytopenia with dangerous microvascular thrombi.[32] Suspicion of heparin-induced thrombocytopenia with thrombosis (HIT) requires immediate termination of heparin therapy.[33] A 40% decrease in platelet count during heparin therapy is an important signal for HIT, but this conclusion is mitigated by the fact that about 30% of patients who receive heparin develop an immediate, benign, limited thrombocytopenia.[34] Because 10% of hospital patients receive heparin during their stay, the laboratory must provide a procedure to confirm HIT and differentiate its types. Tests include aggregometry, washed platelet aggregometry, lumiaggregometry, serotonin release assay, and an enzyme immunoassay for the heparin-dependent anti-PF4 antibody.

Aggregometry or Lumiaggregometry Test for Heparin-Induced Thrombocytopenia

To perform aggregometry or lumiaggregometry testing, the patient must have no heparin for at least 4 hours.[35] Blood is collected into a plain or serum separator tube and allowed to clot. The serum is separated by centrifugation and heated to 56° C for 30 minutes to inactivate residual thrombin and prevent a false-positive test result. The serum is allowed to cool to room temperature before testing.

Whole blood is collected from at least two healthy donors whose platelets are proved to be functional by arachidonic acid–induced aggregometry and proved to be nonresponsive to therapeutic concentrations of heparin. The platelets of many normal individuals aggregate when heparin is added; these donors must be avoided because they give a false-positive result in the test system. Conversely, donors whose platelets are known to be exceptionally responsive to heparin-dependent antiplatelet antibody should be registered and reused because responsiveness varies. Donor whole blood or PRP may be used for the assay.

The clinical laboratory scientist prepares the heparin "agonist" by making dilutions in buffered saline from the same lot of heparin used for the patient's therapy. The dilutions are prepared so that 5-μL aliquots provide heparin concentrations of 0.1 U/mL, 0.5 U/mL, and 100 U/mL of final reaction mixture.

Approximately equal amounts of patient serum and donor whole blood or PRP are mixed, then 500 μL is pipetted to a reaction cuvette containing a plasticized stir bar. Next, 5 μL of heparin dilution or saline (negative control) is added, and the reaction is recorded for 6 to 10 minutes. Either aggregation or ATP release may be used as the marker. Saline and each heparin dilution in turn are mixed with specimen aliquots from each donor in separate cuvettes. For any reaction mixture that generates no response after 10 minutes, arachidonic acid is added to recheck for platelet activity.

A response of 10% or more above control in the 0.1 U/mL and 0.5 U/mL dilutions with no response in the 100 U/mL dilution indicates the presence of a heparin-dependent platelet antibody in the patient serum. The 100 U/mL dilution contains enough heparin to saturate any suspected serum antibody without activating the platelets.

Several conditions must be met for the aggregation test to yield valid results. If the saline control is positive, the patient's serum contains therapeutic heparin, a platelet alloantibody, or a platelet autoantibody. If the patient has been off heparin for at least 24 hours, the response is evidence of an alloantibody or autoantibody, which is confirmed immunometrically. The test depends on the presence of free heparin-dependent antibody in the patient's serum. In some cases of patients who have HIT and are still receiving heparin, the heparin-dependent antibody becomes fixed to their own platelets during clotting, leaving no detectable antibody in the serum. Although aggregometry is specific for HIT, it is only about 50% sensitive.[36]

Serotonin Release Assay for Heparin-Induced Thrombocytopenia

The ^{14}C-serotonin platelet release assay is more sensitive than aggregometry and is used in a few laboratories as a screen for HIT.[37] PRP from healthy donors is incubated with ^{14}C-serotonin and washed to remove the supernatant radioactive solution. Heat-inactivated patient serum or saline (control) is mixed with one of two heparin concentrations, 0.1 U/mL and 100 U/mL (final dilution) and with the ^{14}C-serotonin platelets, and the mixture is allowed to incubate for 60 minutes. EDTA in saline is added to stop the release reaction, and the supernatant is measured for radioactivity in a liquid scintillation counter. The percent release is calculated as follows:

$$\text{Percent release} = \frac{\text{release from test sample} - \text{background} \times 100}{\text{total radioactivity} - \text{background}}$$

Washed Platelet Test for Heparin-Induced Thrombocytopenia

The washed platelet test for HIT, a simplification of the serotonin release assay, also is available. In this test, washed platelets are mixed with test serum and observed for aggregation. This test may be as sensitive as the serotonin release assay.

Immunoassay of Heparin-Dependent Antiplatelet Antibody Based on Platelet Factor 4 Specificity

Amiral et al developed an HIT screening immunoassay based on their discovery that PF4 is the target for the heparin-dependent antiplatelet antibody.[38] Patient plasma is incubated in microtiter plate wells containing a solid-phase complex of highly purified PF4 and heparin or polysulfonate, a plastic molecule that resembles heparin. Heparin-dependent antiplatelet antibodies become bound to the PF4-heparin or PF4-polysulfonate complex. Bound antibodies are detected using enzyme-bound anti-human IgG, IgA, and IgM antibodies and a substrate chromophore. This test is more sensitive than lumiaggregometry or ^{14}C-serotonin platelet release and is able to show antibodies early in the development of HIT, but it may detect antibodies that are accompanied by no clinical symptoms. The immunoassay for heparin-dependent anti-PF4 antibodies is as sensitive and specific for HIT as the serotonin release assay.

QUANTITATIVE MEASUREMENT OF PLATELET ACTIVATION MARKERS

Plasma elevation of the platelet-specific proteins β-thromboglobulin and PF4 may accompany thrombotic stroke or coronary thrombosis.[39] The implication that in vivo platelet activation contributes to the condition or that the measurement of these proteins is of diagnostic or prognostic significance is under investigation.[40] Diagnostica Stago, Inc. (Asnières, France) produces enzyme immunoassay kits for PF4 and β-thromboglobulin under the brand names Asserachrom B-TG and Asserachrom PF4. Special collection techniques are necessary because PF4 and β-thromboglobulin test results may be invalidated by platelet activation during specimen collection.[41] Evacuated tubes containing citrate and the platelet aggregation inhibitors theophylline, adenosine, and dipyridamole (CTAD tubes) are required for specimen collection for these secretions. Plasma must undergo extraction before PF4 and β-thromboglobulin results are accurate because several eicosanoids cross-react with kit antibodies.

Thromboxane A_2, the active product of the eicosanoid pathway, has a half-life of 30 seconds, diffuses from the platelet, and is spontaneously reduced to thromboxane B_2, a stable, measurable plasma metabolite (Chapter 13). Efforts to produce a clinical plasma assay for thromboxane B_2 have been unsuccessful because special specimen management is required to prevent ex vivo platelet activation with factitious unregulated release of thromboxane B_2. Thromboxane B_2 is acted on by liver enzymes to produce an array of soluble urine metabolites, including 11-dehydrothromboxane B_2, which is stable and measurable.[42] Immunoassays of urine 11-dehydrothromboxane B_2 are used to characterize in vivo platelet activation.[43] These assays require no special specimen management and can be performed on random urine specimens. Urinary 11-dehydrothromboxane B_2 also may be used to monitor aspirin and NSAID therapy and to identify cases of therapy failure or antiplatelet therapy resistance.

CORRECTED PLATELET COUNT INCREMENT DURING THERAPY

Effectiveness of platelet concentrate transfusion is assessed using the corrected platelet count increment (CCI) calculation first described by Yankee et al in 1969.[44] The CCI is especially useful when the patient is suspected to be refractory to platelet therapy and provides more reliable and standardized information than the platelet count. To compute the CCI, platelet counts are performed before and 1 hour after administration of the platelet transfusion, and the following calculation is made:

$$\text{CCI at 1 h} = \frac{\text{post-transfusion} - \text{pretransfusion platelet count} \times \text{body surface area (m}^2)}{\text{number of platelets transfused (in multiples of } 10^{11})}$$

Where *CCI* is corrected count increment in platelets/10^{11}/m^2, *body surface area* is computed from height and weight, and *platelets* $\times 10^{11}$ is approximate number of platelets/unit of concentrate. A CCI of 7500 platelets/10^{11}/m^2 is generally regarded as an adequate post-transfusion response using this formula.[45] The body surface area in square meters is estimated from the nomogram of Sendroy and Cecchini[46] based on the weight and height of the recipient.

CLOT-BASED PLASMA PROCOAGULANT SCREENS

The Lee-White whole blood coagulation time test, described in 1913, was the first laboratory procedure designed to assess coagulation.[47] The Lee-White is no longer used, but it was the first in vitro clot procedure to employ a pervasive principle: The time interval from the initiation of coagulation to visible clot formation reflects the condition of the coagulation mechanism. A prolonged clotting time indicates coagulation inadequacy. A 1953 modification, the activated clotting time, supplies a particulate clot activator in the collection tube, speeding the clotting process. The activated clotting time is still used to monitor heparin therapy in high-dosage applications such as cardiac surgery (Chapter 46). The standard clinical battery of clot-based coagulation screening tests, which consists of the PT, PTT, and thrombin clotting time (TCT), uses the clotting time principle of the Lee-White and activated clotting time. Many additional specialized tests, such as coagulation factor assays, tests of fibrinolysis, inhibitor assays, reptilase (Atroxin) time, Russell viper venom time, dilute Russell viper venom time, and tests for circulating anticoagulants, also are based on the relationship between time to clot formation and coagulation function.

Prothrombin Time
Prothrombin Time Principle

PT thromboplastin reagents are prepared from recombinant or affinity-purified tissue factor suspended in phospholipids mixed with a buffered 0.025 M solution of calcium chloride. Some less responsive thromboplastins are organic extracts of emulsified rabbit brain or lung suspended in calcium chloride. When mixed with citrated PPP, the PT reagent triggers fibrin polymerization by activating plasma factor VII (Fig. 45-8). Calcium participates in the formation of the tissue factor–factor VIIa complex, the factor VIIIa–factor IXa complex, and the factor Va–factor Xa complex. The clot is detectable visually or by optical or electromechanical sensors. Although the coagulation scheme implies that the PT would be prolonged in deficiencies of fibrinogen, prothrombin, and factors V, VII, VIII, IX, and X, the procedure is most sensitive to factor VII deficiencies, moderately sensitive to factor V and X deficiencies, sensitive to severe fibrinogen and prothrombin deficiencies, and insensitive to deficiencies of factors VIII and IX.[48,49] The PT is prolonged in multiple factor deficiencies that include deficiencies of factors VII and X and is used most often to monitor the effects of oral anticoagulant warfarin (Coumadin) therapy.

Prothrombin Time Procedure

The thromboplastin–phospholipid–calcium chloride reagent is prewarmed to 37° C. An aliquot of test PPP, 0.05 or 0.1 mL, is transferred to the reaction vessel that also is maintained at 37° C. The PPP aliquot is incubated at 37° C for at least 3 and no more than 10 minutes. Aliquots that are incubated more than 10 minutes deteriorate because of the rapid degradation of factor VIII. They are affected further by evaporation. A premeasured volume of reagent, 0.1 or 0.2 mL, is forcibly added to the PPP aliquot, and a timer is started. As the clot forms, the timer stops, and the elapsed time is recorded. If the procedure is performed in duplicate, the duplicate values must be within 10% of their mean, or the test is repeated. Most

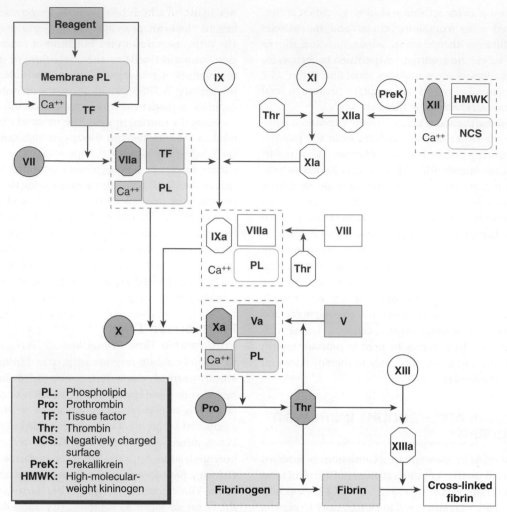

Figure 45-8 The PT reagent consists of tissue factor, phospholipid, and calcium. It activates the extrinsic and common pathways of the coagulation mechanism beginning with factor VII. The PT is affected by deficiencies in VII, X, V, prothrombin, and fibrinogen deficiency when the fibrinogen level is <100 mg/dL. The PT is prolonged in warfarin therapy because warfarin suppresses production of factors VII, X, and prothrombin. Factor VII has a short half-life (6 hours) and has the greatest effect on the PT.

Va, VIIIa	Activated factors V and VIII (cofactors)
XIa, Xa, IXa, VIIa	Activated factors XI, X, IX, VII (serine proteases)
XIIa	Activated factor XII (serine protease, not a procoagulant)
XIIIa	Activated factor XIII (transglutaminase)

laboratory scientists perform PTs using automated instruments with which these steps are strictly controlled. With automated instruments, duplicate testing is unnecessary.

Quality Control for Prothrombin Time and Partial Thromboplastin Time

The clinical laboratory scientist tests normal and prolonged control PPP specimens at the beginning of each 8-hour shift or with each change of reagent.[50] Although lyophilized control PPPs are commercially available, the laboratory manager may choose to collect and pool PPP specimens from designated subjects to make "home-brew" controls. In this case, the speci-

mens must be collected and managed using the same tubes, anticoagulant, and protocol as are used for patient plasma specimen collection. They are pooled, tested, and aliquotted. Whether using commercial or locally prepared controls, the control is tested alongside patient specimens using the protocol for patient PPP testing.

The normal control result should be within the reference interval, and the prolonged control result should be within the therapeutic range for warfarin (PT) and unfractionated heparin (PTT). If the control results fall within the stated limits in the laboratory protocol, the test results are considered valid. If the results fall outside the control limits, the reagents, control, and equipment are checked; the problem is corrected; and the control and patient specimens are retested. The operator records all the actions taken. Control results are recorded and analyzed after regular intervals to determine the long-term validity of results.

Reporting Prothrombin Time Results and International Normalized Ratio

The clinical laboratory scientist reports PT results to the nearest tenth of a second along with the PT reference interval. If the PT is performed in duplicate, the results are averaged, and the average is reported. In view of the inherent variations among thromboplastin reagents, most laboratories report the international normalized ratio (INR) for stably anticoagulated patients using the following formula[51]:

$$INR = \left(PT_{patient}/PT_{geometric\ mean\ of\ normal}\right)^{ISI}$$

Where $PT_{patient}$ is PT of patient in seconds, $PT_{geometric\ mean\ of\ normal}$ is PT of the geometric mean of the reference interval, and ISI is the international sensitivity index. Reagent producers generate the ISI for their thromboplastin by performing an orthogonal regression analysis comparing PT results with the results of the international reference thromboplastin (World Health Organization human brain thromboplastin). Most responsive thromboplastin reagents have ISIs near 1, the assigned ISI of the World Health Organization reagent. Automated coagulation timers "request" the reagent ISI from the operator and compute INR for each test, including specimens from patients who are not stably anticoagulated. INRs are meant only for stably anticoagulated patients. During the first week of warfarin therapy, the physician should interpret PT results in seconds, comparing with the reference interval. For a full discussion of warfarin therapy monitoring, see Chapter 46.

Prothrombin Time Reference Interval

The PT reference interval varies from site to site depending on the patient population, type of thromboplastin used, type of instrument used, and the pH and purity of the reagent diluent. Each center must establish its own range with each new lot of reagents or at least once a year. This may be done by testing a sample of at least 20 specimens from healthy donors of both sexes spanning the adult age range over several days and computing the 95% confidence interval of the results.

Prothrombin Time Used as a Diagnostic Assay

The PT is performed diagnostically in any suspected coagulopathy. Acquired multiple deficiencies, such as disseminated intravascular coagulation (DIC), liver disease, and vitamin K deficiency, all affect factor VII activity and are detected through prolonged PT results. The PT is particularly sensitive to liver disease as factor VII levels become rapidly diminished (Chapters 40 and 41).

Vitamin K deficiency is seen in severe malnutrition, during use of broad-spectrum antibiotics that destroy gut flora, and in malabsorption syndromes. Vitamin K levels are low in newborns, in whom bacterial colonization of the gut has not begun. Hemorrhage is likely in vitamin K deficiency, and the PT is the best indicator. To distinguish between vitamin K deficiency and liver disease, the laboratory scientist performs a factor V and VII level. Both are reduced in liver disease; only factor VII is reduced in vitamin K deficiency. Chapter 41 contains details of liver disease and vitamin K deficiency.

The PT is prolonged in congenital single factor deficiencies of factors X, VII, and V; prothrombin; and fibrinogen when the fibrinogen level is 100 mg/dL or less. When the PT is prolonged but the PTT and TCT results are normal, factor VII activity may be deficient. Any suspected single factor deficiency is confirmed with a single factor assay. The PT is not affected by factor VIII or IX deficiencies because the concentration of tissue factor in the reagent is high, bypassing those factors in fibrin polymerization.

Prothrombin Time Is Minimally Effective as a Screen

Preoperative PT screening of asymptomatic surgical patients to predict intraoperative hemorrhage is not supported by prevalence studies, unless the patient is in a high-risk population.[52,53] No clinical data support the use of the PT as a general screening test for low-risk individuals, and the PT is not useful for establishing baseline values in warfarin therapy.[54] The therapeutic target range is based on the INR, not the baseline PT result or PT control value.

Limitations of Prothrombin Time

Specimen variations profoundly affect PT results (Table 45-8). The ratio of whole blood to anticoagulant is crucial, so collection tubes must be filled within tube manufacturers' specifications and not underfilled. Anticoagulant volume must be adjusted when the hematocrit is greater than 55% to avoid false prolongation of the results. Specimens must be inverted

TABLE 45-8 Factors That Interfere with Prothrombin Time Validity

Problem	Solution
Blood collection volume less than specified minimum	Recollect
Hematocrit ≥55%	Adjust anticoagulant volume and recollect
Clot in specimen	Recollect
Visible hemolysis	Recollect
Icterus or lipemia	Perform test on mechanical coagulometer
Heparin therapy	Use reagent known to be insensitive to heparin or one that includes a heparin neutralizer
Lupus anticoagulant	Use higher therapeutic range or alternative measuré of warfarin therapy
Incorrect calibration of instrument, incorrect dilution of reagents	Correct analytical error and repeat test

four to six times immediately after collection to ensure good anticoagulation, but the mixing must be gentle. Clotted and visibly hemolyzed specimens are rejected because they give unreliable results. Lipemic or icteric plasmas may affect the results of optical instrumentation.

Heparin may prolong the PT. If the patient is receiving therapeutic heparin, it should be noted on the order form and commented on with the results. The laboratory manager selects thromboplastin reagents that are maximally sensitive to oral anticoagulant therapy and insensitive to heparin. Many reagent manufacturers incorporate polybrene in their thromboplastin to neutralize heparin. The clinical laboratory scientist may detect unexpected heparin by using the TCT test described subsequently.

Some thromboplastins are sensitive to lupus anticoagulant, producing prolongation. Lupus anticoagulant is a member of the antiphospholipid antibody family and may partially neutralize PT reagent phospholipids. Warfarin often is prescribed to prevent thrombosis in patients with lupus anticoagulants, but the PT may not be a reliable monitor. Patients taking warfarin who have lupus anticoagulants should be treated to a target INR of 2.5 to 3.5 or should be monitored using an alternative system, such as the chromogenic factor X assay.[55]

Reagents must be reconstituted with the correct diluents and volumes using manufacturer instructions. Reagents must be stored and shipped using manufacturer's instructions and never used after the expiration date.

Partial Thromboplastin Time
Partial Thromboplastin Time Principle
The PTT (also called the *activated partial thromboplastin time*) is performed to monitor the effects of unfractionated heparin therapy and to detect circulating anticoagulants, such as lupus anticoagulant and anti–factor VIII antibody. The PTT also detects all congenital and acquired procoagulant deficiencies except deficiencies of factor VII or XIII.

The PTT reagent contains phospholipid (previously called *partial thromboplastin*) and a negatively charged particulate activator such as kaolin, ellagic acid, or Celite. The activator provides a surface that mediates a conformational change of plasma factor XII, resulting in its activation (Fig. 45-9). Factor XIIa forms a complex with two other plasma components, high-molecular-weight kininogen (or Fitzgerald factor) and prekallikrein (or Fletcher factor). These three plasma glycoproteins, termed the *contact activation factors*, initiate in vitro clot formation but are not involved in in vivo coagulation. Factor XIIa, a serine protease, activates factor XI (XIa), which activates factor IX (IXa) (Chapter 40).

Factor IXa binds calcium, phospholipid, and factor VIIIa to form a complex. In the PTT reaction system, ionic calcium

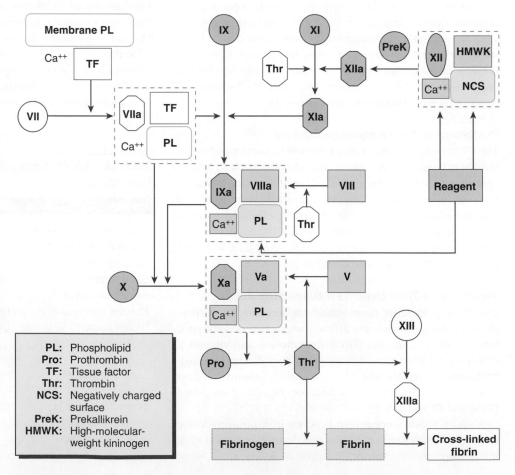

Figure 45-9 The PTT reagent consists of negatively charged particles, phospholipid and calcium. It activates the intrinsic and common pathways of the coagulation mechanism through the contact factors XII, prekallikrein, and high-molecular-weight kininogen (HMWK), none of which are significant in the in vivo coagulation mechanism. The PTT is affected by deficiencies in prekallikrein; HMWK; factors XII, XI, IX, VIII, X, and prothrombin; and fibrinogen, when the fibrinogen level is less than 100 mg/dL. The deficiencies for which the PTT reagent is specifically calibrated are factors VIII, IX, and XI. The PTT is prolonged in heparin therapy because heparin activates plasma antithrombin, which neutralizes all the plasma serine proteases, particularly thrombin (IIa) and activated factor X (Xa). The PTT is prolonged in the presence of lupus anticoagulant because the anticoagulant neutralizes essential reagent phospholipids. For all abbreviations, see Figure 45-8.

PL: Phospholipid
Pro: Prothrombin
TF: Tissue factor
Thr: Thrombin
NCS: Negatively charged surface
PreK: Prekallikrein
HMWK: High-molecular-weight kininogen

and phospholipid are supplied as reagents; synthetic phospholipid replaces partial thromboplastin, an organic extract of rabbit brain tissue. The factor IXa–calcium–factor VIIIa–phospholipid complex catalyzes factor X (Xa). Factor Xa forms another complex with calcium, phospholipid, and factor Va, catalyzing the conversion of prothrombin to thrombin. Thrombin catalyzes the polymerization of fibrinogen and the formation of the fibrin clot.

The factor deficiencies that cause hemorrhage and prolonged PTT results, taken in the order of reaction, are XI, IX, VIII, X, and V; prothrombin; and fibrinogen, when fibrinogen is 100 mg/dL or less. Most PTT reagents are designed so that the PTT is prolonged when the test PPP has less than 0.3 U/mL of VIII, IX, or XI. The PTT also is prolonged in the presence of lupus anticoagulant, an immunoglobulin with affinity for phospholipid-bound proteins, and is prolonged further by anti–factor VIII antibody and heparin. Factor VII and factor XIII deficiencies have no effect on the PTT. Deficiencies of factor XII, prekallikrein, or high-molecular-weight kininogen prolong the PTT but do not cause bleeding.

Partial Thromboplastin Time Procedure

To initiate contact activation, 0.05 or 0.1 mL of prewarmed (37° C) reagent consisting of phospholipid and activator is mixed with an equal volume of prewarmed PPP. The mixture is allowed to incubate for the manufacturer-specified time, usually exactly 3 minutes. Next, 0.1 mL of prewarmed 0.025 M calcium chloride is forcibly added to the mixture, and a timer is started. When a fibrin clot forms, the timer stops, and the interval is recorded. Timing may be done manually or automatically by using an electromechanical or photo-optical device. If the PTT is performed in duplicate, the two results must match within 10%.

Quality Control for Partial Thromboplastin Time

The clinical laboratory scientist tests normal and prolonged control plasma specimens at the beginning of each 8-hour shift or with each new batch of reagent. More frequent use of controls may be required by the laboratory director. Controls are tested using the protocol for patient plasma testing.

The normal control result should be within the reference interval, and the abnormal control result should be within the therapeutic range for unfractionated heparin (Chapter 46). If the control results fall within the stated limits in the laboratory protocol, the test results are considered valid. If the results fall outside the control limits, the reagents, control, and equipment are checked; the problem is corrected; and the control and patient specimens are retested. The operator records each control run and all the actions taken. Control results are recorded and analyzed after regular intervals to determine the long-term validity of results.

Partial Thromboplastin Time Reference Interval

The PTT reference interval varies from site to site depending on the patient population, type of reagent, type of instrument, and the pH and purity of the diluent. One medical center laboratory has established 26 to 38 seconds as its reference interval. This range is typical, but each center must establish its own interval with each new lot of reagent or at least once a year. This may be done by testing a sample of 20 or more specimens from healthy donors of both sexes spanning the adult age range over several days and computing the 95% confidence interval of the results.

Partial Thromboplastin Time Used as a Diagnostic Assay

The PTT is used primarily to monitor unfractionated heparin therapy as described in Chapter 46. The PTT also is used as a diagnostic assay. The physician orders a PTT when a hemorrhagic disorder is suspected or when recurrent thrombosis or the presence of an autoimmune disorder points to the possibility of a lupus anticoagulant. The PTT result is prolonged when there is a deficiency (<30%) of one or more of the following coagulation factors: prothrombin; V, VIII, IX, X, XI, or XII; or fibrinogen when the fibrinogen level is 100 mg/dL or less. The PTT also is prolonged in the presence of a specific inhibitor, such as anti–factor VIII or anti–factor IX; a nonspecific inhibitor, such as lupus anticoagulant; and interfering substances, such as fibrin degradation products (FDPs) or paraproteins.

DIC gives prolonged results because of consumption of procoagulants, but the PTT results alone are not definitive. Vitamin K deficiency results in diminished levels of procoagulant factors II, VII, IX, and X, and the PTT is eventually prolonged. Because factor VII does not affect the PTT, however, and because it is the first coagulation factor to become deficient, the test is not as sensitive to vitamin K deficiency or warfarin therapy as the PT. The PTT is not prolonged in deficiencies of factor VII or XIII. No clinical data support the use of the PTT as a general screening test for low-risk individuals.[56]

Reagents must be reconstituted with the correct diluents and volumes using the manufacturer instructions. Reagents must be stored and shipped using manufacturer instructions and never used after the expiration date.

Partial Thromboplastin Time Mixing Studies for Lupus Anticoagulants and Factor Inhibitors

Lupus Anticoagulants

Lupus anticoagulants are IgG immunoglobulins directed against several phospholipid-protein complexes.[57] Lupus anticoagulants prolong the phospholipid-dependent PTT reaction. Most laboratories employ a moderate-phospholipid PTT reagent to monitor heparin and detect coagulopathies and a second low-phospholipid PTT reagent such as PTT-LA (Stago) as their lupus anticoagulant screen (Chapter 42). Because they have a variety of targets, lupus anticoagulants are called *nonspecific inhibitors*. Chronic lupus anticoagulants confer a 30% risk of arterial or venous thrombosis; every acute care laboratory must provide a means for their detection. Chronic and transient lupus anticoagulants together are found in 1% to 3% of unselected individuals.

Specific Factor Inhibitors

Specific inhibitors are IgG immunoglobulins directed against coagulation factors. Specific inhibitors arise in severe congenital factor deficiencies during factor concentrate treatment. Anti–factor VIII, the most common of the specific inhibitors, is detected in 10% to 20% of severe hemophiliacs, and anti–factor IX is detected in 1% to 3% of factor IX–deficient patients. Auto-anti–factor VIII occasionally may be present in nonhemophiliacs, usually as part of a postpartum bleeding syndrome or in older patients with autoimmune disorders. Allo-anti–factor VIII and autoanti–factor VIII are associated with severe anatomic hemorrhage, and the latter is sometimes called *acquired hemophilia* (Chapter 41).

Detecting and Identifying Lupus Anticoagulants and Specific Inhibitors

Lupus anticoagulant testing is part of every thrombophilia profile (Chapter 42) and is ordered by the physician on suspicion of thrombophilia. An unexpected prolonged screening PTT also may trigger a thrombophilia investigation. Mixing studies are necessary to detect lupus anticoagulants and to distinguish them from specific inhibitors and factor deficiencies.[58,59] First, a TCT is performed to rule out heparin as the cause of the prolonged PTT. If no heparin is present, the patient's PPP is mixed 1:1 with pooled normal PPP, and a PTT is performed on the mixture. If the mixture PTT result is within 10% of the pooled normal PPP result, correction has occurred, and a factor deficiency may be suspected as the cause for the originally prolonged PTT. Before a factor deficiency is confirmed, however, a second aliquot of patient PPP and reagent PPP is incubated for 1 to 2 hours at 37° C. Anti–factor VIII is typically an IgG₄ immunoglobulin whose activity is enhanced by 37° C incubation. If, after the 1- to 2-hour incubation, the PTT result is corrected, the original prolonged PTT is most likely caused by a factor deficiency. The scientist follows up with specific factor assays.

If the initial unincubated mixture PTT result remains prolonged (uncorrected), lupus anticoagulant is suspected. A new aliquot of patient PPP is tested using a kit with a high-phospholipid reagent (Staclot LA, Stago). Shortening of the high-phospholipid reagent arm of the assay by at least 8 seconds compared with the nonphospholipid arm confirms the presence of lupus anticoagulant.

If the unincubated mixture PTT result was normal and the incubated mixture was prolonged (uncorrected), a specific antifactor antibody may be present. The Bethesda titer procedure is used to confirm the presence of specific antifactor antibodies. Antibodies to most coagulation factors have been described; anti–factor VIII is the most common.

Lupus Anticoagulant Test Profiles Require a Second Assay System

Because lupus anticoagulants have multiple targets, it is necessary to employ parallel systems to ensure their detection. The second system most often employed in U.S. laboratories is the dilute Russell viper venom time assay. Russell viper venom triggers coagulation at the level of factor X, depending on factor V, prothrombin, and fibrinogen to generate a normal response. Dilute Russell viper venom is neutralized by lupus anticoagulant and the test is prolonged, DVVtest (American Diagnostica, Inc., Stamford, Conn.). Prolongation is corrected in a high-phospholipid reagent, DVVconfirm (American Diagnostica, Inc., Stamford, Conn.). If the high-phospholipid arm interval is shortened by a ratio of 1:2 compared with the nonphospholipid arm, lupus anticoagulant is confirmed. Two additional assays, the dilute PT and the kaolin clotting time, also may be used in the lupus anticoagulant profile.

Thrombin Clotting Time

Thrombin Clotting Time Reagent and Principle

Commercially prepared bovine thrombin reagent at 2 NIH units/mL cleaves fibrinopeptides A and B from plasma fibrinogen to form a detectable fibrin polymer (Fig. 45-10).

Thrombin Clotting Time Procedure

Reagent thrombin is warmed to 37° C for a minimum of 3 and a maximum of 10 minutes. Thrombin deteriorates during incubation and must be used within 10 minutes of the time incubation is begun. An aliquot, usually 0.1 mL, of normal PPP incubates for a minimum of 3 and a maximum of 10 minutes. The operator forcibly pipettes 0.2 mL of thrombin into the PPP aliquot and starts a timer. TCT tests may be performed in duplicate and the results averaged.

Thrombin Clotting Time Quality Control

The clinical laboratory scientist tests a normal control and an abnormal control with each batch of TCTs and records the results. The normal control results should fall within the laboratory's reference interval. The abnormal control results should be prolonged to the range that TCT results reach in moderate hypofibrinogenemia. If the results fall outside the laboratory protocol's control limits, the reagents, control, and equipment are checked; the problem is corrected; and the control is retested. The actions taken to correct out-of-control tests are recorded. Control results are analyzed after regular intervals (weekly is typical) to determine the long-term validity of the procedure.

Reporting Thrombin Clotting Time Results and Thrombin Clotting Time Clinical Utility

A typical reference interval is 15 to 20 seconds. The TCT is prolonged when the fibrinogen level is less than 100 mg/dL (hypofibrinogenemia) or in the presence of antithrombic materials such as FDPs, paraproteins, or heparin. Afibrinogenemia (absence of fibrinogen) or dysfibrinogenemia (fibrinogen that is biochemically abnormal and nonfunctional) also causes a prolonged TCT. Before a prolonged TCT may be considered to be evidence of diminished or abnormal fibrinogen, the presence of antithrombic activity, such as heparin, FDPs, or paraproteins, must be ruled out.

The fibrinogen assay described subsequently is a simple modification of the TCT. In the fibrinogen assay, the concen-

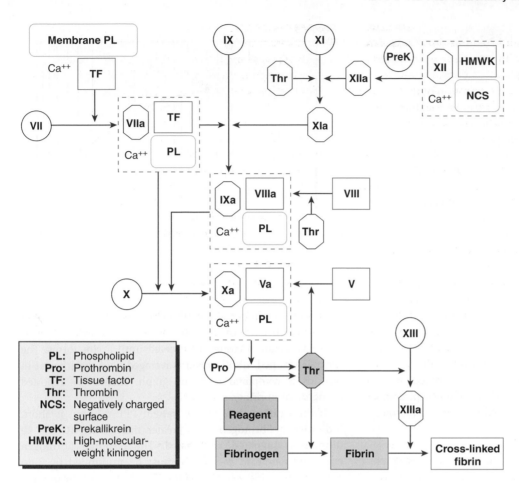

Figure 45-10 Trombin clotting time and reptilase time coagulation pathway. The reagent activates the coagulation pathway at the level of prothrombin and tests for the polymerization of fibrinogen.

PL: Phospholipid
Pro: Prothrombin
TF: Tissue factor
Thr: Thrombin
NCS: Negatively charged
      surface
PreK: Prekallikrein
HMWK: High-molecular-
       weight kininogen

tration of reagent thrombin is about 25 times that of the TCT at 50 NIH units/mL, and the patient specimen is diluted 1:10. This dilution minimizes the effects of heparin or antithrombic proteins. The reptilase time procedure is identical to the TCT except that the reptilase reagent is insensitive to the effects of heparin.

Point of Care Thrombin Clotting Time

The Hemochron Response (International Technidyne, Edison, N.J.) may be used to perform a bedside TCT using a technique similar to the automated activated clotting time. The distributor provides evacuated tubes containing lyophilized thrombin, buffer, calcium chloride, and a plasticized magnet. First, 2 mL of whole blood is collected directly in the tube, the timer is started, and the blood is thoroughly mixed to disperse the reagents. The tube is placed in the instrument test well, where it is continuously monitored for clotting. The interval to clot formation is recorded automatically.

The reference mean of the Hemochron TCT is 45 seconds; although it does not match the PPP TCT time, this gives the advantage of rapid turnaround of results to the physician. A control PPP is provided by the company for quality assurance.

Reptilase Time
Reptilase Time Principle and Reagent

Reptilase is a thrombin-like enzyme isolated from the venom of *Bothrops atrox* that catalyzes the conversion of fibrinogen to fibrin. In contrast to thrombin, the enzyme cleaves only fibrinopeptide A from the fibrinogen molecule, whereas thrombin cleaves fibrinopeptides A and B.[60] The specimen requirements, procedure, and quality assurance protocol for the reptilase time test are the same as for the TCT. Atroxin (Trinity Biotech PLC, Wicklow, Ireland) is reconstituted with distilled water and is stable for 1 month when stored at 2°C to 6° C. Atroxin is a poison that may be fatal if it directly enters the bloodstream.

Reptilase Time Clinical Utility

A prolonged reptilase time indicates decreased functional fibrinogen. Reptilase is insensitive to the effects of heparin and sensitive to dysfibrinogenemia. The reptilase time test is useful for detecting hypofibrinogenemia or dysfibrinogenemia in patents receiving heparin therapy. The reptilase test is prolonged in the presence of FDPs and paraproteins and is insensitive to heparin.

COAGULATION FACTOR ASSAYS

Fibrinogen Assay

Principle of Fibrinogen Assay

The clot-based method of Clauss, a modification of the TCT, is the recommended procedure for estimating the functional fibrinogen level.[61] Reagent bovine thrombin is added to PPP, catalyzing the conversion of fibrinogen to fibrin polymer. In the fibrinogen assay, the thrombin reagent is 25 times more concentrated than in the TCT at 50 NIH units/mL. The PPP to be tested is diluted 1:10 with Owren's buffer, whereas in the TCT the plasma is undiluted. The higher reagent concentration and diluted PPP provide an inverse but linear relationship between interval to clot formation and concentration of functional fibrinogen. The test is linear when the fibrinogen concentration is 100 to 400 mg/dL. Diluting the PPP also minimizes the antithrombotic effects of heparin, FDPs, and paraproteins. Heparin levels less than 0.6 U/mL and FDP levels less than 100 µg/dL do not affect the results of the fibrinogen assay of diluted PPP if the fibrinogen level is 150 mg/dL or greater.

The interval to clot formation is compared with the results of reference plasma. A reference curve is prepared in each laboratory and updated regularly using reference plasma or control plasma that has been calibrated to reference plasma.

Fibrinogen Assay Procedure

Thrombin Reagent.   Most laboratory managers prefer commercially manufactured diagnostic lyophilized bovine thrombin reagent. Pharmaceutical topical thrombin also may be used. The reagent is reconstituted according to manufacturer instructions and used immediately or aliquotted and frozen. If thrombin is to be frozen, it should be prepared in a stock solution of 1000 NIH units/mL and frozen at −70° C until it is ready for use. When thawed, thrombin is stable for only a few hours and cannot be refrozen for later use.

Reference Curve.   A reference curve is prepared with each change of reagent lots, reference plasma, or instrument. The clinical laboratory scientist prepares the curve by reconstituting commercially available lyophilized fibrinogen calibration plasma. Using Owren's buffer, five dilutions of the calibration plasma are prepared: 1:5, 1:10, 1:15, 1:20, and 1:40. An aliquot, usually 0.2 mL, of each dilution is transferred to each of three reaction tubes or cups, warmed to 37° C, and tested by adding 0.1 mL of working thrombin reagent at 50 NIH units/mL. Time from addition of thrombin to clot formation is recorded, duplicates are averaged, and the results in seconds are graphed against fibrinogen concentration (Fig. 45-11). Because patient PPPs are diluted 1:10 before testing, the 1:10 calibration plasma dilution is assigned the same fibrinogen concentration as the undiluted reconstituted calibration plasma value.

Test Protocol.   The clinical laboratory scientist prepares a 1:10 dilution of each patient PPP and control with Owren's buffer. Then 0.2 mL of each of the diluted PPPs is warmed to

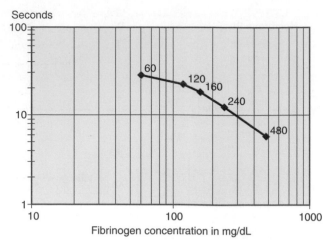

Figure 45-11 Fibrinogen reference table and curve.

37° C in each of two reaction tubes or cups for 3 minutes. After incubation, 0.1 mL of thrombin reagent is added, a timer is started, and the mixture is observed until a clot forms. The timer is stopped, duplicates are averaged, and the interval in seconds is compared with the graph. Results are reported in mg/dL of fibrinogen.

If the clotting time of the patient PPP dilution is short, indicating a fibrinogen level greater than 4 mg/dL, a 1:20 dilution is prepared and tested. The resulting fibrinogen concentration from the graph must be multiplied by 2 to compensate for the dilution. If the clotting time of the original 1:10 patient PPP dilution is prolonged, indicating less than 2 mg/dL of fibrinogen, a 1:5 dilution is prepared. The resulting concentration reading from the graph is divided by 2 to compensate for the concentrated specimen.

Fibrinogen Assay Quality Assurance

All duplicate results must agree within a coefficient of variation of less than 7%. The clinical laboratory scientist tests a normal control and an abnormal control with each batch of fibrinogen levels and records the results. The normal control results should be within the laboratory's reference interval. The abnormal control results should be less than 100 mg/dL. If either control result falls outside the control limits, the reagents, control, and equipment are checked; the problem is corrected; and the control is retested. The actions taken to correct "out-of-control" tests are recorded. Control results are analyzed after regular intervals (weekly is typical) to determine the long-term validity of the procedure.

Results and Clinical Utility of Fibrinogen Assay

One institution's reference interval for fibrinogen concentration is 200 to 400 mg/dL. Hypofibrinogenemia is associated with DIC and severe liver disease. Moderately severe liver disease, pregnancy, and a chronic inflammatory condition may cause an elevated fibrinogen level. Congenital afibrinogenemia gives prolonged clotting times and is associated with a variable hemorrhagic disorder. Dysfibrinogenemia may give the same results as hypofibrinogenemia by this test method because some abnormal fibrinogen species are hydrolyzed more slowly by thrombin than normal fibrinogen. Some forms of dysfibrinogenemia may be associated with thrombosis.[62] Immunologic and turbidimetric (Ellis-Stransky) measures of fibrinogen are normal in dysfibrinogenemia. Although antithrombic effects are minimized by the dilution of PPP specimens, heparin levels greater than 0.6 U/mL and FDP levels greater than 100 μg/mL prolong the results and give falsely lowered fibrinogen results.

Limitations of Fibrinogen Assay

Care must be taken that the thrombin reagent is pure and has not degenerated. Exposure to sunlight or oxidation results in rapid breakdown of thrombin. The working dilution lasts only 1 hour at 2° C to 8° C and should remain cold until just before testing. Specimens with clots, hemolysis, icterus, or lipemia are unacceptable.

Single Factor Assay Using the Partial Thromboplastin Time Test System
Principle of Single Factor Assays Based on Partial Thromboplastin Time

If the PTT is prolonged, the PT and TCT are normal, and there is no ready explanation for the prolonged PTT such as heparin therapy, lupus anticoagulant, or a factor-specific inhibitor, the clinical laboratory scientist may suspect a congenital single factor deficiency. Three factor deficiencies that give this reaction pattern and cause hemorrhage are VIII (hemophilia A); IX (hemophilia B); and XI, which causes a mild intermittent bleeding disorder called *Rosenthal syndrome* primarily found in Ashkenazi Jews.[63] The next step in diagnosis of a congenital single factor deficiency is performance of a one-stage single factor assay based on the PTT system.

Although necessary for diagnosis, PTT-based single-factor assays are most often performed on specimens from patients with previously identified single factor deficiencies. Their purpose is to monitor supportive therapy during bleeding episodes or invasive procedures. Because hemophilia A is the most common single factor deficiency disorder, our discussion is confined to the factor VIII assay; however, the protocol may be applied to factors IX and XI as well.

The clinical laboratory scientist uses the PTT system to estimate the concentration of functional factor VIII by incorporating commercially prepared factor VIII–depleted plasma in the test system. Most factor VIII–depleted plasma is PPP collected from normal donors and immunodepleted using monoclonal anti–factor VIII antibody on a separatory column.[64]

In the PTT system, factor VIII–depleted plasma provides normal activity of all procoagulants but factor VIII. Tested alone, factor VIII–depleted plasma reagent has a prolonged PTT, but when normal PPP is added, the PTT reverts to normal. In contrast, a prolonged result on a mixture of patient and factor VIII–depleted PPP implies that the patient PPP is deficient in factor VIII. The clotting time interval of the patient PPP/factor VIII–depleted PPP mixture may be compared with a previously prepared reference curve to estimate the level of

factor VIII activity in the patient PPP. The quantitative factor assay is performed on a 1:10 dilution of patient PPP, and the reference curve sets the clotting time for a 1:10 dilution of reference plasma at the assayed factor VIII activity percentage from the package insert.

Reference Curve for Factor VIII Assay

To prepare a reference curve for the factor VIII assay, the clinical laboratory scientist obtains a reference plasma such as CAP FVIIIc RM (College of American Pathologists, Northfield, Ill.) and prepares a series of dilutions with buffered saline.[65] Although laboratory protocols vary, most clinical laboratory scientists prepare a series of five dilutions, from 1:5 to 1:500. Each dilution is mixed with reagent factor VIII–depleted plasma and tested in duplicate using the PTT system; the duplicate results are averaged and plotted on log/log or log/linear graph paper (Fig. 45-12). The 1:10 dilution is assigned the factor VIII assay activity value found on the package insert. When patient PPP is tested, the time interval obtained is entered on the vertical coordinate and converted to a percentage.

Procedure for Factor VIII Assay

The clinical laboratory scientist prepares 1:10, 1:20, and 1:40 dilutions of each patient PPP and control, then mixes each dilution with equal volumes of factor VIII–depleted plasma and PTT reagent. In most cases, 0.1 mL of PTT reagent is mixed with 0.1 mL each of patient PPP dilution and factor VIII–depleted plasma. Both dilutions of each specimen or control are tested in duplicate. After incubation for the manufacturer-specified time at 37° C, 0.1 mL of 0.025 N calcium chloride is added, and a timer is started. The interval is recorded in seconds, duplicates are averaged, the mean result is compared with the reference curve, and the percentage of factor VIII activity is reported. Factor activity results of the 1:20 and 1:40 dilutions are multiplied by 2 and 4 to compensate for the dilution factors and should match the results of the 1:10 dilutions within ±10%. If the results of the three dilutions do not match within ±10%, a lupus anticoagulant and the assay

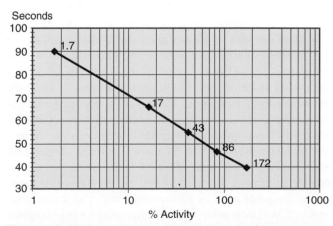

Figure 45-12 Factor VIII assay dilution table and reference curve on linear-log graph form.

cannot provide a reliable estimate of factor VIII activity. This is considered a nonparallel result and is a reliable means for detecting a lupus anticoagulant.

Tests for factors IX and XI are performed using the same approach except that the appropriate factor-depleted plasma is substituted for factor VIII–depleted plasma. Tests for the contact factors XII, prekallikrein, or high-molecular-weight kininogen are seldom requested because deficiencies are not associated with bleeding disorders and are not provided in the laboratories of acute care facilities. Acquired and congenital contact factor deficiencies are relatively common, however, and cause PTT prolongation. These assays are available from hemostasis reference laboratories and may be necessary to account for an unexplained prolonged PTT.

Expected Results and Clinical Utility of Single Factor Assays

The reference range for factor VIII activity is 50% to 150%. Symptoms of hemophilia are evident at activity levels of 10% or less. The test is used most often to estimate the plasma level of factor VIII activity during therapy. Chronically elevated factor VIII predicts an elevated risk of venous thrombotic disease (Chapter 42).

Quality Assurance of Single Factor Assays

All duplicate results must agree within 10%. The clinical laboratory scientist tests a normal and a deficient control with each assay and records the results. The normal control results should fall within the reference interval. The deficient control results should be in the range of 10% factor VIII activity. If either control result falls outside the control limits, the reagents, control, and equipment are checked; the problem is corrected; and the control is retested. The clinical laboratory scientist records all actions taken to correct "out-of-control" tests. Control results are analyzed after regular intervals (weekly is typical) to determine the long-term validity of the procedure.

Limitations of Single Factor Assays

Interlaboratory coefficients of variation for the factor VIII assay reach 80%, implying undesirable variation in the interpretation of therapeutic monitoring results from dissimilar institutions. To reduce inherent variation, the clinical laboratory scientist uses an assayed commercial plasma to prepare the reference curve and selects reference dilutions that comprise only the linear portion of the curve. The laboratory must assay three or more dilutions of patient PPP to check for inhibitors. The scientist also selects a matching reagent-instrument system with a demonstrated coefficient of variation less than 5% and uses factor-depleted substrates with no trace of the depleted factor.[66] As in the PTT test, good specimen management is essential. Clotted, hemolyzed, icteric, or lipemic specimens are rejected because they give unreliable results. Reagents must be reconstituted with the correct diluents and volumes using manufacturer instructions. Reagents must be stored and shipped using manufacturer's instructions and never used after the expiration date. Specimens specifically for factor VIII assays may be stored at 2° C to 4° C to slow factor deterioration.

Bethesda Titer for Anti–Factor VIII Inhibitor

The Bethesda titer is used to confirm and quantify specific anti–factor VIII inhibitor. In this method, 0.2 mL of patient PPP suspected of containing factor VIII inhibitor is incubated with 0.2 mL of reagent normal PPP for 2 hours at 37° C. A control specimen consisting of 0.2 mL of imidazole buffer at pH 7.4 mixed with 0.2 mL of reagent normal PPP is simultaneously incubated. During the incubation period, anti–factor VIII from the patient PPP neutralizes a percentage of normal PPP factor VIII activity. The proportion of factor VIII activity neutralized is related to the level of inhibitor activity. After incubation, residual factor VIII level in the mixture of normal PPP with patient PPP is measured by specific factor assay as described in the section on specific factor assays using the PTT system.

The titer of inhibitor in the specimen is expressed as a percent of the control. If the patient specimen/normal PPP mixture retains 75% of the residual factor VIII of the control, there is no significant factor VIII inhibitor in the patient PPP. If the residual factor VIII level is 25% of control, the patient PPP factor VIII inhibitor level is titered using several dilutions of the patient specimen in reagent normal PPP. One Bethesda unit of activity is the amount of antibody that leaves 50% residual factor VIII in the mixture.

Single Factor Assay Using the Prothrombin Time Test System

If the PTT and the PT are prolonged, the TCT is normal, and there is no ready explanation for the prolonged test results, such as liver disease, DIC, oral anticoagulant therapy, or vitamin K deficiency, the clinical laboratory scientist may suspect a congenital single factor deficiency. Three relatively rare factor deficiencies that give this reaction pattern and cause hemorrhage are prothrombin, factor V, or factor X deficiency. If the PT is prolonged and all other test results are normal, factor VII deficiency is suspected. The next step in diagnosis of a congenital single factor deficiency is performance of a one-stage single factor assay based on the PT test system. The principles and procedure given in the section on single factor assay using the PTT system may be applied, except that tissue thromboplastin reagent replaces the PTT reagent in the test system, and the PT protocol is followed. Prothrombin-depleted and factor V–depleted, factor VII–depleted, and factor X–depleted plasmas are available (Table 45-9).

Factor XIII Assay: 5 mol/L Urea Solubility

Coagulation factor XIII is a transglutaminase that catalyzes covalent cross-links between the α and γ chains of fibrin polymer.[67] Cross-linking strengthens the fibrin clot and renders it resistant to proteases. This is the final event in plasma coagulation, and it is essential for normal hemostasis and normal wound healing. Plasma, platelet, and tissue factor XIII function identically.

TABLE 45-9 Factor Assays Using the Thrombin Clotting Time (TCT), Prothrombin Time (PT), and Partial Thromboplastin Time (PTT) Test Systems

Factor	System
Fibrinogen (I)	TCT
Prothrombin (II)	PT
V	PT
VII	PT
VIII	PTT
IX	PTT
X	PT
XI	PTT
XIII	5 M urea solubility

Inherited factor XIII deficiency, an autosomal recessive disorder, affects both sexes in all races. The first report appeared in 1960, and the frequency is estimated at 1 in 2 million. Factor XIII levels also may be low in chronic DIC secondary to Crohn disease, leukemias, ulcerative colitis, sepsis, inflammatory bowel disease, surgery, and Henoch-Schönlein purpura. In these cases, the factor XIII level decreases to 50% of normal, which is not low enough to create symptoms, although occasionally acquired factor XIII deficiencies do create low enough levels to cause mild bleeding. Acquired factor XIII inhibitors have been described in isoniazid, penicillin, valproate, and phenytoin therapy.[68] Such inhibitors may cause complete absence of factor XIII.

Factor XIII activity levels less than 5% in congenital or acquired disorders result in hemorrhage. In congenital factor XIII deficiency, bleeding is evident in infants with seepage at the umbilical stump. In adults, bleeding is slow but progressive, accompanied by poor wound healing and slowly resolving hematomas. Recurrent spontaneous abortion and post-traumatic hemorrhage are common. Acquired factor XIII inhibitors cause severe bleeding that does not respond to therapy.

Principle and Procedure of Factor XIII Qualitative Test (5 mol/L Urea Solubility)

When a patient presents with bleeding and poor wound healing and the PTT, PT, platelet count, and fibrinogen level are normal, the scientist should consider the time-honored 5 M urea solubility test for factor XIII. The unstable clot that forms in factor XIII deficiency or inhibitor dissolves in a 5 M urea solution, whereas a factor XIIIa–stabilized clot remains intact for at least 24 hours.

The clinical laboratory scientist prepares three tubes. Tube 1 receives 0.3 mL of patient PPP, and tube 3 receives 0.3 mL of normal PPP. Tube 2 receives 0.2 mL of patient PPP and 0.1 mL of normal PPP to test for inhibitor. The clinical laboratory scientist pipettes 0.1 mL of 0.025 M calcium chloride to each tube. After clot formation, all three are incubated at 37° C for 30 minutes. Next, 3 mL of 5 M urea solution is transferred to each tube, and the tubes are tapped gently to dislodge the clots from the sides. The tubes are capped and incubated at ambient temperature for 24 hours but are observed for evidence of clot disintegration at 1, 2, 4, and 24 hours. Decreasing size of clot, fragmentation, and increasing turbidity of the urea solution are evidence for clot disintegration. The clot in the patient plasma tube (tube 1) is compared with the normal plasma tube clot (tube 3), and results are reported as "factor XIII present" or "factor XIII absent." If a factor XIII inhibitor is present in the patient plasma, the clot dissolves in the first tube and the second tube. A clot in normal PPP remains intact for 24 hours.

TESTS OF FIBRINOLYSIS

Quantitative D-Dimer Immunoassay
Physiology of Fibrin Degradation Products and D-Dimers

During coagulation, fibrin polymers become cross-linked by factor XIIIa and bind plasma plasminogen and tissue plasminogen activator (TPA) (Chapter 40). Over several hours, TPA activates bound plasminogen to form plasmin. Bound plasmin cleaves fibrin and yields FDPs D, E, X, and Y and D-dimer. The FDPs represent original fibrinogen domains, and D-dimers are covalently linked D-domains reflecting the cross-linking effects of factor XIIIa. Assays for FDPs, including D-dimer, are convenient for detecting reactive fibrinolysis, indirectly implying the presence of thrombosis. Normally, FDP levels, including D-dimer, remain at plasma concentrations less than 2 ηg/mL. Reactive fibrinolysis yields FDPs at levels greater than 200 ηg/mL. Increased FDP levels are characteristic of acute and chronic DIC, systemic fibrinolysis, deep vein thrombosis, and pulmonary embolism.[69] FDPs, including D-dimer, also are detected in plasma after thrombolytic therapy.[70]

Principle of Quantitative D-Dimer Assay

Several in vitro diagnostics distributors offer automated quantitative immunoassays for plasma D-dimers that are able to yield numerical results within 30 minutes. Microlatex particles in buffered saline are coated with monoclonal anti–D-dimer antibodies. The coated particles are agglutinated by patient plasma D-dimer; the resultant turbidity is measured through turbidometric or nephelometric means. Sensitivity varies by the avidity of the monoclonal anti–D-dimer and the detection method; however, most methods detect 10 ηg/mL.

Clinical Value of Quantitative D-Dimer Assay

The quantitative D-dimer assay is an essential screen for venous thromboembolic disease and an absolute requirement for detecting and monitoring DIC. The D-dimer assay also is helpful in detecting acute myocardial infarction and ischemic stroke. In limited instances, the D-dimer also may be used to monitor the effects of thrombolytic therapy. The various assays possess 90% to 95% negative predictive values and may be used to rule out deep vein thrombosis and pulmonary thrombotic emboli in low-risk patients without resorting to compression ultrasound, tomography, or venous imaging.[71,72] Owing to its sensitivity and specificity values in the 60% to

70% range, physicians do not use the quantitative D-dimer assay to diagnose venous thromboembolic disease definitively. Any chronic or acute inflammation is accompanied by elevated D-dimers; the assay cannot be used to "rule-in" thromboembolic disease. The normal cutoff value for the quantitative D-dimer varies with methodology, ranging from 0 to 250 ηg/mL to 0 to 500 ηg/mL; in DIC, results may reach 10 to 20,000 ηg/mL.

Qualitative D-Dimer Assay

The automated quantitative D-dimer assay has largely replaced manual D-dimer or FDP assays. The SimpliRed D-dimer assay (AGEN Biomedical Ltd., Brisbane, Queensland, Australia) is a manual method that uses monoclonal antibody-coated visible latex particles. SimpliRed D-dimer is suited to low-volume or near-patient applications. The manufacturer reports the clinical sensitivity for pulmonary embolus to be 94% and specificity to be 67%.[73]

Fibrin Degradation Products

Although the assay has largely been replaced by the automated quantitative D-dimer assay, FDPs may be detected using a semiquantitative agglutination immunoassay.[74] One such method is the Thrombo-Wellcotest kit (International Murex Technologies, Toronto, Ontario, Canada). Polystyrene latex particles in buffered saline are coated with anti-D and E fragment–specific polyclonal antibodies calibrated to detect FDPs at 2 mg/mL or greater. The assay usually is performed on serum collected in special tubes that promote clotting and prevent factitious in vitro fibrinolysis, although one FDP kit uses plasma.

Fibrin Degradation Products Protocol

A 1:5 and 1:20 dilution of patient serum or plasma is prepared in buffered saline. One drop each of undiluted specimen, 1:5 and 1:20 dilutions, is placed in three labeled circles on a clean glass slide. One drop of well-mixed latex suspension is added to each drop of specimen or dilution and mixed. The slide is rocked for 2 minutes, and the mixture is observed for agglutination. Negative and positive sera, supplied by the manufacturer, are tested with each unknown patient serum or batch.

Fibrin Degradation Products Assay Results

Results of the FDP test are semiquantitative: If only the undiluted serum mixture shows agglutination, the FDP concentration is reported as 2 μg/mL or greater but less than 10 μg/mL. This is regarded as an equivocal result. If the undiluted and 1:5 dilutions are agglutinated, the result is reported as 10 μg/mL or greater but less than 80 μg/mL, a positive result. If all three circles agglutinate, the result is 80 μg/mL or greater. Control results are observed with each batch, recorded, and reviewed at regular intervals. The FDP test is positive in DIC, deep vein thrombosis, pulmonary embolism, and systemic fibrinolysis in liver disease or after thrombolytic therapy.

Plasminogen Chromogenic Substrate Assay

Plasminogen, the precursor of the trypsin-like proteolytic enzyme plasmin, is produced in the liver and circulates as a single-chain glycoprotein (Chapter 40). When bound to fibrin, plasminogen is converted to plasmin by the action of TPA or urokinase. Bound plasmin degrades fibrin, whereas free plasmin is rapidly inactivated by a circulating inhibitor, α_2-antiplasmin, also called *plasmin inhibitor*.

Congenital plasminogen deficiencies are associated with thrombosis in some families and with hyaline membrane disease in premature infants.[75,76] Acquired plasminogen deficiencies are seen in DIC and acute promyelocytic leukemia.[77] Thrombolytic therapy is ineffective when plasminogen levels are low. Plasminogen is readily measured in PPP using a chromogenic substrate assay, available from several manufacturers.

Principle of Plasminogen Chromogenic (Amidolytic) Substrate Assay

Amidolytic substrates are synthetic polypeptides with amino acid sequences specific for particular enzymes.[78] Plasmin hydrolyzes a bond in the polypeptide sequence Val-Leu-Lys. A fluorophor or a chromophor such as *p*-nitroanaline (pNA) is covalently bonded to the carboxyl end of the polypeptide and may be released on digestion. S-2251, composed of H-D-Val-Leu-Lys-pNA, is a chromogenic substrate for plasmin. On plasmin digestion, the pNA is released and turns yellow (Fig. 45-13).

Streptokinase is an exogenous plasminogen activator derived from beta-streptococcal cultures. Streptokinase is added to patient PPP, where it bonds to and activates plasminogen. The resulting streptokinase-plasmin mixture reacts with a chromogenic substrate such as S-2251 to release a color with an intensity proportional to the original plasminogen concentration. Several analogous chromogenic and fluorogenic substrates are suitable for plasminogen measurement. A control plasma is tested with the unknown, and the results are recorded.

Results and Clinical Utility of Plasminogen Chromogenic Substrate Assay

Normal plasminogen activity is 5 to 13.5 mg/dL. Plasminogen levels are decreased in thrombolytic therapy, DIC, hepatitis, and cancer. Hereditary deficiencies also have been recorded.[79] Decreased plasminogen is associated with thrombotic disorders. Plasminogen increases are seen in inflammation and during pregnancy and may be associated with hemorrhage. Plasminogen levels are elevated in systemic fibrinolysis.[80]

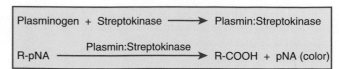

Figure 45-13 Assaying plasma plasminogen using the chromogenic substrate method. Reagent streptokinase activates plasminogen to form plasmin. *R-pNA* designates a chromogenic substrate, where *R* indicates several choices of amide and *pNA* is the chromophore. In the case of plasminogen, the *R* represents H-D-Val-Leu-Lys-pNA. The Val-Leu-Lys amide sequence is recognized and hydrolyzed by plasmin.

Plasminogen assays may be available only from specialty reference laboratories.

Tissue Plasminogen Activator Assay

Physiology and Clinical Significance of Tissue Plasminogen Activator

The two physiologic human plasminogen activators are TPA and urokinase. TPA is synthesized in vascular endothelial cells and released to the circulation, where its half-life is approximately 3 minutes and its plasma concentration averages 5 ηg/mL.[81] Urokinase is produced in the kidney and vascular endothelial cells and has a half-life of approximately 7 minutes and a concentration of 2 to 4 ηg/mL.[82] Both activators are serine proteases that form ternary complexes with bound plasminogen at the surface of fibrin, activating the plasminogen and initiating thrombus degradation. Both are covalently inactivated by the endothelial secretion, plasminogen activator inhibitor-1 (PAI-1).

Tissue Plasminogen Activator Clinical Significance

The upper limit of TPA activity is 1.1 IU/mL. The upper limit for TPA antigen is 14 ηg/mL. TPA is the primary mediator of fibrinolysis. Elevated TPA levels are associated with increased risk of myocardial infarction, stroke, or deep vein thrombosis.[83] Impaired fibrinolysis, in the form of TPA deficiency or PAI-1 excess, also is associated with deep vein thrombosis and myocardial infarction.[84]

Tissue Plasminogen Activator Specimen Collection

TPA levels are influenced by exercise and diurnal variation. TPA may become activated in vitro. Patients should be at rest, tourniquet application should be minimal, and immediate acidification of the specimen in acetate buffer is necessary to stabilize activators.[85] Blood is collected into citrate tubes following the protocol given in the section on hemostasis specimen collection, acidified within 60 seconds of collection, and centrifuged immediately. Acidification may be accomplished using the Stabilyte tube (American Diagnostica, Inc., Greenwich, Conn.). Supernatant PPP is frozen at −70° C until the assay is performed.

Principle of Tissue Plasminogen Activator Assay

TPA antigen may be estimated by enzyme immunoassay. To measure TPA activity, a specified concentration of reagent plasminogen is added to the patient plasma. Plasma TPA activates the plasminogen, and the resultant plasmin is measured with a chromogenic substrate. The resulting color intensity is inversely proportional to TPA activity (Fig. 45-14). The system may incorporate soluble fibrin to increase the TPA activity.

Plasminogen Activator Inhibitor 1 Assay

PAI-1 is produced by vascular endothelial cells and hepatocytes and circulates in plasma bound to vitronectin at an average concentration of 10 μg/L with diurnal variations.[86] An inactive form of PAI-1 circulates in high concentrations in platelets.[87] PAI-1 inactivates TPA by covalent binding. Elevated PAI-1 is strongly associated with venous thrombosis and may be a

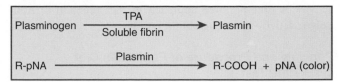

Figure 45-14 Plasma containing TPA is added to plasminogen to produce plasmin. Plasmin activity is measured using the same system as in the plasminogen assay.

cardiovascular risk factor. A few cases of PAI-1 deficiency have been reported; however, hemorrhage apparently occurs only in complete PAI-1 absence.

Citrated plasma is collected from patients at rest and centrifuged immediately to make PPP; this avoids in vitro contamination with PAI-1 from platelets. Several immunometric and chromogenic substrate methods are available for estimation of PAI-1 antigen and PAI-1 activity. One sandwich-type enzyme immunoassay for functional PAI-1 uses urokinase to activate PAI-1. The urokinase–PAI-1 complex is immobilized with solid-phase monoclonal anti-PAI-1 and measured using monoclonal antiurokinase as the detecting antibody.[88]

Most chromogenic substrate approaches are indirect measures using TPA in the plasminogen assay shown in Figure 45-15. Patient PPP is mixed with a measured amount of reagent TPA. Residual activator is assayed in the plasminogen system as shown in Figure 45-15. The resulting intensity of color is inversely proportional to plasma PAI-1.

Confirmation of complete PAI-1 deficiency may be accomplished using the serum PAI-1 assay. In serum, platelet PAI-1 is expressed in excess. In true PAI-1 absence, no PAI-1 is detectable in serum.

Euglobulin Clot Lysis Time Test

Excessive fibrinolytic activity occurs in a variety of conditions. Inflammation and trauma may be reflected in a radical increase in circulating plasmin that causes hemorrhage. Bone trauma, fractures, and surgical dissection of bone as in cardiac surgery may cause increases in fibrinolysis.[89] Fibrinolysis deficiencies occur when TPA or plasminogen levels become depleted or when excess secretion of PAI-1 depresses TPA

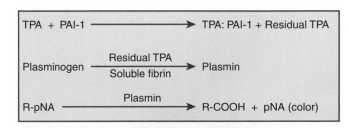

Figure 45-15 To assay PAI-1 activity, plasma containing PAI-1 is added to measured TPA. The residual TPA is assayed as in Figure 45-14. The result is inversely proportional to PAI-1 level.

activity. A time-honored approach to measurement of fibrinolytic activity is the euglobulin lysis test.

Principle and Procedure of Euglobulin Clot Lysis Time Test

The euglobulin clot lysis time is a global screen of the fibrinolytic system. Plasma inhibitors of fibrinolysis are removed chemically, and the reactions of fibrinogen, plasminogen, and plasminogen activators are assayed.

Patient plasma is diluted and acidified with cold 1% acetic acid until the solution reaches the pH of 5.35 to 5.40. On refrigeration for approximately 30 minutes, a precipitate forms that contains fibrinogen, plasminogen, plasmin, and TPA. This precipitate is termed the *euglobulin fraction*. Excluded from the precipitate are α_2-antiplasmin and PAI-1 so that fibrinolysis may proceed unchecked. The tubes are centrifuged, and the supernatant is decanted completely. The precipitate is redissolved in borate buffer, and reagent thrombin or calcium chloride is added. A clot should form within a few minutes. A timer is started at the time of thrombin addition, and the clot is observed periodically for dissolution over 2 to 10 hours. The time required for the intrinsic plasmin to lyse the fibrin clot is the euglobulin lysis time.

Results of Euglobulin Clot Lysis Time Test

If the euglobulin clot dissolves in less than 2 hours, excess fibrinolysis is present. If the clot remains for longer than 10 hours, the fibrinolytic pathway is deficient.

Limitations of Euglobulin Clot Lysis Time Test

Positive and negative plasma controls are included. Fresh or commercial normal PPP is used as the negative control, whereas normal PPP plus streptokinase is used as the positive control. Streptokinase is a nonenzymatic activator of plasminogen. Clot dissolution of the patient fraction is compared with the positive and negative controls.

Another control, the patient-activated control, is also prepared. This is a specimen of the patient's euglobulin fraction with streptokinase. This control ensures against invalid results caused by plasminogen depletion. When patient plasminogen levels are diminished, such as in long-term DIC, clot dissolution extends beyond 10 hours. The patient-activated control indicates when this condition exists because streptokinase-activated plasma from the patient should cause rapid clot dissolution. When plasminogen is depleted, the streptokinase-activated control gives no dissolution, and the euglobulin lysis time is prolonged.

Hypofibrinogenemia and factor XIII deficiency affect the euglobulin lysis time. In hypofibrinogenemia, there is less fibrin to be lysed, and a short lysis time may be seen without a genuine increase in fibrinolytic activity. In factor XIII deficiency, the original clot quality is poor, and dissolution by normal levels of plasmin is more rapid. The euglobulin clot lysis time also may be falsely prolonged in chronic inflammation if the fibrinogen level exceeds 600 mg/dL.

CHAPTER at a GLANCE

- Proper hemostasis specimen collection, management, and centrifugation ensure a valid test result.
- Platelet function tests, particularly the platelet aggregometry profile, determine the source of platelet deficiency–based hemorrhage.
- von Willebrand disease is diagnosed and monitored through the judicious selection and performance of laboratory tests.
- HIT with thrombosis is confirmed through careful laboratory test interpretation.
- Clot-based coagulation screening tests include the activated coagulation time, PT, PTT, and TCT.

- Mixing studies are used to detect factor deficiencies, lupus anticoagulants, and specific factor inhibitors.
- Coagulation factor assays are used to detect and measure coagulation factor deficiencies, and Bethesda titers are used to detect coagulation factor inhibitors.
- Tests of fibrinolysis include FDPs, D-dimer, plasminogen, and plasminogen activators.

Now that you have completed this chapter, go back and read again the case study at the beginning and respond to the questions presented.

REVIEW QUESTIONS

1. What happens if a coagulation specimen collection tube is underfilled?
   a. Clot-based test results are falsely prolonged
   b. Chromogenic test results are falsely decreased
   c. The specimen clots and is useless
   d. The specimen is hemolyzed and is useless

2. If you collect a series of tubes, when in the sequence should the hemostasis (blue-stoppered) tube be collected?
   a. After a lavender-stoppered or green-stoppered tube
   b. First, or after a nonadditive tube
   c. After a serum separator tube
   d. Last

3. You are to perform a PT and PTT on a specimen that is slightly hemolyzed. The patient is not readily available. What should you do?
   a. Retain the specimen, but do not assay; redraw when patient is available.
   b. Test the specimen, but adjust all results by subtracting 10%.
   c. Test the specimen and annotate the results to indicate that the specimen was unacceptable.
   d. Clear the hemolysis with Seroclear.

4. Most coagulation testing must be performed on PPP, which is plasma with a platelet count less than:
   a. 1000/μL
   b. 10,000/μL
   c. 100,000/μL
   d. 1,000,000/μL

5. You wish to collect a 5-mL specimen of whole blood/anticoagulant mixture from a patient whose hematocrit is 65%. What volume of anticoagulant should you use?
   a. 0.5 mL
   b. 0.32 mL
   c. 0.64 mL
   d. 0.68 mL

6. You perform whole-blood lumiaggregometry on a patient who complains of easy bruising. Aggregation and secretion are diminished when the agonists thrombin, ADP, arachidonic acid, and collagen are used. What is the most likely platelet abnormality?
   a. Storage pool disorder
   b. Aspirin-like syndrome
   c. ADP receptor anomaly
   d. Glanzmann thrombasthenia

7. What is the "gold standard" assay for HIT?
   a. Enzyme immunoassay
   b. Serotonin release assay
   c. Platelet lumiaggregometry
   d. Washed platelet aggregation

8. What agonist is used in platelet aggregometry to detect von Willebrand disease?
   a. Arachidonic acid
   b. Ristocetin
   c. Collagen
   d. ADP

9. What single factor deficiency is likely when the PT result is prolonged and the PTT result is normal?
   a. V
   b. VII
   c. VIII
   d. Prothrombin

10. What acquired coagulopathy is reflected in a prolonged PT, a low factor VII level, but a normal factor V level?
    a. Hemophilia
    b. Liver disease
    c. Thrombocytopenia
    d. Vitamin K deficiency

11. The patient has deep vein thrombosis. The PTT is prolonged and is not corrected in an immediate mix of patient plasma with equal parts normal plasma. What is the presumed condition?
    a. Factor VIII inhibitor
    b. Lupus anticoagulant
    c. Factor VIII deficiency
    d. Factor V Leiden mutation

12. You perform a 5-mol/L urea solubility assay on a patient with chronic bleeding and prolonged wound healing. The clot dissolves within 2 hours. What is the presumed cause?
    a. Abnormally increased fibrinolysis
    b. Factor XIII deficiency
    c. Factor IX deficiency
    d. This is normal.

13. What condition causes a pronounced elevation of the quantitative D-dimer assay?
    a. DIC
    b. Deep vein thrombosis
    c. Fibrinogen deficiency
    d. Paraproteinemia

14. What is the name given for the type of assay that uses a synthetic polypeptide substrate that releases a chromophor or fluorophor on digestion by its serine protease?
    a. Clot-based assay
    b. Fluorescence immunoassay
    c. Molecular diagnostic assay
    d. Chromogenic substrate assay

REFERENCES

1. Clinical and Laboratory Standards Institute: Collection, Transport, and Processing of Blood Specimens for Testing Plasma-Based Coagulation Assays: Approved Guideline, 4th ed (CLSI document H21-A4). Wayne, PA: CLSI, 2003.
2. Clinical and Laboratory Standards Institute: Procedures for the Collection of Diagnostic Blood Specimens by Venipuncture: Approved Standard, 5th ed (CLSI document H3-A5). Wayne, PA: CLSI, 2003.
3. Gottfried EL, Adachi MM: Prothrombin time and activated partial thromboplastin time can be performed on the first tube. Am J Clin Pathol 1997;107:681-683.
4. Adcock DM, Kressin DC, Marlar RA: Minimum specimen volume requirements for routine coagulation testing. Am J

Clin Pathol 1998;109:595-599.
5. Ma Z, Monk TG, Goodnough LT, et al: Effect of hemoglobin-and Perflubron-based oxygen carriers on common clinical laboratory tests. Clin Chem 1997;43:1732-1737.
6. Palkuti HS: Specimen collection and quality control. In Corriveau DM, Fritsma GA (eds): Hemostasis and Thrombosis in the Clinical Laboratory. Philadelphia: Lippincott, 1988:67-91.
7. Sunderji R, Gin K, Shalansky K, et al: Clinical impact of point-of-care vs. laboratory measurement of anticoagulation. Am J Clin Pathol 2005;123:184-188.
8. McGlasson DL, Paul J, Shaffer KM: Whole blood coagulation testing in neonates. Clin Lab Sci 1993;6:76-77.
9. Lippi G, Guidi GC: Effect of specimen collection on routine

coagulation assays and D-dimer measurement. Clin Chem 2004;50:2150-2152.

10. van den Besselaar AM, Meeuwisse-Braun J, Schaefer-van Mansfeld H, et al: Influence of plasma volumetric errors on the prothrombin time ratio and international sensitivity index. Blood Coagul Fibrinolysis 1997;8:431-435.

11. Horsti J: Use of EDTA samples for prothrombin time measurement in patients receiving oral anticoagulants. Haematologica 2001;86:851-855.

12. Menssen HD, Melber K, Brandt N, et al: The use of hirudin as universal anticoagulant in haematology, clinical chemistry and blood grouping. Clin Chem Lab Med 2001;39:1267-1277.

13. Ens GE, Newlin F: Spurious protein S deficiency as a result of elevated factor VII levels. Clin Hemost Rev 1995;9:18.

14. Adcock D, Kressin D, Marlar RA: The effect of time and temperature variables on routine coagulation tests. Blood Coagul Fibrinolysis 1998;9:463-470.

15. Dyszkiewicz-Korpanty AM, Frenkel EP, Ravindra Sarode R: Approach to the assessment of platelet function: comparison between optical-based platelet-rich plasma and impedance-based whole blood platelet aggregation methods. Clin Appl Thrombosis/Hemostasis 2005;11:25-35.

16. Pierangeli SS, Harris EN: Clinical laboratory testing for the antiphospholipid syndrome. Clin Chim Acta 2005;357:17-33.

17. Bick RL: Platelet function defects: A clinical review. Semin Thromb Hemost 1992;18:167-185.

18. Lind SE: The bleeding time does not predict surgical bleeding. Blood 1991;77:2547.

19. Duke WW: The pathogenesis of purpura haemorrhagica with especial reference to the part played by the blood platelets. Arch Intern Med 1912;10:445.

20. Ivy AC, Nelson D, Bucher G: The standardization of certain factors in the cutaneous "venostasis" bleeding time technique. J Lab Clin Med 1941;26:1812.

21. Kumar R, Ansell JE, Canoso RT, et al: Clinical trial of a new bleeding device. Am J Clin Pathol 1978;70:642-645.

22. Mielke CH Jr, Kaneshiro MM, Maher IA, et al: The standardized normal Ivy bleeding time and its prolongation by aspirin. Blood 1969;34:204-215.

23. Ingerman-Wojenski CM, Silver MJ: A quick method of screening platelet dysfunction using whole blood lumiaggregometry. Thromb Hemost 1984;51:154-156.

24. Goldenberg SJ, Veriabo NJ, Soslau G: A micromethod to measure platelet aggregation and ATP release by impedance. Thromb Res 2001;103:57-61.

25. Dyszkiewicz-Korpanty AM, Frenkel EP, Sarode R: Approach to the assessment of platelet function: comparison between optical-based platelet-rich plasma and impedance-based whole blood platelet aggregation methods. Clin Appl Thrombosis/Hemostasis 2005;11:25-35.

26. White MM, Foust JT, Mauer AM, et al: Assessment of lumi-aggregometry for research and clinical laboratories. Thromb Haemost 1992;67:572-577.

27. Michiels JJ, Gadisseur A, Budde U, et al: Characterization, classification, and treatment of von Willebrand diseases: a critical appraisal of the literature and personal experiences. Semin Thromb Hemost 2005;31:577-601.

28. Budde U, Drewke E, Mainusch K, et al: Laboratory diagnosis of congenital von Willebrand disease. Semin Thromb Hemost 2002;28:173-190.

29. Allain JP, Cooper HA, Wagner RH, et al: Platelets fixed with paraformaldehyde: a new reagent for assay of von Willebrand factor and platelet aggregating factor. J Lab Clin Med 1975;85:318-328.

30. Gu J, Prastein D, Pierson RN II: Aspirin resistance: an under-recognized risk factor in early vein graft thrombosis after off-pump coronary artery bypass (OPCAB) [abstract]. Presented at American Heart Association, New Orleans, LA, November 7-10, 2004.

31. Manoharan A, Brighton T, Gemmell R, et al: Platelet dysfunction in myelodysplastic syndromes: a clinicopathological study. Int J Hematol 2002;76:272-278.

32. Brace LD: Testing for heparin-induced thrombocytopenia by platelet aggregometry. Clin Lab Sci 1992;5:80-81.

33. Warkentin T: Heparin-induced thrombocytopenia. In Colman RW, Marder VJ, Clowes AW, et al (eds): Hemostasis and Thrombosis, 5th ed. Philadelphia: Lippincott, Williams & Wilkins, 2006:1649-1662.

34. Isenhaart CE, Brandt JT: Platelet aggregation studies for the diagnosis of heparin-induced thrombocytopenia. Am J Clin Pathol 1993;99:324-330.

35. Stewart MW, Etches WS, Boshkov LK, et al: Heparin-induced thrombocytopenia: an improved method of detection based on lumi-aggregometry. Br J Haematol 1995;91:173-177.

36. Messmore HL, Sucha N, Godwin J: Heparin-induced thrombocytopenia and platelet activation in cardiovascular surgery. In Pifarre R (ed): Anticoagulation, Hemostasis, and Blood Preservation in Cardiovascular Surgery. Philadelphia: Hanley & Belfus, 1993:185-200.

37. Sheridan D, Carter C, Kelton JG: A diagnostic test for heparin induced thrombocytopenia. Blood 1986;67:27-30.

38. Amiral J, Bridey F, Dreyfus M, et al: Platelet factor 4 complexed to heparin is the target for antibodies generated in heparin-induced thrombocytopenia. Thromb Hemost 1992;68:95-96.

39. Sadayasu T, Nakashima Y, Yashiro A, et al: Heparin-releasable platelet factor 4 in patients with coronary artery disease. Clin Cardiol 1991;14:725-729.

40. Rapold HJ, Grimaudo V, Declerck PJ, et al: Plasma levels of plasminogen activator inhibitor type 1, beta-thromboglobulin, and fibrinopeptide A before, during, and after treatment of acute myocardial infarction with alteplase. Blood 1991; 78:1490-1495.

41. Papp AC, Hatzakis H, Bracey A, et al: ARIC hemostasis study—I: Development of a blood collection and processing system suitable for multicenter hemostatic studies. Thromb Haemost 1989;61:15-19.

42. Fritsma GA, Ens GE, Alvord MA, et al: Monitoring the anti-platelet action of aspirin. Am Assoc Phys Assist 2001;14:57-62.

43. Eikelboom JW, Hankey GJ: Failure of aspirin to prevent atherothrombosis: potential mechanisms and implications for clinical practice. Am J Cardiovasc Drugs 2004;4:57-67.

44. Yankee RA, Grumet FC, Rogentine GN: The selection of compatible platelet donors for refractory patients by lymphocyte HLA typing. N Engl J Med 1969;22:1208-1212.

45. Friedberg RC, Donnelly SF, Boyd JC, et al: Clinical and blood bank factors in the management of platelet refractoriness and alloimmunization. Blood 1993;81:3428-3434.

46. Sendroy J, Cecchini LP: Determination of human body surface area from height and weight. J Appl Physiol 1954;7:1-12.

47. Lee RI, White PD: A clinical study of the coagulation time of blood. Am J Med Sci 1913;243:279-285.

48. Talstad I: Which coagulation factors interfere with the one-stage prothrombin time? Haemostasis 1993;23:19-25.

49. Biggs R, MacFarlane RG: Reaction of haemophilic plasma to thromboplastin. J Clin Pathol 1951;4:445-459.

50. Clinical Laboratory and Standards Institute: One-Stage Prothrombin Time (PT) Test and Activated Partial Thromboplastin Time (APTT) Test: Approved Guideline (CLSI document H47-A). Wayne, PA: CLSI, 1996.

51. Poller L: Laboratory control of anticoagulant therapy. Semin Thromb Hemost 1986;12:13-19.

52. Eisenberg JM, Clarke JR, Sussman SA: Prothrombin and partial thromboplastin times as preoperative screening tests. Arch Surg 1982;117:48-51.

53. Gravlee GP, Arora S, Lavender SW, et al: Predictive value of blood clotting tests in cardiac surgical patients. Ann Thorac Surg 1994;58:216-221.

54. McKinly L, Wrenn K: Are baseline prothrombin time/partial thromboplastin time values necessary before instituting anticoagulation? Ann Emerg Med 1993;22:697-702.

55. Moll S, Ortel TL: Monitoring warfarin therapy in patients with lupus anticoagulants. Ann Intern Med 1997;127:177-185.

56. McKinly L, Wrenn K: Are baseline prothrombin time/partial thromboplastin time values necessary before instituting anticoagulation? Ann Emerg Med 1993;22:697-702.

57. McNeil HP, Simpson RJ, Chesterman CN, et al: Antiphospholipid antibodies are directed against a complex antigen that includes a lipid-binding inhibitor of coagulation: β-2-glycoprotein I. Proc Natl Acad Sci U S A 1990;87:4120-4124.

58. Brandt JT, Triplett DA, Alving B, et al: Criteria for the diagnosis of lupus anticoagulants: an update. Thromb Haemost 1995;74:1185-1190.

59. Proceedings of the 8th International Symposium on Antiphospholipid Antibodies. Sapporo, Japan, 6-9 October 1998. Lupus 1998;7(Suppl 2):S1-S234.

60. Meh DA, Siebenlist KR, Bergtrom G, et al: Sequence of release of fibrinopeptide A from fibrinogen molecules by thrombin or Atroxin. J Lab Clin Med 1995;125:384-391.

61. Clinical and Laboratory Standards Institute: Procedure for the Determination of Fibrinogen in Plasma: Approved Guideline, 2nd ed (CLSI document H30-A2). Wayne, PA: CLSI, 2001.

62. Comp PC: Overview of the hypercoagulable states. Semin Thromb Hemost 1990;16:158-161.

63. Seligsohn U: High gene frequency of factor XI (PTA) deficiency in Ashkenazi Jews. Blood 1978;51:1223-1228.

64. Rothschild C, Amiral J, Adam M, et al: Preparation of factor VIII depleted plasma with antibodies and its use for the assay of factor VIII. Haemostasis 1990;20:321-328.

65. Arkin CF, Bovill EG, Brandt JT, et al: Factors affecting the performance of factor VIII coagulant activity assays: results of proficiency surveys of the College of American Pathologists. Arch Pathol Lab Med 1992;116:908-915.

66. Hirst CF, Hewitt J, Poller L: Trace levels of factor VIII in substrate plasma. Br J Haematol 1992;81:305-306.

67. Greenberg CS, Sane DC, Lai T: Factor XIII and fibrin stabilization. In Colman RW, Marder VJ, Clowes AW, et al (eds): Hemostasis and Thrombosis, 5th ed. Philadelphia: Lippincott Williams & Wilkins, 2006:317-334.

68. Krumdieck R, Shaw DR, Huang ST, et al: Hemorrhagic disorder due to an isoniazid-associated acquired factor XIII inhibitor in a patient with Waldenstrom's macroglobulinemia. Am J Med 1991;90:639-645.

69. Southern DK: Serum FDP and plasma D-dimer testing: what are they measuring? Clin Lab Sci 1992;5:332-333.

70. Lawler CM, Bovill EG, Stump DC, et al: Fibrin fragment D-dimer and fibrinogen B beta peptides in plasma as markers of clot lysis during thrombolytic therapy in acute myocardial infarction. Blood 1990;76:1341-1348.

71. Heijboer H, Ginsberg JS, Buller HR, et al: The use of the D-dimer test in conjunction with noninvasive testing vs. serial noninvasive testing alone for the diagnosis of deep vein thrombosis. Thromb Haemost 1992;67:510.

72. Stein PD, Hull RD, Patel KC, et al: D-dimer for the exclusion of acute venous thrombosis and pulmonary embolism: a systematic review. Ann Intern Med 2004;140:589-602.

73. Kline JA, Israel EG, Michelson EA: Diagnostic accuracy of a bedside D-dimer assay and alveolar dead-space measurement for rapid exclusion of pulmonary embolism: a multicenter study. JAMA 2001;285:761-768.

74. Drewinko B, Surgeon J, Cobb P, et al: Comparative sensitivity of different methods to detect and quantify circulating fibrinogen/fibrin split products. Am J Clin Pathol 1985;84:58-66.

75. Lottenberg R, Dolly FR, Kitchens CS: Recurring thromboembolic disease and pulmonary hypertension associated with severe hypoplasminogenemia. Am J Hematol 1985;19:181-193.

76. Ambrus CM, Weintraub DH, Dunphy D, et al: Studies on hyaline membrane disease: I. The fibrinolytic system in pathogenesis and therapy. Pediatrics 1963;32:10-24.

77. Walenga JM: Molecular and automated assessments of coagulation. In Corriveau DM, Fritsma GA (eds): Hemostasis and Thrombosis in the Clinical Laboratory. Philadelphia: Lippincott, 1988.

78. Friberger P: Synthetic peptide substrate assays in coagulation and fibrinolysis and their application on automates. Semin Thromb Hemost 1983;9:281-300.

79. Hathaway WE, Goodnight SH: Fibrinolytic defects and thrombosis. In Hathaway WE, Goodnight SH: Disorders of Hemostasis and Thrombosis. New York: McGraw-Hill, 1993:354-361.

80. Booth NA, Bachmann F: Plasminogen-plasmin system. In Colman RW, Marder VJ, Clowes AW, et al (eds): Hemostasis and Thrombosis: Basic Principles and Clinical Practice, 5th ed. Philadelphia: Lippincott, 2006:335-380.

81. Wiman B, Hamsten A: The fibrinolytic enzyme system and its role in the etiology of thromboembolic disease. Semin Thromb Hemost 1990;16:207-216.

82. Patrassi GM, Sartori MT, Casonato A, et al: Urokinase-type plasminogen activator release after DDAVP in von Willebrand disease: different behaviour of plasminogen activators according to the synthesis of von Willebrand factor. Thromb Res 1992;66:517-526.

83. Catto AJ, Grant PJ: Risk factors for cerebrovascular disease and the role of coagulation and fibrinolysis. Blood Coagul Fibrinolysis 1995;6:497-510.

84. Nicholl SM, Roztocil E, Davies MG: Plasminogen activator system and vascular disease. Curr Vasc Pharmacol 2006;4:101-116.

85. Chandler WL, Schmer G, Stratton JR: Optimum conditions for the stabilization and measurement of tissue plasminogen activator activity in human plasma. J Lab Clin Med 1989;113:362-371.

86. Juhan-Vague I, Alessi MC, Raccah D, et al: Daytime fluctuation of plasminogen activator inhibitor 1 (PAI-1) in populations with high PAI-1 levels. Thromb Haemost 1992;67:76-82.

87. Macy EM, Meilahn EN, Declerck PJ, et al: Sample preparation for plasma measurement of plasminogen activator inhibitor-1 antigen in large population studies. Arch Pathol Lab Med 1993;117:67-70.

88. Philips M, Juul A, Selmer J, et al: A specific immunologic assay for functional plasminogen activator inhibitor 1 in plasma standardized measurements of the inhibitor and related parameters in patients with venous thromboembolic disease. Thromb Haemost 1992;68:486-494.

89. Vinazzer H: Basics and practice in evaluating plasminogen. Haemostasis 1988;18(Suppl 1):41-45.

46

Monitoring Anticoagulant Therapy

George A. Fritsma

OBJECTIVES

After completion of this chapter, the reader will be able to:

1. Describe the proper collection and handling of samples for anticoagulant monitoring, and recognize situations in which these criteria have been violated.
2. Describe in general terms the instances or applications of oral anticoagulants (warfarin [Coumadin]), unfractionated heparin, low-molecular-weight heparin (LMWH), direct thrombin inhibitors (DTIs), and platelet inhibitors.
3. Compare the advantages and disadvantages of each treatment listed in terms of mode of administration, necessity or ease of monitoring, and significant side effects (e.g., heparin-induced thrombocytopenia).
4. Monitor various anticoagulant therapies, including selection of appropriate laboratory tests; recognition of appropriate testing frequency or timing relative to dosing; and interpretation of laboratory test indicating adequate, inadequate, or excessive dosage.
5. Describe the principle of each laboratory test used to monitor anticoagulant therapies.
6. Monitor warfarin using the prothrombin time and international normalized ratio.
7. Monitor standard unfractionated heparin using the activated clotting time and the partial thromboplastin time (PTT).
8. Monitor LMWH and pentasaccharide using the chromogenic anti–factor Xa heparin assay.
9. Monitor DTIs using the PTT and the ecarin clotting time.
10. Monitor antiplatelet therapy, aspirin, and clopidogrel using whole-blood aggregometry or a platelet metabolite.

CASE STUDY

After studying the material in this chapter, the reader should be able to respond to the following case study:

In 1996 a 54-year-old clinical laboratory scientist experienced crushing chest pain while exercising and drove himself to the emergency department of a nearby medical center. On arrival, he requested thrombolytic therapy in the form of synthetic tissue plasminogen activator. At the termination of thrombolysis, he was given unfractionated heparin, 8000 U, and was maintained on heparin for 5 days. During heparin therapy, his partial thromboplastin time reached and stabilized at 92 seconds, within the therapeutic range. Shortly after heparin therapy was started, he also was started on warfarin therapy, 5 mg/d. Prothrombin times were started on the second day, and by day 4, his international normalized ratio was 2.3, and on day 5, it was 2.5. On day 2 after admission, he went for percutaneous cardiac intervention (heart catheterization) and had a stent placed. He was discharged on warfarin 5 mg/d, aspirin 81 mg/d, and clopidogrel 75 mg/d. Warfarin and clopidogrel were discontinued after 6 months, and he has experienced no more adverse cardiac events.

1. Why were heparin and warfarin therapy started simultaneously?
2. Why was the heparin terminated at 5 days?
3. What changes to this therapeutic regimen have been instituted since 1996?

Venous or arterial thrombotic disease is managed by anticoagulant and antiplatelet therapy. Venous thromboembolic disease includes superficial and deep vein thrombosis and pulmonary embolism and is treated using warfarin (Coumadin); unfractionated heparin; low-molecular-weight heparin (LMWH); pentasaccharide (Fondaparinux); and the direct thrombin inhibitors (DTIs) argatroban, lepirudin, and bivalirudin. Arterial thrombosis includes acute myocardial infarction, ischemic cerebrovascular accident, and peripheral arterial occlusion and is managed with the heparins, DTIs, and the antiplatelet drugs aspirin, ticlopidine (Ticlid), and clopidogrel (Plavix).

Many lives have been saved through judicious anticoagulant and antiplatelet therapy, and countless more healthy individuals have been spared thrombotic disease through anticoagulant prophylaxis. Anticoagulant and antiplatelet drugs are dangerous, however, because their prophylactic and therapeutic dosage ranges are narrow.[1] Overdose means emergency department visits for uncontrolled bleeding; underanticoagulation leads to additional adverse, often fatal, thrombotic events. Anticoagulant kinetics differ by individual drug because of variations in formulation and metabolism.[2]

Laboratory monitoring, the earliest form of therapeutic drug monitoring, is essential to anticoagulant therapy. Coagulation laboratory scientists perform countless prothrombin times (PTs), partial thromboplastin times (PTTs) or activated partial thromboplastin times, and chromogenic anti–factor Xa heparin assays to monitor anticoagulants, accounting for most of their workload. Antiplatelet drug (aspirin) monitoring, although in its infancy, is likely to surpass the volumes of anticoagulant monitoring assays. Although anticoagulant and antiplatelet monitoring seems routine, vigilance is essential to provide consistently valid results in a dangerous therapeutic world.[3]

WARFARIN THERAPY AND THE PROTHROMBIN TIME

Warfarin Is a Vitamin K Antagonist

As detailed in Chapter 40, coagulation factors II (prothrombin), VII, IX, and X depend on vitamin K for normal production, as do coagulation control proteins C, S, and Z. Vitamin K is responsible for γ-carboxylation of a series of 10 to 20 N-terminus glutamic acids, a post-translational modification that enables the coagulation factors to bind ionic calcium (Ca^{2+}) and cell membrane phospholipids (Fig. 46-1). Vitamin K is extracted from green leafy vegetables and is produced by gut flora; its absence results in the production of noncarboxylated and non-functional factors II, VII, IX, and X and proteins C, S, and Z.

Warfarin sodium (4-hydroxycoumarin) (Coumadin) is a member of the coumarin drug category and is the formulation most often used in North America.[4] Another coumarin is dicumarol (3,3'-methylenebis-[4-hydroxycoumarin]), the original anticoagulant extracted from moldy sweet clover by Link in 1940.[5] Warfarin is a vitamin K antagonist that suppresses γ-carboxylation of glutamic acid (see Fig. 46-1). During war-

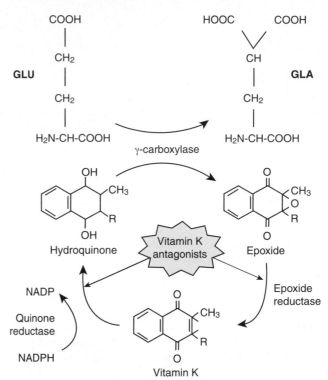

Figure 46-1 The effect of vitamin K antagonists on the γ-carboxylation of glutamic acid. Several copies of glutamic acid (GLU) are located near the N-terminus of coagulation factors II, VII, IX, and X and control proteins C, S, and Z. Hydroquinone catalyzes the γ-carboxylation of glutamic acid (GLA), adding a carboxyl group to the γ carbon. The γ-carboxyl glutamic acid forms a pocket that attracts a calcium ion (Ca^{++}), enabling the molecule to bind phospholipid. Hydroquinone is oxidized to vitamin K epoxide, which is reduced to vitamin K and then reduced further to hydroquinone. Epoxide reductase and quinone reductase activities are suppressed by coumarin-type vitamin K antagonists such as warfarin.

farin therapy, the activities of factors II, VII, IX, and X and proteins C, S, and Z are reduced as nonfunctional molecules are produced. These are called *proteins induced by vitamin K antagonists* (PIVKA); they bind few calcium ions, do not assemble on phospholipid surfaces with their substrates, and do not participate in coagulation. Despite several developmental efforts, coumarins remain the only oral anticoagulants, so warfarin therapy is often called *oral anticoagulant therapy*.

Prophylaxis and Therapy

Warfarin is prescribed prophylactically to prevent strokes in individuals with atrial fibrillation and to prevent thrombosis after trauma, orthopedic surgery, or general surgery. Therapeutic warfarin inhibits recurrence of deep vein thrombosis or pulmonary embolism and controls coagulation after acute myocardial infarction. Warfarin is used after acute myocardial infarction if the event is complicated by congestive heart failure or coronary insufficiency. Warfarin is among the top 20 prescribed drugs in North America.

The standard warfarin regimen begins with a 5- to 10-mg oral dose—less for elderly and small individuals and more for young, well-nourished patients. The activity of the vitamin K–dependent coagulation factors begins to decrease immediately but at different rates (Fig. 46-2), and it takes about

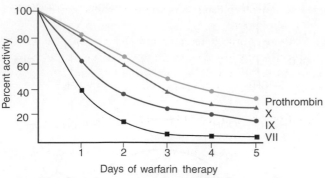

Figure 46-2 Factor VII activity decreases to 50% 6 hours after therapy is begun. This prolongs the factor VIIa–sensitive PT to near the therapeutic range. The half-lives of factors IX, X, and II are longer than VII; prothrombin (II) activity requires at least 3 days to reach 50%. The patient is not fully anticoagulated for at least 3 days after the start of warfarin therapy.

TABLE 46-1 Half-Life, Normal Plasma Level, and Hemostatic Level for the Procoagulant Factors

Factor	Half-Life (h)	Plasma Level	Hemostatic Level
Fibrinogen	100-150	200-400 mg/dL	50 mg/dL
Prothrombin	60	10 mg/mL	20%
V	24	1 mg/mL	25%
VII	6	0.05 mg/mL	20%
VIII	12	0.01 mg/mL	30%
IX	24	1 mg/mL	30%
X	48-52	1 mg/dL	25%
XI	48-84	6 mg/mL	25%
XIII	150	2 mg/mL	2-3%
VWF	30	6 μg/mL	50%

VWF, von Willebrand factor.

5 days for all the factors to reach therapeutic levels. Table 46-1 lists the plasma half-life and level for the coagulation factors.

Control protein activities also are lessened, especially protein C, which has a 6-hour half-life, so for the first 2 or 3 days of warfarin therapy the patient is actually prothrombotic. For this reason, warfarin therapy is "covered" by unfractionated heparin (UFH) or LMWH therapy during initiation. Failure to anticoagulate during this period may result in warfarin skin necrosis.[6]

Warfarin Therapy Monitored Using Prothrombin Time Assay

The PT effectively monitors warfarin therapy because it is sensitive to reductions of factors II, VII, and X, but not IX (Fig. 46-3). PT reagent consists of tissue factor, phospholipid, and ionic calcium, so it triggers the coagulation pathway at the level of factor VII. Owing to the 6-hour half-life of factor

VII, the PT begins to prolong within 24 hours; however, anticoagulation becomes therapeutic only when the activities of factors II and X decrease to less than 50%, in 4 to 7 days.

The first PT is performed 24 hours after therapy is initiated; subsequent PTs are performed daily until consecutive results are therapeutic. Monitoring continues every 4 weeks until therapy is complete, often 6 months. Warfarin therapy for atrial fibrillation is indefinite. Close monitoring is essential to successful warfarin therapy because the therapeutic range is narrow, and out-of-range results signal the danger of thrombosis or hemorrhage.

Reporting Prothrombin Time Results and the International Normalized Ratio

The clinical laboratory scientist reports PT results to the nearest tenth of a second with the PT reference interval (Chapter 45). In view of the inherent variations among thromboplastin

Figure 46-3 The PT reagent activates coagulation beginning with factor VII (extrinsic pathway). The PT is prolonged by deficiencies of factors VII, X, and V; prothrombin; and fibrinogen when the level is less than 100 mg/dL. The PT is prolonged in warfarin therapy, which produces nonfunctional forms of VII, X, and prothrombin. The PTT reagent activates the intrinsic coagulation pathway through the contact factor XII, assisted by prekallikrein (PK), and high-molecular-weight kininogen (HMWK) (not shown). The PTT is prolonged by deficiencies of PK; HMWK; factors XII, XI, IX, VIII, and X; prothrombin; and fibrinogen when the level is less than 100 mg/dL. The PTT is prolonged in heparin therapy because heparin activates plasma antithrombin, which neutralizes the serine proteases XIIa, XIa, Xa, IXa, and thrombin (IIa).

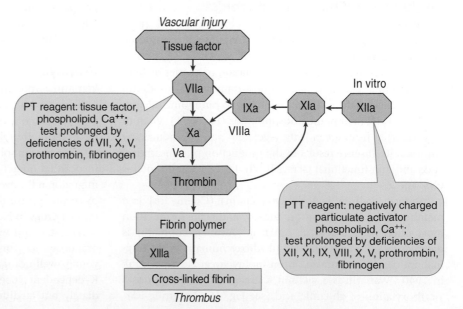

reagents, and to accomplish interlaboratory normalization, all laboratories report the international normalized ratio (INR) for stably anticoagulated patients using the following formula:[7]

$$INR = \left(PT_{patient}/PT_{normal}\right)^{ISI}$$

where *INR* is international normalized ratio, $PT_{patient}$ is PT of the patient in seconds, PT_{normal} is PT of the *geometric mean* of the reference interval in seconds, and *ISI* is international sensitivity index.

A commercial thromboplastin producer generates the ISI by performing an orthogonal regression analysis comparing the PT reagent's results for 50 or more anticoagulated specimens and 10 or more normals with those of the international reference thromboplastin (World Health Organization human brain thromboplastin). Most manufacturers provide ISIs for a variety of coagulometers because each may respond differently to the thromboplastin. Most thromboplastin reagents have ISIs near 1, which is the ISI of the World Health Organization thromboplastin. Automated coagulation timers "request" the reagent ISI from the operator or reagent vial bar code and compute the INR for each assay. Although INRs are meant only for stably anticoagulated patients, they typically are reported for all patients. During the first 5 days of warfarin therapy, the physician should ignore the INR as unreliable and interpret the PT results in seconds, comparing with the reference interval.

Warfarin International Normalized Ratio Therapeutic Range

The physician adjusts the dosage to achieve the desired INR of 2 to 3 or 2.5 to 3.5 if a mechanical heart valve is in place. INRs greater than 4 are associated with increased risk of hemorrhage; an INR of 5 requires immediate communication. Adjustments are conducted conservatively because the INR requires 4 to 7 days to reach the new level.

Pitfalls of Warfarin Therapy

Dietary vitamin K decreases warfarin's effect and reduces the INR. Green vegetables are an important source of vitamin K, but vitamin K also is concentrated in liver, parenteral nutrition formulations, nutrition drinks such as Ensure, multivitamins, red wine, and dietary supplements. A patient taking warfarin is counseled to maintain a regular balanced diet and to follow-up dietary or supplement changes with additional PTs and dosage adjustment if necessary.

Warfarin is metabolized in the mitochondrial cytochrome oxidase P-450 pathway of hepatocytes, the disposal system for at least 80 drugs. Theoretically, any drug so metabolized unpredictably may suppress or enhance warfarin therapy; amiodarone, metronidazole, and cimetidine typically double or triple the INR. Polymorphisms of enzymes in the cytochrome oxidase pathway may slow warfarin catabolism. Individuals with these polymorphisms require a warfarin dosage of about 1 mg/d; the standard dosage leads to the risk of hemorrhage. An enlightened application of the growing science of pharmacogenomics is categorization of cytochrome

oxidase polymorphisms and selection of the corresponding warfarin regimen.[8]

Likewise, warfarin receptor insufficiency may render the patient resistant. Some patients require dosages of 20 mg/d to achieve a therapeutic INR. Warfarin is contraindicated during pregnancy because of its teratogenic fetal effects.

Effect of Direct Thrombin Inhibitors on the Prothrombin Time

The DTIs argatroban, lepirudin, and bivalirudin prolong the PT, although the PTT is the assay typically employed to monitor DTIs. In switching from a DTI to warfarin therapy, the clinician should be aware that the combination of DTI and warfarin nearly doubles the PT for the life of the DTI. Argatroban exerts the greatest effect on the PT, followed by bivalirudin and lepirudin.[9]

Prothrombin Time Point of Care Testing

The following instruments are approved by the U.S. Food and Drug Administration for point of care PTs using a venous whole-blood specimen:

- Actalyke XL and Mini II (Helena Point of Care, Beaumont, Tex.)
- CoaguCheck and CoaguCheck Plus diagnostic coagulation systems (Roche Diagnostics/Boehringer Mannheim Corporation, Indianapolis, Ind.)
- Gem PCL plus (Instrumentation Laboratory, Inc, Lexington, Mass.)
- Hemochron Junior Signature Plus and Signature Elite, Hemochron Response (International Technidyne, Edison, N.J.)
- HMS Plus, ACT Plus (Medtronic, Minneapolis, Minn.)
- I-stat and I-stat 1 (Abbott Point of Care, Inc. East Windsor, N.J.)

Several of these devices also assay capillary specimens of 10 to 50 μL, and a few are portable (Chapter 47).[10]

Point of care instruments permit for near-patient anticoagulation clinic PTs, bedside testing, self-testing, and testing of infants. The operator or patient performs a capillary puncture and captures the free-flowing capillary blood in a cartridge that is transferred to the instrument. Alternatively, a drop of anticoagulated venous whole blood may be transferred to the test cartridge.

Each instrument uses individual patented technology to generate a PT with INR, and each produces reference and therapeutic intervals in INR and seconds that may diverge from plasma-based central laboratory results. In many cases, the manufacturer programs a linear electronic conversion factor so that the readout more closely matches plasma results. The manufacturer also provides internal electronic calibration and whole-blood controls. Before point of care instruments are placed in service, laboratory scientists validate employing plasma-based PTs for the reference method using linear regression and a test of means. Owing to inherent variation, laboratory scientists advise that each point of care analyzer be matched to its own normal and therapeutic interval.

The pharmacists and nurse practitioners who typically manage anticoagulation clinics appreciate point of care instruments

TABLE 46-2 Recommendations for the Reversal of a Warfarin Overdose Based on International Normalized Ratio and Bleeding

Bleeding	INR	Intervention
No significant bleeding	3-5	Lower or omit dose, monitor INR frequently
	5-9	Omit warfarin, monitor INR more frequently, consider oral vitamin K (≤5 mg) if high risk for bleeding (surgery)
	>9	Stop warfarin, give oral vitamin K (5-10 mg), monitor INR frequently
Serious bleeding	Any INR	Stop warfarin, give vitamin K subcutaneously (10 mg), may repeat every 12 h, give fresh frozen plasma, prothrombin complex concentrate, or recombinant factor VIIa
Life-threatening bleeding		Same as serious bleeding except stronger indication for recombinant factor VIIa

for their instantaneous turnaround. Patient waiting time is eliminated, and dosage adjustment is permitted at the time of the patient visit. Clinics thus equipped capitalize on the convenience factor to attract patients and improve their time within therapeutic range.

Portable capillary specimen point of care devices are designed for patient self-testing. Although self-testing seldom duplicates central laboratory precision, properly instructed patients are able to improve on their time within therapeutic range through frequency. In the United States, patients are cautioned not to self-dose, but rather to discuss dosage adjustments with their physician.[11]

Reversal of Warfarin Overdose

Table 46-2 provides recommendations for the reversal of a warfarin overdose based on INR and bleeding.

STANDARD, UNFRACTIONATED HEPARIN THERAPY AND THE PARTIAL THROMBOPLASTIN TIME

Heparin Is a Catalyst That Activates Antithrombin to Neutralize Serine Proteases

Standard UFH is mixture of sulfated glycosaminoglycans (polysaccharides) extracted from porcine mucosa. The molecular weight of UFH ranges from 3000 to 30,000 D. Approximately one third of its molecules present a high-affinity pentasaccharide that binds plasma antithrombin. The anticoagulant action of UFH is indirect and catalytic because pentasaccharide-bound antithrombin undergoes a steric change. This exposes an anticoagulant site that covalently binds and inactivates the coagulation pathway serine proteases IIa (thrombin), IXa, Xa, XIa, and XIIa (Chapter 40). Laboratory scientists call activated antithrombin a *serine protease inhibitor*, and the protease binding reaction yields measurable inactive plasma complexes such as thrombin-antithrombin.

Heparin supports the thrombin-antithrombin reaction through a bridging mechanism (Fig. 46-4). If the heparin molecule exceeds 17 saccharide units, thrombin assembles on the heparin molecule near the activated antithrombin. Bridging drives the thrombin-antithrombin reaction at a rate four times the factor Xa–antithrombin reaction because factor Xa participates only in steric modification (allostery). The anticoagulant action of heparin can be measured within minutes of administration.

Heparin preparations vary in average molecular weight, molecule length, and efficacy. Individual patient pharmacokinetics vary markedly because numerous plasma and cellular proteins bind heparin variably. Consequently, laboratory monitoring is essential.[12]

Unfractionated Heparin Therapy

Physicians administer UFH intravenously to treat deep vein thrombosis, pulmonary embolism, and acute myocardial infarction initially; to prevent reocclusion after stent placement; and to maintain vascular patency during cardiopulmonary bypass with extracorporeal circulation. Therapy begins with a bolus of 5000 to 10,000 U, followed by continuous infusion at approximately 1300 U/h, adjusted to patient weight. UFH is stopped at 5 days to avoid heparin-induced thrombocytopenia with thrombosis (HIT), a morbid, sometimes mortal side effect (Chapter 42). Most UFH therapy is completed at the time of discharge, typically the third day after acute myocardial infarction.

Monitoring Unfractionated Heparin Therapy

Because of its inherent pharmacologic variations and narrow therapeutic range, UFH therapy is diligently monitored using the PTT. Blood is collected before therapy is begun to ensure the baseline PTT is normal.[13] A prolonged baseline may indicate lupus anticoagulant or factor deficiency and confuses the therapeutic interpretation. In this instance, the laboratory scientist switches to the chromogenic anti–factor Xa heparin assay.

A second specimen is collected, and PTT is performed 4 to 6 hours after therapy initiation. The second result should be in the therapeutic range, which is established by the laboratory

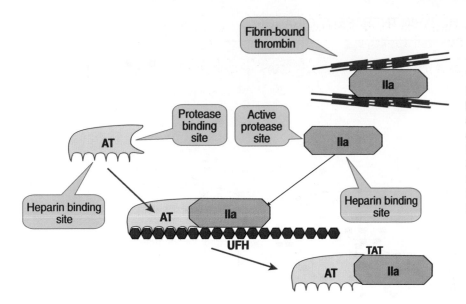

Figure 46-4 The binding site of antithrombin (AT) binds a specific heparin pentasaccharide, producing an allosteric change activating AT. Thrombin (IIa) assembles on the heparin surface if the molecule is at least 17 saccharide units long. AT binds IIa and is released from the heparin to form soluble, measurable thrombin-antithrombin (TAT). The heparin recycles. Fibrin-bound thrombin does not enter the reaction.

scientist (see later) and published with the result. The physician adjusts the infusion rate to ensure the PTT result reaches the target range. The PTT is repeated every 24 hours, and the dosage is continually readjusted until UFH anticoagulation is complete. The physician also monitors the platelet count daily. A 40% or greater reduction, even within the normal range, is evidence of HIT. UFH is immediately replaced with DTI therapy.

Partial Thromboplastin Time Therapeutic Range Determination for Unfractionated Heparin Therapy

The hemostasis laboratory is required to establish and communicate a therapeutic range for PTT management of UFH therapy. The clinical laboratory scientist collects 50 or more plasma specimens from patients taking heparin at all levels of anticoagulation and performs PTTs on all. The specimens must be from patients who are not receiving simultaneous warfarin therapy or whose PTs are normal. Chromogenic anti–factor Xa heparin assays are performed on all specimens, and the paired results are displayed in a linear graph (Fig. 46-5). The range in seconds of PTT results that corresponds exactly with 0.3 to 0.7 chromogenic anti–factor Xa heparin U/mL is the therapeutic range.[14] This is known as the *ex vivo* or *Brill-Edwards method* for establishing the heparin therapeutic range of the PTT and is required by accrediting agencies. Other approaches to the development of the PTT therapeutic range for UFH are disallowed.

Clinical Utility of Partial Thromboplastin Time Monitoring of Unfractionated Heparin and Reporting Results

The clinical laboratory scientist reports the results, the reference interval, and the UFH therapeutic range to the physician, nurse, and pharmacist. Because reagent sensitivity varies among producers and from lot to lot, the clinician must evaluate PTT results in relationship to the institution's therapeutic and reference intervals.[15] No means analogous to the INR exists for normalizing PTT results. The PTT is used mostly to measure the effects of UFH. LMWH selectively catalyzes the neutralization of factor Xa over thrombin and cannot be measured using the PTT. Conversely, the chromogenic anti–factor Xa heparin assay may be used to assay UFH, LMWH, and synthetic heparin pentasaccharide.[16]

Limitations of Partial Thromboplastin Time Monitoring of Unfractionated Heparin

Several interfering conditions affect PTT results, rendering it insensitive to heparin therapy, a circumstance called *heparin resistance*.[17] Inflammation typically is accompanied by hyperfibrinogenemia greater than 400 mg/dL and factor VIII activity greater than 150%. Both tend to shorten the PTT and render it less sensitive to the effects of heparin. In many patients, the antithrombin level becomes depleted as a result of prolonged therapy or an underlying deficiency secondary to chronic inflammation. In this instance, the PTT result remains within the reference interval or becomes only slightly prolonged despite ever-increasing heparin dosages. Inflammation may be reduced through steroids and aspirin or nonsteroidal antiinflammatory drugs, and antithrombin concentrate may be administered. In the interim, however, an alternative monitor such as the chromogenic anti–factor Xa heparin assay is necessary.

Platelets release platelet factor 4, a heparin-neutralizing protein. In specimens from patients on heparin therapy, the PTT begins to shorten only 1 hour after collection because of in vitro platelet factor 4 release, unless the specimen is centrifuged, and the platelet-poor plasma is removed from the cells (Chapter 45).[18] Hypofibrinogenemia, factor deficiencies, lupus anticoagulant, and the presence of fibrin degradation products or paraproteins prolong the PTT independent of heparin levels.[19]

HEPARIN THERAPEUTIC RANGE

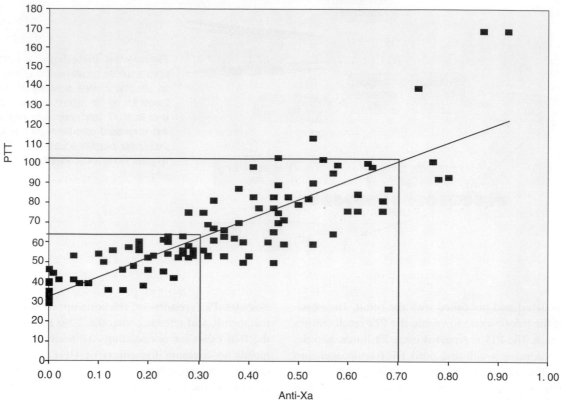

Figure 46-5 Laboratory scientists establish the UFH therapeutic range by collecting specimens from 50 heparinized patients at representative UFH dosages with normal PTs and 20 normal specimens. PTT and chromogenic anti–factor Xa heparin assays are performed on all specimens, and a linear graph of paired results is prepared. The PTT range in seconds is correlated to the chromogenic anti–factor Xa therapeutic range of 0.3 to 0.7 U/mL or the prophylactic range of 0.1 to 0.4 U/mL.

Monitoring Unfractionated Heparin Using the Activated Clotting Time Test in Surgical Suites

The activated clotting time (ACT) is a 1966 modification of the Lee-White whole-blood clotting time test that is used to monitor high-dose heparin therapy (Chapter 45). The ACT is performed at the clinic, inpatient bedside, cardiac catheterization laboratory, or surgical suite.[20]

ACT assay distributors provide evacuated specimen tubes with 12 mg of diatomaceous earth, a particulate clot activator. The tube is calibrated to collect 2 mL of blood. As soon as the specimen is collected, the phlebotomist starts a timer, and the tube is inverted a few times to disperse the activator. The phlebotomist continues to invert the tube until a clot forms. The median of normal ACT results is 98 seconds. Heparin is administered to yield results of 180 to 240 seconds in deep vein thrombosis or 400 seconds during cardiopulmonary bypass surgery or percutaneous cardiac intervention.[21]

The following instruments are designed to provide the ACT[22]:

- Actalyke XL and mini II (Helena Point of Care, Beaumont, Tex.)

- Hemochron Junior, Response, or Signature Elite (International Technidyne, Edison, N.J.)
- HMS Plus, ACT Plus (Medtronic, Minneapolis, Minn.)

After collection, the tube is placed in the instrument, where it is rotated and continuously monitored. When a clot forms, an internal magnet is pulled away from a sensing device. The time interval to clot formation is recorded automatically. The results of the ACT compare with the PTT for UFH monitoring, provided that adequate quality control steps are taken. The ACT is particularly necessary to monitor the high levels of heparin administered during coronary artery bypass surgery.

Reversal of Unfractionated Heparin Overdose Using Protamine Sulfate

Protamine sulfate, a cationic protein extracted from salmon sperm, neutralizes UFH at a ratio of 100 U/mg. The physician administers protamine sulfate slowly through intravenous push. The effect of protamine sulfate may be detected by shortening of the PTT or ACT to within the reference interval. Protamine sulfate also neutralizes LMWH, although the neutralization is incompletely reflected in the results of the chromogenic anti–factor Xa heparin assay described in the following paragraphs.

MONITORING LOW-MOLECULAR-WEIGHT HEPARIN USING THE CHROMOGENIC ANTI–FACTOR XA HEPARIN ASSAY

Low-Molecular-Weight Heparin Is Derived from Unfractionated Heparin

Uncertainty about UFH dose response and worry concerning HIT led to the development of LMWH, which was approved for anticoagulant prophylaxis in the United States and Canada in 1993. LMWH is prepared from UFH using chemical (enoxaparin [Lovenox]) or enzymatic (tinzaparin [Innohep]) fractionation. Fractionation yields a product with a mean molecular weight of 4500 to 5000 D, about one third the size of UFH. LMWH possesses the same active pentasaccharide sequence as UFH; however, the shorter saccharide chains provide little bridging surface, and the antithrombin (IIa) response is reduced (Fig. 46-6). The anti–factor Xa response is unchanged, however, so LMWH provides nearly the same anticoagulant efficacy.

LMWH is administered by subcutaneous injection once or twice per day using premeasured syringes. Prophylactic applications provide coverage during or after general and orthopedic surgery and trauma. LMWH also is used to treat deep vein thrombosis, pulmonary embolism, and unstable angina. LMWH is indicated during pregnancy in patients at risk of venous thromboembolism because warfarin cannot be used.

The advantages of LMWH are rapid bioavailability after subcutaneous injection, making intravenous administration unnecessary; half-life of 3 to 5 hours compared with 1 to 2 hours for UFH; and a fixed dose response that reduces the need for laboratory monitoring. The risk of HIT is reduced by 90%, although owing to cross-reactivity, LMWH is contraindicated in patients who have previously developed HIT after UFH therapy. The risk of LMWH-induced bleeding is equivalent to UFH and is about 10%.

Laboratory Monitoring of Low-Molecular-Weight Heparin

LMWH is cleared by the kidneys and accumulates in renal insufficiency. Laboratory monitoring is necessary when the creatinine clearance is less than 30 mL/min or serum creatinine is greater than 4 mg/dL. Creatinine levels are run periodically to avoid accumulation. Therapy for morbidly obese and pregnant patients also requires LMWH monitoring because of fluid compartment imbalances.

A specimen is collected 4 hours after subcutaneous injection, and the plasma is tested using the chromogenic anti–factor Xa heparin assay because the PTT is insensitive to LMWH. The chromogenic anti–factor Xa heparin assay employs a reagent with a fixed concentration of factor Xa and substrate specific to factor Xa (Fig. 46-7). Some distributors add fixed concentrations of antithrombin; others rely on the patient's plasma antithrombin. The latter formulation provides sensitivity to antithrombin depletion or deficiency. Heparin forms a complex with reagent Xa and antithrombin; excess factor Xa digests the substrate, yielding a colored product whose intensity is inversely proportional to heparin concentration.

To prepare a standard curve, the laboratory scientist obtains characteristic heparin from the pharmacy and computes dilutions to correspond with the therapeutic range. If the chromogenic anti–factor Xa heparin assay is to be used to monitor UFH and LMWH, a single hybrid standard curve may be prepared.[23,24] A separate curve is necessary to monitor pentasaccharide. The therapeutic range for twice-daily regimens is 0.5 to 1 U/mL, and for once-daily regimens, 1 to 2 U/mL.

The chromogenic anti–factor Xa heparin assay is the only assay available to monitor LMWH and pentasaccharide therapy. It also may be used in place of the PTT to assay UFH with little or no modification and substitutes for the PTT when clinical conditions render the PTT unreliable. The chromogenic anti–factor Xa heparin assay is tertiary in the sense that it measures concentration of heparin and not its anticoagulant effects; however, the assay is precise and, in contrast to the PTT,

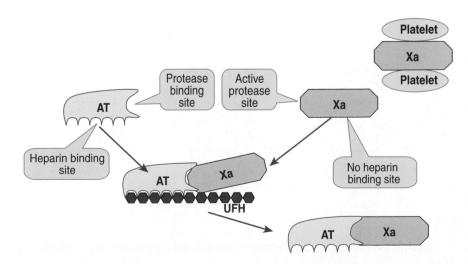

Figure 46-6 The binding site of antithrombin (AT) binds a specific heparin pentasaccharide, producing an allosteric change activating AT. The LMWH molecule is too short to support the thrombin (IIa)-antithrombin reaction; however, factor Xa reacts with AT independent of the bridging phenomenon, producing a soluble AT–factor Xa complex. The heparin recycles. Platelet-bound Xa does not enter the reaction.

Figure 46-7 The chromogenic anti-Xa heparin assay. The reagent for the chromogenic anti–factor Xa heparin assay is a mixture of antithrombin and a measured excess of factor Xa (some kits rely on patient plasma antithrombin). Antithrombin binds heparin, and this complex binds factor Xa. Excess free factor Xa enters a color reaction with its substrate. The color intensity of the product is inversely proportional to plasma heparin. This assay is used for UFH, LMWH, and pentasaccharide (fondaparinux); fondaparinux requires a dedicated standard curve.

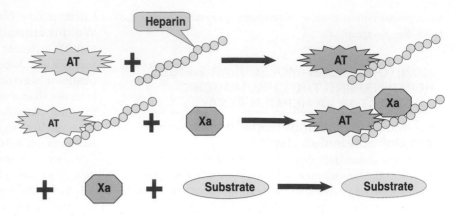

is affected by little interference. The chromogenic anti–factor Xa heparin assay is the reference method for establishing the PTT therapeutic range. On balance, laboratory directors have begun to recognize the merits of the chromogenic anti–factor Xa heparin assay and substitute it for the PTT in UFH therapy monitoring. All that remains is a volume reduction in assay cost and enactment of reasonable reimbursement policies.

MONITORING PENTASACCHARIDE THERAPY USING THE CHROMOGENIC ANTI–FACTOR XA HEPARIN ASSAY

Fondaparinux sodium (Arixtra; GlaxoSmithKline, Research Triangle Park, N.C.) is a synthetic formulation of the active pentasaccharide sequence in UFH and LMWH (Fig. 46-8). Fondaparinux is equivalent in efficacy and safety to UFH and LMWH and has a reproducible dose response and a half-life of 12 to 17 hours, requiring once-a-day subcutaneous injections of 2.5 mg. Fondaparinux is approved for surgical prophylaxis and treatment of deep vein thrombosis and pulmonary embolism and is contraindicated for patients with creatinine clearance less than 30 mL/min or patients with body weight less than 110 lb.

The chromogenic anti–factor Xa heparin assay is used to monitor fondaparinux therapy for infants, children, obese or underweight patients, patients on treatment the past 7 to 8 days, and pregnant women. Blood is collected 4 hours after injection, and the target range is 0.14 to 0.19 mg/L. The laboratory scientist prepares a standard curve using fondaparinux, not UFH, LMWH, or a hybrid standard, because concentrations are expressed in mg/L and not U/dL. The PTT is not sensitive to fondaparinux because fondaparinux reacts with antithrombin and factor Xa but has no activity with thrombin, IXa, XIa, or XIIa. It enhances antithrombin activity 400-fold.

MONITORING DIRECT THROMBIN INHIBITOR THERAPY USING THE PARTIAL THROMBOPLASTIN TIME AND THE ECARIN CLOTTING TIME

Argatroban

The DTIs argatroban, lepirudin, and bivalirudin reversibly bind and inactivate free and clot-bound (argatroban, bivalirudin) thrombin without involving antithrombin (Fig. 46-9). DTIs are substituted for UFH or LMWH when HIT is suspected or confirmed. Even when the only manifestation of HIT is throm-

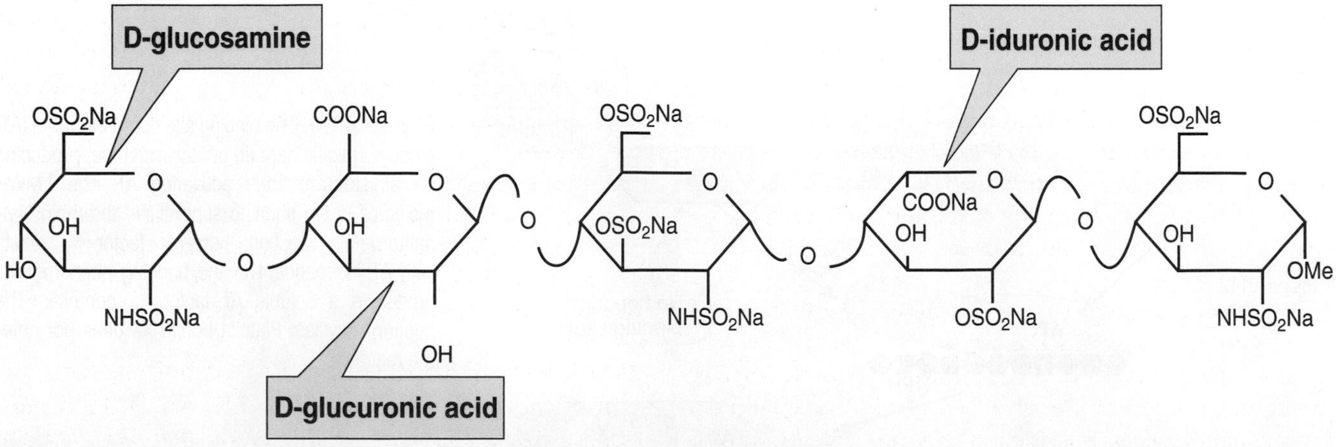

Figure 46-8 The specific saccharide sequence in UFH and LMWH is synthesized to make fondaparinux that binds and activates antithrombin. (From Turpie AGG: Pentasaccharides. Semin Hematol 2002;39:159-171.)

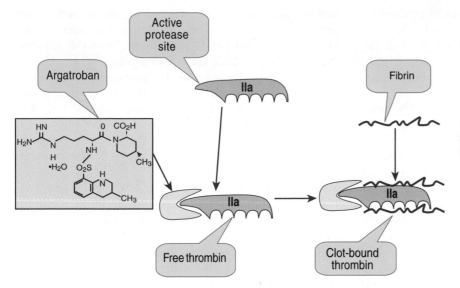

Figure 46-9 Argatroban inhibits the active site of free and clot-bound thrombin. Antithrombin is not involved in this reaction.

bocytopenia, heparin is stopped, and unless a DTI is used, the risk of thrombosis is 50% for the next 30 days.

Argatroban (Novostan; GlaxoSmithKline, Research Triangle Park, N.C.) is a nonprotein L-arginine derivative, molecular weight 527 D. Argatroban was approved in 1997 for anticoagulation in HIT where warfarin, UFH, LMWH, and pentasaccharide are contraindicated.[25] Argatroban is approved for prophylaxis, treatment, and anticoagulation during percutaneous coronary intervention (heart catheterization) for patients with HIT.

The physician initiates argatroban intravenous infusion at 2 µg/kg/min or in hepatic disease at 0.5 µg/kg/min. During percutaneous cardiac intervention, a bolus of 350 µg/kg is given over 3 to 5 minutes followed by 25 µg/kg/min. Argatroban is cleared by the liver and excreted in stool. There is a 5% general bleeding risk and no direct antidote; however, the half-life is 51 minutes, and argatroban clears from the blood in 2 to 4 hours. Argatroban requires laboratory monitoring, particularly in an overdose.

Lepirudin, a Recombinant Analogue of Hirudin

Lepirudin (Refludan; ZLB Behring GmbH, Montville, N.J., and Marburg, Germany) is a synthetic 7000-D protein DTI. Lepirudin is an analogue of natural hirudin, produced in trace amounts by the medicinal leech *Hirudo medicinalis*. Lepirudin is approved for anticoagulation in HIT. Lepirudin binds free but not fibrin-bound thrombin because the molecule is too large and is sterically hindered from binding clot-bound thrombin.

The physician administers a bolus of 0.4 mg/kg up to 110 kg over 15 to 20 seconds followed by 0.15 mg/kg/h as a continuous intravenous infusion for 2 to 10 days. Laboratory monitoring is necessary because the risk of bleeding is 10%. Lepirudin is cleared by the kidney. The dosage must be reduced in accordance with serum creatinine or creatinine clearance and is halted when creatinine clearance is less than 15 mL/min

or serum creatinine is greater than 6 mg/dL. It is necessary to run creatinine levels throughout lepirudin therapy. There is no antidote for lepirudin in overdose, but the plasma half-life is 20 minutes.

Antihirudin antibodies form in about 40% of HIT patients treated with lepirudin. These antibodies may increase the anticoagulant effect owing to delayed renal elimination of active lepirudin-antihirudin complexes. Strict laboratory monitoring is necessary during prolonged therapy, and anaphylaxis may occur during a second administration.[26]

Bivalirudin, a Recombinant Derivative of Hirudin

Bivalirudin (Angiomax; The Medicines Company, Parsippany, N.J.) is a synthetic 20-amino acid peptide derivative of hirudin, molecular weight 2180 D. Bivalirudin inactivates free and clot-bound thrombin. Bivalirudin was approved in 2000 for use as an anticoagulant in patients with unstable angina at risk for HIT undergoing percutaneous coronary intervention.

Bivalirudin is intended for use with aspirin 325 mg/d and has been studied only in patients receiving aspirin. Physicians provide an intravenous bolus dose of 0.75 mg/kg followed by an infusion of 1.75 mg/kg/h for the duration of the percutaneous cardiac intervention. After 4 hours, an additional intravenous infusion may be initiated at a rate of 0.2 mg/kg/h for 20 hours.

The rate of major hemorrhage for bivalirudin is 4%. There is no antidote; however, in normal renal function the half-life is 25 minutes. The dosage is reduced in reduced creatinine clearance or elevated serum creatinine. No antihirudin antibody has been shown in bivalirudin therapy.

Monitoring Direct Thrombin Inhibitors

DTIs affect the thrombin time, PT, PTT, and ACT. In nonsurgical therapy, distributors recommend the PTT with the target therapeutic range 1.5 to 3 times the mean of the laboratory reference interval. For bivalirudin or lepirudin, blood is collected 4 hours after the onset of intravenous therapy, and for argatroban, blood is collected 2 hours later, and the dosage is adjusted to the therapeutic range. The ACT is used during percutaneous cardiac intervention when the dosage is high. Bivalirudin's target ACT is 320 to 400 seconds (median normal 98 seconds).

In instances when the baseline PTT is prolonged by lupus anticoagulant or factor deficiencies, an alternative assay is necessary. The ecarin clotting time (ECT) is an attractive alternative. Ecarin (ecarinase) (Pentapharm, Basel, Switzerland) is an enzyme extracted from *Echis carinatus* venom that converts prothrombin to the intermediate meizothrombin, which converts fibrinogen to fibrin. DTIs bind meizothrombin and yield a linear, dose-dependent prolongation of the ECT. Besides DTIs, the ECT is prolonged only by abnormal low prothrombin and fibrinogen activity. A more recently described ECT reagent enriched with prothrombin and fibrinogen eliminates prolongation caused by variations in patient prothrombin and fibrinogen levels for accurate DTI determinations.[27]

Ecarin reagent requires special handling, and the assay has no prepared calibrators or controls, so the ECT is only slowly becoming available in acute care facility laboratories. Specialized references laboratories such as Esoterix Coagulation in Aurora, Colo., offer the assay.

MONITORING ANTIPLATELET THERAPY WITH PLATELET ACTIVITY ASSAYS

Aspirin, Clopidogrel, and Ticlopidine Reduce the Incidence of Arterial Thrombosis

The most commonly prescribed oral antiplatelet drugs are aspirin, clopidogrel (Plavix; Sanofi-Aventis, Bridgewater, N.J., and Bristol-Meyers Squibb, New York, N.Y.) and ticlopidine (Ticlid; Roche Pharmaceuticals, Nutley, N.J.). Aspirin irreversibly acetylates the platelet enzyme cyclooxygenase at serine 529. The acetyl group sterically hinders the access of arachidonic acid to its reactive site and prevents production of platelet-activating thromboxane A_2 through the eicosanoid synthesis pathway (Chapter 13). Acetylation is irreversible. Clopidogrel and ticlopidine reversibly occupy the platelet membrane adenosine diphosphate receptor P2Y12, suppressing platelet aggregation and secretion response to adenosine diphosphate.

Physicians customarily prescribe aspirin at 81 or 325 mg/d or aspirin plus clopidogrel (75 mg/d) to prevent myocardial infarction and ischemic cerebrovascular disease in patients with stable or unstable angina,[28,29] acute myocardial infarction,[30] transient cerebral ischemia,[31] peripheral vascular disease,[32] and stroke.[33,34] In healthy individuals, aspirin prophylaxis annually prevents 4 thrombotic events per 1000 subjects treated, although it carries a risk of bleeding.[35-37]

Platelet Activity Studies and Variable Antiplatelet Therapy Response

Several investigations confirm that 10% to 15% of individuals taking aspirin generate an inadequate laboratory response as measured in platelet aggregometry using arachidonic acid and collagen, the reference method for determining aspirin sensitivity. Other assays are VerifyNow (Accumetrics, San Diego, Calif.), PFA-100 (Dade-Behring, Deerfield, Ill), and AspirinWorks (Corgenix, Inc., Denver, Colo.).[38,39]

Helgason et al[40] used optical aggregometry to show that 7 of 17 patients with atrial fibrillation achieved partial inhibition of platelet aggregation when taking 325 mg/d of enteric-coated aspirin. Helgason's group further showed that 8.2% of patients with previous ischemic stroke exhibited restoration of platelet aggregation despite escalation of aspirin therapy to ultimately 1300 mg/d.[41]

Eikelboom et al[42] in a case-control retrospective study concluded that the odds for the composite outcome of myocardial infarction, stroke, or cardiovascular death increased with each increasing quartile of urinary 11-dehydrothromboxane B_2, a platelet eicosanoid pathway metabolite derived from thromboxane A_2. Patients in the upper quartile (aspirin resistant) had a 1.8 times higher risk than patients in the lowest quartile (responsive). These investigators concluded, "In aspirin-treated patients, urinary concentrations of 11-dehydrothromboxane B_2 predict the future risk of myocardial infarction or cardiovascular death. These findings raise the possibility that elevated urinary 11-dehydrothromboxane B_2 levels identify patients who are relatively resistant to aspirin and who may benefit from additional antiplatelet therapies or treatments that more effectively block in vivo thromboxane production or activity."

Gum et al,[43] in a prospective randomized control study using optical platelet aggregometry, showed that 5.2% of 326 cardiovascular patients were aspirin resistant. During follow-up, aspirin resistance was associated with a 3.12 times increased risk of death, myocardial infarction, or stroke compared with patients who were aspirin responsive. Although less well defined, the possibility of clopidogrel resistance is reported in several more recent studies.[44]

Laboratory Monitoring of Antiplatelet Resistance

Many models have been developed to explain antiplatelet resistance, and current studies are designed to clarify the mechanism eventually.[45] Many clinicians simply ascribe antiplatelet resistance to patient noncompliance. Nevertheless, coagulation laboratory directors currently are considering the various means of identifying aspirin resistance.[46]

As listed earlier, whole-blood platelet function assays include the following:

- Platelet aggregometry, including optical and whole-blood aggregometry and lumiaggregometry testing platelet response to collagen and arachidonic acid
- Platelet activation assays on specialized instruments—VerifyNow (Accumetrics, San Diego, Calif.) and PFA-100 (Dade-Behring, Deerfield, Ill.).
- AspirinWorks (Corgenix, Inc., Denver, Colo) immunoassay of urinary 11-dehydrothromboxane B_2

The AspirinWorks method assays a urine metabolite of platelet eicosanoid activation. Hepatocyte 11-hydroxythromboxane dehydrogenase acts on platelet-derived plasma thromboxane B_2, spontaneously derived from thromboxane A_2, to produce water-soluble 11-dehydrothromboxane B_2.[47] The urine concentration of 11-dehydrothromboxane B_2 is plentiful and, as platelets seem to be its primary source, proportionally reflects platelet activity within the previous 12 hours.[48] Urine levels of 11-dehydrothromboxane B_2 frequently are

elevated in atherosclerosis, after stroke, transient ischemic attack, intracerebral hemorrhage, and atrial fibrillation.[49] 11-Dehydrothromboxane B_2 levels typically are decreased in aspirin therapy, even in cases of atherosclerosis, myocardial infarction, and atrial fibrillation, but remain normal in aspirin resistance.

CHAPTER at a GLANCE

- Warfarin is the only oral anticoagulant, and it was developed in 1940 by Link. It is used to prevent venous thromboembolism; it has a narrow therapeutic range, and an overdose causes hemorrhage. Warfarin therapy is monitored by the PT assay and reported as an INR. The PT is available on point of care instrumentation.
- UFH is administered intravenously to provide immediate control of coagulation, especially during percutaneous cardiac intervention or coronary artery bypass graft surgery involving extracorporeal circulation. It is monitored using the PTT assay, which requires the scientist to develop a therapeutic range in seconds keyed to the chromogenic anti–factor Xa heparin assay. The PTT is subject to interference. UFH may cause HIT.
- LMWH and pentasaccharide may substitute for UFH and are administered subcutaneously for prophylaxis and therapy. Both provide rapid bioavailability, predictable dose response, and longer half-lives than UFH. LMWH and pentasaccharide are monitored in

renal insufficiency, pregnancy, and morbid obesity, using the chromogenic anti–factor Xa heparin assay.
- The DTIs argatroban, lepirudin, and bivalirudin bind thrombin without involving antithrombin and are substituted for heparin in HIT. Bivalirudin is used only in combination with aspirin. DTIs are monitored using the PTT or ECT, and all affect the PT results during switchover to warfarin therapy.
- The antiplatelet drugs aspirin, clopidogrel, and ticlopidine are used to prevent arterial thrombosis, particularly acute myocardial infarction, stroke, and peripheral artery occlusion. Patients may be resistant to antiplatelet therapy; this may be detected through platelet aggregometry, whole-blood instrumentation, or measurement of urine platelet metabolites.

Now that you have completed this chapter, go back and read again the case study at the beginning and respond to the questions presented.

REVIEW QUESTIONS

1. What is the PT INR therapeutic range for warfarin therapy when a patient has a mechanical heart valve?
   a. 1.0-2.0
   b. 2.0-3.0
   c. 2.5-3.5
   d. Warfarin is not indicated for mechanical heart valves.

2. Monitoring of a patient taking warfarin showed that she seemed stable over about 7 months. The frequency of her visits to the laboratory began to diminish, so the period between testing averaged 6 weeks. This new testing interval is:
   a. Acceptable for a stably anticoagulated patient after 6 months
   b. Unnecessary because testing for patients on oral anticoagulants can be discontinued entirely after 4 months of stable test results
   c. Too long even for a patient with previously stable test results; 4 weeks is the standard
   d. Acceptable as long as the patient performs self-monitoring daily using an approved home testing instrument and reports unacceptable results promptly to her physician

3. What is the greatest advantage of point of care PT testing?
   a. Permits for self-dosing of warfarin
   b. Inexpensive
   c. Convenient
   d. Precise

4. You collect a citrated whole-blood specimen to monitor UFH therapy. What is the longest it may stand before the plasma must be separated from the cells?
   a. 1 hour
   b. 4 hours
   c. 24 hours
   d. Indefinite

5. What test is used to monitor high-dose UFH therapy in the cardiac catheterization operating suite?
   a. PT
   b. PTT
   c. Bleeding time
   d. ACT

6. What test is used most often to monitor UFH therapy in the central laboratory?
   a. PT
   b. PTT
   c. ACT
   d. Chromogenic anti–factor Xa heparin assay

7. What test is used most often to monitor LMWH therapy in the central laboratory?
   a. PT
   b. PTT
   c. ACT
   d. Chromogenic anti–factor Xa heparin assay

8. What is an advantage of LMWH therapy over UFH therapy?
   a. Cheaper
   b. Less bleeding
   c. Stable dose response
   d. No risk of HIT

9. In what situation is a DTI used?
   a. Deep vein thrombosis
   b. HIT
   c. Any situation where warfarin could be used
   d. Uncomplicated acute myocardial infarction

10. What laboratory test may be used to monitor DTIs when the PTT is unreliable?
    a. PT
    b. ECT
    c. Reptilase clotting time
    d. Chromogenic anti–factor Xa heparin assay

11. What is the reference method for detecting aspirin or clopidogrel resistance?
    a. Platelet aggregometry
    b. AspirinWorks
    c. VerifyNow
    d. PFA-100

12. What is the name of the measurable platelet activation metabolite used in the AspirinWorks assay to monitor aspirin resistance?
    a. 11-dehydrothromboxane B_2
    b. Arachidonic acid
    c. Thromboxane A_2
    d. Cyclooxygenase

REFERENCES

1. Levine MN, Raskob G, Beyth RJ, et al: Hemorrhagic complications of anticoagulant treatment: the seventh ACCP conference on antithrombotic and thrombolytic therapy. Chest 2004;126:287S-310S.
2. Francis CW, Berkowitz SD: Antithrombotic and thrombolytic agents. In Kitchens CS, Alving BM, Kessler CM (eds): Consultative Hemostasis and Thrombosis. Philadelphia: Saunders, 2002:375-393.
3. Adverse events and deaths associated with laboratory errors at a hospital—Pennsylvania, 2001. MMWR Morb Mortal Wkly Rep 2001;50:710-711.
4. Ansell J, Hirsh J, Poller L, et al: The pharmacology and management of the vitamin K antagonists: the seventh ACCP conference on antithrombotic and thrombolytic therapy. Chest 2004;126:204S-233S.
5. Kresge N, Simoni RD, Hill RL: Hemorrhagic sweet clover disease, dicumarol, and warfarin: the work of Karl Paul Link. J Biol Chem 2005;280:5-5.
6. Warkentin TE: Coumarin-induced skin necrosis and venous limb gangrene. In Colman RW, Clowes AW, Goldhaber SZ, et al (eds): Hemostasis and Thrombosis: Basic Principles and Clinical Practice. Philadelphia: Lippincott, 2006:1663-1671.
7. Poller L: Laboratory control of anticoagulant therapy. Semin Thromb Hemost 1986;12:13-19.
8. Schalekamp T, Brasse BP, Roijers JF, et al: VKORC1 and CYP2C9 genotypes and acenocoumarol anticoagulation status: interaction between both genotypes affects over-anticoagulation. Clin Pharmacol Ther 2006;80:13-22.
9. Weitz JI, Hirsh J, Samama MM: New anticoagulant drugs: the seventh ACCP conference on antithrombotic and thrombolytic therapy. Chest 2004;126:265S-287S.
10. Coagulation analyzers. CAP Today 2005;March:24-29.
11. Laposata M: Point-of-care coagulation testing: stepping gently forward. Clin Chem 2001;47:801-802.
12. Hirsch J, Raschke R: Heparin and low-molecular-weight heparin: the seventh ACCP conference on antithrombotic and thrombolytic therapy. Chest 2004;126:188S-203S.
13. Olson JD, Arkin CF, Brandt JT, et al (eds): College of American Pathologists conference XXXI on laboratory monitoring of anticoagulant therapy: laboratory monitoring of unfractionated heparin therapy. Arch Pathol Lab Med 1998;122:782-798.
14. Brill-Edwards P, Ginsberg JS, Johnston M, et al: Establishing a therapeutic range for heparin therapy. Ann Intern Med 1993;119:104-109.
15. Brandt JT, Arkin CF, Bovill EG, et al: Evaluation of PTT reagent sensitivity to factor IX and factor IX assay performance. Arch Pathol Lab Med 1990;114:135-141.
16. Tollefsen DM: Laboratory diagnosis of antithrombin and heparin cofactor II deficiency. Semin Thromb Hemost 1990;16:162-168.
17. Bharadwaj J, Jayaraman C, Shrivastava R: Heparin resistance. Lab Hematol 2003;9:125-131.
18. Adcock DM, Kressin DC, Marlar RA: The effect of time and temperature variables on routine coagulation tests. Blood Coagul Fibrinolysis. 1998;9:463-70.
19. Estry DW, Wright L: Laboratory assessment of anticoagulant therapy. Clin Lab Sci 1988;1:161-164.
20. Hattersley P: Activated coagulation time of whole blood. JAMA 1966;136:436-440.
21. Najman DM, Walenga JM, Fareed J, et al: Effects of aprotinin on anticoagulant monitoring: implications in cardiovascular surgery. Ann Thorac Surg 1993;55:662-666.
22. Grill HP, Spero JE, Granato JE: Comparison of activated partial thromboplastin time to activated clotting time for adequacy of heparin anticoagulation just before percutaneous transluminal coronary angioplasty. Am J Cardiol 1993;71:1219-1220.
23. McGlasson DL, Kaczor DA, Krasuski RA, et al: Effects of preanalytical variables on the anti-activated factor X chromogenic assay when monitoring unfractionated heparin and low molecular weight heparin anticoagulation. Blood Coagul Fibrinolysis 2005;16:173-176.
24. McGlasson DL: Using a single calibration curve with the anti-Xa chromogenic assay for monitoring heparin anticoagulation. Lab Med 2005;36:297-299.
25. Yeh RW, Jang IK: Argatroban: update. Am Heart J 2006;151:1131-1138.
26. Cardenas GA, Deitcher SR: Risk of anaphylaxis after re-exposure to intravenous lepirudin in patients with current or past heparin-induced thrombocytopenia. Mayo Clin Proc 2005;80:491-493.
27. Choi TS, Khan AI, Greilich PE, et al: Modified plasma-based ecarin clotting time assay for monitoring of recombinant hirudin during cardiac surgery. Am J Clin Pathol 2006;125:290-295.

28. Juul-Moller S, Edvardsson N, Jahnmatz B, et al: Double-blind trial of aspirin in primary prevention of myocardial infarction in patients with stable chronic angina pectoris. Lancet 1992; 340:1421-1425.

29. The RISC Group: Risk of myocardial infarction and death during treatment with low dose aspirin and intravenous heparin in men with unstable coronary artery disease. Lancet 1990;336:827-830.

30. ISIS-2 Collaborative Group: Randomised trial of intravenous streptokinase, oral aspirin, both or neither among 17,187 cases of suspected acute myocardial infarction: ISIS-2. Lancet 1988;2:349-360.

31. The Dutch TIA Study Group: A comparison of two doses of aspirin (30 mg vs. 283 mg a day) in patients after a transient ischemic attack or minor ischemic stroke. N Engl J Med 1991;325:1261-1622.

32. Hirsh J, Dalen JE, Fuster V, et al: Aspirin and other platelet-active drugs: the relationship among dose, effectiveness, and side effects. Chest 1995;108:247S-257S.

33. International Stroke Trial Collaborative Group: The International Stroke Trial (IST): a randomised trial of aspirin, sub-cutaneous heparin, both, or neither among 19,435 patients with acute ischemic stroke. Lancet 1997;349:1569-1581.

34. CAST (Chinese Acute Stroke Trial) Collaborative Group: CAST: randomised placebo-controlled trial of early aspirin use in 20,000 patients with acute ischemic stroke. Lancet 1997; 349:1641-1649.

35. Antiplatelet Trialists' Collaboration: Collaborative overview of randomized trials of antiplatelet therapy: I. Prevention of death, myocardial infarction, and stroke by prolonged anti-platelet therapy in various categories of patients. BMJ 1994;308:81-106.

36. Hennekens CH, Peto R, Hutchison GB, et al: An overview of the British and American aspirin studies. N Engl J Med 1988;318:923-924.

37. Manson JE, Stampfer MJ, Colditz GA, et al: A prospective study of aspirin use and primary prevention of cardiovascular disease. JAMA 1991;266:521-527.

38. Wu KK, Hoak JC: A new method for the quantitative detection of platelet aggregates in patients with arterial insufficiency. Lancet 1974;2:924-926.

39. McGlasson DL, Chen M, Fritsma GA: Urinary 11-dehydro-thromboxane B2 levels in healthy individuals following a single dose response to two concentrations of aspirin. J Clin Ligand Assay 2005;28:147-150.

40. Helgason CM, Hoff JA, Kondos GT, et al: Platelet aggregation in patients with atrial fibrillation taking aspirin or warfarin. Stroke 1993;24:1458-1461.

41. Helgason CM, Bolin KM, Hoff JA, et al: Development of aspirin resistance in persons with previous ischemic stroke. Stroke 1994;25:2331-2336.

42. Eikelboom JW, Hirsh J, Weitz JI, et al: Aspirin-resistant throm-boxane biosynthesis and the risk of myocardial infarction, stroke, or cardiovascular death in patients at high risk for cardiovascular events. Circulation 2002;105:1650-1655.

43. Gum PA, Kottke-Marchant K, Welsh PA, et al: A prospective, blinded determination of the natural history of aspirin resistance among stable patients with cardiovascular disease. J Am Coll Cardiol 2003;41:961-965.

44. Chen WH: Antiplatelet resistance with aspirin and clopidogrel: is it real and does it matter? Curr Cardiol Rep 2006;8:301-306.

45. Knoepp SM, Laposata M: Aspirin resistance: moving forward with multiple definitions, different assays, and a clinical imperative. Am J Clin Pathol 2005;123:S125-S132.

46. McGlasson DL, Fritsma GA, Chen M, et al: Are different tests of platelet function comparable when taking aspirin? Clin Lab Sci 2006;19:156.

47. Catella F, Fitzgerald GA: Paired analysis of urinary throm-boxane B2 metabolites in humans. Thrombos Res 1987; 47:647-656.

48. Catella F, Fitzgerald GA: Paired analysis of urinary throm-boxane B2 metabolites in humans. Thrombos Res 1987; 47:647-656.

49. Van Kooten F, Ciabattoni G, Koudstaal PJ, et al: Increased platelet activation in the chronic phase after cerebral ischemia and intracerebral hemorrhage. Stroke 1999;30:546-549.

47

Coagulation Instrumentation

Cynthia S. Johns

OBJECTIVES

After completion of this chapter, the reader will be able to:

1. Describe testing methodologies previously considered as specialized that are now routinely available on coagulation analyzers.
2. Identify testing applications employed by various coagulation analyzers.
3. Explain methods of clot detection on each type of coagulation analyzer presented.
4. List common instrument flags to alert operators to specimen and instrument problems.
5. Identify advantages and disadvantages of each method of clot detection.
6. Distinguish the characteristics of manual, semi-automated, and automated coagulation analyzers.
7. Identify key performance characteristics that should be evaluated when selecting the most appropriate coagulation analyzer for an individual laboratory setting.
8. Explain the purpose of incorporating platelet function testing analyzers into the routine coagulation laboratory.
9. Develop a model plan of action to evaluate objectively coagulation analyzers for purchase.
10. Explain the main purpose for point of care coagulation testing.

CASE STUDY

After studying the material in this chapter, the reader should be able to respond to the following case study:

A 35-year-old Caucasian man was admitted to the hospital with abdominal pain, tenderness, malaise, and a low-grade fever. A tentative diagnosis of cholecystitis was made, with possible surgical intervention considered. Previous medical history included tonsillectomy at age 6 and appendectomy at age 18 with no abnormal bleeding symptoms noted. The patient denied taking any medications at this time. In anticipation of surgery, routine coagulation studies were ordered. When the specimen arrived in the laboratory, it was centrifuged and noted to have a whitish, milky appearance to the plasma. The specimen was run on an automated analyzer using photo-optical end point detection methodology with the following results:

Because the laboratory's policy is to rerun all abnormal coagulation results, the prothrombin time and partial thromboplastin time were repeated with similar results obtained.

1. Should the technologist report these test results as obtained from the analyzer to the physician?
2. What action, if any, should be taken to address the lipemia flagging of this specimen?
3. Would you expect this patient to be at risk for bleeding based on these test results?

Test	Results	Flags	Reference Interval
Prothrombin time	16.7 s	Lipemia	10.9-13 s
Partial thromboplastin time	>150 s	Lipemia	30.6-35 s
Fibrinogen	245 mg/dL	Lipemia	190-410 mg/dL

Automation in the coagulation laboratory has brought significant advances in its routine testing capabilities. In the past, the routine coagulation menu consisted of prothrombin time (PT), partial thromboplastin time (PTT) (or activated partial thromboplastin time), fibrinogen, thrombin time, and fibrin degradation products. When necessary, more specialized or complex tests were performed in larger laboratories employing clinical laboratory technologists and technicians who had specialized training in coagulation. With the introduction of new instrumentation and test methodologies, routine coagulation testing capabilities have expanded significantly to the point where many formerly "esoteric" tests can be performed more easily by general clinical laboratory staff who rotate through the coagulation department. The difficulty that is now faced by the laboratory is the ability of the technologists and technicians to recognize preanalytical and analytical variables that can affect the integrity of the test results. Laboratory personnel must develop expertise in interpreting and correlating test results with the patient's diagnosis or condition (i.e., analysis of postanalytical variables). New instrumentation has allowed coagulation testing to become more standardized, consistent, and cost-effective. Automation has not advanced, however, to the point of making coagulation testing a foolproof or exact science. Cognitive ability and theoretical understanding of the hemostatic mechanism is still required to ensure accuracy and validity of test results for the physician to make an informed decision about patient care.

HISTORICAL PERSPECTIVES

Primitive clot detection apparatus were developed in 1910 with the introduction of a detection system called the *coaguloviscosimeter*.[1] The change in viscosity of blood as it clotted was measured by a change in voltage and recorded from a direct read-out system. Voltage changes could be plotted versus time and clot formation measured. In the 1920s, the nephelometer was applied to blood coagulation. Nephelometers use the principles of light dispersion variation in a colloidal suspension. As blood clotted, changes in light scatter of the fluid could be measured over time, a principle that is still in use today.

By the 1930s, the principle of clot detection by photoelectric measurements was developed. This methodology was based on the observation that the optical density of blood changed as it clotted, and the changes could be measured by voltage changes within a photocell as light passed through the specimen. This system has evolved into the photo-optical systems used in many current coagulation analyzers.

The 1950s saw the development of an instrument that still can be found in coagulation laboratories today. This instrument employed an electromechanical clot detection methodology and allowed laboratories to transition from the manual tilt tube or wire loop method to a more accurate semiautomated testing process.

Current coagulation instruments use many of the clot detection principles of these early analytical systems. Although the principles remain the same, the instruments have been dramatically enhanced and improved over the years to eliminate variations in pipetting and end point detection and allow multiple analyses to be performed simultaneously on a single specimen.

GENERAL PRINCIPLES OF END POINT DETECTION

Numerous semiautomated and fully automated instruments are available to perform coagulation testing. Semiautomated equipment requires test plasma and reagents to be delivered manually to the reaction cuvette and limits testing to being performed on only one or two specimens at a time. The advantage is that they are relatively inexpensive and easily operated. Fully automated analyzers contain pipetting systems that automatically add necessary reagents and test plasma to the reaction vessels and measure the end point without further operator intervention (Table 47-1). An additional advantage is that multiple specimens often can be tested simultaneously. These instruments are significantly more expensive to purchase, however, and require increased staff training to operate and maintain. Regardless of the technology selected for use in the laboratory, all semiautomated and automated analyzers have greatly improved coagulation testing accuracy and precision over the traditional manual methods.

Instrument methodologies used for coagulation testing generally are classified into five groups based on the principle of end point detection employed by the analyzer. These five classifications are as follows:
- Mechanical
- Photo-optical (turbidometric)
- Nephelometric
- Chromogenic (amidolytic)
- Immunologic

Historically, coagulation instruments were capable only of providing one type of end point detection, such as mechanical or photo-optical. Photo-optical instruments were designed to read the end point at only one wavelength. Initially, this end point was set at a fixed wavelength between 500 nm and 600 nm and could be used only for detection of clot formation. Later, other instruments were developed to read at 405 nm to measure chromogenic assays. Although this change made it possible to automate advanced coagulation protocols, it required laboratories to purchase and train staff on multiple analyzers if they wanted to offer the wider range of coagulation testing capabilities. Within the past few decades, instrument manufacturers successfully have incorporated multiple detection methods into the same analyzer, allowing a laboratory to purchase and train on only one instrument while still providing specialized testing capabilities on all shifts with multiple operators.

Mechanical End Point Detection Used by Semiautomated and Automated Analyzers

Two methodologies are used for mechanical detection of clot formation. The first, also known as *electromechanical clot detection*, measures a change in conductivity between two metal electrodes immersed in plasma. There is one stationary and

TABLE 47-1 Levels of Coagulation Automation

Level	Description	Examples
Manual	All reagents and specimens are added manually by the operator. Temperature is maintained by a waterbath or heat block; may require external measurement by operator. End point is determined visually by the operator. Timing is initiated and stopped by the operator, most often using a stopwatch	Tilt tube, wire loop
Semiautomated	All reagents and specimens are added manually by the operator. Usually contains a device for maintaining constant 37° C temperature. Analyzer may or may not internally monitor temperature. Has mechanism to initiate timing device automatically on addition of final reagent and internal mechanism for detecting clot formation and stopping the timer	Fibrometer, Start4, KC4 Delta
Automated	All reagents are automatically pipetted by the instrument. Specimens may or may not be automatically pipetted. Contains monitoring devices and internal mechanism to maintain and monitor constant 37° C temperature throughout testing sequence. Timers are initiated, and clot formation is detected automatically	MDA, STA-R, BCS, AMAX, ACL

one moving probe. During clotting, the moving probe enters and leaves the plasma at regular intervals. The current between the probes is broken as the moving probe leaves the plasma. When a clot forms, the fibrin strand conducts current between the two probes even when the moving probe leaves the solution.[2] The current completes a circuit and stops the timer. Electromechanical end point detection has been available since the mid-1950s on an instrument known as the BBL Fibrometer (BD Diagnostic Systems, Sparks, Md.), one of the first "semi-automated" instruments routinely used in the coagulation laboratory.[2]

The second method of mechanical clot detection involves magnetically monitoring the movement of a steel ball within plasma. As the clot forms, the slowing of the ball is detected by the sensor. Two variations are used in current instrumentation. One is based on the detection of increased viscosity of the plasma being tested when fibrin is formed. An electromagnetic field detects movement of a steel ball within the cuvette.[3] The ball oscillates at a constant rate through the plasma-reagent solution. As fibrin strands begin to form, the viscosity starts to increase, slowing the movement (Fig. 47-1). When the oscillation decreases to a predefined rate, the timer stops, which indicates the clotting time of the plasma. This methodology can be found on the Diagnostica Stago analyzers (Fig. 47-2).[3]

In the second variation, a steel ball is positioned in an inclined well. The position of the ball is detected by a magnetic sensor. As the well rotates, the ball remains positioned on the incline. When fibrin forms, the ball is swept out of position. As it moves away from the sensor, there is a break in the circuit, which stops the timer.[4,5] This technology can be found on

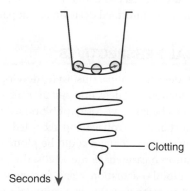

Figure 47-1 Diagram of mechanical clot detection from Diagnostica Stago.

AMAX instruments distributed by Trinity Biotech, Plc (Bray, County Wicklow, Ireland) (Fig. 47-3).

Photo-optical End Point Detection Used by Semiautomated and Automated Analyzers

Detection of a change in optical density is the basis of photo-optical coagulometers. This also is known as *turbidometric methodology*. When a light source of a specified wavelength passes through plasma, a certain amount of light is detected by a photodetector or photocell located on the other side of the solution.[6] The amount of light detected depends on the color and clarity of the plasma specimen and is considered to be the baseline light transmission value. Formation of fibrin strands causes light to scatter, allowing less light to fall on the photodetector.[6] This decreased light reflects the change in optical density. When light decreases to a predetermined deflection from baseline, the timer stops, indicating clot formation (Fig. 47-4). Most automated and semiautomated coagulation instruments developed since 1970 employ photo-optical clot detection (Fig. 47-5).

Nephelometric End Point Detection Used by Automated Analyzers

Nephelometry is an immunometric method for measuring proteins.[7] Antigen-antibody complexes precipitate, causing turbidity that scatters incident light.[7] The nephelometer uses a light-emitting diode producing incident light at greater than 600 nm to detect variations in light scatter at 90 degrees (side) and 180 degrees (forward light scatter) as antigen-antibody

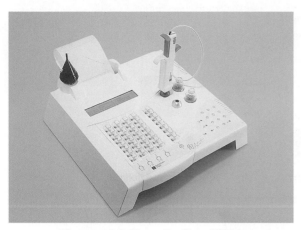

Figure 47-2 Diagnostica Stago STArt 4.

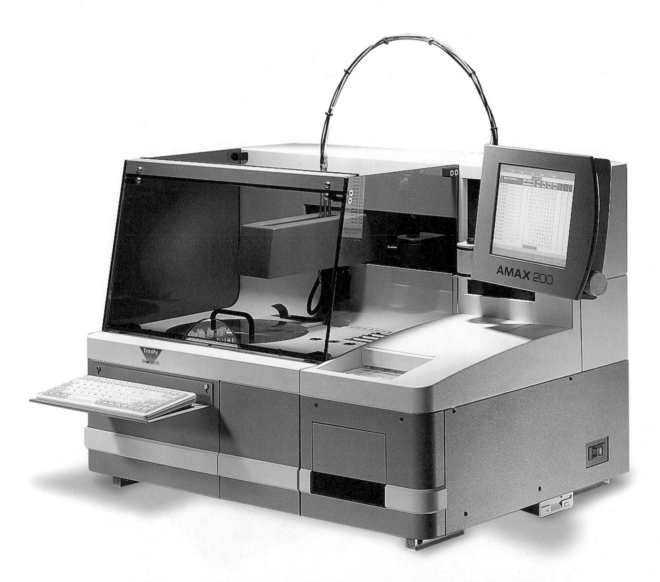

Figure 47-3 AMAX 400 Plus. (Courtesy of Trinity Biotech Plc, Bray, County Wicklow, Ireland.)

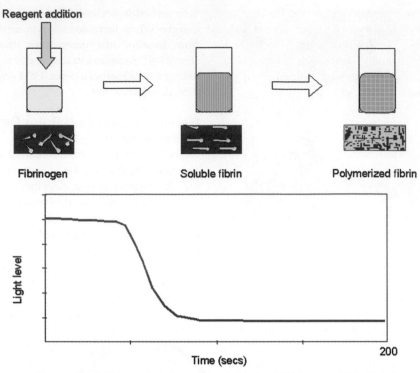

Figure 47-4 Clot waveform from a normal sample—MDA Systems, Trinity Biotech.

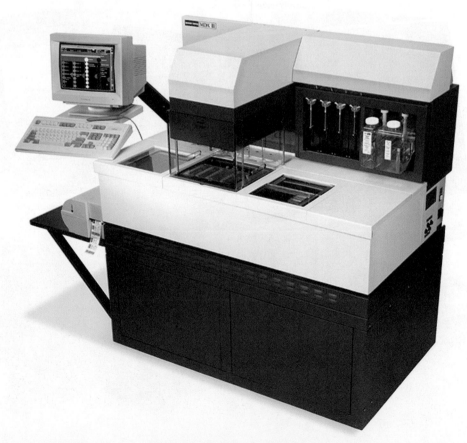

Figure 47-5 MDA II, Trinity Biotech.

complexes form. Nephelometric instruments read the increasing amount of side scatter as agglutinates form (Fig. 47-6).[8] The timer stops when the 90-degree light scatter reaches a predetermined level. This method contrasts with photo-optical systems that record decreased light at the forward 180-degree angle owing to the opacity of the specimen.

In nephelometry, if the immune complexes are too small for detection, the antibodies are attached to latex particles. The coagulation laboratory uses antigen-antibody reactions with coated latex particles to measure specific coagulation proteins.

Chromogenic End Point Detection Used by Automated Analyzers

Chromogenic, or amidolytic, methodology employs a color-producing substance known as a *chromophore*. For the coagulation laboratory, the chromophore used is para-nitroaniline (pNA), which has an absorbance peak at 405 nm. The pNA is bound to a synthetic oligopeptide, a series of amino acids whose sequence matches the structure of the target of the protease being measured.[9] The protease cleaves the chromogenic substrate at the site binding the oligopeptide to the pNA, freeing pNA. Free pNA is yellow; the color intensity of the solution is proportional to protease activity and is measured by a photodetector at 405 nm. As additional pNA is freed, the absorbance is increased. Enzymatic activity of coagulation proteins and other substances can be measured by the chromogenic method in two ways:

- *Direct measurement*—Optical density is proportional to the activity of the substance being measured (e.g., protein C activity assays).
- *Indirect measurement*—The enzyme being measured has an inhibitory effect on another target enzyme that has activity directed toward the synthetic substrate. In this case, the change in optical density is inversely proportional to the concentration or activity of the substance being measured (e.g., heparin anti–factor Xa assays).

Immunologic End Point Detection

Immunologic assays are the newest type of assays available in coagulation laboratories and are based on antigen-antibody reactions similar to nephelometry. Latex microparticles are coated with antibody directed against the selected analyte (antigen). Monochromatic light passes through the suspension of latex microparticles. When the wavelength is greater than the diameter of the particles, only a small amount of light is absorbed.[10] When the coated latex microparticles come into

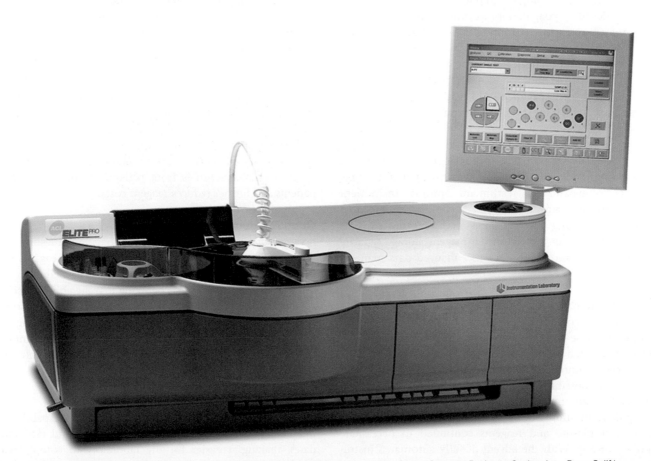

Figure 47-6 ACL ELITE. (Manufactured by Instrumentation Laboratory, Lexington, Mass. Courtesy Beckman Coulter, Inc., Brea, Calif.)

contact with their antigen, however, the antigen attaches to the antibody and forms "bridges," causing the particles to agglutinate. As the diameter of the agglutinates increases to the wavelength of the monochromatic light beam, light is absorbed. The increase in light absorbance is proportional to the size of the agglutinates, which is proportional to the antigen level. This technology has become available on the sophisticated coagulation analyzers introduced to the market in the 1990s and is used to measure a growing number of coagulation proteins, expanding the diagnostic capabilities of the laboratory. Coagulation protein testing, which used to take hours or days to perform via traditional antigen-antibody detection methodologies such as enzyme-linked immunosorbent assay or electrophoresis, now can be done in minutes on an automated analyzer.

The introduction of new coagulation methodologies has improved testing capabilities in the coagulation laboratory. Refinement of these methodologies has allowed the use of synthetic substrates and measurements of single proenzymes, enzymes, and monoclonal antibodies, increasing the ability to recognize the causes of disorders of hemostasis and thrombosis.[11]

ADVANCES IN COAGULATION INSTRUMENTATION

Similar to most technologic equipment developed over the past few decades, coagulation instrumentation has made significant advances in capability and flexibility. Instruments previously required manual pipetting, recording, and calculation of results, necessitating significant operator intervention and time. Current technology allows a "walk away" environment in which, after specimens and reagents are loaded and the testing sequence initiated, the operator can move on to perform other tasks.

In recent years, the methodologies used for clot detection by coagulation analyzers have remained relatively consistent, and multiple methodologies have been incorporated into single analyzers to expand the test menu options. Instrument improvements and advances have been confined to improved technical processing of specimens and reagents such as increased throughput and improved reagent storage capacity and software enhancements such as enhanced data management and result traceability.

Markedly Improved Accuracy and Precision

Previously, coagulation testing was always performed in duplicate because of the large coefficient of variation (often >20%) associated with manual testing. Unless the same experienced technologist performed the tests consistently, it was almost impossible to reproduce results with any degree of accuracy. Semiautomated instruments improved the precision of coagulation testing, but the requirement for manual pipetting of test plasma and reagents continued to necessitate duplicate testing. With the advent of fully automated instruments, precision has improved to the extent that single testing can be performed with confidence. Coefficients of variation of less than 5% and even less than 1% for some tests have been achieved, which allows single testing to become the routine and significantly reduces coagulation reagent and materials costs.

Random Access

The most significant improvement in coagulation analyzers has been the ability to provide random access testing. This means that a variety of tests can be run in any order on the same plasma specimen or many specimens within the same testing sequence. Older analyzers were capable of running only one protocol at a time, so batching of patient specimens within a run was necessary to perform testing in the most efficient manner. The disadvantage was that the patient specimens with multiple orders had to be handled multiple times for each test being run. Coagulation instruments now give the choice of running multiple tests on one specimen, running the same test on multiple specimens, or doing both within the same run. The ability to run multiple tests on one specimen is limited by the number of reagents that can be stored in the analyzer and the instrument's ability to run tests requiring different end point detection methodologies simultaneously (i.e., clotting versus chromogenic versus immunologic).

Improved Reagent Handling
Reduced Reagent/Specimen Volumes

In addition to moving from duplicate to single testing, coagulation analyzers now have the capability to perform tests on decreased sample sizes. Traditionally, PTs used 0.1 mL of patient plasma and 0.2 mL of thromboplastin/calcium chloride reagent. PTTs were tested using 0.1 mL of plasma, 0.1 mL of activated partial thromboplastin, and 0.1 mL of calcium chloride. Newer analyzers can perform the same tests using one half or even one quarter of the traditional volumes for reagents and patient specimens. This decreases the need to draw large volumes of blood on patients for multiple tests and allows one to draw smaller volumes from pediatric or difficult-to-draw patients and further reduces reagent costs.

Open Reagent Systems

A variety of reagents are available for coagulation testing, and laboratories want the flexibility of selecting the reagents that best suit their needs without being restricted in their choice by the analyzers being used. Recognizing that the ability to select reagents independently of the test system is a high priority, instrument manufacturers have responded by developing systems that provide optimal performance with other manufacturer's reagents, provided that the reagents are compatible with the instrument's methodology.

Reagent Tracking

Many fully automated instruments provide the capability of maintaining a record of reagent lot numbers and expiration dates, making it easier for the laboratory to comply with regulatory requirements. Additional features often include on-board monitoring of reagent volumes with flagging systems to alert the operator when an insufficient volume of reagent is detected for the number of specimens programmed to be run.

Improved Specimen Handling
Closed Tube Sampling

Closed tube sampling has improved the safety and efficiency of coagulation testing. After centrifugation, the tube is placed on the analyzer without removing the blue stopper. The cap is pierced by a needle that also aspirates plasma without disturbing the red blood cell layer. Not only does closed tube sampling save staff time, but it also reduces the chances of the operator becoming exposed to the patient specimen through aerosols or spillage.

Primary Tube Sampling

A key feature on many coagulation analyzers is the ability to place the primary collection tube on the instrument after centrifugation without the need to separate the plasma into a secondary tube. Additionally, instruments often allow for multiple sizes of tubes. Significant time savings occur as a result of elimination of the extra specimen preparation step, and errors resulting from mislabeling of the aliquot tube are reduced.

Flagging for Specimen Interferences

Some analyzers monitor the quality of the test specimen for interfering substances or unusual testing characteristics, such as hemolysis, lipemia, bilirubinemia (icterus), abnormal clotting patterns, or results that fall outside the linearity of the reference curve (values above the top curve point or below the bottom curve point). Flags warn the operator of potential errors so that problems can be resolved in a timely manner (see later).

Automatic Dilutions

Many instruments perform multiple dilutions on patient specimens, calibrators, or controls, eliminating the need for the operator to perform this task manually and reducing the potential for error in the testing process.

Expanded Computer Capabilities

Computer technology now incorporates *internal data storage/ retrieval systems* through the use of programs that essentially operate the instruments. Hundreds of results can be stored, retrieved, and compiled into cumulative reports. Multiple calibration curves can be stored and accessed. Quality control files can be stored, eliminating the time-consuming task of manually logging and graphing quality control values. Westgard rules (Chapter 5) can be applied, and failures are automatically flagged. Some analyzers feature automatic repeat testing when failures occur on the initial run. The quality control files can be reviewed or printed on a regular basis to meet regulatory requirements.

Programming flexibility of modern analyzers has enhanced the laboratory's opportunities to provide expanded test menus. Most advanced analyzers are preprogrammed with several routine test protocols ready for use. Specimen and reagent volumes, incubation times, and other testing parameters do not need to be predetermined by the operator but can be changed easily when necessary. Additional tests can be programmed into the analyzer by the user whenever needed, allowing for enhanced flexibility of the analyzer and reducing the need for laboratories to have multiple instruments.

Instrument interfacing to laboratory information systems and specimen bar coding capabilities have become a priorities for even small laboratories as facilities of all sizes endeavor to reduce dependence on manual record keeping. Bidirectional interfaces improve efficiency through the ability of the instrument to send specimen bar code information to the laboratory information systems and receive a response with the tests that have been ordered. This eliminates the need for the operator to program each specimen and test.

Other Features

A few other features offered by modern coagulation analyzers should be mentioned.

- *Improved flagging capabilities* alert the operator when preset criteria have been exceeded (Box 47-1). These flags may indicate instrument malfunction (e.g., cuvette jams, low reagent volume, temperature errors) or a problem with the results of the test (e.g., critical values, inability to detect an end point accurately, values outside of test linearity).
- *Reflex testing* is the automatic ordering of tests based on preset parameters or the results of other tests. Instruments may make additional dilutions if the initial result is outside of the testing limits (i.e., linearity), or supplementary tests can be run automatically if clinically indicated by the initial test result. The first result does not need to wait for review by the operator before follow-up action is taken.
- *Graphing of clot formation* is provided on several analyzers (see Fig. 47-4). The "signature," the shape of the clot formation curve, may correlate to the disease state. Graph evaluation is a troubleshooting tool for unusual results. Figure 47-7 shows examples of a normal (*A*) and multiple

---

BOX 47-1 Flagging Capabilities of Coagulation Instruments

Instrument Malfunction Flags
Temperature error
Photo-optics error
Mechanical movement error
Probe not aspirating

Sample Quality Flags
Lipemia
Hemolysis
Icterus
Abnormal clot formation
No end point detected

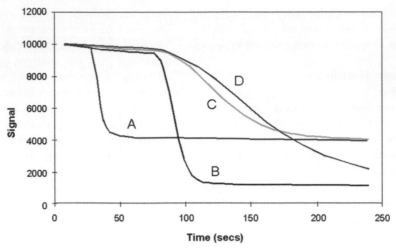

Figure 47-7 Examples of waveform analysis—MDA Systems, Trinity Biotech. Waveform A shows normal clot formation with a normal clotting time. Waveforms *B-D* are examples of abnormal clot formation with prolonged clotting times.

abnormal waveforms (*B-D*). Patients *B*, *C*, and *D* have similar prolonged clotting times, but the clot kinetics are clearly different. Waveform *B* reflects heparin therapy. The lag phase is prolonged, but the clot forms rapidly. Waveforms *C* and *D* show slow-forming clots indicative of factor deficiencies.

Specimen Quality Flags

Specimen quality flags include the following:
- *Lipemia*—may cause falsely prolonged clotting times on optical density instruments because of interference with light transmittance
- *Hemolysis*—may cause falsely shortened clotting times because of premature activation of coagulation factors and platelets
- *Icterus*—an indication of liver dysfunction that may lead to prolonged clotting times because of inadequate clotting factor production; also may interfere with optical density instruments
- *Abnormal clot formation*—may lead to falsely elevated clotting times because of instrument's inability to detect an end point
- *No end point detected*—instrument was unable to detect clot formation, indicating that specimen may need to be tested using an alternate methodology

Instrument Malfunction Flags

Instrument malfunction flags are as follows:
- Temperature error
- Photo-optics error
- Mechanical movement error
- Probe not aspirating
- No end point detected
- Specimen track error

ADVANTAGES AND DISADVANTAGES OF END POINT DETECTION METHODOLOGIES

Several types of end point detection have been developed, and no single methodology can address adequately all specimen conditions or testing circumstances. Each has advantages and disadvantages that should be recognized and understood to ensure the validity of results. Photo-optical end point detection may be confounded by lipemia as the change in optical density is masked by the turbidity of the specimen. Erroneously prolonged clotting times may be obtained. Other coagulation instruments may be unable to employ synthetic reagents because they are more translucent.[13] Table 47-2 summarizes the advantages and disadvantages of each methodology.

NEW INSTRUMENTS FOR PLATELET FUNCTION TESTING

The demand for rapid, cost-effective methods for the evaluation of platelet function has been steadily increasing because of increasing aspirin use for prophylactic treatment of cardiac-related disease. The coagulation laboratory is being asked to provide platelet function testing to evaluate patients who take aspirin, as a means to determine its efficacy. In addition, preoperative evaluation of platelet function is crucial in the hemostatic management of the patient, particularly if the patient has a bleeding history.[14] Platelet function testing always has been a challenge for the clinical laboratory because of the lack of reliable, accurate, and easy-to-perform testing methodologies. Platelet function historically has been assessed by the bleeding time and aggregometry, although both are time-consuming, technically demanding, and lack correlation to bleeding risk.[15,16] In an effort to improve assessment of platelet

TABLE 47-2 Advantages and Disadvantages of End Point Detection Methodologies

Methodology	Advantages	Disadvantages
Mechanical	No interference from specimen lipemia, bilirubinemia, or hemolysis May be able to use small test volumes	Unable to observe graph of clot formation
Photo-optical	Ability to observe graph of clot formation Good precision Multiple wavelength availability may be used for increased test menu flexibility and specimen quality information	Interference from lipemia, hemolysis, bilirubinemia, and increased plasma proteins May have difficulty detecting end point with synthetic reagents[13] Very short clotting times may not be detected owing to high lag phase settings May have difficulty detecting small, delicate clots
Chromogenic	Ability to measure proteins that do not form a fibrin clot as the end point Expands test menu options	Limited by wavelength capabilities of instrument Need large test volume to be cost-effective Cost of instruments and reagents
Immunologic	Ability to automate tests previously available by manual, time-consuming methods Expands test menu capabilities	Limited number of tests available Cost of instruments and reagents May need to have additional instruments available to run routine tests
Nephelometric	Ability to measure antigen-antibody reactions for proteins present in small concentrations	Limited number of tests available Cost of reagents Less familiarity of staff with technology

function, instrumentation has been developed that measures platelet function.

The PFA 100 Platelet Function Analyzer (Dade-Behring, Inc, Deerfield, Ill.) assesses platelet dysfunction.[17] Test cartridges contain membranes coated with collagen/epinephrine or collagen/adenosine diphosphate to stimulate platelet aggregation. Whole blood is aspirated under controlled flow conditions through a microscopic aperture in the membrane. The time required for the platelet plug to occlude the aperture is an indicator of platelet function.[14] Studies indicate that the PFA-100 system is a reliable and cost-effective tool for detecting von Willebrand disease and aspirin-induced bleeding.[18]

The VerifyNow (Ultegra) System (Accumetrics, San Diego, Calif.) is a turbidimetric optical detection system that measures platelet-induced aggregation by microbead agglutination. The system employs a disposable assay device that contains lyophilized fibrinogen-coated beads and a platelet agonist specific for the test. Whole blood is automatically dispensed from the blood collection tube into the assay device by the instrument, with no blood handling required by the user.[19] Assays that can be performed by this instrument include the aspirin assay, glycoprotein IIb/IIIa assay, and P2Y12 (clopidogrel) assay.

The Clot Signature Analyzer (Xylum Corporation, Scarsdale, N.Y.) measures platelet hemostasis time and collagen-induced thrombus formation.[20] Whole, nonanticoagulated blood flows through tubing designed with two holes in separate locations.

Downstream pressure is measured dynamically within the tubing as the blood flows. Hemostatic plug formation within the tube causes a characteristic pattern of pressure changes that is quantified.[21] The time required for the pressure to increase to a predetermined level is measured and is a direct reflection of platelet function.[22]

POINT OF CARE TESTING

Point of care testing represents a growing segment of coagulation testing, primarily resulting from the need to monitor patients on anticoagulant therapy frequently. Also known as *bedside testing*, point of care testing has enhanced the ability of the patient and physician to measure and modify dosing of oral anticoagulants without the delays inherent in conventional testing.

Point of care coagulation analyzers employ capillary or anticoagulated whole blood. For some instruments, a 10-µL to 50-µL sample is transferred to a test cartridge and loaded into the instrument. Other instruments require 500 µL to 2 mL of whole blood. Depending on the technology used, there may be varying degrees of correlation with the same tests performed in the clinical laboratory, and care must be taken to understand the differences in results and ensure that monitoring decisions based on the point of care testing values are made appropriately. Table 47-3 summarizes the variety of point of care instruments that are available.

TABLE 47-3 Summary of Selected Point of Care Analyzers

Manufacturer/Distribution	Instrument	Specimen Requirements	Tests Performed	Special Features
Abbott, East Windsor, N.J.	i-STAT Series	Capillary, venipuncture	PT/INR, ACT	Chemistry testing; quality control and data management program; interface to LIS
Helena, Beaumont, Tex.	Actalyke Series	Venipuncture	ACT	Quality control and data management program; interface to LIS
HemoSense, Inc, San Jose, Calif.	INRatio PT/INR	Capillary	PT/INR	Optional add-on data management program; interface to LIS
Instrumentation Laboratory, Lexington, Mass.	Gem PCL	Capillary, venipuncture	PT/INR, PTT, ACT	Quality control and data management program; interface to LIS
International Technidyne Corp., Edison, N.J.	Protime Microcoagulation System; Hemochron Series	Capillary, venipuncture	PT/INR, PTT, ACT, HITT, Fibrinogen	Quality control and data management program; interface to LIS
Medtronic, Minneapolis, Minn.	HMS Plus; ACT Plus	Venipuncture	ACT	Quality control and data management program; interface to LIS
Roche Diagnostic Corp., Indianapolis, Ind.	CoaguCheck	Capillary, venipuncture	PT/INR	—

From Ford A: Coagulation analyzers (point of care, self-monitoring). CAP Today 20:70-76.
ACT, Activated clotting time; HITT, heparin-induced thrombocytopenia with thrombosis; INR, international normalized ratio; LIS, laboratory information system; PT, prothrombin time.

SELECTING COAGULATION INSTRUMENTATION

In today's laboratory, more than ever before, cost-effectiveness, test capabilities, and standardization are top priorities.[24] As an increasing number of tests become available, laboratories must determine what tests to incorporate to provide guidance to physicians in diagnosis and treatment. Identification of testing needs based on patient population should be the first step in the process. The decisions regarding which tests are the most appropriate for the clinical situations encountered by each laboratory should be made in conjunction with the medical staff. When that input has been obtained, the laboratory can evaluate the availability and cost of instruments that would meet those requirements.

Instrument selection criteria may include, but are not limited to, the following:
- Instrument cost
- Consumables cost
- Reliability and downtime
- Service response time
- Maintenance requirements/time
- Operator ease of use
- Throughput for high-volume testing
- Breadth of testing menu
- Ability to add new testing protocols
- Laboratory information systems interface capabilities
- Footprint (space the instrument occupies on the benchtop)
- Special specifications (water, power, waste drain)
- Flexibility in using other manufacturers' reagents
- Available training program and continued training support

The laboratory director, manager, and technical staff may develop a comparison matrix listing each desired capability. When the choices have been narrowed based on the most desirable criteria, consideration should be given to additional features. Because no instrument has *all* the features, prioritizing helps the laboratory focus on the capabilities that would be the most advantageous for them. Table 47-4 presents a summary of several of these specialized features.

An instrument should be matched to the anticipated workload. It may not be necessary to purchase a highly sophisticated analyzer capable of performing a large menu of tests if the setting is a small hospital laboratory ordering very few of the more "esoteric" test options available on the instrument under consideration. A batch analyzer with high throughput may be more appropriate for this situation.

SUMMARY OF SELECTED INSTRUMENTATION

A variety of coagulation instruments have been developed since the 1990s to address the increasing demand for testing services and capabilities. In general, all analyzers perform routine testing quickly and efficiently. The challenge lies in determining which instruments should be considered for a particular laboratory setting and in developing an organized approach for their evaluation. Table 47-5 summarizes several of the coagulation analyzers currently available, the type of end point detection offered, and selected specialized features highlighted by the manufacturers in their product information.

TABLE 47-4 Specialized Instrument Features

Feature	Description
Random access	A variety of tests can be performed on a single patient specimen in any order as determined by the operator
Primary tube sampling	Test plasma is directly aspirated from an open, previously centrifuged collection tube placed on the analyzer
Cap piercing and closed tube sampling	The analyzer aspirates plasma from the centrifuged primary collection tube with the stopper in place
Bar coding	Reagents and patient specimens are identified through the use of a bar code; eliminates manual information entry
Bidirection LIS interface	Analyzer queries host computer to determine which tests have been ordered. Results are returned to the LIS automatically after verification
Specimen and instrument flagging	Alerts the operator of a potential specimen integrity or instrument malfunction problem
Liquid level sensing	Alerts operator that there may not be enough specimen or reagent volume or that the instrument did not aspirate the entire amount of specimen required. Volume is verified each time a specimen or reagent is aspirated
On-board quality control	Instrument computer programs store and organize quality control data; may include application of Westgard rules for flagging out-of-range results; may transmit quality control data to the LIS
STAT capabilities	Allows operator to interrupt a testing sequence to place a STAT specimen next in line for testing
On-board refrigeration of specimens and reagents	Maintains integrity of specimens and reagents throughout the testing process; allows reagents to be kept on the analyzer for extended periods, reducing setup time for less frequently performed tests
On-board specimen storage capacity	Indicates the number of specimens that can be loaded at a time
Reflex testing capabilities	Allows programming of instrument to perform repeat or additional testing under operator-defined circumstances
Patient data storage	Capacity to store test results for future retrieval; may include clot formation graphs
Reagent volume monitoring	Alerts operator when insufficient reagent volume exists for the number of tests programmed to run; based on initial reagent volumes entered into the system by the operator
Throughput	Number of tests that can be processed within a certain time (usually designated as number of tests per hour); dependent on test mix and methodologies used
Total testing time	Length of time from specimen placement on the analyzer until testing is completed; dependent on type and complexity of test procedure
Graph of clot formation	Allows operator to visualize the formation of the clot within the cuvette; aids in the detection of certain abnormal conditions or disease states or troubleshooting of test results

TABLE 47-5 Summary of Selected Instrumentation

Manufacturer/Distributer	Instrument	Type of Automation	End Point Detection Methodology	Special Features
BBL Microbiology Systems, Sparks, Md.	Fibrometer	Semi	Mechanical	Ease of use, low maintenance, low cost
Trinity Biotech, Plc, Bray, County Wicklow, Ireland	MTX Series; MDA Series	Full	Photo-optical, chromogenic, immunologic	Bar coding, bidirectional interface, primary tube sampling, closed tube sampling, simultaneous performance of end point detection methods, specimen quality flagging, graph of clot formation
Dade Behring, Inc., Deerfield, Ill.	BCS; Sysmex Series	Full	Photo-optical, chromogenic, immunologic	Primary tube sampling, bar coding, specimen quality flagging, graph of clot formation, bidirectional interface
Diagnostica Stago, Parsippany, N.J.	STart Series; STA-R Series	Semi, full	Mechanical, chromogenic, immunologic	Bar coding for reagents and specimens, bidirectional interface, simultaneous performance of end point detection methods, reflex testing, autoprogramming for performance of quality control, user-defined programs
Helena Laboratories, Beaumont, Tex.	Cascade Series	Full	Photo-optical, chromogenic	Bar coding, primary tube sampling, cap piercing, reduced reagent/specimen volumes, reflex testing, automatic application of Westgard rules for quality control
Instrumentation Laboratory/ Beckman Coulter, Brea, Calif.	ACL Series	Full	Nephelometry, photo-optical, chromogenic, immunologic	Primary tube sampling, bar coding, batch analysis, bidirectional interface, graph of clot formation
Trinity Biotech, Plc, Bray, County Wicklow, Ireland	KC Series; AMAX Series	Semi, full	Mechanical, chromogenic, immunologic	Bidirectional interface, reduced reagent/ specimen volumes, liquid level sensing, bar coding, reflex testing

CHAPTER at a GLANCE

- Advanced technology used in semiautomated and automated analyzers has greatly improved coagulation testing accuracy and precision.
- End point detection methodologies employed by modern coagulation analyzers include mechanical, photo-optical, nephelometric, chromogenic, and immunologic.
- Advances in end point detection methodologies have greatly expanded the testing capabilities available in the routine coagulation laboratory.
- Markedly improved instrument precision and reduced reagent volume requirements have led to substantial cost savings in coagulation testing.
- Instrument manufacturers have incorporated many features that have enhanced efficiency, safety, and diagnostic capabilities in hemostasis testing.
- Coagulation analyzer flagging alert functions warn the operator when sample or instrument conditions exist that might lead to invalid test results so that appropriate actions can be taken to ensure test accuracy.

- Each method of end point detection has advantages and disadvantages that must be recognized and understood to ensure the validity of test results.
- Whole-blood analyzers are available to measure platelet function in a more efficient and timely manner compared with traditional methods.
- Coagulation testing has been incorporated into the arena of point of care testing primarily to enhance the patient's and physician's ability to monitor oral anticoagulant therapy.
- A systematic approach for the evaluation and selection of a new coagulation analyzer should be developed and followed to determine the best instrument for a specific laboratory setting.

Now that you have completed this chapter, go back and read again the case study at the beginning and respond to the questions presented.

REVIEW QUESTIONS

1. The photo-optical method of end point detection can be described as:
   a. Measurement of a color-producing chromophor at a wavelength of 405 nm
   b. The change in optical density of a test solution as a result of fibrin formation
   c. Application of an electromagnetic field to the test cuvette to detect the decreased motion of an iron ball within the cuvette
   d. Measurement of the turbidity of a test solution resulting from the formation of antigen-antibody complexes using latex particles

2. Modern coagulation analyzers have greatly enhanced the ability to perform coagulation testing as a result of which of the following?
   a. Maintenance of a similar level of accuracy and precision with manual methods
   b. Increased reagent volume capabilities to improve sensitivity
   c. Automatic adjustment of results for interfering substances
   d. Improved flagging capabilities for sample quality and instrument function

3. Which of the following is considered to be an advantage of the mechanical end point detection methodology?
   a. Not affected by lipemia in the test sample
   b. Has the ability to observe a graph of clot formation
   c. Can incorporate multiple wavelengths into a single testing sequence
   d. Can measure proteins that do not have fibrin formation as the end point

4. Which of the following methods uses the principle of changes in light scatter or transmission to detect the end point of the reaction?
   a. Immunologic, mechanical, photo optical
   b. Photo-optical, nephelometric, mechanical
   c. Photo-optical, nephelometric, immunologic
   d. Chromogenic, immunologic, mechanical

5. Which of the following is a feature of semiautomated coagulation testing analyzers?
   a. The temperature is maintained externally by a heat block or water bath.
   b. Reagents and samples usually are added manually by the operator.
   c. Timers are automatically initiated as soon as the analyzer adds reagents to the test cuvette.
   d. The end point must be detected by the operator.

6. When a sample has been flagged as being icteric by an automated coagulation analyzer, which methodology would be most susceptible to erroneous results because of the interfering substance?
   a. Mechanical clot detection
   b. Immunologic antigen-antibody reactions
   c. Photo-optical clot detection
   d. Chromogenic end point detection

7. Platelet function testing has been incorporated into the routine coagulation laboratory in recent years as a result of:
   a. Increased use of drugs that stimulate platelet production in patients on chemotherapy
   b. The convenience of being able to do the testing on the same instrument that performs the coagulation testing
   c. Increased therapeutic use of aspirin in the treatment of heart disease
   d. Increased outpatient/outreach testing that prevents the laboratory from having access to patients to do bleeding time tests

8. All of the following except one are performance characteristics to consider in the selection of a coagulation analyzer. Select the *exception*:
   a. Location of the manufacturer's home office
   b. Instrument footprint
   c. Ease of use for the operator
   d. Variety of tests the instrument can perform

9. The PFA100 measures platelet function by:
   a. Detecting the change in blood flow pressure along a small tube when a clot impairs blood flow
   b. Aggregation of latex beads coated with platelet activators
   c. Graphing the light transmittance through platelet-rich plasma over time after addition of platelet activators
   d. Detecting the time it takes for a clot to form as blood flows through a small aperture in a tube coated with platelet activators

10. Point of care coagulation testing is used mainly:
    a. To monitor patients on oral anticoagulant therapy
    b. To monitor patients taking platelet inhibitors such as aspirin
    c. To provide a baseline for all subsequent patient test result comparisons when they start any kind of anticoagulant therapy
    d. For obstetric patients at risk of fetal loss

REFERENCES

1. Sabo MG: Coagulation instrumentation and reagent systems. In Triplett DA (ed): Laboratory Evaluation of Coagulation. ASCP Press, Chicago, 1982.
2. BBL FibroSystem Manual. Sparks, MD: BD Diagnostic Systems, 1992.
3. STA-R Operator's Manual,. Parsippany, NJ: Diagnostica Stago, 1998.
4. KC4 Delta Product Information. Bray, County Wicklow, Ireland: Trinity Biotech, Plc., 2001.
5. Thomas LC, Sochynsky CL: Multiple measuring modes of coagulation instruments. Clin Hemost Rev 1999;13:8.
6. MLA Electra 1800C Operator's Manual, Brea, CA: Instrumentation Laboratory/Beckman Coulter, Inc. 1997.
7. Behring Nephelometer 100 Operator's Manual,. Deerfield, IL: Dade Behring, Inc., 1995.
8. ACL 8000 Operator's Manual, Brea, CA: Instrumentation Laboratory/Beckman Coulter Inc., 2003.
9. Miers MK, Exton MG, Daniele C: Cell-counting and

coagulation instrumentation. In Rodak BF (ed): Diagnostic Hematology. Philadelphia: Saunders, 1995, pp 626-631.

10. LIATEST vWF package insert. Parsippany, NJ: Diagnostica Stago, 1997.

11. Gram J, Jespersen J: Introduction to laboratory assays in haemostasis and thrombosis. In Jesperson J, Bertina RM, Haverkate F (eds): Laboratory Techniques in Thrombosis—a Manual, 2nd ed. Boston: Kluwer Academic Publishers, 1999:1-7.

12. MDA 180 Operator's Manual. Bray, County Wicklow, Ireland: Trinity Biotech, Plc., 2002.

13. Aller R, Sheridan B: Service above all. CAP Today 1999; January:39-60.

14. Kundu SK, Heilmann EF, Sio R et al: Characterization of an in vitro platelet function analyzer, PFA-100. Clin Appl Thromb Hemost 1996;2:241-249.

15. Rodgers RPC, Levin J: A critical reappraisal of the bleeding time. Semin Thromb Hemost 1990;16:1-20.

16. Lind DE: The bleeding time does not predict surgical bleeding. Blood 1991;77:2547-2552.

17. Mammen EF, Comp PC, Gosselin R, et al: PFA-100 system: a new method for assessment of platelet dysfunction. Semin Thromb Hemost 1998;24:195-202.

18. News Release, PFA-100 Platelet Function Analyzer. Deerfield, IL: Dade Behring, Inc., August 12, 1999.

19. VerifyNow (Ultegra) product information. San Diego, Calif: Accumetrics, 2005.

20. Clot Signature Analyzer product information. Scarsdale, NY: Xylum Corporation, 1999.

21. Faraday N, Guallar E, Sera VA, et al: Utility of whole blood hemostatometry using the clot signature analyzer for assessment of hemostasis in cardiac surgery. Anesthesiology 2002;96:1115-1122.

22. Li C: The Xylum Clot Signature Analyzer: a novel dynamic measure of global hemostasis testing. Presented at the International Society on Thrombosis and Haemostasis Seminar, Washington, DC, August 17, 1999.

23. Ford A: Coagulation analyzers (point of care, self-monitoring). CAP Today, February 2006;20:70-76.

24. James E: Quality, consistency and cost-effectiveness. Advance for Medical Laboratory Professionals, May 31, 2004.

Material Safety Data Sheet

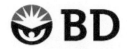 **BD**

Printing Date: 2004-Oct-25

Printing Date: Reviewed on

Product Name: *BD Unopette® Brand Test for Manual WBC/Platelets*

---

1 Identification of substance:

- **Product Details:**
  MSDS Number: VS60326-04
  Issue Date: September 30, 2004
  Supersedes: VS60326-03
  ECO No.: ECO20025
- **Product Name:** *BD Unopette® Brand Test for Manual WBC/Platelets*
- **Catalog Numbers:** 365854, 365855
- **Manufacturer/Supplier:**
  BD Diagnostics, Preanalytical Systems
  1 Becton Drive
  Franklin Lakes, NJ, 07417-1885
- **Information Department:**
  BD Diagnostics, Preanalytical Systems Technical Service, (800) 631-0174
- **Emergency Information:**
  In case of a chemical emergency, spill, fire, exposure, or accident contact BD Diagnostics, Preanalytical Systems, at (308) 423-0300, or ChemTrec at (800) 424-9300

---

2 Composition/Data on components:

- **Description:**
  Chemical name: *Ammonium Oxalate*
  Sorenson's Phosphate
  Synonyms: Ammonium Oxalate: *Diammonium oxalate, monohydrate; Ethanedoic acid, diammonium salt; monohydrate; Oxalic acid, diammonium salt monohydrate*
- **CAS No.:** *Ammonium Oxalate: 6009-70-7*
  Sorenson's Phosphate: 7778-77-0
- **Quantity:** *Ammonium Oxalate: 22.671 mg*
  Sorenson's Phosphate: 1.98 mg
- **Exposure limits:** *None established*

---

3 Hazards identification:

- **Hazard description:**
  EU: *This product contains no hazardous constituents, or the concentration of all chemical constituents are below the regulatory threshold limits described by European Directive 91/155/EEC, and 93/112/EC. This product does not have to be labeled due to the calculation procedure for the "General Classification guideline for preparations of the EU" in the latest valid version.*
  U.S.:
  May cause irritation to the skin and respiratory tract. May cause severe irritation to the eyes. Ingestion may be harmful and possibly fatal.
  Primary route(s) of entry: skin, eyes, inhalation, and ingestion.
- **Health effects:**
  Acute Exposure Effects:
  Eye: Severely irritating to the eyes. May cause redness or pain.
  Skin: May cause redness, pain or swelling.

Courtesy Becton, Dickinson and Company.

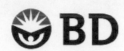

Material Safety Data Sheet
acc. to ISO/DIS 11014

Page 2 of 6

Product Name: *BD Unopette® Brand Test for Manual WBC/Platelets*

Inhalation: May cause irritation of the nose, mouth, or throat, causing coughing or choking.
Ingestion: May cause headache, cramps, muscle pain, drop in blood pressure, poisoning, or coma. May be fatal.

Repeated Exposure Effects:
Skin: May cause dermatitis.
Inhalation: May cause pulmonary edema.
Ingestion: May cause kidney stones or bladder stones.

Medical conditions which might be aggravated: *None identified.*

- **Environmental effects:** *None available*
- **Physical hazards:** *Avoid generating dust.*
- **Classification system:** *The classification was made according to the latest editions of international substances lists, and expanded upon from company and literature data.*
- **NFPA ratings (scale 0-4):**

    Health = 2
    Fire = 0
    Reactivity = 1
    Specific Hazard = 2

- **HMIS ratings (scale 0-4):**

    Health = 2
    Flammability = 0
    Reactivity = 1

---

4   First aid measures:

- **General information:**
  After skin contact: *Immediately flush skin with plenty of soap and water for at least 20 minutes.*
  After eye contact: *Immediately flush with plenty of water for at least 30 minutes.*
  After inhalation: *Move the exposed person to fresh air. Seek medical attention.*
  After Swallowing: *Do not induce vomiting. Immediately give 10 oz. of water to dilute. Immediately seek medical attention.*
  Information for doctor: *Show this label*

---

5   Fire fighting measures:

- **Suitable extinguishing agents:** *Use extinguishing media appropriate for surrounding fire.*

- **Protective equipment:** *Firefighters should wear self-contained breathing apparatus with full face piece operating in positive pressure mode.*

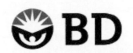 **BD**

Material Safety Data Sheet
acc. to ISO/DIS 11014

Page 3 of 6

Product Name: *BD Unopette® Brand Test for Manual WBC/Platelets*

---

6   Accidental release measures:

- **Person-related safety precautions:** *Avoid overexposure. Wear suitable protective clothing.*
- **Measures for environmental protection:** *None identified*
- **Measures for cleaning/collecting:** *Contain with absorbant material which will not react with material. Place into suitable, covered, labeled container. Flush area with water.*
- **Additional information:** *None*

---

7   Handling and storage:

- **Handling:**
  Information for safe handling: *Avoid generating dust.*

  Information about protection against explosions and fires: *Avoid generating dust.*
- **Storage:**
  Requirements to be met by storerooms and receptacles: *Keep container closed when not in use. Store in a cool, dry, well-ventilated area. Keep out of direct sunlight.*

  Information about storage in one common storage facility: *Store away from incompatible materials.*

  Further information about storage conditions: *Protect from damage.*

---

8   Exposure controls and personal protection:

- **Additional information about design of technical systems:** *Use local exhaust ventilation system.*
- **Components with limit values that require monitoring at the workplace:** *None established*
- **Additional information:** *None*

- **Personal Protective Equipment:**
  General protective and hygienic measures: *Wash thoroughly after handling. Remove contaminated clothing and wash before reuse. Avoid contact with eyes, skin, and clothing. Avoid ingestion and inhalation. Use with adequate ventilation.*
  Breathing equipment: *Use NIOSH/MSHA approved dust respirator if dust levels become high.*
  Protection of hands: *Use impervious gloves.*

  Eye protection: *Use chemical safety goggles.*
  Body protection: *Wear coveralls and long sleeves.*

---

9   Physical and chemical properties:

- **General Information:**
  Form: *Liquid*
  Color: *Colorless*
  Odor: *Odorless*
- **Change in condition:** *Undetermined*

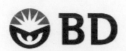

Product Name: *BD Unopette® Brand Test for Manual WBC/Platelets*

Melting point/Melting range: *0°C*

Boiling point/Boiling range: *100°C*

• **Flash point:** *Not applicable*

• **Flammability (solid, gaseous):** *Not applicable*

• **Danger of explosion:** *Product does not present an explosion hazard*

• **Vapor pressure:** *23 hPa*

• **Density:** *$1g/cm^3$*

• **Solubility in/Miscibility w/H_2O:** *Not miscible or difficult to mix*

• **pH-value:** *Not applicable*

• **Solids content:** *1.2%*

---

10   Stability and reactivity:

• **Thermal decomposition / conditions to be avoided**: *No decomposition if used according to specifications.*

• **Materials to be avoided**: *May react violently with strong acids, strong bases, and strong oxidizing agents.*

• **Dangerous reactions**: *Stable; may react violently with incompatible materials.*

• **Dangerous products of decomposition**: *None identified*

---

11   Toxicological information:

• **Acute toxicity**:
   Ingestion: Part of this material caused severe ulcerations of the gastro-intestinal tract when 1000mg was given to monkeys.

• **Primary irritant effect**:
   On the skin: None identified
   On the eye: None identified

• **Sensitization**: *Not established*

• **Additional toxicological information**: *The product is not subject to OSHA classification according to internally approved calculation methods for preparations. When used according to specifications, the product does not have any harmful effects according to our experience and the information provided to us.*

---

12   Ecological information:

• **Ecotoxicological effects:**

• **Other information:** *No data is available on the adverse effects of this material on the environment. Nether COD nor BOD data are available.*

• **General notes:** *None*

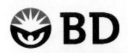 **BD**

Printing Date: 2004-Oct-25

Printing Date: Reviewed on

Product Name: *BD Unopette® Brand Test for Manual WBC/Platelets*

---

13 Disposal considerations:

- **Product:**
  Recommendation
  Smaller quantities may be disposed of with household waste.
  Disposal should be done in accordance with local, state and federal regulations.
  Disposal must be made according to the regulations found in 40 CFR 261.
  This product is not a RCRA hazardous waste.
- **Uncleaned packagings:**
  Recommendation
  Disposal should be done in accordance with local, state and federal regulations.
  Disposal must be made according to the regulations found in 40 CFR 261.
  This product is not a RCRA hazardous waste.
  Recommended cleansing agent
  Water, if necessary with cleansing agents
- **General notes:** *None*

---

14 Transport information:

Note: The information contained in this section only applies to transport of full case cartons
- **DOT regulations:** *Not regulated*

- **Land transport ADR/RID (cross-border):** *Not regulated*
- **Maritime transport IMDG:** *Not regulated*

- **Air transport ICAO-TI and IATA-DGR:** *Not regulated*

---

15 Regulations:

- **SARA Section 355 (extremely hazardous substances):** *Substances not listed*
- **SARA Section 302 (extremely hazardous substances):** *Substances not listed*
- **SARA Section 304 (Reportable Quantity (RQ) under CERCLA):** *5000lbs. (ammonium oxalate)*
- **SARA Section 313 (specific toxic chemical listings):** *Substances not listed*
- **Hazardous chemical(s) under OSHA Hazard Communication Standard (29 CFR 1910.1200):** *None*
- **TSCA (Toxic Substances Control Act) Inventory:** *Substances listed*
- **California Proposition 65 – Chemicals Known to Cause Cancer:** *Substances not listed*
  California Proposition 65 – Chemicals Known to Cause Reproductive Toxicity: *Substance listed:*
  Thimerosal (mercury complex)
- **Carncinogenicity categories**
  IARC (International Agency for Research on Cancer): *Substances not listed*
  NTP (National Toxicology Program): *Substances not listed*
  TLV (Threshold Limit Value established by ACGIH): *Substances not listed*
- **Product related hazard information:** *None*

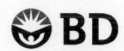

Material Safety Data Sheet
acc. to ISO/DIS 11014

Page 6 of 6

Printing Date: 2004-Oct-25

Printing Date: Reviewed on

Product Name: BD Unopette® Brand Test for Manual WBC/Platelets

---

- **National regulations:** This product is not subject to identification regulations under EU Directives and the Ordinance on Hazardous Materials (German GefStoffV).
- **Water hazard class:** Not Available

---

16   Other information:

To the best of our knowledge, the information contained herein is accurate. However, neither BD or any of its subsidiaries assumes any liabilities whatsoever for the accuracy or completeness of the information contained herein. Final determination of suitability of any material is the sole responsibility of the user. All materials may present unknown hazards and should be used with caution. Although certain hazards are described herein, we cannot guarantee that these are the only hazards that exist.

- **Department issuing MSDS:** Regulatory Affairs

Answers

CHAPTER 2

Case Study

1. This item represents two deficiencies. First, the hematology technologist was not following the lab policy on hand-washing. Hands are washed after removing gloves and before leaving the laboratory. Second, the hematology technologist should have removed the lab coat before going to the meeting. A second lab coat should have been used if it was necessary to wear a lab coat outside the lab.
2. This item represents a deficiency: Storage of food in a specimen refrigerator is prohibited.
3. This item represents a deficiency: Needles should not be recapped unless there is a specific medical procedure that requires recapping. No methods in hematology justify recapping of the syringe.
4. This may or may not be a deficiency. The technologist may have had on a personal lab coat. A second lab coat could have been obtained by the technologist to wear in public areas.
5. No deficiency: Fire extinguishers should be placed every 75 feet.
6. No deficiency: Fire extinguishers should be checked monthly and annually.
7. This item represents a deficiency: Quarterly fire drills should be conducted.
8. This item represents a deficiency: All chemicals should be labeled.
9. This item represents a deficiency: 1:10 bleach solutions should be made fresh daily.
10. No deficiency: Gloves should be worn by all personnel handling specimens.
11. No deficiency: MSDSs can be received electronically.
12. This item represents a deficiency: Chemicals should not be stored under the hood and should not be stored alphabetically.
13. This item represents a deficiency: All staff members should participate in scheduled fire drills.

Review Questions

1. d
2. b
3. c
4. c
5. a
6. b
7. c
8. b
9. b
10. b

CHAPTER 3

Case Study

Case 1

Proper procedure is to ask the patient to state his or her name and confirm by asking birth date or Social Security number. Tubes are *never* pre-labeled. They are labeled after blood is drawn and before leaving the patient.

Case 2

The gel separator tube should not be used for the blood bank because it contains clot activator; it should not be drawn before a tube for coagulation testing because carryover could contaminate the specimen. If K^+ is being tested from a green tube, it must be drawn before the EDTA. EDTA is usually in a K^+ salt, which could falsely elevate blood drawn after it for K^+ levels.

See correct order of draw for evacuated tubes on Page 22, Step 13.

Review Questions

1. c
2. b
3. b
4. b
5. b
6. d
7. b
8. c
9. d
10. b
11. a

CHAPTER 4

Case Study

The following item should be checked:

Is the slide right side up? This is the most common cause of inability to focus a slide under oil when it has been focused under 10× and 40×.

If the slide is right side up, continue with the following steps:
- Is there sufficient oil on the slide? If not, place another drop of oil.
- Is the objective screwed in tightly? If not, tighten the objective.
- If the slide is cover slipped, is there more than one cover slip on the slide? If so, gently remove the top cover slip.
- Has oil seeped into the seal on the oil objective? Examine by removing the objective and using an inverted ocular as a magnifier to check the seal. If the seal is broken, the objective must be replaced.

Review Questions
1. b
2. c
3. a
4. d
5. c
6. d
7. a
8. c
9. d
10. b

CHAPTER 5

Case Study
1. This type of error is constant systematic because the magnitude of error remains constant throughout the range of test measurement.
2. It is not acceptable to continue using the instrument or to simply subtract the constant error from specimens previously run. All samples in question must be rerun after the error is corrected.
3. Look back at the previous hemoglobin control readings to see when the constant systematic error first occurred. Investigate what changes in instrument settings, calibration, reagents, or other changes were made immediately before the error was detected.

Review Questions
1. a
2. b
3. c
4. a
5. a
6. c
7. 7.4
8. 0.17
9. c
10. c

CHAPTER 6

Review Questions
1. b
2. c
3. a
4. b
5. c
6. a
7. d
8. d
9. d
10. b

CHAPTER 7

Review Questions
1. a
2. d
3. c
4. a
5. b
6. c
7. b
8. b
9. a
10. a

CHAPTER 8

Review Questions
1. c
2. a
3. d
4. b
5. b
6. d
7. a
8. d
9. a
10. c
11. b
12. b

CHAPTER 9

Review Questions
1. b
2. a
3. d
4. c
5. a
6. c
7. d
8. c
9. c
10. d
11. a
12. c
13. b
14. d
15. b

16. a
17. d

CHAPTER 10

Case Study

1. Yes. A general reference range for hemoglobin for adult females is 12.0–16.0 g/dL; for newborns, 19.0–23.0 g/dL.
2. Infants have high hemoglobin levels when they are first born. Hemoglobin F does not bind 2,3-BPG well, so a higher level of hemoglobin is needed to provide adequate tissue oxygen. These levels gradually decrease and become similar to adult ranges when infants reach 1 year of age.
3. A hemoglobin test measures the quantitative amount of hemoglobin, and the hemoglobin electrophoresis test measures the types of hemoglobin that are present.
4. Adults and infants have different concentrations of hemoglobins A, A_2, and F. Hemoglobin F (fetal) of the infant consists of two alpha and two gamma chains. A hemoglobin "switch" occurs, and the gamma chains are replaced by the beta chains of hemoglobin A. The mother's results and the newborn's results were within reference range for their respective ages.

Review Questions

1. d
2. a
3. a
4. a
5. b
6. d
7. c
8. b
9. d
10. b
11. c

CHAPTER 11

Case Study

1. The donors had increased iron requirements due to the phlebotomies that were performed on them periodically. The iron in the diet and in the supplements was not enough to offset the loss.
2. For the donors in this age group it would be about 1-2 mg/day.
3. The body can adapt to increased need for iron and increase the amount of iron that is absorbed. When body iron levels decline, hepcidin levels will drop and iron absorption from the intestines will rise.
4. Serum iron, serum TIBC, % saturation, and serum ferritin are common tests done to evaluate iron status. Other tests that can be done include red blood cell protoporphyrin, serum transferrin receptor, unbound iron binding capacity, and bone marrow iron studies.
5. See Table 11-2 and chapter information on the tests.
6. Total serum iron, total iron binding capacity, and the per-

cent transferrin saturation do not provide useful information about iron stores. Serum ferritin is the best test for assessment of iron stores. See Table 11-2.

Review Questions

1. c
2. b
3. d
4. b
5. c
6. b
7. d
8. d
9. b
10. d

CHAPTER 12

Review Questions

1. d
2. b
3. a
4. c
5. c
6. d
7. d
8. c
9. b
10. c

CHAPTER 13

Case Study

1. Bleeding characterized by petechiae, purpura, and ecchymoses is called *mucocutaneous* bleeding, also called *systemic* bleeding. By contrast, *anatomic* bleeding is bleeding into soft tissue, muscles, joints, or body cavities.
2. *Thrombocytopenia*, or low platelet count, is a common cause of mucocutaneous bleeding. Another is diseases that weaken vascular collagen, such as scurvy.
3. No, the bone marrow megakaryocyte estimate is high, indicating an increase in platelet production.
4. *Thrombopoietin* and *interleukin-11* have the greatest effect on recruitment and proliferation of megakaryocytes and their progenitors. Also involved in early progenitor recruitment are interleukin-3 and interleukin-6. Other cytokines and hormones that participate synergistically with TPO and the interleukins are stem cell factor, also called *kit ligand* or *mast cell growth factor*; granulocyte macrophage colony-stimulating factor; granulocyte colony-stimulating factor; and erythropoietin.

Review Questions

1. a
2. d
3. c
4. b

5. a
6. d
7. a
8. a
9. c
10. d

CHAPTER 14

Case Studies

Case 1

1. Hb × 3 = HCT ± 3
   15 × 3 = 45 ± 3 (42–48)
2. Lipemia, increased WBC, abnormal hemoglobin.
3. Lipemia—perform a plasma blank.
   Increased WBC—centrifuge the hemoglobin solution and read the transmittance of the supernatant.
   Abnormal hemoglobin—add potassium carbonate to the prepared dilution of blood and reagent.

Case 2

1. MCV = 59 fL; MCH = 18.1 pg; MCHC = 30.7 g/dL.
2. Microcytic, hypochromic red blood cells.
3. Examine the patient's peripheral blood smear.

Review Questions

1. b
2. c
3. c
4. d
5. d
6. b
7. c
8. c
9. a
10. d

CHAPTER 15

Case Study

1. The platelet count (Plt) and white blood cell count (WBC) should be questioned because of platelet clumping. EDTA-induced pseudothrombocytopenia and pseudoleukocytosis most likely occurred.
2. The specimen should be redrawn in sodium citrate and processed through the automated analyzer. The new WBC and Plt should then be adjusted for the sodium citrate dilution by multiplying the results by the dilution factor 10/9 or 1.1. The following are the new results:
   a. WBC drawn in sodium citrate $(8.4 \times 10^9/L) \times 1.1 = 9.2 \times 10^9/L$ (the corrected WBC)
   b. Plt drawn in sodium citrate $(231 \times 10^9/L) \times 1.1 = 254 \times 10^9/L$ (the corrected Plt)

Review Questions

1. d
2. c

3. a
4. c
5. b
6. c
7. a
8. b
9. Leukocytosis with a relative neutrophilia (includes the young neutrophilic cells). There is a dramatic absolute neutrophilia with a left shift back to blasts but also an absolute lymphocytosis, eosinophilia, and basophilia. RBC morphology is not mentioned and thus is normal.
10. There is a microcytic, hypochromic anemia with anisocytosis. The latter is confirmed in the morphology that also notes poikilocytosis but does not describe any particular cell shape. No mention of polychromasia or inclusions.

CHAPTER 16

Case Study

1. Cellularity is assessed on a core biopsy by comparing the amount of fat to connective tissue (F:C ratio).
2. M:E is 9:1, indicating myeloid hyperplasia.
3. Megakaryocytes are normally seen in bone marrow and are the cells responsible for the production of platelets.

Review Questions

1. c
2. d
3. a
4. d
5. b
6. b
7. c
8. d
9. a
10. b

CHAPTER 17

Case Study

1. A 1:53 dilution with saline is necessary for a satisfactory Cytospin slide.
2. Bacteria.
3. The most likely diagnosis is bacterial meningitis.

Review Questions

1. b
2. b
3. c
4. b
5. a
6. b
7. c
8. d
9. c
10. a

CHAPTER 18

Case Study

1. Anemia is not a disease or diagnosis in itself but is the symptom of an underlying disorder. Complete history and physical examination is necessary to help identify the cause(s) of the anemia. If the underlying cause is not determined and corrected, the patient will continue to be anemic. Questions regarding lifestyle, medications, and bleeding history are only some of the questions that should be asked.

2. The reticulocyte count divides anemias into impaired production (decreased reticulocyte count) or increased destruction (increased reticulocyte count). If the reticulocyte is low, the anemia can be further subdivided on the basis of MCV into normocytic, microcytic, or macrocytic. With that knowledge, appropriate laboratory testing to determine etiology can be ordered.

3. The peripheral blood smear yields valuable information about the size and hemoglobin content of the erythrocytes as well as any abnormal shapes, which may be correlated with specific etiologies. Some anemias are also associated with WBC and/or platelet abnormalities that may be noted on the blood smear.

Review Questions

1. c
2. b
3. a
4. c
5. a
6. b
7. c
8. d
9. b
10. a

CHAPTER 19

Case Study

1. Hypochromic, microcytic anemias would include iron deficiency, thalassemia, sideroblastic anemias, and, possibly, anemia of chronic inflammation.

2. Thalassemia would be eliminated because it would not be an acquired condition late in life. Although iron deficiency is not as common in women after menopause, it is probably the most likely of the remaining possibilities for an anemia this severe.

3. Anemia of chronic inflammation would be eliminated in this case because she is otherwise healthy. Iron deficiency anemia is probably more likely.

4. Iron studies including ferritin would be useful in clarifying the patient's diagnosis. Assuming that she is iron deficient, the ferritin, total serum iron, and percent saturation should all be decreased while the total iron binding capacity would be expected to be increased.

Upon hospitalization, the patient was immediately placed on oxygen while laboratory tests were ordered. With the confirmation by the hospital laboratory of a dangerously low hemoglobin, transfusions were ordered and she received 3 units of packed cells over the first 2 days of hospitalization. They were administered very slowly so as not to stress her cardiovascular system with added volume. Noting the hypochromic, microcytic blood picture, the physician ordered iron studies, which were drawn prior to transfusions. The results were as follows: serum iron decreased, TIBC increased, % saturation decreased, and ferritin decreased. The possibility of gastrointestinal bleeding as a cause for iron deficiency was investigated. Stool guiac tests were negative. The hospital dietitian assessed the patient's usual diet of tea, toast, canned soup, and crackers and determined that it was quite inadequate not only in iron, but also in other important nutrients. The physician concluded that her dietary iron deficiency had developed slowly, thus allowing her to adapt to an exceedingly low hemoglobin. Furthermore, her low level of activity meant that she rarely experienced the effects of the anemia. She was started on a course of oral iron supplementation, and arrangements were made for her to receive one balanced meal daily from the "Meals on Wheels" program sponsored through a community service organization for senior citizens. She was quite responsible about taking her iron supplements, and her hemoglobin was within the reference range within 3 months.

Review Questions

1. b
2. a
3. d
4. a
5. c
6. a
7. d
8. c
9. b
10. d

CHAPTER 20

Case Study

1. The CBC findings for this patient (notably macrocytic, normochromic anemia; pancytopenia; hypersegmentation of neutrophils; and oval macrocytes) were consistent with the physician's suspicion of megaloblastic anemia suggested by the clinical findings.

2. Although the relative reticulocyte count was within the reference range, the calculated absolute count (approximately $40 \times 10^9/L$) was low and clearly inadequate to compensate for a substantial anemia (see Chapter 14), thus indicating ineffective erythropoiesis.

3. The patient's vitamin assays point to a deficiency of vitamin B_{12}, substantiated by an increase in methylmalonic acid.

4. Based on these results, tests for antibodies to parietal cells and intrinsic factor would be appropriate, especially in light of the patient's ethnicity. However, the physician

also inquired further about the patient's dietary habits and learned that he enjoyed dishes of raw fish from the surrounding lakes. Therefore, the physician ordered a stool analysis for ova and parasites. The study indicated the presence in the stool of both eggs and proglottids of the fish tapeworm *Diphyllobothrium latum*. The patient was treated with a suitable purgative, and the scolex of the tapeworm was discovered in a stool sample after a single treatment. The patient was counseled on the proper preparation of fresh fish to avoid reinfection. He received injections of cyanocobalamin for 1 week to replenish his vitamin B_{12} stores. His hemoglobin returned to normal over the next month, and his neurological symptoms subsided.

Review Questions

1. d
2. c
3. c
4. b
5. a
6. b
7. c
8. d
9. a
10. c

CHAPTER 21

Case Study

1. The term used to describe a decrease in all cell lines is *pancytopenia*.
2. Acquired aplastic anemia would be considered due to the pancytopenia, reticulocytopenia, bone marrow hypocellularity, normal vitamin B_{12} and folate levels, absence of blasts and abnormal cells in the bone marrow and peripheral blood, normal myelopoiesis and megakaryopoiesis, and history of a prescribed non-steroidal anti-inflammatory agent.
3. An increase in blasts or reticulin in the bone marrow suggests a diagnosis of myelodysplasia or leukemia.
4. The extent of the patient's bone marrow hypocellularity and her hemoglobin, neutrophil, and platelet counts places her in the non-severe aplastic anemia category.
5. Due to the patient's age, immunosuppression with antithymocyte globulin and cyclosporine is the preferred treatment. In general, red cell transfusion would be administered if the patient had symptoms of anemia, while platelet transfusions would be given if her platelet count fell below $10 \times 10^9/L$.

Review Questions

1. c
2. d
3. b
4. d
5. b
6. d
7. c
8. d

9. c
10. d
11. a

CHAPTER 22

Case Study

1. Intravascular hemolysis with the color due to oxidized hemoglobin in the urine.
2. Haptoglobin, urinary hemoglobin (blood), serum bilirubin, serum lactate dehydrogenase, examination of a blood smear.
3. Due to the likely hemoglobinuria, intravascular hemolysis is expected. Therefore, the haptoglobin would be predicted to be low and the serum lactate dehydrogenase would be elevated. Urine test strip for blood should be positive. The serum bilirubin may not be elevated yet but should rise within several days. The blood smear will probably demonstrate schistocytes.

Review Questions

1. a
2. b
3. d
4. b
5. c
6. a
7. d
8. b
9. c
10. c

CHAPTER 23

Case Study

1. On the basis of morphology in the peripheral smear, the high MCHC, and the predominance of microspherocytes, hereditary spherocytosis should be suspected.
2. Laboratory tests that establish the presence of spherocytic non-immune hemolysis and suggest increased erythrocyte destruction and increased production would be desirable, including:
   - Reticulocyte count (should be elevated)
   - Haptoglobin (should be decreased)
   - Direct antiglobulin test (should be negative)
   - Erythrocyte osmotic fragility (should be increased)
   - Serum bilirubin (should be elevated)
   - Serum lactate dehydrogenase (should be elevated)
3. Hereditary spherocytosis is inherited as an autosomal dominant disease. In this condition there is an intrinsic defect in the RBC membrane. As the cells repeatedly go through the spleen, they suffer loss of membrane and deformability. Excess sodium leaks into the cells, causing formation of microspherocytes.

Review Questions

1. b
2. a

3. a
4. b
5. c
6. d
7. b
8. a
9. b
10. d
11. a
12. c

CHAPTER 24

Case Study

1. The stages of the parasite that were seen on the thin blood smear were ring forms or young trophozoites.
2. On the thick film, the red blood cells were laked (i.e. lysed) by staining with water-based Giemsa stain. There were an extremely large number of rings or early trophozoites. The rings were delicate, and they may frequently collapse and assume a comma shape.
3. The diagnosis was *Plasmodium falciparum* because only rings were found in the thin smear and thick film.

Review Questions

1. b
2. a
3. a
4. d
5. b
6. c
7. d
8. a
9. c
10. d

CHAPTER 25

Case Study

1. Since the patient was previously healthy, this is most likely an acquired problem and thereby extrinsic to the red blood cells. See Table 22-1.
2. A positive DAT denotes an antibody, complement, or both on the RBC surface and is confirmation of an immune hemolytic anemia. The DAT is usually negative in hemolytic anemias from snake and spider bites.
3. Four mechanisms that lead to drug-immune hemolytic anemia are immune complex, drug adsorption (hapten), non-immune protein adsorption, and idiopathic.
4. The drug is nonspecifically bound to or absorbed by the patient's RBCs and remains firmly attached to the cells.
5. In the presence of a hemolytic state, treatment focuses on discontinuation of the drug.

Review Questions

1. b
2. a
3. d

4. c
5. a
6. d
7. d
8. d
9. a
10. a
11. b

CHAPTER 26

Case Study

1. Confirmatory tests that should be performed are a hemoglobin solubility test, expected to be positive, and a citrate agar electrophoresis at a pH between 6.0 and 6.2. On the citrate agar test, hemoglobin C is separated from hemoglobins A, O, and E as a result of mode of migration (cathodally).
2. Characteristically, red blood cells that contain crystallized aggregates of hemoglobin that protrude through the cell membrane are seen.
3. On the basis of the electrophoretic pattern, the diagnosis of presence of hemoglobin SC can be made.
4. According to Mendelian law, the genotype can be depicted by the following chart:

	A	S
A	AA	AS
C	AC	SC

Of the offspring, 25% would be of each genotype: AA, AS, AC, and SC.

Review Questions

1. d
2. b
3. c
4. b
5. d
6. b
7. a
8. b
9. c
10. a

CHAPTER 27

Case Study

1. The family history revealed a Mediterranean ethnic background; both α- and β-thalassemia are common in the Mediterranean. It is a common mistake to treat a thalassemic individual for iron deficiency anemia, especially in areas in which thalassemia is not common in the general population, because both iron deficiency and thalassemia are microcytic, hypochromic anemias. His mother's gallbladder "attacks" were probably caused by pigment stones, which resulted from the mild hemolytic anemia of heterozygous thalassemia. She underwent a cholecystectomy in 1977, which did reveal pigment stones. The student also

had his gallbladder removed in 1983 because of pigment stones. Because Cooley's anemia, which is β-thalassemia major, had been diagnosed in his first cousin's children, it was quite likely that the student had β-thalassemia trait.

2. The elevated level of hemoglobin A_2, which is a marker for β-thalassemia minor, helped establish the diagnosis. Iron studies, which would have revealed normal or increased serum levels of iron in a non–iron-deficient patient with β-thalassemia minor and decreased serum levels of iron in iron-deficiency anemia, would also have differentiated the two conditions. The family history and the elevated Hb A_2 level in this situation made iron studies an unnecessary expense.

3. A microcytic, hypochromic anemia could be α- or β-thalassemia, HbE, iron-deficiency anemia (IDA), or, more rarely, sideroblastic anemia, lead poisoning, or anemia of chronic disease. Iron deficiency is the most common of these, and thalassemia patients often receive misdiagnoses of IDA. This patient's mother had periodically been given iron therapy. In this area of the United States, thalassemia is rather rare because of the small number in the ethnic groups in which this disorder is present, and thus the mistake has been fairly common among these patients.

4. His spouse should have a complete blood count, and microcytosis and anemia should be sought. If they are present, further testing should be conducted. If his spouse is found to carry the thalassemia gene, the couple should be advised that, according to Mendelian law, the genotypes of their offspring would be normal for 25%, thalassemia trait for 50%, and thalassemia major for 25%.

Review Questions

1. b
2. c
3. a
4. d
5. a
6. c
7. a
8. c
9. d
10. a
11. d
12. b
13. c
14. d
15. c

CHAPTER 28

Case Study
Case 1

1. The combination of an elevated WBC count and immature granulocytes, together with the presence of nucleated red cells, is sometimes referred to as an *leukoerythroblastic picture*. This leukoerythroblastic presentation is a common sign of disseminated malignancy.

2. Patients with absolute granulocyte counts below $1.0 \times 10^9/L$ are considered to be at extremely high risk for bacterial infection. This patient's absolute count was approximately $0.35 \times 10^9/L$. Many physicians believe that a patient with fewer than $0.5 \times 10^9/L$ granulocytes should be considered to have a bacterial infection and should be treated appropriately.

3. GM-CSF is one of the cytokines responsible for the commitment and maturation of granulocytes. The use of GM-CSF stimulates the marrow to produce granulocytes, thus lessening the chance of life-threatening infections.

4. The cells most affected by the chemotherapy were the granulocytes because they have a short lifespan. The GM-CSF was used to stimulate production of granulocytes.

Case 2

1. The elevated hemoglobin and hematocrit were caused by the decrease in plasma volume that resulted from the blister formation occurring in second-degree burns. The WBC count and differential were reflective of a stress reaction, perhaps due to the movement of cells within granulocyte pools.

2. Two responses were at work. First, her hemoglobin and hematocrit had been modified by the probable use of intravenous fluids such as saline. This fluid intusion countered the decreases in the plasma volume and may have returned the child's hemoglobin and hematocrit to pre-accident levels or slightly below. Second, the fever and positive wound cultures indicated that an infection was present. The demand for granulocytes to aggressively defend against the bacteria stimulated the productive capacity of the bone marrow that was manifested in the increased numbers of prematurely released granulocytes. This assumption of pre-maturity can be supported by the presence of the Döhle bodies and the toxic granulation, both of which result from stress at the promyelocyte, myelocyte, and metamyelocyte stages of development.

3. Because the mild anemia was still present, either the intravenous fluids were still being used or the hemoglobin and hematocrit reflected her "normal" state. The declining WBC count, coupled with the presence of more mature granulocytes without the toxic granulation or Döhle bodies, indicates that the WBCs together with the antimicrobial agent have prevented the spread of the infection and are in the process of removing it as a significant event in this child's recuperation.

Review Questions

1. c
2. d
3. b
4. d
5. c
6. b
7. c
8. d
9. a
10. b

CHAPTER 29

Review Questions

1. b
2. b
3. c
4. c
5. a
6. d
7. d
8. b
9. c
10. a

CHAPTER 30

Case Study

1. Alpha naphthyl acetate and butyrate esterases stain cells of monocytic origin. Chloroacetate esterase stains neutrophils.
2. The general diagnosis suggested by the elevated WBC count and decreased hemoglobin and platelet count, along with immature cells, is acute leukemia.
3. The most likely diagnosis is acute monocytic leukemia.

Review Questions

1. b
2. c
3. b
4. d
5. d
6. b
7. b
8. c
9. c
10. a

CHAPTER 31

Case Study

1. G-banding utilizes Giemsa to differentiate chromosomes into bands for identification of specific chromosomes. The chromosomes must be pretreated with the proteolytic enzyme trypsin.
2. The mutation is an example of a structural rearrangement between chromosomes 9 and 22, called the *Philadelphia chromosome*. The Philadelphia chromosome represents a balanced translocation between the long arms of chromosomes 9 and 22. At the molecular level, the gene for *ABL*, an oncogene, joins a gene on chromosome 22 named *BCR*. The result of the fusion of these two genes is a new fusion protein.
3. Fluorescence in situ hybridization (FISH) is a molecular technique that uses DNA or RNA probes labeled directly with a fluorescent nucleotide or with a hapten (e.g., dinitrophenyl, digoxygenin, or biotin). Both the probe and either metaphase or interphase cells are made single-stranded (denatured) and then hybridized together. Cells hybridized with a direct-label probe are viewed with a fluorescence microscope. If the probe was labeled with a hapten, antibodies to the hapten, carrying a fluorescent tag, are applied to the cells. Once the antibodies bind to the RNA or DNA probe, the cells can be viewed using a fluorescence microscope. FISH complements standard chromosome analysis by confirming the G-band analysis and by improved resolution, allowing for analysis at the molecular level.

Review Questions

1. c
2. d
3. a
4. d
5. a
6. c
7. d
8. c
9. c
10. b

CHAPTER 32

Case Study

1. DNA isolation for the detection of inherited mutations requires whole blood collected in a lavender top tube containing EDTA, to preserve white blood cells.
2. In the first gel, the correct controls are not present because it lacks a "no DNA" control.
3. Bands in the patient's sample appear at 141, 104, and 82 bp.
4. The following band sizes are expected in factor V DNA analysis:
   - Normal: 104 and 82 bp (37 is sometimes barely visible, as well)
   - Heterozygous: 141, 104, and 82 bp (37 is sometimes barely visible, as well)
   - Homozygous: 141 and 82 bp
5. The initial blood specimen drawn on this patient was in a red top tube for the recovery of serum. Since red top tubes do not preserve the white blood cells needed for DNA isolation, the laboratory requested a redraw of the specimen.
6. After receiving the correct specimen for DNA isolation, the molecular scientist conducted the test resulting in the gel seen in Figure 32-1. However, the supervisor determined this gel was not acceptable and must be repeated. The reason for the rejection is the lack of a no-DNA control. The no-DNA control is essential when conducting any PCR procedure in the clinical laboratory. This control will demonstrate whether cross contamination occurred during the set up of the PCR. The no-DNA control should lack a banding pattern as seen in Figure 32-2. If a banding pattern is present in the no-DNA control or this control is missing, the test must be repeated before reporting patient results.
7. Upon examining the patient's results in Figure 32-2, three bands (141, 104, 82) are present, demonstrating that this patient is heterozygous for the factor V Leiden mutation.

Review Questions

1. a
2. b
3. d
4. b
5. c
6. c
7. a
8. a
9. b
10. c

CHAPTER 33

Case Studies

Case 1

1. The lymphoid population is the most prominent. FSC demonstrates small to medium sized cells. These cells are characterized by low SSC indicative of sparse agranular cytoplasm.
2. The majority of cells expresses CD19, CD10 and kappa light chain. There is also a small population of T-cells positive for CD5 and negative for CD19 antigen.
3. Prominent kappa light chain expression indicates monoclonal B-cell population that is characteristic of lymphoma.

Case 2

1. The low density of CD45 antigen coupled with relatively low SSC is characteristic of blast population. Such a prominent blast population can only be seen in acute leukemias.
2. The expression of immature markers (CD34 and HLA-DR) coupled with positively for myeloid and megakaryoblastic antigen (CD33, CD41 and CD61) is seen in acute megakaryoblastic leukemias.

Review Questions

1. c
2. b
3. a
4. d
5. b
6. a
7. a
8. a
9. c
10. a
11. b

CHAPTER 34

Case Study

1. A myeloproliferative disorder is suggested by the WBC and differential. It would most likely be chronic myeloid leukemia, based on the elevated WBC count and the differential exhibiting a left shift in immature myeloid precursors and elevated basophils.
2. The LAP is low in CML, as opposed to elevated in bacterial infections.

3. The Philadelphia chromosome is present in a large majority of patients with CML.
4. Treatment in CML depends on several factors, including age of the patient, phase of disease, and availability of a matched donor. Therapy may include myelosuppressive agents, such as hydroxyurea, alkylating agents, a multidrug regimen, or interferon–α. Allogeneic stem cell transplant may also be an option. The most recent therapy to be introduced involves a tyrosine kinase inhibitor that targets the BCR-ABL oncogene product.

Review Questions

1. b
2. c
3. d
4. c
5. b
6. c
7. b
8. d
9. a
10. c

CHAPTER 35

Case Study

1. The differential diagnosis of patients with pancytopenia should include megaloblastic anemia (vitamin B_{12} or folate deficiency), aplastic anemia, liver disease, alcoholism, and myelodysplastic syndrome (MDS).
2. The probable diagnosis is MDS.
3. This patient's MDS should be classified as refractory anemia with ringed sideroblasts (RARS).

Review Questions

1. d
2. a
3. b
4. b
5. c
6. c
7. a
8. b
9. d
10. c

CHAPTER 36

Case Study

1. This is a case of acute lymphoblastic leukemia. The chronic leukemias or myeloproliferative disorders usually occur in adults and are rarely associated with thrombocytopenia at presentation. The blasts pictured are small "L1"-type lymphoblasts.
2. This child has clinically good prognostic features: age, female sex, and low white blood count. A poor prognostic finding is the headache, which may represent central nervous system involvement.

3. The most common phenotype of childhood ALL is CD10-positive, TdT-positive immature B lineage ALL, which is also the best phenotype prognostically. T-cell ALL, which usually develops in older male children in association with mediastinal involvement, is a less favorable phenotype, as is surface immunoglobulin–bearing ALL (mature B-cell ALL). Cytoplasmic immunoglobulin is present in pre–B-cell ALL, which carries a prognosis intermediate between those of immature B-cell ALL and B-cell ALL.

Review Questions

1. b
2. a
3. d
4. c
5. a
6. d
7. b
8. c
9. a
10. b

CHAPTER 37

Case Study

1. Diffuse large B-cell lymphoma (DLBCL).
2. This lesion is expected to show exclusive (clonal) kappa or lambda light chain expression. Flow cytometry is particularly sensitive in detecting surface and cytoplasmic immunoglobulin light chains and is commonly used to confirm clonality of lymphoproliferative disorders. In addition, other pan-B-cell markers can be studied by flow cytometry (e.g. CD19, CD22, and FMC7 antigens) to demonstrate B-cell origin of this lymphoma.
3. Most often DLBCL presents as a localized disease involving a group of lymph nodes. The bone marrow involvement is rare at presentation; however, it can occur later in the course of the disease.

Review Questions

1. d
2. c
3. d
4. d
5. b
6. b
7. b
8. a
9. c
10. a

CHAPTER 38

Case Study

1. Yes, typically the hemoglobin is between 17 and 21 g/dL and the hematocrit is 43% to 63%.
2. These values are normal for newborns. Erythrocytes of a newborn are markedly macrocytic. There may be up to

10 NRBCs on the first postnatal day, but they disappear by day 5. The polychromasia reflects the reticulocytosis that persists for about 3 days.

3. These values are normal for newborns. The WBC of a newborn averages 22×10^9/L and may be as high as 30.0×10^9/L without evidence of infection. The differential may show an increase in neutrophils rather than the lymphocyte predominance seen after 2 weeks. In this case the neutrophils and lymphocytes were in equal amounts, but no immature neutrophils were seen.

Review Questions

1. d
2. b
3. a
4. c
5. c
6. d
7. b
8. a

CHAPTER 39

Review Questions

1. a

They appear to be comparable, with each instrument flagging the results for further scrutiny. All four systems performed the WBC count. The Sysmex result is flagged, and the possible causes for the flag are listed below. The Coulter gave a R flag to the WBC, with a suspected Cellular Interference listed to the side. The ADVIA also flagged the WBC; its associated flags are listed as well. The CELL DYN flagged the result with a "WOC" with the interpretation listed below. Even though all the systems flagged the WBC and provided flags, no one WBC seems to be out of line when the four counts are compared with each other.

2. a
3. c

Summary of questions 2 & 3

Instrument	NRBCs	Blasts
Bayer	+++	+
CELL-DYN	Nucleated RBC	No flag
Coulter	No result	No flag
Sysmex	NRBC?	No flag

4. b

All use the same principle for counting platelets. The platelet count is low on all four instruments with the platelet count in the 20,000/µL range. Three of the four systems produced platelet flags, with two of them indicating interference and one indicating platelet clumps. The three systems with flags each counted the platelets using impedance technology and demonstrated various interferences with the count.

5. Yes, a manual differential should be performed based on the presence of NRBC and blast flags. A platelet smear review is indicated as well.

6. c
7. b
8. a
9. b
10. b
11. c
12. d
13. a
14. b
15. c
16. a

CHAPTER 40

Case Study

1. The most likely disorder is hemophilia A. Hemorrhagic disease of the newborn implies a coagulation factor deficiency. While the vitamin K–dependent factors prothrombin, VII, IX, and X are usually diminished at birth, seldom are they low enough to cause bleeding, although they may cause prolonged prothrombin time and activated partial thromboplastin time results. By law in most states, vitamin K is administered at birth to prevent bleeding. Excessive bleeding at birth may be caused by factor VIII deficiency (hemophilia A), a sex-linked disorder that affects boys. Another sex-linked deficiency, factor IX deficiency (Christmas disease), is possible, but factor VIII deficiency is at least four times more common.

2. Treat with factor VIII concentrate. The child should have factor VIII and IX assays performed and a therapeutic regimen of DDAVP and factor concentrate administration initiated.

Review Questions

1. b
2. c
3. b
4. a
5. b
6. a
7. d
8. c
9. a
10. a

CHAPTER 41

Case Study

1. The patient most likely has hemophilia A and has been treated with blood products prior to the advent of purified factor concentrates, which led to infection with one of the hepatitis viruses. Because there was no test to screen for hepatitis C until approximately 12 years ago, and infection with the hepatitis C virus is associated with a high risk of chronic hepatitis, this is the most probable cause of his liver disease. In end-stage liver disease, the liver is scarred and the pressure in the portal circulation causes the spleen to enlarge (splenomegaly). The latter causes platelet sequestration and increased platelet clearance (hypersplenism),

with resultant thrombocytopenia. In addition to low platelets, there is also decreased platelet function, which is caused by the liver disease and is responsible for the epistaxis.

2. His treatment will be dependent on assays of several coagulation factors in the plasma, such as VIII, VII, and V. If he is diagnosed with vitamin K deficiency, a trial of vitamin K may be helpful. However, if the liver is unable to process the vitamin and produce normal levels of prothrombin and factors VII, IX, and X, he may have to receive a transfusion with FFP. In case there is severe hypofibrinogenemia, cryoprecipitate is indicated. Unfortunately, platelet transfusions are not likely to increase his platelet count due to rapid sequestration in the spleen.

Review Questions

1. c
2. b
3. c
4. a
5. b
6. d
7. b
8. b
9. a
10. c

CHAPTER 42

Case Study

1. The following congenital and acquired risk factors are included in a thrombophilia profile. The entries with asterisks are valid when tested at least ten days after termination of a thrombotic event and termination of anticoagulant therapy.
   - Anticardiolipin antibodies—by ELISA
   - Lupus anticoagulant—see below
   - APC Resistance (functional test for Factor V Leiden)
   - Prothrombin 20210 mutation—genetic test
   - Factor VIII—acute phase reactant
   - Protein C—functional; affected by warfarin
   - Protein S—functional; affected by warfarin
   - Antithrombin—functional; affected by heparin
   - Homocysteine

2. The most common risk factor is lupus anticoagulant, and this is the most often implicated in a thrombotic event.

3. When patients are proven to have a thrombosis risk factor, s/he may be instructed to avoid situations that trigger thrombosis, such as immobilization, smoking, the use of oral contraceptives, or hormone replacement therapy. S/he may also be provided with prophylactic anticoagulant therapy under thrombotic circumstances, such as orthopedic surgery.

Review Questions

1. a
2. a
3. d
4. c
5. b

6. b
7. a
8. a
9. d
10. d
11. b
12. d
13. a
14. c

CHAPTER 43

Case Study

1. Yes, the heparin is significant.
2. Heparin-induced platelet aggregation, serotonin release assay, or ELISA should be ordered.

An ELISA assay was performed to look for the presence of heparin-induced antibodies. Results gave an optical density of 0.50, with a reference range of less than 0.400 OD. The patient was found to have clinically significant levels of heparin-induced antibodies.

The patient underwent an above-knee amputation on her left leg. The grafting surgeries were successful, and the patient is now recovering nicely.

Review Questions

1. b
2. d
3. b
4. c
5. b
6. b
7. b
8. c
9. d
10. a

CHAPTER 44

Case Study

1. Storage pool disease, aspirin-like defects, and antiplatelet agents such as aspirin are possibilities.
2. Storage pool disease or aspirin-like defects seem most likely.
3. Based on the results of the quantitative test for ATP release, the likely cause is delta storage pool disease.

These results were confirmed by the results of electron microscopy of the patient's platelets, which revealed the absence of detectable dense granules. Since the patient's bleeding problems are due to an inherited abnormality that typically results in only mild bleeding problems, the patient was counseled to avoid antiplatelet agents, particularly aspirin, because they are known to exacerbate the bleeding problems encountered by patients with dense granule deficiency.

Review Questions

1. d
2. a
3. a

4. b
5. c
6. c
7. d
8. b
9. d
10. a

CHAPTER 45

Case Study

1. The laboratory director questioned the phlebotomist about the problem. The phlebotomist admitted that he had erroneously collected blood in a red- and gray-stoppered "tiger-top" tube and, responding to the patient's remark, had immediately poured the blood into a blue-stoppered tube for analysis. He thought the specimen would be okay because it had not clotted yet.
2. The red and gray "marbleized" stopper designates the serum separator tube. The phlebotomist poured the blood into the blue-stoppered tube before it had begun to clot, however the activator from the "tiger-top" shortened the PT clot time, thus causing an erroneously short prothrombin time and low INR.
3. Unexpectedly shortened prothrombin times during oral anticoagulant therapy are generally indicators of patient non-compliance. The second most common circumstance that affects the prothrombin time is dietary changes, most often an increased intake of vitamin K–rich foods such as green, leafy vegetables, liver, or avocado. In this instance the patient had been fully compliant, carefully adhering to dosage and timing, and her diet had not changed. These facts led the laboratory director to consider a specimen collection error.

Specimens collected in 3.2% sodium citrate may be stored for up to 24 hours at room temperature without a change in the prothrombin time. However, specimens stored at greater than 24° C deteriorate rapidly, causing prolongation of the prothrombin time and an increased INR. Prolonged storage at 2° to 4° C may activate factor VII, slightly shortening the prothrombin time and slightly decreasing the INR.

Many serum separator tubes contain particulate materials that hasten in vitro clotting. Core laboratory managers select these tubes to improve test result turn-around time when the required sample is serum. When collecting a series of tubes including a blue-stoppered tube for hemostasis testing, the blue-stoppered tube should be collected first or should be collected following a non-additive tube. It should not be collected immediately after a serum separator tube with clot activators, as the activators may carry over to the hemostasis specimen and affect test results.

In this instance, an observant patient provided clues that led to the pre-analytical error. The phlebotomist was carefully counseled about the effects of tube additives on hemostasis tests.

Review Questions

1. a
2. b

3. a
4. b
5. b
6. a
7. b
8. b
9. b
10. d
11. b
12. b
13. a
14. d

CHAPTER 46

Case Study

1. The heparin therapy is initiated to prevent further thrombosis and is necessary to prevent warfarin skin necrosis during the first 3 days of warfarin therapy when the patient is prothrombotic.
2. Unfractionated heparin is terminated at five days to avoid triggering heparin-induced thrombocytopenia, which occurs in 2-3% of unfractionated heparin therapy.
3. In current therapy, if the patient is within three hours of a catheterization laboratory at the onset of chest pain, no thrombolytic therapy is started. Stent placement is accomplished within three hours of onset, and the cardiac surgeon does not wish to contend with the anticoagulant properties of the tissue plasminogen activator.

Although the limit for unfractionated heparin therapy is five days, it is usually terminated at 3 days when the patient is discharged. Warfarin therapy has been eliminated from the regimen in favor of aspirin and clopidogrel. Warfarin therapy provides protection from venous thromboembolism but not arterial clotting. Aspirin and clopidogrel are more efficacious.

Review Questions

1. c
2. c
3. c
4. a
5. d
6. b

7. d
8. c
9. b
10. b
11. a
12. b

CHAPTER 47

Case Study

1. No. The description of the sample and the instrument flags indicating lipemia should alert the operator to a potentially invalid test result because lipemia is known to cause erroneous results on most photo-optical coagulation analyzers.
2. Two options can be used to negate the effect of the lipemia and obtain valid test results:
   a. Remove the lipemia from the plasma by high-speed centrifugation or ultracentriguation.
   b. Perform testing using an endpoint detection method that is not susceptible to lipemia in the sample, such as mechanical clot detection.
3. Because the patient history includes previous surgical procedures without bleeding symptoms and there is no other indication of abnormal bleeding tendencies for this patient, it is probably safe to believe that the prolonged PT and APTT results are due to the lipemic nature of the sample. The patient would most likely *not* be at risk for bleeding during the surgery, and it would be anticipated that repeat testing using one of the options listed previously would yield test results within the reference range.

Review Questions

1. b
2. d
3. a
4. c
5. b
6. c
7. c
8. a
9. d
10. a

Glossary

abetalipoproteinemia: An autosomal recessive disorder of lipoprotein metabolism in which lipoproteins containing apolipoprotein B (chylomicrons, very low-density lipoproteins, and low-density lipoproteins) are not synthesized. It is characterized by the presence of acanthocytes in blood and low levels of cholesterol in the plasma.

abluminal: Away from the lumen of a tubular structure, such as a blood vessel.

absolute neutrophil count (ANC): The actual number of neutrophils in a volume of whole blood such as a liter. The ANC is calculated by multiplying the patient's total white blood cell count by the percentage of segmented neutrophils and bands, or can be measured directly.

absolute reticulocyte count (ARC): The actual number of reticulocytes in a volume of whole blood such as a liter. The ARC is calculated by multiplying the patient's reticulocyte percentage times the red blood cell count, or it can be measured directly.

acanthocyte: An erythrocyte with spiny blunt projections of varying lengths distributed irregularly over its surface. Associated with abetalipoproteinemia or abnormalities of lipid metabolism, such as that occurring in liver disease. Also called a *spur cell.*

acanthocytosis: The presence of acanthocytes in the blood.

accuracy: The extent to which a measurement is close to the true value.

achlorhydria: An abnormal condition characterized by the absence of hydrochloric acid in gastric secretions.

acid elution slide test: A test for detecting fetal cells in maternal circulation. Blood smears are immersed in an acid buffer, adult hemoglobin (HbA) is eluted from the erythrocyte, smears are stained, and erythrocytes having fetal hemoglobin (HbF) will take up the stain. Also called *Kleihauer-Betke stain.*

acidified serum test: A test for increased complement sensitivity of red blood cells by placing them in mild acidified fresh serum. Also known as *Ham's test.*

acquired immune deficiency syndrome (AIDS): Suppression or deficiency of cellular immunity. Acquired by exposure to the human immunodeficiency virus (HIV), which attacks the T lymphocyte subgroup known as CD4 cells.

acrocyanosis: A condition marked by symmetrical cyanosis (bluish discoloration of the skin due to excessive concentration of deoxyhemoglobin in the blood) of the extremities, with persistent, uneven blue or red discoloration of the skin of the digits, wrists, and ankles. Also called *Raynaud's phenomenon.*

activated coagulation time (ACT): A whole blood-clotting time test used in operating rooms. Particulate activator is added to blood, and the time to clot is recorded. Used to monitor high-level unfractionated heparin therapy.

activated partial thromboplastin time (APTT): A plasma-clotting time test provided in all coagulation laboratories. Calcium chloride, phospholipid, and activator are added, and the time to clot is recorded. Used to monitor unfractionated heparin therapy and to screen for intrinsic pathway deficiencies.

activated protein C resistance: An inherited thrombosis risk factor in which activated coagulation factor V resists activated protein C digestion.

acute: Describes a disease or disease symptoms that begin abruptly with marked intensity and then subside after a relatively short period.

acute leukemia: Malignant, unregulated proliferation of the cells of the bone marrow, characterized by abrupt onset of clinical signs and, if left untreated, death within months from the time of diagnosis.

acute myocardial infarction: Occlusion of a coronary artery by a clot, causing death of heart tissue. Commonly called a *heart attack.*

acute phase reactant: A serum protein that is produced by the liver and whose blood level is increased by the action of cytokines during inflammation. Examples include C-reactive protein, ferritin, and fibrinogen.

adenopathy: An enlargement of any gland.

adenosine diphosphate (ADP): A molecule involved in energy metabolism; it is produced by hydrolysis of adenosine triphosphate.

adenosine triphosphate (ATP): A molecule involved in energy metabolism and required for metabolic processes. It is produced in all cells and is used to store energy in the form of high-energy phosphate bonds. The free energy derived from hydrolysis of ATP is used to drive metabolic reactions.

adhesion: The property of binding or remaining in proximity; for example, attachment of platelets to such surfaces as subendothelial collagen.

adipocyte: A fat cell.

afibrinogenemia: Lack of fibrinogen (coagulation factor I) in the blood.

agammaglobulinemia: Absence of all classes of immunoglobulins in the blood.

agglutination: The clumping together of cells as a result of interaction with specific antibodies.

aggregation: The clumping of cells to similar particles or cells; e.g., attachment of platelets to other platelets.

agnogenic: Of idiopathic or unknown origin.

agranulocytosis: Any condition involving greatly decreased numbers of granulocytes.

albinism: A congenital, hereditary condition characterized by partial or total lack of melanin pigment in the body. Total albinos have pale skin that does not tan, white hair, and pink eyes.

Alder-Reilly anomaly: An autosomal dominant polysaccharide metabolism disorder in which leukocytes of the myelocytic series, and sometimes all leukocytes, contain coarse azurophilic mucopolysaccharide granules.

allele: One of two or more alternative forms of a gene that occupy corresponding loci on homologous chromosomes. Each allele encodes a certain inherited characteristic. An individual normally has two alleles for each gene, one contributed by the mother and one by the father. If both alleles are the same, the individual is homozygous, but if the alleles are different, the individual is heterozygous. In heterozygous individuals, one of the alleles may be dominant and the other recessive.

alloantibody: An antibody that is produced by one individual and reacts with antigens of another individual of the same species. Also called an *isoantibody*.

alloimmune: Producing antibodies to antigens derived from a genetically dissimilar individual of the same species.

alloimmune hemolytic anemia: Hemolytic anemia caused by antibodies directed against the cells of another person. Examples include hemolytic transfusion reaction and hemolytic disease of the newborn.

alopecia: Lacking hair where it often grows, especially on the head (baldness).

alpha granules: Granules of platelets that store a variety of hemostasis proteins. Visible in Wright-stained platelets.

alpha thalassemia: Thalassemia caused by decreased rate of synthesis of the alpha globin chains of hemoglobin. Also called *phlebotomy*.

amenorrhea: Absence of a menstrual period in a woman of reproductive age. Normal during pregnancy and lactation.

amyloidosis: A disease in which a waxy, starchlike glycoprotein (amyloid) accumulates in tissues and organs, impairing their function.

analog drugs: Drugs that are chemically similar to one another but, because of minor structural differences, may have different physiologic actions.

anaplastic: Characterized by loss of differentiation and growing without structure or form. Anaplasia is a characteristic of cancer.

anemia: A reduction below the normal concentration of hemoglobin in the blood, resulting in diminished oxygen-carrying capacity.

aneuploid: A chromosome number that is not an exact multiple of the normal diploid number. Results in having fewer or more chromosomes than normal.

angiodysplasia: Small vascular deformity of the gut. It can be a basis of gastrointestinal bleeding and anemia.

anisocytosis: Presence in the blood of erythrocytes with excessive variation in volume.

annular diaphragm: A device used in phase microscopy, together with a phase-shifting element, which creates contrast of a cell against its dark background.

anorexia nervosa: Psychiatric diagnosis that describes an eating disorder characterized by low body weight and body image distortion.

anoxia: Absence of oxygen in the tissues.

antagonist: Any agent, such as a drug or muscle, that exerts an opposite action to that of another or competes for the same receptor site.

antecubital fossa: The depression at the bend of the elbow.

antibody (Ab): A specialized protein (an immunoglobulin) produced by lymphocytes in response to bacteria, viruses, or other foreign substances called *antigens*. An antibody is specific to the antigen that stimulated its production.

anticardiolipin antibody (ACA): Part of the antiphospholipid antibody family that includes lupus anticoagulant. An autoantibody detected in a solid-phase immunoassay system in which cardiolipin is the target antigen. Presence of anticardiolipin antibody is related to venous and arterial thrombotic disease.

anticoagulant: A therapeutic that delays in vivo blood coagulation. An additive to blood specimen collection tubes that prevents in vitro blood clotting.

antigen: A substance, usually a protein, that the body recognizes as foreign and that can evoke an immune response.

antihemophilic factor (AHF): Therapeutic concentration of coagulation factor VIII produced through chemical fractionation, immunoaffinity column, or recombinant synthesis. AHF is prescribed in the treatment of hemophilia A, a hereditary deficiency of factor VIII.

antineoplastic: A chemotherapeutic agent that controls or kills cancer cells.

antiphospholipid antibody (APA): Name for the antibody family that includes anticardiolipin antibodies, anti-beta-2-glycoprotein I antibodies, and lupus anticoagulant. These antibodies bind phospholipid-binding proteins, such as beta2-glycoprotein I, annexin, and prothrombin. Presence of an antiphospholipid antibody is related to venous and arterial thrombotic disease.

antiphospholipid syndrome: The series of thrombotic disorders related to the chronic presence of an antiphospholipid antibody, such as anticardiolipin antibody, anti-beta2-glycoprotein I antibody, or lupus anticoagulant. Disorders include migraine, transient ischemic attacks, strokes, acute myocardial infarction, peripheral artery disease, venous thromboembolic disease, and spontaneous abortion.

antithrombin (AT, AT III): Any substance that neutralizes the action of thrombin and thus limits or restricts blood coagulation. Plasma antithrombin III is a circulating serine protease inhibitor produced in the liver and activated by therapeutic heparin.

aperture lever: The lever underneath a microscope condenser that, when moved, changes the angle of light going through the specimen, resulting in greater contrast of cellular detail.

aplasia: A failure of the normal process of cell generation and development.

aplastic anemia: A deficiency of all of the formed elements of blood, representing a failure of the cell-generating capacity of bone marrow.

aplastic crises: Serious complication of infection (human parvovirus B-19) in patients with chronic hemolytic anemia such as sickle cell disease. The bone marrow does not respond to the red blood cell destruction, becoming aplastic.

apoferritin: The protein component of the ferritin molecule.

apoptosis: Programmed cell death; it is a mechanism for cell deletion in the regulation of cell populations.

aspirin (ASA): Acetylsalicylic acid in tablet form; acetylates platelet cyclo-oxygenase and reduces platelet activation. Aspirin is used for its antithrombotic properties.

asynchrony: Occurrence at different times; timing that is not synchronized.

atrial fibrillation (AFIB): An uncontrolled and ineffective atrial heartbeat, present in at least 2 million U.S. citizens, that increases the risk for stroke and is treated with long-term Coumadin therapy.

atypical lymphocytes: Lymphocytes that have been stimulated by antigens. These cells can undergo various nuclear and cytoplasmic morphologic changes (also called *transformed, reactive* or *variant* lymphocytes).

Aüer rod: An abnormal needle-shaped or round inclusion in the cytoplasm of myeloblasts and promyelocytes; composed of condensed primary granules. Stains pink to purple with Wright stain.

autoantibody: An antibody that is produced by an individual that recognizes an antigen on the individual's own tissues (self-antigen).

autoimmune: Pertaining to an immune response to one's own tissues (self-antigen).

autoimmune hemolytic anemia: A complex clinical disorder characterized by premature red blood cell destruction due to autoantibodies that bind to antigens on the red cell surface.

autoinfection: Reinfection by microbes or parasitic organisms that are present on or within the body.

autologous: Related to self or belonging to the same organism, such as blood that is donated by a patient before surgery and is to be returned to the same patient during or after surgery.

autosomal dominant inheritance: A pattern of inheritance in which the transmission of a dominant allele on an autosome causes a trait to be expressed.

autosomal inheritance: A pattern of inheritance in which the transmission of traits depends on the presence or absence of certain alleles on the autosomes.

autosomal recessive inheritance: A pattern of inheritance resulting from the transmission of a recessive allele on an autosome.

autosome: Any of the 22 pairs of chromosomes in humans other than the pair concerned with determination of sex (sex chromosomes).

autosplenectomy: The almost complete disappearance of the spleen through progressive fibrosis and shrinkage.

azurophilic granules: When stained with Wright stain, these appear as large, reddish-purple primary granules that are first seen in promyelocytes and can be seen in lymphocytes. Also called *nonspecific granules* or *primary granules* when seen in promyelocytes.

azurophilic: Staining blue with Giemsa stain. The same structures appear red-purple with Wright's stain.

B cell: A type of lymphocyte that is derived from the bone marrow and functions to produce antibodies. The end product of B (lymphocyte) cell maturation is the plasma cell.

Babesia: A parasite that causes babesiosis in humans. It is transmitted by ticks and infects the erythrocytes. The parasite is described as a small ringlike structure present inside erythrocytes.

band neutrophil: The immediate precursor of the mature segmented neutrophil. Band neutrophils have a nonsegmented, usually curved, nucleus and can be seen in the bone marrow and peripheral blood. Also called a *stab.*

bartonellosis: An acute infection caused by *Bartonella bacilliformis,* transmitted by the bite of a sandfly. The first stage of the disease is associated with severe hemolytic anemia.

base pair: A pair of nucleotides in the complementary strands of a DNA molecule that interact through hydrogen bonding across the axis of the DNA helix. One of the nucleotides in each pair is a purine (either adenine or guanine), and the other is a pyrimidine (either thymine or cytosine). Adenine always pairs with thymine, and guanine always pairs with cytosine.

basophil: A granulocytic leukocyte that is characterized by cytoplasmic granules that stain bluish-black when exposed to a basic dye. Cytoplasmic granules of basophils are of variable size and may obscure the nucleus.

basophilia: An abnormal increase of basophils in the blood.

basophilic normoblast: The second identifiable stage in erythrocyte maturation; it is derived from the pronormoblast. When stained with Wright stain, the basophilic normoblast is a large cell with deep, rich blue cytoplasm and is seen in the bone marrow.

basophilic stippling: The presence of small, dark-blue to purple granules, evenly distributed, within an erythrocyte stained with Wright stain. These inclusions are composed of precipitated ribosomal protein (RNA).

Bence Jones protein: A protein found almost exclusively in the urine of patients with multiple myeloma. The protein constitutes the light chain component of the abnormal immunoglobulins produced.

benign: Noncancerous or not malignant.

Bernard-Soulier syndrome (BSS): A mild to moderate mucocutaneous bleeding disorder caused by one of a series of mutations to platelet GP Ib or GP IX, part of the GP Ib/IX/V von Willebrand factor receptor complex. This is a defect of platelet adhesion.

beta-2-glycoprotein I: Plasma coagulation globulin that is a target of lupus anticoagulant autoantibody.

beta-thalassemia: Thalassemia caused by diminished synthesis of the beta-globin chains that make up hemoglobin.

beta-thromboglobulin: Protein that is stored and secreted by platelet alpha granules and neutralizes heparin.

bifurcation: Separation into two branches

bilirubin: The orange-yellow pigment of bile, formed principally by macrophages from the breakdown of erythrocyte hemoglobin at the end of their life span.

bilirubinemia: The presence of excess bilirubin in the plasma.

2,3-bisphosphoglycerate (2,3-BPG): See *2,3-diphosphoglycerate (2,3-DPG)*.

blast: An immature cell, such as a normoblast, lymphoblast, or myeloblast.

bleeding time: The time required for blood to stop flowing from a wound 2 mm in length and 1 mm deep. The bleeding time test is used to evaluate vascular and platelet function.

Bohr effect: The effect of carbon dioxide and hydrogen ions on the affinity of hemoglobin for oxygen. (Increasing carbon dioxide and hydrogen ions decrease oxyhemoglobin saturation, whereas decreasing concentrations have the opposite effect.)

bone marrow: Specialized semiliquid tissue filling the spaces in spongy bone where white blood cells develop. Red marrow is found in many bones of infants and children and in the spongy bone of the proximal epiphyses of the humerus and femur and the sternum, ribs, and vertebral bodies of adults. Fatty yellow marrow is found in the medullary cavity of most adult long bones.

bone marrow aspirate: A sample of semiliquid red bone marrow obtained by suction through a needle into the marrow cavity. Examined microscopically and used to help diagnose and evaluate patients with hematologic diseases.

bone marrow biopsy: A sample of bone marrow acquired by inserting a needle through the bone into the marrow and then extracting the core sample from the bore of the needle. Examined microscopically particularly to assess cellularity and cell arrangements.

bone marrow examination: A microscopic tissue examination of red bone marrow, used to help evaluate patients with hematologic diseases.

buffy coat: A grayish-white layer of white blood cells and platelets that accumulates on the surface of sedimented erythrocytes when blood is allowed to stand or is centrifuged.

bullae: A defense mechanism of the human body, consisting of a pool of lymph and other bodily fluids beneath the upper layers of the skin (also referred to as a *blister*).

Burkitt lymphoma: A malignant lymphoma that is characterized by Burkitt cells. The Burkitt cell is a mature lymphocyte with multiple vacuoles present in the dark-blue cytoplasm. These characteristic cells can be seen in the bone marrow and peripheral blood.

burst-forming unit (BFU): Similar to colony-forming units. In the hematopoietic theory, erythrocytes are derived from BFU-erythroid (BFU-E) progenitor cells that are less differentiated than the CFU-E.

Cabot rings: Threadlike structures, often appearing as purple-blue loops or rings in erythrocytes by Wright's stain. These inclusions are thought to be composed of remnants of mitotic spindle.

cachectic/cachexia: State of ill health, malnutrition, and wasting. It may occur from malignancies, infections, and chronic disease.

CAP: College of American Pathologists, an agency that accredits medical laboratories.

carboxyhemoglobin: A compound produced by the exposure of hemoglobin to carbon monoxide.

carcinoma: A malignant neoplasm of epithelial origin that tends to invade surrounding tissue and to metastasize to distant regions of the body.

C-banding: A chromosome stain that uses a Giemsa stain to visualize heterochromatic regions near centromeres. Also called a *centromere binding stain*.

CD: Cluster of differentiation; a group of receptors or markers, usually membrane proteins, that characterize cells by their functions. CD profiles can be used to identify cell types.

cell membrane: A lipid bilayer that is the outer covering of a cell.

cellular immunity: The mechanism of acquired immunity characterized by the dominant role of the T lymphocytes.

centriole: An intracellular organelle that is a component of the centrosome. Often occurring in pairs, centrioles are associated with cell division.

cerebrospinal fluid (CSF): Fluid that flows through and protects the four ventricles of the brain, the subarachnoid spaces, and the spinal canal.

cerebrovascular accident (CVA): A stroke; occlusion of an artery of the brain.

CFU-GEMM: A major progenitor cell in the hematopoietic theory, CFU-GEMM is the precursor cell for granulocytes, erythrocytes, monocytes, and megakaryocytes.

chamfered: Having a rounded edge connecting two surfaces. If the surfaces are at right angles, the chamfer will characteristically be symmetrical at 45 degrees.

Charcot-Leyden crystals: Crystalline structures that are shaped like narrow double pyramids and are found in the sputum of persons suffering from asthma and in the feces of dysentery patients. These crystals are formed by the membranes of disintegrating eosinophils.

Chédiak-Higashi anomaly: A congenital, autosomal recessive disorder, characterized by partial albinism, photophobia, and the presence of abnormally large blue granules in leukocytes. Also known as a *Chédiak-Steinbrinck-Higashi anomaly*.

chelation: A chemical reaction in which there is a combination with a metal to form a ring-shaped molecular complex in which the metal is firmly bound and isolated. Chelating agents are used as anticoagulants and in the treatment of lead poisoning or iron overload.

chelosis: A condition in which the lips develop scaling and fissures at the corners of the mouth. Seen in riboflavin deficiencies and iron deficiency anemia.

chemotaxis: Cellular movement toward or away from a chemical stimulus. It is associated particularly with neutrophils and monocytes, whose phagocytic activity is influenced by chemical factors released by invading microorganisms.

chemotherapy: The treatment of disease by chemical agents. In modern usage, chemotherapy usually entails the use of chemicals to destroy cancer cells.

chromogen: A substance that produces color.

chromosome: A threadlike structure in the nucleus of a cell, composed of DNA, that functions in the transmission of genetic information. In humans, there are 46 chromosomes, including 22 homologous pairs of autosomes and 1 pair of sex chromosomes.

chronic: Persisting over a long period of time, often for the remainder of a person's life.

chronic leukemia: Malignant, unregulated proliferation of the cells of the bone marrow, characterized by slow onset and progression of symptoms and death occurring years after diagnosis.

CLIA: Acronym for the Clinical Laboratory Improvement Amendments of 1988, establishing standards for quality testing in the clinical laboratory.

clone: A group of genetically identical cells derived from a single common cell through mitosis.

Clostridium perfringens: Anaerobic, gram-positive bacteria capable of causing gangrene in humans and resulting in intravascular hemolysis and clotting.

CLSI: Clinical Laboratory Standards Institute, a global, non-profit, standards-developing organization that promotes development and use of voluntary consensus standards and guidelines within the healthcare community.

coagulation: The sequential process by which multiple plasma enzymes and cofactors interact in sequence, forming an insoluble fibrin clot.

coagulation cascade: A series of enzymatic reactions beginning with activation of factor VII by tissue factor (extrinsic—in vivo) or factor XII by a negatively charged surface (intrinsic—in vitro) and proceeding through the common pathway to the formation of the fibrin clot.

coagulation factors: One of several plasma proteins, also called *procoagulants*, the interactions of which are responsible for the process of blood clotting.

codocyte: A poorly hemoglobinized erythrocyte seen in hemoglobinopathies and thalassemia. In Wright stain, there is a concentration of hemoglobin in the center and periphery, resembling a target or bull's eye. Also called a *target cell*.

coefficient of variation (CV, CV%): The statistical measure of the deviation of a variable from its mean, expressed as a percentage of the mean.

cold agglutinin: An antibody of uncertain stimulus able to react with red cell membrane in certain diseases; may cause clumping of cells at temperatures below 36° C and hemolysis.

cold agglutinin disease: A rare autoimmune hemolytic disorder resulting from the reaction of cold agglutinins with erythrocytes at temperatures below 30° C.

cold-reacting antibody: An antibody that reacts with erythrocytes at an optimum temperature of 4° C.

colony-forming unit (CFU): Progenitor cells that are derived from the pluripotential hematopoietic stem cell and give rise to the different cell lineages. Also called *committed stem cells*.

colony-stimulating factor (CSF): A cytokine that promotes the division and, sometimes, differentiation of immature blood cells.

common coagulation pathway: The steps in the mechanism of coagulation from the activation of factor X through the conversion of fibrinogen to fibrin. The common pathway begins at the junction of the intrinsic and extrinsic pathways.

complement (C): A system of at least 20 complex, enzymatic serum proteins. In an antigen-antibody reaction, complement causes cell lysis and stimulates chemotaxis of leukocytes.

complementation group: A biochemical cascade of the immune system that assists in clearing pathogens from an organism. It is a result of many small plasma proteins that work together to lyse target cells by disrupting the target cell's plasma membrane. It affects both innate immunity and acquired immunity.

condenser: A device that gathers, organizes, and directs the light from the field diaphragm through the specimen on the microscope stage.

confidence interval (CI): A range of values expected to contain the measured value (parameter), with a predetermined degree of statistical confidence (e.g. 95% CI).

congenital: Present at birth.

Coombs' test: See direct antiglobulin test.

corrected reticulocyte count: A calculation performed on the relative reticulocyte count from specimens with a low hematocrit. In a patient with a low hematocrit, the percentage of reticulocytes may be misleadingly elevated because whole blood contains fewer erythrocytes. A correction factor normalizes the reticulocyte count, using the average normal hematocrit of 0.45 L/L.

cortex: The outermost layer of any organ, as distinguished from the innermost medulla, as in the adrenal gland, thymus, lymph node, etc.

craniofacial dysmorphism: Distortion or misshaping of the head and face.

cryoglobulin: Any of numerous serum globulins, almost always an immunoglobulin, that precipitate at low temperatures (around 4° C) and redissolve at 37° C.

cryoprecipitate (CRYO): A therapeutic rich in fibrinogen, factor VIII, and factor XIII, used to provide fibrinogen or factor XIII for deficiency of either. CRYO is collected from fresh human plasma that has been frozen and thawed slowly.

cyanosis: A bluish discoloration, especially of the skin and mucous membranes, due to excessive concentration of deoxyhemoglobin in the blood.

cytochemistry: The study of chemical elements found in cells; these elements may be enzymatic or nonenzymatic.

Cytochemical staining of cells is a useful tool in differentiating hematopoietic diseases.

cytogenetics: The branch of genetics devoted to the laboratory study of chromosome abnormalities, such as deletions, translocations, and aneuploidy.

cytokine: A cellular product that influences the function or activity of other cells. Cytokines include colony-stimulating factors, interferons, interleukins, and lymphokines.

cytokinesis: The division of the cytoplasm in the cell, generally after mitotic nuclear division.

cytomegalovirus (CMV): A common virus that can cause a variety of clinical syndromes, although the majority of infections are very mild.

cytopenia: A deficiency in numbers of one or more types of blood cells.

cytotoxic: Pertaining to a compound or agent that destroys or damages cells.

dacryocyte: An erythrocyte with a single pointed extension, resembling a teardrop. Also called a *teardrop cell.*

D-dimer (D:D, D-D): One of the fibrin degradation products. D-dimer is composed of two covalently joined fibrin D fragments.

decontamination: Removal or inactivation of an infectious agent from an item or surface so that it no longer causes an infection.

decubitus: The position of a patient who is lying down in bed.

deep venous thrombosis (DVT): The formation of clots in deep leg veins, such as the femoral vein. A manifestation of venous thromboembolic disease that is associated with a number of thrombotic risk factors.

delayed hemolytic transfusion reaction: Hemolysis following days or weeks after a blood transfusion, usually caused by a patient being alloimmunized by a previous pregnancy or transfusion.

delta check: Comparing the result of an analysis of a specimen with the result of the previous specimen for the same analyte for the same patient for the purpose of quality assurance.

deoxyhemoglobin: Hemoglobin not combined with oxygen, formed when oxyhemoglobin releases its oxygen.

deoxyribonucleic acid (DNA): A double-stranded, helical molecule that is the carrier of genetic information and is found in the chromosomes of the nucleus. It is composed of four types of repeating nucleotide bases: adenine, cytosine, guanine, and thymine. Also see *base pairs.*

desmosomes: Cell structures that bind adjacent cells together.

desquamation: The shedding of epithelial elements, chiefly of the skin, in scales or sheets.

Diamond-Blackfan syndrome: A rare, congenital disorder evident in the first 3 months of life, characterized by severe anemia and a very low reticulocyte count but normal numbers of thrombocytes and leukocytes. It is caused by a deficiency of erythrocyte precursors.

diapedesis: The outward passage of blood cells through intact vessel walls as the cells move between the cells lining the vessels.

differential white blood cell count: An examination and enumeration of the distribution of leukocytes in a stained blood smear. The different kinds of leukocytes are counted and reported as percentages of the total examined.

2,3-diphosphoglycerate (2,3-DPG): A substance produced in the glycolytic pathway of the erythrocyte that diminishes the affinity of hemoglobin for oxygen. Also called *2,3-bisphosphoglycerate (2,3-BPG).*

diploid: Having two sets of chromosomes, as normally found in the cells of humans. In humans the normal diploid number is 46.

direct antiglobulin test (DAT): A screening procedure using antihuman globulin to detect antibodies and complement on the surface of erythrocytes that were bound while the cells were in the body.

disseminated intravascular coagulation (DIC): The consumption of plasma coagulation factors by widespread clotting in the capillaries. Although microclots form throughout the body, the primary symptom is widespread mucocutaneous bleeding.

diurnal: Daily, or happening in the daytime.

Döhle bodies: By Wright stain, gray to light-blue round or oval inclusions found singly or in multiples in the cytoplasm of granulocytes. They are composed of ribosomal RNA.

dominant: Capable of expression when carried by only one of a pair of homologous genes.

Donath-Landsteiner (D-L) autoantibody: The IgG autoantibody that attaches to erythrocytes and binds complement at less than 15° C. See *paroxysmal cold hemoglobinuria.*

Donath-Landsteiner (D-L) syndrome: A rare blood disorder marked by hemolysis minutes or hours after exposure to cold. Also called *paroxysmal cold hemoglobinuria.*

drepanocyte: An abnormal crescent-shaped erythrocyte containing hemoglobin S, characteristic of sickle cell anemia. Also called a *sickle cell.*

drug-induced hemolytic anemia: Hemolytic anemia caused directly by a drug or secondary to an antibody-mediated response stimulated by the drug.

DRVVT: See *Russell viper venom time.*

dry tap: The term used when an inadequate sample of bone marrow fluid is obtained during a bone marrow aspiration.

duodenum: The first or proximal portion of the small intestine.

dyscrasia: A condition related to a disease or pathologic state.

dyserythropoiesis: Abnormal erythropoiesis with bizarre bone marrow morphology and ineffective erythropoiesis.

dysfibrinogenemia: A familial disorder in which fibrinogens functions inadequately, resulting in symptoms ranging from bleeding to thrombosis, typically due to abnormal fibrinogen structure.

dysmegakaryopoiesis: Defective megakaryocyte production and maturation characterized by abnormal morphology.

dysmyelopoiesis: Defective myelocytic cell production and maturation characterized by abnormal morphology.

dysplasia: Abnormality of development; an alteration in size, shape, and organization of adult cells.

dyspnea: Difficult or painful breathing.

dystrophic: A disorder state caused by defective nutrition or metabolism.

ecchymosis: A small hemorrhagic spot, larger than a petechia, in the skin or mucous membrane, forming a rounded or irregular blue or purplish patch. Also known as a *bruise*.

echinocyte: A mature red blood cell that is characterized by having short, equally spaced projections; formed during dehydration of the cell and reversible up to a point. May be an artifact, but echinocytes also are seen in association with uremia, pyruvate kinase deficiency, and in some long-distance runners because of an unknown mechanism.

eclampsia: In pregnant women, the convulsive stage of pre-eclampsia. It is a potentially life-threatening disorder characterized by hypertension, generalized edema, and proteinuria.

edema: The accumulation of excess serous fluid in a fluid compartment or tissue.

effusion: The escape of fluid; for example, from blood vessels as a result of rupture or seepage, usually into a body cavity.

Ehrlichia: A genus of small spherical to ellipsoidal nonmotile gram-negative bacteria that cause ehrlichiosis, a tickborne infection, with symptoms similar to, but more severe than, those of Lyme disease.

electrical impedance: Principle of cell counting that is based on the detection and measurement of changes in electrical resistance produced by cells as they transverse a small aperture in a conducting solution.

electrophoresis: The separation of compounds based on differences in their rates of migration in an applied electric field. This technique is widely used to separate and identify hemoglobin types and serum proteins.

elliptocytes: Thin, oval, mature erythrocytes. See also *ovalocytes*.

elliptocytosis: The presence of elliptical or oval erythrocytes on peripheral blood smears. See also *hereditary elliptocytosis*.

Embden-Meyerhof pathway (EMP): A series of enzymatically catalyzed reactions by which glucose and other sugars are broken down to yield lactic acid (anaerobic glycolysis) or pyruvic acid (aerobic glycolysis). The breakdown releases energy in the form of adenosine triphosphate (ATP). Also called *glycolysis*.

embolism: An abnormal condition in which an embolus (foreign object) travels through the bloodstream and becomes lodged in a blood vessel. The obstructing material is most often a blood clot, but it may be a fat globule, air bubble, piece of tissue, or clump of bacteria.

endocytosis: A process in which cells absorb objects by engulfing them with their cell membranes.

endoplasmic reticulum (ER): An extensive network of membrane-enclosed tubules in the cytoplasm of cells. The structure functions in the synthesis of proteins and lipids and in the transport of these metabolites within the cell.

endothelial cell: A cell that lines the inner surface of all blood vessels. Intact endothelial cells prevent thrombosis because they present a smooth, nonactivating surface and secrete antiplatelet and anticoagulant substances. Injured endothelial cells promote clotting through exposure of tissue factor and secretion of coagulation-promoting factors, such as von Willebrand factor.

enterocyte: An intestinal epithelial cell.

eosinophil: A granulocyte that is characterized by large uniform granules that stain orange to pink with the acid dye eosin. Granules usually do not obscure the nucleus.

eosinophilia: An increase in the number of eosinophils in the blood; associated with allergies, parasitic infections, or hematologic disorders.

epiphyses: The ends of long bones.

epistaxis: Hemorrhage from the nose; a nosebleed.

Epstein-Barr virus (EBV): The herpesvirus that causes infectious mononucleosis.

erythroblastosis: Presence of nucleated red blood cells (i.e. erythroblasts) in the blood. Also called *erythroblastemia*.

erythroblastosis fetalis: An alloimmune disease of the fetus and newborn that is characterized by erythroblastosis, hemolytic anemia, hyperbilirubinemia, and extramedullary erythropoiesis. Also known as *hemolytic disease of the newborn*.

erythrocyte sedimentation rate (ESR): The rate at which erythrocytes settle within anticoagulated blood in a certain time period. Elevated sedimentation rates are not specific for any disorder but indicate the presence of inflammation.

erythrocyte survival test: A measure of erythrocyte life span in the blood by labeling with radioactive chromium.

erythrocyte: One of the formed elements in the peripheral blood, constituting the great majority of the cells in the blood. Also called a *red blood cell*.

erythrocytosis: An abnormal increase in the number of circulating erythrocytes.

erythrodontia: Reddish-brown or yellow discoloration of the dentin of the teeth, especially in patients with congenital erythropoietic porphyria.

erythroleukemia: A malignant blood disorder characterized by a proliferation of erythropoietic elements in bone marrow, erythroblasts with bizarre lobulated nuclei, and abnormal myeloblasts in peripheral blood. Also called *di Guglielmo's disease* or *FAB M6 leukemia*.

erythron: The circulating erythrocytes in the blood and their precursors in the bone marrow, considered as a unified tissue.

erythropoiesis: The process of erythrocyte production.

erythropoietin (EPO): A glycoprotein hormone synthesized mainly in the kidneys and released into the bloodstream in response to anoxia. The hormone acts to stimulate and regulate the production of erythrocytes.

essential thrombocythemia: A myeloproliferative disorder characterized by marked thrombocytosis with dysfunctional platelets. Patients may experience bleeding or thrombosis.

etiology: The cause of a disease.

euchromatin: The part of a chromosome that is active in gene expression. It stains most deeply during mitosis when it is coiled and stains lightly when it is partially or fully uncoiled.

euglobulin: One of a class of globulins characterized by being insoluble in water but soluble in saline solutions. This characteristic is useful in classifying proteins.

exogenous: Originating outside the body or produced from external causes, such as a disease caused by a bacterial or viral agent foreign to the body.

exon: The part of an RNA molecule that contains the code for the final messenger RNA.

extracorpuscular: Describes a condition whose source is extracellular.

extramedullary hematopoiesis: The formation and development of blood cells outside the bone marrow, as in the spleen, liver, and lymph nodes.

extranodal: Located outside a lymph node.

extravasated: The movement of fluid or cells from the blood vessels into surrounding tissue. In the case of malignant cancer metastasis, cancer cells exit the capillaries and enter organs.

extravascular hemolysis: Destruction of an erythrocyte outside of a blood vessel, typically by macrophage ingestion.

extrinsic coagulation pathway: The primary in vivo coagulation pathway. Exposure of tissue factor activates factor VII. Factor VIIa activates factors IX and X, triggering the common pathway of coagulation and formation of fibrin.

exudate: An effusion associated with bacterial or viral infections, malignancy, pulmonary embolism, or systemic lupus erythematosus. An exudate is characterized as a cloudy fluid containing cells and a large concentration of protein.

FAB classification: French-American-British; international classification system for acute leukemias, myeloproliferative disorders, and myelodysplastic syndromes, developed in the 1970s and 1980s. In current use being displaced by the World Health Organization (WHO) classification.

factor assay: A test for specific coagulation factor activity.

factor V Leiden mutation: Substitution of factor V Arg 506 with glutamine slows factor V digestion by activated protein C. The factor V Leiden mutation results in increased thrombin production and is a thrombosis risk factor.

Fanconi anemia: A rare, usually congenital disorder transmitted as an autosomal recessive trait, characterized by aplastic anemia in childhood or early adult life, bone abnormalities, and patchy brown discoloration of the skin.

favism: An acute hemolytic anemia caused by ingestion of fava beans or inhalation of the pollen of the plant. Usually occurring due to a deficiency of RBC glucose-6-phosphate dehydrogenase (G6PD).

FEIBA: Factor eight inhibitor bypassing activity. A therapeutic used to bypass factor VIII inhibitor in hemophiliacs. Required to prevent bleeding episodes when therapeutic factor VIII is neutralized by the inhibitor. Also known as *prothrombin complex concentrate.*

ferritin: The iron-apoferritin complex, a major form in which iron is stored in the body.

ferrocheletase: The last enzyme in the synthetic pathway for heme that inserts iron into protoporphyrin IX

ferrokinetics: The study of iron metabolism, including the movement of iron among the storage, transport, and functional iron compartments.

ferroprotein: A protein in the membrane of intestinal enterocytes and macrophages that is able to transfer ferrous iron from the cell cytoplasm to the exterior of the cell.

fibrin: A fibrillar protein produced by the action of thrombin on fibrinogen in the clotting process. Fibrin is responsible for the semisolid character of a blood clot.

fibrin degradation products (FDP): Fragments produced by the action of fibrin-bound plasmin during fibrinolysis. Produces fibrin fragments X, Y, D, E, and D-D. Also called *fibrin split products (FSP).*

fibrinogen: A plasma protein converted into fibrin by thrombin digestion.

fibrinolysis: The continual process of fibrin digestion by bound plasmin. Fibrinolysis is the normal mechanism for the removal of fibrin clots.

fibroblast: Connective tissue cell that produces the extracellular matrix of tissues including ground substance and fibrous connective tissue (i.e. scar tissue).

flammable: The property of igniting and burning easily and rapidly.

flow cytometer: An instrument in which cells suspended in fluid flow one at a time through a focus of exciting light, which is scattered in patterns characteristic to the cells and their components. A sensor detecting the scattered or emitted light measures the size and molecular characteristics of individual cells.

folded cell: Descriptive term for a mature red blood cell whose membrane is folded over.

free erythrocyte protoporphyrin (FEP): A precursor of heme, lacking incorporated iron and found in low concentrations in normal erythrocytes. Elevated levels indicate iron-deficient states or impaired iron insertion into heme.

fresh frozen plasma (FFP): Plasma that is harvested from whole blood donations and contains all of the plasma coagulation factors. FFP is used to correct a number of acquired bleeding problems.

G proteins: Guanine nucleotide binding proteins, a family of proteins involved in second messenger cascades that serve as a general molecular "switch" function to regulate cell processes.

gammopathy: An abnormal condition characterized by the presence of markedly increased levels of gamma globulin (antibodies) in the blood.

Gaucher disease: A rare disorder of fat metabolism caused by a deficiency of glucocerebrosidase. Characterized by widespread reticulum cell hyperplasia in the liver, spleen, lymph nodes, and bone marrow. Also characterized by Gaucher cells, which are lipid-filled macrophages with abnormal cytoplasm resembling crumpled tissue paper.

Gaussian distribution: Also known as a *normal distribution,* which is a symmetrical, bell-shaped curve. The value at the center is the mean, and the distribution of data is expressed as the standard deviations.

gene: A segment of a DNA molecule that contains all the information required for synthesis of a protein, including both coding and noncoding sequences. Each gene has a specific position (locus) on a particular chromosome.

gene microarray: A collection of microscopic DNA spots attached to a surface, such as plastic or glass, that are used for expression profiling or simultaneous monitoring of gene expression levels.

gene mutation: A permanent change in the genetic material transmissable to daughter cells. The change affect the expression of the gene.

gene rearrangement: Reorganization of the DNA sequences of a gene; this rearrangement is known to occur normally in the immunoglobulin and T-cell genes.

gene therapy: A procedure that involves insertion of "healthy" genes or inactivation of mutated genes to cure or treat a genetic disease or similar illness.

gingival: Pertaining to the mucosal tissue that lies over the jawbone.

Glanzmann's thrombasthenia: A severe mucocutaneous bleeding disorder caused by one of a series of mutations to platelet GP IIb or GP IIIa, the components of the arginine-glycine-aspartate (RGD) peptide sequence receptor complex found on fibrinogen and other plasma coagulation factors. This is a defect of fibrinogen-dependent platelet aggregation.

globin: The protein constituent of hemoglobin.

globulin: A class of proteins that are insoluble in water or highly concentrated salt solutions but are soluble in moderately concentrated salt solutions. All plasma proteins are globulins except albumin and prealbumin.

glossitis: Inflammation or infection of the tongue.

glucose-6-phosphate dehydrogenase (G6PD): The first enzyme of the glucose monophosphate shunt; G6PD catalyzes the oxidation of glucose-6-phosphate to a lactone, reducing $NADP^+$ to NADPH.

glucose-6-phosphate dehydrogenase deficiency: An inherited disorder characterized by red blood cells partially or completely deficient in glucose-6-phosphate dehydrogenase. The disorder is associated with episodes of acute hemolysis under conditions of stress, infections, or in response to certain oxidizing chemicals or drugs.

glycocalyx: The glycoprotein and polysaccharide covering that surrounds many cells, such as platelets.

glycolysis: A series of enzymatically catalyzed reactions by which glucose and other sugars are broken down to yield lactic acid (anaerobic glycolysis) or pyruvic acid (aerobic glycolysis). The breakdown releases energy in the form of adenosine triphosphate (ATP). Also called the *Embden-Meyerhof pathway*.

glycophorin: One of a group of proteins that project through the membrane of erythrocytes.

glycoprotein: A conjugated protein containing one or more covalently linked carbohydrate residues.

Golgi apparatus: A complex cellular organelle consisting mainly of a number of flattened sacs and associated vesicles, involved in the post-translational modification and storage of glycoprotein, lipoproteins, membrane-bound proteins, and lysosomal enzymes.

gout: A disorder in which excessive quantities of uric acid in the blood may be deposited in the joints and other tissues.

graft-versus-host disease (GVHD): A condition, including tissue rejection, that occurs when immunologically competent cells or their precursors are transplanted into and react against an immunocompromised host that is not histocompatible with the donor.

granulocytes: A category of leukocytes characterized by the presence of cytoplasmic granules; includes basophils, eosinophils, and neutrophils.

granuloma: A term applied to any small nodular, delimited aggregation of inflammatory cells or a similar collection of modified macrophages usually surrounded by a rim of lymphocytes, often with multinucleated giant cells.

granulomatous: Pertaining to or resembling granulomas.

guaiac test: A test performed on stool samples to detect hemoglobin as evidence of gastrointestinal bleeding. Based on the principle of the peroxidase activity of hemoglobin in blood reacting with guaiac to yield a blue color. The blood may be in small amounts and degraded such that a red color is not apparent; therefore it is known as a test for occult (hidden) blood.

hairy cells: Lymphocytes seen in the peripheral blood and bone marrow, characterized by delicate gray cytoplasm with projections resembling hair. These cells are seen in hairy cell leukemia.

Ham's test: See *acidified serum test*.

haploid: Having half the number of chromosomes characteristically found in the diploid cells of an organism.

haptoglobin: A plasma protein, the only known function of which is to bind free hemoglobin and salvage it.

Heinz bodies: Small, round, blue to purple inclusions present in erythrocytes stained with a vital stain. Heinz bodies may be found singly or in multiples within the erythrocyte and are composed of precipitated hemoglobin.

helmet cell: A fragmented erythrocyte that has been "scooped out" such that it resembles a helmet. A form of schistocyte or fragmented erythrocyte.

hemacytometer (or hemocytometer): A device used in manual blood cell counts. Consists of a slide with a depression, the base of which is marked in grids and into which a measured volume of a diluted blood sample is placed and covered with a cover glass. The number of cells and formed blood elements in the squares is counted under a microscope and used as a representative sample for calculating the number of cells per unit volume. Also called a *counting chamber*.

hemarthroses: Bleeding in joint spaces, often in cases such as hemophilia where the bleeding does not stop.

hematemesis: Vomiting of bright red blood.

hematocrit (Hct): The proportion of the volume of a blood sample that is erythrocytes (packed red blood cells), often expressed as a percentage of the total blood volume.

hematoidin: A yellow-brown or red pigment, apparently chemically identical with bilirubin but with a different site of origin, formed locally in the tissues from hemoglobin, particularly under conditions of reduced oxygen tension.

hematology: The scientific study of blood cells and blood-forming tissues.

hematoma: A localized collection of extravasated (escaped from vessel into tissue) blood, usually clotted, in an organ space or tissue.

hematopathology: The study of the diseases of the blood.

hematopoiesis: The formation and development of blood cells.

hematopoietic stem cell: An actively dividing cell that is the source of all blood cells and is able to renew itself.

hematuria: Abnormal presence of intact red blood cells in the urine.

heme: The pigmented, iron-containing, nonprotein part of the hemoglobin molecule. There are four heme groups in a hemoglobin molecule, each containing an atom of iron in the center. Heme binds and carries oxygen in erythrocytes.

hemochromatosis: A disease of iron metabolism that is characterized by excess deposition of iron in the tissues. The disease may be inherited or develop as a complication of hemolytic anemia, such as sickle cell anemia.

hemoconcentration: An increase in the number of cells in a given volume of whole blood, resulting from a decrease in plasma volume.

hemodialysis: A procedure in which impurities or wastes are removed from the blood. The patient's blood is shunted from the body through a machine for diffusion and ultra-filtration and then returned to the patient's circulation. It is used in treating patients with renal failure and various toxic conditions.

hemodilution: The increase in blood plasma volume that results in reduced concentration of red blood cells.

hemoglobin (Hb): A complex protein-iron compound of erythrocytes that carries oxygen to the cells from the lungs and carbon dioxide away from the cells to the lungs.

hemoglobin CC crystal: A hexagonal crystal, composed of hemoglobin C, formed within the erythrocyte membrane and seen in hemoglobin CC disease.

hemoglobin electrophoresis: A test method that differentiates and measures the types of hemoglobin in the blood. See *electrophoresis.*

hemoglobin SC crystal: A fingerlike crystal composed of hemoglobin S and hemoglobin C; protrudes from the erythrocyte membrane and is seen in hemoglobin SC disease.

hemoglobinemia: The presence of free hemoglobin in the blood plasma; an indication of significant intravascular hemolysis.

hemoglobinopathy: A group of inherited disorders characterized by mutations of the globin gene. Resulting in such conditions as sickle cell anemia or thalassemia.

hemoglobinuria: The presence of free hemoglobin in the urine; indication of intravascular hemolysis.

hemojuvelin: A protein with a role in iron metabolism that is not yet fully defined but appears to regulate hepcidin production; deficiency of hemojuvelin causes excess iron accumulations (i.e. hemochromatosis) beginning in childhood.

hemolysis: Disruption of the integrity of the erythrocyte membrane, causing release of hemoglobin and ultimately the destruction of the erythrocyte.

hemolytic anemia: A condition that occurs because of an increased destruction of erythrocytes accompanied by accelerated production of erythrocytes by the bone marrow. An anemia develops when erythrocyte survival is reduced and the bone marrow cannot provide an adequate compensatory response.

hemolytic disease of the newborn (HDN): An alloimmune disease of the fetus and newborn due to maternal antibodies against fetal antigens; characterized by hemolytic anemia, hyperbilirubinemia, erythroblastosis, and extramedullary erythropoiesis. Also known as *erythroblastosis fetalis.*

hemolytic uremic syndrome (HUS): A severe microangiopathic anemia that is caused by *Escheria coli* serotype 0:157 H7 and causes renal failure, thrombocytopenia, and severe mucocutaneous hemorrhage.

hemopexin: A plasma glycoprotein; it is produced by hepatocytes, and its function is the binding of heme in plasma in the absence of haptoglobin.

hemophilia: A group of hereditary bleeding disorders characterized by a deficiency of one of the factors necessary for coagulation of the blood. The two most common forms of the disorder are hemophilia A and hemophilia B, deficiencies of factors VIII and IX, respectively.

hemophilia A: A sex-linked recessive systemic bleeding disorder caused by deficiency of coagulation factor VIII. Also called *classic hemophilia.*

hemophilia B: A sex-linked recessive systemic bleeding disorder caused by deficiency of coagulation factor IX. Also called Christmas disease.

hemorrhage: A loss of a large amount of blood from the vessels, either externally or internally.

hemorrhagic disease of the newborn: A condition characterized by systemic neonatal bleeding caused by vitamin K deficiency.

hemosiderin: A pigment that is an intracellular storage form of iron, though apparently not metabolically active.

hemosiderinuria: The presence of hemosiderin in the urine seen in hemolytic anemias.

hemosiderosis: A general increase in tissue iron stores without associated tissue damage.

hemostasis: A series of cellular and humoral systems that balances flow of blood within the circulation and blood loss from injuries by formation of thrombi.

heparin: A naturally occurring mucopolysaccharide anticoagulant called a *glycosaminoglycan.* Heparin is produced by basophils and mast cells and catalyses the activity of antithrombin III. Heparin extracted from porcine mucosa is used as a therapeutic anticoagulant.

heparin-induced thrombocytopenia (HIT): A 40% or greater reduction in platelet count within 24 hours during unfractionated heparin therapy. Caused by a platelet factor 4 heparin antibody, HIT is often associated with platelet activation and a severe, often fatal arterial thrombosis.

hepatitis B virus (HBV): A causative agent viral hepatitis. The virus is transmitted by transfusion of contaminated blood or blood products, by sexual contact with an infected person, or by the use of contaminated needles and instruments. Severe infection may cause prolonged illness, destruction of liver cells, cirrhosis, increased risk for liver cancer, or death.

hepatocyte: A liver cell.

hepatomegaly: Abnormal enlargement of the liver; usually a sign of disease.

hepatosplenomegaly: Abnormal enlargement of the spleen and liver.

hepcidin: A hormone produced by the liver that regulates the movement of iron into the blood from intestinal enterocytes or macrophages.

hereditary elliptocytosis: A hereditary defect of the erythrocyte membrane, characterized by the presence of elliptical or oval erythrocytes on peripheral blood smears.

hereditary pyropoikilocytosis: A hereditary defect of the erythrocyte membrane, resulting in a rare disorder that presents in infancy or early childhood as a severe hemolytic anemia with extreme poikilocytosis resembling that seen in burn patients.

hereditary spherocytosis: A hereditary defect of the erythrocyte membrane, producing hemolytic anemia and characterized by numerous microspherocytes on the peripheral blood smear.

hereditary stomatocytosis: A hereditary defect of the erythrocyte membrane, resulting in a complex spectrum of diseases in which the hemolysis is mild to severe and characterized by the presence of stomatocytes on the peripheral blood smear.

hereditary xerocytosis: A hereditary defect of the erythrocyte membrane, resulting in hemolytic anemia with dehydrated erythrocytes and characterized by stomatocytes, target cells, and macrocytes.

heterochromatin: A form of DNA that is generally tightly packed and is not transcribed.

heterozygous: Having two different alleles at corresponding loci on homologous chromosomes. An individual who is heterozygous for a trait has inherited an allele for that trait from one parent and an alternative allele from the other parent. A person who is heterozygous for a genetic disease caused by a dominant allele will manifest the disorder, whereas if it is caused by a recessive allele, the person is asymptomatic or exhibits reduced symptoms of the disease.

high-molecular-weight kininogen (HMWK, Fitzgerald factor): A member of the kinin inflammatory system, digested and activated by kallikrein to form bradykinin. HMWK is one of the in vitro contact activators, which also include prekallikrein and factor XII.

histiocyte: Any of the many forms of mononuclear phagocytes found in tissues, such as Kupffer cells in the liver. Also called a *macrophage*.

histochemistry: The branch of histology that deals with the identification of chemical components in cells and tissues.

histocompatibility: A determination of the similarity of the antigens of a donor and a recipient of transplanted tissue.

histogram: On automated hematology instruments, a graphic display of a frequency distribution that is usually a representation of cell frequencies versus cell volumes.

histology: The science dealing with the microscopic identification of cells and tissues.

histone: A protein that is found in the nucleus of cells, where it forms a complex with DNA in the chromatin and functions in regulating gene activity.

Hodgkin's lymphoma (disease): A malignant disorder characterized by painless, progressive enlargement of lymphoid tissue, usually first evident in cervical lymph nodes. Characterized by splenomegaly and the presence of Reed-Sternberg cells in lymphoid tissue.

homocysteine: Naturally occurring, sulfur-containing amino acid formed in the metabolism of dietary methionine. Homocysteine's concentration in plasma depends on adequate intake of protein, vitamin B_6, vitamin B_{12}, and folate.

homocystinemia: An excess of homocysteine in the blood; it may be an independent risk factor for arterial thrombosis.

homocystinuria: The presence of homocysteine in the urine.

homozygous: Having two identical alleles at corresponding loci on homologous chromosomes. An individual who is homozygous for a trait has inherited from each parent the same allele for that trait. A person who is homozygous for a genetic disease caused by a pair of recessive alleles manifests the disorder.

Howell-Jolly bodies: On Wright stained blood films, these appear as round, blue to purple erythrocyte inclusions composed of DNA. Usually one per affected erythrocyte.

human immunodeficiency virus (HIV): A virus that causes acquired immunedeficiency syndrome (AIDS). HIV is transmitted through contact with an infected individual's blood, semen, breast milk, cervical secretions, cerebrospinal fluid, or synovial fluid. It infects helper T cells of the immune system, resulting in suppression of the immune system.

human leukocyte antigen (HLA): Any one of four significant histocompatibility antigens governed by genes of the HLA complex found on chromosome 6. The HLA system is used to assess tissue compatibility for organ transplant. See *major histocompatibility complex.*

humoral immunity: A form of immunity that responds to bacteria and other foreign antigens. It is mediated by circulating antibodies that coat the antigens and target them for destruction by neutrophils. Circulating antibodies are produced by plasma cells.

hybridization: In molecular biology, association of a partially or wholly complementary nucleic acid strand to a single strand, used to detect and isolate specific nucleic acid sequences.

hydrophobic: Physical property of a molecule that is repelled by water. These molecules tend to be nonpolar and prefer other nonpolar solvents. These molecules also tend to cluster together in water.

hydrops fetalis: Gross edema of the entire body of a fetus or newborn infant, associated with severe anemia, occurring in hemolytic disease of the newborn.

hyperbilirubinemia: Greater than normal amounts of bilirubin in the blood.

hypercellular bone marrow: A state characterized by an abnormal increase in the number of cells present in the bone marrow.

hypercoagulability: Increased thrombotic risk caused by a number of acquired or congenital factors.

hyperplasia: An increase in the number of cells of a body part that results from an increased rate of cellular division. Used to describe the bone marrow. The associated adjective is *hyperplastic.*

hypersegmented neutrophil: A neutrophil having more segments or lobes than usual. Usually classified as hypersegmented when six or more lobes are present.

hypersplenism: A condition characterized by splenomegaly, resulting in exaggeration of the hemolytic function of the spleen, deficiency of peripheral blood elements, and compensatory hypercellularity of the bone marrow.

hypertension: Persistently high blood pressure.

hypertrichosis: A condition of excessive body hair. It can be generalized, affecting most of the torso and limbs, or an area of skin. It is also known as "Werewolf syndrome."

hyperuricemia: An excess of uric acid or urates in the blood.

hyperuricosuria: An excess of uric acid or urates in the urine.

hypocellular bone marrow: A state characterized by an abnormal decrease in the number of cells present in the bone marrow.

hypochromia: An abnormal decrease in the hemoglobin content of erythrocytes such that they appear pale when stained with Wright stain. These cells are called *hypochromic.*

hypoplasia: Underdevelopment of an organ or tissue, usually resulting from the presence of smaller-than-normal numbers of cells. Used to describe the bone marrow. The associated adjective is *hypoplastic.*

hypoxia: Diminished availability of oxygen to the body tissues.

icteric: Pertaining to or resembling jaundice.

idiopathic: Without a known cause.

idiopathic (immune) thrombocytopenic purpura (ITP): A reduced platelet count caused by a platelet-specific autoantibody that reduces the platelet life span. Patients with ITP suffer mucocutaneous bleeding.

immediate transfusion reaction: Hemolysis that begins within minutes or hours of a blood transfusion and is most commonly caused by an incompatibility of the ABO system.

immersion oil: Specific oil placed in the space between the specimen and the objective of the microscope. It is used to increase the refractive index, thus providing high resolution of details.

immune hemolytic anemia: An anemia resulting in a shortened life span of red blood cells, caused by damage of the cells, resulting from binding of antibodies or complement on the surface of the cells.

immunoassay: A biochemical test that detects a substance in a biological fluid using the reaction of an antibody to its antigen.

immunocompromised: Pertaining to an immune response that has been weakened by a disease or an immunosuppressive agent.

immunocytochemistry: The use of antibodies to bind to specific cellular constituents and stimulate a detectable chemical reaction.

immunoglobulin: A protein with known antibody activity.

Synthesized by lymphocytes and plasma cells; a major component of humoral immune response.

immunophenotyping: Analysis of the antigens expressed by cells using antibodies, as in flow cytometry.

immunosuppression: An abnormal condition of the immune system, characterized by markedly inhibited ability to respond to antigenic stimuli; prevents an immune response.

infantile pyknocytosis: Condition in infants in which red blood cells become crenated with surface projections and appear as a spiculed red blood cell.

infectious mononucleosis: An acute herpesvirus infection caused by the Epstein-Barr virus. It is characterized by fever, sore throat, swollen lymph glands, reactive lymphocytes, splenomegaly, hepatomegaly, abnormal liver function, and bruising.

integrin: Any of a family of cell-adhesion receptors that mediate cell-to-cell and cell-to-extracellular matrix interactions.

interferon: A natural glycoprotein formed by cells exposed to a virus or another foreign particle of nucleic acid. It induces the production of translation inhibitory protein (TIP) in noninfected cells. TIP blocks translation of viral RNA, thus giving other cells protection against both the original and other viruses.

interleukin (IL): A group of compounds that are synthesized by lymphocytes, macrophages, and support tissue cells in the marrow. ILs stimulate or influence maturation of blood cells.

international normalized ratio (INR): A method for standardizing prothrombin time results worldwide. Prothrombin time reagent activity is characterized by manufacturers using the international sensitivity index (ISI), which compares the reagent to the international reference thromboplastin preparation provided by the World Health Organization. Local prothrombin times are adjusted using the following formula: INR = patient prothrombin time divided by mean of the prothrombin time normal range raised to the power of the ISI.

interphase: The stage in the cell cycle in which there is an absence of cell division; between phases.

intracorpuscular: Occurring inside the red blood cell.

intracranial hemorrhage (ICH): A stroke caused by rupture of a blood vessel in the brain. Only 15% of strokes are caused by ICH.

intramedullary hematopoiesis: The formation and development of blood cells within the marrow cavity of a bone.

intravascular hemolysis: Destruction of an erythrocyte within a blood vessel.

intrinsic coagulation pathway: A sequence of reactions leading to fibrin formation, beginning with the in vitro contact activation of factor XII, followed by the sequential activation of factors XI and IX and resulting in the activation of factor X, which in activated form initiates the common pathway of coagulation.

intrinsic factor (IF): A substance that is secreted by the gastric mucosa and is essential for the intestinal absorption of vitamin B_{12}. A deficiency of, or antibody to, intrinsic factor causes pernicious anemia.

intron: A sequence of nucleotides in RNA that does not code for amino acids and is typically spliced out of the final RNA.

iron (Fe): A common metallic element essential for the synthesis of hemoglobin.

iron deficiency anemia: A microcytic, hypochromic anemia caused by inadequate supplies of iron needed to synthesize hemoglobin; it is characterized by pallor, fatigue, and weakness.

iron metabolism: The biochemical modification and utilization of iron molecules within the body.

ISI: International Sensitivity Index. See *international normalized ratio.*

isoantibody: An antibody that is produced by one individual and reacts with antigens of another individual of the same species. Also called an *alloantibody.*

jaundice: A yellow discoloration of the skin, mucous membranes, and sclerae (white outer coat of the eyeballs). Caused by greater-than-normal amounts of bilirubin in the blood.

JCAHO: Acronym for the Joint Commission on Accreditation of Healthcare Organizations.

karyorrhexis: Rupture of the cell nucleus, due to cell degeneration, in which the chromatin disintegrates into formless granules that are extruded from the cell.

karyotype: The number, form, and size of chromosomes. A systematic display of the chromosomes of an individual derived from a photomicrograph taken during metaphase of mitosis.

kinectin: An integral transmembrane protein on the endoplasmic reticulum, binding to kinesin, interacting with Rho GTPase, and anchoring the translation elongation factor-1 complex. It also is critical in regard to intracellular membrane trafficking.

kinin: Any of a group of polypeptides with varying inflammatory activities, such as contraction of visceral smooth muscle, vascular permeability, and vasodilation. Examples of kinins include bradykinin and kallidin.

kininogen: Either of two plasma α-2-globulins that are kinin precursors, called *high-molecular-weight kininogen* and *low-molecular-weight kininogen.*

Köhler illumination: Use of the diaphragms and condenser to adjust resolution, contrast, and depth of field and thereby improve illumination of a microscope slide to obtain a field of evenly distributed brightness across the specimen.

koilonychia: A condition of the fingernails in which they are thin, flattened, and concave. Associated with iron deficiency anemia.

Kupffer cells: Macrophages in the liver that can remove severely damaged erythrocytes.

lactate dehydrogenase (LD): An enzyme that catalyzes the interconversion of lactate and pyruvate. It is widespread in tissues and is particularly abundant in the kidney, skeletal muscle, liver, red blood cells, and myocardium.

lactoferrin: A protein produced by neutrophils and stored in the secondary granules that is able to bind iron.

lassitude: Condition of extreme weariness and exhaustion.

leptocyte: An abnormal mature erythrocyte characterized as a thin, flat cell with hemoglobin at periphery and increased central pallor. A hypochromic red blood cell.

leukemia: A broad term given to a group of malignant diseases characterized by diffuse replacement of bone marrow with proliferating leukocyte precursors and abnormal numbers and forms of immature white blood cells in circulation.

leukemoid reaction: A clinical syndrome in which the white blood cell count is elevated, resembling leukemia. A response to an allergy, inflammatory disease, infection, poison, hemorrhage, burn, or severe physical stress.

leukocyte: A white blood cell, one of the formed elements of the blood. The five types of leukocytes are lymphocytes, monocytes, neutrophils, basophils, and eosinophils. Leukocytes function as phagocytes of bacteria, fungi, and viruses; detoxifiers of toxic proteins that may result from allergic reactions and cellular injury; and immune system cells.

leukocytosis: An abnormal increase in the number of circulating leukocytes.

leukoerythroblastic: Characterized by the presence of immature erythrocytes and neutrophils.

leukopenia: An abnormal decrease in the number of circulating leukocytes.

leukoplakia: A condition of the mouth in which white, leathery patches are seen on the tongue and cheek. The spots are smooth and irregular and may become malignant.

leukopoiesis: The process by which leukocytes form and develop.

Levy Jennings chart: A chart used in the clinical laboratory for plotting the results from control specimens. This chart indicates the mean and the first, second, and third standard deviation ranges on both sides of the mean. Deviation from this distribution indicates the occurrence of an analytic systematic error.

lichenoid: Something resembling lichen, a papular skin disease.

ligand: A molecule, ion, or group bound to the central atom of a chemical compound, such as the oxygen molecule in hemoglobin, which is bound to the central iron atom. Or a molecule that binds to another molecule, used especially to refer to a small molecule that specifically binds to a larger molecule.

littoral cells: Macrophages in the spleen that remove aged or damaged erythrocytes.

low-molecular-weight heparin (LMWH): Standard unfractionated heparin that is digested to provide a product with an average MW of 5000-8000. LMWH is used in most prophylaxis of thrombosis, and requires monitoring only in conditions of inadequate metabolism, such as obesity, renal disease, and pregnancy. LMWH is monitored using the chromogenic anti-Xa heparin assay.

lupus anticoagulant: An autoantibody to phospholipid-binding proteins, such as beta2-glycoprotein I, annexin, and prothrombin. Often present in collagen disorders, such as systemic lupus erythematosus, Sjögren syndrome, and rheumatoid arthritis; may be primary. Lupus anticoagulant is associated with venous and arterial thrombosis and spontaneous abortion.

lymphadenitis: Inflammation of one or more lymph nodes, usually the result of systemic neoplastic disease, bacterial infection, or other inflammatory condition.

lymphadenopathy: Any disorder characterized by a localized or generalized enlargement of the lymph nodes or lymph vessels.

lymphoblast: An immature cell found in the bone marrow and not normally in the peripheral blood; the most primitive, morphologically recognizable precursor in the lymphocytic series, which develops into the prolymphocyte.

lymphocyte: Any of the mononuclear, nonphagocytic leukocytes, found in the blood, lymph, and lymphoid tissues, that are the body's immunologically competent cells and their precursors. They are divided into two classes, B and T lymphocytes, responsible for humoral and cellular immunity, respectively.

lymphocytopenia: Reduction in the number of lymphocytes in the blood. Also called *lymphopenia*.

lymphocytosis: Excess of normal lymphocytes in the blood.

lymphoid: Resembling or pertaining to lymph or tissue and cells of the lymphoid system.

lymphokines: Biologic response mediators released by both B and T lymphocytes.

lymphoma: A type of neoplasm of lymphoid tissue that originates in the reticuloendothelial and lymphatic systems. It is usually malignant but in rare cases may be benign.

lymphopoiesis: The formation of lymphocytes.

lymphoproliferative: Pertaining to the proliferation of lymphoid cells.

lyonization: Process by which cells with multiple X chromosomes inactivate one chromosome during mammalian embryogenesis. X-inactivation leads to clumped chromatin termed *Barr bodies*. This formation of Barr bodies is called *lyonization*.

lysosomes: Membrane-bound sacs of varying size found randomly in the cytoplasm of cells and containing hydrolytic enzymes that function in the intracellular digestive system.

macrocyte: An abnormally large mature erythrocyte. The associated adjective is *macrocytic*.

macroglobulin: A plasma globulin with high molecular weight, such as alpha-2-macroglobulin or the IgM. The latter constitutes the abnormal M component of the plasma proteins in Waldenström macroglobulinemia.

macroglobulinemia: A condition characterized by increased macroglobulins in the blood.

macrophage: Any of the many forms of mononuclear phagocytes found in tissues, such as Kupffer cells in the liver. Also called a *histiocyte*.

major histocompatibility complex (MHC): A region on chromosome 6 containing genes that code for proteins that enable the immune system to differentiate tissue or proteins between "self" and "nonself" and govern the human leukocyte antigens. Class I antigens occur on the surface of all nucleated cells and platelets and are important in tissue transplantation. Also called *HLA complex*. If donor and recipient HLA antigens do not match, the nonself antigens are recognized and destroyed by killer T cells.

malaise: A vague feeling of bodily discomfort and fatigue.

malaria: An infectious disease caused by one or more of at least four species of the protozoan genus *Plasmodium*. This disease is transmitted from human to human by a bite from an infected *Anopheles* mosquito.

malignant: Describes a cancerous disease that threatens life through its ability to metastasize.

mast cell: A constituent of connective tissue having large basophilic granules that contain heparin, serotonin, bradykinin, and histamine. These substances are released from the mast cell in response to IgE stimulation.

May-Hegglin anomaly: A rare autosomal dominant inherited blood cell disorder characterized by thrombocytopenia and granulocytes containing cytoplasmic inclusions similar to Döhle bodies.

mean corpuscular hemoglobin (MCH): The average erythrocyte weight in picograms, computed from the erythrocyte count and hemoglobin.

mean corpuscular hemoglobin concentration (MCHC): The average amount of hemoglobin per volume of the erythrocyte, expressed in percent or volume per volume, computed from the hemoglobin and hematocrit. Relates to Wright-stained erythrocyte color intensity.

mean corpuscular volume (MCV): The average erythrocyte volume in femtoliters, computed from the erythrocyte count and hematocrit or directly measured by an impedance or light-activated particle counter. Relates to Wright-stained erythrocyte diameter.

mean: A value that is derived by dividing the total of a set of values by the number of items in the set; the arithmetic average.

medulla: The innermost or central portion of an organ, as distinguished from the outermost cortex.

megakaryoblast: An immature cell found in the bone marrow and not normally in the peripheral blood. It is the earliest, visually identifiable megakaryocyte precursor in the bone marrow.

megakaryocyte: A 30 to 50-micrometer bone marrow cell derived from the megakaryoblast and having a multilobed nucleus. Cytoplasm is composed of platelets, which are released to the peripheral blood through the extension of proplatelet processes.

megakaryopoiesis: The production of megakaryocytes. Also called *megakaryocytopoiesis*.

megaloblast: An abnormally large, nucleated, immature precursor in the erythrocytic series; an abnormal counterpart to the normoblast. In addition to the abnormal size, the nucleus appears more immature than the cytoplasm. Megaloblasts give rise to macrocytic red blood cells.

menorrhagia: Abnormally heavy or prolonged menstrual periods.

mesenteric: Of the mesentery, the membrane that connects part of the small intestine to the posterior wall of the abdomen.

metamyelocyte: A stage in the development of the granulocyte series of leukocytes, between the myelocyte stage and the band stage. Characterized by a mature, granulated cytoplasm and bean-shaped nucleus with slight indentation.

metaphase: The stage in mitosis in which a cell's chromosomes align in the middle of the cell before being divided into two daughter cells.

metaplasia: Conversion of normal tissue cells into another, less differentiated cell type in response to chronic stress or injury.

metastasis: The process by which tumor cells spread to distant parts of the body.

methemoglobin: An abnormal form of hemoglobin in which the iron component has become oxidized from the ferrous to the ferric state. Methemoglobin cannot carry oxygen.

microangiopathic hemolytic anemia (MAHA): A condition in which narrowing or obstruction of small blood vessels by fibrin results in distortion and fragmentation of erythrocytes, hemolysis, and anemia. Causes appearance of schistocytes in the Wright-stained blood film.

microangiopathy: Disease of the small blood vessels (arterioles, venules, and capillaries).

microcyte: An abnormally small erythrocyte.

microfilament: A small solid intracellular structure that gives support to the cytoskeleton and assists with cell motility.

microlocator slide: A glass slide with etched numbers and letters along the x and y axis, which is used to locate previously observed cells.

micrometer reticule: An ocular disc with an arbitrary scale etched on the surface; it is calibrated in conjunction with the known dimensions of the red blood cell area of a hemacytometer to calculate exact measurement in millimeters or microns.

microtubules: Tubulin-based channels that maintain cellular shape, contribute to motility, and comprise mitotic spindle fibers and centrioles.

mitochondria: Round or oval structures found randomly in the cytoplasm of a cell. They serve as the cell's aerobic energy system by producing adenosine triphosphate (ATP).

mitosis: The ordinary process of cell division resulting in the formation of two daughter cells, by which the body replaces dead somatic cells. The daughter cells have identical diploid complements of chromosomes (46).

monoblast: An immature cell found in the bone marrow and not normally in the peripheral blood; the most primitive, morphologically identifiable precursor in the monocytic series, which develops into the promonocyte.

monoclonal: Pertaining to or designating a group of identical cells or organisms derived from a single cell or organism. Also used to describe products from a clone of cells, such as monoclonal antibodies.

monocyte: A mononuclear phagocytic leukocyte having a round to horseshoe-shaped nucleus with abundant gray-blue cytoplasm filled with fine reddish granules. See *reticuloendothelial system*.

monocytopenia: An abnormally low level of monocytes in the peripheral blood.

monocytosis: An increased number of monocytes in the peripheral blood.

mononuclear: Pertaining to one nucleus, such as a monocyte or lymphocyte; distinct from the nucleus of neutrophils that appears to be multiple and hence is called *polymorphonuclear*.

Mott cell: Plasma cells containing cytoplasmic inclusions called *Russell bodies* that appear like vacuoles and containing aggregates of immunoglobulins.

mucocutaneous: Referring to clinical signs affecting both skin and mucous membranes.

multiple myeloma: A malignant neoplasm of plasma cells in which the plasma cells proliferate and invade the bone marrow, causing destruction of the bone and resulting in bone fractures and bone pain and increased production of a monoclonal antibody.

myelo: A prefix relating to bone marrow or spinal cord.

myeloblast: An immature cell found in the bone marrow and not normally in the peripheral blood; the most primitive, morphologically identifiable precursor in the granulocytic series, which develops into the promyelocyte.

myelocyte: A precursor in the granulocytic series, a cell intermediate in development between a promyelocyte and a metamyelocyte; in this stage, differentiation of cytoplasmic granules has begun, so the myelocytes are specifically basophilic, eosinophilic, or neutrophilic.

myelodysplastic syndromes (MDS): A group of acquired clonal hematologic disorders characterized by progressive cytopenias in the peripheral blood, reflecting defects in erythroid, myeloid, and/or megakaryocytic maturation.

myelofibrosis: The replacement of bone marrow with fibrous connective tissue.

myeloid: A general term used for a group of cells including the granulocytes, monocytes, and megakaryocytes (platelets), specifically excluding lymphocytes but may or may not include the erythrocytes, depending on context. May be used synonymously with *nonlymphoid*.

myeloid:erythroid (M:E) ratio: The proportion of myeloid (nonerythroid and nonlymphoid) cells to nucleated erythroid precursors. The M:E ratio is used to evaluate hematologic cell production in a bone marrow sample.

myeloperoxidase: An enzyme that occurs in primary granules of promyelocytes, myelocytes, and neutrophils and exhibits bactericidal, fungicidal, and viricidal properties.

myeloproliferative disorders: A group of conditions characterized by proliferation of myeloid tissue and elevations of one or more myeloid cell types in the peripheral blood; includes myelofibrosis, myeloid metaplasia, essential thrombocythemia, polycythemia vera, and chronic myelocytic leukemia.

myoglobin: The muscle counterpart of hemoglobin. Combines with oxygen released by erythrocytes, stores it, and transports it to the mitochondria of muscle cells, where it generates energy for muscles.

NCCLS: Acronym for the National Committee for Clinical Laboratory Standards. Now the Clinical Laboratory Standards Institute (CLSI).

necrobiotic: Pertaining to or affected by necrosis (cell or tissue death).

necrosis: Localized tissue death that occurs in groups of cells in response to disease or injury.

neonatal: The period of time covering the first 28 days after birth.

neoplasm: Any abnormal growth of new tissue; can be malignant or benign.

neuropathy: A nerve disorder.

neutropenia: An abnormal decrease in the number of neutrophils in the blood.

neutrophil: A mature leukocyte that is polymorphonuclear with cytoplasmic fine granules and is essential for phagocytosis of bacteria and cellular debris.

neutrophilia: An elevated number of neutrophils in the blood.

non-Hodgkin's lymphoma (NHL): One of the two main kinds of lymphomas, a group of malignant tumors involving lymphoid tissue. Diagnosis and type is dependent on results of lymph node biopsy evaluation.

normochromic: Pertaining to a stained erythrocyte having normal color due to having a normal hemoglobin content.

normocyte: A normal, mature red blood cell of average volume.

nuclear-to-cytoplasmic (N:C) ratio: The size of the nucleus in comparison to the amount of cytoplasm present.

nucleated red blood cell (NRBC): A red blood cell that possesses a nucleus; an immature red blood cell.

nucleolus: Located in the nucleus and composed of RNA, it is usually round or irregular in shape and is the site for synthesis and processing of various ribosomal RNA. The plural term is *nucleoli*.

nucleosides: Glycosides of purine and pyrimidine bases. In RNA and DNA, the glycosides incorporate pentoses, ribose and deoxyribose, respectively.

nucleotides: Phosphoric esters of nucleosides. Allow for the formation of phosphodiester bridges between nucleotides to form RNA and DNA.

nucleus: A cellular organelle composed of DNA and RNA. Site of genetic replication.

numeric aperture: The number designating the quality of the microscope objective, stamped on the barrel. The higher the number, the greater the resolution.

objective: The system of microscope lenses closest to the object being examined.

obturator: An object that obstructs a hole or opening.

ocular: The microscope lens, usually 10×, nearest the eye.

oncogene: A gene capable, under certain conditions, of causing the initial and continuing conversion of normal cells into cancer cells. A mutated proto-oncogene.

opsonization: The process by which an antibody or complement attaches itself to foreign material (bacteria), therefore triggering or enhancing phagocytosis by leukocytes.

optical scatter: A basic principle of cell counting and differentiation that uses both laser and nonlaser light. The angle of light scatter correlates to varying cell features, such as size and cellular complexity.

oral anticoagulant therapy (OAT): Treatment involving the use of Coumadin (also called *warfarin*), the only oral anticoagulant, which functions as a vitamin K antagonist to prevent gamma-carboxylation of glutamic acid for coagulation factors II (prothrombin), VII, IX, and X.

OSHA: Acronym for the Occupational Safety and Health Administration.

osmotic fragility test: An assay in which measured volumes of whole blood are pipetted to a series of saline solutions. The series begins with normal saline and decreases in concentration to pure water. The osmotic fragility test is used to detect spherocytosis, in which spherocytes rupture under osmotic stress in saline concentrations near normal saline. It may also detect target cells that, owing to their reduced hemoglobin content, are able to withstand osmotic stress and rupture only at very dilute saline concentrations.

osteoblast: A bone-forming cell.

osteoclast: A large multinuclear cell associated with the absorption and removal of bone.

osteolytic: Promoting osteolysis (dissolution and degeneration of bone).

oval macrocyte: An abnormally large mature red blood cell that is oval or egg shaped. Characteristic of megaloblastic anemia.

ovalocyte: An oblong or oval-shaped mature red blood cell. Thin oval cells are called *elliptocytes*.

oxygen affinity: The ability of hemoglobin to bind oxygen molecules.

oxygen dissociation curve: A graphic expression of the affinity between oxygen and hemoglobin or the amount of oxygen chemically bound at equilibrium to the hemoglobin in blood as a function of oxygen pressure.

oxyhemoglobin: Hemoglobin that contains bound oxygen.

packed cell volume (PCV): The proportion of a given volume of blood that is composed of red blood cells. Determined when the anticoagulated cells are pressed together by the force of being centrifuged. Also called *spun hematocrit*.

palisade: A wall of cells or objects that forms a dividing structure.

pallor: An unnatural paleness or absence of color in the skin.

pancytopenia: A marked reduction in the number of erythrocytes, leukocytes, and thrombocytes.

Pappenheimer bodies: See *siderotic granules*.

paracentric: Located near the center.

parachromatin: Pale-staining portions of the nucleus.

paracortex: Located near the cortex.

parenteral: Pertaining to administration of drugs or other compounds by means other than oral administration; includes intramuscular and intravenous administrations.

paroxysmal cold hemoglobinuria (PCH): An extremely rare form of a cold-reactive antibody autoimmune hemolytic anemia in which the Donath-Landsteiner autoantibody binds to the red blood cells, fixing complements to the surface following exposure to cold. It is characterized by acute episodes of massive hemolysis that occur when the cells warm.

paroxysmal nocturnal hemoglobinuria (PNH): An acquired blood cell membrane defect that causes an increased susceptibility of blood cells to complement, resulting in a hemolytic anemia. It is characterized by intravascular hemolysis and hemoglobinuria, and it occurs in irregular episodes especially at night.

pathogenesis: The development of disease; more specifically, the cellular events and reactions and other pathologic mechanisms occurring in the development of disease.

pathognomonic: Describes a characteristic that is diagnostic of a given disease.

Pelger-Huët anomaly: An inherited condition characterized by granulocytes that have dumbbell-shaped or peanut-shaped nuclei. Normal nuclear segmentation does not occur; however, there is no pathologic consequence.

percutaneous coronary intervention: Angiograms, angioplasty, and stent placement within coronary arteries, performed using cardiac catheterization.

pericentric: Around the center.

peripheral artery occlusion (PAO): Thrombus formation in a noncardiovascular and noncerebrovascular artery; for example, a carotid or brachial artery.

pernicious anemia: A progressive autoimmune disorder that results in megaloblastic macrocytic anemia due to a lack of, or antibodies to, parietal cells or intrinsic factor essential for the absorption of vitamin B_{12}.

pernicious: Very harmful; working in a hidden and harmful way.

personal protective equipment (PPE): Clothing that is used to prevent blood or other potentially infected material from passing through to contacting an employee's work or street clothes, eyes, mouth, or mucous membranes.

petechiae: Pinpoint purple or red spots appearing on the skin as a result of tiny hemorrhages within the dermal or submucosal layers.

phagocyte: A cell that is able to surround, engulf, and digest microorganisms and cellular debris.

phagocytosis: The ingestion of large particles or live microorganisms into a cell.

phagosome: A membrane-bound cytoplasmic vesicle in a phagocyte, containing the phagocytized material.

Philadelphia chromosome: The reciprocal translocation of the long arm of chromosome 22 to chromosome 9, seen in chronic myelocytic leukemia and occasionally in acute lymphoblastic leukemias. Results in fusion of BCR-ABL genes and abnormal tyrosine kinase production.

phlebotomy: Use of a hypodermic needle to puncture a vein and collect blood.

pica: An extended abnormal appetite for non-food items (i.e. paper, dirt, grass, ice, etc.). Most frequently seen in pregnant women or iron deficient individuals.

pinocytosis: Cellular ingestion of small particles or liquids.

pitting: The removal by the spleen of material from within the erythrocytes without damage to the erythrocyte.

PIVKA: Proteins induced by vitamin K absence.

plasma cell: A B-type lymphoid cell found in the bone marrow and sometimes in the peripheral blood. It contains an eccentric nucleus with deeply staining chromatin and dark blue cytoplasm. It is able to produce antibodies.

plasma: The fluid portion of circulating anti-coagulated blood in which the formed elements (leukocytes, erythrocytes, and platelets) are suspended.

plasmin: The active form of plasminogen. Plasmin binds fibrin and, when activated by tissue plasminogen activator, digests fibrin to form fibrin degradation products in the fibrinolytic process.

plasmin activator inhibitor 1 (PAI-1, PAI): An inhibitor of tissue plasminogen activator, it controls fibrinolysis and is secreted by endothelial cells.

plasminogen activator: A substance that cleaves plasminogen and converts it into plasmin; includes urokinase, which is secreted by renal endothelia, and tissue plasminogen activator, which is secreted by all endothelia.

plasminogen: The inactive plasmin precursor.

platelet: The smallest of the formed elements in blood; a disk-shaped, non-nucleated cell formed in the red bone marrow by fragmentation of megakaryocytes. Platelets play an active role in blood coagulation. Also called a *thrombocyte*.

platelet adhesion: Platelet attachment to subendothelial collagen; part of a sequential mechanism leading to the initiation and formation of a thrombus or hemostatic plug. Platelet adhesion requires von Willebrand factor.

platelet aggregation: Platelet-to-platelet binding, part of a sequential mechanism leading to the initiation and formation of a thrombus or hemostatic plug.

platelet factor 4 (PF4): A compound that is released from alpha granules of platelets and inhibits heparin.

platelet-poor plasma (PPP): Plasma centrifuged to achieve a documented platelet count less than $10 \times 10^9/L$. PPP is required for all coagulation testing except routine prothrombin time, partial thromboplastin time, and thrombin time. Non-PPP must be tested immediately subsequent to centrifugation. All special coagulation testing requires PPP, and only PPP may be refrigerated or frozen. A routine spot-check of PPP for acceptable platelet count is required.

platelet production: The creation of platelets through the breaking off of portions of a megakaryocyte cytoplasm in the bone marrow. Controlled by thrombopoeisis.

platelet-rich plasma (PRP): A therapeutic plasma preparation with a platelet count of $200\text{-}300 \times 10^9/L$, used to treat thrombocytopenia. PRP is used for in vitro platelet aggregation testing.

platelet satellitosis: Antibody-mediated in vitro platelet-PMN adhesion. Occurs primarily in EDTA samples and causes pseudothrombocytopenia.

pleomorphic: Occurring in various distinct forms.

plethoric: Containing excessive blood.

pluripotential stem cell: A stem cell that has the potential to develop into several types of mature cells, including lymphocytes, monocytes, granulocytes, megakaryocytes, and erythrocytes. See *hematopoietic stem cell*.

pneumatic tube system: A system of transporting blood specimens or other small materials in hospitals by forced air through tubes.

poikilocytosis: An abnormal degree of variation in the shape of erythrocytes in the blood.

point of care (POC) testing: Clinical tests performed outside of the clinical laboratory at or near the patient and usually performed by nonlaboratory personnel.

polychromatic: A staining quality in which both acid and basic stains are incorporated. Usually used to denote a mixture of pink and blue in Wright's-stained specimens. Also called *polychromatophilic*.

polychromatic normoblast: A precursor in the erythrocytic series, a cell intermediate in development between a basophilic normoblast and an orthochromic normoblast; in this stage, differentiation is based on the decreasing cell size and the gray-blue cytoplasm as hemoglobin first becomes visible. Also called a *polychromatophilic normoblast.*

polychromatophilia: A condition in which the erythrocytes, on staining, show various shades of blue combined with tinges of pink. Due to residual ribosomal RNA. Also called *polychromasia.*

polyclonal: Pertaining to or designating a group of cells or organisms derived from several cells. Each cell is identical to its parent cells (i.e., a clone), but since all cells of the group did not derive from the same cell, the group of cells is mixed.

polycythemia: An abnormal increase in the number of erythrocytes in the blood. Also called *erythrocytosis.*

polycythemia vera (PV): A myeloproliferative disorder in which an acquired mutation leads to a marked increase in the red blood cell count, packed cell volume, hemoglobin, leukocytes, platelets, and total blood volume.

polymerase chain reaction (PCR): A process whereby a strand of DNA can be copied millions of times within a few hours.

polymorphism: Natural differences in the DNA sequence of individuals.

polymorphonuclear leukocyte (PMN): A leukocyte with a multilobed nucleus whose lobules are connected by a filament, such as a segmented neutrophil. Because it appears to have multiple nuclei (i.e., a polymorph), it is distinguished from the mononuclear cells, such as monocytes and lymphocytes. Can apply to any of the granulocytes but is usually reserved for neutrophils.

polyploid: An individual, organism, strain, or cell that has more than twice the haploid number of chromosomes characteristic of the species. The multiple of the haploid is denoted by the appropriate prefix, as in triploid (3X), tetraploid (4X), pentaploid (5X), and so on.

porphyria: A disorder characterized by impaired synthesis of heme with accumulation of porphyrin and its precursors. May be acquired, as with lead poisoning, or inherited, although the term usually refers to the inherited form.

porphyrins: Any of a group of iron- or magnesium-free pyrrole derivatives; the combination with iron forms heme. Heme combines with specific proteins to form hemoproteins, such as hemoglobin.

post-transfusion purpura: Antibody-induced thrombocytopenia in patients who have received multiple transfusions of red cells or platelet concentrate. Antibodies to donor platelets cross-react with patient platelets to cause potentially life-threatening thrombocytopenia.

precision: The extent to which replicate analyses of a sample agree with each other.

precursor: Something that comes before another thing. Used to refer to the young forms of cells that are morphologically identifiable as belonging to a given cell line; for example, pronormoblasts are precursors to reticulocytes in the red blood cell developmental series. Also used to refer to the unactivated form of coagulation factors; for example, prothrombin is a precursor to thrombin.

preeclampsia: A precursor to eclampsia; it is a pathologic condition of late pregnancy characterized by edema, proteinuria, and hypertension.

prekallikrein (PK, Fletcher factor): A member of the kinin inflammatory system, which forms active kallikrein upon digestion by kininogen. Prekallikrein participates in in vitro coagulation contact activation. Prekallikrein deficiency prolongs the PTT but has no clinical consequence.

primary hemostasis: The first stage in coagulation in which the blood vessels contract to seal the wound and platelets fill the open space by forming a platelet plug.

primary standard: A reference material that is of fixed and known composition and capable of being prepared in essentially pure form.

primer: A short piece of DNA or RNA complementary to a given DNA sequence. It acts as a point from which replication can proceed, as in a polymerase chain reaction.

procoagulant: A natural substance necessary for coagulation of blood. Also called *coagulation factors* or *clotting factors.* During the thrombosis process, the procoagulants become activated and produce a localized thrombus.

progenitor: A parent or ancestor. Used specifically to refer to immature bone marrow cells that cannot be morphologically identified as belonging to a particular cell line.

prolymphocyte: A developmental form in the lymphocytic series, intermediate between the lymphoblast and the lymphocyte.

promegakaryocyte: The bone marrow cell stage intermediate between the megakaryoblast and the megakaryocyte.

promonocyte: A precursor in the monocytic series, a cell intermediate in the development between the monoblast and the monocyte.

promyelocyte: A precursor in the granulocytic series, intermediate in development between a myeloblast and a myelocyte, containing primary granules.

pronormoblast: An immature cell found in the bone marrow and not normally in the peripheral blood; the most primitive, morphologically identifiable precursor in the erythrocytic series, which develops into the basophilic normoblast.

prostaglandins: A family of unsaturated 20-carbon fatty acids that are cleaved from a phospholipids and serve as cellular activators and inhibitors. Thromboxane A_2 is a platelet activator, and prostacyclin is an endothelial cell-produced platelet inhibitor.

protein C: A coagulation control protein; the primary control protein of the activated protein C pathway. Activated by thrombin-thrombomodulin, it binds to protein S and controls the coagulation pathway by digesting activated factor V and factor VIII.

protein S: A protein C cofactor necessary for activated protein C digestion of factor V and factor VIII in the protein C coagulation control pathway.

proteolytic: Pertaining to any substance that digests protein by splitting primary peptide bonds.

prothrombin: The plasma precursor of the coagulation factor thrombin. It is converted to thrombin by activated factor X complexed to factor V. Also known as *factor II*.

prothrombin complex concentrate: A therapeutic used to bypass factor VIII inhibitor in hemophiliacs. Required to prevent bleeding episodes when therapeutic factor VIII is neutralized by the inhibitor. Also known as *factor eight inhibitor bypassing activity* or *FEIBA*.

prothrombin time (PT): A test to measure the activity of coagulation factors I, II, V, VII, and X, which participate in the extrinsic and common pathways of coagulation. Widely used to monitor Coumadin therapy.

proto-oncogene: A normal gene controlling cell cycle and cell division.

Prussian blue (PB) reaction: Changing color from blue to white in response to a voltage electrochromically. This is caused by partial oxidation of the Fe(II) to Fe(III), eliminating the intervalence charge transfer that causes PB's blue color.

pseudoleukocytosis: A falsely increased white blood cell count caused by strenuous physical activity or other physical stress. Caused by mobilization of marginal leukocyte pool.

pseudo–Pelger-Huët cells: Hyposegmented, hypogranular neutrophils that resemble Pelger-Huët cells. Seen in leukemia, myeloproliferative disorders, and myelodysplastic syndromes.

pseudothrombocytopenia: A falsely decreased platelet count often related to platelet satellitosis.

pulmonary embolism (PE): An incident in which a fragment of clot from deep venous thrombosis is dislodged and travels through the right side of the heart to the pulmonary circulation, lodging in an artery and causing infarction of the lung. Approximately one third of PEs are fatal within 1 hour.

purpura: A purple skin discoloration of 1 cm or greater diameter seen in mucocutaneous bleeding. Usually caused by thrombocytopenia or vascular disorders, such as scurvy.

pyknosis: Degeneration of a cell in which the nucleus shrinks in size and the chromatin condenses to a solid, structureless mass or masses.

pyridoxine: Part of the vitamin B_6 complex; a cofactor in the conversion of serine to glycine in the folic acid cycle.

pyropoikilocytosis: See *hereditary pyropoikilocytosis*.

pyruvate kinase (PK): An enzyme essential for anaerobic glycolysis in red blood cells.

pyruvate kinase deficiency: A hemolytic anemia caused by a deficiency of pyruvate kinase that leads to reduced red cell life span. It is the most common enzyme deficiency of the Embden-Meyerhof pathway.

Q-banding: A fluorescent chromosome stain useful in identifying DNA polymorphisms and the Y chromosome.

qualitative analysis: The study of a sample of material to determine what chemical substances are present. The amount of the substance is typically not of concern.

quality control: A term used to refer to the control of the testing process to ensure that the test results meet quality requirements. Involves the process of monitoring the characteristics of the testing system.

quantitative analysis: The determination of the amount or concentration of constituents in a sample.

radiotherapy: The treatment of neoplastic disease by using x-rays or gamma rays to deter the proliferation of malignant cells by decreasing the rate of mitosis or impairing DNA synthesis.

Raynaud phenomenon: A condition marked by symmetrical cyanosis of the extremities, with persistent, uneven blue or red discoloration of the skin of the digits, wrists, and ankles. Also called *acrocyanosis*.

R-banding: A chromosome stain method that uses a heated phosphate buffer and Giemsa staining that yields a banding pattern opposite that produced in G-banding.

RBC indices: Numerical representations of average erythrocyte volume (mean corpuscular volume), hemoglobin weight (mean corpuscular hemoglobin), relative hemoglobin concentration (mean corpuscular hemoglobin concentration), and variation in erythrocyte volume *(red cell distribution width)*. Indices are computed from the red cell count, hemoglobin and hematocrit values, or are directly measured by electronic cell counters.

reactive lymphocytes (atypical, transformed, variant): Lymphocytes that have been stimulated by antigens. These cells can undergo various nuclear and cytoplasmic morphologic changes.

recessive: Pertaining to or describing a gene, the effect of which is masked or hidden if there is a dominant gene at the same locus. If both genes are recessive and produce the same trait, the trait is expressed in the individual.

red cell distribution width (RDW): The coefficient of variation of erythrocyte volume. An increased RDW indicates anisocytosis.

red marrow: That portion of the bone marrow that is in use for hematopoiesis.

Reed-Sternberg cell: A giant cell, typically binucleate with the two halves of the cell appearing as mirror images of each other; the nuclei are enclosed in abundant cytoplasm and contain prominent nucleoli. The presence of Reed-Sternberg cells is the definitive histologic characteristic of Hodgkin's disease.

reference interval: The range of test results for a given analyte that is seen in a healthy population of individuals. Each laboratory must define the range for the instrument that is being used and for the population that is being served.

refractive index: The speed at which light travels in air, divided by the speed at which light travels through a substance, such as immersion oil.

relative reticulocyte count: Reticulocyte count reported as a percentage of total RBC count.

reliability: Refers to the extent to which a method is able to maintain both accuracy and precision over a period of time.

remission: The partial or complete disappearance of the clinical characteristics of a chronic or malignant disease.

replication: The duplication of the polynucleotide strands of DNA or the synthesis of DNA. Also refers to the process of cell division.

reptilase: A thrombinlike enzyme, isolated from the venom of *Bothrops atrox*, that catalyzes the conversion of fibrinogen to fibrin in a manner similar to thrombin.

resheathing device: A device that protects the hand or allows a safe one-handed recapping of the needle.

resolution: In microscopy, the smallest distance at which two adjacent objects can be distinguished as separate. It is an important measure of image quality and relates to the smallest item that can be seen with a given set of microscopic lenses.

restriction endonuclease: An enzyme that cleaves (cuts) DNA at a specific nucleotide sequence.

reticulocyte: An immature erythrocyte that is lacking a nucleus but is characterized by a meshlike pattern of threads and particles at the former site of the endoplasmic reticulum, visible with supravital stain.

reticulocyte production index (RPI): A calculation performed to correct for the presence of shift reticulocytes that falsely elevate the relative reticulocyte count.

reticulocytosis: An increase in the number of reticulocytes in the peripheral blood.

reticuloendothelial system (RES): A functional system of the body involved primarily in defense against infection and in disposal of the products of the breakdown of cells. It is composed of the macrophages dispersed throughout the body, including Kupffer cells of the liver and the reticulum cells of the lungs, bone marrow, spleen, and lymph nodes. Also called the *monocyte/macrophage system*.

retinitis pigmentosa: Group of inherited disorders in which abnormalities of the photoreceptors or the retinal pigment epithelium of the retina lead to progressive visual loss.

retroperitoneal: The anatomical space behind the peritoneum and outside the peritoneal cavity

retrovirus: Any of a family of RNA viruses containing the enzyme reverse transcriptase.

reverse transcription PCR (RT-PCR): A PCR amplification process that produces complementary DNA from messenger RNA (mRNA) present in a total RNA sample extracted from a patient's cells.

Rh immune globulin (RhIg): A solution of antibodies with specificity for the Rho(D) antigen given intramuscularly to an Rh-negative mother carrying an Rh-positive fetus or delivering an Rh-positive baby. The antibody will react with fetal cells in maternal circulation, flagging them for rapid removal by macrophages and avoiding stimulation of the maternal production of anti- Rho(D).

Rh: Refers to the Rhesus blood group antigen system.

Rh null disease: Hemolytic anemia in persons who lack all Rh factors (Rh null); it is marked by spherocytosis, stomatocytosis, and increased osmotic fragility.

ribonucleic acid (RNA): A nucleic acid with ribose as the sugar, found in both the nucleus and cytoplasm of cells, that plays several roles in the translation of the genetic code and the assembly of proteins.

ribosomes: Small granules composed of protein and nucleic acid (RNA). They are found free in the cytoplasm or on the surface of rough endoplasmic reticulum and function in protein production.

Richter transformation: The appearance of an aggressive lymphoma in a patient with chronic lymphoid leukemia.

ringed sideroblast: A nucleated erythrocyte precursor with six or more iron granules that circle at least one third of the nucleus; the pathognomonic finding in sideroblastic anemias, visible in iron (Prussian blue) stain.

ristocetin: An antibiotic no longer in clinical use, it facilitates the in vitro interaction of von Willebrand factor with platelet membrane GP Ib. Used as an agonist in platelet aggregation.

roentgenogram: A film made by radiography, such as an x-ray film.

Romanowsky stain: The prototype of the many eosin-methylene blue stains for blood smears and malarial parasites, including Wright stain.

rouleaux: An arrangement of erythrocytes in a stacked formation that may be caused by abnormal proteins.

Russell bodies: Plasma cell cytoplasmic inclusions that appear like vacuoles, containing aggregates of immunoglobulins. Cells with Russell bodies are called *Mott cells*.

Russell viper venom time: A coagulation assay similar to the prothrombin time. Russell viper venom activates the coagulation factor common pathway at the level of factor X. Dilute Russell viper venom time is used routinely in lupus anticoagulant testing. Also called *dilute Russell viper venom time (DRVVT)*.

scatterplot: A plot in rectangular coordinates of paired observations of two random variables, with each observation plotted as one point on the graph; the scatter or clustering of points provides an indication of the relationship between the two variables. A typical scatterplot would graph cell size against cytoplasmic complexity.

schistocyte: A fragmented erythrocyte characteristic of microangiopathic hemolytic anemia, severe burns, disseminated intravascular coagulation, and prosthetic mechanical trauma. Also called a *schizocyte*.

scurvy: A deficiency of vitamin C (ascorbic acid), causing connective tissue breakdown. Marked by weakness, anemia, spongy gums, and a tendency to mucocutaneous bleeding.

secondary hemostasis: The second phase of hemostasis in which enzymatic reaction of plasma coagulation factors result in production of a fibrin clot.

secondary standard: A calibration material in which the analyte concentration has been ascertained by reference to a primary standard.

segmented neutrophil: A mature neutrophil with a multilobed nucleus whose lobules are connected by a filament of chromatin and neutrophilic cytoplasmic granules. Also called a *polymorphonuclear neutrophil*.

selectins: Any of a family of cell adhesion molecules that function to mediate the binding of leukocytes and platelets to the vascular endothelium.

senescent: Aging or growing old.

sensitivity: The conditional probability that a person having a disease will be correctly identified by a clinical test (i.e., diagnostic sensitivity). Also, the lowest level of a substance that can be detected by a laboratory test procedure (i.e., analytical sensitivity).

sepsis: The presence in the blood or other tissues of pathogenic microorganisms or their toxins. Also called *septicemia* or *blood poisoning*.

sequelae: Conditions following and consequential from a disease.

sequestration: A net increase in the quantity of blood within a limited vascular area, such as the spleen. Particular cells may be sequestered, resulting in a decrease in the circulating number of them.

serine protease: Any of a group of proteolytic enzymes with serine in the active site, that include activated procoagulants (thrombin and factors VIIa, IXa, Xa, XIa, and XIIa) and activated inhibitors (plasmin). Serine proteases are synthesized as inactive zymogens; activation occurs when the zymogen is cleaved at one or more specific sites by the action of another protease during the coagulation process.

serine protease inhibitor (SERPIN): Antithrombin, heparin cofactor II, and other coagulation control proteins that function by inhibiting the serine proteases, particularly factors IIa and Xa.

serotonin: The chemical that is released from platelets following damage to the blood vessel walls and acts as a potent vasoconstrictor.

Sézary cell: An abnormal mononuclear cell with a cerebriform (resembling the surface of the brain) nucleus and a narrow rim of cytoplasm. It is a characteristic finding in various T-cell lymphomas.

Sézary syndrome: A form of cutaneous T-cell lymphoma characterized by exfoliative erythroderma; peripheral lymphadenopathy; and Sézary cells present in the skin, lymph nodes, and peripheral blood.

shift reticulocyte: A reticulocyte that is released from the bone marrow prematurely, taking more than 1 day in the peripheral blood to lose its residual RNA. These reticulocytes are shifted from the bone marrow to the peripheral blood in order to compensate for anemia and are the cells reported as contributing polychromasia to the appearance of the cells.

sickle cell: An abnormal crescent-shaped red blood cell containing hemoglobin S, characteristic of sickle cell anemia. Also called a *drepanocyte*.

sickle cell anemia: A severe, chronic, incurable hemoglobinopathy that occurs in people who are homozygous for hemoglobin S. The abnormal hemoglobin results in distortion of erythrocytes (sickle cells) and is characterized by crises of joint pain, anemia, thrombosis, fever, and splenomegaly. Also called *sickle cell disease*.

sickle cell crisis: A broad term that describes several different acute conditions occurring as part of sickle cell disease, such as aplastic crisis, which is temporary bone marrow aplasia; hemolytic crisis, which is acute red cell destruction; and vaso-occlusive crisis, which is severe pain due to blockage of the blood vessels.

sickle cell trait: Heterozygity for sickle hemoglobin, characterized by the presence of both hemoglobin S and hemoglobin A in the red blood cells and without clinical evidence of anemia.

sideroblast: An iron-rich nucleated red blood cell in the bone marrow.

siderocyte: A non-nucleated erythrocyte in which particles of iron are visible by iron stain.

sideropenia: Decreased serum iron levels.

siderotic granules: Red blood cell inclusion bodies composed of ferric iron. With iron stain, they appear as dark-blue granules often seen at the periphery of the cell. With Wright stain they appear as pale blue clusters. Also called *Pappenheimer bodies*.

Southern blot: A technique for transferring DNA fragments separated by gel electrophoresis to a nitrocellulose filter, on which specific fragments can then be detected by their hybridization to probes.

specificity: The conditional probability that a person not having a disease will be correctly identified by a clinical test (i.e., diagnostic specificity). Also used to describe the attribute of antibodies that are able to react only with the antigen that stimulated their production; thus they demonstrate specificity. Also, the quality of laboratory test procedure that is available to detect only the analyte of interest (i.e. analytical specificity).

spectrin: A fibrous protein attached to glycophorin at the cytoplasmic surface of the cell membrane of erythrocytes, providing a skeletal function to the membrane and thus important in maintaining cell shape. A deficiency of spectrin is one cause of hereditary spherocytosis.

spherocyte: An abnormal erythrocyte that has a higher-than-normal concentration of hemoglobin by virtue of a spherocytic shape. Spherocytes are characterized as dense cells lacking central pallor and may be microcytic.

spicule: Pointed skeletal structure found within bone; a fragment or particle of bone marrow. Also pointed projections of red blood cell membranes.

spleen: A large organ in the upper part of the abdominal cavity near the stomach; it is the largest collection of reticuloendothelial cells in the body, responsible for phagocytosis and elimination of senescent red blood cells. Also a lymphoid organ with multiple lymph nodes.

splenectomy: Surgical removal of the spleen.

splenomegaly: Enlargement of the spleen.

standard deviation: A mathematic expression of the dispersion of a set of values or scores from the mean.

standard precautions: A concept of bloodborne disease control, which requires that all human blood and body fluids be treated as if known to be infectious for HIV, HBV, or other bloodborne pathogens, regardless of the perceived low risk of a patient or patient population. Also called *universal precautions*.

steatorrhea: Fat in the stool, usually due to malabsorption.

stem cell: A primitive, multipotential cell whose daughter cells may give rise to a variety of cell types and which is capable of renewing itself, thus maintaining a pool of primitive cells that can differentiate into multiple other cell types.

stenosis (stenotic): The narrowing or constriction of an orifice or passage.

stomatocyte: An abnormal mature erythrocyte that has a slitlike area of central pallor resembling a mouth.

storage pool disease: Mucocutaneous bleeding caused by inadequate platelet delta granule contents. Usually hereditary, related to oculocutaneous albinism conditions, such as Hermansky-Pudlak syndrome, Chédiak-Higashi syndrome, or Wiskott-Aldrich syndrome. Acquired storage pool disorder is sometimes associated with myelodysplastic syndrome.

strike through: A chemical's passage through the protective clothing to the street clothes or skin.

stroma: The supporting tissue or matrix of an organ.

sulfhemoglobin: Hemoglobin with a sulfur atom on one of its porphyrin rings, making it ineffective for transporting oxygen. Results from ingestion of sulfa-type antibiotics.

supernatant: The clear upper liquid part of a suspension after it has been centrifuged.

supernumerary: Exceeding the usual number of something.

suppuration: The formation or discharge of pus.

supravital stain: A stain that colors living tissues or cells. Also called a *vital stain*.

surface-connected canalicular system (SCCS; open canalicular system, OCS): A system of channels that is distributed throughout platelets and extends the plasma membrane inward. The SCCS binds numerous coagulation factors and provides a route for secretion of the protein contents of alpha granules.

syncope: A brief lapse in consciousness; fainting.

syncytium: A large area of cytoplasm that contains many nuclei.

synergy: The action of two or more agents working with each other for a combined function.

systemic lupus erythematosus (SLE): A chronic inflammatory disease manifested in severe vasculitis, renal involvement, and lesions of the skin and nervous system.

T cell: A lymphocyte category that participates in cellular immunity, including cell-to-cell communication, helper cells, and suppressor-cytotoxic cells. Also called a *T lymphocyte*.

tachypnea: Rapid breathing.

target cell: A poorly hemoglobinized erythrocyte seen in hemoglobinopathies and thalassemia. In Wright stain, there is a concentration of hemoglobin in the center and periphery, resembling a target or bull's eye. Also called a *codocyte*.

teardrop cell: An erythrocyte with a single pointed extension, resembling a teardrop. Also called a *dacryocyte*.

telangiectasis: Permanent dilation of preexisting small blood vessels (capillaries, arterioles, and venules), creating focal red lesions, usually in the skin or mucous membranes.

telomerase: An enzyme that adds specific DNA sequence repeats to the 3′ end of DNA strands in the telomere regions located at the ends of eukaryotic chromosomes.

telomeres: A region of non-coding, highly repetitive DNA at the end of a linear chromosome that functions as a disposable end-cap. Telomeres are lost with every cell replication.

thalassemia: A hemolytic hemoglobinopathy anemia characterized by microcytic, hypochromic anemia, caused by deficient synthesis of globin polypeptide chains; classified according to the deficient chain involved, e.g., beta or alpha.

thermocycler: An instrument designed to support the polymerase chain reaction by cycling through selected temperatures.

thrombin clotting time (TCT): A coagulation test that measures the interval to clot formation following addition of thrombin to plasma. Also called *thrombin time*, it is used to test for the presence of heparin.

thrombin: The primary serine protease of coagulation. Factors Xa and V combine to cleave prothrombin to produce thrombin. Thrombin cleaves fibrinopeptides A and B from fibrinogen to initiate fibrin polymerization. Thrombin potentiates coagulation by activating platelets and factors XI, VIII, V, and XIII and also activates the coagulation control protein, protein C.

thrombocyte: A platelet.

thrombocythemia: Thrombocytosis with platelet dysfunction in the myeloproliferative disorder essential thrombocythemia.

thrombocytopathy: A qualitative platelet disorder, such as storage pool disorder, aspirin-like syndrome, or membrane receptor abnormality.

thrombocytopenia: A platelet count below the lower limit of the reference interval.

thrombocytosis: A platelet count above the upper limit of the reference range.

thrombophilia: A condition that increases thrombosis risk; also called *hypercoagulability*.

thrombopoietin: A hormone that is produced by renal tissue and recruits stem cells to the megakaryocyte cell maturation line as well as stimulates megakaryocyte mitosis and maturation in response to thrombocytopenia.

thrombosis: The formation, development, or presence of a clot in a blood vessel (i.e., a thrombus).

thrombospondin: A glycoprotein that is secreted by endothelial cells and by the alpha granules of platelets, interacts with a wide variety of molecules of the coagulation pathways, and plays a role in platelet aggregation.

thrombotic thrombocytopenic purpura (TTP): A congenital or acquired deficiency of endothelial cell von Willebrand factor (VWF)-cleaving protease. Ultra-large VWF multimers activate platelets to form white clots in the microvasculature. This causes severe thrombocytopenia with mucocutaneous bleeding, microangiopathic hemolytic anemia, and neuropathy. Therapy is plasmapheresis with replacement using fresh frozen plasma. Untreated TTP is fatal in 90% of cases.

thrombus: An in vivo blood clot in a blood vessel causing vascular occlusion and tissue ischemia.

tissue factor (TF): A constitutive membrane protein of subendothelium. Exposure to tissue factor activates factor VII of the tissue factor (extrinsic) coagulation pathway. Tissue factor is expressed on monocytes and endothelial cells in chronic inflammation.

tissue plasminogen activator (TPA): Serine protease that is secreted by endothelial cells and binds fibrin. TPA activates nearby plasminogen molecules to trigger fibrinolysis with formation of fibrin degradation products.

total iron-binding capacity (TIBC): The amount of iron that can be bound by transferrin.

toxic granulation: Abnormally large, dark-staining, or dominant primary granules in neutrophils associated with bacterial infections.

trabeculae: Connective tissue that serves as a support for bone marrow cells; extends from cortical bone into the bone marrow space.

transcription: The process by which messenger RNA is formed from a DNA template.

transferrin: A plasma iron-transport protein that moves iron from sites of absorption and storage, to incorporate into rubriblasts and other cells.

translation: The process in which the genetic information carried by nucleotides in messenger RNA directs the amino acid sequence in the synthesis of a specific polypeptide.

translocation: The rearrangement of DNA within a chromosome or the transfer of a segment of one chromosome to a nonhomologous one.

trisomy: The presence of an extra chromosome in a homologous pair.

tublin: The protein of which microtubules are composed.

tungsten halogen light bulb: A bulb used in bright-field microscopy, consisting of a tungsten filament enclosed in a small quartz bulb filled with halogen gas. Tungsten creates a very bright yellow light.

umbilicus: A scar on the abdomen, caused when the umbilical cord is removed from a newborn baby.

unfractionated heparin (UFH, standard heparin): Heparin extracted from porcine mucosa and fractionated to yield MW ranges from 7000-15,000. Is used routinely in cardiac surgery and requires monitoring using the partial thromboplastin time assay.

universal precautions: A concept of bloodborne disease control, which requires that all human blood and body fluids be treated as if known to be infectious for HIV, HBV, or other bloodborne pathogens, regardless of the perceived low risk of a patient or patient population. Also called *standard precautions*.

Unopette system (Becton Dickinson [BD], Franklin Lakes, NJ): A standard self-contained diluting device for manual cell counting.

unsaturated iron-binding capacity (UIBC): The number of unsaturated binding sites for iron located on the transferrin molecules, measured in μmol of iron per L.

urobilinogen: A compound formed in the intestine after the breakdown of bilirubin by bacteria.

urokinase: An enzyme that is produced by the kidney and found in the urine and is a potent plasminogen activator of the fibrinolytic system.

vacuole: Any clear space or cavity formed in the cytoplasm of a cell.

vacuolization: The condition of being vacuolated.

variant: Something that differs in some characteristics from the class to which it belongs.

vasoconstriction: A reactive decrease in blood vessel diameter. Vasoconstriction controls blood pressure, primary hemostasis, and the distribution of blood throughout the body.

venesection: Phlebotomy, but usually used to refer to removal of substantial amounts of blood, often for therapeutic purposes

venipuncture: Use of a hypodermic needle to puncture a vein and collect blood. Also called *phlebotomy*.

verocytotoxin: A heat labile toxin that is produced by some types of *Escherichia coli*.

verrucous: Of, pertaining to, or like a wart or warts.

vertigo: A sensation of rotation or movement of one's self or of one's surroundings; dizziness.

viscosity: The ability or inability of a fluid solution to flow easily.

vital stain: See *supra vital stain*.

vitamin B$_{12}$: Also called *cyanocobalamin*, it is involved in the metabolism of protein, fats, and carbohydrates; normal blood formation; and nerve function.

vitamin K: Natural phylloquinone occurring in green leafy vegetables and liver and produced by intestinal commensals. Vitamin K catalyzes the gamma-carboxylation of glutamic acid in a number of calcium-binding proteins, including the "vitamin K–dependent" proteins of coagulation, factors II (prothrombin), VII, IX, and X, and also the coagulation control proteins C, S, and Z.

von Willebrand disease (VWD): A congenital autosomal dominant variable mucocutaneous bleeding disorder, characterized by deficiency of von Willebrand factor activity and antigen, and subsequent impairment of platelet adhesion.

waived testing: A CLIA test classification; includes tests that are simple and accurate.

Waldenström's macroglobulinemia: A form of monoclonal gammopathy in which immunoglobulin M (IgM) is overproduced by the clone of a plasma B cell. Increased viscosity of the blood may result in circulatory impairment, and normal immunoglobulin synthesis is decreased, leading to increased susceptibility to infections.

warfarin: A vitamin K antagonist that prevents the gamma-carboxylation of glutamic acids of coagulation factors II, VII, IX, and X. Overdose causes risk for hemorrhage, and thus use must be monitored using the prothrombin time test.

warm antibody: An antibody that is usually IgG and reacts with red blood cells at an optimum temperature of 37° C.

warm reactive autoimmune hemolytic anemia (WAIHA): The most common autoimmune hemolytic anemia, which results from the reaction of autoantibodies with red blood cells at an optimum temperature of 37° C.

Wiskott-Aldrich syndrome: An immunodeficiency disorder characterized by oculocutaneous albinism; thrombocytopenia; inadequate T- and B-cell function, and an increased susceptibility to viral, bacterial, and fungal infections.

xanthochromic: Having a yellowish color. Used to describe cerebrospinal fluid. Indicates the presence of bilirubin and thus evidence of a prior episode of bleeding into the brain.

x-linked: Pertaining to genes or to the characteristics or conditions they transmit that are carried on the X chromosome.

x-linked recessive inheritance: A pattern of inheritance in which a recessive allele is carried on the X chromosome; results in the carrier state in females and development of disease characteristics in males, since they do not have a normal X chromosome to compensate.

zymogen: An inactive precursor that is converted to an active form by an enzyme. Inactive coagulation factors, such as prothrombin, are zymogens.

Index

Note: Page numbers followed by f refer to
illustrations; page numbers followed by
t refer to tables.

BODY FLUID CELL COUNT

Fluid	Range
Cerebrospinal fluid	0-10 WBC/µL
Synovial fluid	0-200 WBC/µL
	<25% neutrophils
	0 RBC/µL
Serous fluid	Dependent on source; usually less than 1000 total WBC and <25% neutrophils

COAGULATION TESTING

Monitoring Heparin and Warfarin	Therapeutic Ranges
Anti-Xa heparin assay: therapeutic low MW heparin, U/mL	0.5–1.0
Anti-Xa heparin assay: therapeutic unfractionated heparin, U/mL	0.3–0.7
Anti-Xa heparin assay: prophylactic low MW heparin, U/mL	0.2–0.4
PT warfarin most applications, INR	2–3
PT warfarin, mechanical heart valves, INR	2.5–3.5
PTT unfractionated therapeutic heparin	Always consult local laboratory for range
PTT unfractionated prophylactic subcutaneous heparin	Always consult local laboratory for range

Screening Tests Reference Intervals	
PT, Sec	12.6–14.6
PT, INR	0.93–1.13
PTT, Sec	25–35
TT, Sec	<21

Factor Assays	Reference Intervals
Fibrinogen, mg/dL	220–498
Factor II, V, VII, IX, X, XI, XII, %	50–150
Factor VIII, %	50–186
VWF activity (ristocetin cofactor), %	50–166
VWF antigen, %	50–249
HMWK (Fitzgerald), %	65–135
PK (Fletcher), %	65–135
XIII by urea solubility	Decreased–Normal

Control Proteins	Reference Intervals
Antithrombin activity, %	78–126
Protein C activity, %	70–140
Protein S activity, %	65–140

Other Assays	
Activated protein C resistance, ratio	>1.8
Anti-cardiolipin antibody IgG, GPL	<12
Anti-cardiolipin antibody IgM, MPL	<10
D-dimer, ηg/mL	110–240
Euglobulin clot lysis time, hours	2–6
DRVVT, ratio	<1.3

PT – Prothrombin time
PTT – Partial Thromboplastin time
MW – Molecular weight
INR – International normalized ratio
PK – Prekallikrein
HMWK – High molecular weight kininogen
GPL – IgG anticardiolipin antibody unit
MPL – IgM anticardiolipin antibody unit
DRVVT – Dilute Russell viper venom time